TEXTBOOK OF PALLIATIVE NURSING

Edited by

BETTY ROLLING FERRELL, Ph.D., F.A.A.N.
Research Scientist
Department of Nursing Education and Research
City of Hope National Medical Center
Duarte, California

NESSA COYLE, R.N., M.S., N.P., F.A.A.N.
Director, Supportive Care Program
Pain & Palliative Care Service
Department of Neurology
Memorial Sloan-Kettering Cancer Center
New York, New York

OXFORD
UNIVERSITY PRESS
2001

OXFORD
UNIVERSITY PRESS

Oxford New York
Athens Auckland Bangkok Bogotá Buenos Aires Calcutta
Cape Town Chennai Dar es Salaam Delhi Florence Hong Kong Istanbul
Karachi Kuala Lumpur Madrid Melbourne Mexico City Mumbai
Nairobi Paris São Paulo Shanghai Singapore Taipei Tokyo Toronto Warsaw

and associated companies in
Berlin Ibadan

Published by Oxford University Press, Inc.
198 Madison Avenue, New York, New York 10016

Oxford is a registered trademark of Oxford University Press

Library of Congress Cataloging-in-Publication Data
Textbook of palliative nursing /
edited by Betty Rolling Ferrell, Nessa Coyle.
p. ; cm. Includes bibliographical references and index.
ISBN 0-19-513574-1
1. Palliative treatment. 2. Nursing. 3. Terminal care.
I. Ferrell, Betty. II. Coyle, Nessa.
[DNLM: 1. Nursing Care. 2. Palliative Care. 3. Terminal Care.
WY 152 T355 2001] RT87.T45 T49 2001 616'.029—dc21 00-055060

The science of medicine is a rapidly changing field. As new research and clinical experience broaden our knowledge, changes in treatment and drug therapy do occur. The editors and the publisher of this work have checked with sources believed to be reliable in their efforts to provide information that is accurate and complete, and in accordance with the standards accepted at the time of publication. However, in light of the possibility of human error or changes in the practice of medicine, neither the editors, nor the publisher, nor any other party who has been involved in the preparation or publication of this work warrants that the information contained herein is in every respect accurate or complete. Readers are encouraged to confirm the information contained herein with other reliable sources, and are strongly advised to check the product information sheet provided by the pharmaceutical company for each drug they plan to administer.

9 8 7 6 5 4 3

Printed in the United States of America
on acid-free paper

Foreword by Cicely Saunders

Palliative care stems from the recognition of the potential at the end of life for discovering and for giving, a recognition that an important dimension of being human is the lasting dignity and growth that can continue through weakness and loss. No member of the interdisciplinary team is more central to making these discoveries possible than the nurse. Realizing how little had been written and even less studied in this field, Peggy Nuttall, a former nursing colleague and then editor of the *Nursing Times* in London, invited me to contribute a series of six articles on the care of the dying in the summer of 1959.[1] A registered nurse and qualified medical social worker, I had trained in medicine because of a compulsion to do something about the pain I had seen in patients and their families at the end of life. During 3 years as a volunteer nurse in an early home for such patients, I had persuaded the thoracic surgeon, Norman Barrett, for whom I was working, to follow up a few of his mortally ill patients both there and in their homes. "Go and read medicine," he said. "It's the doctors who desert the dying, and there's so much more to be learned about pain. You'll only be frustrated if you don't do it properly, and they won't listen to you." He was right and I obeyed. After 7 years' work, the first descriptive study of 1100 patients in St. Joseph's Hospice, London, from 1958 to 1965[2] was coupled with visits to clinical pain researchers such as Harry Beecher in Boston and many U.S. homes, social workers, and nurses in 1963. This visit included an all-important meeting with Florence Wald at Yale. A prodigious program of fundraising letters, professional articles, and meetings led to the opening of St. Christopher's Hospice in 1967, the first inpatient, home care, research, and teaching hospice. All of those early contacts and countless other interested people led to the hospice movement and the palliative care that developed within and from it.

Nurses were the first to respond to this challenge and remain the core of the personal and professional drive to enable people to find relief, support, and meaning at the end of their lives. All of the expertise described in this important collection is to this end. The window to suffering can be a window to peace and opportunity. The nurse, in her or his skilled competence and compassion, has a unique place to give each person the essential message "You matter because you are you and you matter to the last moment of your life. We will do all we can to help you, not only to die peacefully but to live until you die."[3]

C.S.
Chair, St. Christopher's Hospice, London

REFERENCES

1. Saunders CM. Care of the dying. *Nurs Times* 1959;
2. Clark D. "Total pain," disciplinary power and the body in the work of Cicely Saunders, 1958–67. Soc Sci Med 1999;49:727–736.
3. Saunders C. Care of the dying. 1. The problem of euthanasia. Nurs Times 1976;72:1003–1005.

Foreword by Florence Wald

Nurses of my generation in the second half of the twentieth century were fortunate to be part of the hospice movement and to respond to an eager public with an alternative way of care for the dying. Medical sociologists' studies of hospital culture showed what many nurses already knew, that when technological intervention failed to stop the course of disease, physicians could not see that the treatment was futile or join the patient in a willingness to cease.

By 1950, nurses began to carry out studies as principal investigators and were on their way to being respected by other disciplines. Two outstanding leaders were Hilde Peplau and Virginia Henderson, both educated nurses in clinical practice who established a foundation for the advanced nurse practitioner to be a valued member of an interdisciplinary team.

This surfaced first in psychiatric nursing, but as hospice care came into being, the nurse became a pivotal part of the interdisciplinary team. "Hospice nursing," Virginia Henderson said, "was the essence of nursing," and because volunteers came quickly into hospice care, proved Henderson's precept, giving the lay individual "the necessary strength, will, and knowledge to contribute to a peaceful death." [1]

Physicians in the forefront of medical ethics, such as Edmund Pellegrino and Raymond Duff, encouraged physicians to recast their roles as decision makers and communicators so that the whole team could keep the patients' values and the families' wants the prime concern.

The works of those who have brought alternative therapies into use, for example, Martha Rogers and Barbara Dossey, have added to the spiritual dimensions of care. The growth of the religious ministry movement and the creative addition of the arts and environment round out the cast of contributors.

Reviewing the progress we nurses have made allows us to proceed more effectively.

F.W.
Branford, Connecticut

REFERENCES

1. Henderson V. Basic Principles of Nursing Care. London: International Council of Nurses, 1961:42.

Foreword by Jeanne Quint Benoliel

At the end of the Second World War in 1945, people in Western societies were tired of death, pain, and suffering. Cultural goals shifted away from war-centered activities to a focus on progress, use of technology for better living, and improvements in the health and well-being of the public. Guided by new scientific knowledge and new technologies, health care services became diversified and specialized and lifesaving at all costs became a powerful driving force. End-of-life care was limited to postmortem rituals, and the actual caregiving of dying patients was left to nursing staff. Palliative nursing in those days depended on the good will and personal skills of individual nurses, yet what they offered was invisible, unrecognized, and unrewarded.

Thanks to the efforts of many people across the years, end-of-life care is acknowledged today as an important component of integrated health care services. Much knowledge has accrued about what makes for good palliative care, and nurses have been in the forefront of efforts to improve quality of life for patients and families throughout the experience of illness. This book is an acknowledgment of the important part played by nurses in helping patients to complete their lives in a context of care and human concern.

J.Q.B.
Professor Emeritus
University of Washington, Seattle

Preface

On reflecting on the evolution of this book, I realized that the story began with my mother's death in 1957 and culminated with my father's death in 1993. In 1957, at the age of 56, my mother died of pancreatic cancer. The time from diagnosis to death was under one month. My mother died on a surgical unit of postoperative complications and left behind 8 children in their teens and twenties. We had not really thought about death before and as a family went through a period of intense bewilderment and grief. My father died in 1993 at home in England. This was a very different experience. He was 99 years old and we were prepared. But he was debilitated and dependent for a long time, and multiple issues surrounding the care of the elderly, division of care among family members, and quality of life surfaced during this period. The death of my parents in these two very different scenarios, as well as the death of a sister, were powerful personal experiences, occurring at the beginning and latter part of my career. These experiences have anchored and influenced an extraordinarily rewarding personal and professional journey of work, addressing the needs of cancer patients and their families. While each patient interaction is a very personal one, perhaps the experiences with our loved ones shape our attitudes towards life and death even more.

The opportunity to edit a comprehensive book on palliative nursing brought these reflections back to mind. I immediately thought of Dr. Betty Ferrell as co-editor. Few people have done as much as Betty to spearhead broad spectrum nursing education in palliative care and to bring about change. Her efforts have been untiring, and those efforts, in combination with the work of so many wonderful nursing colleagues and contributors to a field that is just reaching maturity, have made this book possible.

This book is dedicated to the many patients and families who have allowed us to learn from both their suffering and their courage, as well as to the many nurses who have helped care for them. My personal thanks go to my nursing colleagues in the Pain and Palliative Care Service at Memorial Sloan-Kettering Cancer Center, as well as to Dr. Kathleen Foley, Dr. Russell Portenoy, Dr. William Breitbart, Dr. Nathan Cherny, Dr. Marilyn Bookbinder, and Drs. Mario and Lois Sculco, whose unfailing day-to-day support and encouragement have been an inspiration to me. I am eternally grateful to them.

New York, N.Y. N.C.

Preface

In October, 1998 my mother, Jewel Rolling, died of lung cancer. After 21 years as an oncology nurse, I was given the opportunity to move to the other side and witness cancer and death as a family caregiver. The anguish of losing a mother was balanced by the opportunity to see her life end with peace and dignity in the compassionate and competent care of Mercy Hospice in Oklahoma. I also observed caregiving at its finest through the immaculate care provided by my father, John Rolling. His selflessness reflected the bond of a 55-year marriage and uncompromising dedication to her well-being.

A month after my mother's death, Nessa Coyle contacted me with the idea of co-editing this book. The honor of working with Nessa and the opportunity to contribute to the evolving discipline of Palliative Nursing were compelling. I have read every word of this text with the intent of providing a statement about the kind of care everyone should receive when it is their time to witness life's end for a mother or other loved one.

Nessa and I are grateful to the authors who have contributed to this work and to all nurses whose clinical expertise and commitment have pioneered the specialty of Palliative Nursing. We are also in gratitude to Chel Jacques whose clerical assistance was vital to the text and to Lauren Enck and Susan Hannan from Oxford University Press, whose support was a presence throughout the process.

My personal thanks go to those whose palliative care sustains me—my nursing colleagues at the City of Hope and my own caregivers, Bruce and Annie Ferrell. Through Bruce Ferrell, M.D., an expert spouse, I have learned dedication to a cause, the meaning of quality, and true supportive care. He *is* my quality of life. To Annie, my daughter and inspiration,—this book will be "born" just a few months before your 21st birthday. My wish for you is that you will find your own life work and that it will be as passionate as those whose work is reflected in these pages.

Duarte, California B.R.F.

Contents

Contributors

PAULA ANDERSON, R.N., M.S.N.
Research Specialist
Department of Nursing Research and Education
City of Hope National Medical Center
Duarte, California

SANCHIA ARANDA, R.N., M.N., CERT. ONC., PH.D.
Associate Professor
Center for Palliative Care
Deputy Head
School of Postgraduate Nursing
University of Melbourne and St. Vincent's Hospital
Fitzroy, Victoria, Australia

BARBARA M. BATES-JENSEN, PH.D., M.N., C.W.O.C.N.
Assistant Professor
Department of Nursing
University of Southern California
Los Angeles, California

REVEREND PATRICIA BEIRNE, C.H.T, H.T.P.
Spiritual Counseling, Hypnotherapy and Healing Touch
Private Practice
Honolulu, Hawaii

JEANNE QUINT BENOLIEL, D.N.SC., F.A.A.N.
Professor Emeritus
Psychosocial and Community Health
University of Washington
School of Nursing
Fall City, Washington

PATRICIA BERRY, PH.D., R.N., H.P.N.H., C.S.
Project Coordinator
Institutionalizing Pain Management: A Robert Wood Johnson Foundation Project
University of Wisconsin—Madison
Madison, Wisconsin

MARILYN BOOKBINDER, R.N., PH.D.
Director of Nursing
Department of Pain & Palliative Care
Beth Israel Medical Center
New York, New York

TAMI BORNEMAN, R.N., B.S.N.
Research Specialist
Department of Nursing Research and Education
City of Hope National Medical Center
Duarte, California

GEOFFREY BOWRING
Cancer Relief International
Oxford, United Kingdom

SUSAN BRAJTMAN, R.N., B.N.
Head Nurse
Ina and Jack Kay Hospice
Centre for Supportive Care
Hadassah University Hospital
Mount Scopus, Jerusalem, Israel

CARLEEN BRENNEIS, R.N., M.H.S.A.
Program Director
Regional Palliative Care Program
Grey Nuns Community Hospital and Health Care Centre
Edmonton, Alberta, Canada

KATHERINE BROWN-SALTZMAN, R.N., M.A.
Clinical Nurse Specialist
Assistant Clinical Professor
University of California Los Angeles Medical Center
Los Angeles, California

GILLY BURN, R.G.N., R.C.N.T., R.N.T.
Founder and Director, Cancer Relief India
Cancer Relief International
Oxford, United Kingdom

FERN G. CAMPBELL, R.N., M.S.N., F.N.P.
Pediatric Urology Nurse Practitioner
Department of Urology
University of Virginia
Charlottesville, Virginia

DOUGLAS CLUXTON, M.A., L.P.C.
Spiritual Care Coordinator
The James Hospice
The James Cancer Hospital and Solove Research Institute
The Ohio State University Comprehensive Cancer Center
Columbus, Ohio

INGE B. CORLESS, R.N., PH.D.
Associate Professor
Graduate Program in Nursing
Institute of Health Professionals
Massachusetts General Hospital
Boston, Massachusetts

NESSA COYLE, R.N., M.S., N.P., F.A.A.N. (EDITOR)
Director, Supportive Care Program
Pain and Palliative Care Service
Memorial Sloan-Kettering Cancer Center
New York, New York

PATRICK J. COYNE, R.N., M.S.N., C.S., H.P.N.
Clinical Nurse Specialist
Medical College of Virginia Hospitals of
Virginia Commonwealth University
Richmond, Virginia

CLARA MARIA CULLEN, R.N.
Palliative Care Unit
Tornu Hospital
Buenos Aires, Argentina

CONSTANCE M. DAHLIN, M.S.N., R.N., C.S.
Palliative Care Specialist/ Nurse Practitioner
Palliative Care Service
Massachusetts General Hospital
Boston, Massachusetts

BETTY DAVIES, R.N., PH.D., F.A.A.N
Professor and Chair
Department of Family Health Care Nursing
School of Nursing
University of California—San Francisco
San Francisco, California

GRACE E. DEAN, R.N., M.S.N.
Research Specialist
Nursing Research and Education
City of Hope National Medical Center
Duarte, California

KATHLEEN M. DEFILIPPI, D.N.E., C.H.N.
Director
South Coast Hospice Association
Pain & Palliative Care Service
Port Shepstone, Kwazulu
Natal, South Africa

SUSAN DERBY, R.N. M.A., C.G.N.P.
Nurse Practitioner
Pain and Palliative Care Service
Memorial Sloan-Kettering Cancer Center
New York, New York

ANNA R. DU PEN, A.R.N.P., M.N.
Palliative Care Nurse Practitioner
Pacific Northwest Pain Management Associates
Seattle, Washington

DEBORAH DUDGEON, R.N., M.D., F.R.C.P.C.
Director
Palliative Care Medicine
Queen's University
Kingston, Ontario, Canada

LYNNE EARLY, M.N., C.W.O.C.N., O.N.P.
Enterostomal Therapy Nurse
University of Southern California
Kenneth Norris, Jr. Cancer Center
Hermosa Beach, California

DENICE CARACCIA ECONOMOU, R.N., M.N., A.O.C.N.
Nurse Coordinator
Cancer Pain Management Center
Cedars Sinai Comprehensive Cancer Center
Los Angeles, California

KATHLEEN A. EGAN, M.A., B.S.N., C.H.P.N.
Vice President
Hospice Institute of the Florida Suncoast
Largo, Florida

NANCY ENGLISH, PH.D., R.N.
Palliative Care Consultant
Denver, Colorado

MARY ERSEK, PH.D., R.N.
Associate Research Scientist
Pain Research Department
Swedish Medical Center
Seattle, Washington

BETTY R. FERRELL, R.N., PH.D., F.A.A.N. (EDITOR)
Research Scientist
Department of Nursing Research and Education
City of Hope National Medical Center
Duarte, California

PERRY G. FINE, M.D.
Professor
Department of Anesthesiology
University of Utah Health Sciences Center
Salt Lake City, Utah

REGINA FINK, R.N., PH.D., A.O.C.N.
Research Nurse Scientist
University of Colorado Health Sciences Center
Denver, Colorado

PAMELA E. FOWLER, R.N.
Nursing Services Manager
Hospice Association of the Witwatersrand
Johannesburg, South Africa

WAYNE FURMAN, M.D.
Associate Member
Solid Tumor Team
Department of Hematology-Oncology
St. Jude's Children's Research Hospital
Nashville, Tennessee

RUTH GASSNER, R.N., M.A.
Director
Ina and Jack Kay Hospice
Centre for Supportive Care
Hadassah University Hospital
Mount Scopus, Jerusalem, Israel

ROSE GATES, R.N., M.S.N., A.N.P
Oncology Nurse Practitioner
Private Practice
Colorado Springs, Colorado

ELAINE GLASS, R.N. M.S., A.O.C.N.
Clinical Decisions Program Manager
The James Cancer Hospital and Solove Research Institute
The Ohio State University Comprehensive Cancer Center
Columbus, Ohio

TESSA GOLDSMITH, M.A., C.C.C./S.L.P.
Clinical Specialist/Researcher
Department of Speech-Language Pathology
Massachusetts General Hospital
Boston, Massachusetts

MARCIA GRANT, D.N.SC., F.A.A.N.
Research Scientist and Director
Nursing Research and Education
City of Hope National Medical Center
Duarte, California

MIKEL GRAY, PH.D., C.U.N.P., C.C.C.N., F.A.A.N.
Associate Professor
Department of Urology and School of Nursing
University of Virginia
Charlottesville, Virginia

JULIE GRIFFIE, M.S.N., R.N., C.S., A.O.C.N.
Palliative Medicine Program
Froedtert East Hospital
Milwaukee, Wisconsin

KEIKO HAMAGUCHI, R.N., M.N., C.N.S.C.
Deputy Director of Nursing
Higashi Sapporo Hospital
Sapporo, Japan

SISTER PAULINE A. HANNA, R.N.
Clinical Tutor
Hospice Association of Witwatersrand
Hospice Wits
Johannesburg, South Africa

ANNE HAYES, R.G.N., R.M., R.N.T.
Coordinator
Complementary and Supportive Therapy
Our Lady's Hospice
Harold's Cross
Dublin, Ireland

DEBRA E. HEIDRICH, M.S.N., R.N., A.O.C.N., C.H.P.N.
West Chester, Ohio

PAMELA S. HINDS, PH.D., R.N., C.S.
Coordinator of Nursing Research
Associate Director of Research for Behavioral Medicine
St. Jude's Children's Research Hospital
Memphis, Tennessee

KAREN C. HINTON, R.N.
Education Department Manager
The Highway Hospice Association
Durban, South Africa

ANNE HUGHES, R.N., M.N., F.A.A.N.
Clinical Nurse Specialist
HIV Disease and Oncology
San Francisco General Hospital Medical Center
Montara, California

YASUKO ISHIGAKI, R.N.
Vice President and Director of Nursing
Higashi Sapporo Hospital
Sapporo, Japan

MARTA H. JUNIN, R.N.
Palliative Care Team
Bonorino Udaondo Hospital
Nurse Coordinator
Pallium Rio de la Plata Study Center in Palliative Care
Professor
Postgraduate School of Medicine
Universidad del Salvadore
Buenos Aires, Argentina

DAVID L. KAHN, PH.D., R.N.
Associate Professor and Lucie Baines Johnson Fellow
University of Texas at Austin
School of Nursing
Austin, Texas

PAMELA KEDZIERA, R.N., M.S.N., A.O.C.N.
Clinical Nurse Specialist
Pain Management Center
Fox Chase Cancer Center
Philadelphia, Pennsylvania

CHARLES KEMP, R.N., C.R.N.H.
Lecturer
Baylor University School of Nursing
Dallas, Texas

CYNTHIA R. KING, R.N., N.P., PH.D., F.A.A.N.
Principal and Nurse Consultant
Special Care Consultants
Rochester, New York

ANDREW KNIGHT, R.N.
Director of Nursing
St. Christopher's Hospice
Sydenham, London
United Kingdom

LINDA J. KRISTJANSON, R.N., PH.D
Professor
School of Nursing & Public Health
Associate Dean
Faculty of Communications, Health and Science
Edith Cowan University
Churchlands, Western Australia

KIM K. KUEBLER, R.N., M.N., AN.P.-C.S.
Palliative Care Nurse Practitioner
Adjuvant Therapies, Inc.
Lake, Michigan

MARY J. LABYAK, M.S.W., L.C.S.W.
President and Chief Executive Officer
Hospice of the Florida Suncoast
Largo, Florida

MARGARET ANNE LAMB, PH.D., R.N.
Associate Professor
Department of Nursing
University of New Hampshire
Durham, New Hampshire

MARCIA LEVETOWN, M.D.
Director of the Butterfly Program
Departments of Pediatrics and Internal Medicine
University of Texas Medical Branch at Galveston
Galveston, Texas

LAURIE LYCKHOLM, M.D.
Assistant Professor of Medicine
Division of Hematology Oncology
Medical College of Virginia
Richmond, Virginia

JOAN A. MARSTON, B.SOC.SC. (NURS.)
Executive Director
Bloemfontein Hospice
Bloemfontein, Free State, South Africa

RUTH MCCORKLE, PH.D., F.A.A.N.
Project Director/Chair of Doctoral Program
Center for Excellence in Chronic Illness Care
Yale University School of Nursing
New Haven, Connecticut

MAURA MCDONNELL, M.SC., R.G.N., R.M.
Ward Sister
Our Lady's Hospice
Harold's Cross
Dublin, Ireland

SANDY MCKINNON, R.N., M.N.
Tertiary Palliative Care Unit
Grey Nuns Community Hospital and Health Centre
Edmonton, Alberta, Canada

KATHLEEN MICHAEL, R.N., M.S.N., C.R.R.N.
Coordinator
Rehabilitation Nursing Services
The Johns Hopkins University
Baltimore, Maryland

PAULA MILONE-NUZZO, PH.D., F.A.A.N.
Chair of Doctoral Program
Center for Excellence in Chronic Illness Care
Yale University School of Nursing
New Haven, Connecticut

PAMELA A. MINARIK, M.S., R.N., C.S., F.A.A.N.
Associate Professor
Psychiatric Mental Health Nursing
Yale University School of Nursing
Psychiatric Consultation Liaison Nurse Specialist
Yale New Haven Hospital
New Haven, Connecticut

AUXILIA CHIDEME MUNODAWAFA, R.N., S.C.M., A.N.P., M.S.N.
Department of Nursing Science
Faculty of Medicine
University of Zimbabwe
Harare, Zimbabwe, Africa

NKOSAZANA NGIDI, B.A., S.W.DIP
Social Worker
Highway Hospice Association
Durban, South Africa

LESLIE NIELD-ANDERSON, PH.D., A.P.R.N.
Associate Professor
Psychiatric Mental Health Nursing
Yale University School of Nursing
Psychiatric Consultation Liaison Nurse Specialist
Yale New Haven Hospital
New Haven, Connecticut

LINDA OAKES, M.S.N. R.N., C.C.R.N.
Clinical Nurse Specialist
Intensive Care Unit & Symptom Management Team
St. Jude's Children's Research Hospital
Memphis, Tennessee

SEAN O'MAHONY, M.B.B.CH., B.A.O.
Pain and Palliative Care Fellow
Department of Neurology
Memorial Sloan-Kettering Cancer Center
New York, New York

HOB OSTERLUND, R.N., M.S., C.H.T.P.
Clinical Coordinator
Pain Management Services
The Queen's Medical Center
Clinical Instructor
University of Hawaii
Honolulu, Hawaii

JUDITH A. PAICE, PH.D., R.N., F.A.A.N.
Research Professor of Medicine
Palliative Care and Home Hospice Program
Northwestern Memorial Hospital
Northwestern University
Chicago, Illinois

JEANNIE V. PASACRETA, PH.D., A.P.R.N.
Associate Professor and Director
Psychiatric Mental Health Nursing Specialty
Yale University School of Nursing
New Haven, Connecticut

KATHLEEN PUNTILLO, R.N., D.N.SC., F.A.A.N.
Associate Professor of Nursing
Department of Physiological Nursing
School of Nursing
University of California—San Francisco
San Francisco, California

PATRICE RANCOUR, R.N., M.S., C.S.
Mental Health Clinical Nurse Specialist
The James Cancer Hospital and Solove Research Center
The Ohio State University Comprehensive Cancer Center
Columbus, Ohio

MICHELLE RHINER, R.N., M.S.N., N.P.
Nurse Practitioner/Patient Coordinator
Supportive Care Services
City of Hope National Medical Center
Duarte, California

JEANNE ROBISON, R.N., M.N., A.R.N.P.
Hematology/Oncology Nurse Practitioner
Rockwood Clinic
Spokane, Washington

DAME CICELY SAUNDERS, O.M., D.B.E., F.R.C.P.
Chairman
St. Christopher's Hospice
Sydenham, London
United Kingdom

COLLEEN SCANLON, R.N., J.D.
Senior Vice President, Advocacy
Catholic Health Initiatives
Denver, Colorado

SUSIE SEAMAN, M.S.N., F.N.P., C.E.T.N.
Nurse Practitioner
Grossmont Hospital Wound Healing Center
Sharp Healthcare
San Diego, California

DENICE C. SHEEHAN, R.N., M.S.N.
Coordinator
Palliative Care Program
The Breen School of Nursing
Ursuline College
Pepper Pike, Ohio

DEBORAH WITT SHERMAN, PH.D., R.N., A.N.P., C.S.
Program Coordinator
Advanced Practice Palliative Care Masters Program
New York University
Project on Death in America Faculty Scholar
New York, New York

NEAL E. SLATKIN, M.D., D.A.B.P.M.
Director
Supportive Care and Palliative Medicine
City of Hope National Medical Center
Duarte, California

JEAN K. SMITH, R.N., M.S., O.C.N.
Breast Care Coordinator and Lymphedema Case Manager
Penrose Cancer Center of Centura Health
Colorado Springs, Colorado

THOMAS J. SMITH, M.D., F.A.C.P.
Associate Professor of Medicine and Health Administration
Massey Cancer Center
Virginia Commonwealth University
Richmond, Virginia

KAREN J. STANLEY, R.N., M.S.N., A.O.C.N.
Nursing Consultant, Palliative Care
Claremont, California

DAPHNE STANNARD, R.N., PH.D., C.C.R.N.
Assistant Professor of Nursing
San Francisco State University
San Francisco, California

RICHARD H. STEEVES, PH.D., R.N., F.A.A.N.
Associate Professor
Nursing School
University of Virginia
Charlottesville, Virginia

LIZABETH H. SUMNER, R.N., B.S.N.
Director
Children's Program
San Diego Hospice
Vista, California

ALICIA SUPER, R.N., B.S.N.
President
Pain and Supportive Care Services
Clackamas, Oregon

SIEW TZUH TANG, R.N., M.S.M., O.C.N.
Former Deputy Director
Department of Nursing
Sun Yat-Sen Cancer Center
Taipei, Taiwan

ELIZABETH JOHNSTON TAYLOR, R.N., PH.D.
Associate Professor
School of Nursing
Loma Linda University
Loma Linda, California

MEGUMI TESHIMA, R.N., M.N.
Deputy Director of Nursing
Higashi Sapporo Hospital
Sapporo, Japan

MARY L. S. VACHON, R.N., PH.D.
Consultant, Psychosocial Oncology & Palliative Care
Toronto Sunnybrook Health Regional Cancer Centre
Associate Professor
Departments of Psychiatry and Public Health Sciences
University of Toronto
Toronto, Ontario, Canada

Manuel Mario Vera, R.N.
Palliative Care Unit
Tornu Hospital
Buenos Aires, Argentina

Rose Virani, R.N.C., B.S.N., M.H.A., O.C.N.
Research Specialist
Department of Nursing Research and Education
City of Hope National Medical Center
Duarte, California

Florence Wald, R.N., F.A.A.N.
Branford, Connecticut

Carol M. Wenzl, R.N., M.E.D.
Chaplain
Mercy Health Center
Oklahoma City, OK

Marie Bakitas Whedon, M.S., A.R.N.P., N.P.-C., C.H.R.N., F.A.A.N.
Palliative Care Nurse Practitioner
Team Leader: Palliative Care Coordinators
Robert Wood Johnson Project ENABLE
Norris Cotton Cancer Center
Lebanon, New Hampshire

Sarah A. Wilson, Ph.D., R.N.
Associate Professor
Marquette University College of Nursing
Milwaukee, Wisconsin

Wang Ying, R.N.
Deputy Director
Tianjin Cancer Institute and Hospital He Xi District
Tianjin, People's Republic of China

Anne Marie Zobec, R.N., M.S., N.P.
Oncology Clinical Nurse Specialist
Centura-Penrose Hospital
Colorado Springs, Colorado

Laurie Zoloth-Dorfman, Ph.D., R.N.
Associate Professor
Ethics and Jewish Philosophy
San Francisco State University
College of Humanities
Berkeley, California

Part I

General Principles

1 Introduction to Palliative Nursing Care

NESSA COYLE

I didn't know I could be cared for in this way. I didn't know that there was a team like this. I had made a promise to my husband several months ago, that if he asked I would help him. We spoke with the Hemlock Society. Things were so bad I didn't think that we could manage much more. Things are still bad but I don't feel that way now. I don't feel so alone."

—Spouse

Advances in health care have changed the trajectory of dying. Improved nutrition and sanitation, preventative medicine, widespread vaccination use, the development of broad spectrum antibiotics, and an emphasis on early detection and treatment of disease have resulted in fewer deaths in infancy and childhood and fewer deaths from acute illness.[1,2] The combination of a healthier population in many developed countries and effective treatments for disease has resulted in our ability to prolong life. This has lead to both benefits and challenges for society. For example, in the United States, more than 70% of those who die each year are age 65 or older. The majority of these deaths, however, occur after a long, progressively debilitating chronic illness, such as cancer, cardiac disease, renal disease, lung disease, and acquired immune deficiency syndrome (AIDS).[1] The field of palliative care has expanded in response to this challenge and to the changed trajectory of dying.[1,3] It has built on the long tradition of hospice care so well defined in nursing.

THE "GOOD" AND "BAD" DEATH

Notions of "good" and "bad" deaths are shaped by people's experiences, spiritual beliefs, and culture and by changes in social mores, technology, and options for dying.[1] The National Institute of Medicine Report on improving care at the end of life,[1] suggests that people should be able to achieve a "decent" or "good death"—"one that is free from avoidable distress and suffering for patients, families, and caregivers; in general accord with patients' and families' wishes; and reasonably consistent with clinical, cultural and ethical standard" (p. 24). The report and recommendations focused on the interdisciplinary nature of palliative care, of which nursing is the core discipline. Traditionally, nursing has been at the forefront of the care of patients with chronic and advanced disease, and recent advances in symptom management, combined with the growing awareness of palliative care as a public health issue, have provided the impetus for bringing together this compendium of nursing knowledge.

PALLIATIVE CARE NURSING

It is important to define the field of palliative care nursing and how it differs in essence from other areas of nursing care. In this way, staff can be trained appropriately, and the special nature of such training recognized. Palliative care as a therapeutic approach, however, is appropriate for all nurses to practice. In the acute care or disease-focused model of nursing care, there is much less emphasis on the individuality of the patient or the relationship between patient and nurse. The individual care provider is considered of limited importance within the system.[4–6] In palliative care nursing, however, "the active total care of patients whose disease is not responsive to curative treatment . . . where control of pain, of other symptoms and of psychological distress and spiritual distress is paramount,"[7] the individual counts in the healing relationship. The nurse counts and the nurse's individual relationship with the patient and family counts. The relationship, together with knowledge and skills, is the essence of palliative care nursing.

The palliative care nurse frequently cares for patients experiencing major stressors: physical, psychological, social and spiritual. Many of these patients recognize themselves as dying, and struggle with this role, which they neither sought nor wanted. To be dying and to care for someone who is dying are two side of a complex social phenomenon. There are roles and obligations for each. To be labeled as dying affects how others behave toward the individual and how the individual behaves toward self and others.[5,8,9] The person is dying, or is "becoming dead" (personal communication with Eric Cassell, January 1, 2000), with all that that implies at both an individual and a social level. A feeling of failure and futility may pervade the relationship between the patient and a nurse or physician not well versed in hospice or palliative care, and the potential for growth may be lost. This experience is beyond their ken, they are made uncomfortable by it and may therefore disengage and step aside.

The following case illustrates the distress experienced by a nurse and physician who did not know how to transition and care for a patient when the goals of care changed from a life-prolonging focus to care at the end of life. That the patient and family struggled during this time of transition is made clear.

Case Study: Mr. George, a Patient with Gastric Cancer

Mr George, a 41-year-old man dying at home of gastric cancer, had been ill for 2 years and supported on total parenteral nutrition (TPN) for 6 months. He had severe pain and multiple other symptoms. Initially well controlled, the pain rapidly escalated, and distress surrounding lack of options for life prolonging therapies made communication with his physician and office nurse difficult. Telephone calls to the physician increased in frequency and urgency, and the patient's wife, his caregiver at home, became more and more distraught. The physician, who had developed a close relationship with this patient and family, felt overwhelmed, ineffective and guilty. At the advice of the office nurse, he consulted a palliative care nurse, almost in desperation. She became a sounding board for both the physician's and the wife's frustration and worries, which helped them to refocus on achievable goals of care for this man as a person. The physician came to an understanding of success and healing as something other than cure; he was kept in the palliative care "loop," and his role and importance to the patient and wife were supported. The phone calls decreased in number and became less cure-focused and less stressful. The relationship between administering TPN and increased pain was noted by the patient, and he asked that the TPN be stopped. The goal of comfort rather than nutrition became foremost in the patient's mind. Limited hydration continued at the wife's request. The patient expressed comfort that he was getting water. Although symptom control remained difficult and required constant vigilance, the physician and palliative care nurse shared this responsibility, and the patient was able to die at home with some comfort. The physician made home visits and maintained his fidelity to the patient.

While ineffective life-prolonging treatments were stopped, intensive palliative care continued, with a focus on relationships, rigorous symptom control, a life shared and sorrow that it was to end, and hope for the future.[10] Central to the ability of the nurse to evaluate the core of the distress of the physician, patient and family, and to intervene appropriately were assessment skills, ability to listen, communication skills, comfort in talking about spirituality, and knowledge regarding symptom control and healing at the end of life.[5,6,11] Each of these aspects of care is covered in different chapters of this book.

THE NURSE AND THE INTERDISCIPLINARY TEAM/ COLLABORATIVE PRACTICE

The composition of teams providing palliative care vary tremendously, depending on the needs of the patients and the resources available.[12] The common denominator is the presence of a nurse and a physician on the team. Regardless of the specific type of palliative care team, it is the nurse who serves as a primary liaison between the team, patient and family and who brings the team plan to the bedside, whether in the home or in the hospital. Because of the close proximity of the nurse to the patient and family through day-to-day observation and care, there is often a shift in the balance of decision making at the end of life from physician to nurse.[12] However, continued involvement of the physician in palliative care should be fostered and encouraged. It is a myth that physicians need be less involved as the goal of care shifts from cure to comfort. As illustrated in the case of Mr. George, a physician oriented toward life-prolonging therapies who had provided care for a patient over a number of years may feel lost, helpless, overwhelmed and uncertain of his or her role in the care of the dying; yet the patient and family may be very bonded to that physician and have a great need for him or her at this time. Fear of abandonment by the physician and the physician not wanting to abandon but to "do everything" may result in inappropriate and harmful treatment being offered and accepted. A nurse trained in palliative care and end of life care can do much to guide and support the physician during this transition and to redirect the interventions from "doing everything" toward doing everything to provide comfort and healing.

There may, however, be reasons that patients want to continue aggressive, life-prolonging interventions in the face of impending death. Understanding why aggressive medical care and life-prolonging measures are sought is an integral part of the role of the nurse on the palliative care team. This is illustrated in the following case example:

Case Study: Mr. Ray, a Patient with Prostate Cancer

Mr. Ray, a 57-year-old man with far advanced prostate cancer and rapidly failing pulmonary status, wanted every measure to be used to maintain life, including a tracheostomy and respirator. He had a wonderful and caring family who wanted whatever he wanted. Staff felt they were doing harm by introducing these extraordinary measures but complied with the patient's wishes. Mr Ray had fought "the odds" on several previous occasions and expected to do so again. He remained on a respirator for 6 weeks, during which time he was alert and cognitively intact. What the staff did not realize was that during this time the man was completing important work. He sold his business, which he wanted to do before he died so that his wife would not be burdened with this task after his death. Once this goal was completed Mr Ray gave his physician the "thumbs up" sign and indicated that he was ready to come off the respirator. The family were at peace with this decision, but the young physician who was responsible for his care and had become very close to the patient and family struggled with the concept of prolonging death versus hastening death if the respirator was withdrawn. Some of the nursing staff were similarly troubled. It would have been easier not to have started the treatment then to withdraw it. An experienced palliative care nurse mentored the young physician and nurses through their personal ethical struggles, and stayed by the physician's side as he administered a sedative drug and withdrew the respirator. The patient died 2 days later, a family member was with him all the time. The young physician expressed relief that the patient had not died "right away" as he felt more comfortable as having "not crossed the line."

Although other members of the interdisciplinary team, including the chaplain and social worker, were involved with this patient and family's care and in family and staff "de-briefing" and bereavement follow-up, the palliative care nurse played a central role coordinating and mentoring to meet the needs of the patient, family, and staff. No single discipline can meet the needs of most patients and their families; a team is required.[12]

How little we know about patients and their families, their aspirations, is also illustrated by this case. What seems to be an irrational choice to health care providers may be eminently sensible to the patient and family. The frequent struggle and suffering of nurses and physicians as they grapple with their own mortality and with being asked to provide care that they think is inappropriate or harmful is also demonstrated. The importance of assessment and communication skills, as well as a firm foundation on the ethical principles of palliative care and end-of-life care when treating such patients, is clear. This text provides such a foundation.

THE SCOPE AND AIMS OF THIS TEXT ON PALLIATIVE NURSING CARE

As illustrated through the previous discussion and case reports, palliative nursing care is a world of many connections. To see the world of the individual, a multidimensional, multi-lens perspective is needed. Often, this complexity is best conveyed through simple stories.[13–15] This duality of complexity and simplicity is incorporated into the structure of this volume. Each chapter is introduced by a quotation from a patient or family member to illustrate the content of the chapter. In addition, brief case examples are used to anchor the theoretical and practical content of the chapter in real-life situations.

The text, which includes an international perspective, is intended as a resource for nurses in the emerging field of palliative care. The approach has been to incorporate the principles of palliative care nursing throughout the course of a chronic, progressive, incurable disease rather than only at the end of life. The scope is broad. The content, contributed by more than 80 national and international nurse experts and divided into 63 chapters in nine parts, covers the world of palliative care nursing.

Part I provides a general introduction to palliative nursing care and a brief overview of the text; an exploration of the influence of palliative care on quality of life in progressive medical illness; an in-depth review of the principles and practice of hospice care; and a survey of palliative care planning and effectiveness based on careful patient evaluation and family assessment. Clinically useful assessment tools are provided.

Part II, moves into the critical area of symptom assessment and management. Each chapter addresses the assessment and pathophysiology of the symptom, pharmacologic interventions, non-drug treatments, and patient/family teaching within the goals of palliative care. Part III addresses psychosocial support at the end of life. Here the focus is on communication, the meaning of hope at the end of life, bereavement, family support, complementary therapies, and planning for the death and death rituals. Spiritual care and meaning in illness are addressed in Part IV. The impact of spiritual distress on quality of life at the end of life has become increasingly clear. The ability of the nurse to recognized such distress in patients and their families and to make appropriate interventions and referrals are essential components of palliative care.

In Part V the needs of special populations are addressed. Included are the elderly and the cognitively impaired, children, the poor and underserved, and individuals with AIDS. Part VI, focuses on improving the quality of end-of-life care across settings. After a practical overview on monitoring quality and development of pathways and standards in end-of-life care, subsequent chapters discuss long-term care, home care, hospice care, pediatric palliative care, hospital care, intensive care, and care in the outpatient or office setting. Part VI concludes with a discussion of the construct of rehabilitation within the context of palliative care and hospice care.

Part VII leads into a discussion of nursing issues that influence end-of-life care, giving voice to the nurse who provides care at the end of life and exploring the special issues encountered. Included are responsibility without power, responsibility with inadequate training, witness to difficult deaths without the opportunity to debrief and mourn, and coping with one's own loss and grief. This proceeds to an exploration of ethical considerations in end-of-life care, including accountability and quality, truth telling, medical futility, withdrawal of treatment, euthanasia and physician assisted-suicide, ethical decision making, and the function of ethics committees. The concluding chapters cover nursing education, including undergraduate, graduate and continuing education, as well as the palliative care nurse as researcher. Instruments to measure end-of-life outcomes and areas for future research are included in this section.

An international perspective is presented in Part VIII. Diverse models, with the multifactorial political and cultural factors that influence the development of palliative care, are illustrated through a variety of countries, including Australia, New Zealand, Japan, Canada, Israel, Great Britain, Ireland, China, India, South America, Africa and Taiwan. Part IX gives voice to the patient and family, exploring the concept of "a good death" through a detailed case discussion. The appendices provide a variety of useful community and professional resources.

The purpose of this text is to organize and disseminate the existing nursing knowledge of experts in palliative care nursing and to provide a scientific underpinning for practice. The focus is on assessment and management of the wide range of physical, psychosocial, and spiritual needs of patients, their families, and staff in palliative care across clinical settings. Topics frequently cited as challenges in nursing care at the end of life, including terminal sedation, communication, ethics, research, and providing care for the underserved and homeless, are addressed. As illustrated throughout, the world of palliative care nursing is complex, scientifically based, and immensely rewarding.

REFERENCES

1. Field M, Cassel C, Committee on Care at the End of Life, Institute of Medicine. Approaching Death: Improving Care at the End of Life. Washington DC: National Academy Press, 1997.

2. Corr C. Death in modern society. In: Doyle D, Hanks WC, MacDonald N, eds. Oxford Textbook of Palliative Medicine, 2nd Ed. Oxford: Oxford University Press, 1998:31–40.

3. Doyle D. The provision of palliative care. In: Doyle D, Hanks WC, MacDonald N, eds. Oxford Textbook of Palliative Medicine, 2nd Ed. Oxford: Oxford University Press, 1998:41–53.

4. Weissman DE, Block SD, Blank L, Cain J, Cassem N, Danoff D, Foley K, Meier D, Schyve P, Theige D, Wheeler HB. Recommendations for incorporating palliative care education into the acute care hospital setting. Acad Med 1999;74: 871–877.

5. Cassell EJ. Diagnosing suffering: a perspective. Ann Intern Med 1999;131:531–534.

6. Cassell EJ. The Nature of Suffering and the Goals of Medicine. New York: Oxford University Press, 1991.

7. World Health Organization. Cancer Pain Relief and Palliative Care. Technical Report Series 804. Geneva: WHO, 1990:11.

8. Aries P. Western Attitudes Towards Death: From the Middle Ages to the Present. Baltimore: Johns Hopkins University Press, 1974.

9. Cherny N, Coyle N, Foley KM. Suffering in the advanced cancer patient. Part I: A definition and taxonomy. J Palliat Care 1994;10: 57–70.

10. Nekolaichuk CL, Bruera E. On the nature of hope in palliative care. J Palliat Care 1998;14:36–42.

11. Kearney M. Mortally Wounded. New York: Scribner, 1996.

12. Ingham J, Coyle N. Teamwork in end of life care: a nurse–physician perspective on introducing physicians to palliative care concepts. In: Clark D, Hockley J, Ahmedzai S, eds. New Themes in Palliative Care. Buckingham: Open University Press, 1997:255–274.

13. Steeves RH. Loss, grief and the search for meaning. Oncol Nurs Forum 1996;23:897–903.

14. Ferrell BR. The quality of lives: 1525 voices of cancer. Oncol Nurs Forum 1996;23: 907–915.

15. Coyle, N. Suffering in the first person. In: Ferrell BF, ed. Suffering. Boston: Jones and Bartlett, 1996:29–64.

2 Hospice Care: A Model for Quality End-of-Life Care

KATHLEEN A. EGAN and MARY J. LABYAK

We thought this was going to be the most difficult time of our lives. With the support, love, and care provided by our hospice team, it became a time to treasure, even though it was difficult. We experienced the love, compassion, and skill of the hospice team. The care and dignity they provided allowed my husband and me to travel this last journey together and become closer than at any other time through our 50 years of marriage.

—Spouse of a hospice patient

Hospice is a program of care provided across a variety of settings, based on the understanding that dying is part of the normal life cycle. As people experience this last phase of life, a hospice provides comprehensive palliative medical and supportive services, compassion, and care with the goals of comfort and quality of life closure. A hospice supports the patient through the dying process and the family through the dying and the bereavement. Understanding that the last phase of life is as individual as each person who experiences it, a hospice advocates so that people may live the remainder of their lives with dignity and die in a manner that is meaningful to them.

HOSPICE IN THE UNITED STATES

As sickness progresses toward death, measures to minimize suffering should be intensified. Dying patients require palliative care of an intensity that rivals even that of curative efforts even though aggressive curative techniques are no longer indicated, professionals and families are still called on to use intensive measures—extreme responsibility, extraordinary sensitivity and heroic compassion.[1]

Hospice began in the United States as a grassroots effort to improve the quality of the dying experience for patients and their families. Historically, health care delivery systems have been disease-driven, with the focus on cure and rehabilitation. Approaches have focused on scientific knowledge of diseases driving the care processes. When cure is the goal, approaches to care are different from when cure is no longer possible. End-stage disease progression and resulting symptoms present different physiologic responses as well as different emotional responses. Hospice care began as a grassroots effort in communities where the traditional medical model fell short of addressing those differences.

In 1999, the National Hospice and Palliative Care Organization (NHPCO; formerly the NHO) described hospice philosophy as follows:

> Hospice provides support and care for persons in the last phases of incurable disease so that they may live as fully and as comfortably as possible. Hospice recognizes dying as part of the normal process of living and focuses on enhancing the quality of remaining life. Hospice affirms life and neither hastens nor postpones death. Hospice exists in the hope and belief that through appropriate care, and the promotion of a caring community sensitive to their needs that individuals and their families may be free to attain a degree of satisfaction in preparation for death. Hospice recognizes that human growth and development can be a lifelong process. Hospice seeks to preserve and promote the inherent potential for growth within individuals and families during the last phase of life. Hospice offers palliative care for all individuals and their families without regard to age, gender, nationality, race, creed, sexual orientation, disability, diagnosis, availability of a primary caregiver, or ability to pay.
>
> Hospice programs provide state-of-the-art palliative care and supportive services to individuals at the end of their lives, their family members and significant others, 24 hours a day, seven days a week, in both the home and facility-based care settings. Physical, social, spiritual, and emotional care are provided by a medically-directed interdisciplinary team consisting of patients and their families, professionals and volunteers during the
>
> 1. Last phase of an illness;
> 2. Dying process; and
> 3. Bereavement period.[2]

The Hospice Holistic Approach to Care

Understanding the need for a better way to care for the dying, the hospice movement began to provide alternatives to the traditional curative model. Hospice expanded the traditional model not only to address end-stage disease management but also to provide for the emotional, social, and spiritual dimensions of the patient's and family's dying experience.

The beginning of the contemporary hospice movement is credited to Dame Cicely Saunders. Beresford describes her pioneering work: "Her concept of hospice was to combine the most modern medical techniques in terminal care with the spiritual commitment of the medieval religious orders that had once created hospices as way stations for people on pilgrimages." [3]

The experience of the last phase of

life is an individual journey involving one's mind, body, and spirit. Cassell[4] describes a theory of personhood whereby each person is a holistic being with dynamic, interrelated dimensions that are affected by the changes and adaptations experienced with progressive illness and dying. These dimensions involve the physical experience of end-stage disease, the emotional experience of one's relationships, and how one defines spiritual existence.[4] As the disease progresses and the physical dimensions decline, the other dimensions (i.e., interpersonal, spiritual) take on added meaning and purpose. What one defines as quality of life changes substantially for people with life-limiting illnesses. Life perspectives, goals, and needs change. It is a time of reflection on a broader sense of meaning, purpose, and relationships based on each individual's values.

Hospice grew from this understanding of full personhood and is designed to offer expert end-of-life care to patients and families addressing all of these dimensions through an interdisciplinary team approach. Each patient and family is supported by an interdisciplinary team consisting of physicians, nurses, social workers, counselors, chaplains, therapists, home health aides, and volunteers. These disciplines reflect the expertise needed to address the varied dimensions affected through the course of illness, dying, and bereavement.

Aging in the United States and End-of-Life Care

The aging of America has changed the nature and needs of people who are dying. The hospice Medicare benefit was designed to provide substantial professional and material support (medications, equipment) to families caring for the dying at home during their last 6 months of life. The benefit was designed for, and lends itself well to, the predictable trajectory of end-stage cancers but not as well to unpredictable chronic illnesses like congestive heart failure, chronic lung disease, stroke, and dementing illnesses.[5] An examination of hospice care and the delivery of quality end-of-life services must reflect this societal change in aging demographics and the varied needs in our end-of-life care models.

In our society, the overwhelming majority of dying people are the elderly, who typically die of a slowly progressing, chronic disease or of multiple coexisting problems resulting in multisystem failure. Their final phase of life, often lasting several years prior to death, is marked by a progressive functional dependence and associated family and caregiver burden. Hospice programs in demographic areas that represent the future of our aging society, such as Florida, have expanded care and service options to more fully respond to the frail elderly in their communities dying of chronic, progressive illnesses. These newer delivery models are applying hospice philosophy and services in the care of patients and their families long before the last 6 months of life, recognizing the slow dying process, allowing people to age in place, and providing an array of services so that they may stay in their own homes until death.

Hospice, therefore, neither hastens nor postpones death but, rather, affirms life. The focus is on quality of life closure, which begins with the patient's and family's definitions of their choices, goals, and dreams during this time.

HOSPICE PHILOSOPHY

Hospice philosophy supports the long-term objective of creating a personalized experience with each patient at the end of life whereby in the face of suffering there is opportunity for growth and quality end-of-life closure for both the patient and family. Promoting quality of life and death with dignity, hospice emphasizes that the patient and family live each day as fully as possible with the "hope of making the very best of today when . . . tomorrows are limited." [6]

The Patient and Family Experience

The dying experience has significant and profound effects on both the patient and family. Therefore, hospice philosophy supports both the patient and family as the unit of care. Family is defined as not only the biologic relatives but also those people identified by the patient as significant.

Hospice patients and families face many changes and losses. Patients often become concerned about the burden they may cause their family and how their family will survive after they are gone. Families become concerned over how to care for the patient, how to adapt to role changes, their reactions to their losses, and how their lives will change after the death.

Hospice philosophy, therefore, promotes the patient and family as one unit of care. Care does not stop after the death of the patient. Just as the patient's death experience involves the physical, emotional, spiritual, and social dimensions, survivors' reactions to loss are also experienced through all dimensions. Bereavement-support services are continued for family and caregivers for a year or more after the death of the patient.

Care Is Directed by Patient and Family Values

Hospice philosophy supports the understanding that dying is the patient's and family's experience. Nurses providing hospice care are challenged to approach the care process differently from other situations. Hospice care begins with a facilitated discussion with the patient and family, to discern their values, choices, wishes, and needs for the remaining life and death. This information becomes the foundation that directs the team in the provision of care. Goals become patient/family-directed rather than nurse-directed. It is not about what nurses feel is best but about what the patient and family choose and decide. The care plan becomes the "patient/family care plan" and the care process is defined by the patient and family values, goals, and wishes.

A patient/family value–directed care process begins to differentiate the specialty of hospice nursing with an overall goal of quality of life closure as defined by the patient and family. Quality of life closure refers to the possibilities for positive experiences in the face of suffering where patient and family may grow, find meaning, and reach personal goals prior to and after the death.

Palliative Care versus Curative Care

Hospice philosophy emphasizes palliative care, which can be as aggressive as curative care, but with a focus on comfort, dignity, quality of life closure, and patient/family choice. When a patient's disease process is no longer curable or reversible, aggressive curative treatment becomes increasingly inappropriate. An aggressive curative approach to care can actually cause more suffering when cure is no longer possible or simply extend the period of suffering needlessly. As a patient advocate, the hospice nurse is responsible for understanding the differences between curative and palliative interventions, to avoid futile care and prevent unnecessary suffering.

The curative model of care has an inherent problem orientation. Practitioners are often trained to assess and identify "problems" and then determine how to reverse the problem effects. Palliative care moves beyond problem identification. The specialty of hospice nursing involves the expert management of end-stage disease symptomatology as a prerequisite to providing the opportunity for patients and families to experience growth and find meaning and value in the dying and bereavement experience. Hospice has moved from a problem orientation to a quality of life closure orientation that reflects the full scope of the patient's and family's dying experience.

By anticipating and preventing the negative effects of physical symptoms, suffering can be decreased, which allows the patient and family the energy to address their personal life closure goals. Moving ahead of a simple problem orientation, the focus has become one of prevention of suffering and opportunity for growth rather than simply the physical reaction to disease.

A search for meaning and purpose in life is a common experience for dying patients and their families. From the individual experience of suffering, death can be a time for personal growth, interpersonal relationship growth, and enrichment of meaning.

Autonomy and Choice

Hospice philosophy promotes patient autonomy in which dying is in accordance with the patient's and family's desires. Hospice philosophy strongly believes in patient choice regarding all aspects of living, dying, and grieving including where they will die, how they will die, and with whom they will die. Respecting the patient's and family's choices is paramount to quality hospice care.

One of the dying patient's and family's greatest concerns is the fear of loss of control. Many losses are anticipated and experienced by terminally ill patients and their families, including loss of bodily functions, loss of independence and self-care, loss of income with resulting financial burdens, loss of the ability to provide for loved ones, loss or lack of time to complete tasks and mend relationships, and loss of decision making. Dying patients have a right to remain in control of their lives and their deaths. They are often concerned that their wishes will not be honored, that their requests will not be answered, and that when they are too ill, control of their lives will be taken from them. It is critical to provide continued opportunities for choice, input, informed decision making, and ability to change decisions as situations change.

Informed Decisions and Autonomy

Hospice philosophy also supports the ethical principle of veracity, or truth telling. Patients' wishes for information about their condition are respected. Patients have the right to be informed about their condition, treatment options, and treatment outcomes so that they can make autonomous, informed choices and spend the rest of their life the way they choose.

Truth telling is the essence of open, trusting relationships. A sense of knowing often relieves the burden of the unknown. A large majority of the American population state that they would want to know their diagnosis and information that concerns them.[6] Knowing and talking about diagnosis and prognosis aids in informed decisions. Patients who have not been told about their illness naturally suspect that something is wrong or being hidden from them, which can result in frustrating, unanswered questions. When patients and families are not told the truth or information is withheld, they can no longer make informed choices about the end of their life.

The hospice philosophy of autonomy results in empowerment of the patient and family in making their own informed decisions regarding life and death. Hospice encourages the discussion of advance directives but does not influence those decisions. Hospice nurses educate on these issues and offer support while the patient and family discuss and choose what is best for them. Their choices may change over time, as the disease progresses, the patient becomes more dependent, or they accomplish their life closure goals.

Advance directives such as living wills, health care surrogacy, durable power of attorney, and do-not-resuscitate orders allow for the patient's wishes to be carried out when he or she is no longer able to communicate or make health care decisions. With advance preparation, these directives can act in place of the patient's verbal requests and assure that end-of-life decision making is in accordance with the patient's wishes. When patient and family members discuss advance directives together, there is often less conflict over decisions and family members are more comfortable supporting the patient's choices. When advance directives are combined with hospice philosophy, they can serve as preventive measures to assure that patient's choices will be carried out without ethical dilemmas.

Hospice care supports sensitivity in truth telling to the degree that the patient and family choose, with open communication between the patient, family, physicians, and hospice team. Preparation for death becomes difficult when communication is not open and truthful. With a truthful understanding and freedom of informed choice, patients are more able to control their own death instead of being controlled by the disease and/or treatment plan. They can put their affairs in order, say their good-byes, and prepare spiritually in a way that promotes quality and dignity.

Dignity and Respect for Patients and Families

Quality end-of-life care is most effective from the patient/family perspective when the patient's lifestyle is maintained and his or her philosophy of life is respected. Individual patient's and family's needs vary depending on values, cultural orientation, personal characteristics, and environment. The hospice approach allows for individual lifestyles to be supported and respected. This requires respect for ethnicity, cultural orientation, social and sexual preferences, and varied family structures. Hospice nursing requires the provision of nonjudgmental, unconditional, positive regard when caring for terminal patients and families, treating each person as unique.

Each person and family has individual coping skills, varied dynamics, and strengths and weaknesses. It is our responsibility to "accept patients and families where they are," approaching living and dying in their way. Patients should be encouraged to express any emotion, including anger, denial, or depression. By listening without being judgmental, the hospice nurse accepts the patient's and family's coping mechanisms as real and effective.

Dying patients have their own needs and wants, and hospice nurses must be open to accept patients' direction. Patients' focus may include saving all their energy for visits from loved ones, loving and being loved, sharing with others their own philosophy of life and death, reviewing their life and family history, and sharing thoughts and prayers with their family and/or caregivers. Their goal may also include looking physically attractive or intrinsically exploring the purpose and meaning of their lives. Being open and prepared to accept and support the patient's and family's direction on any given visit will facilitate and respect their goals. The patient's and family's own frame of reference for values, preferences, and outlook on life and death is considered and respected without judgment.

Respecting patients requires hospice nurses to communicate a sense of what is important to the patient/family by allowing them to express their values and opinions, participating in care planning, making decisions regarding their care and how they choose to spend their time, and participating in their own care. Fostering an environment that allows the patient and family to retain a sense of respect, control, and dignity is the foundation of hospice nursing.

The Hospice Nurse as Advocate

Enhancing quality of life is the primary goal of hospice and palliative care. Patients who, in the later stages of their life, have chosen to receive palliative care have a right to have their wishes honored and respected at all points of entry into and across the health care system. Optimizing quality of life and respecting patient's and family's wishes involve a great deal of commitment, collaboration, and communication. In promoting patient autonomy, hospice nurses participate as patient advocates across all care settings, supporting the patients' and their family's choices and goals for the remainder of their lives.

By integrating the hospice philosophies and values described above, the hospice nurse acts as advocate for the patient/family, to preserve their rights and protect the goals of their palliative care plan. The hospice nurse's role of professional advocacy involves collaboration with physicians, health care institutions, and health care systems. She or he may be involved in advocating for appropriate symptom management, identifying valuable resources, gaining access to these resources, and coordinating the utilization of resources and services.

The patient, family, hospice interdisciplinary team, physician, hospice organization, other health and human service providers, and legal institutions are all impacted by patient choices. It is the responsibility of every care provider to respect and insure the rights of dying patients and their families.

HOSPICE CARE DELIVERY SYSTEMS

Hospice care is not defined by a distinct physical setting or individual organizational structure. It is provided in a variety of settings. Although 90% of hospice patient time is spent in a personal residence, some patients live in long-term care facilities, assisted living facilities, hospice care centers, or other group quarters. In addition, some hospices provide day-care programs.[7]

As identified by the NHPCO, the following organizational structures of hospice programs exist, with ever-expanding care and service designs to meet the needs of varied communities:

1. *Community-based, independent hospice programs* represent approximately 28% of hospice programs. *Community-based* is defined as being independent of affiliation to a hospital, home health care agency, or other care agency.
2. *Hospices as divisions of a corporation other than a hospice* are managed as departments or divisions of a hospital or health system. Approximately 59% of hospice programs are of this type.
3. The remaining 13% are unidentified.[8]

Hospice Care and Service Sites

Patient's and Family's Private Home. Encompassing the philosophical principle of autonomy, hospice supports patients and families wherever they choose to die. The majority of hospice care is provided in the patient's private home setting. According to a Gallup poll commissioned by the NHPCO and released in 1996, hospice care coupled with a wish to die at home have widespread support among the public. In perhaps the most striking response in the survey, a significant majority of 88% of those polled said they would prefer to die in the comfort of their own home, surrounded by family and friends, rather than in any health care institution.[9] Therefore, hospice supports patients staying at home until death if that is where they choose to die.

With so many people choosing to stay at home with family, hospice emphasizes the need to empower families so that they can participate to the level they are able in providing care to the patient. Hospice's ability to involve the family in caregiving often improves their perspectives and experience. Research has shown significant differences in favor of hospice in four measures used to evaluate the quality of life of the primary caregiver (family). Primary caregivers for hospice patients were found to be less anxious and more satisfied with their involvement in care than were their nonhospice counterparts.[10]

Long-Term Care Settings. As our population ages, we are challenged to provide care and services in different ways. Hospices are increasingly serving elderly people, many over 75 years of age, who live alone or with a frail family caregiver. As evidenced by the recent expansion of elder care communities, the definition of "home" has also changed for many elderly and can include a variety of residential settings with various levels of assistance. Another part of our population receiving hospice care is the homeless. Each of these differences has posed challenges for hospice programs to expand service delivery options and provide care in all of these homes.

Hospice seeks to affirm life while assuring continuity of palliative care in long-term care settings. Some hospice patients are referred while residing in long-term care, while others may be transferred into long-term care after being admitted to a hospice program at home. As patient and family needs change at the end of life, hospice home care patients may find long-term care placement a chosen, necessary alternative care setting.

Many hospice programs also have arrangements to admit a hospice home patient into a long-term care facility for respite care. *Respite care* is care for a limited period of time that provides a break for the family while the patient is cared for in another setting. Wherever the patient resides, hospice philosophy can be incorporated and care provided by the full interdisciplinary team (IDT) in collaboration with the long-term care staff.

The hospice IDT again supports autonomy in decision making by providing information on many alternative care options to the patient and family when home care is no longer appropriate. The hospice nurse and team have the responsibility to educate the family about patient care needs and respect and support the family's ability to set limits and acknowledge their own needs in placing their loved ones in other care settings.

Assisted-Living Settings. With the aging of our population, there are a variety of elder care living settings where people may be dying. Recent expansion of adult living facilities (ALFs) has presented the challenge to care for people while allowing them to "age in place" and to "die in place." In the past, facilities licensed as ALFs were required to transfer a resident out of their facility if they could not independently provide care. For many people, this removed them from their home environment as they came closer to death, often losing all sense of control over their lives. These residents were prevented from aging in place and dying in place.

Due to recent recognition of the detrimental effects of moving people at this time in their lives, residents in ALFs in many parts of the country are now able to stay in the ALF until death, as long as hospice is involved. The end result supports hospice philosophy by allowing for autonomy of where and how someone chooses to die. Just as in other care settings, the hospice team remains the care manager in collaboration with the ALF staff to advocate for the patient/family palliative care goals.

Hospice Residences. Emerging as another alternative setting for people who can no longer stay in their own home is hospice residential care. Residential hospice care refers to the care provided in a facility that is staffed and owned by hospice programs. Patients are usually admitted to a hospice residential setting when they are no longer able to care for themselves and do not have a caregiver, their caregiver is frail, or their caregiver is working and unable to provide care at home. Patients may also be admitted to hospice residential care when their care needs (especially highly skilled technical ones) are more than the family can handle. The same hospice services are available at the residence as in private homes. Family of patients at hospice residences are encouraged to participate in their care to their level of comfort, but hospice staff and volunteers are available 24 hours a day to provide needed care. The number of hospice residences is growing as communities are realizing their value in filling a care need not provided in the same way in other settings.

Children, adolescents, young adults, and the elderly can be cared for in this setting. Consistent with hospice philosophy, admittance to residential care should not depend on race, color, creed, or ability to pay. Admission to hospice residences is based on the needs and preferences of the patient and family. Some hospice programs have admission guidelines that maintain their residential care option to those closer to death, for example, within 2 months. Most programs, however, have found this option of care to be beneficial for many different reasons and have not limited its use or length of stay to a specific time frame.

Hospice seeks to create a community of caring within its residences, striving to be flexible and home-like. Patients may follow their own personal schedule, and their visitors have unlimited access. Patients are usually free to come and go as they please and are encouraged to bring some of their belongings to create an environment that is most comforting to them. The residential setting promotes community and affirms life by offering group activities, group meals, events, and celebrations that promote socialization. Patient choice in participation is respected.

Palliative Care Units. More recently in the United States, hospice programs have created partnerships with acute and long-term care settings to open palliative care units as a service offered within those facilities. The expertise of acute care professionals coupled with that of hospice professionals allows for the combined benefits of both systems in care of the patient at the end of life. Generally, there are patients in palliative care units who are placed there as hospice patients needing acute interventions or as transfers from the acute care setting when a transition to hospice is expected but not yet indicated.

Many people access acute care settings during an episode of exacerbated symptomatology related to an end-stage and/or chronic disease process. Depending on the response to care and prognostic indicators, patients, families, and physicians begin to realize that conventional curative care is no longer beneficial. Palliative care units are a more realistic option, allowing attention to acute symptomatology by expert end-of-life clinicians while encouraging comfort and dignity for the patient's and family's experience. Palliative care units provide the opportunity for a smooth transition from the curative model of care to a palliative model for these patients.

Some hospice programs have contracted with hospitals or skilled nursing facilities to develop palliative care units for the treatment of acute episodes for hospice patients. The advantage for the patient and family is that they are cared for by staff and volunteers who are competent in skilled medical care and end-of-life care. The patient's palliative plan of care continues to be paramount to care decisions and interventions.

Hospital Settings and Hospice. Inpatient hospital care is an option for patients and families, usually to meet their acute care needs. Most hospice patients admitted to the hospital setting are considered to be inpatients, as defined by the Medicare levels of care, receiving skilled care. While most patients want to live out the remainder of their lives in their home, there are times when inpatient hospitalization is requested or necessary to meet the changing needs of patients and families.

The reasons for hospitalization can vary. For some patients, the physician may request hospitalization for acute problems, including exacerbation of symptoms that are difficult to control in a home care setting. The patient may also require hospitalization for palliative surgical intervention. At times, hospice patients are admitted to the hospital for a condition that is not related to their terminal diagnosis. Physical needs resulting in hospitalization vary from patient to patient and should be an option in response to patient need and choice.

Some patients may request hospitalization for a fracture repair, while others may request to stay at home with medication for pain control. In situations involving possible hospitalizations, it is important for the hospice nurse and IDT to be available to explore with the patient his or her choices in care and care setting before the hospitalization. The patient and family should also remain involved in the plan of care, to determine how to best meet their changing needs. It is vital that the team provide the patient and family with other available services and care options, to prevent hospitalization if that is the patient's and family's wishes.

While assessing the changing needs of patients and families, it is also important that the hospice nurse with the IDT support patient and family choice regarding care setting and that they continue to honor the patient's and family's requests.

Hospice Nurse's Responsibilities in Facility-Based Care Settings

Regardless of the type of setting, the hospice nurse and IDT are responsible for continuity of the patient's and family's palliative plan of care. When a patient is admitted to a facility, the hospice IDT remains the patient's care manager. Regulations also require collaborative care planning as well as documentation of mutually developed goals and interventions in some settings, such as between long-term care facilities and hospice.

To assure the highest level of patient/family autonomy, hospice nurses have a responsibility to educate the facility staff about philosophy, principles, and practices of hospice care. The staff should be able to integrate into their practice a dying patient's rights and their responsibility in allowing the patient to make his or her own decisions. The specialty of end-of-life symptom management is still elusive to most nurses; therefore, hospice nurses are often involved in nonhospice settings, educating staff about protocols for pain and symptom management. Education of the staff improves the delivery of palliative care and makes the staff feel more confident and comfortable in caring for dying patients and their families rather than the avoidance that sometimes comes from feelings of inadequacy.

To provide continuity of care for the patient and family, the hospice nurse should be in contact with the facility staff to assure the patient's and family's physical, psychosocial, and spiritual status; their goals and wishes; and that their decisions regarding advance directives are communicated. While respecting the policies and procedures of each setting, the hospice IDT must communicate and collaborate with the patient, family, physician, and facility staff to assure continuity of the patient/family plan of care.

HOSPICE CARE PROVIDED THROUGH AN INTERDISCIPLINARY TEAM

The Patient/Family Value–Based End-of-Life Care Model

Nurses caring for patients and their families at the end of life need to first comprehend the basic differences between curative approaches and palliative end-of-life approaches based on a patient/family value model.

Within the foundation of hospice philosophy, one of the significant differences in hospice nursing revolves around the concept of the patient and family directing care. Such issues as dignity and quality can be defined only subjectively by those who are experiencing life changes associated with dying.

The *patient/family value–based end-*

of-life model is founded on the following principles:

1. Dying is a personal experience.
2. People experience the last phase of their lives through many related dimensions.
3. The last phase of life provides continued opportunity for positive growth and development in the face of suffering.[11]

Principle 1: Dying is a personal experience.

Respecting patients' individuality is the foundation of humane care. It requires confronting the fullness of the human context in which illness and aging occur. Individual patients must be the focus of attention, and their particular values, concerns, and goals must be recognized and addressed.[12]

Just as earlier stages of life for each individual are different, so is dying. How one adapts to changes brought on as a result of an end-stage disease process or changes brought on by the normal slowing of systems associated with aging is a very personal response. These responses reflect the diversity of an individual's life experience, beliefs, and values. Looking to the future in end-of-life care and understanding the vast differences among those individuals who are in the final phase of life, nurses must provide care that results in individualized, customized relationships that respect patient's and family's values, preferences, and expressed needs in the final phase of life.

What one person defines as quality of life in the final phase may differ drastically from the next person or differ at points in the life continuum. For one patient, self-determined life closure may mean not being dependent on life-sustaining machines or having a living will. For another patient, it may mean being able to die at home, with family at the bedside. For the patient who has spent the last 3 years confined to a wheelchair, it may involve dying on the screened porch of a mobile home.

The hospice philosophy of care most closely attends to respecting the individuality of dying. Nurses providing quality end-of-life care must use the guiding principles of autonomy/choice, advocacy, and acceptance to best meet the goal of supporting individualized dying experiences.

Principle 2: People experience the last phase of their lives through many related dimensions.

The dying experience is one that impacts all dimensions of a person. To comprehend the nature of suffering among the dying, it is essential to know and understand the person. Eric Cassell[13] describes a model for understanding suffering in his "topology" of personhood. In his multidimensional model of personhood, each person exists as a dynamic matrix of dimensions, or realms, of the self. Each dimension has a significant and dynamic impact on and relationship with the other dimensions. Applying this dynamic relationship of dimensions to the last phase of life will guide the nurse in providing excellence in service and an optimal end-of-life experience for the patient and family.

Ira Byock and Melanie Merriman,[14] authors of the Missoula-VITAS Quality of Life Index (the only assessment tool designed to evaluate quality of life closure as an interdimensional, subjective experience of the patient), have developed an end-of-life construct based on Cassell's topology of personhood. The basis for this construct is that people experience the last phase of life as multidimensional beings. As a person's physical and functional dimensions decline, quality of life can be enhanced by attention to their interpersonal, well-being, and transcendent dimensions. Each dimension is briefly described below:

Physical Dimension: one's experience of the physical discomfort associated with progressive illness, perceived level of physical distress.

Function Dimension: one's perceived ability to perform accustomed functions and activities of daily living, experienced in relation to expectations and adaptations to declining functionality.

Interpersonal Dimension: degree of investment in personal relationships and perceived quality of one's relations with family, friends, and others.

Well-Being Dimension: self-assessment of internal condition; subjective sense of "wellness" or "dis-ease," contentment or lack of contentment, personal sense of well-being, how they feel within themselves.

Transcendent Dimension: one's experienced degree of connection with an enduring construct; one's relationship on a transpersonal level may involve, but does not have to involve, spiritual or religious values; can involve one's perception of the meaning of life, suffering, death, afterlife, etc.[14]

Nurses must approach end-of-life care with the understanding that a change in one of these dimensions affects the other dimensions. Examining pain as a physical dimension without being prompted to determine how this has affected all other dimensions (interpersonal, functional, etc.) of that person's experience would not attend to the full dying experience.

An example of a hospice nurse's assessment of a patient's pain from an interdimensional perspective is illustrated in the following:

Case Study: Mr. Carey, a Patient with Cancer of the Bone

The patient has suffered a pathological fracture to his dominant arm (*physical dimension*). Due to this pain, he is confined to his bed and unable to fully bathe and toilet independently (*function dimension*). Because any movement is too difficult, he is no longer able to leave his room and is isolated from family and friends (*interpersonal dimension*). He is feeling depressed and guilty because he cannot be self-sufficient (*well-being dimension*). As a result, he begins questioning "Why is this happening to me?", "What did I do to deserve this?" (*transcendent dimension*).

Continuing with the understanding that hospice cares for the patient and family, the nurse's assessment of the family (his wife) may be illustrated in the following:

Mr. Carey's wife cannot stand watching his suffering, feeling helpless to change it and asking God, "Why are you allowing him to suffer?" (*spiritual dimension*). Since he can no longer care for himself independently, she is doing all his personal care and is becoming exhausted (*physical dimension*). She is no longer able to rationalize his angry outbursts and lashes back at him (*interpersonal dimension*). When she does stop to think about his suffering, she feels guilty for lashing out and feels like she is inadequate (how could she blame him?) (*well-being dimension*).

Referred to as interdimensional care, this approach respects the full scope of the dying experience and is the basis for optimally affecting quality of life closure. The challenge within hospice nursing is to approach all interactions with patients and families with an understanding of this dynamic dimensional relationship. By approaching and assessing this patient's situation from a singular symptom dimension and medical/physical perspective, opportunities to improve the quality of life for the patient and family in all of the other dimensions are neglected.

When all dimensions are assessed and the individual is able to direct his or her own care, an extraordinary possibility for growth, healing, dignity, and positive life closure occurs. There is opportunity for review, restitution, amends, exploration, development, insight affecting all dimensions, and therefore end-of-life growth.

Principle 3: The last phase of life provides continued opportunity for positive growth and development in the face of suffering.

In his book, *Dying Well*, Ira Byock[15] has written about the opportunities for growth and development at the end of life. As a hospice physician, he shares his observations of patients and families at the end of life. He explains how people in the face of suffering are able to personally develop a sense of completion, to find meaning in their lives, to experience love of self and others, to say their goodbyes, and to surrender to the unknown.

Hospice nursing involves incorporating the first two principles, dying as an individual experience and the interdimensional experience of dying, with end-of-life developmental landmarks and tasks. The ultimate goal is to provide the opportunity for growth and to improve the quality of life closure for patients and families through the accomplishment of these life closure tasks.

In addition to the potential for physical distress and suffering, terminal illness presents a final opportunity to complete landmarks and tasks of life-long development. Quality of life is enhanced as the tasks are completed and the landmarks achieved. Hospice protects and amplifies the opportunity for personal growth in the final stage of life, thereby enhancing quality of life among patients and families.[16]

Dying is a part of living. The period of time referred to as dying can therefore be considered a stage in the life of the individual person and the family. Developmental psychology involves the study of life stages and the related tasks to be accomplished and opportunities for growth associated with each stage. Within our current culture, there seems to be an assumption that once given a terminal diagnosis meaningful life has ended, yet dying is a specific stage with related growth tasks and accomplishments.

As reflected in *The Quest to Die with Dignity: An Analysis of Americans' Values, Opinions and Attitudes Concerning End-of-Life Care*,[17] people tend to see the last phase of life as one awaiting death, hoping minimally for some measure of comfort and not being a burden to others. This limited perspective devalues and separates this last stage of life from the continuum of a person's existence while minimizing hopes and goals.

Byock[16] has conceptualized dying as a stage of the human life cycle that inherently holds opportunities to broaden the personal experience, determine "what matters most," influence the outcome for improved quality of life closure, and in so doing, reveal new sources of hope. He believes that individuality extends through the very end of life, characteristic challenges and meaningful developmental landmarks can be discerned, and representative tasks toward the achievement of goals for life completion and life closure can be identified.[16]

During this last phase of life, Byock[16] has elucidated the opportunity for uncovering new or deeper sources of meaning in people's lives and in their dying. It is important that a developmental approach to the end of life not be misconstrued as a set of prescribed requirements. Rather, these landmarks and tasks can become part of a conceptual framework in which to approach end-of-life care processes, systems, and relationships. They can provide a common language and approaches to assure patient/family value–directed care that optimizes quality of life closure. How each patient/family chooses to attend to or accomplish these tasks will be specific to their values, goals, and needs.

The developmental landmarks and taskwork for life completion and life closure that Byock[16] has defined provide direction for care in the final phase of life (Table 2–1). They reflect the gradual process of life transition from worldly and social affairs to individual relationships to intrapersonal and transcendent dimensions.

These tasks and landmarks can offer a guide for professionals caring for people at the end of life. By first opening dialogue about the possibility of meaningful experiences related to these landmarks and tasks, we acknowledge and validate the patient/family experience. As with other developmental stages in life, developmental tasks are best accomplished with optimal interventions and a supportive environment, such as a toddler learning to walk or talk. Stimulation of a safe, encouraging, and nurturing environment is essential for a toddler to be able to safely accomplish these tasks of development. Hospice approach to the patient/family/caregiver relationships becomes one of providing interventions that create optimal, safe, nurturing environments to facilitate work on end-of-life tasks to the extent that a patient/family chooses, is interested, and is able to engage.

As nurses, we have the responsibility to attend to the physical and functional dimensions of care while supporting issues of life closure in the other dimen-

Table 2–1. Developmental Landmarks and Taskwork for Life Completion and Life Closure

Landmark	Task Work
Sense of completion with worldly affairs	Transfer of fiscal, legal, and formal social responsibilities
Sense of completion in relationships with community	Closure of multiple social relationships (employment, business, organizational, congregational)
	Components include expression of regret, expressions of forgiveness, acceptance of gratitude and appreciation
	Leave-taking, saying good-bye
Sense of meaning about one's individual life	Life review
	The telling of "one's stories"
	Transmission of knowledge and wisdom
Experience of love of self	Self-acknowledgment
	Self-forgiveness
Experience love of others	Acceptance of worthiness
	Acceptance of forgiveness
Sense of completion in relationships with family and friends	Reconciliation, fullness of communication, and closure in each of one's important relationships
	Component tasks include expression of regret expressions of forgiveness and acceptance, expressions of gratitude and appreciation, expressions of affection
	Leave-taking, saying good-bye
Acceptance of the finality of life, of one's existence as an individual	Acknowledgment of the totality of personal loss represented by one's dying and experience of personal pain of existential loss
	Expression of depth of personal tragedy that dying represents
	Decathexis (emotional withdrawal) from worldly affairs and cathexis (emotional connection) with an enduring construct
	Acceptance of dependence
Sense of a new self (personhood) beyond personal loss	Acceptance of new definition of self
	Acknowledgment of the value of that new self
Sense of meaning about life in general	Achieving sense of awe
	Recognition of transcendent realm
	Developing/achieving a sense of comfort with chaos
Surrender to the transcendent, to the unknown, "letting go"	Will to die
	Acceptance of death
	Saying good-bye
	Withdrawal from family, friends, and professional caregivers

Source: Byock (1996), reference 16.

sions so that patients and families can accomplish the end-of-life developmental landmarks to the extent that they choose. Accordingly, the hospice nurse's initial role in end-of-life care is to work with the patient and family to prevent and/or minimize suffering resulting from the physical and functional deterioration of advancing age and/or end-stage disease progression. It is when these dimensions are addressed and managed that the patient and family can attend to life-closure tasks and landmarks they feel are important and that involve the other dimensions of their interpersonal, well-being, and transcendent experience.

Although each patient approaches these landmarks and associated task work in his or her own way, there are some common aspects. Generally, patients will first accomplish the few landmarks/tasks which relate to separating and/or settling worldly affairs and community relationships prior to moving or separating from friends and family and finally move to those tasks marked by introspection. As people get closer to death, it is common to observe a gradual withdrawal from worldly relationships, friends, and family as they begin the transition on their individual journey from life to death. Our goal is to explain and normalize this experience, thereby recruiting the IDT and family members to help preserve the patient's opportunities to experience peace and comfort within themselves during their personal encounter with death.

NORMALIZING THE DYING–NURSING PROCESS FROM A HOSPICE PERSPECTIVE

Hospice nursing involves three broad areas: (1) approaching care from a patient/family-based, interdimensional care focus as described above; (2) expertise in end-stage disease and symptom management; and (3) applying the nursing process as a member of the hospice IDT through a critical thinking approach.

End-stage disease and symptom management present a unique challenge for many nurses when they begin hospice nursing. This challenge involves incorporating norms for disease progression and symptom management different from those applied in a curative model. Symptoms considered abnormal in a curative approach may become the expected norm for a person who is dying.

Pharmacologic interventions for pain and symptom management are emerging as a body of knowledge that has not yet been integrated well into the nursing curriculum. Nonpharmacologic interventions considered appropriate for a patient on a curative path may actually increase suffering for a patient who is dying. An example may be encouraging food and fluids. For a curative approach, this is appropriate, to increase strength and healing. When a patient approaches death, however, the systems are slowing. This slowing results in a decreased caloric requirement as well as a slowing of fluid perfusion. By forcing food and fluids, we could increase the demands on the gastrointestinal as well as circulatory systems, thereby creating increased discomfort. It becomes the responsibility of any nurse caring for patients at the end of life to gain specific knowledge and competence in end-stage disease and symptom management.

Critically Thinking Through the End-of-Life Nursing Process

Suffering, dying, and death evoke many interdimensional changes and reactions not only for the patient but for the family as well. By looking at a patient/family from this perspective, we begin to move away from a traditional problem-oriented approach to a quality of life closure–oriented approach. All of our care processes and tools must therefore prompt a different critical thought process.[19]

Each step of the hospice interdimensional care process (assessment, care planning, goal setting, interventions, and evaluation) must involve three critical questions:

1. Are we approaching care based on the patient/family values, goals, and choices?
2. How does an issue/problem/opportunity in one dimension affect the other dimensions of the patient and family?
3. How does an issue/problem/opportunity affect the patient's and/or family's quality of life closure?

The main steps of the hospice interdimensional care process are similar to the nursing process but with a focus on quality of life closure rather than rehabilitation or cure. Nurses must also look beyond problem identification as they apply the interdimensional care process and anticipate changes to prevent suffering while preserving opportunity for growth. At each step of the care process (assessment, planning, intervention, and evaluation), the three critical thinking questions must be applied.

Integrating the Nursing Process with the Hospice Interdimensional Care Process

Incorporating the nursing process into an interdimensional care process further defines the specialty of hospice nursing in that it involves the nurse working as a collaborative member of the IDT and expanding the picture of the nursing process to an interdisciplinary interdimensional care process. All disciplines on the hospice team are valued and their expertise combined to apply the hospice interdimensional care process. The steps of the hospice interdimensional care process are outlined below.

Step 1: Interdimensional Assessment

Assessment begins with discussion soliciting information about the patient/family situation, including their values, wishes, and dreams, that they identify as important. Data collection assesses all dimensions of a person and family as well as how changes in those dimensions affect the quality of life closure. Traditional nursing physical assessment is accomplished during this step, utilizing norms for end-stage disease and symptom management.

Subjective and objective data are collected from a palliative, comfort care perspective and based on what patients and families define as important to them at this time. Their identified goals become the focus and driving force for the hospice team.

Step 2: Identifying Specific Issues/ Problems/Opportunities and Etiology

The next step involves identifying specific issues, which is comparable to developing the nursing diagnosis. A specific issue, problem, or opportunity is defined from a palliative perspective and the etiology identified. In this step, hospice differentiates between definitions of problems that are expected norms for the dying process and those that are unexpected or may cause secondary suffering for the patient and/or family.

For example, a patient may become incontinent as his or her systems fail and death is imminent. This is an expected physical change during the dying process. If this situation was assessed using an interdimensional approach, we might determine the problem to be the potential for skin breakdown (with an etiology of incontinence) rather than incontinence being the primary problem secondary to advanced disease. Another problem/issue may be that the "spouse is exhausted from being awake all day and night changing the patient's linens secondary to incontinence of the patient." What a nurse may instinctively identify as a problem in a curative model often becomes the etiology of a problem in end-of-life care.

Another important difference in hospice nursing is to assess and identify problems, issues, or opportunities beyond the physical and functional dimensions, including the following:

1. Physical symptoms/prevention of related suffering
2. Psychosocial symptoms/prevention of related suffering
3. Spiritual symptoms/prevention of related suffering
4. Accomplishment of developmental tasks of life completion and closure to the extent that the patient/family chooses to participate
5. Family dynamics/relationship issues/opportunities
6. Grief/loss/bereavement issues
7. Functional status/environmental status

This step also involves determining etiology/cause of the problem, issue, or opportunity. Etiology of medical problems can often be identified through physiologic changes, but nurses must also take into consideration other causes related to all of the dimensions. For example, a patient with end-stage chronic obstructive pulmonary disease may complain of shortness of breath. Initial reactions would be to identify the problem as shortness of breath "secondary to ineffective air exchange in the lung." Again, in end-stage chronic obstructive pulmonary disease, this is an expected norm. With further interdimensional assessment, the patient identifies episodes of shortness of breath secondary to "anticipated fear of being alone at night." Obviously, the interventions for each would be different when the full dimensions are assessed and the patient's experience directs the process.

Etiology of problems that are not physiologically based can often be attributed to a patient's and/or family's adaptation to the current situation or unfinished personal conflict. In this step, opportunities can also be identified where problems or issues could be prevented or situations presented that would enhance personal growth and completion of life-closure tasks.

For example, a patient with chronic obstructive pulmonary disease who was imminently dying was becoming progressively anxious with increased episodes of shortness of breath despite all medical interventions. Upon assessing this problem, the patient shared that he had a son whom he had not spoken to for over 20 years. The patient was afraid of dying before mending that relationship, apologizing to his son, and letting him know he loved him. The hospice team assisted in locating his son and arranging for a visit. The patient and son were able to spend time together, give and receive forgiveness, and in so doing mend their relationship. The patient's unfinished relationship issues were the etiology of his physical episodes of shortness of breath. Hospice nursing involves a holistic approach that realizes the potential effect one dimension (interpersonal, transcendence, etc.) can have on all other dimensions (physical, well-being) and assures that the nursing assessment gathers and utilizes all dimensional changes for optimal interventions.

Step 3: Interdisciplinary Team Care Planning

Interdisciplinary care planning is a process that occurs from the time the patient is referred through the family's bereavement period. It occurs both in formal IDT care planning meetings and between meetings as patient/family needs change and members of the IDT collaborate on care. Patients and families are assessed by the nurse and a psychosocial professional upon admission. As the care plan is developed, each discipline blends its own area of expertise with other team members to formulate shared interventions that support the patient's and family's goals.

Similar to the nursing process, this step involves planning the care, including goal setting with patient, family, IDT, and staff of facilities; determining the best interventions; and devising a team plan for providing services. The key components in this process include the following:

1. collaboration
2. patient/family-directed goal setting
3. IDT planning of interventions

Collaboration. Collaboration builds an interdisciplinary awareness of interdependence with a common mission, values, and goals of optimal care for the patient and family. Collaboration is essential for all hospice professionals as they stimulate each other and innovative ideas and interventions are formulated. One of the key reasons for IDT collaboration is to share assessment data and feedback that each member was able to solicit from patients and families so that a comprehensive interdimensional care plan can be established and mutually understood by all team members caring for that patient and family. The hospice nurse therefore collaborates first with the patient and family to determine goals, then with other IDT members to assure a holistic approach to continuity of care. If the patient is residing in a facility, the nurse must also include the staff of that facility in care planning. Collaboration assures continuity of care.

Patient/Family-Directed Goal Setting. A comprehensive plan develops and goals are identified in three areas: (1) patient family goals, (2) life-closure goals, and (3) clinical obligation goals.

Primarily, the care plan should be directed by what the patient and family have defined as their goals. The hospice plan of care belongs to the patient and family; therefore, goals should be articulated from their perspective, not the nurse's perspective of how things "should happen." Some goals articulated by hospice patients and families may include things such as being able to care for a spouse while he or she is bedridden and ranking pain as 3 out of 10 at meal times so that the patient can join the family at the table. By articulating goals from the patient/family perspective, it becomes apparent what direction each member of the IDT should take to collaboratively help them meet their goals. It also becomes apparent that the IDT as a group, not one discipline, is equipped to deal with complex issues associated with dying and bereavement.

Life completion and life-closure goals relate to the end-of-life accomplishments, the completion of unfinished business, landmarks and tasks of dying, and the emotional/spiritual separation of dying. Hospice nurses, as part of the IDT, add their expertise to support the patient and family in accomplishing life-closure goals through disease and symptom management as well as emotional and spiritual support. An example of a life-closure goal as defined by the patient may be to take one last trip to visit and say good-bye to family and friends. The nurse may be involved by teaching energy conservation, the use of portable oxygen, transfer techniques to the family for car transportation, or titration of medications to assure comfort. Life-closure goals may also include "creating a memory book for my grandchildren to have when I'm gone" or being forgiven for a life transgression. Again, the focus becomes the patient's and family's goals as they relate to life-closure tasks, and the nurse collaborates with other team members, such as the psychosocial counselor or chaplain, to help the patient/family accomplish these goals.

Clinical obligation goals are identified by the IDT only in those situations where the patient or family is unable to identify the problem or issues. These goals are strictly related to clinical obligation situations such as neglect or suicide, where the team must establish goals to insure the patient's or family's safety.

Interdisciplinary Team Planning of Interventions. Interventions are based on interdimensional assessment with the overall goals of reducing or preventing suffering and accomplishing life closure. Directed by patient/family goals and with their input and approval, the hospice nurse and the other IDT members collaborate to determine the optimal interventions that would move the patient/family closer to their goals.

The interdisciplinary planning process involves determining which discipline, or combination of disciplines, is most appropriate to assist patients/families in accomplishing their goals. Some patients and families may allow only one or two disciplines to be involved in their care. Some individuals expect nurses to provide care and are not always open to visits from social workers or chaplains. The nurse in these situations may be the sole team representative, incorporating the expertise of all disciplines. When this happens, it becomes crucial that members of the IDT collaborate and share expertise so that interdisciplinary care can still be delivered and patient's and family's goals can still be addressed. The nurse's role may then include facilitating the involvement of the team to the degree that the patient/family is comfortable.

Step 4: Providing Interventions to Meet Patient and Family Goals

The hospice care plan involves interventions in four areas:

1. Palliative therapeutic interventions
2. Education interventions
3. Collaboration interventions
4. Assessment interventions

Palliative Therapeutic Interventions. Palliative therapeutic interventions include those that have been identified to be conducive to meeting the patient/family goals. These include both pharmacologic as well as nonpharmacologic interventions to best address the interdimensional adaptation and goals of the patient/family.

Hospice nurses must always be aware of not only the traditional medical interventions but also those interventions specific to the specialty of end-of-life care that support quality of life closure. An example is a patient who had a stroke, leaving him aphasic of both spoken and written word. During his lifetime, he kept a scrapbook of national newspaper articles, including articles and current events journals. In the scrapbook, he would write his perception of how an event may have been significant to his daughter's life. To assist this patient in finding meaning and purpose in his life, the nurse requested a volunteer to help the patient engage in life review. The volunteer would visit the patient, reading the articles and the patient's philosophical messages to his daughter related to each event in the history of their life together. Through the reading of these scrapbooks, the patient was able to sense his contribution and value as a parent.

Again, hospice nursing is based on a holistic approach and the understanding that life closure is an interdimensional experience for both the patient and family.

Educational Interventions. As with all nursing practice, patient and family education is a cornerstone of hospice nursing. Since most patients followed by hospice do stay in their homes until death, the primary role of the hospice team is to empower the patient and family so that they can develop the skills to comfortably provide care and find meaning and purpose in the experience.

The nurse becomes involved in patient/family education as it relates to personal care, prevention of problems such as skin breakdown, administration and management of medications, nonpharmacologic interventions such as therapeutic touch, application of heat, breathing exercises, and functional assistance with activities of daily living. As the patient's disease progresses, the hospice nurse is also involved in educating the family about expected changes. Common responses to each stage of the disease and related interventions to decrease suffering are taught so that they are optimally prepared prior to changes. When patients and families know what to expect, hospice can help to prevent or reduce anxiety related to the unknown.

Another crucial goal of patient/family education is to provide information and support so that patients and families can advocate for themselves in all care settings, with other providers, and with other family members.

Collaboration Interventions. Crucial to assuring unified delivery of care to patients and families is the practice of collaboration. When planning interventions, it is crucial to assure that the patient, family, and professional caregivers are involved. Caregivers include IDT members, facility staff, attending and consulting physicians, therapists, and the family. For example, the hospice nurse collaborates with the attending physician about the need for medication for symptom management or with facility nurses to educate and assure around-the-clock administration of pain medications. If a hospice patient is residing in a nursing facility, the hospice nurse must collaborate with the nursing facility staff, communicating and documenting the outcome of that collaboration. Communication of these interventions is paramount to assure continuity of care between and among team members, caregivers, and care settings.

Assessment Interventions. The final type of hospice nursing intervention is ongoing assessment necessary to determine if continuation of the care plan is effective or optimal. For hospice nursing, this may include closely monitored titration of opioids for pain control or respiratory status to determine effective doses as symptoms change or the patient's needs change throughout the trajectory of illness.

Step 5: Evaluating Interventions and Continuation or Revision of the Care Plan

With the patient and family as the core of the hospice team, evaluation begins with their perspective of the effectiveness of the care plan interventions. Do the interventions help them to reach their goals? What has been most beneficial from their perspective? What do they want to continue or discontinue? As with all other steps in the care process, the patient and family direct the care. Therefore, it is crucial that the hospice nurse involve the patient and family in evaluating the effectiveness of the care plan interventions on an ongoing basis.

By evaluating and documenting the effects of interventions, the hospice nurse shares his or her expertise as a valued member of the IDT. If the current care plan is effective at meeting the patient's and family's palliative care goals, then interventions continue. If interventions do not meet the patient/family goals, then the hospice nurse collaborates with the IDT for additional assessment.

Dying, death, and bereavement are experienced in such personal ways. Hospice care allows for the patient and family to direct the care based on their own values, goals, and needs. A significant difference between traditional nursing and hospice care is the involvement of the patient/family as they guide the hospice IDT in providing palliative care and services that are most meaningful to them.

KEY ELEMENTS OF A HOSPICE PROGRAM

Purpose and Process of Interdisciplinary Team Care Management

In *The Hospice Handbook*, Larry Beresford states, "The glue that holds together this hospice approach to care is the interdisciplinary team."[3] The primary purpose of the IDT model of care management is to build a caring community between the patient, family, and hospice team. This integrated community is responsible for responding to patients' and families' dynamic needs 24 hours a day, seven days a week. The entire IDT is accountable for the physical, psychosocial, spiritual, and bereavement needs of both the patient and family, assuring that the palliative care plan is carried out across all care settings.

Because the physical, psychosocial, spiritual, and bereavement needs of patients and families are inseparable, the interdisciplinary approach is also the hospice approach to care. The team, not just the hospice nurse, becomes the care manager. The patient, family, and IDT are equally important in problem solving and goal formulation, collaborating with each other for expertise and input into care planning. The hospice approach is a holistic care process directed by the patient and family to best meet their interdimensional needs.

Care management by the IDT is a process, not an event. This process begins at the time the patient is admitted to the hospice program and continues until well after the death of the patient, through bereavement services for the survivors. Effective IDT care management promotes daily, ongoing collaborative practice that incorporates shared goals, care planning, role blending, and shared leadership.

Interdimensional Care Delivered by an Interdisciplinary Team

Terminal illness affects patients and families not only physically but psychologically, emotionally, spiritually, and financially. To provide effective, quality hospice care, all of these dimensions of the dying experience should be addressed. An IDT, incorporating the expertise of members from several disciplines who are trained to meet these varied needs of patients and families, provides the most effective holistic approach to end-of-life care.

In a traditional multidisciplinary approach to patient care, a member representing each discipline visits the patient and formulates goals depending on his/her own area of expertise. Patient's and family's goals may not always be considered together as a unit of care, and the specific goals of one discipline are not always shared by the other disciplines caring for the patient. Often, one discipline is the "case manager," having more direction and input than the others in the care- planning process. This lack of collaborative care planning and goal setting can create an inconsistent approach that lacks cohesion and continuity and often frustrates those receiving care. The focus is on the "discipline" (nurse, social worker, etc) rather than the patient and family. In the interdisciplinary approach to care, the nurse coordinates the plan of care with the patient, family, and other members of the IDT to "effectively mobilize each other's skills to meet patients' needs in a variety of healthcare settings."[20]

The hospice IDT model improves upon the multidisciplinary approach with a process that allows for the following:

1. patient and family involvement in decision making in all aspects of care
2. determination of patient/family value–directed care plan goals
3. collaboration of expertise by varied disciplines
4. identification of appropriate interventions
5. role blending of expertise among disciplines

The IDT model provides optimal interdimensional care by jointly assessing and determining goals and sharing ideas for interventions with the patient, family, and all team members working toward common goals and interventions. The success of the hospice IDT model lies in the partnership between professionals that best reflects the full scope and experience of dying, focusing on the choices, goals, wishes, and experiences of the patient and family.

The Hospice Interdisciplinary Team Structure and Role Blending

The structure of the hospice IDT is designed to meet the interdimensional needs of patients and families. The IDT includes direct and consultative team

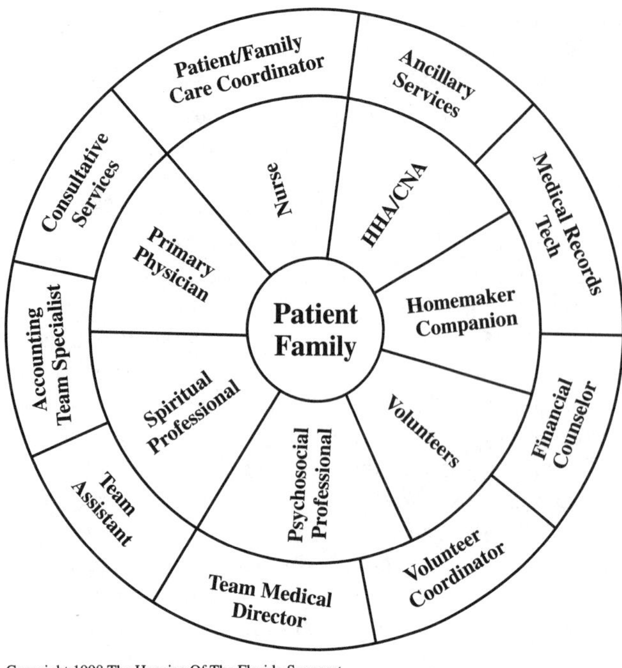

Fig. 2–1. The hospice interdisciplinary team. HHA, home health aide; CNA, certified nursing assistant. ©1998 The Hospice Institute of the Florida Suncoast.

members, as shown in Figure 2–1. While each discipline of the IDT involves special areas of expertise, responsibilities, and duties, the IDT approach to care management requires that each team member expand and blend the traditional roles with those of other disciplines to provide a holistic approach to patient and family care.

One must be an expert in his or her own discipline and have the basic competence to provide physical, psychosocial, spiritual, and bereavement care. Assessment, planning, intervention, and evaluation are ongoing responsibilities of all team members, implying that each is attentive to all dimensions of patient and family care. Role blending is essential for providing coordinated, comprehensive hospice services. As such, roles need to be dynamic, changing, growing, and overlapping.

Direct Responsibilities of Patient/Family Care Team Members

Registered Nurse. The registered nurse is primarily responsible for physical care, including the patient's physical condition and comfort, yet must also possess some level of expertise in psychosocial and spiritual aspects of care, to address the patient and family from a holistic perspective. He or she must be highly skilled in end-stage physical assessment, disease progression, and pain and symptom management. The nurse is also responsible for educating the patient and family on physical care, which includes such things as medication administration, equipment use, skin care, nutrition, catheter care, and transfers.

For those hospice programs that are hospice Medicare-certified, regulations require the coordination of care by a registered nurse and primary physician. As a member of the IDT, the nurse's expertise related to disease and symptom management is one of the critical aspects of providing competent end-of-life care. The nurse's primary role involves managing and preventing the physical and functional decline to reduce suffering so that the patient and family can attend to activities that promote quality of life closure.

The hospice nurse is also responsible for supervising related nursing personnel, including licensed practical nurses, certified nursing assistants, and home health aides. Communicating care plan goals and interventions and monitoring and evaluating the care provided by these other IDT members are the responsibilities of the hospice registered nurse.

Psychosocial Professionals. Psychosocial professionals may include social workers and counselors who are competent in psychosocial assessment, family dynamics, social/emotional therapeutic interventions, grief and bereavement, and group work. They provide support to patients and families, assisting with psychological issues, emotional responses, and the overall adaptation of the patient, family, and significant others through counseling and utilization of community resources. They may also be involved with financial issues, legal issues, advance directives, and funeral arrangements. Overall, the psychosocial professional helps the patient and family as they adapt to and cope with a terminal illness and the survivors as they adjust to life during the bereavement process. It is crucial for the nurse to possess expertise in end-of-life psychosocial issues as they too will be involved in addressing and supporting the patient's and family's psychosocial needs as a member of the IDT.

Spiritual Care Professionals. Spiritual care is a significant component in end-of-life care. The spiritual caregiver, also known as the chaplain, clergy person, or pastoral care worker, can be a paid hospice professional or a resource volunteer from the community. Hospice spiritual care is nonsectarian, nondenominational, and all-inclusive, with the goal of supporting the patient's and family's spiritual and/or religious practices. The hospice philosophy to spiritual care is nonjudgmental and focuses on healing, forgiveness, and acceptance. Spiritual care is provided through direct spiritual counseling and support by collaborating with the patient's and family's own clergy or by working with patients who do not have a clergy person and request spiritual care. Spiritual interventions can include prayer, rites, rituals, assistance in planning and performing funerals and memorial services, and assistance with ethical dilemmas. Again, the nurse must have some level of expertise in the spiritual aspects of care to address the patient's and family's spiritual needs.

Patient's Primary Physician. The patient's primary physician is also part of the IDT. The primary physician is responsible for the overseeing patient care. The physician often refers the patient to hospice; certifies the patient's terminal condition; and provides the admitting diagnosis and prognosis, current medical findings, dietary orders, and orders for medications, treatments, diet, and symptom management.

Hospice Medical Director. The hospice medical director is a member of the IDT. She or he is responsible for the overall medical management of all patients. Depending on the structure of the hospice program she or he may also become a patient's primary physician. The role of the hospice medical director is to participate in the team care planning process as a collaborative member of the IDT. He or she is also responsible for the oversight of medical services provided by the hospice.

Certified Nursing Assistant or Home Health Aide. Certified nursing assistants provide basic physical and functional care where there is a need as well as patient and family support. They provide and educate caregivers on personal care assistance with activities of daily living, which may include bathing, grooming, mouth care, skin care, transfers, repositioning, and sometimes light housekeeping, shopping, cooking, and laundry. Visits vary depending on patient and family needs and what is most important to the patient at each visit. At times, a walk in the garden is more therapeutic than a bath.

Homemaker/Companion. The homemaker/companion assists the patient and family by doing light housekeeping, meal planning and preparation, laundry, and shopping and by acting as a companion to the patient. The homemaker/companion does not provide direct hands-on care. For elderly patients living alone, it is often the addition of a homemaker/companion that allows them to remain independent in their home until they die.

Patient Care Volunteer. Volunteers play an integral role in providing hospice care and are fundamental to the hospice philosophy. Hospice patient care volunteers are trained to work in a variety of roles. The most common role is working with a single patient and family in providing support through companionship, listening, diversion, delivering medications, running errands, taking patients to appointments or on outings, shopping, or preparing a special meal. They may provide companionship to patients in extended care facilities or respite time for the home patient's caregiver. Specialized volunteer roles may include bereavement volunteers who work exclusively with grieving families and friends or those who sit at the bedside during the dying process. The scope of volunteers' duties are all-inclusive, depending on the patient and family needs and quality-of-life goals.

Roles and Responsibilities of Consultative Team Members

Consultative team members participate in direct patient care as needed to meet the palliative care goals of the care plan. Consultative team members can include the hospice team medical director; consulting physician; psychologist or psychiatrist; nutritional counselor; community clergy; clinical pharmacist; occupational, physical, respiratory, speech, and language therapists; intravenous infusion nurse; and pharmacy, x-ray, lab, and durable medical equipment services.[21]

COPING WITH CUMULATIVE LOSS: THE NURSE AS CAREGIVER

The hospice philosophy of care, emphasizing intense interpersonal care and active involvement with the dying patient and family, creates more intense and intimate relationships between the nurse, patient, and family than exist in traditional health care settings. Like families who grieve the loss of their loved ones, the hospice nurse also grieves over the loss and, in fact, may need to grieve on a continuous basis due to the number of deaths that occur. As the hospice nurse adjusts to caring for dying patients and their families, the stress of coping with death on a daily basis can trigger many emotional feelings, reactions, and behaviors.

Other factors may also influence the nurse's successful adaptation to caring for dying patients and their families. If the nurse has experienced death on a personal level or experienced life changes that signify loss, such as children leaving home or a divorce, caring for dying patients and families may trigger issues of unresolved grief. The nurse's ability to verbalize his or her feelings regarding death and loss with other members of the IDT are important for support and for normalizing these feelings.

If the hospice nurse is unable to process these losses through appropriate grief and personal death awareness, he or she may begin to distance himself or herself from emotional involvement with the patient and family. This withdrawal may negatively affect not only the coping ability of the professional but also the quality of compassionate delivery of care and the ability to meet the needs of dying patients and their families during the terminal phases of an illness.

Stages of Adaptation for the Hospice Nurse

Hospice nurses go through many stages when they begin caring for dying patients and their families. Successful progression through these stages and the support systems in place to facilitate successful progression are vitally important in determining if the nurse will be comfortable and effective in caring for the dying.

As proposed by Bernice Harper,[22] an expert in anxiety issues in the professional caregiver, there are six stages of adaptation that characterize the hospice nurse's normal progression, adaptation, and coping in caring for the dying:

1. Intellectualization
2. Emotional survival
3. Depression
4. Emotional arrival
5. Deep compassion
6. The Doer

Five of these stages and the emotions, behaviors, and reactions of each stage are shown in Figure 2–2 and Table 2–2.

Intellectualization. Intellectualization usually occurs during the first 1 to 3 months of caring for the dying. During this time, professional caregivers are usually confronted with their first experience of a hospice death. Nurses in this initial stage spend much of their energy learning the facts, tasks, policies, and procedures of the job. Emotional involvement in the dying and death of the patient may be inadvertently avoided, and the hospice nurse seldom reacts on an emotional level to the death.

Emotional Survival. Emotional survival generally occurs within 3 to 6 months of employment. Emotional involvement and a deeper connection with the patient and family occur. The nurse begins to confront the reality of the patient's death, to face his or her own mortality, and to feel sadness about the patient's situation and/or the loss of the patient. Often during this stage, the nurse begins to fully understand the magnitude of his or her role and responsibilities and to question his or her abilities and desire to continue caring for dying patients and their families. This is a crucial time, and the nurse needs to be reassured and given support and resources to feel competent and confident so that he or she can progress successfully in the field.

Depression. Depression occurring at 6 to 9 months, is often a time when hospice nurses process the losses rather than avoid them or remain emotionally detached. They begin to explore their own feelings about death, accept their own mortality, and accept death as a natural part of life.

It is in this stage that hospice professionals move toward positive resolution of death and loss and accept the reality of death and dying or negatively resolve death and loss by choosing to avoid the emotional pain. In positive resolution, hospice professionals emotionally arrive at a comfortable place in caring for dying patients and their families.

Emotional Arrival. Emotional arrival occurs within 9 to 12 months of caring for the dying. With positive resolution of the last stage, hospice professionals become sensitive to the emotional needs and issues associated with dying and death. They can now cope with and accept loss, participate in healthy grieving, experience and conceptually work within the principles of hospice philosophy by advocating for the patient and family, and become involved with patients and families on a deeper level.

Deep Compassion. Deep compassion occurs after the first year as a hospice nurse. In this stage, hospice professionals begin to refine their knowledge and skills and are comfortable in providing compassionate, physical, psychosocial, and spiritual care to dying patients and their families. This stage is characterized by personal and professional growth and development.

The Doer. The final stage, the doer, characterizes hospice professionals who are efficient, vigorous, knowledgeable, and able to understand and comprehend humankind. Death has an inner meaning embedded in caring. Doers have grown and developed personally and professionally through the experiences of caring for the terminally ill.

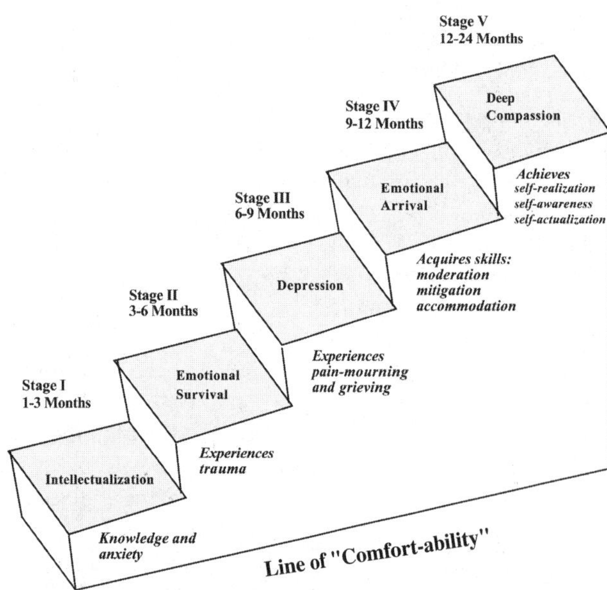

Figure 2–2. Cumulative Loss and the Caregiver. Five stages experienced by the hospice nurse while caring for the dying. Source: Harper BC. Death: The Coping Mechanism of the Health Professional. Greenville, SC: Swiger Associates Inc., 1994.

Support Systems

In caring for dying patients and their families, the hospice nurse is vulnerable to emotions, reactions, and behaviors that can ultimately affect his or her personal well being and the delivery of quality palliative care. To effectively care for patients and families, the nurse must also be responsible for attending to his or her own emotional, physical, and spiritual needs. Successfully coping with and adapting to dying, death, and cu-

Table 2–2. Cumulative Loss and the Professional Caregiver

Stage I 0–3 months *Intellectualization*	Stage II 3–6 months *Emotional Survival*	Stage III 6–9 months *Depression*	Stage IV 9–12 months *Emotional Arrival*	Stage V 12–24 months *Deep Compassion*
Professional knowledge	Increasing professional knowledge	Deepening professional knowledge	Acceptance of professional knowledge	Refining professional knowledge
Intellectualization	Less intellectualization	Decreasing intellectualization	Normal intellectualization	Refining intellectual base
Anxiety	Emotional survival	Depression	Emotional arrival	Deep compassion
Some uncomfortableness	Increasing uncomfortableness	Decreasing uncomfortableness	Increasing comfortableness	Increased comfortableness
Agreeableness	Guilt	Pain	Moderation	Self-realization
Withdrawal	Frustration	Mourning	Mitigation	Self-awareness
Superficial acceptance	Sadness	Grieving	Accommodation	Self-actualization
Providing tangible services	Initial emotional involvement	More emotional involvement	Ego mastery	Professional satisfaction
Utilization of emotional energy on understanding the setting	Increasing emotional involvement	Overidentification with the patient	Coping with loss of relationship	Acceptance of death and loss
Familiarizing self with policies and procedures	Initial understanding of the magnitude of the area of practice	Exploration of own feelings about death	Freedom from concern about own death	Rewarding professional growth and development
Working with families rather than patients	Overidentification with the patient's situation	Facing own death	Developing strong ties with dying patients and families	Development of ability to give of one's self
		Coming to grips with feelings about death	Development of ability to work with, on behalf of, and for the dying patient	Human and professional assessment
			Development of professional competence	Constructive and appropriate activities
			Productivity and accomplishments	Development of feelings of dignity and self-respect
			Healthy interaction	Ability to give dignity and self-respect to dying patient
				Feeling of comfortableness in relation to self, patient, family, and the job

Source: Harper (1994), reference 22.

mulative loss is possible only if a system is in place that provides support to the nurse. Support systems may include personal death awareness exercises, time to verbalize in one-on-one counseling and/or with the IDT, supervisor support, preceptors/mentors, spiritual support, funeral or memorial services for closure, joint visits with members of other disciplines, and educational opportunities. The nurse should also explore individually facilitated support systems through journal writing, exercise, relaxation, meditation, and socialization with family and friends. By exploring and accessing support systems, the hospice nurse can find satisfaction, fulfillment, and growth and development in his or her personal and professional lives as he or she provides compassionate end-of-life care to patients and their families.[23]

BARRIERS TO HOSPICE CARE

A Death-Defying Society

The prevailing attitude of our society toward death continues to be "death-defying." Unquestionable acceptance of innovation, efficiency, science, technological advances, and the ability to prolong life reflects the current perspective on health care. Therefore, acceptance of death as a natural process is difficult and offensive. Even with the growing hospice movement, most deaths happen in hospitals, often with uncontrolled pain.[24] As experts in the care of patients and families at the end of life, hospices will continue to shape the way in which people view dying and death.

Access Barriers

As a result of dissatisfaction with care afforded the dying over 20 years ago, community members introduced the vision of hospice care. Congress adopted this vision through the creation of the Medicare Hospice Benefit in 1982. Millions of Americans have benefited from care under this act, but it has fallen short of meeting current needs of the dying.

At the request of the National Hospice and Palliative Care Organization, the Committee on the Medicare Hospice Benefit and End-of-Life Care spent nearly a year addressing issues related to hospice and end-of-life care. As part of the committee's review and recommendations, barriers to achieving the characteristics of the ideal future hospice and extending hospice to more Americans were identified. The specific recommendations of the report were wide-ranging, from improving the Medicare Hospice Benefit to changing the education of health and human service professionals to raising the expectations for performance by hospice programs. All are important, but the following steps were identified as having the highest priority:

- eliminating the 6-month prognosis under the Medicare Hospice Benefit and identifying alternative eligibility specifications;
- collecting and analyzing comprehensive data on the cost of meeting patient and family needs through hospice with the intent to address inadequacies in Medicare payments;
- developing outcome measures for assessing the quality of end-of-life care;
- engaging the public in a campaign to create wider understanding and utilization of hospice care.[25]

Prognostic Limitations

One of the significant factors limiting access to hospice care is the determination of when hospice care should begin. There is mounting clinical evidence of the appropriateness of palliative care but few documented, valid, and reliable prognostic indicators of when palliative care should begin, especially with the chronic noncancer and aging multisystem failure diagnosis. This ambiguity can cause delay in referral to hospice or toward any palliative care focus. Further development and research of practice protocols for the care of patients with terminal disease is needed. Recommendations of the NHPCO Committee on the Medicare Hospice Benefit and End-of-Life Care include developing criteria to trigger an advance care planning evaluation that includes consideration of desire and eligibility for hospice care. Once developed, these criteria should be incorporated into practice guidelines.[25]

THE FUNDING OF HOSPICE PROGRAMS

The original hospices, which began as grassroots community efforts, were funded almost exclusively by charitable support, grants, and volunteer efforts. Some components of care were supported by Medicare or insurance, such as skilled nursing visits, medications, or durable medical equipment on a per-unit fee-for-service basis allowed under an acute care model. In 1980, Congress authorized a 2-year demonstration program in 27 hospices around the nation to study the outcomes of hospice care and the costs associated with it. The demonstrations included researchers at each site who collected both field data from patients and families and cost data from each organization. Ultimately, the demonstration was continued for 1 additional year. Based on very preliminary findings, Congress created the Hospice Medicare Benefit as a 2-year endeavor and then subsequently approved it as a permanent part of the Medicare program in August of 1982.

The Hospice Medicare Benefit was a landmark event under Medicare in that it was the first formal recognition of the unique needs of dying patients and their families. It was also the first form of what ultimately became managed care. It included provisions never before included as health care benefits, such as spiritual support, volunteers, and bereavement support for family members.

It was an all-inclusive benefit in which all services related to the terminal illness were to be provided, coordinated, and paid for through the hospice program. While this is now frequently viewed as a strategy to control costs, it was at the time designed in this manner because surviving family members cited the complexity of bills and the financial toll of a terminal illness as one of the greatest stressors.

The benefit included the following core hospice services: nursing care, medical and social services, physician services, counseling/pastoral services, short-term inpatient and respite care, medical appliances and supplies including drugs and biologicals, home health aide and homemaker services, therapies (physical, occupational, speech), bereavement counseling, and drugs for symptom management and pain control.[10] It also had a provision for four levels of care depending on the intensity and place of care rendered any given day. Continuity across all care settings with hospice professional management of care was and continues to be a strong underpinning of the benefit.

Following the Hospice Medicare Benefit demonstration and benefit development, Medicaid and private insurance hospice benefits began to emerge. Ultimately, most states developed Medicaid benefits, which are mandated to be no less than the Medicare benefit. Private insurers frequently model their benefit based on the Medicare benefit, although they are under no mandate to do so.

Most hospices are committed to providing care regardless of ability to pay and continue to be dependent on charitable dollars to provide such care. Additional supportive services, above the benefit, such as children's programs, in-home caregiver programs, hospice residences, and community bereavement and education programs, are provided in many hospice communities.

While a small portion of the people receiving health care are at the end of life and receiving terminal care, the terminally ill consume a disproportionate percentage of all health care expenditures. There are several studies on the cost savings in hospice versus traditional health care at the end of life. Hospice has remained a positive example of integrating a managed care model with proven cost savings while meeting patients' and families' needs and receiving high quality scores.

Initially, hospices were slow to seek certification for Medicare status, but this has grown steadily as hospices have become more comfortable with assuming the risk of total costs of care. There were also financial reimbursement and other utilization caps in the program which concerned many. Today most hospices are Medicare-certified, and the number of recipients of hospice in America has grown commensurately to over 500,000 patients and their families receiving hospice care in 1998.

The Medicare Hospice Benefit

The different levels of care outlined in the Medicare Hospice Benefit reflect the variations in care intensity to meet patient/family needs in the last phase of life. Medicare provides coverage for hospice care to Medicare beneficiaries who have elected the hospice benefit and who have been certified as terminally ill with a prognosis for a life expectancy of 6 months or less. Once elected, Medicare pays one of four prospective, per diem rates for hospice care: routine home care, continuous home care, respite care, general inpatient care. Each of these payment categories is defined below. Changing the level of care is determined through a collaborative effort by the hospice IDT, patient, family, and primary physician.

Routine Home Care. Routine home care is provided in the patient's home, nursing home, or residential care setting or wherever the patient and family reside. The hospice core services provided at this level include nursing care, home health aide care, social services, therapies, medical appliances and supplies, and drugs.

Continuous Care. Continuous care covers patients in brief periods of crisis, during which 8 or more hours per day of care is provided to the patient at home, with at least 50% of the care delivered by a registered nurse or licensed practical nurse.

Inpatient Respite Care. Inpatient respite care covers patients in an approved inpatient facility for the relief of the patient's primary caregiver, for a maximum of 5 days per episode. It includes coverage of drugs, supplies, and equipment as well.

General Inpatient Care. General inpatient care covers patients in a participating hospice inpatient unit of a hospital, skilled nursing facility, intermediate care facility, or freestanding hospice for medically necessary days for the control of pain or acute or chronic symptom management which cannot be managed in other settings. It includes coverage for ancillary services (oxygen, laboratory, pharmacy, etc.).[10]

The Medicaid Hospice Benefit

Medicaid coverage for hospice is patterned after the Medicare benefit, including both patient eligibility requirements and coverage for specific services. States do have some flexibility in developing their hospice benefit.

Private Insurance Reimbursement and Managed Care

Private insurance companies have begun to realize the benefits of hospice care and are including a hospice benefit in their services. As with Medicaid, many private insurers pattern their benefit after Medicare. Some insurers have negotiated services with hospices. Many managed care companies have also reflected the Medicare benefit in services provided to their members either through their own hospice programs or under contract with programs serving the patient's community.

CONCLUSION

Hospice is more than a program of health services. It is an approach and philosophy of care and services that strives to encompass and support the full experience of the dying process for both the patient and family. Although a difficult time, with sensitive support, the last phase of life can be a time of tremendous growth and opportunity for the person who is dying and for loved ones, such as in the finding of meaning and purpose of one's suffering, the value of one's life accomplishments, the deepening of relationships, and the personal spiritual significance of the experience.

Nurses can positively affect this experience for others by allowing the patient's and family's personal values and goals to guide the support and care they offer as they are invited to share in this intimate time of life. Regardless of the site of care or type of program or services, nurses providing end-of-life care must be proficient in end-stage disease and symptom management. However, nurses must be guided by dignity, compassion, love, and individual acceptance of patient and family values and choices to assure quality end-of-life care.

REFERENCES

1. Cassell EJ. The nature of suffering and the goals of medicine. N Engl J Med 1982;306: 639–642.

2. Standards and Accreditation Committee. Hospice Standards of Practice. Arlington, VA: National Hospice and Palliative Care Organization, 1999.

3. Beresford L. The Hospice Handbook: A Complete Guide. Boston: Little, Brown, 1993.

4. Cassell EJ. The Nature of Suffering and the Goals of Medicine. Oxford: Oxford University Press, 1991.

5. Meier DE, Morrison RS. Old age and care near the end of life. J Am Soc Aging 1999; 23:7.

6. Schneidman E. Death: Current Perspectives. Mountain View, CA: Mayfield, 1994.

7. Lattanzi-Licht M, Mahoney JJ, Miller GW. The Hospice Choice: In Pursuit of a Peaceful Death. New York: Simon and Schuster, 1998.

8. National Hospice Organization. NHO Hospice Fact Sheet. Arlington, VA: National Hospice Organization. 1999.

9. Mooney B (Ed). Poll shows Americans prefer to die at home. In: Hot Topics in Hospice, Atlanta: Hospital Management Advisor, 1997:167–170.

10. Manard B, Perrone C. (1994). Hospice Care: An Introduction and Review of the Evidence. Arlington, VA: National Hospice Organization, 1994.

11. Egan K. A Patient–Family Value Based End-of-Life Care Model. Largo, FL: Hospice Institute of the Florida Suncoast, 1998.

12. Gerteis M, Edgman-Levitan S, Daley J, Delbanco TL (Eds). Through the Patient's Eyes: Understanding and Promoting Patient-Centered Care. San Francisco: Jossey-Bass, 1993:20.

13. Cassell EJ. The Nature of Suffering and the Goals of Medicine. Oxford: Oxford University Press, 1991.

14. Byock I, Merriman MP. Measuring quality of life for patients with terminal illness: the Missoula–VITAS® Quality of Life Index. Palliat Med 1998;12:231–244.

15. Byock I. Dying Well: The Prospect for Growth at the End of Life. New York: G.P. Putnam's Sons, 1997.

16. Byock I. The nature of suffering and the nature of opportunity at the end-of-life. Clin Geriatr Med 1996;2:237–251.

17. Tyler BA, Perry MJ, Lofton TC, Millard F. The Quest to Die with Dignity: An Analysis of Americans' Values, Opinions and Attitudes Concerning End-of-Life Care. Atlanta, GA: American Health Decisions, 1997.

18. Egan KA, Brandt K. Hospice, the final song in the rhythm of life: opportunities for growth and development at the end of life. Presented at the American Society on Aging 45th Annual Meeting, Orlando, FL. 1999.

19. Egan KA, Walsh T. Interdimensional care at the end of life: a quality of life model for end-of-life care. Paper presented at Institute for Quality Healthcare University of Iowa. Dec. 1998.

20. Sherman DW. Training advanced practice palliative care nurses. J Am Soc Aging 1999;23:88.

21. Lo KA, Egan KA. Interdisciplinary Team Case Management. Largo, FL: 1996. Hospice Institute of the Florida Suncoast.

22. Harper BC. Death: The Coping Mechanism of the Health Professional. Greenville, SC: Swiger Associates Inc. Southeastern University Press, 1994.

23. Lo KA, Egan KA. Creating and Maintaining a Healthy Balance. Largo, FL: Hospice Institute of the Florida Suncoast, 1996.

24. SUPPORT Principal Investigators. A controlled trial, to improve care for seriously ill hospitalized patients. JAMA 1995;274:1591–1598.

25. Committee on the Medicare Hospice Benefit and End-of-Life Care. Final Report to the Board of Directors. Arlington, VA: National Hospice Organization, 1998:23–25.

3 The Context of Palliative Care in Progressive Illness

ALICIA SUPER

Palliative nursing care in the new millennium is unique because it strives to intervene at the time of diagnosis, is driven by individual and family needs, and remains consistent through initial curative attempts, beginning palliative medicine, comfort care, terminal care, and bereavement.

—Alicia Super

The emerging technology of the 1950–1970s made diagnosing and treating illnesses more achievable. Accordingly, society's expectations took a giant leap about what modern health care could accomplish for the ill person. The breakthrough inventions and interventions of the medical establishment meant more efficient and more effective care for those with curable illnesses. The medical team was looked to as leader and ultimate authority on what was beneficial for the ill person.

Without discrimination, society's expectations about the medical establishment's ability to care for those with incurable illness made the same giant leap. Whereas, previously, dying persons were cared for by loved ones in their own homes, more and more families opted to return their dying relatives to the hospital environment for care. Battling the perceived enemy, death, health care professionals continued to play the lead role and often applied curative therapies and technology even to those whose death was inevitable. Attempting to avoid or delay inevitable death, most individual, health care, and societal resources are exhausted in a frantic search for the elusive "cure," often at the expense of living in meaningful ways according to individual values and goals.[1]

Times have changed, and society is now recognizing the limitations of the health care system. National studies demonstrate a growing gap between what people with life-threatening illness desire and what they experience from health care systems and providers.[2] Until now, there has been limited systematic assessment of the needs and experiences of individuals with life-threatening illness and their families. Most programs and services available for those experiencing life-threatening illness are based on the assumptions of health care providers rather than the experience of the persons involved. A distorted perspective of the place for medical intervention in the last phase of life means that most health care and research dollars continue to go to inpatient institutions and technology.[3] Although beginning to change, communities still expect the health care system to take care of individuals with life-threatening illness in social, emotional, and spiritual ways as well as the obvious physical aspects.[4–6]

Within the current health care system, individual, family, and community energies and resources for the last phase of life also focus on medical issues and events, often to the detriment of the meaning of this phase of life and the natural process of dying. Referrals to important supports during this time of life (e.g., hospice programs) are often based on prognosis and/or evidence of imminent death. There has been less acknowledgment that end-of-life goals are important and that end-of-life care should also include aggressive management of symptoms (Fig. 3–1).

Persons with more ambivalent prognostic illnesses (e.g., heart disease) have been less frequently referred to hospice programs, continuing instead to be cared for in an acute care or rehabilitation setting.

With the view that most of the ill person's time, energy, and resources are spent in the health care system, current research and development efforts focus on what medicine does (Figs. 3–2, 3–3).[7] Myriad organizations, systems, and institutions are researching the medical care issues pertinent to the time of dying.[1,8,9] A major effort has been spent on medical care documentation such as do-not-resuscitate (DNR) orders, advance directives, and other newly developed documents regarding life-sustaining treatment.[10] While important tools for stimulating discussions about end-of-life medical care, these documents tell us what medicine will *not* do. They do not guarantee that the person with life-threatening illness and his or her loved ones will receive state-of-the-art palliative care and meaningful support in the emotional, spiritual, and social dimensions.

Studies show that the values and goals of ill people and their families are often not assessed or honored.[10] While good medical care is imperative to control pain and symptoms, this care should also include attention to *healing and growth regardless of physical diminishment.*[11,12] Good medical care must support, and not obstruct, living fully until death.

People with life-threatening illness emphasize their focus on living in community, continuing in relationships with relatives and friends. This is an important phase of life during which even the most physically debilitated often report a sense of well-being. Now, their "well-

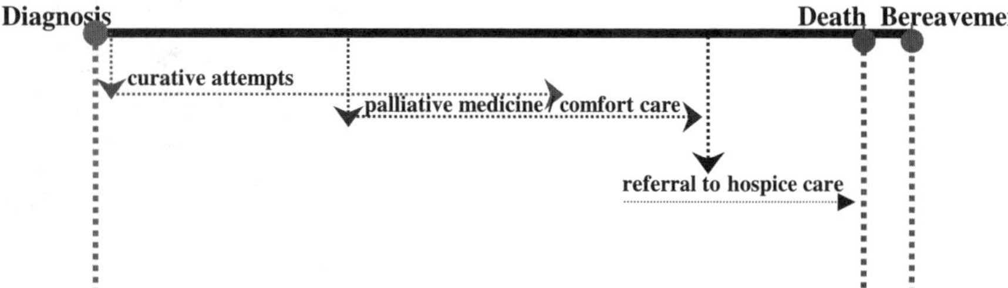

Fig. 3–1. Trajectory of illness and typical timing of services.

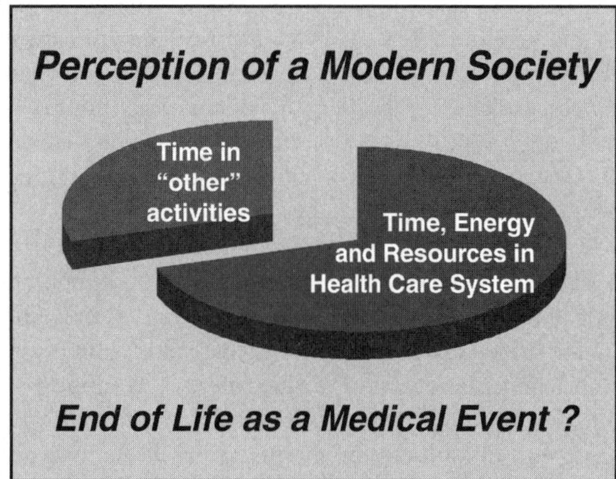

Fig. 3–2. Perception of modern society.

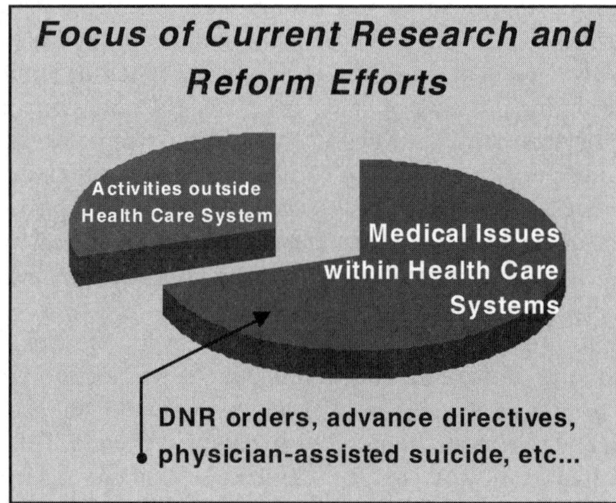

Fig. 3–3. Current focus on end-of-life care.

ness" has to do with dimensions of life other than the physical, such as the emotional, spiritual, and/or social.[11–13]

Recent research[11,12] reveals that people with life-threatening illnesses repeatedly emphasize that they are not so much afraid of dying as they are afraid they will not be able to *live* until they die. Their desire is to be treated as living human beings up until the time of death. They want to be fully integrated in their community, focusing on the issues of living and participating in work, hobbies, or family/community activities that are meaningful to them.[11,12]

Often, people in the last phase of life relate a sense of healing, growth, and "wellness" that transcends the purely physical issues of life.[11–13] Their surviving family and friends demonstrate improved coping and function when living, rather than dying, is the focus of care and support in their loved one's last phase of life.[11,12]

The proportion of time spent in the health care system is actually much smaller than would have been imagined prior to this research (Fig. 3–4).[11,12] While good medical care is important, it is a significantly smaller portion of the last phase of life than previously believed. With this new perspective, we can see that most current research in health care focuses on this one part of the last phase of life. Additionally, this research illustrates the distressing fact that medical competence and confidence are lacking even in the things we say we will do, such as pain and symptom management, respect for patient wishes (as outlined in advance directives, etc.), and assurance of "death with dignity." [12]

This chapter presents some available statistics and a case study to demonstrate the roles of nurses and others who incorporate the individual's desire to remain integrated in meaningful ways. It illustrates the phenomenon of healing and growth in emotional, spiritual, and relational or social dimensions even as the physical body diminishes in the last phase of life.

This chapter examines the impact of goal assessment and interventions on

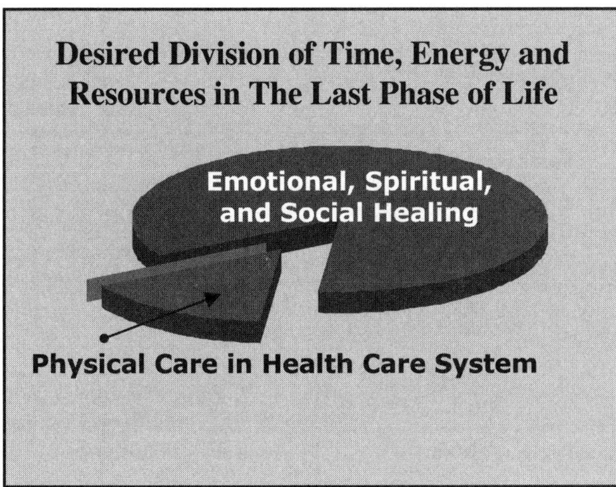

Fig. 3–4. Care needs at the end of life.

persons with life-threatening illness, their caregivers, primary health care providers, and community support networks. Public policy ideas that facilitate or obstruct goal assessment and achievement in the last phase of life will come to light. In these ways, the "why" for continued evolution and quality improvement in palliative nursing care across the nation will be understood. Appropriate health care system and interdisciplinary provider roles and resource allocation will be viewed in the context of community opportunities to resume important roles in the support of persons in the last phase of life.

PALLIATIVE CARE IN EVOLUTION

In the first state known for enacting legislation allowing physician-assisted suicide, Oregon is reported to use 70% more morphine today than it did in 1994.[14] It has a governor-appointed task force on pain and symptom management[15] and innovations in use of advance directives.[16] Hospices of this state report an average 20% increase in referrals over the last few years, leading the nation in referral rates and growth.[17] Without looking deeper, one might assume the state of Oregon was most progressive in end-of-life care. Without understanding why every state must continue to push forward for change, Oregon's health care leaders could feel satisfied that these statistics are proof of quality and a job well done.

Upon closer inspection, the health care leaders of Oregon discover that palliative care in the state is in the early stages of evolution. Oregon is moving in the right direction but far from "done." Physicians in Oregon are, indeed, prescribing more opioids since the passage of physician-assisted suicide legislation in 1994. They are in "phase I" of the evolution of their pain management practice.[18] Never before were physicians so ready to prescribe these analgesics in doses required to relieve malignant pain. Increasingly, however, Oregon patients and their families are complaining about the side effects of these potent drugs and continued, unrelieved pain. Pain management experts recognize that opioids alone are often being prescribed for pain which is opioid-resistant or only partially responsive to opioids (e.g., bone pain, neuropathic pain),[19–21] and patients are suffering the consequences. Phase II of the evolution in pain management practice will emphasize the imperative for skillful assessment, re-evaluation, and use of adjuvant analgesic therapies[18,19] in an effort to support individual and family goal achievement in the last phase of life. It is important to understand why we need to evolve before the resources and effort will be made available for this continued improvement.

Case Study: Harold, a Patient with Prostate Cancer

Harold was a 74-year-old man with end-stage prostate cancer. He was widowed 6 years before, when his wife of 46 years died of ovarian cancer. Today, Harold lives in his home with one of his six children, Nancy, and her spouse, Nathan, because he needs help with all activities of daily living.

Harold's son, Mike, is alarmed at how sedated his father has become as increasing doses of opioids have been prescribed for Harold's pain. Mike witnessed the death of his mother 6 years ago and says his mother died in a great deal of pain. He does not want that for his father, but he does not like what the opioid is doing to Harold's mentation. While Mike and his siblings acknowledge that Harold is coming to the end of his life, the family feels that this sedation is drug-induced, and they want more time and clarity with their father before he dies.

A palliative care nurse was contacted by the family and agreed to assess the situation. After a complete initial physical assessment was accomplished (Table 3–1), short-term goals were established for Harold, Mike, and Nancy (Table 3–2). A total of ten sites of pain of various types (muscle, bone, nerve, etc.) were assessed, and Harold's analgesic regimen was changed in collaboration with his physician (Table 3–3). In addition, the nurse taught Mike and Nancy to do light trigger point pressure and massage to loosen Harold's tight muscles and to give them a means to provide their father some hands-on, healing touch.

Within 2 days, Harold was alert, ambulatory, and interacting with family and friends (Table 3–1). He lived for an additional 2 months, his pain was controlled to his satisfaction throughout, and his level of consciousness was maintained until just 24 hours before his death, when he entered the expected somnolent stage of the active dying process. Harold died very peacefully with his children and granddaughter present and prepared.

It was apparent that Harold met his third goal (Table 3–2) when Mike described the last few days of his father's life:

> Dad saw an angel standing quietly in the corner 4 days before his death. As each day ensued, the angel moved to a position closer to his bed. One day as he was talking with Nancy, Dad asked if she could see the angel standing just beside her. He said the angel was telling him it was time

Table 3–1. Harold's New Physical Assessment

Area	Initial Assessment (before intervention)	Final Assessment (after intervention)
	Pain	
Location 1: buttocks, bilaterally	Location 1: intensity 4–5, "aching," intermittent	Location 1: none
Location 2: toes, bilaterally	Location 2: intensity 1–2, "aching" with light pressure	Location 2: none
Location 3: right shoulder	Location 3: intensity 8–9, "sharp, shooting," with touch or movement of right upper extremity	Location 3: none
Location 4: right anterior chest wall (changes over time to bilateral posterior and anterior)	Location 4: intensity 8–9, "sharp, like being stuck with the pin of a medal," intermittent	Location 4: none
Location 5: right thigh, anterior (changes over time bilateral)	Location 5: (no intensity rating) "deep aching," intermittent	Location 5: "some soreness there, but it's nothing really," intermittent
Location 6: left ankle	Location 6: "horrible," "deep aching" upon awakening	Location 6: none
Location 7: right posterior rib cage (changes over time to bilateral and centered at approximately T4–T5 spine)	Location 7: "terrible," "deep aching" upon awakening (changes over time to "sharp, shooting" and bilateral)	Location 7: (no intensity rating) "aching" when moving from supine to side-lying position, intermittent
Location 8: pelvis	Location 8: (no intensity rating) "deep aching" upon awakening	Location 8: none
Location 9: left shoulder	Location 9: intensity 5, "tender" to moderate palpation, associated with "trigger point" acuity and relief	Location 9: none
Location 10: right upper extremity at deltoid area	Location 10: intensity 5, "aching"	Location 10: none
	Mental Status	
	Sedated: dysphoric, unable to track conversation, confused at time, "semi-comatose" in afternoon and evening per Mike	Clear, conversant, full range of emotions, appropriate
	Sleep	
	Nighttime: "semi-comatose" per Mike	Nighttime: regular "night-owl" pattern (to bed/sleep about 2 AM and awakening about 9–10 AM)
	Daytime: limited alertness in early morning, then semi-comatose for remainder of day.	Daytime: regular afternoon nap; otherwise awake, alert, and active.
	Ambulation	
	Bedbound except for in wheelchair for assessment (somnolent in chair)	Ambulatory with cane; makes trips outside home and onto front porch to visit with friends
	Appetite	
	Poor: nausea/vomiting and taste changes.	Excellent, occasionally asks for seconds
	Fluid Intake	
	Poor: son must force fluids due to patient's "semi-comatose" state	Good intake of all types beverage
	Bowel/Bladder	
	Constipated (×4 days) with intermittent bleeding from rectum, urinary catheter with small amount of concentrated urine	Normal daily bowel movement, no bleeding; urinary catheter as before with ~2000 cc clear, yellow urine per day

Table 3–2. Initial Short-Term Goal Assessment

Goal	Initial Assessment
Harold's Goals	
Goal 1: "Get back to the studio (he was a water-color artist) to finish that painting for Nathan." Goal 2: "I sure wish I could see that baby (first grandchild due in 3 weeks)." Goal 3: "I've got some hard work to do with God."	Goals not met: Harold sedated, "semi-comatose," dysphoric, confused at times and nonambulatory
Mike's Goal	
"I can't stand to see Dad hurting. I want to finish the book we were reading together and to talk over some important things about the old days."	Goal not met: Harold too sedated and unable to track reading or conversation
Nancy's Goal	
"I want Dad to be more comfortable and to be able to see my baby be born (Harold's first grandchild)."	Goal not met: Harold has significant pain and is nonambulatory, anorexic, and developing pneumonia due to immobility

to go. Dad assured Nancy that this was true and that the angel was a comfort and most welcome. The next day, Dad slipped into a very sleepy and peaceful state. He would occasionally open his eyes, look upward and smile. When Nathan asked Dad what he was smiling at, Dad whispered that the angels were numerous now and coming closer. He told my family that they were the most beautiful creatures he had ever seen, so exquisite that he could barely describe them. Moments later, Dad slowly moved his hands over his body from hips to chin as he smiled and whispered, 'They're here; they're just coming all over me.' He sighed and never breathed again.

The nurse received the following letter some time later:

> The whole family wants you to know how much we appreciate what you did for our father in managing his pain. He never painted the picture for Nathan, not because he hurt, but because he just lacked the muscle. But he was able to see his granddaughter and even attend her baptism. And those trips out of the house to church, which he accomplished without too much difficulty, gave him confidence enough to demand to be taken to his eye doctor for his annual check-up and to get a new prescription so that he could read and watch television.
>
> Also, he spent many happy hours smoking expensive cigars on the front porch with Nathan and other friends and relatives who happened by. He has long been an anti-tobacco advocate, but you know, he did enjoy a good cigar in the past on occasion before the anti-tobacco stance was developed. This seemed like the perfect opportunity to enjoy them again. My brother said he might have just enjoyed being a 'bad boy' for once. Also, many people were able to come by and chat with him. They talked about the years gone by, and my father told them how much he enjoyed their friendship.
>
> And he ate! He really enjoyed his food again. My sister says he was even developing a 'gut.'
>
> Anyway, in his final months, he was able to enjoy so many things he would have been unconscious through if you hadn't listened to us. When I left that last time, I thought that might be the last time I saw him and so we had a really good, good-bye and he was fully aware. I had hoped to see him again, but he died while I was on the plane home.
>
> My brother from California and my sister from Florida were able to spend several weeks with him and, despite the physical care he needed towards the end, were able to enjoy some special times with him.
>
> One thing I especially want to thank you for is that he was able to enjoy his

Table 3–3. Harold's Analgesic Regimen

Current Regimen	New Regimen
Sustained-release oxycodone, 280 mg (PO) q AM Sustained-release oxycodone, 320 mg (PO) q PM	Sustained-release oxycodone, 40 mg (PO) q AM (this reduced dose was achieved over time to prevent opioid-withdrawal symptoms) Sustained-release oxycodone, 80 mg (PO) q PM (this reduced dose was achieved over time to prevent opioid-withdrawal symptoms) Choline magnesium trisalicylate, 1000 mg (PO) q 12 h Dexamethasone, 8 mg (PO) q 8 h Gabapentin, 100 mg (PO) q AM, 100 mg (PO) q mid-afternoon, then 200 mg (PO) q hs Baclofen, 5 mg (PO) q 12 h

granddaughter. We have one priceless video my sister took of him singing 'Where Go the Boats?' to her. It's a poem by Robert Louis Stevenson that Dad used to sing to us when we were kids. I could go on and on, but the main thing is, he wouldn't have been able to do any of these things if it weren't for what you did.

You made my Father's final months so much better not only for him, but also for all of us. We all thank you so much.

Sincerely,

(signatures of all the adult children of Harold)

The ultimate goal for dying individuals is not simply relief of pain but the ability to have the kind of quality of life in which they can achieve meaningful goals. This case study clearly demonstrates supportive roles for health care professionals. By assessing patient and family goals and following the lead of those who are truly managing end-of-life care (in this case, Harold's children), the nurse provided specialized care which allowed Harold and his family to make meaning of the last phase of life and to heal and grow in emotional and spiritual ways. By virtue of the time nurses typically spend with patients and their families (in all settings), nurses have excellent opportunities to heighten their skills in assessing and supporting end-of-life goal achievement.

PALLIATIVE CARE AND HOSPICE

The apparent success of Oregon's hospices is reflected in rapidly rising referral rates.[22] However, a deeper look at these statistics shows an alarming decline in length of stay,[22] meaning that home hospices across the state and across the nation often operate in crisis mode (Fig. 3–5). Patients admitted within 10 to 14 days of death are in dire need of pain and symptom management. Their families rarely have time to develop therapeutic relationships with their home hospice caregivers. By all accounts, overwhelming evidence of imminent death is the primary stimulus for hospice referral. Hospice programs report that as many as 9% of referred patients die before they can be admitted, even though admission occurs within 24 hours of referral.[22] This has enormous implications for quality and efficacy of care and program viability. Hospice programs suffer staff and financial stressors as their teams struggle to provide effective palliation to patients admitted to their program so close to death.[17,22] Until we comprehend the life goals of individuals and family caregivers, we will continue to make last-minute transitions that stress all involved.

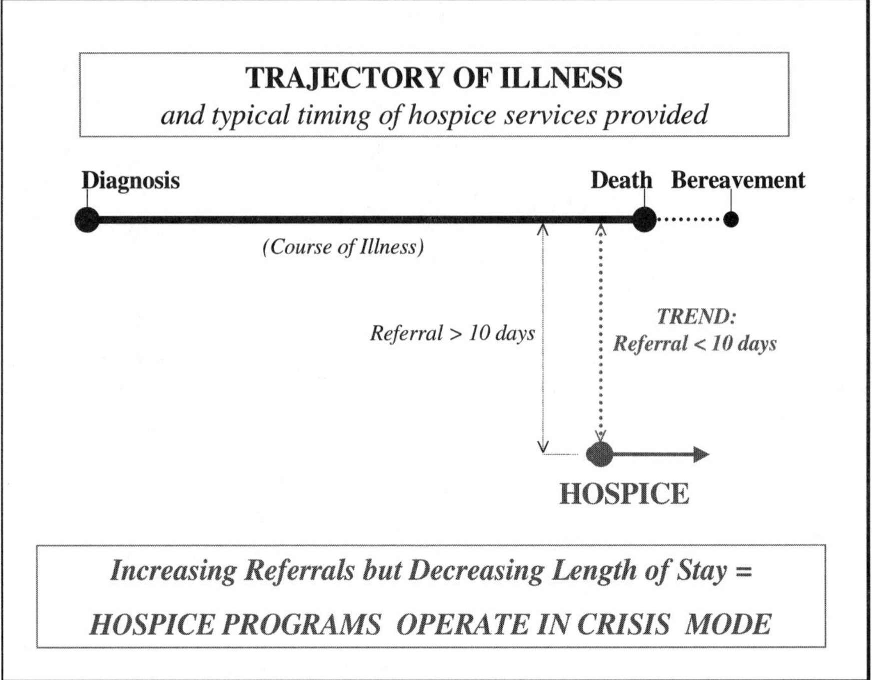

Fig. 3–5. Trajectory of illness and typical timing of hospice referrals.

Until recently, health care systems and providers have not spent time defining how people utilize the majority of their time, energy, and resources outside of health care systems. Accordingly, we do not know what role we play in the community assisting people to achieve that sense of wellness above the physical plane.[12] Additionally, we are just beginning to understand how poor quality or absent palliative care or futile curative therapies can actually obstruct a person's ability to achieve a sense of wellness and healing. Nurses have a particularly keen opportunity to invest in this discovery. With leadership and research, we are illustrating and defining the last phase of life: its tasks, its potential opportunities for healing and growth, the supportive roles for the community and health care providers. Nurses are challenging the current concept that care for persons with life-threatening illness is provided continuously by and within health care systems. We are learning that, while most people with life-threatening illness want more frequent contact and seamless palliative care, they actually receive only episodic and fragmented care from all health care systems and professionals.[11,12] Nurses can play an important role in mentoring colleagues in holistic care and reinforcing the resulting changes in behaviors and skill in order to affect not only community support of ill persons and their families but also how the entire interdisciplinary health care team behaves when cure is not achievable.

In this regard, nurses must join forces with all of the community to plan, develop, and test the tools and processes which

1. emphasize living before death and demonstrate the opportunities of the last

phase of life for persons, families, and communities;
2. reduce the emphasis and sole focus on medical issues in the last phase of life by assisting health care providers, payers, and systems to find their appropriate roles in supporting the goals of patients and families;
3. return control to persons with life-threatening illnesses and their families;
4. empower the community to integrate people with illness in meaningful ways;
5. identify and institute policy changes to support the above.

GOALS FOR PALLIATIVE NURSING CARE IN THE NEW MILLENNIUM

Nursing has a unique leadership opportunity to reform end-of-life care, but education alone has not been shown to change clinician practice, particularly in the area of palliative care.[23] By applying evolving concepts in end-of-life care (Table 3–4), nurses have the influence and ability to create and implement a sustainable mentor program[24] for persons with life-threatening illnesses, their families (of origin and/or choice), health care providers, health care systems, payers, state and federal legislators, workplace administrators, and the community at large. The mentor program would involve clinicians in a longitudinal process with the person with life-threatening illness, their family, and others who support meaningful, integrated living in community. In this way, the clinician experiences first-hand the wholeness of the ill person's life and values, the tasks and gifts of the last phase of life, and a community of caring individuals accompanying that person on this important journey. With coaching, insight, and reinforcement, this profound, personal experience will guide clinician practice with subsequent patients and their loved ones. Such an effort would achieve the following goals:

1. Illustrate the last phase of life as an important developmental stage of human healing and growth (in dimensions other than the purely physical):
   A. Educate regarding the tasks and gifts of the last phase of life.
   B. Develop the community tool(s) and construct for setting goals for the emotional, spiritual, and social dimensions of life.
   C. Facilitate persons with life-threatening illness and their families in setting goals for the last phase of life according to individual values and beliefs.
   D. Connect person and family with others dealing with the last phase of life.
2. Identify the appropriate roles[26] and resource allocations for health care systems and providers:
   A. Facilitate health care providers' understanding that the last phase of life is *not* solely a medical event; rather, it is an important *living*, human developmental phase with abundant opportunity for growth and healing in dimensions other than the purely physical.
   B. Train and build confidence in physicians for the skills and behaviors of comprehensive, supportive care and

Table 3–4. Evolving Concepts in End-of-Life Care: A Nursing Opportunity

Current	Evolving	Reformed
"Terminal" diagnosis means patient is dying.	Diagnosis of life-threatening illness means therapies may prolong life. Focus is on battling disease.	Diagnosis of life-threatening illness integrated into living. Focus is on living, clarifying values, setting and achieving goals, and finding meaning for person and family.
Death occurs as a "complication" and signifies "failure" of medical care.	Death is anticipated and acknowledged in last 48 hours when burdensome technology is removed and comfort measures are instituted. Physician refers to chaplain or social worker for support for family.	Last phase of life is acknowledged and considered an important developmental stage for the ill person and loved ones. Goals are actively assessed; tasks valued by person/family are accomplished; gifts are realized. Collegial health care team provides flexible support according to person/family values and priorities. The "last days" (days to weeks) are sacred for person/family unit and health care team. Life and death are inseparable.
Patient's illness is managed by physician.	Patient's health is managed by physician. Preventive medicine is valued. Futile care is discouraged.	Person and family manage life, illness, and dying in community with others. Flexible, interdisciplinary health care team plays supportive role according to person/family values and goals. Holistic growth and healing are valued for both person and family.
Physician care ends when cure cannot be achieved.	Physician leadership role continues in palliation of pain and symptoms with some assistance from interdisciplinary team until patient dies. Hospice provide support to the survivors of enrolled patients. Bereavement acknowledgement and support are limited in community.	Interdisciplinary team joins community in supportive roles that focus on healing and growth for ill person and family unit in emotional, relational, and spiritual realms. Community continues to care for survivors in all settings (industry, schools, political bodies, neighborhoods, etc.) during extended and flexible bereavement period.

interdisciplinary collaboration in customary environments.

C. Assure the clinical competence and confidence of all professional caregivers in the following areas of responsibility: pain assessment and skillful intervention, symptom control, values assessment, goal-setting facilitation, holistic guidance and support, and communication.

D. Empower palliative care "champions" with provision of time and financial and human resources to integrate services and assure clinical competence.

E. Educate and advocate for health care providers and systems to identify ill persons' and family caregivers' goals, outlining possible legislative/policy issues along the way.

F. Provide real-life mentoring experiences whereby health care providers and systems comprehend the wholeness of an individual's life and the potential for growth and healing through goal achievement. These experiential activities will help the medical establishment discern when their efforts facilitate goal achievement in the final phase of life and when they obstruct the individual's ability to grow and heal in other dimensions.

G. Adopt productivity standards that embrace the healing and integration of individuals, families, and communities.

H. Challenge the working definition of "healthier communities" to integrate the natural processes of illness, dying, and death.

I. Recognize the opportunity to embrace and improve hospice programs by assuring excellence in provider training and skills.

J. Replace traditional medical hierarchies with collaborative teams which function from the knowledge that spiritual, emotional, and relational healing take precedence in the last phase of life for persons with life-threatening illness and their families.

K. Replace provider-centric protocols, which perpetuate the myth of system and professional control over patients with life-threatening illness, with flexible professional capacities to respond to and follow individuals and families according to their unique values.

L. Initiate hands-on, experiential learning programs that teach and encourage holistic, supportive care skills and behaviors for professional caregivers.

M. Position health care systems within communities to share knowledge and resources which create effective support networks for both persons with life-threatening illness and their families in traditional settings (e.g., hospitals, hospice programs, long-term care facilities) and nontraditional settings (e.g., schools, industries, prisons, homeless shelters, and spiritual centers).

3. Outline community responsibilities and opportunities:
   A. Facilitate the person and family to achieve their goals by providing education, resources, support, and advocacy in appropriate arenas (e.g., workplace, neighborhoods, and religious/spiritual groups).
   B. Recognize support opportunities and the long-term benefits of integrating ill persons and their families into society.
   C. Outline policy issues that support the above goals (e.g., flexible leave policies for the ill and/or caregiving individuals, bereavement benefits that acknowledge that grief and mourning take more than 3 days).
4. Monitor individual and family caregiver communication and achievement of goals and measure the impact on health care systems, providers, and the community.
5. Urge local and global media to increase awareness in the following areas:
   A. Palliative care reform efforts, progress, and study findings,
   B. The positive focus on living and the value of the last phase of life,
   C. Cooperation between state and communities to improve quality of life in the final phase,
   D. Society's silence on the meaning and value of life even as the physical body diminishes.

TARGET POPULATION FOR HOLISTIC END-OF-LIFE CARE

Utilizing statistics from the state of Oregon again as an example, we can examine what has been done to assist those with life-threatening illness and where improvements can be made.

About 28,900 residents of Oregon died in 1996;[25] 77% of these deaths were the direct result of a life-threatening illness or condition (Table 3–5).[27] While more than 99% of Oregonians have access to hospice in their communities, only 36% of those with life-threatening illnesses or conditions were referred to a hospice in 1996:[22]

Table 3–5. Oregon Data:[27] Causes of Death Related to Illness in 1996

Diseases of the heart
Malignant neoplasm
Cerebrovascular disease
Chronic obstructive pulmonary disease
Alzheimer's disease
Diabetes mellitus
Alcoholism, alcoholic cirrhosis, and alcoholic psychosis
Perinatal conditions
Other diseases of the arteries
Arteriosclerosis
Parkinsonism
Acquired immune deficiency syndrome
Hypertension with/without renal disease
Nephritis/nephrosis
Congenital anomalies

- 64% of hospice enrollees had a diagnosis of cancer (even though cancer accounted for only 30% of illness-related deaths in the state)
- 1.5% had human immunodeficiency virus or acquired immune deficiency syndrome
- 12% had heart-related illnesses or stroke (even though 50% of illness-related deaths in the state were caused by heart disease and stroke)
- 6% had respiratory disease
- 4% had a neurological disease
- 5% had kidney or liver disease[27]

Nurses can impact individual and family healing and growth in the last phase of life by being aware of statistics such as these in their own states and working to identify persons with life-threatening illness of any diagnosis when cure is not expected. The trigger for identification would be the diagnosis itself (Fig. 3–6) rather than prognosis or impending death (as occurs for referral to hospice programs). Beginning holistic palliative care as soon as diagnosis is made allows individuals and their families to set and achieve goals in the last phase of life and to influence the

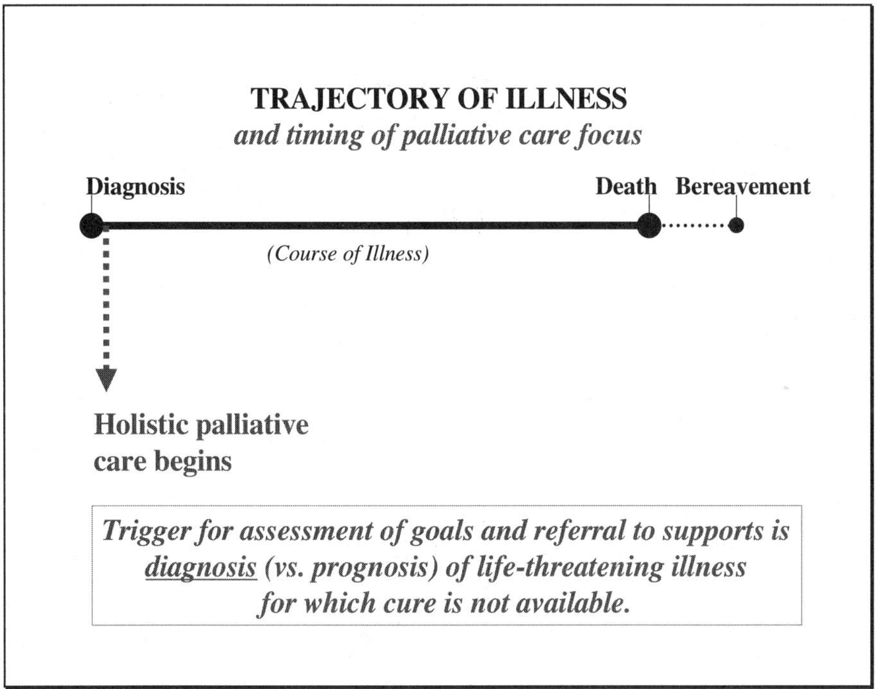

Fig. 3–6. Trajectory of illness and timing of palliative care focus.

appropriateness and quality of palliative care and support received.

While clearly some individuals and families may yet pursue experimental therapies aimed at cure, early nursing identification and communication of individual and family goals will influence this practice over time as such therapy often interferes with the achievement of meaningful goals. Likewise, this nursing effort will impact increasing home hospice length of stay, reversing the current trend (Fig. 3–5). Integral to any effort will be keeping the person with illness and his or her personal/family caregiver at the center of all reform.

Although health care providers will discover new roles for themselves while caring for persons who cannot be cured of illness, it is anticipated that the traditional "captain of the ship" role of physicians will diminish in favor of a supporting role. In addition, expectations about the role of health care providers and systems will be reconsidered to facilitate broader, supportive roles for the community.

Health care systems will need to negotiate partnerships with their communities, where systems may learn the proper place of medicine in end-of-life care. It is in these partnerships that system leaders and professionals will learn that life-threatening illness holds abundant opportunity for healing and growth regardless of physical status. It is in community that health care systems and professionals will witness the living emphasis and healing potential in emotional, spiritual, and relational dimensions of life for individuals and families.

Positioning health care systems in proper perspective with communities will require the system to relinquish control and power to the community. The capacity of community to care for its own will grow when health care systems acknowledge the findings of recent studies[11–13] and recognize the value of a more humble system influence.

Nurses have a unique opportunity to enhance palliative care by leading the reform effort for care of persons with life-threatening illness. We must actively promote and share our work with others so that the values we hold about care for the suffering, vulnerable, and dying are demonstrated across all settings.

Caring for persons with life-threatening illness, their loved ones, caregivers, and communities requires a team approach and the commitment of persons and resources that effectively deliver holistic, compassionate, and skillful care. Palliative care in the new

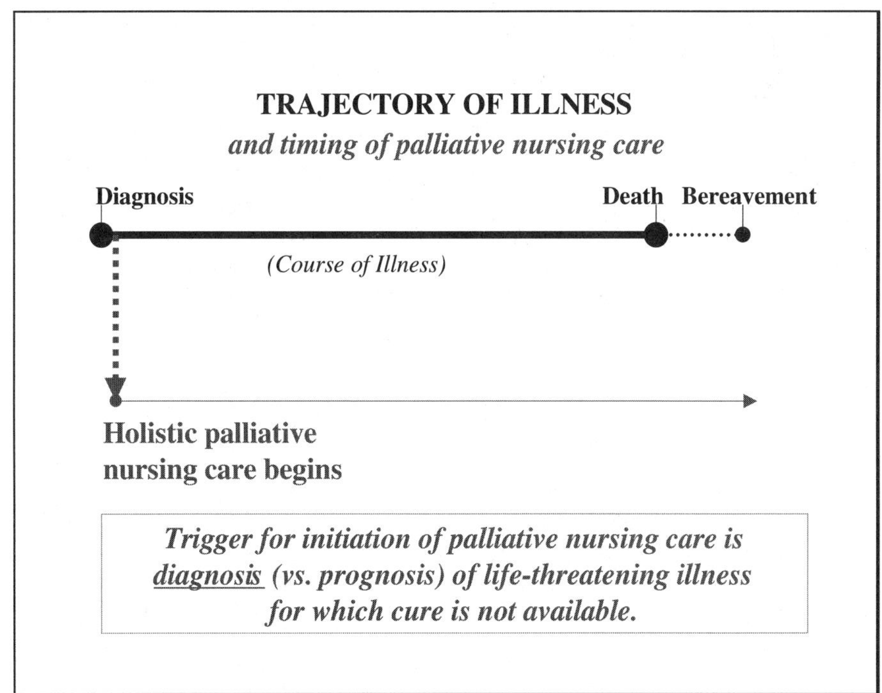

Fig. 3–7. Trajectory of illness and provision of palliative nursing care.

millennium will provide information, services, and support to individuals with life-threatening illness of any type, from the time of diagnosis through the trajectory of illness, dying, death, and bereavement. Excellence in palliative nursing care will require close collaboration with individuals, their loved ones, and the broader community in a manner that respects the integrity of caregivers. This service must provide holistic care with a multidimensional focus on the spiritual, relational, emotional, as well as physical realms, to affirm life at all stages. The fundamental nursing values of human dignity, human solidarity and interdependence, sensitivity to the poor, stewardship, compassion, justice, and excellence guide the care of individuals with life-threatening illness in the context of the opportunities, challenges, and barriers posed by today's pluralistic society.

Palliative nursing care in the new millennium is unique because it strives to intervene at the time of diagnosis, is driven by individual and family needs, and remains consistent through initial curative intervention attempts, beginning palliative medicine, comfort care, terminal care, and bereavement (Fig. 3–7). This model acknowledges the uncertainties of science and medicine and holds as its ultimate goal the growth and healing of individuals, whether that be into wellness or unto death.

REFERENCES

1. Extreme Care, Humane Options (ECHO). Community Recommendations for Appropriate, Humane Medical Care for Dying or Irreversibly Ill Patients. Carmichael, CA: Sacramento Healthcare Decisions, 1997.

2. Institute of Medicine. Initiatives to improve care at the end of life. In: Field MJ, Cassel CK, eds. Approaching Death: Improving Care at the End of Life. Washington DC: National Academy Press, 1997:18–20.

3. Groopman J. The Measure of Our Days: New Beginnings at Life's End. New York: Viking Press, 1997.

4. McKnight J. The Careless Society: Community and Its Counterfeits. New York: BasicBooks, 1995.

5. Carlson KL. Maximizing health through lifestyle changes and community partnerships. California Hosp 1995;8–12.

6. Conklin M. Improving community health depends on widespread involvement. Health Care Strat Manage 1994;12:6.

7. Institute of Medicine. Research leadership. In: Field MJ, Cassel CK, eds. Approaching Death: Improving Care at the End of Life. Washington DC: National Academy Press, 1997: 253–258.

8. Lynn J. Unexpected returns: insights from SUPPORT. In: Isaacs SL, Knickman JR, eds. To Improve Health and Health Care 1997: The Robert Wood Johnson Anthology. San Francisco: Jossey-Bass, 1997:161–186.

9. The Robert Wood Johnson Foundation. The Last Acts Campaign. Princeton, NJ: Robert Wood Johnson Foundation, 1997.

10. SUPPORT Principal Investigators. A controlled trial to improve care for seriously ill hospitalized patients: the study to understand prognoses and preferences for outcomes and risks of treatments (SUPPORT). JAMA 1995;274:1591–1598.

11. McSkimming S, Hodges MO, Super A, et al. The experience of life-threatening illness: patients' and their loved ones' perspective. J Palliat Med 1999;2:173–184.

12. McSkimming SA, Super A, Driever MJ, et al. Living and Healing During Life-Threatening Illness. St. Louis: Catholic Health Association of the United States, 1997.

13. Longaker C. Facing Death and Finding Hope: A Guide to the Emotional and Spiritual Care of the Dying. New York: Doubleday, 1997.

14. Office of Diversion Control. DADS Quarterly Report. Arlington, VA: US Department of Justice, 1996.

15. Oregon State Legislative Policy, Research and Committee Services. 69th Oregon Legislative Assembly, 1997–98 Interim. Salem: Oregon State Legislative Publications and Distribution, 1998.

16. Tolle SW. Care of the dying: clinical and financial lessons from the Oregon experience. Ann Intern Med 1998;128:567–568.

17. Jackson A. Oregon Hospice Statistics and Trends (draft of 3/3/98). Portland: Oregon Hospice Association, 1998.

18. Super A. Going one step further: skilled pain assessment and the art of adjuvant analgesia. Am. J. Hospice Palliat Care 1997;14:279–284.

19. Portenoy RK. Adjuvant analgesics in pain management. In: Doyle D, Hans G, MacDonald N, eds. Oxford Textbook of Palliative Medicine. New York: Oxford University Press, 1993:187–203.

20. American Pain Society. Principles of Analgesic Use in the Treatment of Acute Pain and Cancer Pain, 4th Ed. Skokie, IL: American Pain Society, 1999.

21. Jacox A, Carr DB, Payne R, et al. Management of Cancer Pain. Clinical Practice Guideline No. 9. Rockville, MD: US Public Health Service, Agency for Health Care Policy and Research 94-0592, 1994.

22. Oregon Hospice Association. Hospice in Oregon—a profile. In: 1998 Fact Sheet. Portland: Oregon Hospice Association, 1998.

23. Super A. Improving pain management practice. Health Prog 1997;70:50–54.

24. Forbes JF. Towards an optimal teaching programme for supportive care. Support Care Cancer 1994;2:7–15.

25. Oregon Health Division, Center for Health Statistics. Table 20—Deaths by Age, Sex, and County of Residence, Oregon. Portland: Oregon Health Division, 1996.

26. Zablocki E. Improving community health status: strategies for success. Qual Lett 1996;2:2–12.

27. Oregon Health Division, Center for Health Statistics. Table 21—Leading Causes of Death by County of Residence, Oregon. Portland: Oregon Health Division, 1996.

4 Principles of Patient and Family Assessment

ELAINE GLASS, DOUGLAS CLUXTON, and PATRICE RANCOUR

What we see depends mainly on what we look for.

—John Lubbock

An effective assessment is key to establishing an appropriate nursing care plan for the patient and family. The initial palliative care nursing assessment varies little from a standard nursing assessment.[1] In order to assess effectively, members of the health care team need to maximize their listening skills and minimize quick judgments. Medical experts contend that during a medical assessment interview, in which a physician mostly listens and gently guides the patient's story, the physician can accurately diagnosis the patient's problem 70% to 80% of the time.[2]

The goals of the palliative care plan that evolve from the initial and ongoing nursing assessments focus on enhancing quality of life. Ferrell's quality-of-life framework[3] is used to organize the assessment. The four quality-of-life domains in this framework are physical, psychological, social, and spiritual well-being. For the purpose of this chapter, the psychological and social domains are combined into one, the psychosocial domain.

Because the needs of patients and families change throughout the course of a chronic illness, these quality-of-life assessments are examined at four times during the illness trajectory:

- Diagnosis
- Treatment
- Posttreatment: long-term survival or terminal phase
- Active dying

Maria, a fictitious patient, serves as a case example throughout her illness experience with breast cancer.

NONMALIGNANT TERMINAL DISEASES

As the authors of this chapter work primarily with oncology patients, much of the assessment content is based on the cancer experience. The experiences of terminally ill patients with diseases other than cancer can be equally dynamic in terms of the continuous or episodic declines they face throughout the illness trajectory.

A primary difference between patients with malignant and nonmalignant illness lies in the current acceptance by the medical establishment that efforts toward cure are unavailable for many nonmalignant diseases. Thus, from the start, the focus of medical care for these patients is palliative rather than curative: reduction of symptoms, improvement of quality of life, and optimization of the highest level of wellness. Examples of these kinds of illness today include acquired immune deficiency syndrome (AIDS); refractory cardiovascular, hepatic, and renal diseases; brittle diabetes; and neurological disorders such as multiple sclerosis, cerebral palsy, amyotrophic lateral sclerosis, Parkinson's disease, and Alzheimer's disease. For some of these diseases, the focus of medical care may include attempting to extend life through research with the hope of finding a cure.

In contrast, medical professionals and the public are continually looking and hoping for a cure for cancer. Thus, the oncology patient may repeatedly alter his or her expectations about the future. Words describing the status of the disease during a cancer illness include "no evidence of disease," "remission," "partial remission," "stable disease," "recurrence," and "relapse." Patients report experiencing a "roller-coaster ride," in which the hopeful points in remission are often followed by a crisis with relapse or disease progression. Patients may be told, more than once, that they will probably die within a short time. Then, they recover and do well for awhile. As a result, the reality of death may be more difficult when it does occur.

INTRODUCTION TO PHYSICAL ASSESSMENT

Before beginning the assessment interview and physical exam, it is important for the nurse to establish a relationship with the patient by doing the following:

- Introducing himself or herself to the patient and others in the room.
- Verifying that this is the correct patient.
- Determining how the patient would like to be addressed: first name? last name? a nickname?
- Explaining the purpose of the interaction and the approximate length of time that he or she intends to spend with the patient.
- Asking the patient's permission to proceed with the assessment, giving the patient an opportunity to use the restroom, and excusing others whom the patient does not wish to be present during the interview and exam. (Some patients may want significant others to be present during the interview to assist with recall but may not want these people present during the exam; therefore, the nurse needs to modify the assessment routine to accommodate the patient's preferences.)
- Taking a seat near the patient, being re-

spectful of the patient's cultural norms for physical closeness and eye contact.
- Inviting the patient to tell about how the current problem or diagnosis came to light.
- Taking care not to interrupt the patient too often; using communication techniques such as probing, reflecting, clarifying, responding empathetically, and asking open-ended questions to encourage greater detail if the patient is brief or sketchy in describing his or her history of the illness.

INTRODUCTION TO PSYCHOSOCIAL ASSESSMENT

Tables 4–1 through 4–3 provide a framework for three key elements of assessment, including conducting a psychosocial assessment, distinguishing normal grief and depression, and doing a general mental status assessment. Throughout the illness trajectory, the nurse can use these tools to monitor the patient's response to illness and treatment.

Anyone diagnosed with a serious or life-threatening illness experiences many losses. However, responses to illness vary tremendously among individuals. In addition, the same person may respond differently at various times during an illness. How a particular patient copes depends on the severity of the illness, the patient's history of coping with stressful life events, and available supports. Some individuals develop coping styles that are more helpful than others when facing a life-threatening illness.

The nurse needs to assess two very important parameters in order to assist the patient in coping in the most functional way possible: the patient's need for information and need for control in making decisions. Observers of "exceptional" patients, like Bernie Siegel,[4] note that patients who are proactive, assertive, information seekers often appear to have better outcomes than patients who are passive in decision-making. Indicators of a person's need for control may include:

- Comfort in asking questions.
- Willingness to assert own needs and wishes relative to the plan of care.
- Initiative taken to research print and internet resources on the illness and treatment.

Table 4–1 provides details for doing a psychosocial assessment. More detailed information on the psychosocial aspects of oncology can be found in Holland's *Psycho-oncology*.[5]

Grief is a normal reaction to loss, especially a major loss like one's health. In chronic illness, grief is likely to be recurrent as losses accumulate. This does not make it pathological, but it does form the basis of the "roller-coaster" phenomenon that many patients describe. Some patients with advanced disease have been able to integrate their losses in a meaningful way, and others have managed to reconcile and transcend them. An example of such a person is Morrie Schwartz, who wrote about his illness in *Letting Go: Morrie's Reflections on Living While Dying*.[6]

Table 4–2 contrasts and compares normal grief with depression, to assist the nurse in determining when a patient needs to be referred for counseling. For further information, consult John Schneider's classic work "Clinically Significant Differences between Grief, Pathological Grief and Depression." [7]

In some cases, patients may appear to be having difficulties in coping but the nurse may be unable to easily identify the specific problem. The nurse may need to make a more thorough mental health assessment to determine the most appropriate referral. Key elements in such an assessment are found in Table 4–3. For more detailed psychosocial information, consult Holland's *Psycho-oncology*.[5]

Table 4–1. Framework for Psychosocial Assessment

Determining the types of losses

Physical	*Psychosocial*	*Spiritual*
Energy	Autonomy	Illusion of predictability/certainty
Mobility	Sense of mastery	Illusion of immortality
Body parts	Body image alterations	Illusion of control
Body function	Sexuality	Hope for the future
Freedom from pain and other forms of physical dysfunction	Relationship changes	Time
Sexuality	Lifestyle	
	Work changes	
	Role function	
	Money	
	Time	

Observing emotional responses

Anxiety, anger, denial, withdrawal, shock, sadness, bargaining, depression

Identifying coping styles

Functional: normal grief work and problem-solving
Dysfunctional: aggression, fantasy, minimization, addictive behaviors, guilt, psychosis

Assessing the need for information

Wants to know details
Wants the overall picture
Wants minimal information
Wants no information, but wants the family to know

Assessing the need for control

Very high
High
Moderate/average
Low
Absent, wants others to decide

Table 4–2. Differentiating Normal Grief from Depression

Normal Grief / Response to Loss of Health	Depression
Self-limiting but recurrent with each additional loss	Frequently not self-limiting, lasting longer than 2 months
Preoccupied with loss	Self-preoccupied, rumination
Emotional states variable	Consistent dysphoria or anhedonia, absence of pleasure
Episodic difficulties sleeping	Insomnia or hypersomnia
Lack of energy, slight weight loss	Extreme lethargy, weight loss
Identifies loss	May not identify loss or may deny it
Crying is evident and provides some relief	Crying absent or persists uncontrollably
Socially responsive to others	Socially unresponsive, isolated
Dreams may be vivid	No memory of dreaming
Open expression of anger	No expression of anger
Recovery does not require professional intervention	Recovery requires professional treatment

Table 4–3. General Mental Health Assessment

Appearance	**Psychomotor Behavior**
Hygiene	Gait
Grooming	Movement
Posture	Coordination
Body Language	Compulsions
	Energy
	Observable Symptoms (tics, perseveration)
Mood and Affect	**Speech**
Interview Behavior	Pressured, slow, rapid
Specific Feelings expressed	Goal-oriented, rambling,
	Incoherent, fragmented, coherent
Facial Expressions	Relevant, irrelevant
	Poverty of speech
	Presence of latencies (delayed ability to respond when conversing)
Intellectual Ability	**Thought Patterns**
Attention	Loose, perseverating
Concentration	Logical, illogical, confused
Concrete/Abstract thinking	Oriented, disoriented
	Tangential, poorly organized, well-organized
Comprehension	Preoccupied
Insight	Obsession
Judgment	Paranoid ideas of reference
Educational Level	Delusions
	Hallucination, illusions
	Blocking, flight of ideas
	Neologisms (made up words)
	Word salad (meaningless word order)
	Presence of suicidal or homicidal ideation
Sensorium/Level of Consciousness	
Alert	
Somnolent	
Unresponsive	

INTRODUCTION TO SPIRITUAL ASSESSMENT

Although Chapter 29 provides a more detailed discussion of spiritual assessment, the following illustrates the importance of assessing the spiritual domain as a component of a comprehensive evaluation.

Attempts to define spirituality can often result in feelings of dismay and inadequacy. It is like trying to capture the wind or grasp water. Therefore, assessing and addressing the spiritual needs of patients can be a formidable challenge. Spirituality may include one's religious identity, beliefs, and practices but it involves much more. The person without an identified religious affiliation is no less spiritual. Indeed, the desire to speak one's truth, explore the meaning of one's life and illness, and maintain hope are fundamental human quests which reflect the depth of the spirit. Haase and co-workers[8] concluded that the spiritual perspective is "an integrating and creative energy based on belief in, and feeling of interconnectedness with, a power greater than self." Amenta[9] views spirituality as "the life-force springing from within that pervades our entire being." Hay[10] defines it as "the capacity for transcending in order to love or be loved, to give meaning, and to cope." Doyle[11] writes, "Spiritual beliefs may be expressed in religion and its hallowed practices, but a person can and often does have a spiritual dimension to his or her life that is *totally* unrelated to religion and not expressed or explored in religious practice." He further notes that "a prerequisite to discussion of spiritual issues with a patient is to create a situation which permits speaking of spiritual problems, i.e. environment, ambience, and attitude." [11]

The spiritual issues that arise following the diagnosis of a serious/life-threatening illness are abundant and varied. As a person progresses through the phases of an illness (diagnosis, treatment, posttreatment, and active dying), he or she is confronted with mortality, limitations, and loss. This frequently leads to questions such as "What is my life's purpose?", "What does all this mean?", "What is the point of my suffering?", "Why me?", and "Is there life after death?" Indeed, Victor Frankl,[12] in his classic *Man's Search for Meaning*, affirmed that the quest to find meaning is one of the most characteristically human endeavors. To find meaning in suffering enhances the human spirit and fosters survival.

Following Abraham Maslow's[13] theory, human needs can be placed on a hierarchy that prioritizes them from the most basic physical and survival needs to the more transcendent. Thus, a patient's ability and willingness to dialogue about issues of meaning, to discuss successes and regrets, and to express his or her core values may occur only after more fundamental needs are addressed. This reality in no way diminishes the spiritual compared with the physical; rather, it supports the need for an interdisciplinary approach that provides holistic care of the entire person. For example, if a physician relieves a young woman's cancer pain and a social worker secures transportation for her to treatments, she and her family may be more able to address the vital concerns of her soul.

The sensitivity of the nurse to a patient's spiritual concerns improves the quality of palliative care throughout the illness trajectory. When members of the health care team serve as "companions" to a patient and family during their journey with an illness, they offer vital and life-affirming care.

Responding to the spiritual needs of patients and families is not solely the domain of the chaplain, clergy, or other officially designated professionals. All members of the health care team share the responsibility of identifying and being sensitive to spiritual concerns.

It is vital that a patient is viewed not in isolation but in the context of those who are affected by the illness. Thus, the focus of spiritual assessment includes both the patient and the family or significant others. This perspective affirms the power of a systems view, which sees the patient and family as mutually dependent and connected. Providing support to the family members will not only assist them directly but may also contribute to the patient's comfort secondarily as he or she sees loved ones being cared for as well.

The purpose of a spiritual assessment is to increase the health care team's knowledge of the patient's and family's sources of strength and areas of concern in order to enhance their quality of life and the quality of care provided. The methods of assessment include direct questioning, acquiring inferred information, and observing. This is most effectively accomplished when a basis of trust has been established. Fitchett[14] noted that spiritual assessments consist of both "substantive" and "functional" information. Table 4–4 examines these categories of spiritual assessment.

One of the fundamental principles underlying spiritual assessment and care is the commitment to the value of telling one's story. Alcoholics Anonymous, a very successful program with spiritual tenets, acknowledges the power of story. This might be paraphrased as follows: in the hearing is the learning, but in the telling of one's story is the healing.

Similarly, Thompson and Janigan[15] developed the concept of "life schemes," which provides a sense of order and purpose for one's life and promotes a perspective on the world, oneself, events, and goals. Simple, open-ended questions such as "How is this illness affecting you?" and "How is the illness affecting the way you relate to the world?" provide the opportunity for validation and exploration of the patient's life scheme.

CULTURAL COMPETENCE

It is unrealistic to expect that health care professionals will know all of the customs, beliefs, and practices of patients from every culture for whom they care. There are useful reference compendiums to assist in gaining cultural competence.[16] However, all providers should strive for some degree of cultural competence, which has been defined as "an educational process, which includes the ability to develop working relationships across lines of difference. This encompasses self-awareness, cultural knowledge about illness and healing practices, intercultural communication skills and behavioral flexibility." [17]

The members of the health care team can increase their cultural competence by concentrating on the following:

- Being aware of one's own ethnocentrism.
- Assessing the patient's and family's beliefs about illness and treatments.

Table 4–4. Categories of Spiritual Assessment

Substantive Information
The "**what**" of spiritual life
Present religious affiliation or past religious background
Beliefs about God, the transcendent, an afterlife
Present devotional practices and spiritual disciplines, like praying, attending worship services, meditation, yoga, etc.
Significant religious rituals
Identification of membership in a faith community and the degree of involvement and level of support
Functional Information
The "**how**" of spiritual life
Making meaning
Retaining hope
Securing a source of inner strength and peace
Exploring the relationship between beliefs, practices, and health
Surviving losses and other crises

Table 4–5. Meeting the Need for Translator Services

A child or family member should not be used as a translator for major explanations or decision-making about health care. Even adult children may feel uncomfortable speaking with their parents or grandparents about intimate topics. Furthermore, many lay people do not know or understand medical terms in their language. Informed consent requires that the patient receive accurate information that he or she can understand, before making a health care decision.

It is recommended that the health care team:

- Obtain the services of a certified medical translator, if possible.
- In the absence of an on-site certified translator, use **AT&T** translators. In the United States or Canada, call 1-800-752-6096 to set up an account and obtain a password.

- Conveying respect, such as saying "I am unfamiliar with your culture. Please help me understand why you think you got sick and what you think will make you better."
- Soliciting the patient and family as teachers and guides regarding cultural practices.
- Asking the patient's personal preferences and avoiding expecting any individual to represent his or her whole culture.
- Respecting cultural differences regarding personal space and touch, such as requesting "Whom do I ask for permission to examine you?" and "May I touch you here?"
- Determining needs and desires regarding health-related information, such as asking "When I have information to tell you, how much detail do you want to know and to whom do I give it?"
- Noting and affirming the use of complementary, alternative, and integrative medical practices.
- Incorporating the patient's cultural healing practices into the plan of care.
- Responding to resistance from the patient and family about the recommended treatment plan with understanding, negotiation, and compromise.
- Being sensitive to the need for translator services (Table 4–5 contains more information on translator services).

ASSESSMENT AT THE TIME OF DIAGNOSIS

The goals of a palliative care nursing assessment at the time of diagnosis are as follows:

1. Determine the baseline health of the patient and family.
2. Document problems and plan interventions with the patient and family to improve their quality of life.
3. Identify learning needs to guide teaching that promotes optimal self-care.
4. Recognize patient and family strengths to reinforce healthy habits and behaviors for maximizing well-being.
5. Discern when the expertise of other health care professionals is needed, for example, social worker, registered dietician, etc.

PHYSICAL ASSESSMENT AT DIAGNOSIS

When the patient has finished telling his or her story about the illness, the nurse needs to do a head-to-toe physical assessment. This assessment utilizes the general categories of head and neck, shoulders and arms, chest and spine, abdomen, pelvis, legs and feet, and general. The nurse obtains data by observing, interviewing, and examining the patient. The forms, policies, procedures, and expectations of the health care agency in which the assessment occurs guide the specific details that are collected and documented. Figure 4–1 shows cues to guide the physical assessment.

Because the family is so important to the palliative care focus on quality of life, the overall health of other family members needs to be documented. Identification of the major health problems, physical limitations, and physical strengths of family members serves as a basis for planning. The physical capabilities and constraints of the caregivers available to assist and support the patient may impact the plan of care, especially related to the most appropriate setting for care. This information also provides direction for the types of referral that may be needed to provide care.

PSYCHOSOCIAL ASSESSMENT AT DIAGNOSIS

The primary psychosocial feature of a new diagnosis is the trigger of anticipatory grief. Patients' responses to receiving bad news range from shock, disbelief, and denial to anger and fatalism. As further losses occur along the illness continuum, this grief mechanism is retriggered so that losses become cumulative. Statements such as "I can't believe this is happening to me" or "Why is this happening to us?" are signals to the health care professional that the patient and family are grappling heavily with this threat to their equilibrium. There is already a sense that life will be forever changed. A longing emerges to return to the way things were.

In response to these emotional states, the health care team is most helpful when they do the following:

- Normalize the patient's and family's experiences.
- Use active listening skills to facilitate grief work.
- Create a safe space for self-disclosure, build a trust relationship.
- Develop a collaborative partnership to establish a mutual plan of care.
- Respect the patient's and/or family's use of denial in the service of coping with harsh realities: "It must be hard to believe this is happening."
- Assess the patient's and family's coping styles: "When you have experienced hard times in the past, how did you get through them?"
- Reinforce strengths.
- Maximize a sense of control, autonomy, and choice.
- Assess the patient's need for information: "What do you know about your illness?", "Are you the kind of person who likes to know as much as possible or as little as possible?", "What would you like to know about your illness now?"
- Check the need for clarification: "What did you hear?" or "Summarize in your own words how you understand your situation now."
- Avoid "medspeak," which is medical terminology unfamiliar to the average person.
- Mentor patients and families who have had little experience with the health care system, including coaching them in conversations with their physicians and teaching them ways to be wise consumers.

Head & Neck:

Hair- Texture, fullness, shine, dandruff, well-kept, bald? Complexion- Skin condition? Scars? Make-up?

Mind- Alert & Oriented x3? MMSE needed? Capacity for decision-making? Speech, language, vocabulary? Education? Ability to read? Memory & attention span? General mood? Stress level? Hx of anxiety, depression, phobias? Hx headaches? Seizures? Knowledge & experience with illness? Perception of illness? Meds?

Senses-Sight - PERRLA? Visual acuity? Glasses/contacts? Redness, itching, puffiness, icterus? Eye drops?
Hearing - Deficits? Use of aids? Tinnitus? Dizziness? Pain? Inspect for excess wax, signs of infection.
Smell - Ability? Sensitivities? Taste - Flavor dislikes?

Nose- Hx of sinusitis or other sinus problems? Nose bleeds? Frequency of URIs? Pain? Meds?

Mouth-Inspect condition of teeth, gums, & mucous membranes? Dryness? Sores? Infection? Brushing & flossing habits? Semi-annual cleanings & dental exams? Dentures, bridges? Hx of sore throats? Pain?

Lips- Dry or cracked? Hx of fever blisters?

Neck- Quality & clarity of voice? Full ROM? Hx of problems- swallowing, laryngitis, esophagitis, reflux? Swollen lymph nodes? Venous distension? Carotid pulses? Pain?

Shoulders & Arms:

Full ROM? Strength? Dexterity? Coordination? Crepitus? Deformities? Swelling? Joint/muscle pain or stiffness? Neuropathies? Changes in sensation? Reflexes? Venous access?

Chest & Spine:

Lungs-Respiratory rate; SOB? DOE? Orthopnea? Lung sounds? Cough? Sputum? CXR? Shape of chest? Smoking hx? Hx of infections, asthma, or night sweats? Pain? Meds?

Heart-Heart rate & rhythm? Murmurs? BP? EKG? Hx of palpitations, CP, MI? CAD/CHF? Pedal edema? Meds?

Breasts-Appearance, lumps, discharge? BSE? Mammogram? Regular HCP Exam? Pain/tenderness?

Spine-Hx back pain, problems, or injuries? Flexibility? Deformities?

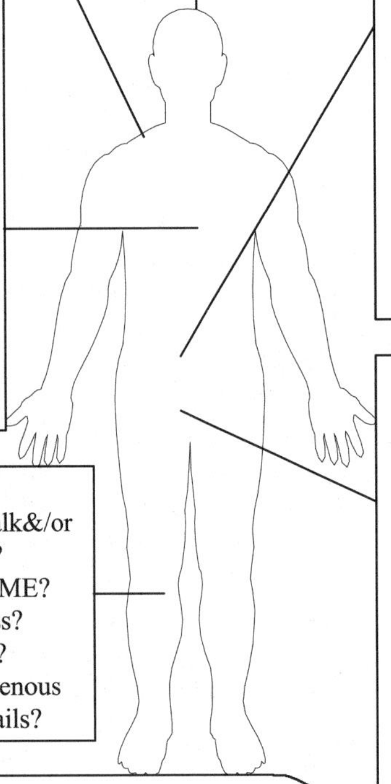

Legs & Feet:

Full ROM? Strength? Crepitus? Ability to walk&/or run? How far? Gait? Coordination? Balance? Weakness? Paralysis? Deformities? Use of DME? Hx of problems? Muscle/joint pain or stiffness? Reflexes? Change in sensation? Temperature? Edema? Pedal pulses? Dryness? Cellulitis? Venous stasis? Skin discoloration? Condition of toenails?

Abdomen:

General- Appearance? Ascites? Masses? Tenderness? Surgery scars?

Stomach- Usual diet? Appetite? Caffeine intake? Vitamin use? Hx of problems?- PUD? Belching? Pain? Motion sickness? N & V with pregnancy?

Liver- Alcohol intake? Hx hepatitis? LFTs?

GB- Hx of indigestion? Pain?

Pancreas-Hx of diabetes?

Bowels- Normal habits? Recent changes? Color, form? Diarrhea? Incontinence? Constipation? Laxative use? Gas? Pain? Fat & fiber diet? Hemorrhoids? Rectal bleeding? Hemocult tests? Regular HCP rectal exams? Sigmoidoscopy?

Pelvis:

Kidneys- /Urine Color, frequency? Nocturia? Pain? Hx of UTIs? Incontinence? Other problems?

Male= TSE? DRE? PSA? Hx BPH? Meds? Hernia? Sexually active? Hx STDs? Contraception? Circumcised? Sexual function concerns? Impotence? Importance to self concept, relationships, & quality of life?

Female= Gx Px-x-x-x? Contraception? LMP? Menarche age? Usual menses cycle? Break through bleeding? Menses pain or problems? Menopause - age? ERT? Pelvic exam & PAP smear? Vaginal discharge, dryness, odor, infection? Sexually active? Sexual function concerns? Importance to self concept, relationships, & quality of life?

General:

Allergies? Temperature? Height? Weight? -loss, gain, ideal?

Functional Status? Exercise tolerance? Needs related to ADLs?

Appearance- Personal hygiene, dress, posture, body language, sweating? Intolerance to heat or cold?

Skin- Color, turgor, bruising, rashes, itching? Moles? - ABCD? Wounds? Previous surgical sites healed?

General- Aches, pains? Muscle twitching, tingling, cramps? Hx broken bones? Hx of major illness, injuries, surgeries? Family hx of illnesses? Past health & well-being? Sleep patterns/problems? Prevention habits? Rest, relaxation, recreation? Immunizations? Use of alternative therapies?

The nurse must remember that while the patient is feeling strong emotions, the family is also experiencing intense feelings. Similar assessments of family members will help to mobilize resources at critical times. Family members will experience their grief reactions at their own individual rates throughout the course of the illness. Each family member will vary in his or her particular coping style and need for information.

The nurse and other members of the health care team assist the patient and family when they do the following:

- Observe changes in family members' roles and responsibilities, for example, the breadwinner becomes a caregiver, the homemaker begins working outside the home.
- Identify external community support systems.
- Assist the patient and family in identifying coping strategies when awaiting test results, which is one of the most stressful times, and which recurs throughout the illness.
- Help the patient and family explore the benefits and burdens of different treatment options when changes are needed in the plan of care.
- Assess parental readiness to assist children with their adaptation needs: "How do you plan to tell your children?"

Assess the coping of children within the family by being aware of their fears and concerns. Table 4–6 describes some common responses of children to having an adult loved one who is ill.

Assisting in the process of making initial treatment decisions can be an opportunity to begin a relationship that will continue to grow. Members of the health care team may ask questions such as, "What is most important to you in life?" and "Is quality of life or quantity of life most meaningful?" Assisting the patient and family in identifying and expressing their values will guide them in subsequent decision-making.

Table 4–6. Common Responses of Children to Serious Illness in the Family

Concrete, magical thinking that results in feelings of guilt, e.g., "I once told Mommy I wished she were dead."
Fears of abandonment, especially in younger children
Fears of contracting the disease
Anger, withdrawal, being uncooperative, especially in adolescents
Acting out behavior with lack of usual attention
Frustrations with an altered lifestyle because of decreased financial resources and less family fun activities because of the ill person's inability to participate, etc.
Inability to concentrate and focus, especially regarding schoolwork

SPIRITUAL ASSESSMENT AT DIAGNOSIS

The diagnosis of a serious illness generally brings with it a sense of shock to the patient and family. It may threaten many of their assumptions about life, disrupt their sense of control, and cause them to ask "Why?" The health care team can be most helpful at this time if they do the following:

- Determine the patient's and family's level of hopefulness about the future: "What are you hoping for?" or "How do you see the future at this time?"
- Inquire about how the patient and family have dealt with past crises of faith, meaning, or loss: "What helped you get through that?"
- Determine the comfort level with talking about the spiritual life: "Some people need or want to talk about these things, others don't. How is it for you?"
- Inquire about spiritual support persons available to them, e.g., pastor, rabbi, counselor, or spiritual advisor.
- Determine the patient's or family's need or desire to speak with a spiritual support person.
- Ask about spiritual self-care practices to promote healthy coping: "How are you taking care of *you* at this time?"
- Listen for comments from the patient and family regarding the importance of their religious traditions and practices.

Spiritual goals at this phase are to normalize initial concerns, provide information to foster positive coping, and encourage the patient and family to seek supportive spiritual resources.

Case Study: Maria at the Time of Diagnosis of Breast Cancer

Maria is a 56-year-old Latino woman who came to the United States from Mexico when she was 25, to pursue a career in music. She married David, an Anglo-American orchestra member, when she was 30 and he was 35. They have four children: Rachel, 23; Jose, 20; Juan, 16; and Juanita, 14. Maria and her family are practicing Roman Catholics. Maria had been in fairly good health with a past medical history of hypertension diagnosed at age 35, type II diabetes diagnosed at age 50, and mild obesity since the birth of her last child.

During a routine gynecological visit, Dr. Jane Smith felt a suspicious lump in Maria's

Fig. 4–1. Assessment at the time of diagnosis. Obtaining a baseline of the patient's health status. Abbreviations: ABCD = How to assess a skin mole (**A**symmetry; **B**orders, regular or irregular; **C**olor, multicolored; **D**iameter, generally > 6 mm); ADLs = activities of daily living; BP = blood pressure; BPH = benign prostatic hypertrophy; BSE = Breast self-exam; CAD = coronary artery disease; CHF = congestive heart failure; CP = chest pain; CXR = chest x-ray; DOE = dyspnea on exertion; DME = durable medical equipment (e.g., wheelchairs, walkers, hospital beds, etc.); DRE = digital rectal exam; EKG = electrocardiogram; ERT = estrogen replacement therapy; Gx Px-x-x-x = gravida (number of pregnancies), parity = (number of deliveries past 20 weeks, number of abortuses, number of premature deliveries, number of living children); GB = gallbladder; HCP = health care provider/professional; Hx = history; LFTs = liver function tests; LMP = last menstrual period; Meds = medications; MI = myocardial infarction; MMSE = Mini Mental Status Exam; N & V = nausea and vomiting; PAP = Papanicolao test for cervical cancer; PERRLA = pupils equal, round, react to light, accommodation; PSA = prostate-specific antigen; PUD = peptic ulcer disease; ROM = range of motion; SOB = shortness of breath; STD = sexually transmitted disease; TSE = testicular self-exam; URIs = upper respiratory infections; UTIs = urinary tract infections.

right breast. Maria had not been doing breast self-exams, in part because of a cultural taboo about self-touching. A mammogram confirmed the presence of a lump. Maria and her husband scheduled an appointment to learn the results of the breast x-ray. Maria was then referred to an oncology surgeon.

Maria's mother, who remains influential in her life, urges Maria to consider the services of a *curandero*, a traditional healer. This creates conflict in the family, especially with David and the children who are native-born U.S. citizens. They insist on conventional treatment, which they hope will provide a cure. Maria's mother is emphatic in her point of view. She believes that any serious disease has both a physical and a spiritual component. Both aspects must be brought into harmony by a *curandero*. To keep peace in the family and to demonstrate respect for her mother, Maria agrees to keep her appointment with the surgeon and to see a *curandero*.

GOALS

- Acknowledge the validity of each family member's coping styles and beliefs.
- Seek ways to integrate the family's beliefs and alternative practices into the medical treatment plan.

ASSESSMENT DURING TREATMENTS

The goals of a palliative care assessment during active treatment are as follows:

1. Assess the patient's systems in all domains that are at risk for problems considering both the patient's baseline problems and any side effects of the treatments.
2. Record the current and potential problems and plan early interventions with the patient and family.
3. Ascertain the need for teaching to prevent, minimize, and manage problems with the goal of maximizing quality of life.
4. Reinforce patient and family strengths, healthy habits, and behaviors to maximize well-being.
5. Recognize when other health care professionals' expertise is needed and make appropriate referrals, for example, physical therapist, pharmacist, etc.

PHYSICAL ASSESSMENT DURING TREATMENTS

Reassessments during treatment determine the changes that have occurred from the initial assessment. Knowledge of the usual disease process and the side effects of treatment will assist the nurse in focusing reassessments on the body systems most likely to be affected.

In addition to the patient's physical assessment, the nurse should make periodic observations and inquiries about the health of other family members. It is important to document any changes in their health problems or physical limitations and physical strengths that might have an impact on the patient's care and the family's overall quality of life.

PSYCHOSOCIAL ASSESSMENT DURING TREATMENTS

Once a treatment plan has been initiated, patients often express relief that "something is finally being done." Taking action frequently reduces anxiety. The most important psychosocial intervention at this stage is the amelioration of as many treatment side effects as possible. When basic needs for physical well-being are assessed and symptoms are controlled, the patient is able to explore and meet higher needs. These higher needs include belonging, self-esteem, and self-actualization.[13] Patients who are preoccupied with pain and nausea or vomiting have no energy or ability to explore the significance of the illness or their feelings about it. Effective management of physical symptoms is mandatory before the patient can begin to work on integrating the illness experience into the tapestry of his or her life.

After several months or years of treatment, the wear and tear of having a chronic illness may exhaust even the hardiest person. Patients may begin to weigh the benefits versus the burdens of continuing aggressive therapies. Initially, patients will endure almost anything if they believe a cure is possible. As time unfolds, their attitude may change as they watch their quality of life erode with little prospect of a more positive outcome. Patients may also reprioritize what is most important to them; for example, the workaholic may find less satisfaction at the office, or the homemaker may experience less fulfillment from daily routines around the house. Change, transition, and existential questioning characterize this phase. The nurse and other members of the health care team will assist the patient and family when they do the following:

- Inquire about the patient's newly emerging identity as a result of the illness: "What activities and which relationships bring you the most joy and meaning?" or "Have you been able to define a new purpose for yourself?"
- Assess for signs of anxiety and depression, which remain the two most common psychosocial problems associated with severe illness (Table 4–7 contains an outline of the characteristics of anxiety and depression; for more information contrasting anxiety and depression, consult Holland's *Psycho-oncology*.[5]
- Screen for suicidal ideation in cases of depression: "Have you been feeling so bad that you've been thinking of a way to hurt yourself?" and "Do you have a plan for how to do it?"
- Refer for counseling and possible psychotropic medication to enhance positive coping and comfort.

SPIRITUAL ASSESSMENT DURING TREATMENTS

With the treatment of a serious illness comes the introduction of an additional stressor to the patient and family. It is important to assess how they incorporate the demands of treatment into their daily routine and how these changes have impacted the meaning of their lives. The nurse and other members of the care team will be helpful to the patient and family if they normalize the stress of treatment and:

- Inquire about the patient's and family's hopes about the future.
- Assess the level and quality of support they are receiving, for instance, from other family members, faith community, and neighbors.
- Invite expressions of anxiety and fear by asking "What is concerning you the most at this time?"
- Assess patient's and family's coping with the rigors of treatment: "What is the most challenging part of this for you?" and "What is helping you day by day?" Consider referrals as needed.

Table 4–7. Assessment of Anxiety and Depression

Signs and Symptoms of Anxiety	Signs and Symptoms of Depression
Excessive worry	Depressed mood
Trouble falling or staying asleep	Insomnia or hypersomnia
Irritability, muscle tension	Anhedonia (absence of pleasure)
Restlessness, agitation	Psychomotor retardation
Unrealistic fears (phobias)	Feelings of worthlessness or inappropriate guilt
Obsessions (persistent painful ideas)	Diminished ability to concentrate, make decisions or remember
Compulsions (repetitive ritualistic acts)	Recurrent thoughts of death, suicidal ideation (lethality assessed by expressed intent, presence of a plan and the means to carry it out, previous attempts, and provision for rescue)
Frequent crying spells, headaches, gastrointestinal upsets, palpitations, shortness of breath	
Self-medication	
Anorexia or overeating	Marked weight loss or weight gain
Interference with normal activities of daily living	Fatigue

- Inquire about the patient's and family's definitions of quality of life and the impact of treatment on these aspects of their lives: "What is most important to you in life?"
- Determine their use of spiritual practices and offer assistance in developing these, for example, meditation, relaxation, prayer.
- Ask how the patient or family members feel about their current practices: "Are these helpful, inadequate?"

The health care team's goals are to reinforce positive coping, mobilize existing spiritual resources, invite the patient and family to develop new skills for self-care, and continue disclosures in an atmosphere of trust.

Case Study: Maria During Treatments for Breast Cancer

The oncology surgeon recommends that Maria have a biopsy. Knowing that some women in Maria's culture sometimes defer decision-making to their husbands, the surgeon asks Maria how he should disclose information about the results of the biopsy. Maria says that she wants to know about her illness in general, but she does not wish to learn the details. She wants her husband, David, to be present during any information-giving discussions. Maria is more comfortable relating to the nurse. If David wants more information, Maria tells the nurse to tell David but not her. Based on Maria's wishes, the nurse schedules Maria for a return visit with her husband 3 days after the biopsy is done.

Maria's biopsy is positive. After the surgeon explains the options, Maria and David decide on a lumpectomy with a sentinel node dissection, followed by radiation and chemotherapy.

Listening to her favorite orchestral recordings on audiotape seems to comfort and relax Maria during her 3-hour chemotherapy infusions. Maria is stoic regarding side effects from the chemotherapy. The clinic nurse soon learns that she has to actively inquire about each possible side effect because Maria is uncomfortable volunteering this information.

Maria completes chemotherapy 9 months after her diagnosis. The small scars from her surgery and the mild skin changes from the radiation leave Maria's breast looking much better than she had imagined. She experiences severe fatigue, which leads to moderate depression from not being able to participate in family activities. Maria's libido is also diminished. David is patient and understanding, but Maria struggles with guilt feelings. Dr. Smith offers her an antidepressant, but Maria politely refuses. She decides to intensify her prayers, instead, and to counsel with her priest.

GOALS

- Respect individual communication styles.
- Assist Maria and her family in identifying and using any coping mechanisms that help her deal with her illness and its treatment.
- Continue to assess Maria to determine interventions that may improve symptom management and quality of life.

ASSESSMENT AFTER TREATMENTS

Long-term Survival or Terminal Phase

The goals of a palliative care assessment after treatments are as follows:

1. Examine the benefits and burdens of all interventions to manage the residual symptoms remaining from the treatments and/or disease process.
2. Determine the current physical problems that are most distressing to the patient and family and plan rehabilitative interventions.
3. Assess learning needs to provide teaching to aggressively manage problems with the goal of maximizing quality of life.
4. Continue to reinforce patient and family strengths, healthy habits, and behaviors to enhance well-being and to prevent problems.

Survivors are defined as those patients whose diseases are cured or go into long remissions. These individuals may require some degree of palliative care for the rest of their lives. Examples of survivors likely to require palliative care include those with graft-versus-host disease (GVHD), irreversible peripheral neuropathies, or structural alterations of the integumentary, gastrointestinal, and genitourinary systems.

Psychosocial issues for survivors include fear of recurrence as well as practical considerations, such as insurance and job discrimination. Many patients make major life changes regarding work and relationships as a result of their illness experiences. These patients, though cured, live with the ramifications of the disease and its treatment for the rest of their lives.

Some patients begin to explore, in new ways, the spiritual foundations and assumptions of their lives. Often, patients relate that in spite of the crisis of an illness and its treatment, the experience resulted in a deepened sense of meaning and gratitude for life. Examples of such growth experiences as a result of surviving cancer can be found in *Cancer as a Turning Point: A Handbook for People with Cancer, Their Families and Health Professionals*[20] and *Silver Linings: The Other Side of Cancer.*[21]

PHYSICAL ASSESSMENT AFTER TREATMENTS

Reassessments after treatments are finished determine changes from previous assessments, focusing on the systems that have been affected and altered by the treatments. Thorough assessment of these residual problems and changes in the patient's body are critical to successful symptom management. Effective management of symptoms with rehabilitative interventions achieve the goal of maximizing the patient's and family's quality of life, whether in long-term survival or during the terminal phase. Two examples of functional assessment tools used in physical rehabilitation are the Functional Assessment of Cancer Therapy (FACT) Scale[22] and the Rotterdam Symptom Checklist.[23]

In addition to the patient's physical assessment, the nurse should continue to make periodic observations and inquiries about the health of other family members. Noting changes in family members' health problems, physical limitations, and physical strengths is important to ascertain impact on the patient's care and the family's life-style.

An emerging issue that relates to family members' health is genetic testing for familial diseases. The health care team needs to ask patients who have diseases that could have a genetic origin if they would be interested in receiving more information. Patients or family members desiring more facts will benefit from written materials and referral to an experienced genetic counselor. Table 4–8 provides resource information on genetic counseling.

Table 4–8. Genetic Counseling Information

To locate a genetic counselor in a particular region of the United States, contact
National Society of Genetic Counselors
610-872-7608
www.nsgc.org

Table 4–9. Assessment of Family Members' Risk Factors for Complicated Bereavement

Concurrent life crises
History of other recent or difficult past losses
Unresolved grief from prior losses
History of mental illness or substance abuse
Extreme anger or anxiety
Marked dependence on the patient
Age of the patient and the surviving loved ones, developmental phases of the patient and the family members
Limited support within the family's circle or community
Anticipated situational stressors, e.g., loss of income, financial strain, lack of confidence in assuming some of the patient's usual responsibilities
Illnesses among other family members
Special bereavement needs of children in the family
The patient's dying process is difficult, e.g., poorly controlled symptoms such as pain, shortness of breath, agitation, delirium, anxiety, etc.
Absence of helpful cultural and/or religious beliefs

PSYCHOSOCIAL ASSESSMENT AFTER TREATMENTS

Recurrence is most often signaled by the appearance of advancing physical symptoms. When this happens, the patient's worst nightmare has been realized. A recurrence is experienced differently from an initial diagnosis as the patient is now a veteran of the patient role and understands all too well what the recurrence means. Attention to concerns at this phase of illness include the following:

- Revisiting the quality versus quantity of life preferences as the patient and family weigh the benefits and burdens of treatment.
- Being sensitive to the patient's readiness to discuss a transition from curative to palliative care. The patient often signals his or her readiness by statements like "I'm getting tired of spending so much time at the hospital" or "I've had it with all of this" Ask: "What has your physician told you that you can expect now?" or "How do you see your future?"
- Exploring the setting of new goals of treatment.
- Considering a referral to hospice when the patient begins to question the efficacy of treatments.
- Discussing the completion of advance directives: "Have you thought about what you would like us to do if your heart stops beating or if you stop breathing?"
- Determining the patient's and family's interest or need for education about death and dying.
- Discerning risk factors for complicated bereavement in family members as described in Table 4–9.

SPIRITUAL ASSESSMENT AFTER TREATMENTS

Following treatment, the patient will embark on a journey leading to long-term survival or recurrence and the terminal phases of the illness. The nurse and other caregivers can provide valuable spiritual support at these junctures when they do the following:

- Determine the quality and focus of the patient's and family's hopes for the future. Listen for a transition of hoping for a cure to another hope, for example, of a remission or to live until a special family event occurs. For an in-depth, practical, and inspiring discourse on hope, refer to *Finding HOPE: Ways to See Life in a Brighter Light.*[24]
- Listen for comments suggesting a crisis of belief and meaning; for example, at recurrence, a patient may feel abandoned or experience an assault on his or her faith. Questions such as "Why?" and "Where is God?" and "Why are my prayers not being answered?" are very common. The nurse can best respond to these questions by normalizing them and emphasizing that to question God or one's faith can indicate a vitality of faith, not an absence.
- Assess the patient's and family's use of spiritual practices: "What are you doing to feel calmer and more peaceful?" Consider a chaplain referral if the patient or family are interested and open to such an intervention.

- Inquire regarding the desire for meaningful rituals like communion or anointing. Consult with local clergy or a hospital chaplain to meet these needs.
- Assess the level and quality of community supports: "Who is involved in supporting you and your family at this time?"
- Encourage referral to hospice for end-of-life care.
- Listen for indicators of spiritual suffering, for example, unfinished business, regrets, relationship discord, diminished faith, or fears of abandonment: "What do you find yourself thinking about at this time?" and "What are your chief concerns or worries?"
- Assess the need and desire of the patient and family to talk about the meaning of the illness, the patient's declining physical condition, and possible death. Ask questions to foster a review of critical life incidents, to allow grieving and explore beliefs regarding the afterlife.
- Determine the need and desire for reconciliation: "Are there people with whom you want or need to speak?" and "Do you find yourself having any regrets?"
- Invite a discussion of the most meaningful, celebratory occurrences in life to foster integrity, life review, and a sense of meaning
- Assess the patient's and/or family's readiness to discuss funeral preferences and plans and desired disposition of the body, as noted in Table 4–10.

The main spiritual goal of this phase of illness is to provide the patient and family a "place to stand" in order to review the past and look toward the future. This encourages grieving past losses, creating a sense of meaning, and consolidating strengths for the days ahead.

Table 4–10. Assessment of Funeral Plans and Preferences

Has the patient and/or family selected a funeral home?
Has the patient and/or family decided about the disposition of the body, for example, organ, eye, and/or tissue donation; autopsy; earth burial (above ground or below ground); cremation; simple disposition?
Has the decision been made regarding a final resting place?
Does the patient want to make his or her wishes known regarding the type of service, or will the family decide this?

Case Study: Maria after Completion of Treatments for Breast Cancer

Within a year after the cancer treatments are complete, Maria feels fully recovered. However, to please her mother, she continues to take several herbs. Her hair grows back, her energy returns, and she and David enjoy a renewed sensuality in their married life.

Five years after her diagnosis, Maria starts to experience low back pain while gardening. She delays going to the doctor until she develops shortness of breath and her children insist that she go see her doctor.

Dr. Smith suspects recurrent breast cancer and schedules Maria for a computerized axial tomography (CAT) scan of her chest and spine to rule out metastatic disease. When the results of the scan are available, Maria asks Dr. Smith to talk with her and her family and allow them to help her decide about further treatment if it is needed. The scans confirm metastatic breast cancer to the lungs and spine. Maria's family urges her to return to the hospital for more chemotherapy. Maria is not convinced that aggressive treatments will help. To keep peace, Maria agrees to take tamoxifen pills at home. However, she is far more interested in the services of *yerbalistas* (herbalists) and *sobadoras* (masseuses). The *curandero* visits her often. Because of her respiratory distress, Maria has to stop playing the flute, a major coping loss for her, because she relied on music for self-expression.

As Maria becomes weaker from the progression of the disease; she needs assistance with her activities of daily living. She does not want to disturb the family life of her children, so she asks her sister to move in to help provide care for her in her home. Dr. Smith's nurse recommends hospice services, and Maria agrees. Her children continue to urge more aggressive treatments but finally defer to Maria and their grandmother.

Maria likes the focus on the family provided by the hospice team. Hospice home care is also compatible with Maria's traditional belief that if a person dies at home, his or her soul will not get lost.

Maria's older belief systems emerge as the dominant coping mechanism in the final stages of her life. The social worker observes that there are rosary beads as well as a statue of the Virgin of Guadelupe on Maria's nightstand. The priest has recently administered the Sacrament of the Anointing of the Sick. Maria is sipping teas made by the *curandero*. Maria's mother continues to pray that "the Virgin will intercede for my baby." Extended family members are intensely involved in Maria's care at home.

GOALS

- Assist the family to resolve conflicts about choosing treatment options so that Maria will feel supported.
- Support the patient's chosen methods of coping.
- Attentively listen and affirm all family members as they are coming to terms with Maria's impending death in their different ways, reflecting relationship, generational and cultural dynamics.
- Validate the reliance on all therapies that lend support to the patient and family.

ASSESSMENT DURING ACTIVE DYING

The goals of a palliative care assessment when the patient is actively dying are as follows:

1. Observe for signs and symptoms of impending death, aggressively managing symptoms and promoting comfort.
2. Determine the primary source of the patient's and family's suffering and plan interventions to provide relief.
3. Identify the primary sources of strength for the patient and family members so that these can be used to provide support.
4. Ascertain the patient's and family's readiness and need for teaching about the dying process.
5. Look for ways to support the patient and family to enhance meaning during this intense experience.
6. Determine if the family members and friends who are important to the patient have had the opportunity to visit in person or on the phone, as desired by the patient and family.

PHYSICAL ASSESSMENT DURING ACTIVE DYING

Physical assessment during the active dying process is very focused and limited to determining the cause of suffering and identifying sources of comfort. Figure 4–2 shows common areas to assess in the last few days of a person's life.

In addition to the patient's physical assessment, the nurse should monitor the health of other family members to prevent and minimize problems that could compromise their health during this very stressful time.

Head & Neck:
Mind- How important is level of alertness versus control of pain and anxiety which may cause sedation?
Senses-Sight - What objects at the bedside provide comfort when seen by the patient? Family photos? Children's drawings? Special objects? Pets? Loved ones sitting nearby? What degree of lighting does the patient prefer? Does darkness increase anxiety? Would scented candles provide solace?
Hearing - What sounds most comfort the patient? Music? Family chatting nearby? The TV or radio on in the background? Someone reading to him or her? Silence?
Smell - What scents does the patient enjoy? Would aromatic lotions be soothing?
Taste - What are the patient's favorite flavors? Would mouth care to relieve dryness be more acceptable with fruit punch or apple juice?
Mouth /Lips - Does the family/caregiver understand how to provide good, frequent mouth and lip care, especially if the patient is a mouth -breather?

Shoulders & Arms:
Does the family/caregiver understand good body alignment and several ways to position the patient comfortably? Are they following good body mechanics when repositioning the patient?
Would applying aromatic lotion to hands and arms comfort the patient and give family members something meaningful to do?

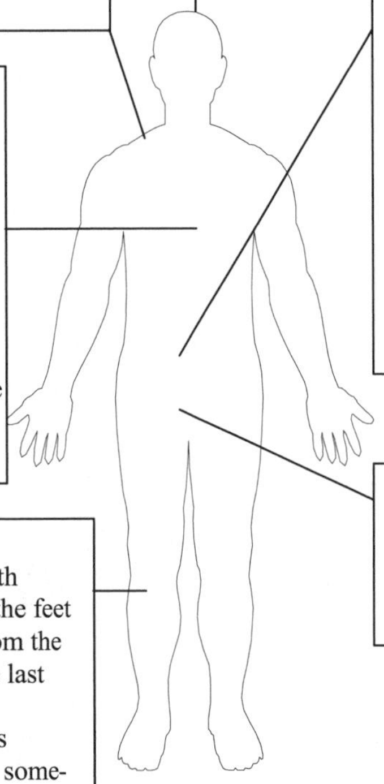

Chest & Spine:
Lungs-Is the patient at high risk for death rales? Is there a scopolamine patch in the home for immediate use if noisy respirations begin?
Would oxygen help the patient breathe easier?
Heart-If pt at home,is the family prepared for the moment of death? E.g., do they know NOT to call 911? Do they have a neighbor close by to come and be with them until a HCP arrives?

Abdomen:
Bowels- If the patient is incontinent of stool, do family members know how to provide personal hygiene?
Do family members know how to use protective pads, adult diapers, pull sheets to keep the patient clean?
Does the family know how to make an occupied bed, using good body mechanics?
Are protective ointments needed to decrease skin breakdown if the incontinence is frequent?
If stools are frequent, can anti-diarrheals be given?

Pelvis:
Kidneys-If incontinence is present, would /Urine inserting a Foley catheter prevent skin irritation & conserve the patient's & family's energies?

Legs & Feet:
Are family members interested/concerned with learning the assessment technique of feeling the feet and limbs for coolness slowly progressing from the periphery to the center of the body during the last few hours of life?
Would applying aromatic lotion to feet & legs comfort the patient and give family members something meaningful to do?

General:
- Are the patient's pain & other symptoms well controlled?
- Are family members capable & comfortable with continuing to provide physical care for the patient? Are family members getting enough sleep and rest to maintain their own health? Are additional resources needed to support the family?
- Is the home the best place for the patient to die? Has the family thought about their comfort in living in the house if their loved one dies there?
- Does the family know whom to call on a 24-hour basis for advice and support?

Fig. 4–2. Assessment when the patient is actively dying: Determining causes of pain and discomfort and identifying sources of comfort. See Figure 4–1 for key to abbreviations.

Hospice team members have excellent skills in making palliative care assessments at the end of life. The goal of hospice is to support the terminally ill patient and family at home, if that is their wish. Many hospice teams also provide palliative care in acute care settings and nursing homes. Unfortunately, many patients die without the support of hospice services in any of these settings.

PSYCHOSOCIAL ASSESSMENT DURING ACTIVE DYING

The transition from life to death is as sacred as the transition experienced at birth. Keeping this in mind, the nurse can help to create a safe environment in which patients and families are supported in their relationships and the creation of meaningful moments together. The patient may also still be reviewing his or her life. Common psychosocial characteristics of the person who is actively dying include social withdrawal, decreased attention span and decreasing ability to concentrate, resulting in gradual loss of consciousness. Behaviors normally considered to be psychotic in Western culture, such as visions and visitations, are often experienced as transcendent—and normal—at this stage of life by those with strong spiritual beliefs.

Members of the health care team can assist the patient and family in the following vital ways:

- Normalize the patient's report of seeing deceased loved ones or visions of another world.
- Encourage continued touching and talking to the patient, even when he or she is unconscious.
- Assist communication among the patient, family members, and close friends.
- Invite family members to "give permission" to the patient "to let go," providing reassurance that the family will be all right and remain intact.
- Assess the patient's and family's need for continued education about death and dying.
- Observe family members for evidence of poor coping and consider making referrals for additional support.
- Encourage family members to consider "shift rotation" in the face of lengthy, exhausting vigils at the bedside.

SPIRITUAL ASSESSMENT DURING ACTIVE DYING

When the patient enters the phase of active dying, spiritual realities often increase in significance. The nurse and other members of the care team can facilitate adaptation during the process of dying and provide much valuable support when they do the following:

- Determine the need for different or more frequent visits by their spiritual support person: "Is there anyone I can call to be with you at this time?" and "Are there any meaningful activities or rituals you want to do?"
- Inquire about dreams, visions, or unusual experiences, for example, seeing persons who have died. Normalize these if they are disclosed. Ask if these experiences are sources of comfort or fear. Encourage further discussion if the patient is interested.
- Foster maintenance of hope by asking "What are you hoping for at this time?" Reassure the patient and family that they can be hopeful and still acknowledge that death is imminent. Moving toward a transcendent hope is vital. Observe that earlier the focus of hope may have been on cure, remission, or an extension of time. Now, hope may be focused on an afterlife, the relief of suffering, or the idea of living on in loved ones' memories.
- Listen for and solicit comments regarding the efficacy of spiritual practices; for instance, if the patient is a person who prays, ask "Are your prayers bringing you comfort and peace?"
- Realize that expressions of fear, panic attacks, or an increase in physical symptoms like restlessness, agitation, pain, or shortness of breath may indicate intense spiritual distress. A chaplain's intervention may provide spiritual comfort and assist the patient in reaching peace. This may reduce the need for medications.
- Determine the need and desire of the patient and family to engage in forgiveness, to express feelings to one another, and to say their good-byes.
- Recognize that a prolonged dying process may indicate that the patient is having difficulty "letting go," perhaps due to some unfinished business or fears related to dying. Assist the patient and family in exploring what these issues might be. A referral to a chaplain may be very helpful.
- Encourage the celebration of the life of the loved one by acknowledging his or her contributions to family members, close friends, and the community.
- Explore the need and desire for additional comfort measures in the environment, for example, soothing music, devotional readings, gazing out a window at nature, or increased quiet.
- Ask the family about their anticipated needs and preferences at the time of death: "Is there anyone you will want us to call for you?" "What can the health care team do to be most supportive?" "Are there specific practices regarding the care of the body that you want the team to respect?"

The goals of spiritual care at this phase of illness are as follows:

- Facilitate any unfinished business among the patient and significant others, for example, expressions of love, regret, forgiveness, and gratitude.
- Promote integrity of the dying person by honoring his or her life. One way to do this is by encouraging reminiscence at the bedside of the patient, recalling the "gifts" the patient bestowed on the family, that is, his or her legacy of values and qualities passed on to survivors.
- Assist the patient and family in extracting meaning from the dying experience.
- Provide sensitive comfort by being present and listening.
- Provide information regarding bereavement support groups and/or counseling if indicated.

Case Study: Maria's Death

Maria remains at home for 4 months with hospice care. Fentanyl patches keep her comfortable. Her family members rub Maria's hands, legs, and feet with her favorite lilac-scented lotion and play her favorite music.

As Maria's death approaches, both the priest and the *curandero* are in attendance for various family members. As Maria dies, family and friends wail in mourning. After a period of time, members of her family care for the body. Maria's mother teaches her granddaughters these traditions. Maria's body remains in the house until hours later when family members can properly take leave of it.

GOALS

- Affirm the sensitive and holistic care provided by the family.
- Respect and support the family's right to grieve in whatever ways they wish.
- Allow the family to give post-mortem care to the body. It is a valued practice of many Latinos to show respect and honor for the deceased by washing and

preparing the body. Due to the great deference and respect demonstrated for the dead person, the hospice nurse chooses not to discuss organ donation and autopsy with this family.

(In death, the body is sacred for many older, more traditional Latinos. In the United States, however, younger, more acculturated Latino patients and families may or may not object to organ donation.)

SUMMARY OF A COMPREHENSIVE PALLIATIVE CARE ASSESSMENT

A comprehensive assessment of the patient and family provides the foundation for mutually setting goals, devising a plan of care, implementing interventions, and evaluating the effectiveness of care. Reassessments are done throughout the patient's illness, to ensure that quality of life is maximized. Colleen Scanlon[25] reminds the nurse and other health care team members that two of the most important assessment questions to ask the patient and family members, regardless of the phase or focus of the assessment, are "What is your greatest concern?" and "How can I help?"

REFERENCES

1. Bates B. A Guide to Physical Examination and History Taking, 5th Ed. Philadelphia: J.B. Lippincott, 1991.

2. Cassell EJ, Coulehan JL, Putnam SM. Making good interview skills better. Patient Care 1989;3:145–166.

3. Ferrell BR. The impact of pain on quality of life; a decade of research. Nurs Clin North Am 1995;30:609–624.

4. Siegel BS. Love, Medicine and Miracles. New York: Harper and Row, 1986.

5. Holland J, Ed. Psycho-oncology. New York: Oxford University Press, 1998.

6. Schwartz M. Letting Go: Morrie's Reflections on Living while Dying. New York: Delta, 1997.

7. Schneider JM. Clinically significant differences between grief, pathological grief and depression. Patient Counsel Health Educ 1980;4: 267–275.

8. Haase J, Britt T, Coward D, Leidy N, Penn P. Simultaneous concept analysis of spiritual perspective, hope, acceptance, and self-transcendence. Image J Nurs Sch 1992;24:143.

9. Amenta M. Nurses as primary spiritual care workers. Hospice J 1988;4:47–55.

10. Hay MW. Principles in building spiritual assessment tools. Am J Hospice Care 1989;6: 25–31.

11. Doyle D. Have you looked beyond the physical and psychosocial? J Pain Symptom Manage 1992;7:303.

12. Frankl V. Man's Search for Meaning. Boston: Beacon Press, 1959.

13. Maslow, AH. Motivation and Personality, 3rd Ed. Hummelstown, PA: Scott Foresman-Addison Wesley, 1987.

14. Fitchett, G. Assessing Spiritual Needs. Minneapolis: Augsburg, 1993.

15. Thompson S, Janigan A. Lifeschemes: a framework for understanding the search for meaning. J Soc Clin Psychol 1988;7:260–280.

16. Lipson J, Dibble SL, Minarik PA, eds. Culture and Nursing Care: A Pocket Guide, San Francisco: University of California Nursing Press, 1996.

17. Andrews M, Boyle J. Competence in transcultural nursing care. Am J Nurs 1997;8:16AAA–16DDD.

18. Noyes, R, Holt, CS, Massie, MJ. Anxiety disorders. In: Holland J, ed. Psycho-oncology. New York: Oxford University Press, 1998: 548–563.

19. Massie MJ. Depressive disorders. In: Holland J, ed. Psycho-oncology. New York: Oxford University Press, 1998:518–540.

20. Shehan, L. Cancer as a Turning Point: A Handbook for People with Cancer, Their Families and Health Professionals. Long Beach, CA: Plume, 1994.

21. Gullo S, Glass E, Gamiere M. Silver Linings: The Other Side of Cancer. Pittsburgh: Oncology Nursing Press, 1997.

22. Cella DF, Tulsky DS, Gray G, et al. The Functional Assessment of Cancer Therapy Scale: development and validation of the general measure. J Clin Oncol 1984;11:570–579.

23. de Haes JCJM, van Knippenberg FCE, Neijt JP. Measuring psychological and physical distress in cancer patients: structure and application of the Rotterdam Symptom Checklist. Br J Cancer 1990;62:1034–1038.

24. Jevene RF, Miller JE. Finding Hope: Ways to See Life in a Brighter Light. Fort Wayne, IN: Willowgreen, 1999.

25. Scanlon C. Creating a vision of hope: the challenge of palliative care. Oncol Nurs Forum 1989;16:491–496.

APPENDIX A: PALLIATIVE CARE BIBLIOGRAPHY

Carroll-Johnson, Rosemary. *Psychosocial Nursing Care Along the Cancer Continuum,* Pittsburgh: Oncology Nursing Press, Inc., 1998.

Baird, Susan, Editor. *A Cancer Source Book for Nurses.* Atlanta: American Cancer Society, 1991.

Bolen, Jean Shinoda, *Close to the Bone, Life Threatening Illness and the Search for Meaning,* New York: Scribner, 1996.

Byock, Ira. *Dying Well: Peace and Possibilities at the End of Life.* New York: Riverhead Books, 1998.

Hutchinson, J. and Rupp, J. *May I Walk You Home? Courage and Comfort for Cargivers of the Very Ill.* Notre Dame, Indiana: Ave Maria Press, 1999.

Kramp, E. and Kramp, D. *Living with the End in Mind, a Practical Checklist for Living Life to the Fullest by Embracing Your Mortality,* New York: Three Rivers Press, 1998.

Lynn, J. and Harrold, J. *Handbook for Mortals: Guidance for People Facing Serious Illness,* New York: Oxford University Press, 1999.

MCR. *Let the Choice Be Mine: A Personal Guide to Planning Your Own Funeral.* Standpoint, Indiana: MCR, 1995.

Miller, James E. *One You Love Is Dying: 12 Thoughts to Guide You On the Journey.* Fort Wayne, Indiana: Willowgreen Publishing, 1997.

Miller, James E. *When You Know You're Dying: 12 Thoughts to Guide You Through the Days Ahead.* Fort Wayne, Indiana: Willowgreen Publishing, 1997.

National Selected Morticians Resources, Inc. *A Helpful Guide to Funeral Planning.* Evanston, Illinois: NSMR, Revised, 1985.

Ohio State University Medical Center. *Consumer Health Education Materials.** Columbus, Ohio. The following materials are available on the OSU Web site: www.osumedcenter.edu → Health and Wellness → Health Information → Patient Education Materials from OSU Experts → Click on bottom of page where there is an agreement to a disclaimer—Choose among the options below.

→ General Information → End of Life
Autonomic Hyperreflexia
Choices for the Critically Ill: Focusing on the Goal of Treatment
Coma
Coping When a Loved One Has a Serious Illness
Coping When a Loved One in the ICU
Coping with Kidney Failure
Depression
Grief
Helping Children Understand Death
Making Decisions About Life Support
Should I Have a DNR Order?
Suggestions For Making Each Day Count
Understanding Pain Control and Pain Medicine
Using a Resuscitation Bag
Ventilators
Where To Begin After A Death

Rancour, P. Those Tough Conversations. *American Journal of Nursing: Critical Care Supplement,* 2000; 100:24HH—24LL.

Stoll, R. Guidelines for Spiritual Assessment. *American Journal of Nursing,* 1979;79:1574–1577.

Taylor, Rosemarie. Check Your Cultural Competence, *Nursing Management,* 1998;3:30–32.

*For information on purchasing the rights to use and/or adopt these materials for your organization, contact Dr. Sandy Cornett/Consumer Health Education/13-5-522 BTL/1375 Perry Street/ Columbus OH 43201/614-293-3191.

Part II

Symptom Assessment and Management

5 Pain Assessment

REGINA FINK and ROSE GATES

If we cannot assess pain, we will never be able to relieve pain.
—Betty Ferrell, City of Hope Duarte, California

Pain is a common companion of birth, growth, death, and illness; it is intertwined intimately with the very nature of human existence. Most pain can be palliated, and patients can be relatively pain-free. To successfully relieve pain and suffering, accurate and continuous pain assessment is mandatory. However, evidence demonstrates that pain is undertreated in the palliative care setting, contributing significantly to patient discomfort and suffering at the end of life. Recent studies suggest that as many as 30% to 40% of cancer patients at the time of diagnosis and 65% to 80% undergoing treatment or in the terminal phase of disease have unrelieved pain.[2–9] One study reported that more than 50% of cancer patients have increased suffering requiring sedation in the last days of life.[10] Coyle and colleagues[11] reported that 100% of their patients had pain and 37% had increased opioid requirements of 25% or more during the last month of life. In the Palliative Care Consultation Service at the Medical College of Wisconsin, pain and end-of-life decisions were the most frequent reasons for consultation.[12] Additionally, many persons with chronic, life-threatening illness experience moderate to severe pain. It is also estimated that 9% of the U.S. adult population suffers from moderate to severe noncancer-related chronic pain.[13]

This chapter considers various types of pain, describes barriers to optimal pain assessment, and reviews current clinical practice guidelines for the assessment of pain in the palliative care setting. A multifactorial model for pain assessment is proposed, and a variety of instruments and methods that can be used to assess pain in patients at the end of life are discussed.

TYPES OF PAIN

According to the International Association for the Study of Pain, *pain* is defined as "a sensory or emotional experience associated with tissue damage."[14] *Pain* has also been clinically defined as "whatever the experiencing person says it is, existing whenever the experiencing person says it does."[15] The categorization of pain along a continuum of duration is commonly how pain is described. Acute pain is usually associated with tissue damage, inflammation, a disease process that is relatively brief, or a surgical procedure. Regardless of intensity, acute pain is of relatively brief duration: hours, days, weeks, or a few months.[16] Acute pain serves as a warning that something is wrong and is generally viewed as a time-limited experience.[17] In contrast, chronic pain worsens and intensifies with the passage of time and persists for extended periods: months, years, or a lifetime. Chronic pain has been further subclassified into chronic malignant and chronic nonmalignant pain and can accompany a disease process including cancer, human immunodeficiency virus (HIV) and acquired immune deficiency syndrome (AIDS), arthritis, chronic obstructive pulmonary disease, neurological disorders (e.g., multiple sclerosis and cerebrovascular disease), fibromyalgia, sickle cell disease, cystic fibrosis, and diabetes. It can also be associated with an injury that has not resolved within an expected period of time: low back pain, trauma, spinal cord injury, reflex sympathetic dystrophy, and phantom limb pain.

BARRIERS TO OPTIMAL PAIN ASSESSMENT

Inadequate pain control is not the result of a lack of scientific information. Over the last two decades, a plethora of research on pain management has generated knowledge about pain and its management. Reports that document the inability or unwillingness of health care professionals to use knowledge from research and advances in technology continue to appear in the nursing and medical literature. The armamentarium of knowledge is available to assist professionals in the successful assessment and management of pain; the problems lie in its misuse or lack of use. Undertreatment of pain is often due to clinicians' failure or inability to evaluate or appreciate the severity of the patient's problem. Although accurate and timely pain assessment is the cornerstone to optimal pain management, studies of nurses and other health care professionals continue to demonstrate the contribution of suboptimal assessment to the problem of inadequate pain management.[2,18–22]

Multiple barriers to the achievement of optimal pain assessment and management have been identified (Table 5–1).[8,18,23–25] The knowledge and attitudes of health care professionals toward pain assessment are extremely important because these factors influence the priority placed on pain treatment.[26]

Table 5–1. Barriers to Optimal Pain Assessment

Health care professional barriers
Lack of identification of pain assessment and relief as a priority in patient care
Inadequate knowledge about how to perform a pain assessment
Perceived lack of time to conduct a pain assessment
Inability of clinician to empathize or establish rapport with patient
Prejudice and bias in dealing with patients
Health care system barriers
A system that fails to hold health care professionals accountable for pain assessment
Lack of criteria or availability of instruments for pain assessment in health care settings
Lack of institutional policies for performance and documentation of pain assessment
Patient/family/societal barriers
The highly subjective and personal nature of the pain experience
Lack of patient and family awareness about the importance of pain assessment
Lack of patient communication with health care professionals about pain
Presence of unfounded beliefs and myths about pain and its treatment

Recognition of the widespread inadequacy of pain assessment and management has prompted corrective efforts within multiple health care disciplines, including nursing, medicine, pharmacy, and pain management organizations. Representatives from various health care professional groups have convened to develop clinical practice guidelines and quality assurance standards for the assessment and management of acute, cancer, and end-of-life pain.[5,27–31] The establishment of a formal monitoring program to evaluate the efficacy of pain assessment and interventions was encouraged. The Agency for Health Care, Policy, and Research (AHCPR) Acute and Cancer Pain Practice Guidelines, The American Pain Society (APS) Quality Assurance Standards, The Oncology Nursing Society Position Paper on Cancer Pain Management, and The APS Position Statement on Treatment of Pain at the End of Life are reflective of the national trend in health care to assess quality of care in high-incidence patients by monitoring outcomes as well as assessing and managing pain. The AHCPR recommends the following "ABCDE" mnemonic list as a summary of the clinical approach to pain assessment and management:

A. Ask about pain regularly. Assess pain systematically.
B. Believe the patient and family in their reports of pain and what relieves it.
C. Choose pain control options appropriate for the patient, family, and setting.
D. Deliver interventions in a timely, logical, and coordinated fashion.
E. Empower patients and their families. Enable them to control their course to the greatest extent possible.

Members of the Joint Commission on Accreditation of Healthcare Organizations (JCAHO) routinely inquire about pain assessment and management practices and quality assurance activities designed to monitor patient satisfaction and outcomes within institutions. Revised JCAHO standards for assessing and managing pain in hospital, ambulatory, home care, and long-term care have been recently released.[32] The JCAHO supports "institutionalizing pain management" and using an interdisciplinary approach to effect change in health care organizations. Additionally, it recommends that culturally sensitive pain rating scales appropriate to a patient's age be available and that new or existing assessment forms include pain as the "fifth vital sign." The continuous quality improvement (CQI) process is *continuous* with the achievement of low levels of reported pain severity and of pain-related behaviors as an appropriate objective.[33,34] Providing health care systems within a CQI perspective of patient-centered care requires that health care professionals seek opportunities to improve pain management by improving assessment processes to produce the desired outcome of decreased pain for patients.

Additionally, health care reform processes such as managed care require that patients be discharged sooner without adequate time to assess pain and evaluate newly prescribed pain management regimens. Thus, the prevalence of inadequate pain assessment and management may be even greater than reported, secondary to more persons suffering silently in their homes. An adequate pain assessment may not have been done or documented. Health care professionals may not believe patients' reports of pain and may not take time to communicate, care, or understand the meaning of the pain experience for the patient. With the influences and increasing demands of managed care and changes in the delivery of health care, pain assessment and management may not be a priority.

PROCESS OF PAIN ASSESSMENT

Accurate pain assessment is the basis of pain treatment and a continuous process encompassing multidimensional factors. To formulate a pain management plan of care, an assessment is crucial in identifying the pain syndrome or the cause of pain. A comprehensive assessment addresses each type of pain and includes the following: a detailed history, including an assessment of the pain intensity and its characteristics (Figure 5–1); a physical examination with pertinent neurological exam, particularly if neuropathic pain is suspected; a psychosocial and cultural assessment; and appropriate diagnostic work-up to determine the cause of pain.[5] Attention should be paid to any discrepancies between patients' verbal descriptions of pain and their behavior and appearance. The physical exam should focus on an examination of the painful areas as well as common referred pain locations. In frail or terminally ill patients, physical exam maneuvers and/or diagnostic tests should be performed only if the findings will potentially change or facilitate the treatment plan. The burden and potential discomfort of any diagnostic tests must be weighed against the potential benefit of the information.[35] Ongoing and subsequent evaluations are necessary to determine the effectiveness of

PAIN ASSESSMENT GUIDE

TELL ME ABOUT YOUR PAIN

Words to describe pain

aching	throbbing	shooting
stabbing	gnawing	sharp
tender	burning	exhausting
tiring	penetrating	nagging
numb	miserable	unbearable
dull	radiating	squeezing
crampy	deep	pressure

Pain in other languages

itami	Japanese	dolor	Spanish
tong	Chinese	douleur	French
dau	Vietnamese	bolno	Russian

Intensity (0-10)

If 0 is no pain and 10 is the worst pain imaginable, what is your pain now? ... in the last 24 hours?

Location

Where is your pain?

Duration

Is the pain always there?
Does the pain come and go? (Breakthrough Pain)
Do you have both types of pain?

Aggravating and Alleviating Factors

What makes the pain better?
What makes the pain worse?

How does pain affect

sleep	energy	relationships
appetite	activity	mood

Are you experiencing any other symptoms?

nausea/vomiting	itching	urinary retention
constipation	sleepiness/confusion	weakness

Things to check

vital signs, past medication history, knowledge of pain, and use of noninvasive techniques

REFERENCES: Jacox A, Carr DB, Payne R, et al. Management of Cancer Pain. Clinical Practice Guideline No. 9. AHCPR Publication No. 94-0592. Rockville, MD. Agency for Health Care Policy and Research, U.S. Department of Health and Human Services, Public Health Service, March 1994. — Wong, D, and Whaley, L: Clinical Handbook of Pediatric Nursing, ed. 2, The C.V. Mosby Company, St. Louis, 1986, p. 373.

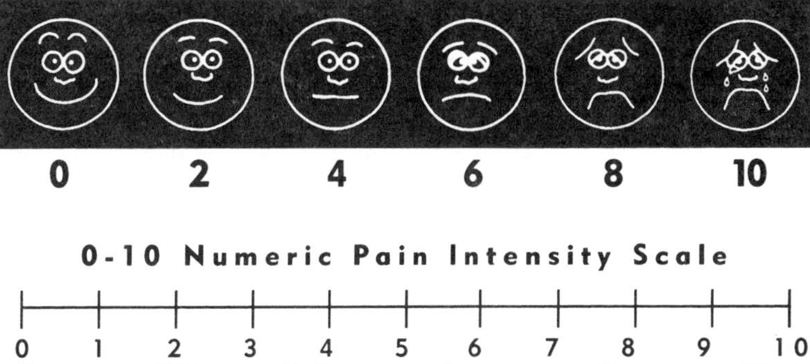

Fig. 5–1. A pocket pain assessment guide for use at the bedside. The health care professional can use this guide to help the patient identify the level and intensity of pain and to determine the best approach to pain management in the context of overall care. (©1996 Regina Fink, University of Colorado Health Science Center; used with permission.)

pain relief measures and to identify any new pains.

Pain assessment should be performed at regular intervals, if there is a change in the pain, after analgesic administration, and after any modifications in the pain management plan. Pain assessment should be individualized and documented so that all multidisciplinary team members involved will have an understanding of the pain problem. Information about the patient's pain can be obtained from multiple sources: observations, interviews with the patient and significant others, reviews of medical data, and feedback from other health care providers.

While pain is uniquely personal and subjective, its management necessitates certain objective standards of care and practice. The first opportunity to understand the subjective experience is at the perceptual level. Perception incorporates the patient's self-report and the pain assessment accomplished by the health care provider. *Perception* is "the act of perceiving, to become aware directly in one's mind, through any of the senses; especially to see or hear, involving the process of achieving understanding or seeing all the way through," and *assessment* is defined as "the act of assessing, evaluating, appraising, or estimating by sitting beside another."[36] Perception is an abstract process where the person doing the perceiving is not just a bystander but is immersed in the understanding of the other's situation. Perception is influenced by "higher-order" processes that characterize the cognitive and emotional appraisal of pain, what people feel and think about their pain and their future with the pain. Perception also includes the interpersonal framework in which the pain is experienced (with family, friends, or alone), the meaning or reason for the pain, the person's coping pattern or locus of control, the presence of additional symptoms, and others' concerns (e.g., family members' depression or anxiety). Alternatively, assessment is a value judgment that occurs by observing the other's experience.

Assessment and perception of the patient's pain experience at the end of life is essential prior to planning interventions. However, the quality and usefulness of any assessment is only as good as the ability of the assessor to be thoroughly patient-focused. This means listening empathetically, maintaining open communication, and validating and legitimizing the patient's and family/significant other's concerns. A clinician's understanding of the patient's pain and accompanying symptoms confirms that there is genuine personal interest facilitating a positive pain management outcome.

Pain does not occur in isolation. Other symptoms and concerns experienced by the patient compound the suffering associated with pain. *Total pain* has been described as the sum of all of the following interactions: physical, emotional/psychological, social, spiritual, bureaucratic, financial (Fig. 5–2).[37] At times, patients describe their whole life as painful. The provision of palliative care to relieve pain and suffering is based on the conceptual model of this whole person experiencing "total pain."

It is not always necessary or relevant to assess all dimensions of pain in all patients or every setting.[38] At the very least, both the sensation of pain and the response to pain must be considered during an assessment.[39] The extent of the assessment should be dictated by its purpose, the patient's condition or stage of illness, clinical setting, feasibility, and relevance of a particular dimension to the patient or health care provider. For example, a comprehensive assessment may be appropriate for a patient in the early stage of palliative care, while only a pain intensity score is needed when evaluating a patient's response to an increased dose of analgesic. Incorporating the following multidimensional factors into the pain assessment will ensure a comprehensive approach to understanding the patient's pain experience.

Factors Influencing Perception of Pain

Other symptoms
Adverse effects of treatment
Insomnia and chronic fatigue
PHYSICAL

PSYCHOLOGICAL
Anger at delays in diagnosis
Anger at therapeutic failure
Disfigurement
Fear of pain and/or death
Feelings of helplessness

TOTAL PAIN

SOCIAL
Worry about family and finances
Loss of job prestige and income
Loss of social position
Loss of role in family
Feelings of abandonment and isolation

SPIRITUAL
Why has this happened to me?
Why does God allow me to suffer like this?
What's the point of it all?
Is there any meaning or purpose in life?
Can I be forgiven for past wrongdoing?

Fig. 5–2. Factors influencing the perception of pain. Pain intensity is modulated by psychological, social, and spiritual factors as well as by tissue damage and other physical influences. (Reproduced with permission from Twycross, reference 37.)

MULTIFACTORIAL MODEL FOR PAIN ASSESSMENT

Pain is a complex phenomenon involving many interrelated factors. The multifactorial pain assessment model is based on the work of a number of individuals over the last three decades.[38,40–44] An individual's pain is unique and actualized by the multidimensionality of the experience and the interaction among the factors within each person and in interaction with other individuals.

Melzack and Casey[40] suggested that pain was determined by the interaction of three components: the sensory/discriminative (selection and modulation of pain sensations), the motivational/affective (affective reactions to pain via the brain's reticular formation and limbic system), and the cognitive (past or present experiences of pain).[40] Evidence presented by Ahles and co-workers[41] supported the usefulness of a multidimensional model for cancer-related pain by describing the following theoretical components of the pain experience: physiologic, sensory, affective, cognitive, and behavioral. McGuire[43,45] expanded the work of Ahles and colleagues by proposing the integration of a sociocultural dimension to the pain model. This sociocultural dimension, comprised of a broad range of ethnocultural, demographic, spiritual, and social factors, influences an individual's perception of and responses to pain. Bates[42] proposed a biocultural model, combining social learning theory and the gate control theory, as a useful framework for studying and understanding cultural influences on human pain perception, assessment, and response. She believed that different social communities (ethnic groups) have different cultural experiences, attitudes, and meanings for pain that may influence pain perception, assessment, tolerance, neurophysiological, psychological, and

Table 5–2. Multifactorial Pain Assessment

Factors	Question
Physiologic/sensory	What is happening in the patient's body to cause pain? How does the patient describe his or her pain?
Affective	How does the patient's emotional state affect the patient's report of pain? How does pain influence the patient's affect or mood?
Cognitive	How does the patient's knowledge, attitudes, and beliefs about pain affect the pain experience? How does the patient's past experience with pain influence the pain?
Behavioral	How do you know the patient is in pain and what is the patient doing that tells you that pain is being experienced? What is the patient doing to decrease his or her pain?
Sociocultural	How does the patient's sociocultural background affect pain expression?
Environmental	How does the patient's environment affect pain expression?

behavioral responses to pain sensation. Hester[44] proposed an environmental component referring to the setting, environmental conditions, or stimuli that affect pain assessment and management. Excessive noise, lighting, or adverse temperatures may be sources of stress for individuals in pain and may negatively impact the pain experience.

Given the complexity of the interaction between the factors, if a positive impact on the quality of life of patients is the goal of palliative care, then the multifactorial perspective provides the foundation for assessing and ultimately managing pain. Some questions that can guide the nurses' multifactorial pain assessment are reviewed in Table 5–2.

Physiologic and Sensory Factors

The physiologic and sensory factors of the pain experience explain the etiology and characterize the person's pain. Patients should be queried about their description of pain to include its quality, intensity, location, temporal pattern, and aggravating/alleviating factors. The five key factors included in the pain assessment are outlined in Figure 5–1. In the palliative care setting, the patient's cause of pain may have already been determined. However, changes in pain location or character should not always be attributed to these preexisting causes but should instigate a reassessment. Treatable causes, such as infection or fractures, may be the cause of new or persistent pains. A comprehensive pain assessment revealed different causes of pain in 64% of oncology patients with new complaints of pain.[46]

Words. Patients are asked to describe their pain using words or qualifiers. Neuropathic or deafferentation pain can be described as burning, shooting, numb, radiating, or lancinating pain; visceral pain is poorly localized and can be described as squeezing, cramping, or pressure; somatic pain is described as achy, throbbing, and well-localized pain. Identifying the qualifiers will enhance the understanding of the pain's etiology and should optimize pain treatment. Not doing so may result in an incomplete pain profile. Table 5–3 summarizes various pain types, qualifiers, etiological factors, and choice of analgesia based on pain type.

Intensity. Although an assessment of intensity captures only one aspect of the pain experience, it is the most frequently used parameter in clinical practice. Asking for the patient's pain intensity or

Table 5–3. Pain Descriptors

Pain Type	Qualifiers	Etiological Factors	Analgesic Choice
Neuropathic or deafferentation	Burning, shooting, tingling, numbness, radiating, "fire-like" or electrical sensations	Nerve involvement by tumor (cervical, brachial, lumbosacral plexi), postherpetic neuralgia, diabetic neuropathies, poststroke pain	Antidepressants, anticonvulsants, benzodiazepines ±opioids ±steroids
Visceral (poorly localized)	Squeezing, cramping, pressure, distention, deep, stretching bloated feeling	Bowel obstruction, venous occlusion, ischemia, liver metastases, ascites, thrombosis, postabdominal or thoracic surgery, pancreatitis	Opioids (caution must be used in the administration of opioids to patients with bowel obstruction) ±nonsteroidal antiinflammatory drugs (NSAIDs)
Somatic (well localized)	Dull, achy, throbbing, sore	Bone or spine metastases, fractures, arthritis, injury to deep musculoskeletel, structures or superficial cutaneous tissues	NSAIDs, steroids, muscle relaxants, bisphosphonates ± opioids

pain score will objectively measure how much pain a person is experiencing. Pain intensity should be evaluated not only at the present level, but also at its least, worst, and with movement. A review of the amount of pain after the administration of analgesics and adjuvant drugs can also add information about the patient's level of pain. Pain intensity can be measured quantitatively using a visual analogue scale, numeric rating scale, verbal descriptor scale, or faces scale. During instrument selection, the nurse must consider the practicality, ease, and acceptability of the instrument's use by terminally ill patients (for a description of these instruments, refer to the section Quantitative Assessment of Pain, below).

Location. Greater than 75% of persons with cancer have two or more sites of pain;[47] thus, it is crucial to ask questions about the pain's location. Using an assessment sheet with a figure demonstrating anterior and posterior views or encouraging the patient to point or place a finger on the area involved will be more specific than verbal self-report. Separate pain histories should be acquired for each major pain complaint since their etiologies may differ and the treatment plan may need to be tailored to the particular pain type.

Duration. Learning if the pain is either persistent or intermittent, or both, will guide the nurse in the selection of interventions. Patients may experience "breakthrough" or an intermittent, transitory flare of pain.[48] This type of pain will require a fast-acting opioid, whereas persistent pain is usually treated with long-acting, continuous-release opioids. Patients with progressive diseases, such as cancer and AIDS, may experience chronic pain that has an ill-defined onset and unknown duration.

Aggravating/Alleviating Factors. If the patient is not receiving satisfactory pain relief, inquiring about what makes the pain better or worse, the alleviating or aggravating factors, will assist the nurse and other health care professionals in determining what diagnostic tests need to be ordered or what nonpharmacological approaches can be incorporated into the plan of care. This is also an important aspect of the initial pain assessment as it helps to determine the etiology of the pain. Total pain must be assessed by determining the pain's effects on sleep, appetite, energy, activity, relationships, sexuality, and mood.

Affective Factor

Assessing the affective factor includes the emotional responses associated with the pain experience and, possibly, such reactions as depression, anger, distress, anxiety, decreased ability to concentrate, mood disturbance, and loss of control. A person's feelings of distress, loss of control, or lack of involvement in the plan of care may impact outcomes of pain intensity and patient satisfaction with pain management.

Cognitive Factor

The cognitive factor of pain refers to the way pain influences the person's thought processes; the way the person views himself or herself in relation to the pain; the knowledge, attitudes, and beliefs the person has about the pain; and the meaning of the pain to the individual. Past experiences with pain may influence one's beliefs about pain. Whether a person feels another person believes his/her pain also contributes to the cognitive dimension.

Patients' knowledge and beliefs about pain play an obvious role in pain assessment, perception, function, and response to treatment.[49] Patients may be reluctant to tell a nurse when they have pain, may attempt to minimize its severity, may not know they can expect pain relief, and may be concerned about taking pain medications for fear of deleterious effects. A comprehensive approach to pain assessment includes evaluating the patient's knowledge and beliefs about pain and its management and common misconceptions about analgesia (Table 5–4).

Behavioral Factor

Pain behavior may be a means of expressing pain or a coping response.[52] The behavioral factor describes actions the person exhibits related to the pain, such as verbal complaints, moaning, groaning, crying, facial expressions, posturing, splinting, lying down, pacing, rocking, or suppression of the expression of pain. Other cues can include anxious behaviors, insomnia, boredom, inability to concentrate, restlessness, and fatigue.[53,54] Unfortunately, some of these behaviors, or cues, may relate to causes or symptoms other than pain. For example, insomnia may be due to depression, thus complicating the pain assessment.

Nonverbal expression of pain can

Table 5–4. Common Patient Concerns and Misconceptions About Pain and Analgesia

Pain is inevitable. I just need to bear it.
If the pain is worse, it must mean my disease (cancer) is spreading.
I had better wait to take my pain medication until I really need it or else it won't work later.
My family thinks I am getting too "spacey" on pain medication; I'd better hold back.
If it's morphine, I must be getting close to the end.
If I take pain medicine (such as opioids) regularly, I will get hooked or addicted.
If I take my pain medication before I hurt, I will end up taking too much. It's better to "hang in there and tough it out."
I'd rather have a good bowel movement than take pain medication and get constipated.
I don't want to bother the nurse or doctor; they're busy with other patients.
If I take too much pain medication, it will hasten my death.
Good patients avoid talking about pain.

Sources: Cleeland (1993), reference 23; Fink (1997), reference 50; Gordon and Ward (1995), reference 51.

complement, contradict, or replace the verbal complaint of pain.[55] (refer to Pain Assessment in Nonverbal Patients or Patients with Cognitive Failure, below, for a more complete discussion of assessment parameters). "Actions do not always speak louder than words," [39] but words do not always tell the complete story. Observing a patient's behavior or nonverbal cues, understanding the meaning of the pain experience to the patient, and collaborating with family members and other health care professionals to determine their thoughts about the patient's pain are all part of the process of pain perception.

The behavioral dimension also encompasses the unconscious or deliberate actions taken by the person to decrease the pain. Pain behaviors include, but are not limited to, analgesic use, both prescribed and over-the-counter; seeking medical assistance; use of nonpharmacological approaches; and other coping strategies such as removal of aggravating factors (e.g., noise and light). Behaviors used to control pain in patients with advanced-stage disease include special positions, immobilizing or guarding a body part, rubbing, and adjusting pressure to a body part.[56]

Sociocultural Factor

The sociocultural factor encompasses all of the demographic variables of the patient experiencing pain. The impact of these factors (e.g., age, gender, ethnicity, spirituality, marital status/social support) on pain assessment, treatment, and outcomes has been examined in the literature. While many of the studies promote each individual dimension, few have concentrated on the highly interactive nature of these components with the other dimensions. Ultimately, all of these factors can influence pain assessment.

Age. Much of the pain literature has called attention to the problem of inadequate pain assessment and management in the elderly in a palliative care setting. Elderly patients suffer disproportionately from chronic painful conditions and have multiple diagnoses with complex problems and accompanying pain. Elders have physical, social, and psychological needs distinct from younger and middle-aged adults and present particular challenges for pain assessment and management. Pain assessment may be more problematic in elderly patients because their reporting of pain may differ from that of younger patients due to their increased stoicism.[24] Elderly people often present with failures in memory, depression, and sensory impairments that may hinder history taking; they may also underreport pain because they expect pain to occur as a part of the aging process.[57] Moreover, dependent elderly people may not report pain because they are concerned that they will cause more distress in their family caregivers.[58]

Studies have documented the problem of inadequate pain assessment in the elderly.[59] Cleeland and colleagues[2] studied 1308 metastatic cancer outpatients and found that those 70 years or older were more likely to have inadequate assessment and analgesia. Approximately, 40% of elderly nursing home patients with cancer experience pain every day, according to Bernabei and colleagues,[60] who reviewed Medicare records of more than 13,625 cancer patients aged 65 or older discharged from hospitals to nearly 1500 nursing homes in five states. Pain assessment was based on patient self-report and determined by a multidisciplinary team of nursing home personnel involved with the patients. Of the over 4000 patients who complained of daily pain, 16% were given a non-opioid, 32% were given codeine or other weak opioids, 26% received morphine, and 26% received no analgesic medication at all. As age increased, a greater proportion of patients in pain received no analgesic drugs (21%, 26%, and 30% of patients aged 65–74, 75–84, and 85 and older, respectively, $P < 0.001$). Thus, it is imperative to pay particular attention to assessing pain in the elderly patient so that the chance of inadequate analgesia is decreased.

Gender. Gender differences affect sensitivity to pain, pain tolerance, pain distress, willingness to report pain, exaggeration of pain, and nonverbal expression of pain.[61–65] Multiple studies demonstrate that men show more stoicism than women, women exhibit lower pain thresholds and less tolerance to noxious stimuli than men, and women respond better to kappa-opioid analgesics than do men.[63,66–68] Whether women are more willing to report pain than men or experience pain differently from men is unclear. However, beliefs about gender differences may affect nurses' interpretation and treatment of patients' pain. Nurses and other health care professionals need to be mindful of possible gender differences when assessing pain and planning individualized care for persons in pain.

Ethnicity. Ethnicity is a predictor of pain expression and response. While assessing pain, it is important to remember that certain ethnic groups and cultures have strong beliefs about expressing pain and may hesitate to complain of unrelieved pain.[69] The biocultural model of Bates and associates[70] proposed that culturally accepted patterns of ethnic meanings of pain may influence the neurophysiological processing of nociceptive information responsible for pain threshold, pain tolerance, pain behavior, and expression. Thus, the manner in which a person reacts to the pain experience is strongly related to cultural background. An individual's memories and cultural beliefs may influence whether pain impulses reach the level of awareness and impact the person's perception of pain and response to it.[39] The biocultural model hypothesizes that social learning from family and group membership can influence psychological and physiological processes, which in turn can affect the perception and modulation of pain. Bates and colleagues[70] stressed that all individuals, regardless of ethnicity, have basically similar neurophysiological systems of pain perception. Early clinical studies of pain expression and culture concluded that the preferred values and traditions of culture affected an individual's handling and communication of pain.[71–73] As stated by Fabrega,[74] "there is no culture-free way of apprehending pain in its essence."

Marital Status. The degree of family or social support in a patient's life should be assessed as these factors may influence the expression, meaning, and perception of pain and the ability to comply with therapeutic recommendations. Few studies have examined the influence of marital status on pain experience and expression. Dar, and co-workers[75] studied 40 patients (45% women, 55% men) with metastatic cancer pain and found that patients minimized their pain when their spouses were present. When asked if and how their pain changed in the presence of spouses, 40% of the patients said the pain was better and 60% reported no change; none reported that the pain was worse. The majority (64%) of patients agreed that they conceal their pain so that their spouses will not be upset, even though spouses were generally accurate in their estimates of the patients' pain levels. Almost all patients reported a very high degree of satisfaction with the way their spouses helped them cope with pain.

Spirituality. Spross and Wolff Burke[76] believe that the spiritual dimension mediates the person's holistic response to pain and pain expression and influences how the other aspects of pain are experienced. While pain refers to a physical sensation, suffering refers to the quest for meaning, purpose, and fulfillment. Although pain is often a source of suffering, suffering may occur in the absence of pain. Many patients believe that pain and suffering are meaningful signs of a higher being's presence and must be endured; others are outraged by the pain and suffering they must endure and demand alleviation. The nurse must verify the patient's beliefs and give permission to verbalize their personal points of view. Assessing the patient's existential view of pain and suffering is important as it can affect the healing and dying processes. Spiritual assessment is covered in greater detail in Chapter 29.

Environmental Factor

The environmental factor refers to the context of care, setting, or environment where the person receives pain management. Creating a peaceful environment free from bright lights, extreme noise, and excessive heat or cold may assist in alleviating the patient's pain.

Additionally, particular nurse or physician specialists may perceive an individual's pain differently. A review of the literature suggests that nurses and other health care professionals are inconsistent in their reliance on patient self-report as a major component in the assessment process. Agreement between patients' perceptions and health care professionals' perceptions were relatively low and are generally an inadequate substitute for a patient's reporting of pain.[77–79] Ferrell and colleagues[80] found that 91% of nurses surveyed reported asking patients about the intensity of their pain, yet only 45% believed that a patient's report of pain was the most important factor in determining pain intensity. It is not apparent if this was due to a deficiency of information, lack of time to perform an assessment, or interference of values or bias in the decision-making process. Health care providers' ratings corresponded more with patients' ratings when pain was severe.[78,81] Additionally, when nurses' pain assessment was documented over time, early assessments were more accurate than later ones.[82] Werner and colleagues[83] suggested that patients who are cognitively intact might have better pain assessments.

A multifactorial framework describing the influences of the above factors on the assessment of pain and the pain experience is desirable to attain positive pain outcomes. The factors comprising the framework are assumed to be interactive and interrelated. Using this framework for pain assessment has clear implications for clinical practice and research.

QUANTITATIVE ASSESSMENT OF PAIN

Although pain is a subjective, self-reported experience of the patient, the ability to quantify the intensity of pain is essential to monitoring a patient's responsiveness to analgesia.

Pain Intensity Assessment Scales

The four most commonly used scales, the visual analogue scale (VAS), the numeric rating scale (NRS), the verbal rating scale (VRS), and the faces scale, are reviewed in Table 5–5, with advantages and disadvantages delineated. These scales have proven to be a very effective, reproducible means of measuring pain and other symptoms and can be universally implemented and regularly applied in many care settings.[84] How useful these tools are in the assessment of pain in the palliative care patient is a question that needs to be answered.

Although no one scale is appropriate or suitable for all patients, Dalton and McNaull[104] recommend a universal adoption of a 0–10 scale for clinical assessment of pain intensity in adult patients. Standardization may promote collaboration and consistency in evaluation among caregivers in multiple settings: inpatient, outpatient, and home care or hospice environments. This standardization would facilitate multiple studies of pain across sites. Collection of comparative data would be enabled, allowing for simplification of the analytic process when conducting research. Detailed explanation of how to use the pain scales is necessary prior to use by patients in any clinical care area.

The VAS has been evaluated comprehensively by many researchers over the years and has usually been found to be valid and reliable.[93,94,104–109] However, some patients have found it difficult to convert a subjective sensation to a straight line.[110] Herr and Mobily[96] studied 49 senior citizens aged >65 years and reporting leg pain, to determine the relationships among various pain intensity measures, to examine the ability to use the tools correctly, and to determine elderly people's preferences. The VAS used were 10 cm horizontal and vertical lines; a Verbal Descriptor Scale (VDS) had six numerically ranked choices of word descriptors, including no pain, mild pain, discomforting, dis-

Table 5–5. Pain Intensity Assessment Scales

Scale	Graphic of Scale	Advantages	Disadvantages
Numeric Rating Scale (NRS)	The number that the patient gives represents his or her pain intensity from 0 to 5, 0 to 10, or 0 to 100 with the understanding that 0 = no pain and 5, 10, or 100 is the worst pain imaginable. Numerical Graphic Rating Scale No Pain ______________ Worst pain imaginable 0 1 2 3 4 5 6 7 8 9 10	Validity and demonstrated sensitivity to treatments which impact pain intensity.[85,86] Verbal administration to patients allows those by phone or who are physically and visually disabled to quantify pain intensity.[87] Ease in scoring, high compliance, high number of response categories.[85,87] Scores may be treated as interval data and are correlated with VAS (see below).[88]	Lack of research comparing sensitivity to VAS. Different word anchors may yield different pain reports.
Verbal Rating Scale (VRS) or Verbal Descriptor Scale (VDS)	Adjectives reflecting extremes of pain are ranked in order of severity. Each adjective is given a number which constitutes the patient's pain intensity. Verbal Graphic Rating Scale No ______________ Worst pain Pain Mild Moderate Severe imaginable	Ease of administration to patients, easily comprehended, and high compliance.[85] Validity is established.[89] Sensitivity to treatments that are known to impact pain intensity.[90]	Less reliable among illiterate patients and persons with limited English vocabulary.[91] Patients must choose one word that describes their pain even if no word accurately describes it.[85] Variability in use of verbal descriptors is associated with affective distress.[92] Scores on VRS are considered ordinal data; however, the distances between its descriptors are not equal but categorical. Thus, parametric statistical procedures may be suspect.[87] Different word anchors may yield different pain reports.
Visual Analogue Scale (VAS)	Line of 10 cm or 100 mm anchored at each end by verbal descriptors (0 = no pain and 10 or 100 = worst pain imaginable). Patients are asked to make a slash mark or X on the line at the place that represents the amount of pain experienced. Visual Analogue Scale No Pain ______________ Worst pain imaginable	Positive correlation with other self-reported measures of pain intensity and observed pain behavior.[85,90] Sensitive to treatment effects and distinct from subjective components of pain.[89,93] Qualities of ratio data with high number of response categories make it more sensitive to changes in pain intensity.[90,94]	Scoring may be more time-consuming, involve more steps, and be less reliable.[85] Patients may have difficulty understanding and using VAS measure.[92] Too abstract for many adults, and difficult to use with geriatric patients, non-English-speaking patients, and patients with physical disability, immobility, or reduced visual acuity, which may limit their ability to place a mark on the line.[92,95,96] Different word anchors may yield different pain reports.
Faces Scale	Cartoon-type faces. The "no pain" face shows a widely smiling face, and the "most pain" face shows either a face with tears[97] or a grimacing, sad face.[98] 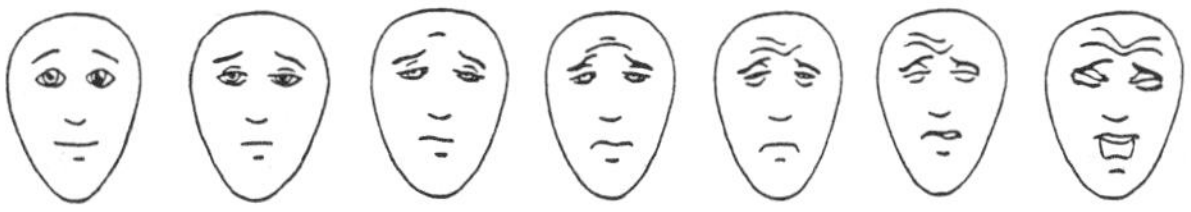 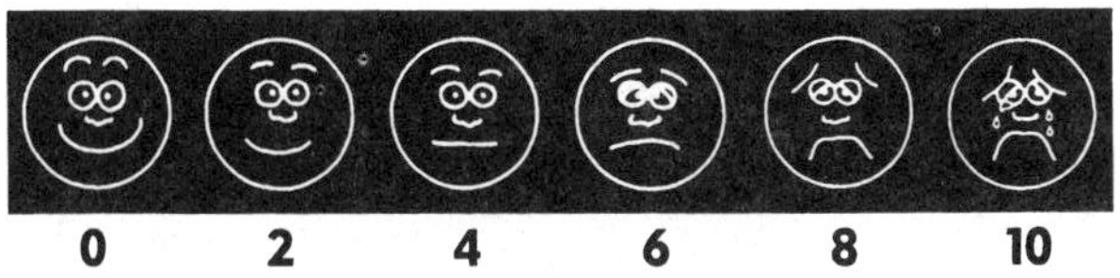 0 2 4 6 8 10	Validity is supported by research reporting that persons from many cultures recognize facial expressions and identify them in similar ways.[99] Oval-shaped faces without tears are more adult-like in appearance, possibly making the scale more acceptable to adults.[98] Simplicity, ease of use, and correlation with VAS makes it a valuable option in clinical settings.[101,102] Short, requires little mental energy and little explanation for use.[103]	Presence of tears on the "most pain" face may introduce a cultural bias when the scale is used by adults from cultures not sanctioning crying in response to pain.[100]

tressing, horrible, and excruciating; the NRS had numbers from 1 to 20; and a pain thermometer had seven choices ranging from no pain to pain as bad as it could be. The scale preferred by most respondents was the VDS. Of the two VAS scales, the vertical scale was chosen most often because the elderly had a tendency to conceptualize the vertical presentation more accurately. Elderly patients may have deficits in abstract ability that makes the VAS difficult to use.[111] Other researchers have noted that increased age is associated with an increased incidence of incorrect response to the VAS.[110]

Paice and Cohen[87] used a convenience sample of 50 hospitalized adult cancer patients with pain to study their preference in using the VAS, the VDS, and the NRS.[87] Fifty percent of the patients preferred using the NRS. Fewer patients preferred the VDS (38%), with the VAS chosen infrequently (12%). Twenty percent of the patients were unable to complete the VAS or had difficulty in doing so. Problems included needing assistance with holding a pencil, making slash marks that were too wide or not on the line, marking the wrong end of the line, and asking to have instructions read repeatedly during the survey.

Additional problems exist with use of the VAS. When using multiple horizontal scales to measure different aspects or dimensions such as pain intensity and distress or depression, subjects tend to mark all of the scales down the middle. Pain intensity has been noted to be consistently higher on each scale for depressed–anxious patients compared to nondepressed–nonanxious patients.[111,112] Photocopying VAS forms may result in distortion so that the scales may not be exactly 10 cm and the reliability of measurement may be in question. Physical disability or decreased visual acuity may limit the palliative care patient's ability to mark the appropriate spot on the line. The VAS also requires pencil and paper; the VDS requires the patient to be knowledgeable about various English pain adjectives.

The Faces Pain Scales have been used to assess pain in both pediatric and adult populations.[97,98] Findings from various studies indicate that patients used the Faces Scale to measure pain appropriately and that the scales should be considered an alternative to the NRS or VAS in various populations.[97–103] Carey and colleagues[113] asked patients which of several scales they preferred to use: modified Wong-Baker Faces Scale (tears were removed), NRS, and a vertical VAS. They found that less educated adults, both African American and Caucasian, preferred the Faces Scale. More educated patients preferred the number scale.

In summary, there are a variety of scales that have been used to assess pain in many different patient populations. Each has been widely used in clinical research and practice. Little research has been done on the appropriateness of pain scales in the palliative care setting. Intellectual understanding and language skills are prerequisites for such pain assessment scales as the VAS and VDS. These scales may prove to be too abstract or difficult for patients in the palliative care setting. Since most dying patients are elderly, simple pain scales, such as the NRS or Faces Scale, may be more advantageous for use.

Pain Instruments

There are several pain measurement instruments that can be used to standardize pain assessment, incorporating patient demographic factors, pain severity scales, pain descriptors, and other questions related to pain.[114] Four instruments have been considered short enough for routine clinical use with cancer patients. All of these instruments provide a quick way of measuring pain subjectively; however, their use in seriously ill, actively dying patients needs further study (see the AHCPR Acute and Cancer Pain Guidelines for a description of many of these instruments).

Short Form McGill Pain Questionnaire. A short form of the McGill Pain Questionnaire[115] has been developed and includes 15 words to describe pain. Each word or phrase is rated on a four-point intensity scale (0 = none and 3 = severe). Three pain scores are derived from the sum of the intensity rank values of the words chosen for sensory, affective, and total descriptors.

Brief Pain Inventory. The Brief Pain Inventory (BPI)[116,117] asks patients to rate the severity of their pain at its worst, least, and average and at present. Using an NRS (0–10), the patient is also asked for ratings of how much pain interferes with mood, physical activity, work, social activity, sleep, and relationships. The BPI also asks patients to represent the location of their pain on a drawing and asks about the cause of pain and duration of pain relief.

Memorial Pain Assessment Card. The Memorial Pain Assessment Card[118] consists of three VASs for pain intensity, pain relief, and mood and one VDS to describe the pain.

City of Hope Patient Pain Questionnaire. The City of Hope Patient Pain Questionnaire[119] was designed to measure the knowledge, attitudes, and experience of patients with chronic cancer pain. The 14-item survey, using an ordinal scale format, can be administered to inpatients or outpatients.

Because terminally ill patients have multiple symptoms, it is impossible to limit an assessment to only the report of pain. Complications or symptoms related to the disease process may exacerbate pain, or interventions to alleviate pain may cause side effects that result in new symptoms or a worsening of other symptoms, such as constipation or nausea. In a prospective study of 1635 cancer patients referred to a pain clinic, patients experienced pain plus an average of three other symptoms,[120] including insomnia (59%), anorexia (48%), constipation (33%), sweating (28%), nausea (27%), dyspnea (24%), dysphagia (20%), neuropsychiatric symptoms (20%), vomiting (20%), urinary symptoms (14%), dyspepsia (11%), paresis (10%), diarrhea

(6%), pruritis (6%), and dermatological symptoms (3%). Therefore, pain assessment must be accompanied by assessment of other symptoms. Various surveys or questionnaires not only assess pain but also incorporate other symptoms into the assessment process. Many of these instruments are discussed in other chapters.

PAIN ASSESSMENT IN NONVERBAL PATIENTS OR PATIENTS WITH COGNITIVE FAILURE

The gold standard of pain assessment is the patient's self-report. However, pain instruments relying on verbal self-report that were very useful in the early stages of palliative care may not be practical for use on dying patients who cannot verbalize pain or on patients with advanced disease when delirium or cognitive failure is prevalent. Furthermore, the current definition of pain, from the International Association of Pain (IASP), has been challenged because of the its reliance on verbal report and exclusion of nonverbal beings (e.g., neonates or nonverbal adults).[121] It is also thought that the current definition contributes to a lack of ethical justice for nonverbal patients.[122] Anand and Craig[121] propose that "the behavioral alterations caused by pain are the infantile forms of self-report and should not be discounted as 'surrogate measures' of pain." They suggest that behavioral alterations have meaning within the biobehavioral milieu of the newborn infant and in all succeeding developmental stages. The definition of pain should be improved by recognizing that nonverbal beings have conscious perception of pain and that behavioral or emotional reactions are just as important as verbal information.[123]

The potential for unrelieved and unrecognized pain is greater in patients who cannot verbally express their discomfort. The inability to communicate effectively due to impaired cognition and sensory losses is a serious problem for many patients with terminal illnesses. Cognitive failure develops in the majority of cancer patients before death, and delirium is the most common psychiatric complication of patients with advanced cancer.[124,125] Loss of consciousness occurs in almost half of dying patients during the final 3 days of life.[126] Clearly, pain assessment techniques and tools are needed that conform to patients, whether mentally incompetent or nonverbal, who communicate only through their unique behavioral responses. Interpretation of the meaning of specific biobehavioral response patterns during episodes of pain could potentially reduce barriers to optimal pain assessment and management in nonverbal patients.[121] An instrument that could detect a reduction in pain behaviors could assess the effectiveness of a pain management plan. However, because pain is not just a set of behaviors, absence of certain behaviors would not necessarily mean that the patient was pain-free.[127] It is important for nurses and other health care professionals to remember that pain is communicated through both verbal and nonverbal behaviors. Verbal self-reports, whenever possible, are still important to reflect the individual's perception of pain. Because nonverbal pain behaviors may or may not concur with verbal reports, caution is necessary when assessing pain based solely on any single parameter.

Pain Behaviors in the Nonverbal Patient

It may be more complicated to assess nonverbal cues in the palliative care setting because, in contrast to patients with acute pain, terminally ill patients with chronic pain may not demonstrate any specific behaviors indicative of pain. It is also not satisfactory and even erroneous to assess pain by reliance on involuntary physiologic bodily reactions, such as increases in blood pressure, pulse, or respiratory depth. Elevated vital signs may occur with sudden, severe pain but not with persistent pain when the body reaches physiologic equilibrium.[128] However, absence of behavioral or involuntary cues does not negate the presence of pain.[5] Nonverbal patients should be empirically treated for pain if there is pre-existing pain or evidence that an individual in a similar condition would experience pain.[129] Likewise, palliative measures should be considered in non-verbal patients with behavior changes potentially related to pain. In a study assessing pain in elderly nonverbal patients, Simons and Malabar[130] reported that pain behavior was modified by interventions and adjustments in analgesia. The questions and suggestions in Table 5–6 can be used as a template for assessment of pain in the nonverbal patient.

Table 5–6. Assessment and Treatment of Pain in the Nonverbal Patient

Is there a reason for the patient to be experiencing pain?
Was the patient being treated for pain? If so, what regimen was effective (include pharmacologic and nonpharmacologic interventions)?
How does the patient usually act when he or she is in pain? (Note: the nurse may need to ask family/significant others or other health care professionals.)
What is the family/significant others' interpretation of the patient's behavior? Do they believe the patient is in pain? Why do they feel this way?
Try to obtain feedback from the patient, e.g., ask patient to nod head, squeeze hand, move eyes up or down, raise legs, or hold up fingers to signal presence of pain.
If appropriate, offer writing materials or pain intensity charts that patient can use or point to.
If there is a possible reason for or sign of acute pain, treat with analgesics or other pain-relief measures.
If a pharmacologic or nonpharmacologic intervention results in modifying pain behavior, continue with treatment.
If pain behavior persists, rule out potential causes of the behavior (delirium, side effect of treatment, symptom of disease process); try appropriate intervention for behavior cause.
Explain interventions to patient and family/significant other.

It is not known whether patients with cognitive failure or dementia experience pain in the same way as cognitively intact individuals. Most studies suggest that pain reports in cognitively impaired individuals describe decreased intensity and frequency, which may be related to a decreased capacity to report pain.[131] Behavior or responses caused by noxious stimuli in a cognitively impaired or demented individual may not necessarily reflect classic pain behaviors. In a study of 26 patients with painful conditions from a nursing home Alzheimer's unit, Marzinski[132] reported diverse responses to pain that were atypical of conventional pain behaviors. For example, pain changed the behavior of a patient who normally moaned and rocked to one who became quiet and withdrawn. Pain in another nonverbal patient caused rapid blinking. Other patients who normally exhibited disjointed verbalizations could, when experiencing pain, give accurate descriptions of their pain.

Instruments Used to Assess Pain in Nonverbal Patients or Patients with Cognitive Failure

Research studies and instruments are lacking in assessment of pain in nonverbal patients and those with cognitive failure. This lack of information potentially results in several problems regarding the treatment of pain. Pain may not be relieved because it is not recognized. Pain could be overtreated with opioids because it is mistaken with other signs, such as delirium or cognitive failure, thus negatively impacting on potentially reversible causes of cognitive failure.[133] Conflicts and dissatisfaction could occur among staff members and between staff members and family because agitated cognitive failure or delirium may be interpreted as a sign of pain.[124]

It is difficult to use an instrument to quantitatively measure pain in patients who are not verbal or have cognitive failure. The following are examples of instruments used to measure pain behaviors in nonverbal patients or persons with cognitive failure.

Discomfort Scale. Hurley and colleagues, based on behaviors observed by nurses, developed an objective scale for assessing discomfort in nonverbal patients with advanced Alzheimer's disease.[134] The investigators defined discomfort as "a negative emotional and/or physical state subject to variation in magnitude in response to internal or environmental conditions." The negative states they referred to could be a condition other than pain, such as anguish and suffering. After testing for reliability, a scale of nine items was retained from an original list of 26 behavioral indicators for discomfort. Items retained were noisy breathing, negative vocalization, absence of a look of contentment, looking sad, looking frightened, having a frown, absence of relaxed body posture, looking tense, and fidgeting (Table 5–7). Research needs to determine the generalization of this scale to palliative care patients who cannot verbally communicate their pain or discomfort.

Edmonton Symptom Assessment System. When patients are incapable of reporting their own pain, observer judgments of pain become necessary. Eighty-three

Table 5–7. Discomfort Scale (DS-DAT)

Discomfort Scale Items	Behavioral Indicators
Noisy breathing	Negative-sounding noise on inspiration or expiration Breathing looks strenuous, labored, or wearing Respirations sound loud, harsh, or gasping Difficulty breathing or trying hard to achieve a good gas exchange Episodic bursts of rapid breaths or hyperventilation
Negative vocalization	Noise or speech with a negative or disapproving quality Hushed, low sounds, e.g., constant muttering Gutteral tone, monotone, subdued, or varying pitched noise Faster rate than a conversation Moan or groan Repeating the same words with a mournful tone Expressing hurt or pain
Content facial expression	Pleasant, calm-looking face Tranquil, at ease, or serene Relaxed facial expression, an unclenched jaw Overall look is one of peace
Sad facial expression	Troubled-looking face; looking hurt, worried, lost, or lonesome; tears, crying; distressed appearance; sunken "hang dog" look with lackluster eyes
Frightened facial expression	Scared- or concerned-looking face; looking bothered, fearful, or troubled; alarmed appearance with open eyes and pleading face
Frown	Face looks strained, stern, or scowling; displeased expression with a wrinkled brow and creases in the forehead; corners of mouth turned down
Relaxed body language	Easy, open-handed position; look of being in a restful position and may be cuddled up or stretched out; muscles look of normal firmness and joints are without stress; look of being idle, lazy, or laid back; appearance of "just killing the day," casual
Tense body language	Extremities show tension; wringing hands, clenched fist, knees pulled up tightly; look of being in a strained, inflexible position
Fidgeting	Restless, impatient motion; acts squirmy or jittery; appearance of trying to get away from hurt area; forceful touching, tugging, rubbing of body part

Source: Reprinted with permission from Hurley et al. (1992), reference 134.

percent of symptom assessments were done by nurses or patients' relatives for 101 consecutive patients hospitalized in a palliative care unit.[135] The Edmonton Symptom Assessment System (ESAS) is a validated tool for use in the palliative care setting. The ESAS is a brief and reproducible scale consisting of separate VASs and NRSs that evaluate nine symptoms (pain, activity, nausea, depression, anxiety, drowsiness, appetite, sensation of well-being, and shortness of breath). The tool is completed twice a day by palliative care unit patients, daily by hospice patients, and several times a week by home care patients. If patients are unable to complete the form, a space is provided for whoever completes the assessment. When patients are unresponsive and during the final hours or days of life, the main caregiver and/or nurse completes the Edmonton Comfort Assessment and Symptom Assessment Form (Fig. 5–3). The scores on either assessment can be transferred to a graph to present a visual display of trends in patients' symptoms and discomfort. Lower scores designate better symptom control (the highest possible score is 900 on the ESAS). Although the ESAS has been considered useful to display incidence of symptoms, some investigators have found it to be impractical in patients with a poor performance status.[136] To evaluate pain and other symptoms, an individualized approach may be more appropriate than completing health-related checklists.

Other Scales. Many chronic pain programs systematically observe and measure the frequency of pain behaviors and use scales such as the UAB (University of Alabama in Birmingham) Pain Behavior Scale,[137] The West Haven-Yale Multidimensional Pain Inventory (WHYMPI),[138] and The Checklist for Interpersonal Pain Behavior (CHIP).[139] Examples of observed and measured behaviors include, but are not limited to, verbal and nonverbal vocal complaints, facial grimaces, use of supportive equipment, vegetative signs such as sleep and appetite alterations, quantity of medications taken, activity level, and social interactions.[140] Four distinct facial actions that have been consistently identified in pain expression include brow lowering, eye narrowing or closure, and raising the upper lip.[141] Although facial expressions are related to pain intensity ratings on sensory and affective scales,[142,143] facial assessment tools, such as the Facial Action Coding System (FACS),[144] are currently too time-consuming and laborious for use in the clinical setting. Furthermore, observations of facial expressions may not be valid in patients with conditions that result in distorted facial expressions, such as Parkinson's disease or strokes.

Health Care Professional Assessment of Pain in the Nonverbal Patient

Just as the experience of pain is subjective, "witnessing another in pain is a subjective experience." [122] Without verbal validation from the patient, the clinician must rely on behavioral observations, as well as intuition and personal judgment. It is also particularly important to elicit the opinions of the individuals closest to the patient, which are also subjective. While some health care providers may assign greater importance to nonverbal expression of pain than to self-report, many observers would find that the patient's pain might be incomprehensible without words to help interpret behavior.

Nurses or other health care providers reflect the difficulty of accurately assessing pain in nonverbal patients in studies that show low concurrence between patients' self-ratings of pain and ratings of the same patients.[145–147] Other findings are equivocal, with some studies on family caregivers'/significant others' perceptions of patients' pain suggesting that family members accurately estimated the amount of pain cancer patients experience[75,80] whereas other studies propose that family caregivers overestimated the patient's pain.[148–150] Pain in patients with chronic malignant and nonmalignant disease affects family/significant others, with patients routinely underestimating stress, depression, and anxiety in their caregivers.

Because of changing patient conditions, patients' "typical pain behaviors" should be documented for future reference. Patients should also be asked while they are mentally competent "If you couldn't tell me how much pain you were having, how would I know you were having pain?"[151] When patients are no longer able to verbally communicate whether they are in pain or not, the best approach is to assume that their underlying disease is still painful and to continue pain interventions.[152]

SUMMARY

In summary, multiple factors should be incorporated into the assessment of the pain experience. The following case example includes some of the pain assessment techniques discussed in this chapter and may prove beneficial in applying this content for nurse clinicians.

Case Study: M.B., a Man with Metastatic Prostate Cancer

M.B. was a 72-year-old man diagnosed with metastatic prostate cancer to his bones and spine. Various hormonal manipulations had failed M.B., and he noticed changes in his lifestyle and activities he once enjoyed. Sometimes the imposition of pain can trigger losses that will affect quality of life as one has known it before the pain. M.B. had a very supportive family, who always accompanied him to clinic appointments. He loved to take his family on trips. He also had a contracting business; his sons and daughters worked side-by-side with their father. M.B. was in the midst of retiring and turning the business over to his family. He complained of new pain in his spine and lower back. He was reluctant to stop hormone and chemotherapy; he was anxious to see if radiation therapy would help this new pain. He described his pain as "achy, throbbing, continuous with muscle spasms that grab me. Whenever I bend over the pain catches me from behind in my lower back. I would rate the pain a 7 out of 10."

When asked about how his pain affected his life, he said, "a part of me is lost. I used to, me and my son, used to go fly fishing on the weekends and during the summer. Now I just do, you know, some things around the

Capital Health

CARITAS HEALTH GROUP

Edmonton Symptom Assessment: Numerical Scale

Please circle the number that best describes:

No Pain	0	1	2	3	4	5	6	7	8	9	10	Worst Possible Pain
Not Tired	0	1	2	3	4	5	6	7	8	9	10	Worst Possible Tiredness
Not Nauseated	0	1	2	3	4	5	6	7	8	9	10	Worst Possible Nausea
Not Depressed	0	1	2	3	4	5	6	7	8	9	10	Worst Possible Depression
Not Anxious	0	1	2	3	4	5	6	7	8	9	10	Worst Possible Anxiety
Not Drowsy	0	1	2	3	4	5	6	7	8	9	10	Worst Possible Drowsiness
Best Appetite	0	1	2	3	4	5	6	7	8	9	10	Worst Possible Appetite
Best Feeling of Wellbeing	0	1	2	3	4	5	6	7	8	9	10	Worst Possible Feeling of Wellbeing
No Shortness of Breath	0	1	2	3	4	5	6	7	8	9	10	Worst Possible Shortness of Breath
Other Problem	0	1	2	3	4	5	6	7	8	9	10	

Name: ______________
Date: ______________
Time: ______________
Assessed By: ______________

A

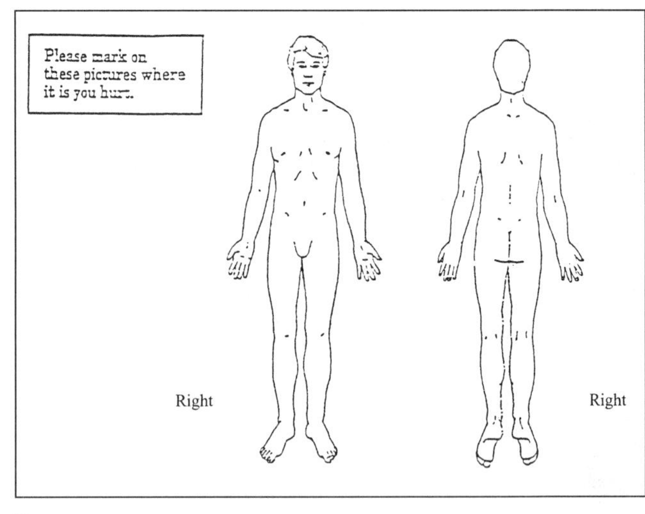

B

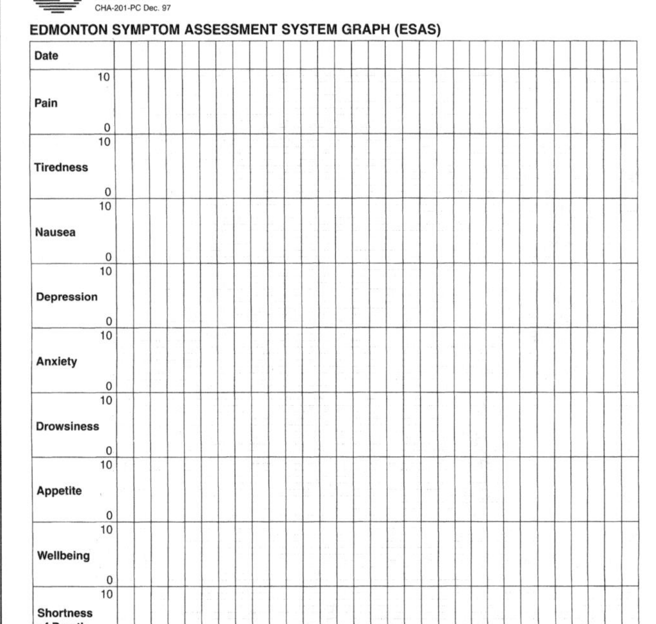
Capital Health

CHA-201-PC Dec. 97

EDMONTON SYMPTOM ASSESSMENT SYSTEM GRAPH (ESAS)

Date	
Pain	10 / 0
Tiredness	10 / 0
Nausea	10 / 0
Depression	10 / 0
Anxiety	10 / 0
Drowsiness	10 / 0
Appetite	10 / 0
Wellbeing	10 / 0
Shortness of Breath	10 / 0
Mini-Mental Normal	
Modified EFAT	
Assessed by	

Cage Score ________ **Level of Education** ________

C

Fig. 5–3. The Edmonton Comfort and Symptom Assessment Form. Instructions for the use of this multipart form are presented in Appendix A. (Reprinted with permission of Capital Health.)

Capital Health
CARITAS HEALTH GROUP

Edmonton Comfort Assessment Form (ECAF)
GRAPH

DATE		
ADMISSION DAY		
HOUR (End of Shift)		
1. Caregiver Comfort VAS		10 9 8 7 6 5 4 3 2 1 0
Caregiver VAS		
2. Caregiver Reason (✓)	Pain	
	Nausea	
	Confusion / restlessness	
	Urinate / defecate	
	Shortness of breath	
	Hunger / thirst	
	Unknown	
	Other	
1. Nurse Score (0-24)		
2. Nurse Reason (✓)	Pain	
	Nausea	
	Confusion / restlessness	
	Urinate and / or defecate	
	Dyspnea	
	Hunger / Thirst	
	Unknown	
	Other	
3. RN VAS		
4. MD VAS		

D

Capital Health
CARITAS HEALTH GROUP

Edmonton Comfort Assessment Form (ECAF)

(Please ask caregivers to complete first) Date Completed: ______ Time: ______

Regular Family Caregiver (if present) ______ ☐ Not Applicable

1. How comfortable has the person been during the last day? *(Please circle the appropriate number)*

Very comfortable 0 1 2 3 4 5 6 7 8 9 10 Very Uncomfortable

2. Why do you think the patient is uncomfortable today? (Check the reason-You may check more than one)

☐ Pain ☐ Nausea ☐ Confusion / Restlessness ☐ Need to Urinate / Defecate
☐ Shortness of Breath ☐ Hunger / Thirst ☐ Unknown
☐ Other *(please specify)* ______

Nurse Score:					
1. Behaviour Observed Today *(Please check only 1 scale for Behaviour)*	Not Observed During Shift 0	Observed only upon Stimulation 1	Occasional Spontaneous 2	Frequent *(most of the time)* 3	Continuous 4
A. Grimacing					
B. Groaning-Isolated Words					
C. Shouting					
D. Touching-Rubbing Area					
E. Purposeless Movements					
F. Laboured Noisy Breathing					
SCORE					
				TOTAL SCORE (0-24)	

2. Suspected Reason *(Check more than one)*

☐ Pain ☐ Nausea ☐ Confusion / Restlessness ☐ Urinary Retention / Defecation
☐ Dyspnea ☐ Hunger / Thirst ☐ Unknown
☐ Other *(please specify)* ______

3. RN Global Comfort Assessment Score: 0 - 10 scale ______ *(0 = very comfortable; 10 = very uncomfortable)*

E

Fig. 5–3. (*continued*) The Edmonton Comfort and Symptom Assessment Form. Instructions for the use of this multipart form are presented in Appendix A.

house. Just last week, I went fishing with my son but I told him, 'Son, I'm not going to be able to fish with you today.' I said, 'my back . . . it's too hard for me. I'm not the man I used to be.'" After assessing M.B.'s pain characteristics and their impact on his lifestyle, his medication regimen was adjusted to include a long-acting opioid for his continuous pain and a short-acting opioid for breakthrough pain coupled with a nonsteroidal anti-inflammatory drug for somatic pain. His pain scores dramatically decreased, and he was able to fish with his son and continue to engage in some of the activities that gave him enjoyment and quality of life.

Because nurses have sustained contact with patients across all care settings, they are in positions to identify undertreated and untreated pain and to advocate for its relief. As members of interdisciplinary teams involved in practice, education, administration, and research, nurses are pivotal to improving the relief of pain. The overlapping and complementary aspects of caregivers' roles in assessing and managing pain clearly point to the need for a multidisciplinary, collaborative approach to the care of persons experiencing pain in the palliative care setting. The unfolding of the concept of pain from a unidimensional to a multifactorial experience has the potential to open new opportunities for the study of pain that may dramatically influence pain outcomes and the way pain is assessed and managed in the future.

REFERENCES

1. Ferrell BR. Personal communication, 1998.

2. Cleeland CS, Gonin R, Hatfield AK, et al. Pain and its treatment in outpatients with metastatic cancer N Engl J Med 1994;330:592–596.

3. Desbiens NA, Wu AW, Broste SK, et al. Pain and satisfaction with pain control in seriously ill hospitalized adults: findings from the SUPPORT research investigations. Crit Care Med 1996;24:1953–1961.

4. Desbiens NA, Wu AW, Yasui Y, et al. Patient empowerment and feedback did not decrease pain in seriously ill hospitalized adults. Pain 1998;75:237–246.

5. Jacox A, Carr DB, Payne R, et al. Management of Cancer Pain. Clinical Practice Guideline No. 9. AHCPR Publication 94-0592. Rockville, MD: Agency for Health Care Policy and Research, U.S. Department of Health and Human Services, Public Health Service, 1994.

6. Payne R, Weinstein SM, Hill CS. Assessment and management of pain. In: Levin V, ed. Cancer in the Nervous System. New York: Churchill-Livingstone, 1996.

7. Portenoy RK. Cancer pain: epidemiology and syndromes. Cancer 1989;63:2298–2307.

8. Von Roenn JH, Cleeland CS, Gonin R, Hatfield AK, Pandya KA. Physician attitudes and practice in cancer pain management: a survey from the Eastern Cooperative Oncology Group. Ann Intern Med 1993;119:121–126.

9. Zhukovsky DS, Gorowski E, Hausdorff J, Napolitano B, Lesser M. Unmet analgesic needs in cancer patients. J Pain Symptom Manage 1995;10:113–119.

10. Ventafridda V, Ripamonti C, DeConno F, Tambarini M, Cassileth BR. Symptom prevalence and control during cancer patient's last days of life. J Palliat Care 1990;6:3–4.

11. Coyle N, Adelhardt J, Foley KM, Portenoy RK. Character of terminal illness in the advanced cancer patient: pain and other symptoms during the last four weeks of life. J Pain Symptom Manage 1990;5:83–93.

12. Weissman DE, Griffie J. The palliative care consultation service of the Medical College of Wisconsin. J Pain Symptom Manage 1994; 9:474–479.

13. Chronic pain in America: roadblocks to relief. Study conducted by Roper Starch Worldwide, Inc., January 1999.

14. International Association for the Study of Pain. Pain terms: a list with definitions and notes on usage. Pain 1979;6:249.

15. McCaffery M. Nursing Practice Theories Related to Cognition, Bodily Pain, and Man–Environment Interactions. Los Angeles: UCLA Press, 1968:95.

16. Turk DC, Melzack R. The measurement of pain and the assessment of people experiencing pain. In: Turk DC, Melzack R, eds. Handbook of Pain Assessment. New York: Guilford Press, 1992: 3–14.

17. Vasudevan SV. Impairment, disability, and functional capacity assessment. In: Turk DC, Melzack R, eds. Handbook of Pain Assessment. New York: Guilford Press, 1992:100–110.

18. Ferrell BR, Dean GE, Grant M, Coluzzi P. An institutional commitment to pain management. J Clin Oncol 1995;13:2158–2165.

19. Larue F, Colleau SM, Fontaine A, Brasseur L. Oncologists and primary care physicians' attitudes toward pain control and morphine prescribing in France. Cancer 1995;76:2375–2382.

20. Schmitt RM, Gates RA, Slover R, et al. A Comprehensive Multidisciplinary Education and Research Program to Assess and Improve Outcomes of Patients with Pain. Denver: University of Colorado. Hospital Authority Grants Program.

21. Weissman DE, Dahl JL. Attitudes about cancer pain: a survey of Wisconsin's first year medical students. J Pain Symptom Manage 1990;5: 345–349.

22. Wilson JF, Brockopp GW, Kryst S, Steger H, Witt WO. Medical students' attitudes toward pain before and after a brief course on pain. Pain 1992;50:251–256.

23. Cleeland CS. Documenting barriers to cancer pain management. In: Chapman CR, Foley KM, eds. Current and Emerging Issues in Cancer Pain: Research and Practice. New York: Raven Press, 1993:321–330.

24. Foley KM. The treatment of cancer pain. N Engl J Med 1985;313:84–95.

25. National Center for Nursing Research. National Nursing Research Agenda, Vol. 1. Developing Knowledge for Practice: Challenges and Opportunities. NIH Publication 93-2416. Bethesda, MD: National Institutes of Health, U.S. Public Health Service, U.S. Department of Health and Human Services, 1993.

26. Cleeland CS. The impact of pain on the patient with cancer. Cancer 1984;58:2635–2641.

27. Acute Pain Management Guidelines Panel. Acute Pain Management: Operative or Medical Procedures and Trauma. Clinical Practice Guideline. AHCPR Publication 92-0032. Rockville, MD: Agency for Health Care Policy and Research, Public Health Service, U.S. Department of Health and Human Services, 1992.

28. American Pain Society Committee on Quality Assurance Standards. In: Bond MR, Charlton JE, Wolff CJ, eds. Proceedings of the Sixth World Congress on Pain. New York: Elsevier, 1991:185–189.

29. American Pain Society Quality of Care Committee. Quality improvement guidelines for the treatment of acute pain and cancer pain. JAMA 1995;1874–1880.

30. Spross J, McGuire DB, Schmitt RM. Oncology Nursing Society position paper on cancer pain. Oncol Nurs Forum 1990;17:595–614.

31. Max M, Cleary J, Ferrell BR, Foley K, Payne R, Shapiro B. Treatment of pain at the end of life: a position statement from the American Pain Society. APS Bull 1997;7:1–3.

32. JCAHO standards. http://www.jcaho.org/standard/pm 1999.

33. Miaskowski C. Pain management: quality assurance and changing practice. In: Gebhardt GF, Hammond DL, Jensen TS, eds. Proceedings of the 7th World Congress on Pain, Progress in Pain Research and Management, Vol. 2. Seattle: IASP Press, 1994:75–96.

34. Miaskowski C. Commentary. J Pain Symptom Manage 1996;12:331–333.

35. Peyerwold M. Pain assessment. In: Comprehensive Pain Management in Terminal Illness. Coluzzi PH, Volker B, Miashowski C, eds. Sacramento: California State Hospice Association, 1996:29–34.

36. Morris W, ed. American Heritage Dictionary of the English Language. Boston: Houghton Mifflin, 1996:79, 428, 972.

37. Twycross RG. Oral Morphine in Advanced Cancer, 3rd Edition. Beaconsfield, Bucks, UK: Beaconsfield Publishers, 1997:1–42.

38. McGuire D. The multiple dimensions of cancer pain: a framework for assessment and management. In: McGuire D, Yarbro CH, and Ferrell BR, eds. Boston: Jones and Bartlett, 1995:1–17.

39. Meinhart NT, McCaffery M. Pain: A Nursing Approach to Assessment. Norwalk, CT: Appelton-Century-Crofts, 1983.

40. Melzack R, Casey KL. Sensory, motivational, and central control determinants of pain: a new conceptual model. In: Kenshalo, D, ed. The Skin Senses. Springfield, IL: Charles C. Thomas, 1968:423–439.

41. Ahles TA, Blanchard EB, Ruckdeschel JC. The multidimensional nature of cancer-related pain. Pain 1983;17:277–288.

42. Bates, MS. Ethnicity and pain: a biocultural model. Soc Sci Med 1987;24:47–50.

43. McGuire DB. The multidimensional phenomenon of cancer pain. In: McGuire DB, Yarbro CH, eds. Cancer Pain Management. Philadelphia: WB Saunders, 1987:1–20.

44. Hester NO. Assessment of acute pain. Baillieres Clin Paediatr 1995;3:561–577.

45. McGuire DB. Comprehensive and multidimensional assessment and measurement of pain. J Pain Symptom Manage 1992;7:312–319.

46. Gonzales GB, Payne R, Foley KM, Portenoy RK. Prevalence and characteristics of brachial plexopathy in a large cancer center: a retrospective study. Presented at Third Annual Bristol-Myers Pain Research Symposium, Seattle, WA, 1992.

47. Twycross RG & Fairfield S. Pain in far-advanced cancer. Pain 1982;14:303–310.

48. Portenoy RK, Hagen NA. Breakthrough pain: definition, prevalence, and characteristics. Pain 1990;41:273–281.

49. Williams DA, Robinson ME, Geisser ME. Pain beliefs: assessment and utility. Pain 1994;59:71–78.

50. Fink RM. Pain assessment: the cornerstone to optimal pain management. Analgesia 1997;9:17–25.

51. Gordon DB, Ward SE. Correcting patient misconceptions about pain. Am J Nurs 1995; 95:43–45.

52. Keefe FJ, Dunsmore J. Pain behavior: concepts and controversies. APS J 1992;1:92–100.

53. Turk DC, Matyas TA. Pain-related behaviors: communication of pain. APS J 1992;1: 109–111.

54. Vlaeyen JWS, Van Eek H, Groenman NH, Schuerman JA. Dimensions and components of observed chronic pain behavior. Pain 1987;31: 65–75.

55. Craig KD. The facial expression of pain: better than a thousand words? APS J 1992;1:153–162.

56. Wilkie DJ, Lovejoy N, Dodd M, Tesler M. Cancer pain control behaviors: description and correlation with pain intensity. Oncol Nurs Forum, 1988;15:723–731.

57. Ferrell BA. Overview of aging and pain. In: Ferrell BR, Ferrell BA, eds. Pain in the Elderly. Seattle, WA: IASP Press, 1996:1–10.

58. Ferrell BR. Patient education and non-drug interventions. In: Ferrell BR, Ferrell BA, eds. Pain in the Elderly. Seattle, WA: IASP Press, 1996;35–44.

59. Cleeland CS. Undertreatment of cancer pain in elderly patients. JAMA 1998;279:1914–1915.

60. Bernabei R, Gambassi G, Lapane K, et al. Management of pain in elderly patients with cancer. JAMA 1998;279:1877–1882.

61. McCaffery M, Ferrell BR. Does the gender gap affect your pain-control decisions? Nursing 1992;22:48–51.

62. Vallerand AH. Gender differences in pain. Image J Nurs Sch 1995;27:235–237.

63. Miaskowski C. Women and pain. Crit Care Nurs Clin North Am 1997;9:453–458.

64. Berkley KJ. Sex, drugs and. . . . Nat Med 1996;2:1184–1185.

65. Unruh AM. Gender variations in clinical pain experience. Pain 1996;65:123–167.

66. Dubreuil D, Kohn P. Reactivity and response to pain. Person Indiv Diff 1986;7:907–909.

67. Robin O, Vinard H, Varnet-Maury E, Saumet JL. Influence of sex and anxiety of pain threshold and tolerance. Func Neurol 1987;2: 73–179.

68. Walsh N, Schoenfield L, Ramamurthy S, Hoffman J. Normative model for cold pressor test. Am J Phys Med Rehabil 1989;68:6–11.

69. Fink RS, Gates R. Cultural diversity and cancer pain. In: McGuire DB, Yarbro CH, Ferrell BR, eds. Cancer Pain Management, 2nd ed. Boston: Jones and Bartlett, 1995:19–39.

70. Bates MS, Edwards WT, Anderson KO. Ethnocultural influences on variation in chronic pain perception. Pain 1993;52:101–112.

71. Lipton JA, Marbach JJ. Ethnicity and the pain experience. Soc Sci Med 1984;19:1279–1298.

72. Zborowski M. People in Pain. San Francisco: Jossey-Bass, 1969.

73. Zola IK. Culture and symptoms: an analysis of patients' presenting complaints. Am Soc Rev 1996;31:615–630.

74. Fabrega H Jr. Language, culture and the neurobiology of pain: a theoretical exploration. Behav Neurol 1989;2:235–259.

75. Dar R, Beach CM, Barden PL, Cleeland CS. Cancer pain in the marital system: a study of patients and their spouses. J Pain Symptom Manage 1992;7:87–93.

76. Spross J, Wolff Burke M. Nonpharmacological management of cancer pain. In: McGuire DB, Yarbro CH, Ferrell BR, eds. Cancer Pain Management. Boston: Jones and Bartlett, 1995: 159–205.

77. Brunelli C, Costantini M, Di Giulio P, et al. Quality of life evaluation: when do terminally ill cancer patients and health-care providers agree? J Pain Symptom Manage 1998;15:151–158.

78. Grossman SA, Sheidler VR, Swedeen K, Mucenski J, Piantadosi S. Correlation of patient and caregiver ratings of cancer pain. J Pain Symptom Manage 1991;6:53–57.

79. Ketovuori H. Nurses' and patients' conception of wound pain and the administration of analgesics. J Pain Symptom Manage 1987;2: 213–218.

80. Ferrell BR, Eberts M, McCaffery M, Grant M. Clinical decision making and pain. Cancer Nurs 1991;14:289–297.

81. Carpenter JS, Brockopp D. Comparison of patients' ratings and examination of nurses' responses to pain intensity rating scales. Cancer Nurs 1995;18:292–298.

82. Puntillo KA, Miaskowski C, Kehrle K, Stannard D, Gleeson S, Nye P. Relationship between behaviorial and physiological indicators of pain, critical care patients, self-reports of pain, and opioid administration. Crit Care Med 1997;25: 1159–1166.

83. Werner P, Cohen-Mansfield J, Watson V, Pasis S. Pain in participants of adult day care centers: assessment by different raters. J Pain Symptom Manage 1998;15:8–17.

84. Bruera E, Pareira J. Recent developments in palliative cancer care. Acta Oncol 1998;37: 749–757.

85. Jensen MP, Karoly P. Self-report scales and procedures for assessing pain in adults. In: Turk DC, Melzak R, eds. Handbook of Pain Assessment. New York: Guilford Press, 1992:135–151.

86. Wallenstein SL, Heidrich G, Kaiko R, Houde RW. Clinical evaluation of mild analgesics: the measurement of clinical pain. Br J Clin Pharmacol 1980;10:319S–327S.

87. Paice JA, Cohen FL. Validity of a verbally administered numeric rating scale to measure cancer pain intensity. Cancer Nurs 1997;20: 88–93.

88. Downie WW, Leatham PA, Rhind VM, Wright V, Brancho JA, Anderson JA. Studies with pain rating scales. Ann Rheum Dis 1978;37: 378–381.

89. Ahles TA, Ruckdeschel JC, Blanchard EB. Cancer-related pain. II. Assessment with visual analogue scales. J Psychosom Res 1984;28: 121–124.

90. Ohnhaus EE, Adler R. Methodological problems in the measurement of pain: a comparison between the verbal rating scale and the visual analogue scale. Pain 1975;1:379–384.

91. Ferraz MB, Quaresma MR, Aquino LRL, Atra E, Tugwell P, Goldsmith CH. Reliability of pain scales in the assessment of literate and illiterate patients with rheumatoid arthritis. J Rheumatol 1990;17:1022–1024.

92. Kremer E, Atkinson J. Pain language: affect. J Psychosom Res 1984;28:125–132.

93. Scott J, Huskisson EC. Graphic representation of pain. Pain 1976;2:175–184.

94. Revill SI, Robinson JO, Rosen M, Hogg MIJ. The reliability of a linear analogue for evaluating pain. Anaesthesia 1976;31:1191–1998.

95. Shannon MM, Ryan MA, D'Agostino N, Brescia FJ. Assessment of pain in advanced can-

cer patients. J Pain Symptom Manage 1995;10: 274–278.

96. Herr KA, Mobily PR. Comparison of selected pain assessment tools for use with the elderly. Appl Nurs Res 1993;6:39–49.

97. Wong DL, Baker CM. Pain in children: comparison of assessment scales. Pediatr Nurs 1988;14:9–17.

98. Bieri D, Reeve R, Champion GD, Addicoat L, Ziegler JB. The Faces Pain Scale for the self assessment of the severity of pain experienced by children: development, initial validation, and preliminary investigation for ratio scale properties. Pain 1990;41:139–150.

99. Matsumoto D. Ethnic differences in affect intensity, emotion judgments, display rule attitudes, and self-reported emotional expression in an American sample. Motiv Emot 1993;17: 107–123.

100. Casas JM, Wagenheim BR, Banchero R, Mendoza-Romero J. Hispanic masculinity: myth or psychological schema meriting clinical consideration. Hisp J Behav Sci 1994;16:315–331.

101. Frank AJM, Moll JMH, Hort JF. A comparison of three ways of measuring pain. Rheumatol Rehabil 1982;21:211–217.

102. Wilson JS, Cason CL, Grissom NL. Distraction: an effective intervention for alleviating pain during venipuncture. J Emerg Nurs 1995; 21:87–94.

103. Stuppy DJ. The Faces Pain Scale: reliability and validity with mature adults. Appl Nurs Res 1998;11:84–89.

104. Dalton JA, McNaull F. A call for standardizing the clinical rating of pain intensity using a 0 to 10 rating scale. Cancer Nurs 1998; 21:46–49.

105. Gift AG. Visual analogue scales: measurement of subjective phenomena. Nurs Res 1989;38:286–288.

106. Grossi E, Borghi C, Montanari M. Measurement of pain: comparison between visual analog scale and analog chromatic continuous scale. In: Fields HL, Dabner R, Cervera F, eds. Advances in Pain Research and Therapy, Vol. 12, Issues in Pain Measurement. New York: Raven Press, 1985: 391–493.

107. Grossman SA, Sheidler VR, McGuire DB, Geer C, Santor D, Piantadosi S. A comparison of the Hopkins pain rating instrument with standard visual analogue and verbal descriptor scales in patients with cancer pain. J Pain Symptom Manage 1992;7:196–203.

108. Lee KA, Kieckhefer GM. Measuring human responses using visual analogue scales. West J Nurs Res 1989;11:128–132.

109. Wewers ME, Lowe NK. A critical review of visual analogue scales in the measurement of clinical phenomena. Res Nurs Health 1990;13: 227–236.

110. Jensen MP, Karoly P, Braver S. The measurement of clinical pain intensity: a comparison of six methods. Pain 1986;27:117–126.

111. Kremer E, Hampton Atkinson J, Ignelzi RJ Measurement of pain: patient preference does not confound pain measurement. Pain 1981;10: 241–248.

112. Shacham S. Anxiety or pain: what does the scale measure? J Consult Clin Psychol 1981; 49:468–469.

113. Carey SJ, Turpin C, Smith J, Whatley J, Haddox D. Improving pain management in an acute care setting: The Crawford Long Hospital of Emory University experience. Orthopaedic Nursing 1997;16:29–36.

114. Cleeland CS, Syrjala KL. How to assess cancer pain. In: Turk DC, Melzack R, eds. Handbook of Pain Assessment. New York: Guilford Press, 1992:362–390.

115. Melzak R. The short-form McGill Pain Questionnaire. Pain 1987;30:191–197.

116. Cleeland C. Measurement of pain by subjective report. In: Chapman CR, Loeser JD, eds. Advances in Pain Research and Therapy, Vol. 12, Issues in Pain Measurement p. 391–403.

117. Daut RL, Cleeland CS, Flanery R. Development of the Wisconsin Brief Pain Inventory to assess pain in cancer and other diseases. Pain 1983;17:197–210.

118. Fishman B, Pasternak S, Wallenstein SL, Houde RW, Holland JC, Foley KM. The Memorial Pain Assessment Card: a valid instrument for the evaluation of cancer pain. Cancer 1987;60:1151–1158.

119. Ferrell B. Patient Pain Questionnaire. Available at: http:/prc.coh.org

120. Grond S, Zech D, Diefenbach C, Bischoff A. Prevalence and pattern of symptoms in patients with cancer pain: a prospective evaluation of 1635 cancer patients referred to a pain clinic. J Pain Symptom Manage 1994;9:372–382.

121. Anand KJS, Craig KD. New perspectives on the definition of pain. Pain 1996;67:3–6.

122. Cunningham N. Primary requirements for an ethical definition of pain. Pain Forum 1999;8:93–99.

123. Anand KJS, Rovnaghi C, Walden M, Churchill J. Consciousness, behavior, and clinical impact of the definition of pain. Pain Forum 1999;8:64–73.

124. Bruera E, Fainsinger RL, Miller MJ, Kuehn N. The assessment of pain intensity in patients with cognitive failure: a preliminary report. J Pain Symptom Manage 1992;7:267–270.

125. Stiefel F, Fainsinger R, Bruera E. Acute confusional states in patients with advanced cancer. J Pain Symptom Manage 1992;7:94–98.

126. Lynn J, Teno JM, Phillips RS, et al. Support investigators, study to understand prognosis and preferences for outcomes and risks of treatment. Ann Intern Med 1997;126:97–106.

127. Keefe FJ, Dunsmore J. Pain behavior: concepts and controversies. APS J 1992;1:92–100.

128. McCaffery M, Ferrell BR. How vital are vital signs? Nursing 1992;22:43–46.

129. Coluzzi PH, Volker B, Miaskowski C. Comprehensive Pain Management in Terminal Illness. Sacramento: California State Hospice Association, 1996.

130. Simons W, Malabar R. Assessing pain in elderly patients who cannot respond verbally. J Adv Nurs 1995;22:663–669.

131. Farrell MJ, Katz B, Helme RD. The impact of dementia on the pain experience. Pain 1996;67:7–15.

132. Marzinski LR. The tragedy of dementia: clinically assessing pain in the confused nonverbal elderly. J Gerontol Nurs 1991;17:25–28.

133. Fainsinger R, Young C. Palliative care round: cognitive failure in a terminally ill patient. J Pain Symptom Manage 1992;6:492–494.

134. Hurley AC, Volicer BJ, Hanrahan PA, Houde S, Volicer L. Assessment of discomfort in advanced Alzheimer patients. Res Nurs Health 1992;15:369–377.

135. Bruera E, Kuehn N, Miller MJ, Selmser P, MacMillan K. The Edmonton Symptom Assessment System (ESAS): a simple method for the assessment of palliative care patients. J Palliat Care 1991;7:6–9.

136. Rees E, Hardy J, Ling J, Broadley K, A'-Hearn R. The use of the Edmonton Symptom Assessment Scale within a palliative care unit in the UK. Palliat Med 1998;12:75–82.

137. Richards JS, Neopomuceno C, Riles M, Suer Z. Assessing pain behavior: the UAB Pain Behavior Scale. Pain 1982;14:393–398.

138. Kerns RD. Turk DC, Rudy TE. The West Haven-Yale Multidimensional Pain Inventory (WHYMPI). Pain 1985;23:345–356.

139. Vlaeyen JW, Pernot DF, Kole SA, Schuerman JA, Van EH, Groenman NH. Assessment of the components of observed chronic pain behavior: the Checklist for Interpersonal Behavior (CHIP). Pain 1990;43:337–347.

140. Hebben N. Psychodynamics and psychotherapy of the chronic pain syndrome. In: Aronoff GM, ed. Evaluation and Treatment of Chronic Pain. Baltimore: Williams & Wilkins, 1992:384–393.

141. Prkachin KM. Measurement in the face of pain. APS J 1992;1:167–169.

142. LeResche L, Dworkin SF. Facial expressions of pain and emotions in chronic TMD patients. Pain 1988;35:71–78.

143. Prkachin KM, Mercer SR. Pain expression in patients with shoulder pathology: validity, properties and relationship to sickness impact. Pain 1989;39:257–265.

144. Ekman P, Friesen WV. Facial Action Coding System: A technique for the Measurement of Facial Movement. Palo Alto, CA: Consulting Psychologists Press, 1978.

145. Choiniere M, Melzack R, Girard N, et al. Comparisons between patients' and nurses' assessments of pain and medication efficacy in severe burn injuries. Pain 1990;40:143–152.

146. Teske K, Daut RL, Cleeland CS. Relationships between nurses' observations and patients' self-reports of pain. Pain 1983;16:289–296.

147. Van der Does AJW. Patients' and nurses' ratings of pain and anxiety during burn wound care. Pain 1989;39:95–101.

148. Clipp EC, George LK. Patients with

cancer and their spouse caregivers. Cancer 1992; 69:1074–1079.

149. Madison JL, Wilkie DJ. Family members' perceptions of cancer pain. Comparisons with patient sensory report and by patient psychologic status. Nurs Clin North Am 1995;30:625–645.

150. Yeager KA, Miaskowski C, Dibble SL, Wallhagen M. Differences in pain knowledge and perceptions of the pain experience between outpatients with cancer and their family caregivers. Oncol Nurs Forum 1995;22:1235–1241.

151. Peyerwold M. Pain assessment. In: Coluzzi PH, Volker B, Miashowski C, eds. Comprehensive Pain Management in Terminal Illness. Sacramento: California State Hospice Association, 1996:29–34.

152. Levy M. Pain management in advanced cancer. Semin Oncol 1985;12:394–410.

APPENDIX

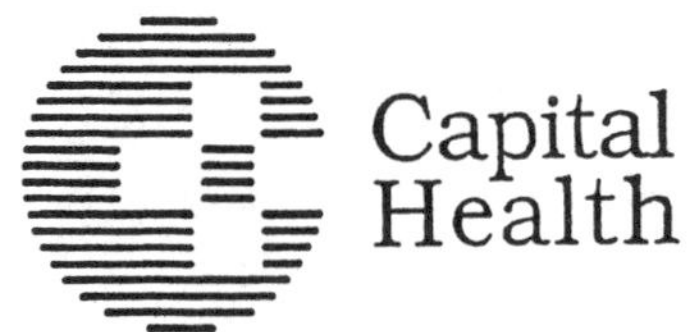

Regional Palliative Care Program Guideline

Title: Edmonton Comfort Assessment Form (ECAF) - Instructions for Use

Date: June 8, 1998 **Approved By:** Program Director

Purpose: Patient assessment is required throughout the palliative care process. The majority of patients will experience confusion and delirium before death. In these patients, who are unable to communicate, primary caregivers, and staffs input is important for assessment and for the opportunity to explain to the caregiver how to interpret the discomfort of the patient. This evaluation may decrease the caregivers concerns regarding the comfort of their family/friend

Procedure:

1. ECAF vs. ESAS: When to use: All patients admitted to all the palliative programs within the Edmonton region are assessed using the ESAS. When patients reach the unresponsive state of their illness, the ESAS will be discontinued and replaced by the ECAF. If patients present with brief periods of confusion or somnolence, then expect it to be reversible. The assessment should continue with ESAS. When the patient is considered to have reached the last hours or days of life the assessment will be changed to the ECAF.

   The decision to change the assessment system will be determined by the physicians and/or team leaders in the Acute Palliative Care Unit, it will be written by the Unit Managers in the 3 hospices, by the physician or nurse consultants at the Regional Palliative Care Program, and the Referral Centre palliative care program. In Home Care, the decision to change from ESAS to ECAF will be made by the Palliative Home Care Coordinator.

2. Frequency of Completion: At the end of the day/evening shift in the (Acute Palliative Care Unit), day shift in the (Hospices) or the nursing visit for patients assessed at home or in the referral centres.

3. Method of Completion: Please note that the form has two parts.

   a) Main Caregiver: This part should only be completed by the caregiver that is at the bedside most of the time; at home, in hospice, or in the palliative care unit. If no caregiver is present most of the time at the bedside checkmark not applicable . If there is a caregiver, he or she should be presented with the upper portion of the form and asked to circle the item #1 (comfort) and to check the appropriate reasons under item #2.

b) Nurse Score: The nurse will complete the form regarding behaviors. Please notice that these also have three items:
   i) Observed behavior: Rate the observed behavior according to the graph by placing an X in the appropriate box. Calculate the total score by adding the corresponding number for each X together. Maximum score is 24.
   ii) Checkmark the suspected reason(s).
   iii) Enter the global comfort assessment score from 0-10 (same as caregiver scale above).

4. After completing the form the information will be transcribed to the ECAF Graph. The ECAF Graph has the following components:

   a) Date and admission day: Please notice that there is enough room for two daily assessments (Acute Palliative Care Unit). Patients admitted to the hospices will undergo one assessment a day. Patients seen by the other teams will have one assessment done on occasion of each visit.

   b) Caregiver VAS (Item 1): Fill the bar up to the number across by the caregiver in the same way as we graph the results of the ESAS. If no caregiver enter N for not applicable.

   c) Caregiver Reason (Item 2): Simply check the reason(s) that have been checked in the ECAF form by the caregiver.

   d) Nurse Score (0-24): Write down on the space the number that results from adding each of the 6 line items for the observed behaviour (Item 1 of the Nursing Score).

   e) Nurse Reason: Check the suspected reason(s) identified by the nurse during the assessment.

   f) RN VAS: Enter the number of the nurse's assessment of the level of comfort (0-10).

   g) Physician VAS: Upon every visit (once a day on acute unit), on each visit in acute care, hospice and home) the physician assesses the level of comfort and enters the global comfort assessment score (0-10).

GUIDELINES FOR USING THE EDMONTON SYMPTOM ASSESSMENT SHEET (ESAS VISUAL ANALOGUE, NUMERICAL SCALE AND GRAPH)

1. This tool is designed to assist the patient in the assessment of his/her symptoms. Those symptoms include pain, activity, nausea, depression, anxiety, drowsiness, appetite, wellbeing and shortness of breath. The patient and family should be taught how to complete the scales. It is the patients opinion of the severity of the symptoms that is the "gold standard" for symptom assessment.

2. There are two formats for the ESAS. The first is a visual analogue scale (ESAS) that is 100mm long. The patient marks the line to indicate where the symptom is between the two extremes. (See Tool) This tool is used on the acute palliative care units, and referral hospital sites.

3. The other format, ESAS numerical is a scale from 0 to 10 where the patient circles the most appropriate number to indicate where the symptom is between the two extremes. This tool is used in all other settings, such as home care and continuing care. This tool is considered easier for a patient to complete with minimal assistance.

No pain	0	1	2	3	4	5	6	7	8	9	10	worst possible pain

The circled number on the continuum is then transcribed onto the symptom assessment graph. (ESAS graph) (See #12)

4. Synonyms for words that may be difficult for the patients to comprehend include the following:

Depression	-	blue or sad
Anxiety	-	nervous or restless
Drowsy	-	sleepy
Wellbeing	-	overall comfort both physical and psychological, truthfully answering the question, how are you?

5. For Home Care, during each telephone or personal contact, the ESAS scale should be completed and the values transferred to the ESAS graph. If the patient's symptoms are in good control, and there are no predominant psychosocial issues, the ESAS can be completed 2 to 3 times a week.

In continuing care settings the ESAS should be completed daily. Referral hospital site consultants will utilize the tool in their assessment on every visit. The ESAS is completed twice (~1000h, 1800h) on the acute palliative care unit.

6. In the home, or hospice, if the patient's symptoms are not in good control (>5/10), the nurse should be notifying the family doctor, and visiting the patient on a daily basis, until the symptoms are back within good control. (See #8)

7. If symptom management is not attained, or consultation about possible care options is needed, a consult to the Regional Palliative Care Program should occur. (***Family doctor must agree***). Informal consultation with the Regional program nurses and physicians can occur at any time.

8. A patient may consistently score high on an isolated symptom, and treatment has been actively pursued, until no resolution is possible. If at this point, consensus is reached between the coordinator and the family practitioner and/or consultant that a symptom cannot be modified, visits may return to their normal pattern for that patient.

9. Ideally, the patient should fill out their own assessment (ESAS). However, if there is cognitive impairment (ie: patient's mini-mental score below normal for their age and education) or lack of understanding on how to mark the continuum, the assessment becomes family assisted, or nurse.

10. The person who did the assessment must be identified on the symptom control graph. (ESAS graph)

P	=	Patient
N	=	Nurse/Health Care Worker
NA	=	Nurse/Health Care Worker Assisted
F	=	Family/Primary Caregiver

11. If the assessment is done by the nurse and she/he is unable to communicate with the patient (ie: cognitively impaired and cognition level might be reversible) she/he assesses the following areas only: pain, activity, nausea, drowsiness, appetite and shortness of breath.

NB: **<u>ACTIVITY</u> IS A PURPOSEFUL VOLUNTARY ACTION BY THE PATIENT. CONSIDER THE PATIENT NOT ACTIVE IF HE/SHE IS RESTLESS OR AGITATED**

<u>APPETITE</u> BECOMES THE ABSENCE OR PRESENCE OF EATING

<u>NAUSEA</u> BECOMES THE ABSENCE OR PRESENCE OF RETCHING, VOMITING, ETC.

12. The nurse can document her assessment directly on the Symptom Assessment Graph (ESASII). She does not have to fill out the ESAS scale. The ESAS graph is kept in the patient home envelope, and a copy on the patient chart. The chart copy should be brought to the home and updated with the home copy, on each visit.

13. A patient has the right to refuse the symptom assessment or any question on it. In the event the patient refuses to do his/her own assessment, it becomes a nurse assessment (see # 10,11)

15. The ESAS is available in Cantonese, German, French and in faces, for those patients who do not read.

16. The ESASII (graph) provides an excellent clinical "picture" or "snapshot" of how a patient is feeling in various physical or psychological areas. You may see a symptom increase or decrease over time. On rare occasions, a patient may score everything as 9 or 10 out of 10. The graph looks very black and shows a picture of total pain or total suffering. A patient with this picture requires interdisciplinary support.[1]

17. The Graph also contains space to add the patient's mini mental state exam score. The "normal" box refers to the normal range for the patient, based on age and education level (see Instructions for MMSE).

18. Modified EFAT score can be entered on this form (as applicable).

19. A new assessment tool for patients who are not able to complete their own ESAS is currently being developed. (Edmonton Discomfort Assessment Tool).

6 Pain at the End of Life

JUDITH A. PAICE and PERRY G. FINE

If I have to die—do I have to die in pain too?

—A patient

Of the many symptoms experienced by those at the end of life, pain is one of the most common and most feared.[1] However, this fear is largely unfounded as the majority of patients with terminal illness can obtain relief. Nurses are critical members of the palliative care team, particularly in providing pain management. The nurse's role begins with assessment, continuing throughout the development of a plan of care and its implementation. During this process, the nurse provides education and counsel to the patient, family, and other team members. Nurses also are critical to the development of institutional policies and the monitoring of outcomes that ensure good pain management to all patients within their palliative care program. To provide optimal pain control, all health care professionals must understand the frequency of pain at the end of life, the barriers that prevent good management, the assessment of this syndrome, and the treatments used to provide relief.

PREVALENCE

The prevalence of pain in the terminally ill varies by diagnosis and other factors. Approximately one-third of persons who are actively receiving treatment for cancer and two-thirds of those with advanced malignant disease experience pain.[2–6] Individuals at particular risk for undertreatment include the elderly, minorities, and women.[7–9] Almost three-quarters of patients with advanced cancer admitted to the hospital experience pain upon admission.[10] In a study of cancer patients very near the end of life, pain occurred in 54% and 34% at 4 weeks and 1 week prior to death, respectively.[5] In other studies of patients admitted to palliative care units, pain often is the dominant symptom, along with fatigue and dyspnea.[1,11]

More recently, an attempt has been made to characterize the pain experience of those with human immunodeficiency virus (HIV) disease, a disorder frequently seen in palliative care settings. In a retrospective chart review of 50 patients with acquired immune deficiency syndrome (AIDS) at the end of life (prognosis of 6 months or less), the "present" pain averaged 7.47 (using a 0–10 scale).[12] Activity was reduced in 16% of patients, and 15% reported depressed mood as a result of pain. Headache, abdominal pain, chest pain, and neuropathies were the most frequently reported types of pain. Lower $CD4^+$ cell counts were associated with higher rates of neuropathy.[13] Numerous studies have reported undertreatment of persons with HIV disease.[14–17]

Unfortunately, there has been very little characterization of the pain prevalence and experience of patients with other life-threatening disorders. However, those working in palliative care are well aware that pain frequently accompanies many of the neuromuscular and cardiovascular disorders, such as multiple sclerosis and stroke, seen at the end of life.[18,19] Furthermore, many patients seen in hospice and palliative care are elderly and more likely to have existing chronic pain syndromes, such as osteoarthritis.[20]

Additional research is needed to fully characterize the frequency of pain and the type of pain syndromes seen in patients at the end of life. This information will lead to improved detection, assessment, and ultimately treatment. Unfortunately, pain continues to be undertreated, even when prevalence rates and syndromes are well understood. The undertreatment is largely due to barriers related to health care professionals, the system, and patients and their families.

BARRIERS

Barriers to good pain relief are numerous and pervasive. Often, due to lack of education, misconceptions, and attitudinal issues, these barriers contribute to the large numbers of patients who do not get adequate pain relief.[21] The Agency for Health Care Policy and Research guidelines differentiate these barriers by the health care professional, the health care system, and the patient (Table 6–1).[22] Careful examination of these barriers provides a guide for changing individual practice, as well as building an institutional plan within the palliative care program to improve pain relief. These barriers specifically address cancer pain. The barriers facing individuals with other disorders commonly seen in palliative care have not been as thoroughly studied. One might suggest that these individuals are affected to an even greater extent as biases may be more pronounced in those with noncancer diagnoses.

Health Care Providers

Fears held by professionals related to opioids lead to underuse of these analgesics. Numerous surveys have revealed that physicians and nurses express concerns about addiction, tolerance, and side effects of morphine and related compounds.[23–25] Inevitability of pain is also expressed, despite evidence to the contrary.[26] Not surprisingly, lack of at-

Table 6–1. Barriers to Cancer Pain Management

Problems related to health care professionals
Inadequate knowledge of pain management
Poor assessment of pain
Concern about regulation of controlled substances
Fear of patient addiction
Concern about side effects of analgesics
Concern about patients becoming tolerant to analgesics
Problems related to the health care system
Low priority given to cancer pain treatment
Inadequate reimbursement
Restrictive regulation of controlled substances
Problems of availability of treatment or access to it
Problems related to patients
Reluctance to report pain
Concern that distracting physicians from treatment of underlying disease
Fear that pain means disease is worse
Concern about not being a "good" patient
Reluctance to take pain medications
Fear of addiction or of being thought of as an addict
Worries about unmanageable side effects
Concern about becoming tolerant to pain medications.

Source: Jacox et al. (1994), reference 22.

tention to pain and its treatment during basic education is frequently cited.[27,28] Those providing care at the end of life must evaluate their own knowledge and beliefs and strive to educate themselves and colleagues.

Health Care Settings

Lack of availability of opioids is pervasive, affecting not only sparsely populated rural settings but also inner-city pharmacies reluctant to carry these medications. Pain management continues to be a low priority, although the new Joint Commission on Accreditation of Healthcare Organizations (JCAHO) standards on pain management will help to alleviate this problem.[29] All JCAHO-certified clinical settings must evaluate their procedures to ensure that pain is appropriately assessed, treated, and documented.

Patients

Understanding these barriers will lead the professional to better educate and counsel patients. Since these fears are pervasive, patients and family members or support persons should be asked if they are concerned about addiction and tolerance (often described as becoming "immune" to the drug by laypersons). Studies have suggested that these fears lead to undermedication and increased intensity of pain.[30–32] Concerns about being a "good" patient or belief in the inevitability of cancer pain lead patients to hesitate in reporting pain.[30,33–35] In these studies, less educated and older patients were more likely to express these beliefs.

At the end of life, patients may need to rely on family members or other support persons to dispense medications. Each person's concerns must be addressed or provision of medication may be inadequate. Studies suggest that little concordance exists between patients' and family members' beliefs regarding analgesics.[36] The interdisciplinary team is essential, with nurses, social workers, chaplains, physicians, volunteers, and others providing exploration of the meaning of pain and possible barriers to good relief. Education, counseling, reframing, and spiritual support are imperative. Ersek[37] provided an excellent review of the assessment and interventional approaches indicated for specific patient barriers.

EFFECTS OF UNRELIEVED PAIN

Although many professionals and laypersons fear that opioid analgesics lead to shortened life, there is significant evidence to the contrary. Inadequate pain relief hastens death by increasing physiological stress, potentially diminishing immunocompetence, decreasing mobility, worsening proclivities toward pneumonia and thromboembolism, and increasing work of breathing and myocardial oxygen requirements. Furthermore, pain may lead to spiritual death as the individual's quality of life is impaired. Therefore, it is the professional and ethical responsibility of clinicians to focus on and attend to adequate pain relief for their patients and to properly educate patients and their caregivers about opioid analgesic therapies.[38–45]

ASSESSMENT AND COMMON PAIN SYNDROMES

Comprehensive assessment of pain is imperative. This must be conducted initially, regularly throughout the treatment, and during any changes in the patient's pain state.[22,46] A recent randomized controlled trial using algorithms found that the comprehensive pain assessment integral to these algorithms contributed to reduced pain intensity scores.[47] For a complete discussion of pain assessment, see Chapter 5.

PHARMACOLOGICAL MANAGEMENT OF CONTINUOUS AND EPISODIC PAIN IN ADVANCED AND END-STAGE DISEASE

A sound understanding of pharmacotherapy in the treatment of pain is of great importance in palliative care nursing. First, this knowledge allows the nurse to contribute to and fully understand the comprehensive plan of care. Thorough understanding also allows the nurse to recognize and assess medication-related adverse effects, understand drug–drug and drug–disease interactions, and educate patients and caregivers regarding appropriate medication usage. This will assure a comfortable process of dying for the well-being of the patient and for the sake of those in attendance.

This section provides an overview of

the most commonly used and some of the newer pharmaceutical agents available in the United States for the treatment of unremitting and recurrent pain associated with advanced disease. The intent of this section is to arm the reader with a fundamental and practical understanding of the medications that are (or should be) available in most contemporary care settings, emphasizing those therapies for which there is clear and convincing evidence of efficacy. For an extensive review of mechanisms of pain and analgesia, pharmacological principles of analgesics, and more detailed lists of all drugs used for pain control throughout the world, the reader is referred to recent comprehensive reviews.[38,39,48–60]

Non-opioid Analgesics

Acetaminophen. Acetaminophen has been determined to be one of the safest analgesics for long-term use in the management of mild pain or as a supplement in the management of more intense pain syndromes.[61–63] It is especially useful in the management of non specific musculoskeletal pains or pain associated with osteoarthritis, but acetaminophen (also abbreviated as APAP) should be considered an adjunct to any chronic pain regimen. It is often forgotten or overlooked when severe pain is being treated, so a reminder of its value as a "co-analgesic" is warranted. However, acetaminophen's limited antiinflammatory effect should be considered when selecting a nonopioid. Reduced doses or avoidance of acetaminophen is recommended in the face of renal insufficiency or liver failure.[64,65]

Nonsteroidal Antiinflammatory Drugs. Nonsteroidal antiinflammatory drugs (NSAIDs) affect analgesia by reducing the biosynthesis of prostaglandins, thereby inhibiting the cascade of inflammatory events that cause, amplify, or maintain nociception. These agents also appear to reduce pain by influences on the peripheral or central nervous system independent of their antiinflammatory mechanism of action. This secondary mode of analgesic efficacy is poorly understood.[66] The "classic" NSAIDs (e.g., aspirin) are relatively nonselective in their inhibitory effects on the enzymes that convert arachidonic acid to prostaglandins.[67] As a result, gastrointestinal ulceration and renal dysfunction are common.[68,69] A new class of NSAIDs selectively blocks the cyclooxygenase-2 (COX-2) enzymatic pathway, which is induced by tissue injury or other inflammation-inducing conditions. It is for this reason that there appears to be less risk of gastrointestinal bleeding, renal dysfunction, and generalized bleeding with continuous or prolonged use of the COX-2 NSAIDs.[67,70] These COX-2 NSAIDs include celecoxib (Celebrex) and refocoxib (Vioxx). Because there is cross-sensitivity, patients allergic to sulfa-containing drugs should not be given celecoxib (Table 6–2).

The NSAIDs, as a class, are very useful in the treatment of many pain conditions mediated by inflammation, including those caused by cancer.[71,72] There are insufficient data to determine whether the newly available COX-2 agents have any specific advantages over the nonselective NSAIDs in the management of pain due to conditions such as metastatic bone pain. The NSAIDs do offer the potential advantage of causing minimal nausea, constipation, sedation, or other effects on mental functioning, although there is evidence that short-term memory in older patients can be impaired by them.[73] Therefore, depending on the cause of pain, NSAIDs may be very useful for moderate to severe pain control, either alone or as an adjunct to opioid analgesic therapy. The addition of NSAIDs to opioids has the benefit of potentially allowing the reduction of the opioid dose when sedation, obtundation, confusion, dizziness, or other central nervous system effects

Table 6–2. Acetaminophen and Selected Nonsteroidal Antiinflammatory Drugs

Drug	Dose if patient >50 kg	Dose if patient <50 kg
Acetaminophen*†	4000 mg/24 h q 4–6 h	10–15 mg/kg q 4 h (oral) 15–20 mg/kg q 4 h (rectal)
Aspirin*†	4000 mg/24 h q 4–6 h	10–15 mg/kg q 4 h (oral) 15–20 mg/kg q 4 h (rectal)
Ibuprofen*†	2400 mg/24 h q 6–8 h	10 mg/kg q 6–8 h (oral)
Naproxen*†	1000 mg/24 h q 8–12 h	5 mg/kg q 8 h (oral/rectal)
Choline magnesium trisalicylate*§	2000–3000 mg/24 h q 8–12 h	25 mg/kg q 8 h (oral)
Indomethacin†	75–150 mg/24 h q 8–12 h	0.5–1 mg/kg q 8–12 h (oral/rectal)
Ketorolac‡	30–60 mg IM/IV initially, then 15–30 mg q 6 h bolus IV/IM or continuous IV/SQ infusion; short-term use only (3–5 days)	0.25–1 mg//kg q 6 h short-term use only (3–5 days)
Celecoxib§¶	100–200 mg PO up to b.i.d.	No data available
Refocoxib§¶	25–50 mg po q day	No data available

* Commercially available in a liquid form.
† Commercially available in a suppository form.
‡ Potent antiinflammatory (short-term use only due to gastrointestinal side effects).
§ Minimal platelet dysfunction.
¶Cyclooxygenase-2-selective nonsteroidal antiinflammatory drug.

of opioid analgesic therapy alone become burdensome.[73] As with acetaminophen, decreased renal function and liver failure are relative contraindications for NSAID use. Similarly, platelet dysfunction or other potential bleeding disorders contraindicate use of the nonselective NSAIDs due to their inhibitory effects on platelet aggregation, with resultant prolonged bleeding time.

Table 6–3. Definitions

Tolerance: Reduced effect from repeated doses of the same drug class.
Physical Dependence: A pharmacological phenomenon associated with repeated doses of the same drug class, characterized by an abstinence syndrome when abrupt drug discontinuation occurs or an antagonist is administered.
Addiction: A compulsive or overpowering drive to take a drug in order to experience psychological effects, even in the face of known potential self-harm.
Pseudoaddiction: The mistaken assumption of addiction in a patient who is seeking relief from pain.
*Pseudotolerance:*The misconception that the need for increasing doses of drug is due to tolerance rather than disease progression or other factor.

Source: Jacox et al. (1994), reference 22.

Opioid Analgesics

As a pharmacological class, the opioid analgesics represent the most useful agents for the treatment of pain associated with advanced disease. The opioids are nonspecific insofar as they decrease pain signal transmission and perception throughout the nervous system, regardless of the pathophysiology of the pain.[74] Moderate to severe pain is the main clinical indication for the opioid analgesics. Other indications include the treatment of dyspnea, use as an anesthetic adjunct, and as a form of prophylactic therapy in the treatment of psychological dependence to opioids (e.g., methadone maintenance for those with a history of heroin abuse).

The only absolute contraindication to the use of an opioid is a history of a hypersensitivity reaction (rash, wheezing, edema). Allergic reactions are almost exclusively limited to the morphine derivatives. In the rare event that a patient describes a true allergic reaction, one might begin therapy with a low dose of a short-acting synthetic opioid (e.g., intravenous fentanyl) or try an intradermal injection as a test dose. The rationale for using a synthetic opioid (preferably one without dyes or preservatives since these can cause allergic reactions) is that the prevalence of allergic reactions is much lower. If the patient does develop a reaction, using a low dose of a short-acting opioid will produce a reduced response for a shorter period of time when compared to long-acting preparations.

Because misunderstandings lead to undertreatment, it is incumbent upon all clinicians involved in the care of patients with chronic pain to clearly understand and differentiate the clinical conditions of tolerance, physical dependence, addiction, pseudoaddiction, and pseudotolerance (Table 6–3).

It is also critically important for clinicians who are involved in patient care to be aware that titration of opioid analgesics to affect pain relief is rarely associated with induced respiratory depression and iatrogenic death.[75] In fact, the most compelling evidence suggests that inadequate pain relief hastens death by increasing physiological stress, decreasing immunocompetence, diminishing mobility, increasing the potential for thromboembolism, worsening inspiration and thus placing the patient at risk for pneumonia, and increasing myocardial oxygen requirements.[38–45] Furthermore, in a recent survey of high-dose opioid use (>299 mg oral morphine equivalents) in a hospice setting, there was no relationship between opioid dose and survival.[76]

In a study of patients with advanced cancer, no reliable predictors for opioid dose were identified.[10] There is significant inter-and intraindividual variation in clinical responses to the various opioids, so in most cases, a dose-titration approach should be viewed as the best means of optimizing care. This implies that close follow-up is required to determine when clinical end points have been reached. Furthermore, idiosyncratic responses may require trials of different agents in order to determine the most effective drug and route of delivery for any given patient.[77] Table 6–4 lists more specific suggestions regarding optimal use of opioids.

Another factor that needs to be continually considered with opioid analgesics is the potential to accumulate toxic metabolites, especially in the face of decreasing drug clearance and elimination as disease progresses and organ function deteriorates.[78] Due to its neurotoxic metabolite, normeperidine, me-

Table 6–4. Guidelines for the Use of Opioids

Clinical studies and experience suggest that adherence to some basic precepts will help optimize care of patients who require opioid analgesic therapy for pain control:

- Intramuscular administration is highly discouraged except in "pain emergency" states when nothing else is available.
- New noninvasive drug delivery systems that "bypass" the enteral route (e.g., the transdermal and the oral transmucosal routes for delivery of fentanyl for treatment of continuous pain and breakthrough pain, respectively) may obviate the necessity to use parenteral routes for pain control in some patients who cannot take medications orally or rectally.
- Anticipation, prevention, and treatment of sedation, constipation, nausea, psychotomimetic effects, and myoclonus should be part of every care plan for patients being treated with opioid analgesics.
- Changing from one opioid to another or one route to another is often necessary, so facility with this process is an absolute necessity. Remember the following points:
  - Incomplete cross-tolerance occurs, leading to decreased requirements of a newly prescribed opioid.
  - Use morphine equivalents as a "common denominator" for all dose conversions in order to avoid errors.

peridine use is specifically discouraged for chronic pain management.[79] As well, the mixed agonist–antagonist agents, typified by butorphanol, nalbuphine, and pentazocine, are not recommended for the treatment of chronic pain. They have limited efficacy, and their use may cause an acute abstinence syndrome in patients who are otherwise using pure agonist opioid analgesics.[80]

Morphine. Morphine is most often considered the "gold standard" of opioid analgesics and is used as a measure for dose equivalence (Table 6–5).[81] Some patients cannot tolerate morphine due to itching, headache, dysphoria, or other adverse effects.[82] However, common initial dosing effects such as sedation and nausea often resolve within a few days. In fact, one should anticipate these adverse effects, especially constipation, nausea, and sedation, and prevent or treat appropriately (see below). The metabolites of morphine (morphine-3-glucuronide and morphine-6-glucuronide) are active and may contribute to sedation, myoclonus, and psychotomimetic effects.[78] Side effects and metabolic effects can be differentiated by the time course. Side effects generally occur soon after the drug has had time to absorb, whereas there is a delay of several doses of the drug administered over several days associated with metabolite effects. If adverse effects exceed the analgesic benefit of the drug, convert to an equianalgesic dose of a different opioid. Because cross-tolerance is incomplete, reduce the calculated dose by one-third to one-half and titrate upward based on the patient's pain intensity scores.[40]

Morphine's bitter taste may be prohibitive, especially if "immediate-release" tablets are left in the mouth to dissolve. When patients have dysphagia, several options are available. The 24-hour, long-acting morphine capsule can be broken open and the "sprinkles" placed in applesause or other soft food.[83] Oral morphine solution can be swallowed, or small volumes (0.5 to 1 ml) of a concentrated solution (e.g., 20 mg/ml) can be placed in the mouth of patients whose voluntary swallowing capabilities are more significantly limited.[84] Transmucosal uptake of morphine is slow and not very predictable due to its hydrophilic chemical nature. In fact, most of the analgesic effect of a morphine tablet or liquid placed buccally or sublingually is due to drug trickling down the throat and the resultant absorption through the gastrointestinal tract. Furthermore, again due to the hydrophilic nature of morphine, creams and patches that contain morphine provide little if any analgesic effect. Another useful route of administration when oral delivery is unreasonable is the rectal route.[84] Commercially prepared suppositories, compounded suppositories, or microenemas can be used to deliver drug into the rectum or stoma.[85–87] Sustained-release morphine tablets have been used rectally, with resultant delayed time to peak plasma level and approximately 90% of the bioavailability achieved by oral administration.[88]

Table 6–5. Approximate Equianalgesic Doses of Most Commonly Used Opioid Analgesics

Drug	Parenteral Route	Enteral Route
Morphine†	10 mg	30 mg
Codeine	130 mg	200 mg (not recommended)
Fentanyl‡ ††	50–100 mcg	OTFC available‡
Hydrocodone	Not available	30 mg
Hydromorphone§	1.5 mg	7.5 mg
Levorphanol¶	2 mg acute, 1 chronic	4 mg acute, 1 chronic
Methadone¶	10 mg acute, 2–4 chronic	20 mg acute, 2–4 chronic
Oxycodone††	Not available	20–30 mg

*Dose conversion should be closely monitored since incomplete cross-tolerance may occur.
†Available in continuous and sustained-release pills and capsules, formulated to last 12 or 24 hours. Interindividual variation in duration of analgesic effect is not uncommon, signaling the need to increase the dose or shorten the dose interval.
‡Also available in transdermal and oral transmucosal forms, see package insert materials for dose recommendations. OTFC = oral transmucosal fentanyl citrate.
§Available soon as a continuous-release formulation lasting 24 hours.
¶These drugs have long half-lives, so accumulation can occur; close monitoring during first few days of therapy is very important.
**Available in several continuous-release doses, formulated to last 12 hours. Interindividual variation in duration of analgesic effect is not uncommon, signaling the need to increase the dose or shorten the dose interval.
††Fentanyl 100 mcg patch ≅ 4 mg IV morphine/h.

Transdermal Fentanyl. Transdermal fentanyl, often called the fentanyl patch, is particularly useful when patients cannot swallow, do not remember to take medications, or have adverse effects to other opioids.[89] Opioid-naive patients should start with a 25 mcg/h patch (currently the lowest available dose) after evaluation of effects with immediate-release opioids (Table 6–6). Patients should be monitored by a responsible caregiver for the first 24 to 48 hours of therapy until steady-state blood levels are attained. Fever, diaphoresis, cachexia, morbid obesity, and ascites may have a significant impact on the absorption, predictability of blood levels, and clinical effects of transdermal fentanyl; thus, this form of administration may not be appropriate in these conditions.[90] The specific effects of body mass and temperature on absorption have not been studied. Some believe the changes in fat stores (seen with cachexia) alter the fat depot needed for absorption of this lipid-soluble compound. There is some suggestion that transdermal fentanyl may produce less constipation when compared to long-acting morphine.[91] Further study is needed to confirm these findings.

Some patients experience decreased analgesic effects after only 48 hours of applying a new patch; this should be accommodated by determining if a higher dose is tolerated with increased duration of effect or a more frequent (q 48 h) patch change should be scheduled. As with all long-acting preparations, break-

Table 6–6. Fentanyl Patch Instructions to Patients and Caregivers

1. Place patch on the upper body in a clean, dry, hairless area (clip hair, do not shave).
2. Choose a different site when placing a new patch, then remove the old patch.
3. Remove the old patch or patches and fold sticky surfaces together, then flush down the toilet.
4. Wash hands after handling patches.
5. All unused patches (patient discontinued use or deceased) should be removed from wrappers, folded in half with sticky surfaces together, and flushed down the toilet.

through pain medications should be made available to patients using continuous-release opioids such as the fentanyl patch. Several reports have documented the safe and effective use of subcutaneous fentanyl when the transdermal approach could no longer provide relief or side effects occurred to other opioids.[92] However, parenteral fentanyl is commercially available in a 50 mcg/ml concentration. Higher doses may preclude the subcutaneous route. When this occurs, the intravenous route is warranted.

Oral Transmucosal Fentanyl Citrate. Oral transmucosal fentanyl citrate (OTFC or Actiq) is composed of fentanyl on an applicator that patients rub against the oral mucosa to provide rapid absorption of the drug.[93] This formulation of fentanyl is particularly useful for breakthrough pain, described later in this chapter. One example of OTFC use would be pain relief of rapid onset or during a brief but painful dressing change. Adults should start with the 200 mcg dose and monitor efficacy, advancing to higher dose units as needed.[94] Clinicians must be aware that, unlike other breakthrough pain drugs, the around-the-clock dose of opioid does not predict the effective does of OTFC. Pain relief can usually be expected in about 5 minutes after beginning use.[94] Patients should use OTFC over a period of 15 minutes as too rapid use will result in more of the agent being swallowed rather than absorbed transmucosally. Any remaining partial units should be disposed of by placing under hot water or inserting the unit in a child-resistant temporary storage bottle provided when the drug is first dispensed.

Levorphanol, Methadone. Levorphanol and methadone are potentially useful in selected patients as second-line opioid analgesics due to their somewhat long durations of effect, making dosing intervals (q 6 h) relatively convenient compared with other immediate-release opioids (although some patients require 4-hour dosing).[95,96] Also, methadone is much less costly than comparable doses of proprietary continuous-release formulations, making it potentially more available for patients without sufficient financial resources for more costly drugs.[97,98] The dose ratio between morphine and methadone remains unclear, ranging from 1:1 to 4:1 (4 mg of oral morphine is approximately equal to 1 mg of methadone).[99] Based on newer studies and experiences with methadone, the American Pain Society[40] recommends the equianalgesic dose of 20 mg oral methadone equal 10 mg parenterally when used in acute situations and 2 to 4 mg po approximately equal to that dose parenterally when given chronically. Thus, caution is warranted when converting from another opioid to methadone. Clinical experience suggests cutting back as much as 75% to 80% of the equianalgesic dose when converting to methadone from a short half-life drug such as morphine or hydromorphone.

The long half-lives of both levorphanol (12–16 hours) and methadone (24–36 hours or longer) increase the potential for drug accumulation prior to achievement of steady-state blood levels, putting patients at risk for oversedation and respiratory depression.[40] This might occur on day 2 to 3 of levorphanol administration and after 2 to 5 days of treatment with methadone. Close monitoring of these potentially adverse or even life-threatening effects is required.

Other Opioids. Hydromorphone (Dilaudid) is a useful alternative when synthetic opioids provide an advantage. Available in oral tablets, liquids, suppositories, and parenteral formulations, hydromorphone will soon be available in the United States in a long-acting formulation. Oxycodone is available in a long-acting formulation (OxyContin), as well as immediate-release tablets (alone or with acetaminophen) and liquid. As synthetic opioids, hydromorphone and oxycodone provide an advantage when patients have true allergic responses to morphine or inadequate pain control or intolerable side effects or when renal function is poor and morphine metabolites accumulate.

Alternative Routes. Many routes of administration are available when patients can no longer swallow or when other dynamics preclude the oral route or favor other routes. These include transdermal, transmucosal, rectal, vaginal, topical, epidural, and intrathecal. In a study of cancer patients at 4 weeks, 1 week, and 24 hours before death, the oral route of opioid administration was continued in 62%, 43%, and 20% of patients, respectively. Over half of these patients required more than one route of opioid administration. As patients approached death and oral use diminished, the use of intermittent subcutaneous injections and intravenous or subcutaneous infusions increased.[5]

Thus, in the palliative care setting, nonoral routes of administration must be available. Enteral feeding tubes can be used to access the gut when patients can no longer swallow. The size of the tube should be considered when placing long-acting morphine "sprinkles," to avoid obstruction of the tube. The rectum, stoma, or vagina can be used to deliver medication. Thrombocytopenia or painful lesions preclude the use of these routes. Additionally, delivering medications via these routes can be difficult for family members, especially when the patient is obtunded or unable to assist. Because the vagina has no sphincter, a tampon covered with a condom or an inflated urinary catheter balloon may be used to prevent early discharge of the drug.[86] As previously discussed, transdermal fentanyl is a useful alternative to these techniques.

Parenteral administration includes subcutaneous and intravenous delivery (intramuscular opioid delivery is inappropriate in the palliative care setting). The intravenous route provides rapid drug delivery but requires vascular access, placing the patient at risk for infection. Subcutaneous boluses have a slower onset and lower peak effect when compared with intravenous boluses.[40] Subcutaneous infusions may include up to 10 ml/h (although most patients absorb 2 to 3 ml/h with least difficulty). Volumes greater than these are poorly absorbed. Hyaluronidase has been reported to speed absorption of subcutaneously administered drugs.[100]

Intraspinal routes of administration have a limited role in end-of-life care. The epidural or intrathecal route may allow delivery of drugs, such as opioids, local anesthetics, and/or α-adrenergic agonists, which may provide relief in pain refractory to conventional routes.[101] However, the equipment used to deliver these medications is complex, requiring specialized knowledge for health care professionals and potentially greater caregiver burden. Risk of infection is also of concern. Furthermore, cost is a significant concern related to high-technology procedures. See Chapter 22 for a review of high-technology procedures for pain relief.

Preventing and Treating Adverse Effects

Constipation. Always begin a prophylactic bowel regimen when commencing opioid analgesic therapy.[102] Avoid bulking agents (e.g., psyllium) since these tend to cause a larger, bulkier stool, increasing desiccation time in the large bowel. Furthermore, debilitated patients can rarely take in sufficient fluid to facilitate the action of bulking agents. Fluid intake should be encouraged whenever feasible. Senna tea and fruits may be of use. For a more comprehensive review, refer to Chapter 11.

Sedation. Excessive sedation may occur with the initial doses of opioids.[103] If sedation persists after 24 to 48 hours and other correctable causes have been identified and treated if possible, the use of psychostimulants may be beneficial. These include dextroamphetamine 2.5 to 5 mg PO q morning and mid-day or methylphenidate 5 to 10 mg PO q morning and 2.5 to 5 mg mid-day (although higher doses are frequently used). Adjust both the dose and timing to prevent nocturnal insomnia and monitor for undesirable psychotomimetic effects (such as agitation, hallucinations, and irritability).

Respiratory Depression. Respiratory depression is rarely a clinically significant problem for opioid-tolerant patients in pain.[41,51] When respiratory depression occurs in a patient with advanced disease, the cause is usually multifactorial. Therefore, other factors beyond opioids need to be assessed, although opioids are frequently blamed for the reduced repirations. When undesired depressed consciousness occurs along with a respiratory rate <8/min or hypoxemia (O_2 saturation <90%) associated with opioid use, cautious and slow titration of naloxone should be instituted. Excessive administration may cause abrupt opioid reversal with pain and autonomic crisis. Dilute 1 ampule of naloxone (0.4 mg/ml) in 10 ml of injectable saline (final concentration 40 mcg/ml) and inject 1 ml every 2 to 3 minutes while closely monitoring the level of consciousness and respiratory rate. Because the duration of effect of naloxone is approximately 30 minutes, the depressant effects of the opioid will recur at 30 minutes and persist until the plasma levels decline (often 4 or more hours) or until the next dose of naloxone is administered.[40]

Nausea and Vomiting. Nausea and vomiting are common with opioids due to activation of the chemoreceptor trigger zone in the medulla, vestibular sensitivity, and delayed gastric emptying, but habituation occurs in most cases within several days.[104,105] Assess for other treatable causes. In severe cases or when nausea and vomiting are not self-limited, pharmacotherapy is indicated. The doses of nausea-relieving medications and antiemetics listed below are to be used initially but can be increased as required. See Chapter 9 for a thorough discussion of the assessment and treatment of nausea and vomiting.

Myoclonus. Myoclonic jerking occurs more commonly with high-dose opioid therapy.[97,127,165,166] If this should develop, switch to an alternate opioid, especially if using morphine, since evidence suggests this symptom is associated with metabolite accumulation. A lower relative dose of the substituted drug may be possible, due to incomplete cross-tolerance, which might result in decreased myoclonus. Clonazepam 0.5 to 1 mg PO q 6 to 8 h, to be increased as needed and tolerated, may be useful in treating myoclonus in patients who are still alert, able to communicate, and take oral preparations. Lorazepam can be given sublingually if the patient is unable to swallow. Otherwise, parenteral administration of diazepam is indicated if symptoms are distressing. Grand mal seizures associated with high-dose parenteral opioid infusions have been reported and may be due to preservatives in the solution.[106] Preservative-free solutions should be used when administering high-dose infusions.

Pruritus. Pruritus[107] appears to be most common with morphine, in part due to histamine release, but can occur with most opioids. Fentanyl and oxymorphone may be less likely to cause histamine release.[40] Most antipruritus therapies cause sedation, so this side effect must be viewed by the patient as an acceptable trade-off. Antihistamines (such as diphenydramine) are the most common first-line approach to this opioid-induced symptom when treatment is indicated. Ondansetron has been reported to be effective in relieving opioid-induced pruritus, but no randomized controlled studies exist.[108]

Adjuvant Analgesics

A wide variety of nonopioid medications from several pharmacological classes have been demonstrated to reduce pain caused by various pathological conditions (Table 6–7). As a group, these drugs have been called analgesic "adjuvants," but this is something of a misnomer since they often reduce pain when used alone. However, under most circumstances, when these drugs are indicated for the treatment of severe neuropathic pain or bone pain, opioid analgesics are used concomitantly to provide adequate pain relief.

Antidepressants. The mechanism of the analgesic effect of tricyclic antidepressants appears to be related to inhibition

Table 6–7. Adjuvant Analgesics

Drug Class	Daily Adult Starting Dose* (Range)	Routes of Administration	Adverse Effects	Indications
Tricyclic antidepressants	Amitriptyline 10–25 mg Nortriptyline 10–25 mg Desipramine 10–25 mg	PO	Anticholinergic effects	Neuropathic pain, such as burning pain, poor sleep
Anticonvulsants	Clonazapam 0.5–1 mg hs, bid or tid	PO	Sedation	Neuropathic pain, such as shooting pain
	Carbamazapine 100 mg q day or tid	PO		
	Gabapentin 100 mg q day or tid	PO		
Corticosteroids	Dexamethasone 2–4 mg tid, qid, or q day; may give up to 100 mg IV bolus for pain crises	PO/IV/SQ	"Steroid psychosis," dyspepsia	Cerebral edema, spinal cord compression, bone pain, neuropathic pain, visceral pain
	Prednisone 15–30 mg tid, qid	PO		
Local anesthetics	Mexiletine 150 mg tid	PO	Lightheadedness, arrhthymias	Neuropathic pain
	Lidocaine 1–5 mg/kg hourly	IV or SQ infusion		
N-Methyl-D-aspartate antagonists	Dextromethorphan, effective dose unknown	PO	Confusion	Neuropathic pain
	Ketamine (see Pain Crises)	IV		
Bisphosphonates	Pamidronate 60–90 mg over 2 h every 2–4 weeks	IV infusion	Pain flare	Osteolytic bone pain
Calcitonin	25 IU/day	SQ/nasal	Hypersensitivity reaction, nausea	Neuropathic pain, bone pain
Capsaicin	0.025–0.075%	Topical	Burning	Neuropathic pain
Baclofen	10 mg q day or qid	PO	Muscle weakness, cognitive changes	
Calcium channel blockers	Nifedipine 10 mg tid	PO	Bradycardia, hypotension	Ischemic pain neuropathic pain, smooth muscle spasms with pain

*Pediatric doses for pain control not well established.

of norepinephrine and serotonin.[109,110] Amitriptyline and nortriptyline produce more sedation than desipramine; therefore, the first two should be given at bedtime and the latter in the morning. Cardiac arrhythmias, conduction abnormalities, narrow-angle glaucoma, and clinically significant prostatic hyperplasia are relative contraindications to the tricyclic antidepressants.[111] The delay in onset of pain relief, from days to weeks, may preclude the use of these agents for pain relief in end-of-life care. However, their sleep-enhancing and mood-elevating effects may be of benefit.

Anticonvulsants. The older anticonvulsants, such as carbamazepine and clonazepam, relieve pain by blocking sodium channels.[112] Often referred to as membrane stabilizers, these compounds are very useful in the treatment of neuropathic pain, especially those with episodic, lancinating qualities. The newest anticonvulsant, gabapentin, has a different, as yet unclear mechanism of action. Formerly believed to act on the γ-aminobutyric acid system, this drug may have N-methyl-D-aspartate (NMDA) antagonist and other analgesic activities.[113] The analgesic doses of gabapentin reported to relieve pain in non-end-of-life pain conditions ranged from 900 to 3600 mg/day in divided doses.[114–116]

Corticosteroids. Corticosteroids inhibit prostaglandin synthesis and reduce edema surrounding neural tissues.[117,118] This category of drug is particulary useful for neuropathic pain syndromes, including plexopathies and pain associated with stretching of the liver capsule due to metastases. Corticosteroids are also highly effective at treating bone pain due to their antiinflammatory effects. Dexamethasone produces the least amount of mineralocorticoid effect, leading to reduced potential for Cushing's syndrome. The standard dose is 16 to 24 mg/day and can be administered once daily due to the long half-life of this drug.[22] Doses as high as 100 mg may be given with severe pain crises. Intravenous bolus doses should be pushed slowly, to prevent uncomfortable perineal burning and itching.

Local Anesthetics. Local anesthetics work in a manner similar to the older anticonvulsants, by inhibiting the movement of ions across the neural membrane. They are useful for relieving neuropathic pain. Local anesthetics can be given orally, topically, intravenously, subcutaneously, or spinally. Mexiletine has been reported to be useful when anticonvulsants and other adjuvant therapies have failed. Doses start at 150 mg/day and increase to levels as high as 900 mg/day in divided doses.[119,120] Local anesthetic gels and patches have been used to prevent the pain associated with needle stick and other minor procedures. Both gel and patch (Lidoderm) versions of lidocaine have been shown to reduce the pain of postherpetic neuropathy.[121–123] Intravenous lidocaine at 1 to 5 mg/kg (maximum 500 mg) administered over 1 hour has been reported to reduce chronic neuropathic pain with little effect on cardiovascular function.[124–126] Epidural or intrathecal lidocaine or bupivacaine delivered with an opioid can reduce neuropathic pain.

N-*Methyl*-D-*Aspartate Antagonists.* Antagonists to NMDA are believed to block the binding of excitatory amino acids, such as glutamate, in the spinal cord. Ketamine, a dissociative anesthetic, relieves severe neuropathic pain by blocking NMDA receptors (see the section Pain Crisis, below). Routine use is limited by cognitive changes and other adverse effects. Oral compounds containing dextromethorphan have been tested. Unfortunately, dextromethorphan was ineffective at relieving cancer pain.[127]

Bisphosphonates. Bisphosphonates inhibit osteoclast-mediated bone resorption and alleviate pain related to metastatic bone disease and multiple myeloma.[128–131] Pamidronate disodium reduces pain, hypercalcemia, and skeletal morbidity. The optimal dosing schedule is not known; however, 60 mg every 2 or 4 weeks and 90 mg every 4 weeks have been shown to be safe and effective.[129] Serum levels of calcium, phosphate, magnesium, and potasium should be evaluated regularly. Analgesic effects occur in 2 to 4 weeks. Clodronate, olpadronate (which is not available in the United States), and sodium etidronate appear to provide little or no analgesia.[132–134]

Calcitonin. Subcutaneous calcitonin may be effective in the relief of neuropathic or bone pain, although studies are inconclusive.[135,136] The nasal form of this drug may be more acceptable in end-of-life care when other therapies are ineffective. Usual doses are 100 to 200 IU/day subcutaneously or nasally.[137]

Radiopharmaceuticals. Radiolabeled agents such as strontium 89 and samarium 153 have been shown to be effective at reducing metastatic bone pain.[138,139] Thrombocytopenia and leukopenia are relative contraindications since strontium-89 causes thrombocytopenia in as many as 33% of those treated and leukopenia up to 10%.[140] Because of the delayed onset and timing of peak effect, only those patients with a projected life span of greater than 3 months should be considered for treatment. Patients should be advised that a transitory pain flare is reported by as many as 10% of individuals treated, and additional analgesics should be provided in anticipation.

Other Adjunct Analgesics. Topical capsaicin is believed to relieve pain by inhibiting the release of substance P.[141] This compound has been shown to be useful in relieving pain associated with postmastectomy syndrome, postherpetic neuralgia, and post-surgical neuropathic pain in cancer.[142] A burning sensation experienced by patients is a common reason for discontinuing therapy.

Baclofen is useful in the relief of spasm-associated pain. Doses begin at 10 mg/day, increasing every few days. A generalized feeling of weakness and confusion or hallucinations often occurs with doses above 60 mg/day.[101]

Calcium channel blockers are believed to provide pain relief by preventing conduction. Nifedipine 10 mg orally may be useful to relieve ischemic or neuropathic pain syndromes.

NONPHARMACOLOGICAL THERAPIES

Nondrug therapies, including cognitive–behavioral techniques and physical measures, can serve as adjuncts to analgesics in the palliative care setting. This is not to suggest that when these therapies work the pain is of psychological origin.[143] The patient's and caregivers' abilities to participate must be considered when selecting one of these therapies, including their fatigue level, interest, cognition, and other factors.

Cognitive–behavioral therapy often includes strategies to improve coping and relaxation. In a randomized clinical trial of patients undergoing bone marrow transplantation, pain was reduced in those patients who received relaxation and imagery training and in those who received cognitive–behavioral skill development with relaxation and imagery.[144] Patients who received treatment as usual or those randomized to receive support from a therapist did not experience pain relief.

Physical measures produce relaxation and relieve pain. In a study of massage in hospice patients, relaxation resulted as measured by blood pressure, heart rate, and skin temperature.[145] A 10-minute back massage was found to relieve pain in male cancer patients.[146] Rhiner and colleagues[147] employed a comprehensive nondrug program for cancer patients that included education; physical measures such as heat, cold, and massage; and cognitive–behavioral strategies such as distraction and relaxation. All therapies were rated as useful, with distraction and heat scoring highest. More research is needed in the palliative care setting regarding nondrug therapies that might enhance pain relief.

DIFFICULT PAIN SYNDROMES

The above therapies provide relief for the majority of patients (Table 6–8). Unfortunately, complex pain syndromes may require additional measures. These syndromes include breakthrough pain, pain crises, and pain control in the patient with a past or current history of substance abuse.

Breakthrough Pain

Intermittent episodes of moderate to severe pain that occur in spite of control of baseline continuous pain are very common in patients with advanced disease. Studies suggest that although breakthrough pain in cancer patients at home is common, short-acting analgesics are frequently not provided and patients do not take as much as is allowed.[148] Mostly described in cancer patients, there is evidence that patients with other pain-producing and life-limiting diseases commonly experience breakthrough pains a few times a day, lasting moments to many minutes.[149–151] The risk of increasing the around-the-clock or continuous-release analgesic dose to cover breakthrough pains is that of increasing undesirable side effects, especially sedation, once the more short-lived, episodic breakthrough pain has remitted. Guidelines for categorizing, assessing, and managing breakthrough pain are described below:

Incident Pain. Incident pain is predictably elicited by specific activities. Use a rapid-onset, short-duration analgesic formulation in anticipation of pain-eliciting activities or events. Use the same drug that the patient is taking for baseline pain relief for incident pain whenever possible. In 1998, OTFC was approved specifically for this indication in cancer patients.[94] Clinical experience is being gained on its efficacy in other clinical situations. Adjust and titrate the breakthrough pain medication dose to the severity of anticipated pain or the intensity and duration of the pain-producing event. Past experience will serve as the best prescriptive guide.

Spontaneous Pain. Spontaneous pain is unpredictable and not temporally associated with any activity or event. These pains are more challenging to control. Use of pain-attenuating drugs ("adjuvants") for neuropathic pains may help to diminish the frequency and severity of these types of pain (Table 6–7). Otherwise, immediate treatment with a potent, rapid-onset opioid analgesic is indicated.

End-of-Dose Failure. End-of-dose failure describes pain that occurs toward the end of the usual dosing interval of a regularly scheduled analgesic. This results from declining blood levels of the around-the-clock analgesic prior to administration or uptake of the next scheduled dose. Appropriate questioning and use of pain diaries will assure rapid diagnosis of end-of-dose failure. Increasing the dose of around-the-clock medication or shortening the dose interval to match the onset of this type of breakthrough pain should remedy the problem. For instance, a patient who is taking continuous-release morphine every 12 hours and whose pain "breaks through" after about 8 to 10 hours is experiencing end-of-dose failure. The dose should be increased by 25% to 50%, if this is tolerated, or the dosing interval should be increased to every 8 hours.

Pain Crisis

Most nociceptive (i.e., somatic and visceral) pain is controllable with appropriately titrated analgesic therapy.[152] Some neuropathic pains, such as invasive and compressive neuropathies, plexopathies, and myelopathies, may be poorly responsive to conventional analgesic therapies, short of inducing a nearly comatose state. Widespread bone metastases or end-stage pathological fractures may present similar challenges. When confronted by a pain crisis, the following considerations will be helpful:

- Differentiate terminal agitation or anxiety from "physically" based pain, if possible. Terminal symptoms unresponsive to rapid upward titration of an opioid may respond to benzodiazepines (e.g., diazepam, lorazepam, midazolam).
- Make sure that drugs are getting absorbed. The only *guaranteed* route is the intravenous route. Although invasive routes of

Table 6–8. Guidelines for Pain Management in Palliative Care

- Sustained-release formulations and around-the-clock dosing should be used for continuous pain syndromes.
- Immediate-release formulations should be made available for breakthrough pain.
- Cost and convenience (and other identified issues influencing compliance) are highly practical and important matters that should be taken into account with every prescription.
- Anticipate, prevent, and treat predictable side effects and adverse drug effects.
- Titrate analgesics based on patient goals, requirements for supplemental analgesics, pain intensity, severity of undesirable or adverse drug effects, measures of functionality, sleep, emotional state, and patients'/caregivers' reports of impact of pain on quality of life.
- Monitor patient status frequently during dose titration.
- Discourage use of mixed agonist–antagonist opioids.
- Be aware of potential drug–drug and drug–disease interactions.
- Recommend expert pain management consultation if pain is not adequately relieved within a reasonable amount of time after applying standard analgesic guidelines and interventions.
- Know the qualifications, experience, skills, and availability of pain management experts (consultants) within the patient's community *before* they may be needed.

These basic guidelines and considerations will optimize the pharmacologic management of patients in the palliative care setting with debilitating pain.
Sources: Jacox et al. (1994), reference 22; American Pain Society (1999), reference 40; American Geriatric Society Panel on Chronic Pain in Older Persons (1998), reference 61; World Health Organization (1996), reference 81.

drug delivery are to be avoided unless necessary, if there is any question about absorption of analgesics or other necessary palliative drugs, parenteral access should be established.

- Preterminal pain crises which are poorly responsive to basic approaches to analgesic therapy merit consultation with a pain management consultant as quickly as possible. Radiotherapeutic, anesthetic, or neuroablative procedures may be indicated.

Table 6–9. Protocol for Using Ketamine to Treat an Opioid Nonresponsive Pain Crisis

1. *Bolus:* ketamine 0.1 mg/kg IV. Double the dose if no clinical improvement in 5 minutes. Repeat as often as indicated by the patient's response. Follow the bolus with an infusion. Decrease opioid dose by 50%.
2. *Infusion:* ketamine 0.015 mg/(kg/min) IV (about 1 mg/min for a 70 kg individual). Subcutaneous infusion is possible if IV access is not attainable. In this case, use an initial IM bolus dose of 0.3–0.5 mg/kg. Decrease opioid dose by 50%.
3. It is advisable to administer a benzodiazapine (e.g., diazapam or lorazapam) concurrently to mitigate against the possibility of hallucinations or frightful dreams since many moribund patients under these circumstances may not be able to communicate such experiences.
4. Observe for problematic increases in secretions; treat with glycopyrrolate, scopolomine, or atropine as needed.

Source: Fine (1999), reference 154.

Management of Refractory Symptoms at the End of Life

Sedation at the end of life is an important option for patients with intractable pain and suffering. The literature describing the use of sedation at the end of life, however, is largely anecdotal and refers to the use of opioids, neuroleptics, benzodiazepines, and barbiturates. The anesthetic propofol is also used. In the absence of controlled relative efficacy data, guidelines for drug selection are empirical. Irrespective of the agent or agents selected, administration initially requires dose titration to achieve relief, followed by ongoing therapy to maintain effect. The depth of sedation necessary to control symptoms varies greatly. Once adequate relief is obtained, the parameters for ongoing monitoring are determined by the goal of care. If the goal of care is to ensure comfort until death, the salient parameters to monitor are those pertaining to comfort of the patient, family, and staff.

Parenteral administration of ketamine is also useful for some patients with refractory symptoms at the end of life. Ketamine is a potent analgesic at low doses and a dissociative anesthetic at higher doses. Its use under conditions of terminal crescendo-type pain may not only provide greatly improved pain relief but also allow a significant decrease in the dose of concurrent analgesics and sedatives, allowing in some cases increased interactive capability. Ketamine is usually reserved for terminal situations, due to rapidly developing tolerance and psychotomimetic effects (hallucinations, dysphoria, nightmares) that may occur with higher doses and drug accumulation (Table 6–9).[153,154] Long-term intravenous or subcutaneous use of ketamine (for example over 2 months) has been reported to be effective in intractable pain states not relieved by large doses of opioids and other adjuncts.[155] Haloperidol can be used to treat the hallucinations, and scopolamine may be needed to reduce the excess salivation seen with this drug.

Substance Abuse

The numbers of patients entering palliative care with a current or past history of substance abuse are increasing. Caring for these patients can be extremely challenging. Thorough assessment of the pain and their addiction is critical. Patients can be categorized in the following manner: *(1)* individuals who used drugs in the past but are not now using them, *(2)* patients in methadone maintenance programs, and *(3)* patients who are actively abusing drugs.[156] Treatment is different for each group.

A frequent fear expressed by professionals is that they will be "duped," or lied to, about the presence of pain. One of the limitations of pain management is that pain, and all its components, cannot be proven.[157] Therefore, complaints of pain must be believed.[158]

As with all aspects of palliative care, an interdisciplinary team approach is indicated. This may include inviting addiction counselors, representatives from Narcotics Anonymous, and experts in this field.[167] Realistic goals must be established.[159] For example, recovery from addiction is impossible if the patient does not seek this rehabilitation. The goal in that case may be to provide a structured and safe environment for patients and their support persons. Comorbid psychiatric disorders are common, particularly depression, personality disorders, and anxiety disorders.[159] Treatment of these underlying problems may reduce relapse or aberrant behaviors and may make pain control more effective. Consistency is essential. Inconsistency can increase manipulation and lead to staff frustration.[157] Setting limits is a critical component of the care plan, and medication contracts may be indicated.[160] In fact, one primary clinician may be designated to handle the pharmacological management of pain.[167] Weekly team meetings provide a forum to establish the plan of care and discuss negative attitudes regarding the patient's behavior.

The pharmacological principles of pain management in the substance abuser are not unlike those in a person without an abuse history. Tolerance must be considered; thus, opioid doses may require more rapid titration and may be higher than for patients without a history of substance abuse.[167] Requests for increasing doses may be due to psychological suffering, so this possibility must also be explored. Nonopioids may be used, including antidepressants, anticonvulsants, and other adjuncts. However, psychoactive drugs with no analgesic effect should be avoided in the treatment of pain.

Withdrawal from drugs of abuse

must be prevented or minimized. These may include cocaine, benzodiazepines, and even alcohol.[159] Alcoholism in palliative care has been underdiagnosed.[161] Thus, a thorough assessment of the drugs of abuse, including alcohol, must be conducted. Urine toxicology studies may be necessary.

Patients in recovery may be extremely reluctant to consider opioid therapy. Patients may need reassurance that opioids can be taken for medical indications, such as cancer or other illnesses. If patients currently are treated in a methadone maintenance program, continue the methadone but add another opioid to provide pain relief.[157] Communicate with the program to ensure the correct methadone dose. Nondrug alternatives may also be suggested.

OUTCOMES AND DOCUMENTATION

Quality improvement measures to relieve pain in the palliative care setting include setting outcomes, developing strategies to maintain or meet these outcomes, then evaluating effectiveness.[162] Some suggested goals and outcome measures that can be listed in each patient's care plan are listed in Table 6–10.

Documentation is also essential to ensure continuity of care. Recommendations for documentation in the medical record include the following:

- Initial assessment, including findings from the comprehensive pain assessment; the current pain management regimen; prior experience with pain and pain control; patient and caregiver understanding of expectations and goals of pain management; elaboration of concerns regarding opioids; and a review of systems pertinent to analgesic use, including bowels, balance, memory, etc.
- Interdisciplinary progress notes, including ongoing findings from recurrent pain assessment; baseline pain scores; breakthrough pain frequency and severity with associated causes and timing of episodes; effect of pain and pain treatment on function, sleep, activity, social interaction, mood, etc.; types and effects (outcomes) of intervention, including adverse effects (bowel function, sedation, nausea/vomiting assessments); documentation of specific instructions, patient/caregiver understanding, and compliance; and patient/caregiver coping.

Comprehensive strategies to improve pain outcomes in the hospice setting have included improving professional education, developing policies and procedures, enhancing pain documentation, and instituting other performance-improvement measures.[163,164] These have resulted in reduction of pain intensity scores and other changes. More research is needed in the development of quality improvement strategies that most accurately reflect the needs of patients and families in palliative care settings.

CONCLUSION

Pain control in the palliative care setting is feasible in the majority of patients. For patients whose pain cannot be controlled, sedation is always an option. Understanding the barriers that limit relief will lead to improved education and other strategies to address these obstacles. Developing comfort and skill with the use of pharmacological and nonpharmacological therapies will enhance pain relief. Quality improvement efforts within a palliative care setting can improve the level of pain management within that organization and ultimately the pain relief experienced by these patients. Together, these efforts will reduce suffering, relieve pain, and enhance the quality of life of those at the end of life.

Table 6–10. Outcome Indicators for Pain Control in the Palliative Care Setting

- *Initial Evaluation:* Pain that is not well controlled (patient self-report of >3 out of 10 or greater than the patient's acceptable comfort level) is brought under control within 48 hours of a patient's initial evaluation.
- *Ongoing Care:* Pain that is out of control is assessed and managed with effective intervention(s) within a predetermined time frame in all patients (set an appropriate time limit).
- *Terminal Care:* No patient dies with pain out of control.
- *Adverse Effects:* Analgesic adverse effects and side effects are prevented or effectively and quickly managed in all patients.

REFERENCES

1. Ng K, von Gunten CF. Symptoms and attitudes of 100 consecutive patients admitted to an acute hospice/palliative care unit. J Pain Symptom Manage 1998;16:307–316.
2. Daut RC, Cleeland CS. The prevalence and severity of pain in cancer. Cancer 1982;50:1913–1918.
3. Donovan MI, Dillon P. Incidence and characteristics of pain in a sample of hospitalized cancer patients. Cancer Nurs 1987;10:85–92.
4. Dorrepaal KL, Aaronson NK, van Dam FSAM. Pain experience and pain management among hospitalized cancer patients. A clinical study. Cancer 1989;63:593–598.
5. Coyle N, Adelhardt J, Foley KM, et al. Character of terminal illness in the advanced cancer patient: pain and other symptoms during the last four weeks of life. J Pain Symptom Manage 1990;5:83–93.
6. Paice JA, Mahon SM, Faut-Callahan M. Factors associated with adequate pain control in hospitalized postsurgical patients diagnosed with cancer. Cancer Nurs 1991;14:298–305.
7. Cleeland CS, Gonin R, Hatfield AK, et al. Pain and its treatment in outpatients with metastatic cancer. N Engl J Med 1994;330:592–596.
8. Cleeland CS, Gonin R, Baez L, Loehrer P, Pandya KJ. Pain and treatment of pain in minority patients with cancer. The Eastern Cooperative Oncology Group Minority Outpatient Pain Study. Ann Intern Med 1997;127:813–816.
9. Ferrell BR, Ferrell BA. Pain in the Elderly. A Report of the Task Force on Pain in the Elderly of the International Association for the Study of Pain. Seattle: IASP Press, 1996.
10. Brescia FJ, Portenoy RK, Ryan M, Krasnoff L, Gray G. Pain, opioid use, and survival in hospitalized patients with advanced cancer. J Clin Oncol 1992;10:149–155.
11. Jenkins CA, Taube AW, Ken T, Hanson J, Bruera E. Initial demographic, symptom, and medication profiles in patients admitted to continuing palliative care units. J Pain Symptom Manage 1998;16:163–170.
12. Eldridge AD, Severance-Lossin L, Nicholas PK, Leuner JD. Prevalence and characteristics of pain in persons with terminal-stage AIDS. J Adv Nurs 1994;20:260–268.
13. Hewitt DJ, McDonald M, Portenoy RK, Rosenfeld B, Passik S, Breitbart W. Pain syndromes and etiologies in ambulatory AIDS patients. Pain 1997;70:117–123.
14. Breitbart W, Rosenfeld BD, Passik S, Mc-

Donald MV, Thaler H, Portenoy RK. The undertreatment of pain in ambulatory AIDS patients. Pain 1996;65:243–249.

15. Breitbart W, Rosenfeld B, Passik S, Kaim M, Funesti-Esch J, Stein K. A comparison of pain report and adequacy of analgesic therapy in ambulatory AIDS patients with and without a history of substance abuse. Pain 1997;72:235–243.

16. McCormack JP, Li R, Zarowny D, Singer J. Inadequate treatment of pain in ambulatory HIV patients. Clin J Pain 1993;9:279–283.

17. Larue F, Fontaine A, Colleau SM. Underestimation and undertreatment of pain in HIV disease: multicentre study. BMJ 1997;314:23–28.

18. Archibald CJ, McGrath PJ, Ritvo PG, et al. Pain prevalence, severity and impact in a clinic sample of multiple sclerosis patients. Pain 1993; 58:89–93.

19. Casey KL. Pain and Central Nervous System Disease: the Central Pain Syndromes. New York: Raven Press, 1991.

20. Crook J, Hideout E, Brown G. The prevalence of pain complaints in a general population. Pain 1984;18:299–314.

21. Pargeon KL, Hailey BJ. Barriers to effective cancer pain management: a review of the literature. J Pain Symptom Manage 1999;18:358–368.

22. Jacox A, Carr DB, Payne R, et al. Management of Cancer Pain: Clinical Practice Guideline, 9. AHCPR Publication 94–0592. Rockville, MD: Agency for Health Care Policy and Research, US Department of Health and Human Services, Public Health Service, 1994.

23. Elliott TE, Elliott BA. Physician attitudes and beliefs about use of morphine for cancer pain. J Pain Symptom Manage 1992;7:141–148.

24. Elliott TE, Murray DM, Elliott BA, et al. Physician knowledge and attitudes about cancer pain management: a survey from the Minnesota Cancer Pain Project. J Pain Symptom Manage 1995;10:494–504.

25. Fife BL, Irick N, Painter JD. A comparative study of the attitudes of physicians and nurses toward the management of cancer pain. J Pain Symptom Manage 1993;8:132–139.

26. Rawal N, Hylander J, Arner S. Management of terminal cancer pain in Sweden: a nationwide survey. Pain 1993;54:169–179.

27. MacDonald N, Findlay HP, Bruera E, Dudgeon D, Kramer J. A Canadian survey of issues in cancer pain management. J Pain Symptom Manage 1997;14:332–342.

28. Warncke T, Breivik H, Vainio A. Treatment of cancer pain in Norway: a questionnaire study. Pain 1994;57:109–116.

29. Lowers J. To improve pain management: measure, educate, change habits. Qual Lett 1999; 11:2–10.

30. Ward SE, Goldberg N, Miller-McCauley V, et al. Patient-related barriers to management of cancer pain. Pain 1993;52:319–324.

31. Paice JA, Toy C, Shott S. Barriers to cancer pain relief: fear of tolerance and addiction. J Pain Symptom Manage 1998;16:1–9.

32. Ersek M, Kraybill BM, Du Pen AR. Factors hindering patients' use of medications for cancer pain. Cancer Prac 1999;7:226–232.

33. Berry PE, Ward S. Barriers to pain management in hospice: a study of family caregivers. Hospice J 1995;10:19–33.

34. Riddell A, Fitch MI. Patients' knowledge of and attitudes toward the management of cancer pain. Oncol Nurs Forum 1997;24:1775–1784.

35. Elliott BA, Elliott TE, Murray DM, Braun BL, Johnson KM. Patients and family members: the role of knowledge and attitudes in cancer pain. J Pain Symptom Manage 1996;12: 209–220.

36. Ward SE, Berry PE, Misiewicz H. Concerns about analgesics among patient and family caregivers in a hospice setting. Res Nurs Health 1996;19:205–211.

37. Ersek M. Enhancing effective pain management by addressing patient barriers to analgesic use. J Hospice Palliat Nurs 1999;1:87–96.

38. Portenoy RK. Inadequate outcome of opioid therapy for cancer pain: influences on practitioners and patients. In: Patt RB, ed. Cancer Pain. Philadelphia: JB Lippincott, 1993:119–128.

39. Lipman AG, Gauthier ME. Pharmacology of opioid drugs: basic principles. In: Portenoy RK, Bruera E, eds. Topics in Palliative Care, vol 1. New York: Oxford University Press, 1997:137–162.

40. American Pain Society. Principles of Analgesic Use in the Treatment of Acute Pain and Cancer Pain. Glenview, IL: American Pain Society, 1999.

41. Twycross RJ. Misunderstandings about morphine. In: Twycross R, ed. Pain Relief in Advanced Cancer. New York: Churchill Livingstone, 1994:333–347.

42. Page GG, Ben-Eliyahu S, Yirmiya R, Liebeskind JC. Opioids attenuate surgery-induced enhancement of metastatic colonization in rats. Pain 1993;54:21–28.

43. Sklar LS, Anisman H. Stress and coping factors influence tumor growth. Science 1979;205: 513–515.

44. Liebeskind JC. Pain can kill. Pain 1991; 44:3–4.

45. Cousins MJ. Prevention of postoperative pain. In: Bond MR, Charlton JE, Woolf CJ, eds. Pain Research and Clinical Management, vol 4. Amsterdam: Elsevier, 1991:45–52.

46. American Pain Society Quality of Care Committee. Quality improvement guidelines for the treatment of acute pain and cancer pain. JAMA 1995;274:1874–1880.

47. Du Pen SL, Du Pen AR, Polissar N, et al. Implementing guidelines for cancer pain management: results of a randomized controlled clinical trial. J Clin Oncol 1999;17:351–370.

48. Fine PG, Ashburn MA. Functional neuroanatomy and nociception. In: Ashburn M, Rice LJ, eds. The Management of Pain. New York: Churchill Livingstone, 1998:1–16.

49. Lipman AG. Pharmacological approaches to pain management: nontraditional analgesics and analgesic adjuvants. In: Ashburn M, Rice LJ, eds. The Management of Pain. New York: Churchill Livingstone, 1998:99–110.

50. Zuckerman LA, Ferrante FM. Nonopioid and opioid analgesics. In: Ashburn MA, Rice LJ, eds. The Management of Pain. New York: Churchill Livingstone, 1998:111–140.

51. Hanks G, Cherny N. Opioid analgesic therapy. In: Doyle D, Hanks GWC, MacDonald N, eds. Oxford Textbook of Palliative Medicine, vol 2. New York: Oxford University Press, 1998: 331–355.

52. Rawlins MD. Non-opioid analgesics. In: Doyle D, Hanks GWC, MacDonald N, eds. Oxford Textbook of Palliative Care, vol 2. New York: Oxford University Press, 1997:355–361.

53. Portenoy RK. Adjuvant analgesics in pain management. In: Doyle D, Hanks GWC, MacDonald N, eds. Oxford Textbook of Palliative Care, vol. 2. New York: Oxford University Press, 1998:361–390.

54. Stambaugh J. Role of nonsteroidal anti-inflammatory drugs in the management of cancer pain. In: Patt RB, ed. Cancer Pain. Philadelphia: Lippincott Company, 1993:105–117.

55. Hill CS Jr. Oral opioid analgesics. In: Patt RB, ed. Cancer Pain. Philadelphia: JB Lippincott, 1993:129–142.

56. Bruera E, Ripamonti C. Adjuvants to opioid analgesics. In: Patt RB, ed. Cancer Pain. Philadelphia: JB Lippincott, 1993:143–159.

57. Bruera E, Ripamonti C. Alternate routes of administration of opioids. In: Patt RB, ed. Cancer Pain. Philadelphia: JB Lippincott, 1993:160–184.

58. Ellison NM. Opioid analgesics for cancer pain: toxicities and their treatments. In: Patt RB, ed. Cancer Pain. Philadelphia: JB Lippincott, 1993:185–194.

59. Ruzicka DR, Gates RA, Fink R. Pain management. In: Gates RA, Fink RM, eds. Oncology Nursing Secrets. Philadelphia: Hanley & Belfus, 1997:284–303.

60. Waller A, Caroline NL. Pain control (general considerations and principles and techniques of pharmacologic management). In: Waller A, Caroline NL, eds. Handbook of Palliative Care in Cancer. Boston: Butterworth-Heinemann, 1996:3–41.

61. American Geriatric Society Panel on Chronic Pain in Older Persons. The management of chronic pain in older persons. J Am Geriatr Soc 1998;46:635–651.

62. Bradley JD, Brandt KD, Katz BP, et al. Comparison of an antiinflammatory dose of ibuprofen, an analgesic dose of ibuprofen and acetaminophen in the treatment of patients with osteoarthritis of the knee. N Engl J Med 1991; 325:87–91.

63. Avorn J, Gurwitz JH. Drug use in nursing homes. Ann Intern Med 1995;123:87–91.

64. Sandler DP, Smith JC, Weinberg CR, et al. Analgesic use and chronic renal disease. N Engl J Med 1989;320:1238–1243.

65. Shiodt FV, Rochling FA, Casey DL, Lee WM. Acetaminophen toxicity in an urban county hospital. N Engl J Med 1997;337:1112–1117.

66. Vane JR, Botting RM. Mechanism of action of aspirin-like drugs. Semin Arthritis Rheumatology 1997;26 (Suppl):2–10.

67. Cryer B, Feldman M. Cyclooxygenase-1 and cyclooxygenase-2 selectivity of widely used nonsteroidal anti-inflammatory drugs. Am J Med 1998;104:413–421.

68. Allison MC, Howatson AG, Torance CJ, Lee FD, Russell RI. Gastrointestinal damage associated with the use of nonsteroidal antiinflammatory drugs. N Engl J Med 1992;327:749–754.

69. Kaufman DW, Kelly JP, Sheehan JE, et al. Nonsteroidal anti-inflammatory drug use in relation to major upper gastrointestinal bleeding. Clin Pharmacol Ther 1993;53:485–494.

70. Garcia RLA. Nonsteroidal antiinflammatory drugs, ulcers and risk: a collaborative meta-analysis. Semin Arthritis Rheum 1997;26(Suppl): 16–20.

71. Lipsky PE, Isakson PC. Outcome of specific COX-2 inhibition in rheumatoid arthritis. J Rheumatol 1997;24(Suppl 49):9–14.

72. Foley KM. The treatment of cancer pain. N Engl J Med 1985;313:84–95.

73. Goodwin JS, Regan M. Cognitive dysfunction associated with naproxen and ibuprofen in the elderly. Arthritis Rheum 1982;25:1013–1016.

74. Twycross RG. Opioids. In: Wall PD, Melzack R, eds. Textbook of Pain. Edinburgh: Churchill Livingstone, 1999:1187–1214.

75. Dahl JL. Effective pain management in terminal care. Clin Geriatr Med 1996;12:279–300.

76. Bercovitch M, Waller A, Adunsky A. High dose morphine use in the hospice setting: a database survey of patient characteristics and effect on life expectancy. Cancer 1999;86:871–877.

77. Watanabe S, Intraindividual variability in opioid response: a role for sequential opioid trials in patient care. In: Portenoy RK, Bruera E, eds. Topics in Palliative Care, vol 1 New York: Oxford University Press, 1997:195–203.

78. Sjogren P. Clinical implications of morphine metabolites. In: Portenoy RK, Bruera E, eds. Topics in Palliative Care, vol 1. New Yord: Oxford University Press, 1997:163–176.

79. Kaiko RF, Foley KM, Grabinski PY. Central nervous system excitatory effects of meperidine in cancer patients. Ann Neurol 1983;13:180–185.

80. Hoskin PJ, G.W.H. Opioid agonist antagonist drugs in acute and chronic pain states. Drugs 1991;41:326–344.

81. World Health Organization. Cancer Pain Relief. Geneva: WHO, 1996.

82. Twycross RJ. Oral morphine. In: Twycross R, ed. Pain Relief in Advanced Cancer. New York: Churchill Livingstone, 1994:307–332.

83. O'Brien T, Mortimer P, McDonald C, Miller A. A randomised crossover study comparing the efficacy and tolerability of a novel once-daily morphine preparation (MXL capsules) and MST continuous tablets in cancer patients with severe pain. Palliat Med 1997;11:475–482.

84. Ripamonti C, Bruera E. Rectal, buccal and sublingual narcotics for the management of cancer pain. J Palliat Care 1991;7:30–35.

85. De Conno F, Ripamonti C, Saita L, MacEachern T, Hanson J, Bruera E. Role of rectal route in treating cancer pain: a randomized crossover clinical trial of oral versus rectal morphine administration in opioid-naive cancer patients with pain. J Clin Oncol 1995;13:1004–1008.

86. McCaffery M, Martin L, Ferrell BR. Analgesic administration via rectum or stoma. J Enterostomal Therapy Nurs 1992;19:114–121.

87. Cole L, Hanning CD. Review of the rectal use of opioids. J Pain Symptom Manage 1990; 5:118–126.

88. Kaiko RF, Fitzmartin RD, Thomas GB, et al. The bioavailability of morphine in controlled-release 30-mg tablets per rectum compared with immediate-release 30-mg rectal suppositories and controlled-release 30-mg oral tablets. Pharmacotherapy 1992;12:107–113.

89. Simmonds MA. Transdermal fentanyl: long-term analgesic studies. J Pain Symptom Manage 1992;7(Suppl):36–39.

90. Newshan G. Heat-related toxicity with the fentanyl transdermal patch. J Pain Symptom Manage 1998;16:277–278.

91. Ahmedzai S, Brooks D. Transdermal fentanyl versus sustained-release oral morphine in cancer pain: preference, efficacy, and quality of life. J Pain Symptom Manage 1997;13:254–261.

92. Watanabe S, Pereira J, Hanson J, Bruera E. Fentanyl by continuous subcutaneous infusion for the management of cancer pain: a retrospective study. J Pain Symptom Manage 1998;16:323–326.

93. Fine PG, Streisand JB. A review of oral transmucosal fentanyl citrate: potent, rapid and noninvasive opioid analgesia. J Palliat Med 1998;1: 55–63.

94. Fine PG. Clinical experience with Actiq® (oral transmucosal fentanyl citrate) for the treatment of cancer pain. J N Dev Clin Med 1999;17:1–11.

95. Wallenstein SL, Rogers AG, Kaiko RF, Houde RW. Clinical analgesic studies of levorphanol in acute and chronic cancer pain. In: Foley K, Inturrisi CE, eds. Advances in Pain Research and Therapy, vol 1. New York: Raven Press, 1986:211–215.

96. Fainsinger R, Schoeller T, Bruera E. Methadone in the management of cancer pain: a review. Pain 1993;52:137–147.

97. Mercadante S, Casuccio A, Agnello A, Serretta R, Calderone L, Barresi L. Morphine versus methadone in the pain treatment of advanced cancer patients followed up at home. J Clin Oncol 1998;16:3656–3661.

98. De Conno F, Groff L, Brunelli C, Zecca E, Ventafridda V, Ripamonti C. Clinical experience with oral methadone administration in the treatment of pain in 196 advanced cancer patients. J Clin Oncol 1996;14:2836–2842.

99. Ripamonti C, Groff L, Brunelli D, Polastri D, Stavrakis A, De Conno F. Switching from morphine to oral methadone in treating cancer pain: what is the equianalgesic dose ratio? J Clin Oncol 1998;16:3216–3221.

100. Storey P, Hill HH, St. Louis RH, et al. Subcutaneous infusions for control of cancer symptoms. J Pain Symptom Manage 1990;5:33–41.

101. Gianino JM, York MM, Paice JA. Intrathecal drug therapy for spasticity and pain. New York: Springer, 1996.

102. Curtis E, Krech R, Walsh T. Common symptoms in patients with advanced cancer. J Palliat Care 1991;7:25–29.

103. Bruera E, Brenneis C, Paterson AH, MacDonald N. Use of methylphenidate as an adjuvant to narcotic analgesics in patients with advanced cancer. J Pain Symptom Manage 1989; 4:3–6.

104. Campora E, Merlini L, Pace M, et al. The incidence of narcotic-induced emesis. J Pain Symptom Manage 1991;6:428–434.

105. Lichter I. Results of anti-emetic management in terminal illness. J Palliat Care 1993; 9:19–25.

106. Gregory RE, Grossman S, Sheidler VR. Grand mal seizures associated with high-dose intravenous morphine infusions: incidence and possible etiology. Pain 1992;51:255–258.

107. Bernard JD. Mechanisms and management of pruritus. New York: McGraw-Hill, 1994.

108. Larijana GE, Goldberg ME, Rogers KH. Treatment of opioid-induced pruritus with ondansetron: report of four patients. Pharmacotherapy 1996;16:958–960.

109. Max MB, Lynch SA, Muir J, Shoaf SE, Smoller B, Dubner R. Effects of desipramine, amitriptyline, and fluoxetine on pain in diabetic neuropathy. N Engl J Med 1992;326:1250–1256.

110. Onghena P, Van Houdenhove B. Antidepressant induced analgesia in chronic nonmalignant pain: a meta-analysis of 39 placebo-controlled studies. Pain 1992;49:205–219.

111. Watson CPN. Antidepressant drugs as adjuvant analgesics. J Pain Symptom Manage 1994;9:392–405.

112. McQuay H, Carroll D, Jadad A, Wiffeh P, Moore A. Anticonvulsant drugs for management of pain: a systematic review. BMJ 1995;311:1047–1052.

113. Taylor CP, Gee NS, Su T-Z, et al. A summary of mechanistic hypothesis of gabapentin pharmacology. Epilepsy Res 1998;29:233–249.

114. Rowbotham M, Harden N, Stacey B, Bernstein P, Magnus-Miller L, Group GPNS. Gabapentin for the treatment of postherpetic neuralgia. JAMA 1998;280:1837–1842.

115. Backonja M, Beydoun A, Edwards KR, et al. Gabapentin for the symptomatic treatment of painful neuropathy in patients with diabetes mellitus: a randomized controlled trial. JAMA 1998;280:1831–1836.

116. Merren MD. Gabapentin for treatment of pain and tremor: a large case series. South Med J 1998;91:739–744.

117. Watanabe S, Bruera E. Corticosteroids as adjuvant analgesics. J Pain Symptom Manage 1994;9:442–445.

118. Ettinger AB, Portenoy RK. The use of corticosteroids in the treatment of symptoms associated with cancer. J Pain Symptom Manage 1988; 3:99–103.

119. Dejgard A, Petersen P, Kastrup J. Mex-

iletine for treatment of chronic painful diabetic neuropathy. Lancet 1988;i:9–11.

120. Backonja MM. Local anesthetics as adjuvant analgesics. J Pain Symptom Manage 1994; 9:491–499.

121. Rowbotham MC, Davies PS, Fields HL. Topical lidocaine gel relieves postherpetic neuralgia. Ann Neurol 1995;37:246–253.

122. Rowbotham MC, Davies PS, Verkempinck C, Galer BS. Lidocaine patch: double-blind controlled study of a new treatment method for post-herpetic neuropathy. Pain 1996;65:39–44.

123. Galer BS, Rowbotham MC, Perander J, Friedman E. Topical lidocaine patch relieves postherpetic neuralgia more effectively than a vehicle topical patch: results of an enriched enrollment study. Pain 1999;80:533–538.

124. Ferrante FM, Paggioli J, Cherukuri S, Arthur GR. The analgesic response to intravenous lidocaine in the treatment of neuropathic pain. Anesth Analg 1996;82:91–97.

125. Rowbotham MC, Reisner-Keller LA, Fields HL. Both intravenous lidocaine and morphine reduce the pain of postherpetic neuralgia. Neurology 1991;41:1024–1028.

126. Brose WG, Cousins MJ. Subcutaneous lidocaine for treatment of neuropathic cancer pain. Pain 1991;45:145–148.

127. Mercadante S, Casuccio A, Genovese G. Ineffectiveness of dextromethorphan in cancer pain. J Pain Symptom Manage 1998;16:317–322.

128. Purohit OP, Anthony C, Radstone CR, Owen J, Coleman RE. High-dose intravenous pamidronate for metastatic bone pain. Br J Cancer 1994;70:554–558.

129. Glover D, Lipton A, Keller A, et al. Intravenous pamidronate disodium treatment of bone metastases in patients with breast cancer. Cancer 1994;74:2949–2955.

130. Berenson JR, Lichtenstein A, Porter L, et al. Long-term pamidronate treatment of advanced multiple myeloma patients reduces skeletal events. J Clin Oncol 1998;16:593–602.

131. Koeberle D, Bacchus L, Thuerlimann B, Thuerlimann, Senn HJ. Pamidronate treatment in patients with malignant osteolytic bone disease and pain. Support Care Cancer 1999;7:21–27.

132. Ernst DS, MacDonald RN, Paterson AH, Jensen J, Brasher P, Bruera E. A double-blind, crossover trial of intravenous clodronate in metastatic bone pain. J Pain Symptom Manage 1992;7:4–11.

133. Pelger RC, Hamdy NA, Zwinderman AH, Lycklama a Nijeholt AA, Papapoulos SE. Effects of the bisphosphonate olpadronate in patients with carcinoma of the prostate metastatic to the skeleton. Bone 1998;22:403–409.

134. Smith JA. Palliation of painful bone metastases from prostate cancer using sodium etidronate: results of a randomized, prospective, double-blind, placebo-controlled trial. J Urol 1089;141:85–87.

135. Mystakidou K, Befon S, Hondros K, Kouskouni E, Vlahos L. Continuous subcutaneous administration of high-dose salmon calcitonin in bone metastasis: pain control and beta-endorphin plasma levels. J Pain Symptom Manage 1999;18:323–330.

136. Roth A, Kolaric K. Analgesic activity of calcitonin in patients with painful osteolytic metastases of breast cancer. Results of a controlled randomized study. Oncology 1986;43:283–287.

137. Lyritis G, Paspati I, Karachalios T, Ioakimidis D, Skarantavos G, Lyritis PG. Pain relief from nasal salmon calcitonin in osteoporotic vertebral crush fractures: a double blind, placebo-controlled clinical study. Acta Orthop Scand 1997;68:112–114.

138. Robinson RG, Preston DF, Schiefelbein M, Baxter KG. Strontium 89 therapy for the palliation of pain due to osseous metastases. JAMA 1995;274:420–424.

139. Serafini AN, Houston SJ, Resche I, et al. Palliation of pain associated with metastatic bone cancer using samarium-153 lexidronam: a double-blind placebo-controlled clinical trial. J Clin Oncol 1998;16:1574–1581.

140. Porter AT, McEwan AJ, Powe JE, et al. Results of a randomized phase-III trial to evaluate the efficacy of strontium-89 adjuvant to local field external beam irradiation in the management of endocrine resistant metastatic prostate cancer. Int J Radiat Oncol Biol Phys 1993;25:805–813.

141. Watson CPN. Topical capsaicin as an adjuvant analgesic. J Pain Symptom Manage 1994;9:425–433.

142. Ellison N, Loprinzi CL, Kugler J, et al. Phase III placebo-controlled trial of capsaicin cream in the management of surgical neuropathic pain in cancer patients. J Clin Oncol 1997; 15:2974–2980.

143. Turk DC, Feldman CS. Noninvasive approaches to pain control in terminal illness: the contribution of psychological variables. Hospice J 1992;8:1–23.

144. Syrjala KL, Donaldson GW, Davis MW, Kippes ME, Carr JE. Relaxation and imagery and cognitive-behavioral training reduce pain during cancer treatment: a controlled clinical trial. Pain 1995;63:189–198.

145. Meek SS. Effects of slow stroke back massage on relaxation in hospice clients. Image J Nurs Sch 1993;25:17–21.

146. Weinrich SP, Weinrich MC. The effect of massage on pain in cancer patients. Appl Nurs Res 1990;3:140–145.

147. Rhiner M, Ferrell BR, Ferrell BA, Grant MM. A structured nondrug intervention program for cancer pain. Cancer Pract 1993;1:137–143.

148. Ferrell BR, Juarez G, Borneman T. Use of routine and breakthrough analgesia in home care. Oncol Nurs Forum 1999;26:1655–1661.

149. Portenoy RK, Hagen NA. Breakthrough pain: definition, prevalence, and characteristics. Pain 1990;41:273–281.

150. Fine PG, Busch MA. Characterization of breakthrough pain by hospice patients and their caregivers. J Pain Symptom Manage 1998;16:179–183.

151. Portenoy RK, Payne D, Jacobsen P. Breakthrough pain: characteristics and impact in patients with cancer pain. Pain 1999;81:129–134.

152. Hagen NA, Elwood T, Ernst S. Cancer pain emergencies: a protocol for management. J Pain Symptom Manage 1997;14:45–50.

153. Mercadante S. Ketamine in cancer pain: an update. Palliat Med 1996;10:255–230.

154. Fine PG. Low-dose ketamine in the management of opioid nonresponsive terminal cancer pain. J Pain Symptom Manage 1999;17: 296–300.

155. Luczak J, Dickenson AH, Aleksandra K-L. The role of ketamine, an NMDA receptor antagonist, in the management of pain. Prog Palliat Care 1995;3:127–134.

156. Passik SD, Portenoy RK. Substance abuse issues in palliative care. In: Berger AM, Portenoy RK, Weissman DE. Principles and Practice of Supportive Oncology. Philadelphia: Lippincott-Raven, 1998:513–529.

157. McCaffery M, Vourakis C. Assessment and relief of pain in chemically dependent patients. Orthop Nurs 1992;11:13–27.

158. Gonzales GR, Coyle N. Treatment of cancer pain in a former opioid abuser: fears of the patient and staff and their influence on care. J Pain Symptom Manage 1992;7:246–249.

159. Passik S, Portenoy RK, Ricketts PL. Substance abuse issues in cancer patients. Part 2: Evaluation and treatment. Oncology 1998;12:729–734.

160. Hoffman M, Provatas A, Lyver A, Kanner R. Pain management in the opioid-addicted patient with cancer. Cancer 1991;68:1121–1122.

161. Bruera E, Moyano J, Siefert L, Fainsinger RL, Hanson J, Suarez-Almazor M. The frequency of alcoholism among patients with pain due to terminal cancer. J Pain Symptom Manage 1995;10:599–603.

162. Higginson I. Clinical and organizational audit in palliative care. In: Doyle D, Hanks GWC, MacDonald N, eds. Oxford Textbook of Palliative Medicine. Oxford: Oxford University Press, 1998:67–81.

163. Holzheimer A, McMillan SC, Weitzner M. Improving pain outcomes of hospice patients with cancer. Oncol Nurs Forum 1999;26:1499–1504.

164. Duggleby W, Alden C. Implementation and evaluation of a quality improvement process to improve pain management in a hospice setting. Am J Hospice Palliat Care 1998:209–216.

165. Tiseo PJ, Thaler HT, Zapin J, et al. Morphine-6-glucuronide concentrations and opioid-related side effects: a survey in cancer patients. Pain 1995;61:47–54.

166. Eisele JH, Grisby EJ, Dea G. Clonazepam treatment of myoclonic contractions associated with high-dose opioids: case report. Pain 1992;49:213–232.

167. Hanks G, Cherny N. Opioid analgesic therapy. In: Doyle D, Hanks GWC, MacDonald N, eds. Oxford Textbook of Palliative Care, 2nd ed. Oxford: Oxford University Press, 1998:331–355.

7 Fatigue

GRACE E. DEAN and PAULA R. ANDERSON

Fatigue means my whole being is tired. This tiredness penetrates the whole bone structure; you feel it in the very marrow of your bone. It is total physical tiredness, and on top of that is mental tiredness. It's like an undercurrent that undermines your thinking. Your body is wearing out. The weight of fatigue is 'in the shadows.' If I rest, the fatigue will overwhelm me.[1]

—A patient

Fatigue knows no strangers. It spans the entire trajectory of illness and end-of-life experience. Sparing no one, fatigue holds many patients with advanced cancer firmly in its grip through the last days of life. Leisure activities are relinquished, usually the first activities to go.[2] Progressing fatigue makes taking a shower an all-day event because of the exhaustion. Even the most basic functions, such as brushing one's teeth or shaving, become overwhelming. The effort of flushing the toilet can become a major challenge. Climbing the stairs is out of the question. Patients report inability to hold their eyes open, and conversations become monosyllabic. When walking or sitting, the weight of their own bodies works against them. Patients describe a sensation of heaviness, like trying to walk through wet cement. However, as critical a symptom as it may be, fatigue remains invisible in a way, without objective measure.

DEFINITIONS OF FATIGUE

Some authors distinguish between the concepts of fatigue and weakness, while others see them as accompanying each other and comprising a syndrome known as asthenia.[3] Most of the existing research, however, uses "fatigue" as a broadly defined term, which includes such descriptors as weary, exhausted, worn-out, done for, tired, slow body, listless, lack of motivation, bone-tired, and rubber knees.[1,4]

Fatigue is an example of a complex phenomenon that has been studied by many disciplines but has no widely accepted definition.[5] The discipline of nursing is no exception. Even within different specialties of nursing, there has been little agreement on a definition of fatigue. In oncology, for example, different stages of cancer show fatigue in various situations. The newly diagnosed patient retrospectively views fatigue as a warning symptom of the diagnosis. The patient undergoing initial treatment for cancer experiences fatigue as a side effect of treatment. The patient who has finished treatment and is in recovery discovers a "new normal" level of energy. The patient who has experienced a recurrence of cancer considers fatigue to be as much an enemy as the diagnosis itself. Finally, the patient who is in the advanced stage of cancer interprets fatigue as the end of a very long struggle to be endured.

Historically, during the study of fatigue, several characteristics emerged that were fundamental to the development of the concept.[6] These characteristics are included in the following list of provisional criteria identifying fatigue: *(1)* the subjective perception of fatigue, *(2)* an alteration in neuromuscular and metabolic processes, *(3)* a decrease in physical performance, *(4)* a decrease in motivation, and *(5)* a deterioration in mental and physical activities. Several well-known definitions of fatigue were evaluated according to these five criteria. The North American Nursing Diagnostic Association (NANDA) defined fatigue as "an overwhelming, sustained sense of exhaustion and decreased capacity for physical or mental work." [7] This definition includes two of the five provisional criteria: *(1)* the subjective perception of fatigue and *(2)* a deterioration in mental and physical activities. Piper's[8] definition of fatigue is "an unusual, abnormal or excessive whole body tiredness, disproportionate to or unrelated to activity or exertion." [8] This definition includes only one of the criteria, the subjective perception of fatigue. More recently, investigators from the University of Kansas School of Nursing defined fatigue as "the awareness of a decreased capacity for physical and/or mental activity due to an imbalance in the availability, utilization, and/or restoration of resources needed to perform activity." [9] This definition includes three of the five criteria: *(1)* the subjective perception of fatigue, *(2)* a deterioration in mental and physical activities, and *(3)* an alteration in neuromuscular and metabolic processes. Overall, this definition seems to be the most comprehensive, including the fatigue experienced when diagnosed and then experienced in palliative care.

Although fatigue research in adults is gaining momentum, fatigue research in children and adolescents has received little attention. A definition of fatigue for children has not yet been developed. Additionally, early research involving focus groups of pediatric patients with cancer, their parents, and health care staff related that perceptions of fatigue were complicated by the fact that the fatigue existed within the greater context of the child's developmental stage.[10] For example, the definition of fatigue derived from a group of 7- to 12-year-old pediatric oncology patients consisted of "a profound sense of being weak or tired, or of having difficulty with movement such as using arms or legs, or opening eyes." [10] While in the same study, 13- to 18- year-old pediatric oncology patients' fatigue was described as "a complex, changing state of exhaustion that at times seems to be a physical condition, at other times a mental state, and still other times to be a combination of physical and mental tiredness." [10] The children's definition emphasizes a physical sensation (weakness), whereas the adolescents' definition accentuated both physical and mental exhaustion. Developmental stage may have a greater impact when evaluating fatigue than has yet been appreciated.

PREVALENCE

Cancer-related fatigue is reported by 60% to 99% of cancer patients and is a significant quality-of-life issue in cancer care.[5,11,12] The knowledge base concerning this number one reported side effect, although increasing continually, remains one of the least explained phenomena of advanced disease.[12,13] Significant research has contributed to the body of knowledge about cancer-related fatigue in the adult population[2,8,9,14–17] as well as in the pediatric and adolescent groups.[18,19]

Research in the palliative care arena has focused primarily on adults.[16,20,21] A prospective study of fatigue compared advanced cancer patients to age- and sex-matched controls. The control group had a moderate excess of women (57%), with 49% (48/98) who were overweight and 50% having at least one concomitant medical problem, such as arthritis, airflow limitation, or hypertension.[20] Although both patients and controls complained of a degree of fatigue, the severity of symptoms in patients was much worse. The prevalence of severe subjective fatigue (which was defined as a score on the fatigue scale of greater than the 95th percentile of controls) was 75% in the advanced cancer group. In this patient group, there were a variety of cancer diagnoses (breast, lung, and prostate) and many of the patients were also taking opioid medications.[20]

Another relevant study, conducted by the World Health Organization, included 1840 palliative care patients.[22] The prevalence of nine symptoms (pain, nausea, dyspnea, constipation, anorexia, weakness, confusion, insomnia, and weight loss) was examined in seven palliative care centers from the United States, Europe, and Australia. With the exception of moderate to severe pain, weakness was the most common symptom, reported by 51% of patients.[22]

Cancer is only one of several diseases in which fatigue is a common symptom. Fatigue has been a frequent experience in patients with end-stage renal disease. One study of 191 patients on dialysis reported that tiredness was the most frequently reported somatic symptom, experienced by 72% of hemodialysis patients and 68% of chronic ambulatory peritoneal dialysis patients.[23] Another study asked 137 ambulatory dialysis patients about their fatigue.[24] The same amount of fatigue was reported by equal numbers of those receiving dialysis for less than 4 years (short-term) and those receiving long-term dialysis. However, the investigators reported that patients receiving short-term dialysis had a greater amount of moderate fatigue. The authors suggested that there may be a pattern of adjustment over time to end stage renal disease. Interestingly, no correlation between fatigue scores and other laboratory values (blood urea nitrogen and creatinine) was found.[24]

Fatigue exists in all gradations of rheumatoid arthritis (RA), which affects approximately 7.5 million Americans.[25] The prevalence of fatigue severity, distress, and impact was evaluated in 133 older adults with RA.[25] Participants averaged 67 years of age and had a mean disease duration of 18 years. Fatigue was reported to occur every day, remained constant during the week, and affected walking and household chores.[25]

Coronary artery disease affects nearly 13 million Americans, and according to research, fatigue is a significant side effect.[26,27] Fatigue was identified as a precoronary symptom during interviews of 142 relatives of people who died a sudden, unexpected death from coronary artery disease.[26] The investigators found a history of tiredness and decreased energy in 41% of patients, as reported by the relatives. In acute infarct survivors (n = 40), 77% had increasing and abnormal fatigue for 6 months to 3 years prior to the infarct. Fatigue was also examined in 80 women who had been hospitalized with known heart failure in the previous 12 twelve months.[27] According to the authors, fatigue demonstrated the greatest increase over time and was experienced more than any other symptom.

Patients with human immunodeficiency virus (HIV) infection or acquired immune deficiency syndrome (AIDS) are plagued with fatigue.[28,29] In one study of three separate groups, one with AIDS [Centers for Disease Control (CDC) stage IV], one with lymphadenopathy (CDC stage III), and one group who were HIV-seronegative, fatigue was problematic in more than half of the stage IV patients. Those with more advanced disease experienced more hours of daily fatigue and slept more hours at night, even though they napped more frequently during the day.[28]

Reported fatigue research in the pediatric population has been scarce. One multiinstitutional study examined the effects of cancer treatment on 75 school-aged children with cancer.[30] Fatigue was a common symptom, reported by more than 50% of participants. Fatigue was expressed by the children as being tired, not sleeping well, and not being able to do the things they wanted to do. More than half the children were not as active as before the illness and reported playing less. No studies on fatigue in children with advanced cancer were identified.

PATHOPHYSIOLOGY

Models to explain the causes of fatigue have been developed by different disciplines in the basic sciences and by clinicians. Table 7–1 represents a variety of

Table 7–1. Fatigue Theories, Models, and Frameworks

Theory/Model/Framework	Description
Accumulation hypothesis	Accumulated waste products in the body result in fatigue.
Depletion hypothesis	Muscular activity is impaired when the supply of substances such as carbohydrate, fat, protein, adenosine triphosphate, and protein is not available to the muscle. Anemia can also be considered a depletion mechanism.
Biochemical and physiochemical phenomena	Production, distribution, use, equalization, and movement of substances such as muscle proteins, glucose, electrolytes, and hormones may influence the experience of fatigue.
Central nervous system control	Central control of fatigue is placed in the balance between two opposing systems: the reticular activating system and the inhibitory system, which is believed to involve the reticular formation, the cerebral cortex, and the brain stem.
Adaptation and energy reserves	Each person has a certain amount of energy reserve for adaptation, and fatigue occurs when energy is depleted. This hypothesis incorporates ideas from the other hypotheses but focuses on the person's response to stressors.
Psychobiologic entropy	Activity, fatigue, symptoms, and functional status are associated based on clinical observations that persons who become less active as a result of disease or treatment-related symptoms lose energizing metabolic resources.
Aistar's organizing framework[64]	This framework is based on energy and stress theory and implicates physiologic, psychologic, and situational stressors as contributing to fatigue. Aistar attempts to explain the difference between tiredness and fatigue within Selye's general adaptation syndrome.[63]
Piper's integrated fatigue model[8]	Piper suggests that fatigue mechanisms influence signs and symptoms of fatigue. Changes in biologic patterns such as host factors, metabolites, energy substrates, disease, and treatment, along with psychosocial patterns, impact a person's perception and lead to fatigue manifestations. The fatigue manifestations are expressed through the person's behavior.
Attentional fatigue model	Use of attentional theory linked to attentional fatigue. When increased requirements or demands for directed attention exceed available capacity, the person is at risk for attentional fatigue.

Source: Barnett (1997), reference 61.

theories, models, or frameworks to explain cancer-related fatigue that have been reported in the literature. The three most prominent theories are presented in more detail below. While these models were developed with the cancer patient in mind, the depletion model may also be applied to end-stage renal disease and the central peripheral model may be applied to multiple sclerosis.

The *accumulation theory* suggests that fatigue may be related to the abnormal accumulation of muscle metabolites, such as lactate, that interfere with normal cellular functioning based on limited muscle function studies.[31,32] One of the most intensively studied examples of the accumulation model is the production of cytokines in response to the development of cancer. Tumor necrosis factor has been linked to a reduction in skeletal muscle protein stores, resulting in muscle wasting associated with cachexia, observed in some patients with cancer and AIDS.[33,34] Interleukin-1β has been associated with the fatigue resulting from localized radiation treatment.[35] In addition, fatigue often accompanies the exogenous administration of biological response modifiers, such as interferon or interleukin-2, when used as cancer therapy.[4,36,37] These data suggest that similar mechanisms may be involved in the pathogenesis of certain types of fatigue.[38] However, to date, there is no direct evidence to support a causal relationship between any cytokine and the occurrence of fatigue.[13]

Anemia, a deficiency of red blood cells or lack of hemoglobin that leads to a reduction in oxygen-carrying capacity of the blood, is an example of the *depletion theory*. Anemia is a common occurrence in patients with advanced disease or those receiving aggressive therapy.[39,40] Although there is reliable evidence that fatigue can be caused by anemia,[41] little is known about the relationship between the degree or rate of hemoglobin loss and the development of fatigue. One study described results of a new questionnaire that was tested on a sample of 50 patients with either solid tumors or hematological malignancies.[42] The fatigue subscale, a new addition to the Functional Assessment of Chronic Illness Therapy Measurement System, was able to distinguish patients with a hemoglobin level greater than 12 g/dl from those with a level less than 12 g/dl. Research on patients with end-stage renal disease indicates no relationship between hematocrit and subjective fatigue, even though anemia is a major side effect of the disease.[24,43] While one study demonstrated some association between subjective fatigue and anemia, it is by no means conclusive and suggests that further research is needed.[43]

The *central nervous system model* suggests integration between central and peripheral mechanisms that lead to fatigue.[32] At the peripheral nervous system level, a decline in intracellular calcium in peripheral nerves, for example, leads to the failure to maintain required or expected muscle force, resulting in reduced performance. The chemoreceptors in fatigued muscles send sensory impulses back to the reticular formation in the central nervous system. These sensory impulses can inhibit motor pathways anywhere from the voluntary centers in the brain to the spinal motor neurons.

The search for foundational causes of fatigue continues because no one theory thoroughly explains the basis for fatigue in the patient with advanced disease. The search for such a theory is complicated. Fatigue, like pain, is not only explained by physiological mechanisms but must be understood as a multicausal, multidimensional phenomenon that includes physical, psychological, social, and spiritual aspects. As such, factors influencing fatigue are beginning to be addressed.

FACTORS INFLUENCING FATIGUE

Characteristics that may predispose patients with advanced disease to develop fatigue have not been comprehensively studied. Oncology research has placed importance on patient characteristics in treatment-related fatigue. Table 7–2 provides a list of factors that have been associated with cancer-related fatigue. Several of these factors have been studied and are presented in some detail below.

Age is one factor that has been examined in several studies of treatment-related fatigue in oncology. The majority of completed research indicates that younger adult patients with cancer report more fatigue than older patients with cancer.[42,43] This suggests that reported fatigue may be influenced by the developmental level of the adult. For example, young adults may have heavy responsibilities of balancing career, marriage, and child-rearing, while older adults may be at the end of their careers or retired with empty nests. Additionally, the older adult often has more than one medical condition and may even attribute the fatigue to advancing age, thereby not viewing it as abnormal. These may partially explain why fatigue is reported more frequently by younger adults.

Psychological depression has been linked to patients with cancer-related fatigue.[44–46] Depression and fatigue are two related concepts. Fatigue is part of the diagnostic criteria for depression,[47] and depression may develop as a result of being fatigued.[48] While depression is less frequently reported than fatigue, feelings of depression are common in patients with cancer, with a prevalence rate in the range of 20% to 25%.[49,50] In addition, with cancer, depression and fatigue may coexist without having a causal relationship because each can originate from the same pathology.[48,51]

Recent information derived from the scientific literature supports the notion that advanced stage of disease compounds the level of fatigue. Evidence demonstrates that the more advanced the cancer, the greater the occurrence of subjective fatigue.[52] Fobair and colleagues[52] interviewed 403 long-term survivors of Hodgkin's disease who had completed their initial therapy between 1 and 21 years before. Patients were asked if their energy had changed, and if it had changed, how long it took to return to normal. Patients whose energy level had not returned to normal were more frequently found to be in the later stages of the disease.

As illustrated by the following case reports, patient perceptions may be influenced by *other symptoms*.

Table 7–2. Predisposing Factors in Developing Fatigue

Personal factors
Age
Marital status
Menopausal status
Psychosocial factors (depression, fear, anxiety, unfinished business, unresolved family/friend conflicts, unmet goals)
Culture/ethnicity
Income/insurance
Physical living situation
Spiritual factors
Disease-related factors
Anemia
Stage of disease/presence of metastases
Pain
Sleep patterns/interruptions
Permanent changes in energy "new normal"
Continency
Cachexia
Dyspnea
Treatment-related factors
Medication side effects (nausea, vomiting, diarrhea, weight loss or gain, taste changes)
Permanent physiologic consequences (altered energy or sleep pattern)
Care factors
Number/cohesiveness of caregivers
Commitment of doctor/nurse (involvement and availability)

Case Study: Mrs. Edwards

Mrs. Edwards, a 52-year-old white woman, married with adult children, worked as a secretary in a hospital, transcribing dictation. Mrs. Edwards is a self-proclaimed "burn the candle at both ends" type of person. She had recently had bilateral hip replacement, which she had postponed until she could stand the pain no longer. During the recovery phase, she did not bounce back as quickly as she had expected and kept blaming the fatigue on her age and the slow healing process. A chest x-ray a few months later revealed a mediastinal mass. It was biopsied and proved to be positive for lung cancer. Her cancer was inoperable. She was offered both palliative radiation and chemotherapy to shrink the tumor and buy some time. She opted for radiation only and continued to work during treatment. She described her fatigue as follows:

"The radiation fatigue was a gradual descent. I began to feel more fatigued and nauseated. I also had pain. I couldn't eat because my esophagus was so inflamed. The radiation just wore away gradually at my energy level. I zonked out after not eating for 3 or 4 days and still tried to do radiation. I finally stopped it and said 'no more.' The reason I held on for as long as I could was that I didn't want to alarm my husband. I am very poor about letting other people do for me. We had an established pattern. He comes home, we talk; and I didn't want to break that pattern. So I would fight to stay up . . . just trying to keep my eyes open. . . . It was like the sand fairy came and spread all the sleep granules and you just keep pushing them away and the cobwebs, and brushing them away . . . you want to use toothpicks to keep your eyeballs open. I knew that when he came home I would revive a little bit. I don't know how much of that was for him and how much was for me. I think, in my mind, I think the mental process is 'Keep doing it because you still can do it and to give it up means the decline is more advanced,' and I think that's one part of it, is that mental process.

"Fatigue is the worst symptom because it's chronic and the edge of it is always there even when I'm doing things and I'm feeling pretty good; it's like the dark edge creeps in all the time. As the day goes by, it begins to overtake you and pretty soon it makes you absolutely inert."

FATIGUE ASSESSMENT

Assessing Mrs. Edwards's fatigue included measuring the intensity/severity (0–10 scale), location, duration, general appearance, muscle strength, aggravating/alleviating factors, knowledge/meaning of fatigue, use of medications that may cause fatigue, level of current activity, affect, physical exam based on symptoms and lab results (anemia, malnutrition, electrolyte imbalance).

FATIGUE INTERVENTION

Mrs. Edwards was somewhat familiar with self-care in chronic and terminal illness because of working in a hospital setting. She was able to incorporate what she had learned about other patients into her own situation. She stopped smoking, worked at improving her nutritional status by using supplemental protein drinks, planned how to spend her energy, but chose not to exercise. "I've never been a walker; I don't like to walk. If it has wheels or hooves on it, that's always been my mode of transportation."

Family meetings helped her adult children to rally and share responsibilities of home, shopping, meal preparation, and care for Mrs. Edwards, thus reducing her fatigue.

Fatigue in patients undergoing cancer treatment has been closely linked with other distressing symptoms, such as pain, dyspnea, anorexia, constipation, sleep disruption, depression, anxiety, and other mood states.[9,11,53] Research on patients with advanced cancer has demonstrated that fatigue severity was significantly associated with similar symptoms.[20]

Like patients with cancer, patients with end-stage renal disease on chronic dialysis complained of a high level of fatigue that was associated with other symptoms.[54] The other symptoms identified were headaches, cramps, itching, dyspnea, sleep disruption (highest mean score), nausea, chest pain, and abdominal pain. However, there was no relationship found between other symptoms and any of the demographic variables.

One hundred patients with RA were asked to identify factors that contributed to their fatigue.[55] Results indicated that the rheumatoid disease process itself was the primary cause of fatigue, with specific mention of joint pain. Disturbed sleep was the second most frequent factor, and physical effort to accomplish daily tasks ranked third. Patients with RA indicated that they had to exert twice the effort and energy to accomplish the same amount of work. Another study of patients with RA reported that women experienced more fatigue than men.[25] The authors explained this variance by the female patients' higher degrees of pain and poor quality of sleep.

Other symptoms were also identified as impacting fatigue in a study of 80 women with congestive heart failure.[27] The women were interviewed if hospitalized in the previous 12 months for heart failure, and a second interview occurred 18 months after the first interview. Sleep difficulties, chest pain, and weakness each explained a unique variance in fatigue during the first interview. Dyspnea was the only symptom that explained the variance in fatigue at the second interview.[27]

Fatigue in children and adolescents with advanced cancer has not been addressed. However, research has begun on pediatric oncology patients' reports of factors influencing their fatigue.[10,18] In one study, for example, 7- to 12-year- old patients with cancer viewed hospital noises, new routines, changing sleep patterns, getting treatment, and low blood counts as contributing factors to the development of fatigue.[18] In the same study, 13- to 18-year-old patients reported that going for treatment, noisy nurses and inpatient children, changes in sleep position, boredom, being fearful or worried, and treatment side effects led to their fatigue.

Little research on factors influencing fatigue in patients with advanced cancer has been conducted. However, results from treatment-related fatigue research do give direction for assessment and management of fatigue in the palliative care setting.

ASSESSMENT

Fatigue assessment of the whole person remains paramount and includes the consideration of the body as well as the mind and spirit. When assessing fatigue, one may refer to the current literature regarding pain assessment for assistance. In pain assessment, the patient is the one whose opinion is most highly regarded. Pain is whatever the patient says it is; so, too, it should be with fatigue. Caregiver or staff perceptions may be very different from those of the person experiencing fatigue. There is no agreement as to the perfect definition for fatigue; therefore, it is most efficient to use an individual patient's definition or descriptions of fatigue. This personal fatigue may include any reference to or decrease in energy, weakness, or feeling tired or wiped out.

There are numerous methods of assessing fatigue. Many scales have been developed to measure fatigue in the adult, with varying levels of research-related validity and reliability. Current fatigue measurement tools include the Multidimensional Assessment of Fatigue, the Symptom Distress Scale, the Fatigue Scale, the Fatigue Observation Checklist, and a Visual Analogue Scale for Fatigue.[9] These scales are available for use in research and may be used in the clinical area. One scale that has been used extensively in the oncology population is the Piper Fatigue Scale.[56]

This questionnaire has 22 items that measure four dimensions of fatigue: affective meaning, behavioral/severity, cognitive/mood, and sensory. This scale measures perception, performance, motivation, and change in physical and mental activities.[4]

In clinical practice, however, a verbal rating scale may be the most efficient. Fatigue severity may be quickly assessed using a 0 (no fatigue) to 10 (extreme fatigue) scale. As with the use of any measure, consistency over time and a specific frame of reference are needed. During each evaluation, the same instructions must be given to the patient. For example, the patient may be asked to rate the level of fatigue for the past 24 hours.

Fatigue, as with any symptom, is not static. Changes take place daily and sometimes hourly in the patient with advanced disease. As such, fatigue bears repeated evaluation on the part of the health care provider. One patient, noticing the dramatic change in his energy level, remarked "Have I always been this tired?" He seemed unsure whether there had ever been a time when he did not feel overwhelmed by the impact of fatigue. The imperative for palliative care nursing is simply to ask the patient and continue to ask, while keeping in mind that the ultimate goal is the patient's comfort. An example of a thorough assessment of the symptom of fatigue is found in Table 7–3.

Fatigue assessment tools in the pediatric population have not been developed. Many questionnaires developed for the adult patient with cancer may provide a framework for use in pediatrics. Until then, a simple assessment of fatigue severity may be incorporated.

INTRODUCTION TO THE MANAGEMENT OF FATIGUE

When considering palliative care, the management of fatigue is extremely challenging. By its very definition, palliative care may encompass a prolonged period prior to death, when a person is still active and physically and socially participating in life, to a few weeks before death, when participatory activity may be minimal. With fatigue interventions, the wishes of the patient and family are paramount. One must consider management in the context of the extent of disease, other symptoms (pain, nausea, diarrhea, etc.), whether palliative treatment is still in process, age and developmental stage, and emotional "place" of the patient.

Interventions for fatigue have been suggested to occur at two levels: managing symptoms that contribute to fatigue and the prevention of additional or secondary fatigue by maintaining a balance between restorative rest and restorative activity.[5] Fatigue interventions have been grouped into four broad categories: active exercise, attention restoration, preparatory education, and psychosocial interventions.

Several investigators have reported on the benefits of a consistent exercise regime in breast cancer patients.[57,58] They have found that exercise decreased perceptions of fatigue and indicated that those patients who exercised reported half the fatigue level of those not exercising. The generalizability of these findings to palliative care is unknown.

When attention-restoring interventions were used with cancer patients, it was found that attentional capacity was enhanced and fatigue was reduced.[14] These activities are based on a program that required patients to select and engage in a favorite activity three times a week for 30 minutes. The use of this technique seemed to provide restorative distraction and replace boredom and understimulation. Included in the activities were spending time in a natural environment, participating in favorite hobbies, writing, fishing, music, and gardening. Regardless of the limitations of the patients with advanced disease, incorporation of some of these activities may prove helpful.

Another broad category for fatigue intervention includes taking advantage of every educational opportunity over the advanced disease course. With education of both the patient and family a constant theme, every attempt should

Table 7–3. Fatigue Assessment

Location: Where on the body is the fatigue located: Upper/lower extremities? All muscles of the body? Mental/attentional fatigue? Total body fatigue?
Intensity/severity: Does the fatigue interfere with activities (work, role/responsibilities at home, social, things the patient enjoys)?
Duration: How long does the fatigue last (minutes, hours, days)? Has it become chronic (more than 6 months' duration)? What is the pattern (wake up from a night's sleep exhausted, evening fatigue, transient, unfading, are circadian rhythms affected)?
Aggravating factors: What makes it worse (rest, activity, other symptoms, environmental heat, noise)?
Alleviating factors: What relieves it (a good night's rest, food, listening to music)?
Patient's knowledge of fatigue: What meaning does the patient assign to the symptom of fatigue (getting worse, disease progression, dying)?
Medications: Is the patient taking any medications that could cause the fatigue (for pain or sleep)?
Physical exam based on subjective symptom: Is there anything obvious on exam that could account for the fatigue (nerve damage, malnourished, dehydrated)?
Muscle strength: Tests to elicit muscle strength are available (Jamar grip strength, nerve conduction studies).
General appearance: Often, there is nothing in a patient's general appearance to indicate how fatigued he or she is; however, some patients do exhibit signs such as appearing pale or having a monotone voice, slowed speech, short of breath, obvious weight loss, dull facial expression.
Vital signs: Anything out of the ordinary to explain their fatigue (fever, low blood pressure, weak pulse)?
Laboratory results: Oxygenation status (blood gases, hemoglobin, hematocrit, electrolytes, other hormones such as thyroid)?
Level of activity: Have usual activities changed?
Affect: What is the patient's mood (anxious, depressed, flat)?

Table 7–4. Nursing Management of Cancer-Related Fatigue

Problem	Intervention	Rationale
Lack of information/ lack of preparation	Explain complex nature of fatigue and importance of communication with health care professionals. Explain causes of fatigue in advanced cancer: • Fatigue can increase in advanced disease. • Cancer cells can compete with body for essential nutrients. • Palliative treatments, infection, and fever increase body's need for energy. • Worry or anxiety can cause fatigue as well as depression, sadness, or tension. • Changes in daily schedules, new routines, or interrupted sleep schedules contribute to the development of fatigue. Prepare patients for all planned activities of daily living (eating, moving, bath)	Preparatory sensory information reduces anxiety and fatigue. Realistic expectations decrease distress and decrease fatigue.
Disrupted rest/sleep patterns	Establish or continue regular bedtime and awakening. Obtain as long sleep sequences as possible, plan uninterrupted time. Rest periods or naps during the day, if needed, but do not interfere with nighttime sleep. Use light sources to cue the body into a consistent sleep rhythm. Pharmacologic management of insomnia should be used only when behavioral and cognitive approaches have been exhausted.	Curtailing time in bed, unless absolutely necessary, helps patient feel refreshed and avoids fragmented sleep; strengthens circadian rhythm.
Deficient nutritional status	Recommend nutritious, high-protein, nutrient-dense food to make every mouthful of food "count." Suggest more small, frequent meals. Use protein supplements to augment diet. Encourage adequate intake of fluids, recommend 8–10 glasses or whatever is comfortably tolerated unless medically contraindicated to maintain hydration. Frequent oral hygiene. Corticosteriods may be prescribed to assist with appetite stimulation.	Food will help energy levels; less energy is needed for digestion with small, frequent meals.
Symptom management	Control contributing symptoms (pain, depression, nausea, vomiting, diarrhea, constipation, anemia, electrolyte imbalances, dyspnea, dehydration). Assess for anemia and evaluate for the possibility of medications or transfusion.	Managing other symptoms requires energy and may interfere with restful sleep.
Distraction/ restoration	Encourage activities to restore energy: spending time in the natural environment, listening to music, praying, meditating, engaging in hobbies (art, journaling, reading, writing, fishing), spending time with family and friends, joining in passive activities (riding in car, being read to, watching meal preparation).	Pleasant activities may reduce/relieve mental (attentional) fatigue.
Decreased energy	Plan/schedule activities: Choose someone to be in charge (fielding questions, answering the phone, organizing meals). Determine where energy is best spent and eliminate or postpone other activities.	Energy conservation helps to reduce burden and efficiently use energy available.

(continued)

Table 7–4. Nursing Management of Cancer-Related Fatigue (*continued*)

Problem	Intervention	Rationale
	Utilize optimal times of the day: • Save energy for most important events. • Learn to listen to the body; if fatigued, rest. Let things go around the house.	
Physical limitations	Engage in an individually tailored exercise program approved by the health care team. Enjoy leisure activities (sitting outside, music, gardening, etc.) Be receptive to the patient's pace, and move slowly when providing care. Mild physical therapy may be helpful in maintaining joint flexibility and preventing potential pain from joint stiffness.	Exercise reduces the deleterious effects of immobility and deconditioning.

be made to forewarn of changes in disease progression, procedures, treatment, medication side effects, or scheduling. Even a personnel change can be enough to impact the physical and emotional energy reserves. Nurse-initiated and planned educational sessions with both the patient and family give a forum in which to field forgotten questions, reinforce nutritional information, and together manage symptoms.

Psychosocial techniques are the last broad category of fatigue intervention. One review of 22 studies of psychosocial treatment with cancer patients reported findings that indicate that psychosocial support and individualized counseling have a fatigue-reducing effect.[59] If deemed appropriate, encourage the patient and/or family to participate in disease-specific support groups or to use telephone or the internet if unable to travel. Individual counseling by professionals in nursing, social work, or psychology are also helpful to many.

Table 7–4 includes a list of common fatigue-related problems the patient

Table 7–5. Rules for Sleep Hygiene

Rule	Rationale
Sleep just long enough	Each patient should sleep as much as needed to feel refreshed during the following day; some people seem to need more sleep than others. Sleep no longer than is necessary. Limiting time in bed seems to solidify sleep; excessively long times in bed seem to be related to fragmented and shallow sleep.
Wake up and go to bed at the same time every day	Regulating the sleep schedule seems to strengthen circadian cycles and will help lead to regular sleep onset. Weekends should not be an exception to the schedule.
Exercise regularly	A consistent amount of daily exercise helps to deepen sleep over the long haul, but occasional sporadic exercise may not. Do not exercise right before retiring as this will interfere with sleep onset.
Get light exposure every day (open shades, walk, work outdoors)	Sets the circadian clock.
Eliminate noise	Occasional loud noises (e.g., aircraft flyovers, sirens, others up and moving about, dogs barking) disturb sleep even when people do not awaken because of them and do not remember them in the morning. The use of ear plugs may be helpful.
Regulate room temperature	Excessive cold or heat disturbs sleep. Regulate the temperature for comfort.
Eat a bedtime snack	A light snack and something warm to drink helps many people sleep.
Know the effect that daytime napping has on you	Some people sleep better at night, and others have sleep disruption following daytime napping. The time used to take a nap should be limited to 30 minutes in the early afternoon.
Avoid stimulants	Many poor sleepers are sensitive to stimulants. Caffeine takes at least 8 hours to metabolize. No stimulant drinks should be taken after lunchtime.
Limit alcohol consumption	Alcohol initially helps stressed people to fall asleep, but the sleep is fragmented and not restful or restorative.
Do not try too hard	If unable to fall asleep after 15–20 minutes, get out of bed and go into another room. Read with a dim light and avoid watching TV (because of light exposure). Return to bed only when sleepy.
Chronic use of tobacco can be disruptive to sleep	Nicotine acts as a stimulant.

Source: Hu and Silverfarb (1991), reference 62.

with advanced disease may encounter, along with suggestions for interventions and rationales for their use. Sleep disruption is one common problem encountered by the patient with advanced cancer. Sleep cycles may be negatively affected by innumerable internal and external factors whose effect should not be underestimated. Simple changes in environment and habits may improve sleep distress tremendously. Table 7–5 provides practical suggestions for the management of disturbed sleep.

Fatigue-management interventions need to be considered within the cultural context of the patient and family. For some cultures, this may include only the "nuclear" family, whereas in other cultures, there are ritual or extended relatives. When information is shared and decisions are made regarding intervention, the "family" is acknowledged formally, and care should be made inclusive of these variations.[60]

Management of and interventions for fatigue in pediatric oncology, in general, have not yet been defined. Additionally, what helps the pediatric patient with fatigue depends on his or her developmental stage.[10] Children with cancer up to 13 years old view fatigue-alleviating factors as taking a nap or sleeping, having visitors, and participating in fun activities. Adolescent patients with cancer add their perceptions of what helps their fatigue by including going outdoors, protracted rest time, keeping busy, medication for sleep, physical therapy, and receiving blood transfusions.[10] Regardless of the perceptions of the contributing or alleviating factors in the younger patient, knowing the results of this research emphasizes the importance of including all members of the team (patient, parent, and staff) in designing approaches to intervene in solving the problem of fatigue.

SUMMARY

This chapter has provided an overview of fatigue as it spans the illness trajectory and end-of-life experience. While fatigue is a complex phenomenon that has been widely studied, there is no universally accepted definition. Fatigue is experienced by individuals with various chronic diseases; is influenced by many factors such as age, depression, stage of disease and other concurrent symptoms; and has numerous causes. The authors have provided a fatigue-assessment checklist that can be used to identify potential sources and/or antecedents for the patient's fatigue. Because there is no instant cure for fatigue, the patient experiencing it may be frustrated and reluctant to use the practical interventions provided in Table 7–4. Nurses are challenged to provide current information about fatigue, its reversable causes, and its normal occurrence with various illnesses and to encourage patients to actively participate in fatigue-management strategies.

REFERENCES

1. Schaefer KM, Potylycki MJ. Fatigue associated with congestive heart failure: use of Levine's conservation model. J Adv Nurs 1993;18:260–268.
2. Ferrell BR, Grant M, Dean G, Funk B, Ly J. "Bone tired": the experience of fatigue and its impact on quality of life. Oncol Nurs Forum 1996;23:1539–1547.
3. Richardson A, Ream E. Fatigue in patients receiving chemotherapy for advanced cancer. Int J Palliat Nurs 1996;2:199–204.
4. Dean GE, Ferrell BF. Fatigue. In: Johnson BL, Gross J, eds. Handbook of Oncology Nursing, 3rd ed. Boston: Jones and Bartlett, 1998:360–376.
5. Winningham ML, Nail LM, Burke MB, et al. Fatigue and the cancer experience: the state of the knowledge. Oncol Nurs Forum 1994; 21:23–36.
6. Hart LK, Freel. Fatigue. In: Norris CM, ed. Concept Clarification in Nursing. Rockville, MD: Aspen, 1982:251–261.
7. Tiesinga LJ, Dassen TWN, Halfens RJG. Fatigue: a summary of the definitions, dimensions and indicators. Nurs Diagn 1996;7:51–62.
8. Piper B. Fatigue. In: Carrieri-Kohlman V, Lindsey A, West C, eds. Pathophysiological Phenomena in Nursing: Human Responses to Illness, 2nd ed. Philadelphia: WB Saunders, 1993:279–302.
9. Aaronson LS, Teel CS, Cassmeyer V, et al. Defining and measuring fatigue. Image J Nurs Sch 1999;31:45–50.
10. Hinds PS, Hockenberry-Eaton M, Gilger E, et al. Comparing patient, parent, and staff descriptions of fatigue in pediatric oncology patients. Cancer Nurs 1999;22:277–289.
11. Blesch K, Paice J, Wickman R, et al. Correlates of fatigue in people with breast or lung cancer. Oncol Nurs Forum 1991;18:81–87.
12. Vogelzang N, Breitbart W, Cella D, et al. Patients, caregivers and oncologists perception of cancer related fatigue: results of a tripart assessment survey [abstract]. Proc Am Soc Clin Oncol 1997;16:53A.
13. Portenoy RK, Miakowski C. Assessment and management of cancer-related fatigue. In: Berger AM, Portenoy RK, Weissman DE, eds. Principles and Practice of Supportive Oncology. Philadelphia: Lippincott-Raven, 1998:109–118.
14. Cimprich B. Attentional fatigue following breast cancer surgery. Res Nurs Health 1992; 15:199–207.
15. Haylock PJ, Hart LK. Fatigue in patients receiving localized radiation. Cancer Nurs 1979;2: 461–467.
16. Maltoni M, Nannie O, Pirovano M, et al. Successful validation of the palliative prognostic score in terminally ill cancer patients. J Pain Symptom Manage 1999;17:240–247.
17. Smets EMA, Visser MRM, Willems-Groot AF, et al. Fatigue and radiotherapy: (A) experience in patients undergoing treatment. Br J Cancer 1998;78:899–906.
18. Hinds PS, Hockenberry-Eaton M, Quargnenti A, et al. Fatigue in 7- to 12-year old patients with cancer from the staff perspective: an exploratory study. Oncol Nurs Forum 1999;26: 37–45.
19. Hockenberry-Eaton M, Hinds P. Developing a conceptual model for fatigue in children [abstract]. Oncol Nurs Forum 1999;25:332.
20. Stone P, Hardy J, Broadley K, Tookman A, Kurowska A, Hern R. Fatigue in advanced cancer: a prospective controlled cross-sectional study. Br J Cancer 1999;79:1479–1486.
21. Priovano M, Maltoni M, Nanni O, et al. A new palliative prognostic score: a first step for the staging of terminally ill cancer patients. J Pain Symptom Manage 1999;17:231–239.
22. Vainio A, Auvinen A. Prevalence of symptoms among patients with advanced cancer: an international study. J Pain Symptom Manage 1996; 12:3–10.
23. Barnett B, Varasour A, Major A, Parfrey P. Clinical and psychological correlates of somatic symptoms in patients on dialysis. Nephron 1990; 55:10–15.
24. Cardenas D, Kutner N. (1982). The problem of fatigue in dialysis patients. Nephron 1982;30:336–340.
25. Belza B, Henke C, Yelin E, Epstein W, Gilliss C. Correlates of fatigue in older adults with rheumatoid arthritis. Nurs Res 1993;42:93–109.
26. Nixon P, Bethell H. Preinfarction ill health. Am J Cardiol 1974;33:446–449.
27. Friedman M, King K. Correlates of fatigue in older women with heart failure. Heart Lung 1995;24:512–518.
28. Darko D, McCutchan J, Kripke D, Gillin J, Golshan S. Fatigue, sleep disturbance, disability and indices of progression of HIV infection. Am J Psychiatry 1992;149:514–520.
29. Grady C, Anderson R, Chase GA. Fatigue in HIV-infected men receiving investigational interleukin-2. Nurs Res 1999;47:227–234.

30. Bottomley S, Teegarden C, Hockenberry-Eaton M. Fatigue in children with cancer: clinical considerations for nursing. J Pediatr Oncol Nurs 1995;13:3.

31. Burt ME, Aoki TT, Gorschboth CM, Brennan MR. Peripheral tissue metabolism in cancer-bearing man. Ann Surg 1983;198:685–691.

32. Gandevia SC. Some central and peripheral factors affecting human motoneuronal output in neuromuscular fatigue. Sports Med, 1992;13: 93–98.

33. Billingsly KG, Alexander HR. The pathophysiology of cachexia in advanced cancer and AIDS. In: Bruera E, Higginson I, eds. Cachexia–Anorexia in Cancer Patients. New York: Oxford University Press, 1996:1–22.

34. St Pierre B, Kasper C, Lindsey A. Fatigue mechanisms in patients with cancer: effects of tumor necrosis factor and exercise on skeletal muscle. Oncol Nurs Forum 1992;19:419–425.

35. Greenberg DB, Sawicka J, Eisenthal S, Ross D. Fatigue syndrome due to localized radiation. J Pain Symptom Manage 1992;7:38–45.

36. Mannering GJ, Deloria LB. The pharmacology and toxicology of the interferons: an overview. Ann Rev Pharmacol Toxicol 1986;26: 455–515.

37. Wills RJ, Dennis S, Spiegel HE, Gibson DM, Nadler PI. Interferon kinetics and adverse reactions after intravenous, intramuscular, and subcutaneous injection. Clin Pharmacol Ther, 1984; 35:722–727.

38. Neuenschwander H, Bruera E. Asthenia–cachexia. In: Bruera E, Higginson I, eds. Cachexia–Anorexia in Cancer Patients. New York: Oxford University Press, 1996:57–75.

39. Cella DF. Methods and problems in measuring quality of life. Support Care Cancer 1995;3:11–22.

40. Glaspy J. The impact of therapy with Epoetin alfa on clinical outcomes in patients with nonmyeloid malignancies during cancer chemotherapy in community oncology practice. J Clin Oncol 1997;15:1218–1234.

41. Cella D. The Functional Assessment of Cancer Therapy–Anemia (FACT-An) Scale: a new tool for the assessment of outcomes in cancer anemia and fatigue. Semin Hematol 1997;3(Suppl 2):13–19.

42. Ashbury FD, Findlay H, Reynolds B, McKerracher K. A Canadian survey of cancer patients' experiences: are their needs being met? J Pain Symptom Manage 1998;16:298–306.

43. Woo B, Dibble SL, Piper BF, Keating SB, Weiss MC. Differences in fatigue by treatment methods in women with breast cancer. Oncol Nurs Forum 1998;25:915–920.

44. Hardman A, Maguire P, Crowther D. The recognition of psychiatric morbidity on a medical oncology ward. J Psychosom Res 1989;33: 235–239.

45. Kathol RG, Noyes R, Williams J. Diagnosing depression in patients with medical illness. Psychosomatics 1990;31:436–449.

46. Valente SM, Saunders JM, Cohen MZ. Evaluating depression among patients with cancer. Cancer Pract 1994;2:65–71.

47. American Psychiatric Association. Diagnostic and Statistical Manual of Mental Disorders, (4th ed.) Washington DC: American Psychiatric Association, 1994:317–391.

48. Visser MRM, Smets EMA. Fatigue, depression and quality of life in cancer patients: how are they related? Support Care Cancer 1998;6: 101–108.

49. Hayes JR. Depression and chronic fatigue in cancer patients. Prim Care 1991;18:327–339.

50. Ibbotson T, Maguire P, Selby P, Priestman T, Wallace L. Screening for anxiety and depression in cancer patients: the effects of disease and treatment. Eur J Cancer 1993;30:37–40.

51. Redd WH, Jacobson PB. Emotions and cancer. Cancer 1988;62:1871–1879.

52. Fobair P, Hoppe RT, Bloom J, Cox R, Varghese A, Spiegel D. Psychosocial problems among survivors of Hodgkin's disease. J Clin Oncol 1986;4:805–814.

53. Gift A, Pugh G. Dyspnea and fatigue. Nurs Clin North Am 1993;28:373–384.

54. Brunier G, Graydon J. The influence of physical activity on fatigue in patients with ESRD on hemodialysis. Am Nephrol Nurses Assoc J 1993;20:457–461.

55. Crosby L. Factors which contribute to fatigue associated with rheumatoid arthritis. J Adv Nurs 1991;16:974–981.

56. Piper BF, Dibble SL, Dodd MJ. The revised Piper Fatigue Scale: confirmation of its multidimensionality and reduction in number of items in women with breast cancer [abstract]. Oncol Nurs Forum 1996;23:352.

57. Winningham M, MacVicar M, Burke C. Exercise for cancer patients: guidelines and precautions. Physician Sportsmed 1986;14:125.

58. Mock V, Dow KH, Meares CJ, et al. Effects of exercise on fatigue, physical functioning, and emotional distress during radiation therapy for breast cancer. Oncol Nurs Forum 1997;24:991–1000.

59. Trijsburg R, van Knippengerg F, Rijpma S. Effects of psychological treatment on cancer patients: a comparison of strategies. Psychosom Med 1992;54:489–517.

60. Kagawa-Singer M. A multicultural perspective on death and dying. Oncol Nurs Forum 1998;25:1752–1756.

61. Barnett ML. Fatigue. In: Otto SE, ed. Oncology Nursing, 3rd ed. St. Louis: Mosby, 1997; 670.

62. Hu DS, Silverfarb PM. Management of Sleep Problems in Cancer Patients. Oncology 1991;5:23–27.

63. Selye H. Forty Years of Stress Research: Principal remaining problems and misconceptions. Can Med Assoc J 1976;115:53–56.

64. Aistars J. Fatigue in the cancer patient: a conceptual approach to a clinical problem. Oncol Nurs Forum 1987;14:25–30.

8 Anorexia and Cachexia

CHARLES KEMP

I have no appetite. I know it upsets my family, but I just can't eat. It scares me sometimes; you have to eat to live.

—A patient

Anorexia, the "lack or loss of appetite, resulting in the inability to eat," and resulting weight loss are common in many illnesses. At least in the early stages, anorexia usually resolves with resolution of the illness and any weight lost is replaced with nutritional supplements or increased intake.[1,2] Unchecked, anorexia (or decreased nutritional intake from other causes such as lack of available food) leads to protein calorie malnutrition (PCM) and weight loss, primarily of fat tissue but also of lean muscle mass. These conditions are virtually universal among patients with advanced cancer and acquired immune deficiency syndrome (AIDS).[3,4]

Cachexia, a condition distinct from anorexia, also is common in cancer and AIDS, as well as other conditions, including congestive heart failure, severe sepsis, tuberculosis, and malabsorption.[2] The word "cachexia" is derived from the Greek *kakos*, meaning bad, and *hexis*, meaning condition. *Cachexia* is defined as a state of "general ill health and malnutrition, marked by weakness and emaciation; it occurs in more than 80% of patients with cancer before death and is the main cause of death in more than 20% of such patients.[5,6] In contradistinction to anorexia or starvation, in cachexia, there is approximately equal loss of fat and muscle, significant loss of bone mineral content, and no response to nutritional supplements or increased intake.[1,7] Weight loss, regardless of etiology, has a decidedly negative effect on survival; and loss of lean body mass has an especially deleterious effect.[8]

In patients with cancer, weight loss is most common in cancers of digestive organs (stomach, pancreas, colon) and is also common in (but not limited to) lung cancer and non-Hodgkin's lymphoma. However, even in digestive organ cancers, the weight loss is not due solely to decreased digestive function but also to other metabolic processes, as described below.[8]

Cachexia was previously considered to result from tumor energy demands and/or an advanced state of anorexia, but there is now convincing evidence that in advanced disease, such as cancer and AIDS, anorexia is often "an almost universal characteristic of cachexia"[9] and that cachexia develops from a low-level, lengthy, systemic inflammatory response (metabolic imbalance) related especially to the presence of proinflammatory cytokines.[1] Simply stated, the inflammatory response and metabolic imbalance(s) of cachexia lead to anorexia. In other cases, however, anorexia results from, or is a symptom of, exogenous processes such as primary eating disorders, psychiatric illnesses, or unpleasant aspects of illness like pain or nausea.[1]

The basic etiologies of primary anorexia/cachexia syndrome (ACS) are metabolic imbalances resulting from the action of cytokines, tumor by-products, and the catabolic state. These result in derangement of function (mechanisms) with negative effects on survival and quality of life. There is within some of these mechanisms a mutually reinforcing aspect; for example, anorexia leads to fatigue, fatigue increases anorexia, anorexia increases fatigue, and so on. Table 8–1 summarizes the mechanisms and effects of ACS.

ETIOLOGIES AND PROCESS

Common causes of anorexia and/or ACS are described below.[1,3,4,10,11] Anorexia or ACS may be considered secondary if resulting from symptoms or exogenous etiologies such as pain, depression, nausea, or obstruction, and primary if resulting from endogenous metabolic abnormalities such as cytokine production stimulation.

METABOLIC ALTERATIONS AS THE PRIMARY CAUSE OF ANOREXIA/CACHEXIA SYNDROME

Metabolic alterations are common (and in many respects similar) in cancer and AIDS[3] and due in large part to the systemic inflammatory response and stimulation of cytokine production[1] [principally tumor necrosis factor (TNF) and interleukin-1 and interleukin-6 (IL-1 and IL-6)]. As noted earlier, at least initially, the metabolic alterations cause the anorexia rather than the anorexia causing the metabolic alterations. Indeed, major metabolic alterations may include glucose intolerance, increased glucose turnover, insulin resistance, increased lipolysis, increased skeletal muscle catabolism, negative nitrogen balance, and in at least some patients increased basal energy expenditure.[11] Table 8–2 lists metabolic abnormalities in ACS.

PARANEOPLASTIC SYNDROMES

Metabolic paraneoplastic syndromes, such as hypercalcemia or hyponatremia (syndrome of inappropriate antidiuretic hormone) may also cause anorexia or symptoms such as fatigue that contribute to anorexia. Some consider ACS to be a paraneoplastic syndrome, and others describe it as a "distant effect" of

Table 8–1. Mechanisms and Effects of Anorexia/Cachexia Syndrome

Mechanisms	Effect
Loss of appetite	Generalized host tissue wasting, nausea or "sick feeling," loss of socialization and pleasure at meals
Reduced voluntary motor activity	Skeletal muscle wasting and inanition (fatigue)
Reduced rate of muscle protein synthesis	Skeletal muscle wasting and asthenia (weakness)
Decreased immune response	Increased susceptibility to infections
Decreased response to therapy	Earlier demise and increased complications of illness

Sources: Bistrian (1999), reference 1; Grant and Rivera (1995), reference 19; Seligman et al. (1998), reference 21.

tumor.[8,12] Paraneoplastic gastrointestinal tract syndromes, such as esophageal achalasia or intestinal pseudoobstruction, result in decreased intake and, thus, PCM.[13]

PHYSICAL SYMPTOMS

A number of physical symptoms of advanced disease may contribute to, or cause, anorexia, including pain, *dysguesia* (abnormalities in taste, especially aversion to meat), *ageusia* (loss of taste), *hyperosmia* (increased sensitivity to odor), *hyposmia* (decreased sensitivity to odor), *anosmia* (absence of sense of smell), stomatitis, dysphagia, odynophagia, dyspnea, hepatomegaly, splenomegaly, gastric compression, delayed emptying, malabsorption, intestinal obstruction, nausea, vomiting, diarrhea, constipation, inanition, asthenia, various infections (see below), and early satiety. Alcoholism or other substance dependence may also contribute to, or cause, anorexia. Primary or metastatic disease sites have an effect on appetite, with cancers, such as gastric and pancreatic, having direct effects on organs of alimentation.

Table 8–2. Metabolic Abnormalities in Cachexia

Metabolic Dimension	Parameter	Usual Effect
Carbohydrate	Body glycogen mass	Decreased
	Glucose tolerance	Decreased
	Glucose production	Increased
	Glucose turnover	Increased
	Serum glucose level	Unchanged
	Insulin resistance	Increased
	Serum insulin level	Unchanged
Protein	Body (lean) muscle mass	Decreased
	Body protein synthesis	Increased
	Nitrogen balance	Negative
	Urinary nitrogen excretion	Unchanged
Lipid	Body lipid mass	Decreased
	Lipoprotein lipase activity	Decreased
	Fat synthesis	Decreased
	Fatty acid oxidation	Increased
	Serum lipid levels	Increased
	Serum triglyceride levels	Increased
Energy	Voluntary motor activity	Decreased
	Energy expenditure	Increased or decreased
	Energy stores	Decreased
	Energy balance	Negative

Sources: Bistrian et al. (1999), reference 1; Tisdale et al. (1997), reference 2; Ma and Alexander (1997), reference 8; Rivadeneira et al. (1998), reference 11.

Each of these should be ruled out as a primary or contributing cause of anorexia and, if present, treated as discussed elsewhere in this book. In general, people who are seriously ill and/or suffering distressing symptoms have poor appetites. Many cancer or human immunodeficiency virus (HIV) treatments have deleterious effects on appetite or result in side effects leading to anorexia and/or weight loss (see Medication Side Effects, below). Patients with HIV disease may also develop primary muscle disease, leading to weight loss.

MEDICATION SIDE EFFECTS

Side effects of medications (especially those used to treat HIV infection, such as acyclovir, ethambutol, foscarnet, ganciclovir, isoniazid, interferon, pyrimethamine, zidovudine, and others) may directly result in anorexia or have side effects such as nausea, taste changes, and diarrhea that lead to anorexia and PCM. While aggressive curative treatment is seldom appropriate for patients with terminal illness, it is not always possible to discern who is terminal, who is not terminal, and, if terminal, how much time remains.[14] Moreover, palliative care is not restricted to patients who are expected to die. Cytotoxic drugs that tend to be most emetic are cisplatin, dactinomycin, anthracyclines, dacarbazine, nitrosoureas, nitrogen mustard, and high-dose cyclophosphamide.[15]

PSYCHOLOGICAL AND/OR SPIRITUAL DISTRESS

Psychological and/or spiritual distress is an often overlooked cause of anorexia. The physical effects of the illness and/or treatment coupled with psychological responses (especially anxiety and/or depression) and/or spiritual distress, such as feelings of hopelessness, may result in little enthusiasm or energy for preparing or eating food. As weight is lost, changes in body image occur, and as energy decreases, changes in self-image occur. Moreover, appetite and the ability to eat are key determinants of physical and psychological quality of life.[2] In some cultures, for example, Southeast and East Asian, some degree of obesity is perceived as a sign of good health and weight loss is seen as a clear sign of declining health.[16] For many patients, the net result of ACS and the resulting weight loss constitute a negative-feedback loop of ever-increasing magnitude and increased suffering in multiple dimensions.

OTHER PHYSICAL CHANGES

The fit of dentures may change with illness, or already poorly fitting dentures may not be as well tolerated in advanced disease. Dental pain may be overlooked in the context of terminal illness. Oral (and sometimes esophageal) infections and complications increase with disease progression and immunocompromise. Aphthous ulcers, mucositis, candidiasis, aspergillosis, herpes simplex, and bacterial infections cause oral or esophageal pain and, thus, anorexia.

ASSESSMENT

Assessment parameters in anorexia and ACS are summarized in Table 8–3.

Anorexia and weight loss may begin insidiously with slightly decreased appetite and slight weight loss characteristic of virtually any illness. As the disease progresses and comorbid conditions increase in number and severity, anorexia and PCM increase and a mutually reinforcing process may emerge. For example, along with the metabolic abnormalities of ACS, fatigue leads to more pronounced anorexia and PCM, which in turn leads to increased fatigue and weakness that may in turn accelerate the metabolic processes of ACS.

With ACS common, and in many cases inevitable among patients with terminal illness, identifying specific causes is an extremely challenging and, in far advanced disease, ultimately futile task. Moreover, there are no clear and widely accepted diagnostic criteria for ACS. Nevertheless, anorexia from some etiologies is treatable; hence, assessment of the possible presence of etiologies noted above is integral to quality palliative care. Other assessment parameters are used according to the patient's ability to tolerate and benefit from the assessment. At some point in the illness, even basic assessments, such as weight, serve only to decrease the patient's quality of life. Assessment parameters of nutritional status include decreased intake, decreased weight, muscle wasting, decreased fat, loss of strength, and changes in laboratory values. The patient is likely to report anorexia and/or early satiety and to experience a decline in mental acuity.

Assessment also includes usual intake patterns, food likes and dislikes, and determining the meaning of food or eating to the patient and family. Too often, a family member attaches huge significance to nutritional intake and exerts pressure on the patient to increase intake: "If he would just get enough to eat." Giving sustenance is a fundamental means of caring and nurturing, and it is no surprise that the presence of devastating illness often evokes an almost primitive urge to give food.

Table 8–3. Assessment Parameters in Anorexia and Cachexia

The patient is likely to report anorexia and/or early satiety.
Weakness (asthenia) and fatigue are present.
Mental status declines, with decreased attention span and ability to concentrate. Depression may increase concurrently.
Inspection/observation may show progressive muscle wasting, loss of strength, and decreased fat. There often is increased total body water, and edema may thus mask some wasting.
Weight may decrease. Weight may reflect nutritional status or fluid accumulation or loss. Increased weight in the presence of heart disease suggests heart failure.
Triceps skinfold thickness decreases with protein calorie malnutrition (PCM, skinfold thickness and mid-arm circumference vary with hydration status).
Mid-arm muscle circumference decreases with PCM.
Serum albumin concentrations decrease as nutritional status declines. Albumin has a half-life of 20 days; hence, it is less affected by current intake than other measures.
Other lab values associated with anorexia/cachexia syndrome include anemia, increased triglycerides, decreased nitrogen balance, and glucose intolerance.[8,26]

Sources: Ottery et al. (1998), reference 3; Rivadeneira et al. (1998), reference 11; Casciato (1995), reference 15.

INTERVENTIONS

There are few credible reports of nutritional interventions that reverse ACS in advanced disease. Nevertheless, the process may be slowed to some extent in early and even late disease stages, especially with the use of multimodal approaches (nutritional, combined drug therapy, and exercise).[3,9] There are, of course, interventions that are efficacious in treating anorexia from exogenous etiologies such as nausea or esophageal stricture. Interventions are divided into exogenous symptom management, nutritional support, enteral and parenteral nutrition, pharmacological management, and multimodal approaches.

(EXOGENOUS) SYMPTOM MANAGEMENT

The presence or absence of symptoms that may cause or contribute to anorexia and weight loss should be evaluated. If anorexia is due to an identifiable problem or problems, such as pain, nausea, fatigue, depression, taste disorder, etc., then intervene as discussed elsewhere in this book.

NUTRITIONAL SUPPORT

Nutritional support, especially oral, to increase intake overall or to maximize nutritional content may be helpful to some extent, especially early in the disease process.[11,17] As noted earlier, some degree of obesity is thought by some cultures to be a sign of good health and any weight loss to be a sign of ill health. Helping family members understand nutritional needs and limitations in terminal situations is essential. General guidelines for altering diet include the following:[4,17–21]

- Determine the meaning to the patient and family of giving, taking, and refusing food. In families in which dying is experienced to some extent as a time of personal growth or closeness, redirection of food-related personal values from symbolic nurturing to symbolic sharing is possible. Thus, even half a bite of food shared in "sacred meals" eaten with loved ones is a kind of victory over the disease or hopelessness.[22] Usually, however, strong and even unconscious beliefs about food are difficult to modify, and many families require education and frequent support in the face of helplessness and frustration related to ever-diminishing intake.
- Culturally appropriate or favored foods should be encouraged. In some cases, certain traditional foods may be thought especially nutritious and some foods with good nutritional content, harmful. Some commercial supplements (called "milk"), for example, are thought by many Southeast Asians to have highly desirable, almost magical healing properties.
- Small meals, on the patient's schedule and according to the taste and whims of the patient, are helpful, at least emotionally, and should be instituted early in the illness so that eating does not become burdensome.[4]
- Foods with different tastes, textures, temperatures, seasonings, degrees of spiciness, degrees of moisture, colors, etc. should be tried; but the family should be cautioned against barraging the patient with a constant parade of foods to try. Room temperature and less spicy foods are preferred by many patients.[21]
- Different liquids should also be tried. Cold, clear liquids are usually well tolerated and enjoyed, except that cultural constraints may exist; for example, patients with illnesses that are classified as "cold" by some Southeast Asians and Latinos are thought to be harmed by taking cold drinks (or foods).[21]
- The nutritional quality of intake should be evaluated and, if possible and appropriate, modified to improve the quality. Patients who are not moribund may benefit from supplementary sources of protein and calories, though "taste fatigue" may result from too frequent intake of these.[11]
- Measures as basic as timing intake may also be instituted. Patients who experience early satiety, for example, should take the most nutritious part of the meal first (usually without fluids other than nutritional supplements).
- Procedures, treatments, psychological upsets (negative or positive), or other stresses or activities should be limited prior to meals.

ENTERAL AND PARENTERAL NUTRITION

Enteral feeding (via nasoenteral tube, gastrostomy, jejunostomy) is indicated in a "small subset" of terminally ill patients, including those with weight loss due to, or exacerbated by, fistulas, mechanical bowel obstruction, dysphagia, odynophagia, vomiting, or malabsorption due to tumor or treatment.[23] For short-term feeding (<4 weeks), nasoenteral feeding is commonly used, while for long-term enteral feeding (>4 weeks), gastrostomy or jejunostomy is the preferred means.[11] A wide variety of feeding formulas exist, with many providing complete nutrition. The primary sources of nutrients are usually as follows:

- Calories from carbohydrates
- Protein from casein or whey
- Fat from triglycerides or vegetable oils
- Various nutrients (fish oil, glutamine, arginine, and RNA are sometimes added)

Specific formulas are based on various body functions (usually decreased), for instance, heart, liver, kidneys, as well as other factors.[11]

Table 8–4. Pharmacological Options in Anorexia/Cachexia Syndrome

Medication and Common Dosing	Effects and/or Indications	Side Effects and Other Considerations
Progestational agents, especially megestrol acetate 480–800 mg PO qid in liquid suspension	Improves appetite and reduces nausea/vomiting and taste alterations, most useful for patients expected to live for weeks or months	Fluid retention, menstrual irregularities, and tumor flare in patients with breast cancer; contraindicated in patients with thrombophlebitis; sudden discontinuation can induce hypertension, thromboembolism, vaginal bleeding, peripheral edema, hyperglycemia, Cushing's syndrome, and adrenal dysfunction
Prokinetic agents, especially metoclopramide 10 mg PO tid	Early satiety from delayed gastric emptying or gastric paresis	Dystonic reactions (trismus, torticollis, facial spasm, oculogyric crisis, anxiety), akathisia, and tardive dyskinesia (involuntary chewing, vermicular tongue movements)
Corticosteroids, e.g., dexamethasone 4–8 mg q AM	Improved sense of well-being; most useful in patients with limited life expectancy or when rapid effect is needed	Euphoria, other mood changes, fluid retention, gastrointestinal irritation
Cannabinoids, e.g., dronabinol 2.5–5 mg PO q 3–6 h; some patients prefer to smoke marijuana rather than take oral medications as a source of cannabinoid	Improves appetite and decreases nausea; when smoked with others, serves as a social event	Sedation, euphoria, difficulty concentrating; older patients may have unpleasant feelings from cannabinoids

Sources: Kempt (1999), reference 20; Fainsinger (1997), reference 22; Bruera and Fainsinger (1998), reference 24; Brant (1998), reference 26; Waller and Caroline (1996), reference 27.

Total parenteral nutrition (TPN) clearly has a place early in the process of cancer, for example, during some treatment regimes such as bone marrow transplantation and under circumstances noted above (dysphagia, etc.). It has greater potential for complications than does enteral nutrition, seldom improves outcome, and thus is very seldom indicated in terminally ill patients with advanced disease.[1,23,24]

PHARMACOLOGICAL INTERVENTIONS

Pharmacological options to address ACS in the palliative setting are limited and, in the final stages of terminal illness, futile. Pharmacological options with indications and notable side effects are presented in Table 8–4.

Medications under investigation for the treatment of ACS include thalidomide (inhibits cytokine production), melatonin (decreases levels of circulating TNF), clenbuterol (improves muscle strength), anabolic androgenic steroids (enhance protein synthesis), and omega-3 fatty acids (decrease IL-6).[5] Medications that have not shown efficacy in the treatment of ACS include cyproheptadine, pentoxifylline, and hydrazine sulfate.[5]

MULTIMODAL APPROACH

The devastating consequences, complexities, and resistance to the treatment of ACS lead inevitably to consideration of a multimodal approach.[1,3] Such an approach could include some or all of the following:

- Prevention or early recognition and treatment of exogenous symptoms that may contribute to anorexia
- Recognition and early intervention in the nutritional needs of patients with potentially life-threatening illnesses or illnesses associated with ACS
- Pharmacological therapy that combines appetite stimulants such as progestational agents or cannabinoids with anabolic agents such as androgenic steroids; anticytokine agents may also become part of the armamentarium for the treatment of ACS
- Resistance training to increase lean muscle mass is effective at least early in the disease process

Clearly, the involvement of several disciplines (medicine, nursing, nutrition, physical therapy, and perhaps others) is required in this approach. The following case study illustrates some of the issues commonly associated with ACS.

Case Study: The Patient with ACS and Alcohol Addiction

A 58-year-old woman with a diagnosis of advanced cervical carcinoma was cared for at home by family and the services of a home care agency. Despite careful symptom management and nutritional support, she continued to lose weight and suffer from increasing weakness and fatigue. She had refused several opportunities for inpatient treatment, but when she developed fever, diarrhea, and dehydration, she agreed to go to the hospital.

Within several hours of admission, she became agitated and disoriented. Her condition deteriorated rapidly; she developed chest pain and became extremely fearful and paranoid, and she began hallucinating. She was started on intravenous haloperidol with little effect. A consulting psychiatrist called from the emergency department, determined that she was experiencing acute alcohol withdrawal. Although the patient and family had previously denied alcohol use, when confronted with her deteriorating condition, the family admitted that the patient was a heavy drinker.

She was switched to intravenous diazepam and within several days was lucid. She also was septic, requiring hospitalization for 6 weeks for treatment of her sepsis and nutritional status. In the third week, she began to gain weight. She continued to gain weight throughout the hospitalization and experienced a slight increase in strength. Within a few weeks of discharge, she, unfortunately, began losing weight, and it was clear that she was again drinking. She died in an emaciated state at home several months later.

SUMMARY

Increasingly, ACS is recognized as a serious aspect of advanced or terminal illness and as an area requiring further research, especially with respect to *(1)* the pathophysiology of cachexia and *(2)* increasing treatment options. Current understanding of ACS includes the following:

- Anorexia and cachexia are distinct syndromes but clinically are difficult to differentiate.
- Anorexia is characterized by decreased appetite, may result from a variety of causes (including unmanaged symptoms such as nausea and pain), results primarily in loss of fat tissue, resultant weight loss is reversible.
- Cachexia is a complex metabolic syndrome thought to result from the production of proinflammatory cytokines such as TNF and IL-1. In cachexia, there is approximately equal loss of fat and muscle and significant loss of bone mineral content. Weight loss from cachexia does not respond to nutritional interventions.
- Assessment and treatment of ACS include determination of whether exogenous etiologies such as nausea or pain are involved, vigorous treatment of any such etiologies, and nutritional support if indicated.
- Treatment of cachexia is unsatisfactory, but some temporary gains may occur with progestational agents, especially megestrol acetate, prokinetic agents such as metoclopramide, corticosteroids, or cannabinoids.

Progress is being made in understanding and treating the problem, but ACS is not yet completely understood nor is treatment optimized.

REFERENCES

1. Bistrian BR. Clinical trials for the treatment of secondary wasting and cachexia. J Nutr 1999;129 (Suppl):290S–294S.

2. Tisdale MJ. Biology of cachexia. J Natl Cancer Inst 1979;89:1763–1773.

3. Ottery FD, Walsh D, Strawford A. Pharmacologic management of anorexia/cachexia. Semin Oncol 1998;25(Suppl 6):35–44.

4. Ungvarski PJ, Angell J, Lancaster DJ, Manlapaz JP. Adolescents and adults: HIV disease care management. In: Ungvarski PJ, Flaskerud JH, eds. HIV/AIDS: A Guide to Primary Care Management. Philadelphia: WB Saunders, 1999:131–193.

5. Bruera E. Pharmacological treatment of cachexia: any progress? Support Care Cancer 1998;6:109–113.

6. Mosby's Medical Dictionary. St. Louis: Mosby Year-Book, 1998.

7. Anker SD, Clark AL, Teixeira MM, Hellewell PG, Coats AJ. Loss of bone mineral in patients with cachexia due to heart failure. Am J Cardiol 1999;83:612–615.

8. Ma G, Alexander HR. Prevalence and pathophysiology of cancer cachexia. In: Bruera E, Portenoy RK, eds. Topics in Palliative Care, vol 2. New York: Oxford University Press, 1997:91–129.

9. Bruera E, Neumann CM. Management of specific symptom complexes in patients receiving palliative care. Can Med Assoc J 1998;158:1717–1726.

10. Casey KM. Malnutrition associated with HIV/AIDS: definition and scope, epidemiology, and pathophysiology. J Assoc Nurses AIDS Care 1997;8:24–32.

11. Rivadeneira DE, Evoy D, Fahey TJ, Lieberman MD, Daly JM. Nutritional support of the cancer patient. CA Cancer Clin 1998;48: 69–80.

12. Haapoja IS. Paraneoplastic syndromes. In: Groenwald SI, Frogge MH, Goodman M, Yarbro CH, eds. Cancer Nursing: Principles and Practice, 4th Ed. Boston: Jones and Bartlett, 1997: 702–720.

13. Tabbarah HJ, Lowitz BB. Abdominal complications. In: Casciato DA, Lowitz BB, eds. Manual of Clinical Oncology, 3rd Ed. Boston: Little, Brown, 1995:498–506.

14. Vigano A, Dorgan M, Bruera E, and Suarez-Almazor ME. The relative accuracy of the clinical estimation of the duration of life for patients with end of life cancer. Cancer 1999; 86:170–176.

15. Casciato DA. Symptom care. In: Casciato DA, Lowitz BB, eds. Manual of Clinical Oncology, 3rd Ed. Boston: Little, Brown, 1995:76–97.

16. Kemp CE. Laotian refugees and immigrants. In: Kemp C, Rasbridge L, eds. Refugee and Immigrant Health. Austin: Texas Department of Health, 1999:123–130.

17. Staats JA, Sheran M, Herr R. Adolescents and adults: care management of AIDS-indicator diseases. In: Ungvarski PJ, Flaskerud JH, eds. HIV/AIDS: A Guide to Primary Care Management. Philadelphia: WB Saunders, 1999:194–254.

18. Casey KM. Malnutrition associated with HIV/AIDS: assessment and interventions. J Assoc Nurses AIDS Care 1997;8:39–48.

19. Grant MM, Rivera LM. Anorexia, cachexia, and dysphagia: the symptom experience. Semin Oncol Nurs 1995;11:266–271.

20. Kemp CE. Terminal Illness: A Guide to Nursing Care, 2nd Ed. Philadelphia: Lippincott-Williams & Wilkins, 1999.

21. Seligman PA, Fink R, Massey-Seligman EJ. Approach to the seriously ill or terminal cancer patient who has a poor appetite. Semin Oncol 1998;25(Suppl 6):33–34.

22. Fainsinger R. The modern management of cancer related cachexia in palliative care. Prog Palliat Care 1997;5:191–195.

23. Abrahm JL. Promoting symptom control in palliative care. Semin Oncol Nurs 1998;14:95–109.

24. Bruera E, Fainsinger RL. Clinical management of cachexia and anorexia. In: Doyle D, Hanks GWC, MacDonald N, eds. Oxford Textbook of Palliative Medicine, 2nd Ed. Oxford: Oxford University Press, 1998:548–557.

25. Jaskowiak NT, Alexander HR. The pathophysiology of cancer cachexia. In: Doyle D, Hanks GWC, and MacDonald N, eds. Oxford Textbook of Palliative Medicine, 2nd Ed. Oxford: Oxford University Press, 1998:534–548.

26. Brant JM. The art of palliative care: living with hope, dying. Oncol Nurs Forum 1998; 25:995–1004.

27. Waller A, Caroline NL. Handbook of Palliative Care in Cancer. Boston: Butterworth-Heinemann, 1996.

9 Nausea and Vomiting

CYNTHIA R. KING

Lewis suffered from constant nausea and stomach distress the last few weeks of his life. He said it was the worst part of dying. He was thirsty and hungry at times but would not take anything because he was afraid of upchucking. I called his primary care physician repeatedly for help, but nothing was done until we entered a hospice program. They started him on medicine, and he was finally comfortable the last few days. He even ate a few of his favorite foods before he died.

—Wife

Nausea and vomiting are symptoms commonly experienced by cancer patients. They are symptoms experienced secondary to the underlying malignancy as well as frequent side effects of the medications used to treat the cancer. To date, most research has focused on treatment-induced nausea and vomiting in patients receiving chemotherapy for cure or control of disease. Unfortunately, there is a paucity of literature about nausea and vomiting in cancer patients who are not receiving chemotherapy or who are in the terminal phase of their illness.[1]

Nausea and vomiting are frequent and distressing symptoms experienced by patients with advanced cancer who are receiving palliative care. Research has shown that 40% to 60% of patients with advanced cancer experience nausea and/or vomiting. Additionally, research has shown that these symptoms are more common in patients under 65 years old, in women, and in patients with cancer of the stomach or breast. For stomach cancer, the high frequency may be due to local causes such as obstruction. For breast cancer the causes may be multifactorial and include hypercalcemia, brain metastases, medications, and gender.[2–5] Sadly, this symptom complex of nausea and vomiting in advanced cancer has not been reduced in the past decade.

The level of distress associated with nausea and vomiting may be profound. If these symptoms are left untreated, they can interfere with usual daily activities, increase anxiety and other symptoms, and impair quality of life (QOL). It is essential that these symptoms be adequately treated throughout the trajectory of cancer care and across all settings. As more palliative care is provided in outpatient settings, homes, and hospices, it is important to involve the patient and family in the management of nausea and vomiting. Nurses who provide palliative care to cancer patients of any age and in any setting need to adequately assess for nausea and vomiting, provide appropriate drug and nondrug interventions, provide essential teaching of self-care to patients and families, and evaluate all interventions and self-care. The approach must be practical, with the goal being relief of symptoms as soon as possible. The treatment may be directed at the cause, at the symptom, or at both. This disruption in QOL can be of particular significance to patients facing the end of life.

NAUSEA AND VOMITING AND QUALITY OF LIFE

The distress and disruption in daily activities caused by nausea and vomiting can impair QOL for patients with advanced disease. Although there is controversy over the number and exact dimensions of QOL, the City of Hope National Medical Center QOL model includes the four dimensions of physical well-being, psychological well-being, social well-being, and spiritual well-being.[6] The distress caused by nausea and vomiting can affect one or all of the four dimensions of QOL (Fig. 9–1).[7] Adequate management of nausea and vomiting can positively affect all dimensions of a patient's QOL. The control of nausea and vomiting can provide patients with a sense of control over their body and life, decrease anxiety and fear, decrease caregiver burden, and allow patients to carry out some of their usual daily acitivities.[7]

CONCEPTUAL CONCERNS RELATED TO NAUSEA AND VOMITING

To thoroughly examine the problem of nausea and vomiting in palliative care, it is important to be clear about certain concepts. Symptoms such as nausea and vomiting are composed of subjective components and dimensions unique to each patient. Symptoms are different from signs, which are objective and can be observed by the health care professional.[8] *Symptom occurrence* is comprised of the frequency, duration, and severity with which the symptom presents.[9] Symptom *distress* involves the degree or amount of physical and mental or emotional upset and suffering experienced by an individual. This is different from symptom occurrence.[8] Lastly, symptom *experience* involves the individual's perception and response to the occurrence and distress of the symptom.[8]

The terms "nausea" and "vomiting" represent clearly distinct concepts. Un-

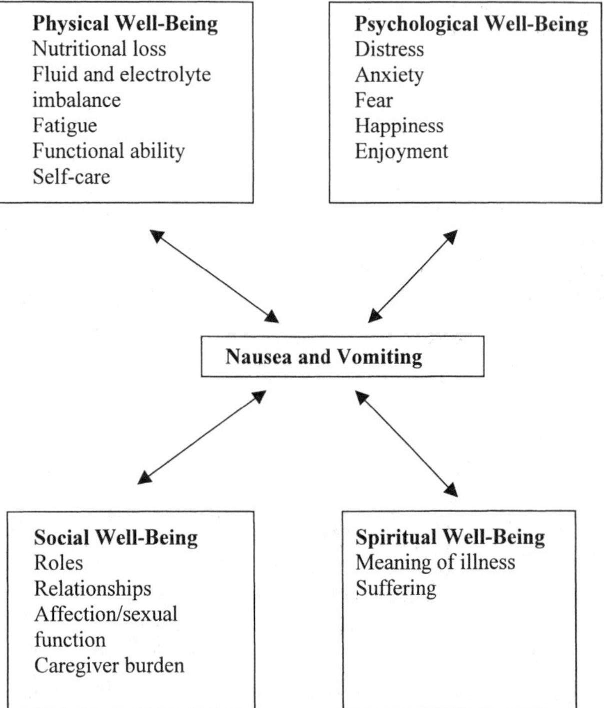

Fig. 9–1. The effect of nausea and vomiting on the domains of quality of life. From Grant (1997), reference 7, with permission.

fortunately, terms used to describe them are frequently used interchangeably. This may result in confusion during assessment, measurement, treatment, or patient and family education. *Nausea* is a subjective symptom involving an unpleasant sensation experienced in the back of the throat and the epigastrium, which may or may not result in vomiting.[8,10] Other terms used by patients include "sick at stomach," "butterflies," and "fish at sea." The symptoms of increased salivation, dizziness, lightheadedness, difficulty swallowing, and tachycardia may accompany the feeling of nausea. Patterns of nausea include acute, delayed, and anticipatory. Acute nausea occurs within minutes or hours after such events as having chemotherapy. Delayed nausea generally occurs at least 24 hours after events like chemotherapy and may last for several days. Anticipatory nausea occurs before the actual stimulus and develops only after an individual has had a prior bad experience with an event such as chemotherapy that resulted in nausea or vomiting.[8,10,11]

Vomiting is often confused with nausea but is, in fact, a separate phenomenon. It is frequently described as "throwing up," "pitching," "barfing," or "upchucking." It may or may not occur in conjunction with nausea. It is a self-protective mechanism by which the body attempts to expel toxic substances. It involves the expulsion of gastric contents through the mouth, caused by forceful contraction of the abdominal muscles. Retching involves the spasmodic contractions of the diaphragm and abdominal muscles.[8,10,11]

PHYSIOLOGICAL MECHANISMS OF NAUSEA AND VOMITING

After thoroughly understanding the concepts of nausea and vomiting, it is important to understand the physiological mechanisms and causes of this symptom complex. Vomiting is controlled by stimulation of the vomiting center (VC) or emetic center, which is an area of the brainstem. There are multiple central and peripheral pathways that can stimulate the VC. It is important for nurses to understand these pathways in order to determine a cause and select appropriate treatments. The various pathways include the peripheral pathways of the vagal afferents, the pharyngeal afferents, and the vestibular system (Fig. 9–2). The central pathways include the midbrain afferents and the chemoreceptor trigger zone (CTZ) (Fig. 9–2).[10–14]

The vagal afferent pathway involves fibers located in the wall of the stomach and proximal small intestine, which sense mechanical or chemical changes in the upper gastrointestinal tract. The pharyngeal afferent pathway involves mechanical irritation of the glossopharyngeal nerve. Excessive coughing may irritate this. The vestibular system involves stimulation starting in the inner ear. This involves nausea and vomiting resulting from such causes as motion sickness. If a patient has a prior history of motion sickness, he or she may have an increased incidence of nausea and vomiting with treatments such as chemotherapy.[11,12,14]

The central pathways include the midbrain and the CTZ. Intracranial pressure, stress, anxiety, sights, sounds, or tastes may stimulate the midbrain afferent pathway. The CTZ is located at the area postrema of the fourth ventricle of the brain. Once the CTZ is exposed to various neurotransmitters, such as serotonin, dopamine, histamine, or prostaglandins, nausea and vomiting may result. The vagal afferents also enter the CTZ.[11–14]

In the past, it was hypothesized that chemotherapy-induced nausea and vomiting occurred as a result of stimulation of the CTZ by the chemotherapy or other drugs. Although it is now known that exposure of the CTZ to the neurotransmitters is the most important factor, there is more emphasis being placed on understanding other mechanisms, such as the 5-hydroxytryptamine$_3$ (5-HT$_3$) receptor sites in the small intestine. In newer theories, it appears that for patients receiving chemotherapy, radiation to the duodenum, or other drugs, the enterochromaffin cells of the mucosa of the duodenum lead to the release of 5-HT$_3$. When 5-HT$_3$, or serotonin, is re-

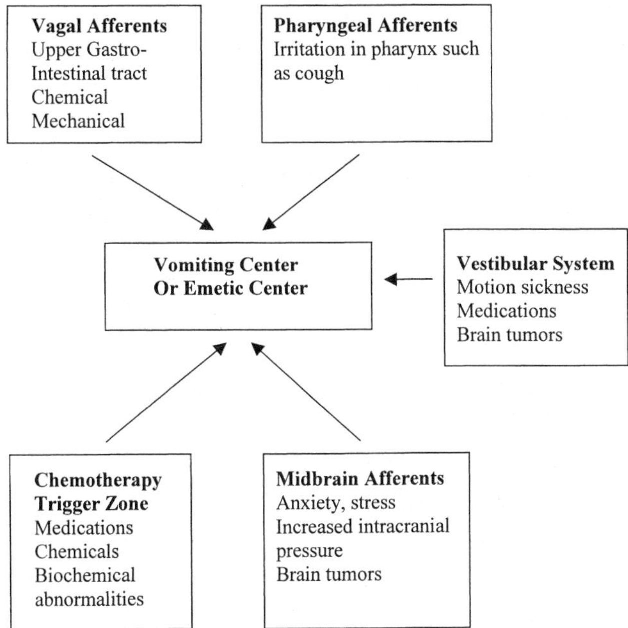

Fig. 9–2. Physiological mechanisms of nausea and vomiting.

Table 9–1. Causes of Nausea and Vomiting

Irritation/Obstruction of Gastrointestinal Tract	**Biochemical Abnormalities**
Cancer	Hypercalcemia
Chronic cough	Hyponatremia
Esophagitis	Fluid and electrolyte imbalances
Peptic ulcer	Volume depletion
Gastric distension	Adrenocorticol insufficiency
Gastric compression	Liver failure
Delayed gastric emptying	Renal failure
Bowel obstruction	
Constipation	**Drugs**
Hepatitis	Chemotherapy
Biliary obstruction	Opioids
Chemotherapy	Digoxin
Radiation	Antibiotics
	Anticonvulsants
Sepsis	Aspirin and NSAIDs
Metastases	
CNS	**Increased Intracranial Pressure**
Brain	Cerebral edema
Meninges	Intracranial tumor
Liver	Intracranial bleeding
	Skull metastases
Psychological	
Fear	
Anxiety	

CNS = central nervous system; NSAIDs = nonsteroidal antiinflammatory drugs.

leased from these cells, it binds to specific 5-HT_3 receptors and these afferent impulses travel to the VC.[11,15]

CAUSES OF NAUSEA AND VOMITING

There are numerous potential causes of nausea and vomiting in terminal cancer patients requiring palliative care. These are presented in Table 9–1 and are useful to remember when dealing with advanced disease. Reversible causes (e.g., constipation) may be found, and it is crucial to abolish nausea and vomiting as quickly as possible. Often, the cause for nausea and vomiting is multifactorial.[5,11,13,16] For instance, there may be a physiological imbalance, such as a fluid and electrolyte imbalance, occurring at the same time as nausea is provoked by addition of opioids or nonsteroidal anti-inflammatory drugs (NSAIDs) to control pain. In the 2-year experience of the World Health Organization with the analgesic ladder in cancer pain, nausea and vomiting were present in 22% of the days during the three-step treatment.[17] Additionally, when considering nausea and vomiting from a QOL perspective (Fig. 9–1),[7] psychological, social, and spiritual distress can cause or exacerbate nausea and vomiting.

ASSESSMENT OF NAUSEA AND VOMITING

Assessment is an important process and the foundation of all treatment-related decisions. It should be an ongoing process that begins with the initial patient contact regarding nausea and vomiting. Without a complete and ongoing assessment, nausea and vomiting may be mismanaged. This can result in unnecessary anxiety, suffering, and a decrease in QOL for the patient and family. Nurses working in all settings and with all age ranges of patients need to use skillful observation along with effective data collection techniques during assessment. It is rare that patients present with nausea and vomiting as a first sign of advanced cancer. Generally, patients who complain of this symptom complex have a well-documented history of their disease, including diagnosis, prior treatment, and sites of metastases. If this information is not available, nurses should obtain a complete medical/surgical history, including previous episodes of nausea and vomiting, effectiveness of previous treatments for this symptom complex, and any current treatment that might be contributing to these symptoms. Information obtained by questionnaires or self-report tools such as diaries, journals, or logs is crucial for the identification and management of this symptom complex and for improving the patient's QOL.[8,13,14] Goodman[18] provided examples of a chemotherapy treatment diary that could be adapted for use with terminally ill patients to record nausea and vomiting (Fig. 9–3).

Assessment and evaluation of nausea and vomiting also must include the pattern, what triggers the symptom complex, assessment of the mouth, assessment of the abdomen and bowel sounds, assessment of the rectum, possible laboratory studies (e.g., renal and liver function, ionized calcium, electrolytes, white blood cell count and differential, serum drug levels), and possible radiographic studies (e.g., computed tomography, magnetic resonance imaging scan, abdomen flat plate). Specifically, nurses should try to determine if there is a pattern to the nausea after certain drugs, after meals, on movement, in certain situations, or with certain smells. It is also important to ask if there is epigastric pain (? gastritis), pain on swallowing (? oral thrush), pain on standing (? mesenteric traction), thirst (? hypercalcemia), hiccups (? uremia), heartburn (? small stomach syndrome), or constipation.[19]

There are several measurement tools that may be used to assess one or more of the components of nausea and vomiting.[10,20–23] Some tools measure multiple components, while others measure a single component or a global measure of the nausea/vomiting. Instruments may involve checklists, visual analogue scales, patient interviews, or Likert scales. Almost all involve self-report by the patient.[8]

Whatever tool nurses use should be evaluated and chosen carefully. Rhodes[8] recommends the following points when using an instrument to measure nausea and vomiting: *(1)* use self-report tools instead of observational assessments; *(2)* determine and describe the symptoms and components; *(3)* consider the clarity, cultural sensitivity, and understandability of the tool; *(4)* check reliability and validity; *(5)* use an instrument with an easy-to-read format; *(6)* consider the purpose of the tool, the target population, and whether it is for acute, delayed, or anticipatory nausea and vomiting or for patients with advanced cancer; and *(7)* consider the type of score obtained (total versus subscale scores) and the ease of scoring.

Name

Medications to take For Nausea & Vomiting

Medication	Time to take	How to take

Special instructions:

If you have difficulty drinking fluids or your nausea and/or vomiting does not go away, you must call your doctor or hospice.

Doctor's phone

Hospice phone

Nausea Log

Date	Drug	Time	Degree of Nausea*	Vomiting (# of times)	Effect Of Drug**

*0 = no nausea; 1 = slight nausea; 2 = moderately severe nausea; interferes with activities and eating; 3 = severe nausea; intolerable.
** Effect of drug: 1 – very effective, 2=moderately effective, 3 =not effective

Fig. 9–3. Nausea diary. From Goodman (1997), reference 18, with permission

Case Study 1: Acute Onset of Nausea

A 55-year-old hospice patient with metastatic breast cancer complains of severe nausea. She is receiving 100 mg of sustained-release morphine three times per day and oral transmucosal fentanyl citrate 400 mcg four times per day as needed for pain. As the hospice nurse, you know this is a new symptom. You perform a thorough assessment of this new symptom by *(1)* asking the patient/family about the severity/intensity of the nausea, duration of nausea, frequency of nausea, pattern of nausea, triggers (e.g., with movement, after eating or drinking), and presence of vomiting; *(2)* asking the patient/family about epigastric pain, pain on swallowing, pain on standing, thirst, hiccups, heartburn, constipation, and any changes in medications; and *(3)* performing a thorough assessment of the abdomen and bowel sounds, and of the rectum.

Your assessment determines that the patient/family cannot remember when the patient last had a stool; bowel sounds are decreased in all quadrants, and the abdomen is firm and distended. Additionally, the patient reports that she stopped taking the stool softener and laxative prescribed by the hospice team.

With the assistance of the family, you prepare and give the patient an enema of molasses, skim milk, and warm water and follow this by 8 ounces of warm water. The patient has two large bowel movements and restarts a bowel regimen with Senokot-S. You choose this product because it has a stool softener and mild stimulant in one pill rather than the multiple pills the patient was taking previously. The hospice physician also prescribes 10 mg of metoclopramide every 6 hours with additional 10 mg doses as needed for severe nausea. Within 2 days the patient's nausea is under control and she is able to take some fluids, food, and medications by mouth.

PHARMACOLOGICAL PALLIATIVE MANAGEMENT OF NAUSEA AND VOMITING

Progress has been made in managing chemotherapy-induced nausea and vomiting but not necessarily in nausea and vomiting experienced by patients with advanced disease requiring end-of-life care. The challenge is to provide appropriate antiemetic protocols for these patients in the setting in which they are receiving palliative care, while appreciating the demand for cost containment in health care delivery. Individuals with advanced cancer range from pediatric patients to elderly patients and receive end-of-life care in many health care settings (e.g., home, hospitals, inpatient hospice units, hospice houses, and outpatient and ambulatory units). The array of antiemetics available has increased (Table 9–2),[2,5,13,16,18] which now allows for individualized protocols. Thus, it is important for nurses to continually ask the patient and family about nausea and vomiting and the effectiveness of the treatment. Additionally, it is essential that nurses utilize nonpharmacological methods to prevent and decrease nausea and vomiting.

According to Kaye[19] the overall plan of management for palliative care of nausea and vomiting should be as follows:

1. Assessment
2. Consider the causes
3. Choose the antiemetic(s)
4. Choose the route
5. Change the protocol if it is not working
6. Consider steroids
7. Consider ranitidine
8. Decrease or change the opioid for pain
9. Remember that anxiety can cause nausea

Woodruff[12] adds that pharmacological management should include adequate doses of antiemetics; combinations of antiemetics; and use of intravenous (IV) and rectal routes if necessary. If nausea and vomiting continue, consider psychological factors, reassess for missed physical causes, and try different combinations of antiemetics.

Successful pharmacological management of nausea and vomiting in advanced cancer is related to the frequency, dose, and type of antiemetic. Successful management is also related to providing antiemetics around the clock.

Classes of Antiemetics

There are currently nine classes of drugs used as antiemetics in palliative care: butyrophenones, prokinetic agents, cannabinoids, phenothiazines, antihistamines, anticholinergics, steroids, benzodiazepines, and 5-HT_3 receptor antagonists.

Mannix[5] recommends seven steps to choosing an appropriate antiemetic protocol for palliative care. The first step involves identifying the likely cause(s) of the symptoms. In the second step, the health care professional should try to identify the pathway by which each cause is triggering nausea and vomiting (Fig. 9–2). In step three, it is helpful to identify the neurotransmitter receptor that may be involved in the pathway, such as the 5-HT_3 receptor. Once the receptor is identified, step four requires selection of the most potent antagonist to that receptor. Step five involves selecting a route of administration that will ensure that the drug will reach the site of action. Once the route is chosen, step six is to titrate the dose carefully and give the antiemetic around the clock. Lastly, in step seven, if symptoms continue, then review the likely cause(s) and consider additional treatment that may be required for an overlooked cause.

Butyrophenones are dopamine antagonists. Haloperidol and droperidol are the drugs in this class, and they are most potent at the CTZ (Fig. 9–2). Butyrophenones are major tranquilizers, whose mode of action, other than dopamine blockade, is not well understood. In general, these drugs are less effective at controlling nausea and vomiting than other drugs, except for the phenothiazines. They are effective, however, when used in combination with other drugs, especially with the 5-HT_3 receptor antagonists. Butyrophenones can be effective when anxiety and anticipatory symptoms aggravate the intensity of a patient's nausea and vomiting. They can have severe side effects (Table 9–2), including extrapyramidal effects.[5,12,18]

Prokinetic agents (Table 9–2) include metoclopramide and domperidone. They are also called "substituted benzamides." Metoclopramide is the most commonly used drug in this category. It has some antidopaminergic activity at the CTZ and stimulates 5-HT_4 receptors, which helps to bring normal peristalsis in the upper gastrointestinal tract and to block 5-HT_3 receptors in the CTZ and gut. Extrapyramidal side effects are common. Infusing the drug over 30 minutes and administering diphenhydramine 25 to 50 mg at the same time may lessen these side effects. Metoclopramide also enhances gastric emptying, decreases the sensation of fullness caused by gastric stasis, decreases the heartburn caused by chemotherapy, and slows the colonic transit time caused by the 5-HT_3 receptor antagonists. Although initially used as a single agent, metoclopramide is now the main component of several combination protocols.

Cannabinoids (Table 9–2), such as dronabinol, are options for patients who are refractory to other antiemetics. Marijuana is the best known cannabinoid, but dronabinol is the preparation available for prescriptive use. Marijuana, however, may be more effective. The actual site of action is not known but thought to be at the cortical level. Cannabinoids are especially helpful in younger adults who do not have a history of cardiac or psychiatric illness. Younger patients may have a more positive experience. Older adults tend to have more hallucinations, feeling "high" and sedation. Although these side effects may be decreased by low-dose phenothiazines. Because the central sympathomimetic activity may increase with the use of

Table 9–2. Antiemetic Drugs in Palliative Care

Drug	Indication	Dosage, Route, and Schedule	Side Effects	Comments
Butyrophenones Haloperidol	Opioid-induced nausea, chemical and mechanical nausea	Oral: 0.5–5 mg every 4–6 h IM: 5 mg/ml every 3–4 h IV: 0.5–2 mg every 3–4 h	Dystonias, dyskinesia, akathisia	Side effects are less at low doses. Butyrephenones may be as effective as phenothiazines, may have additive effects with other CNS depressants. Use when anxiety and anticipatory symptoms aggravate intensity of nausea and vomiting.
Droperidol		IV, IM: 1.25–2.5 mg every 2–4 h		
Prokinetic agents Metoclopramide	Gastric stasis, ileus	Oral: 5–10 mg every 2–4 h IV: 1–3 mg/kg every 2–4 h	Dystonias, akathisia, oesophageal spasm, colic if gastrointestinal obstruction, headache, fatigue, abdominal cramps, diarrhea	Infuse over 30 min to prevent agitation and dystonic reactions; use diphenhydramine to decrease extrapyramidal symptoms.
Domperidone		Oral: 10–30 mg every 2–4 h PR: 30–90 mg every 2–4 h		
Cannabinoids Dronabinol	Second-line anti-emetic	Oral: 2–10 mg every 4–6 h	CNS sedation, dizziness, disorientation, impaired concentration, dysphoria, hypotension, dry mouth, tachycardia	More effective in younger adults.
Phenothiazines Prochlorperazine	General nausea and vomiting, not as highly recommended for routine use in palliative care	Oral: 5–25 mg every 3–4 h PR: 25 mg every 6–8 h IM: 5 mg/ml every 3–4 h IV: 20–40 mg every 3–4 h	Drowsiness, irritation, dry mouth, anxiety, hypotension, extra-pyramidal side effects	May cause excessive drowsiness in elderly, IM route is painful.
Thiethylperazine		Oral: 10 mg every 3–4 h IM: 10 mg/2 ml every 3–4 h PR: 10 mg every 6–8 h		
Trimetho-benzamide		Oral: 100–250 mg every 3–4 h PR: 200 mg every 3–4 h IM: 200 mg/2 ml every 3–4 h		

(*continued*)

Table 9–2. Antiemetic Drugs in Palliative Care (*continued*)

Drug	Indication	Dosage, Route, and Schedule	Side Effects	Comments
Antihistamines				
Diphenhydramine	Intestinal obstruction, peritoneal irritation, vestibular causes, increased ICP	Oral: 25–50 mg every 6–8 h IV: 25–50 mg every 6–8 h	Dry mouth, blurred vision, sedation	Cyclizine is the least sedative, so it is a better choice.
Cyclizine		Oral: 25–50 mg every 8 h PR: 25–50 mg every 8 h SQ: 25–50 mg every 8 h		
Anticholinergics				
Scopolamine	Intestinal obstruction, peritoneal irritation, increased ICP, excess secretions	Sublingual: 200–400 mcg every 4–8 h SQ: 200–400 mcg every 4–8 h Transdermal: 500–1500 mcg every 72 h	Dry mouth, ileus, urinary retention, blurred vision, possible agitation	Useful if nausea and vomiting co-exist with colic.
Steroids				
Dexamethasone	Given alone or with other agents for nausea and vomiting	Oral: 2–4 mg every 6 h IV: 2–4 mg every 6 h	Insomnia, anxiety, euphoria, perirectal burning	Compatible with 5-HT_3 receptor antagonists or metoclopramide. Taper dose to prevent side effects.
Benzodiazepine				
Lorazepam	Effective for nausea and vomiting as well as anxiety	Oral: 1–2 mg every 2–3 h IV: 2–4 mg every 4–8 h	Sedation, amnesia, pleasant hallucinations	Use with caution with hepatic or renal dysfunction or debilitated patients.
5-HT_3 receptor antagonists				
Ondansetron	Chemotherapy, abdominal radiotherapy, postoperative nausea and vomiting	Oral, IV: 0.15–0.18 mg/kg every 12 h	Headache, constipation, diarrhea, minimal sedation	Indicated for moderate to highly emetogenic chemotherapy. Ideal for elderly and pediatric patients. Effectiveness is increased if used with dexamethasone.
Granisetron		Oral: 1 mg every 12 h IV: 10 mcg/kg every 12 h		
Miscellaneous				
Octreotide acetate	Nausea and vomiting associated with intestinal obstruction	SQ (recommended), IV bolus (emergencies), 100–600 mcg SQ in 2–4 doses/day	Diarrhea, loose stools, anorexia, headache, dizziness, seizures, anaphylactic shock	May interfere as others with insulin and β-adrenergic blocking agents; watch liver enzymes.
Dimenhydrinate	Nausea, vomiting, dizziness, motion sickness	Oral: 50–100 mg q 4 h not >400 mg/day IM, IV: 50 mg prn	Dry mouth, blurred vision, sedation	Geriatric clients may be more sensitive to dose.

IM = intramuscular; SQ = subcutaneous; IV = intravenous; PR = per rectum; ICP = intracranial pressure; prn = as required; 5-HT = 5-hydroxytryptamine.
Sources: Baines (1997), reference 2; Mannix (1998), reference 5; Fallon (1998), reference 13; Enck (1994), reference 16; Goodman (1997), reference 18.

cannabinoids, these drugs should be used with caution in patients with hypertension or heart disease or in those who are receiving psychomimetic drugs.[5,12,18,24,25]

Phenothiazines (Table 9–2) were once considered the mainstay of antiemetic therapy. These drugs, like prochlorperazine and thiethylperazine, are primarily dopamine antagonists. They have tranquilizing as well as antiemetic effects. They have been used as single agents and in combination protocols. One advantage has been that they are available in several preparations (oral, rectal suppository, parenteral, and sustained release preparation). The phenothiazines are especially effective for acute or delayed nausea. Because they have a different mechanism of action, they may be combined with 5-HT_3 receptor antagonists and dexamethasone. There is a high risk for extrapyramidal side effects (e.g., dystonia, akathisia, dyskinesia, akinesia). These symptoms appear to be greater in patients who are less than 30 years old. Frequently, 25 to 50 mg of diphenhydramine is given to prevent the extrapyramidal side effects.[5,12,18,24]

Antihistamines act on histamine receptors in the VC and on the vestibular afferents. Diphenhydramine is often used in combination protocols to minimize the development of extrapyramidal side effects. Cyclizine is less sedative than scopolamine (an anticholinergic) and can be given subcutaneously (SQ). These are rarely used as single agents for nausea and vomiting in palliative care.[5,12,24,26]

Anticholinergics currently are not used as frequently in antiemetic therapy. They do have an advantage in that they can be given sublingually, SQ, and transdermally. They have an anticholinergic effect at or near the VC. Parasympathetic side effects, like drying secretions, may sometimes by beneficial or troublesome because they cause dry mouth, ileus, urinary retention, and blurred vision. These drugs are effective at reducing peristalsis and inhibiting exocrine secretions and, thus, contribute to the palliation of colic and nausea.[5,12]

Corticosteroids, especially dexamethasone, are frequently a component of aggressive antiemetic regimens.[24,27–29] The use of steroids remains controversial. They appear to exert their antiemetic effect as a result of their antiprostaglandin activity. Dexamethasone has an advantage because it is in oral and parenteral forms and is compatible in solution with 5-HT_3 receptor antagonists and metoclopramide. In general, corticosteroids are most effective in combination with other agents. The efficacy of ondansetron, granisetron, and metoclopramide can be enhanced by adding dexamethasone.[30] Use of corticosteroids over 4 to 5 days can prevent delayed nausea and vomiting. However, the dose should be tapered after several days to decrease or prevent insomnia, anxiety, euphoria, and other side effects common to corticosteroids. A trial of high-dose steroids should be considered if there is increased intracranial pressure, hypercalcemia, or malignant pyloric stenosis. They also should be tried for advanced cancer when nausea is resistant to other antiemetics.[12,18,19,24,26]

The site of action for benzodiazepines, like lorazepam (Table 9–2), is the central nervous system. Lorazepam may be used alone but is more commonly used in combination protocols. Additionally, lorazepam is a potent anxiolytic and amnesic. The temporary amnesic effect may be useful in patients with anticipatory nausea and vomiting.[5,12,18,24] Malik and Khan[31] found that lorazepam decreased the incidence of anticipatory nausea and vomiting as well as acute emesis. Pediatric patients may experience sedation and pleasant hallucinations. Lorazepam should be used with caution in debilitated patients or those with hepatic or renal dysfunction.

Since 1986, when the selective blockade of 5-HT "m" receptors was shown to block vomiting associated with cisplatin, there has been a rapid creation of new drugs and increased knowledge of the sites and roles of 5-HT receptors. The 5-HT_3 receptors have been discovered in the CTZ, in the VC (centrally), and in the terminals of the vagal afferents in the gut (peripherally). The activities of these 5-HT_3 receptor antagonists (Table 9–2), like ondansetron and granisetron, appear to be limited to serotonin inhibition. Therefore, the extrapyramidal side effects associated with dopamine antagonists are eliminated. Granisetron is the most specific 5-HT_3 receptor antagonist and has the highest potency and a longer duration of action than ondansetron. All of these medications can be given to children and the elderly and have few side effects. They, however, have had little testing related to nausea and vomiting in advanced cancer patients who are receiving palliative care.[5,12,18,24]

There are some additional miscellaneous agents that may be helpful for terminally ill patients. Octreotide acetate is a somatostatin analogue. Thus, it mimics the actions of the natural hormone somatostatin and is long-acting. It may be helpful for nausea and vomiting associated with intestinal obstruction. Specifically, it inhibits gastric, pancreatic, and intestinal secretions and reduces gastrointestinal motility. Another agent is dimenhydrinate, which contains both diphenhydramine and chlorotheophylline. It is not known how dimenhydrinate alleviates nausea and vomiting. It is helpful for nausea, vomiting, and dizziness.

Combination Protocols

Currently, combining antiemetic drugs appears to improve efficacy, decrease side effects, and increase QOL. This practice is based on the theory is that blocking different types of neurotransmitter receptor may offer better management of nausea and vomiting. In some instances, single agents, such as granisetron, ondansetron, and prochlorperazine, may be used for this symptom complex. However, the combination of a 5-HT_3 receptor antagonist and a corticosteroid may be the most effective antiemetic regimen.[5,18,24,32] The various agents used in combination are adjusted according to the individual's tolerance to specific agents.

Routes of Administration

Nausea and vomiting may be treated with a combination of oral medications. If tolerated by the patient, this may be the most cost-effective treatment and provide the best prophylaxis. Unfortunately, other routes are needed if the patient has severe vomiting or is unable to swallow. If the patient has IV access, IV medications are appropriate. Some drugs may be given by intramuscular (IM) injection, but this can be painful and, thus, is usually avoided. Other options are to give drugs by a continuous SQ infusion, rectal suppository or tablet in the rectum, sublingually, or by a transdermal patch. A continuous SQ infusion is useful for severe nausea and vomiting, to avoid repeated injections. It is also important to remember nondrug methods in combination with antiemetic agents.[19]

NONPHARMACOLOGICAL PALLIATIVE MANAGEMENT OF NAUSEA AND VOMITING

Some literature exists related to nonpharmacological management of chemotherapy-induced nausea and vomiting,[33] but little concerning nonpharmacological techniques for patients receiving end-of-life care. Nonpharmacological management of nausea and vomiting may involve simple self-care techniques (Table 9–3)[14,16] or uniting the body and mind using psychological interventions to control physiological responses.[34] There are many different nonpharmacological techniques available today.

Many nonpharmacological techniques used to control nausea and vomiting in patients with advanced cancer are classified as behavioral interventions. This involves the acquisition of new adaptive behavioral skills. These techniques may include relaxation, biofeedback, self-hypnosis, cognitive distraction, guided imagery, and systematic desensitization. Other therapies that are gaining in popularity are acupuncture, acupressure, and music therapy (Table 9–4).[33]

Behavioral interventions can be used alone or in combination with antiemetic drugs to prevent and control nausea and vomiting. All of these techniques attempt to induce relaxation as a learned response. They differ only in the manner in which they induce relaxation.[33]

Behavioral interventions have been found to be effective for the following reasons: *(1)* they produce relaxation, which can decrease nausea and vomiting; *(2)* they serve as a distraction from the stimulus causing nausea and vomiting; *(3)* they enhance feelings of control and decrease feelings of helplessness as patients are actively involved in decreasing nausea and vomiting; *(4)* they have no side effects; and *(5)* they are easily self-administered.[33–36] There is currently no definitive research that indicates which method is most effective; rather, it appears to depend on individual preference.

Self-Hypnosis

Self-hypnosis was the first behavioral technique tested to control the symptom complex of nausea and vomiting. With this intervention, individuals learn to invoke a physiological state of altered consciousness and total-body relaxation. This results from the individual's intensified attention receptiveness, and increased receptiveness to a specific idea.[33] As with many of the behavioral techniques, there have been few controlled studies on self-hypnosis. Most of the research has been performed with children and adolescents as they are more easily hypnotized than adults.[37–41] Additionally, this research has been with individuals receiving chemotherapy and not individuals with advanced cancer receiving palliative care. The results of the research have been mixed, with only some patients having a decrease in the frequency, severity, amount, and duration of vomiting as well as duration of nausea. Unfortunately, hypnotic methods are not standardized, but all include relaxation and relaxation imagery. The advantages include an absence of side effects, no need for equipment, minimal physical effort, and minimal training. Health care professionals, including nurses, have successfully taught patients self-hypnosis techniques.[37–40] Research is desperately needed to evaluate which behavioral interventions are most effective in patients of all ages with advanced disease receiving end-of-life care.

Progressive Muscle Relaxation

Progressive muscle relation (PMR) is also called active relaxation and involves individuals learning to relax by progressively tensing and then relaxing different muscle groups in the body. Passive relaxation is considered relaxation that does not involve active tensing of the muscles. Often, PMR is used in combination with guided imagery, and research has shown that it can decrease chemotherapy-induced nausea and vomiting as well as depression and anxiety.[33,35,42–45] However, research has not been conducted on terminally ill patients receiving palliative care. When reviewing the research that has been performed on chemotherapy-induced nausea and vomiting, PMR has been shown to decrease: anxiety and nausea during chemotherapy, physiological indices of arousal (e.g., heart rate and blood pressure), anxiety after treatment, depression

Table 9–3. Nonpharmacological Self-Care Activities for Nausea and Vomiting

Self-Care Activities
Oral care after each episode of emesis
Apply a cool damp cloth to the forehead, neck, and wrists
Decrease noxious stimuli like odors and pain
Restrict fluids with meals
Eat frequent small meals
Eat bland, cold or room-temperature food
Lie flat for 2 h after eating
Wear loose-fitting clothes
Have fresh air with a fan or open window
Avoid sweet, salty, fatty, and spicy food
Limit sounds, sights, and smells that precipitate nausea and vomiting

Sources: Ladd (1999), reference 14; Enck (1994), reference 16.

Table 9–4. Nonpharmacological Interventions for Nausea and Vomiting

Techniques	Description	Comments
Behavioral interventions		
Self-hypnosis	Evocation of physiological state of altered consciousness and total body relaxation. This technique involves a state of intensified attention receptiveness and increased receptiveness to an idea.	Used to control anticipatory nausea and vomiting Limited studies, mostly children and adolescents Easily learned No side effects Decreases intensity and duration of nausea Decreases frequency, severity, amount, and duration of vomiting
Relaxation	Progressive contraction and relaxation of various muscle groups.	Often used with imagery Can use for other stressful situations Easily learned No side effects Decreases nausea during and after chemotherapy Decreases duration and severity of vomiting Not as effective with anticipatory nausea and vomiting
Biofeedback	Control of specific physiological responses by receiving information about changes in response to induced state of relaxation.	Two types: electromyographic and skin temperature Used alone or with relaxation Easily learned No side effects Decreases nausea during and after chemotherapy More effective with progressive muscle relaxation
Imagery	Mentally take self away by focusing mind on images of a relaxing place.	Most effective when combined with another technique Increases self-control Decreases duration of nausea Decreases perceptions of degree of vomiting Feel more in control, relaxed, and powerful
Distraction	Learn to divert attention from a threatening situation and to relaxing sensations.	Can use videos, games, and puzzles No side effects Decreases anticipatory nausea and vomiting Decreases postchemotherapy distress
Desensitization	Three-step process involving relaxation and visualization to decrease sensitization to aversive situations.	Inexpensive Easily learned No side effects Decreases anticipatory nausea and vomiting
Other interventions		
Acupressure	Form of massage using meridians to increase energy flow and affect emotions.	Inconclusive literature support Acupressure wrist bands may be helpful to decrease nausea and vomiting
Music therapy	Use of music to influence physiological, psychological, and emotional functioning during threatening situations.	Often used with other techniques No side effects Decreases nausea during and after chemotherapy Decreases perceptions of degree of vomiting

Source: King (1997), reference 33.

after treatment, and the occurrence of vomiting.[45]

Interestingly, as many as 65% of patients who learned PMR while undergoing chemotherapy continued to use it even after chemotherapy.[46] It can also be easily taught to health care professionals and to patients, to apply on their own.[35,47] However, there remains much to be learned about the use of PMR with terminally ill cancer patients suffering from nausea and vomiting.

Biofeedback

Biofeedback is a behavioral technique by which patients learn to control a specific physiological response (e.g., muscle tension) by receiving information about moment-to-moment changes in that response. Two specific types of biofeedback include electromyography (EMG) and skin temperature (ST). The purpose of EMG biofeedback is to induce a state of deep muscle relaxation from tense muscles. The purpose of ST is to prevent skin temperature changes, which precede nausea and vomiting.[33,35,39]

Recently, research has shown that biofeedback may help individuals achieve a state of generalized relaxation.[35,39,48,49] However, research has not shown EMG or ST biofeedback to be as effective as PMR alone or biofeedback with PMR at decreasing chemotherapy-induced nausea and vomiting.[48] Therefore, little definitive data exist regarding biofeedback as a behavioral technique for chemotherapy-induced nausea and vomiting and even fewer data to demonstrate that either EMG or ST is effective at decreasing this symptom complex with terminally ill patients.

Guided Imagery

Guided imagery allows individuals with nausea and vomiting to mentally take themselves away from their current site to a place that is relaxing. Individuals may choose a vacation spot, a safe place, a specific place at home, or any pleasant place. It is believed that when individuals imagine what they would usually feel, hear, see, taste, and smell at their pleasant spot, they can mentally block the negative conditioned stimuli from the cerebral cortex and prevent nausea and vomiting. It is possible that the body physiologically responds to the created image rather than to the negative conditioned stimuli.[33,34]

Research has suggested that guided imagery, or visualization, can facilitate relaxation, decrease anxiety, decrease anticipatory nausea and vomiting, and increase self-control.[38,50–52] Guided imagery has also been assessed in combination with music therapy.[51] When the results were compared to the pretest measures of nausea and vomiting, the duration of nausea was shorter with music therapy combined with guided imagery than preintervention. Interestingly, the subjects' perceptions of the occurrence of nausea remained unchanged. The degree of vomiting was also reduced significantly, and there was a trend toward a decreased duration of vomiting observed with the music therapy/guided imagery intervention. In a more recent study[53] patients who received guided imagery plus the standard antiemetic therapy exhibited a significantly more positive response to chemotherapy. Unfortunately, guided imagery did not have an effect on patients' perceptions of the frequency of nausea and vomiting or the distress associated with these symptoms. The subjects did, however, express that they felt more prepared, in control, powerful, and relaxed when using guided imagery.

From the limited research, it appears that guided imagery may be most effective at decreasing nausea and vomiting associated with chemotherapy and only when it is combined with another nonpharmacological technique, such as PMR or music therapy. There is little research that has examined guided imagery alone or in combination with another behavioral technique for patients receiving palliative care. Certainly, oncology nurses could instruct patients with advanced cancer in all settings regarding guided imagery alone or with another technique.

Cognitive Distraction

Cognitive distraction is also known as attentional diversion. This behavioral technique is thought to act by focusing an individual's attention away from nausea, vomiting, and the stimuli associated with these phenomena.[33,35,39,54] Research has shown that simply distracting children and adolescents by video games can decrease anticipatory nausea and vomiting.[54,55] Research with adults has demonstrated that cognitive distraction can significantly decrease postchemotherapy nausea, whether patients have low or high anxiety.[56] Whether cognitive distraction, such as video games, would be effective at decreasing nausea and vomiting in patients receiving end-of-life-care requires further research. Certainly, it is worth discussing this technique with patients.

Systematic Desensitization

Systematic desensitization is a standardized intervention that has been used to counteract anxiety-laden maladaptive responses such as phobias. There are three key steps to the desensitization process. First, the individual is taught a response, such as PMR, that is incompatible with the current maladaptive response (e.g., chemotherapy-induced nausea and vomiting). After this first step, the individual and teacher create a hierarchy of anxiety-provoking stimuli related to the feared situation (events related to receiving chemotherapy such as driving to the clinic, entering the treatment room, and seeing the chemotherapy nurse). This hierarchy of anxiety-provoking stimuli range from the least to the most frightening. In the last step, the individual uses the alternative response while systematically visualizing the increasingly aversive scenes related to chemotherapy and nausea and vomiting.[33,39,57–59]

Early studies demonstrated that systematic desensitization can be effective with anticipatory nausea and vomiting associated with chemotherapy.[57,60–62] Specifically, systematic desensitization has decreased the frequency, severity, and duration of anticipatory nausea and vomiting. Additionally, systematic desensitization significantly decreased the duration and severity of posttreatment nausea. Research has also shown that this particular behavioral technique can be effectively implemented by a variety of trained health care professionals (e.g., nurses, physicians, and clinical psychologists).[57] Currently, research supports the use of this technique as an inexpensive, effective, nonpharmacological treatment for chemotherapy-induced nausea and vomiting; but there is little research with health care professionals effectively implementing this as a palliative care technique. It is important for trained nurses to begin to teach this technique to patients who might benefit when terminally ill and suffering from nausea and vomiting.

Other Nonpharmacological Interventions

Acupuncture and acupressure are Eastern health care therapies that are gaining awareness in oncology nursing and palliative care. Acupressure is a form of massage that uses specific energy channels known as meridians. *Tsubos*, are acupuncture/acupressure points. *Tsubos* are points of decreased electrical resistance running along the body's energy pathways that form the meridian system.

It is believed that stimulating the *tsubo* improves energy flow, affects organs distant from the area being stimulated, and positively affects emotions.[33,63] Results have been mixed regarding the effectiveness of acupuncture/acupressure at decreasing nausea and vomiting. Most studies have been performed with chemotherapy-induced nausea and vomiting and not as palliative care techniques for nausea and vomiting.[64–68] Some studies have shown acupuncture on P6 (Neiguan point) to be effective at decreasing nausea and vomiting for 8 hours, and if acupressure is applied immediately after P6 acupuncture, there is a prolonged antiemetic effect.[65–67] Aglietti and colleagues[69] treated women receiving cisplatin with metoclopramide, dexamethasone, and diphenhydramine with and without acupuncture. Patients had a temporary acupuncture needle for 20 minutes during the infusion of chemotherapy and then a more permanent needle 24 hours after chemotherapy. Acupuncture did decrease the intensity and duration of nausea and vomiting, but the investigators commented that it was difficult to perform acupuncture in daily practice. One study was done on terminally ill patients. Unfortunately, the investigators found that acupressure wristbands were ineffective at decreasing the intensity or frequency of nausea and vomiting.[70] The investigators experienced difficulty in obtaining complete data and found subject recruitment a problem. Thus, studies on terminally ill patients need to be repeated and extended to confirm the usefulness of acupuncture or acupressure, even though research with terminally ill patients is difficult to conduct.

Music therapy has been used with patients to prevent or control nausea or vomiting. This involves the application of music to produce specific changes in behavior. The main objective in the past has been to influence the patient's physiological, psychological, and emotional and behavioral well-being.[71] Music therapy has most often been used in combination with other nonpharmacological techniques. Few studies have been conducted on the ability of music therapy to decrease nausea and vomiting in cancer patients. Most of the studies have not used music therapy as a single intervention and have assessed nausea and vomiting only related to chemotherapy. Frank[51] combined music therapy with guided imagery. The duration of nausea and the patients' perceptions of the degree of vomiting were decreased; however, the patients' perceptions of nausea did not change, and there was only a slight decrease in the duration of vomiting. Standley[72] used music therapy alone as an intervention and assessed the effects on the frequency and degree of anticipatory nausea and vomiting, as well as vomiting during and after chemotherapy. The individuals who received the music intervention reported less nausea and a longer time before nausea began. Ezzone and colleagues[73] evaluated whether a music intervention would decrease bone marrow transplant patients' perceptions of nausea and number of episodes of vomiting while receiving high-dose chemotherapy. Significant differences were found, with the music therapy patients having less nausea and fewer episodes of vomiting. Generally, music such as classical, folk, pop, or jazz is best. The music should be quiet and should create a calm background rather than being disruptive.[74] Music therapy is an intervention that can be initiated independently by nurses in all settings for all oncology patients and individualized for each patient. Additionally, music as an intervention for patients with advanced cancer receiving end-of-life care would require less time and energy to implement than relaxation or guided imagery and, therefore, may be less taxing for the terminally ill patient. Certainly, music therapy in combination with antiemetic therapy warrants further study as a way to significantly decrease the distressing symptoms of nausea and vomiting.

PATIENT AND FAMILY EDUCATION

Family caregivers are also involved with managing nausea and vomiting, as with all aspects of end-of-life care. They often are responsible for overall symptom management, emotional support, support of daily activities, administering medications, providing nutrition, and performing other aspects of care. Additionally, the family is frequently the communication link between the patient and the nurse. Nurses depend heavily on family members for information about patients, especially when patients deteriorate. Thus, it is essential that family be involved in any education given to the patient. Education is an important tool for family members to have if they are to function effectively as a team.[75]

First, patients and family need to be taught how to systematically assess the patient's nausea and vomiting. They may use a log, such as the one developed by Goodman[18] (Fig. 9–3). It is helpful to teach the patient and family members to rate the distress caused by these symptoms on a scale of 0 to 10. This provides more accurate information regarding the intensity and/or relief of symptoms. The patient and family need to be taught problem-solving skills for specific situations (e.g., when they can give an extra dose of antiemetic) and self-care activities (Table 9–3). The importance of taking antiemetics on a schedule and as prescribed should be reinforced. Information regarding medications and instructions for self-care should be provided in written form. Specific instruction should be given as to when to call the physician or nurse. Lastly, it is helpful to teach nonpharmacological methods for decreasing nausea and vomiting (e.g., music therapy or relaxation).

Case Study 2: The Patient Who Wants to Be at Home

A 62-year-old man with metastatic lung cancer is admitted to a palliative care unit because his family "can no longer care for him at home." He has severe bone pain, severe nausea, anorexia, anxiety, and panic attacks. He has told the hospice team and his family that he wants to be at home when he dies. He currently has three 100 mcg fentanyl patches placed every 3 days and takes two hydrocodone (7.5 mg hydrocodone with 750 mg acetaminophen) tablets every 3 to 4 hours for breakthrough pain. He takes one prochloraperazine every 8 hours as needed for nausea. He has nothing prescribed for anxiety. You do a thorough assessment of his pain, nausea, and anxiety and learn the following: *(1)* his persistent pain is a 6 to 9 out of 10, his breakthrough pain level is 8 to 10 out of 10, his fentanyl patches give pain relief for 48 to 52 hours (pain level decreases to 2 to 3 out of 10 for the first 40+ hours of the patch), his nausea is a 10 out of 10; *(2)* many years ago, he had learned transcendental meditation but has not practiced in 20 years; *(3)* his anxiety and panic attacks are precipitated by planning his funeral and will; *(4)* he is "allergic" to morphine; and *(5)* he refuses anything for pain, nausea, or anxiety that will involve needles or invasive procedures. After a hospice team discussion and talking to the patient and family, several changes are made. The order for the fentanyl transdermal patch is changed to three 100 mcg patches every 48 hours. The hyrocodone tables are changed to fentanyl oral transmucosal fentanyl citrate (Actiq). This is started at 200 mcq orally four times per day as needed for breakthrough pain and titrated upward to 600 mcg. Prochlorperazine is changed to metoclopramide 10 mg every 6 hours around the clock with an additional 10 mg as needed for severe nausea. Dexamethasone is added at 4 mg three times per day to help with nausea and anorexia. Lorazepam is ordered at 1 mg every 6 hours as needed for anxiety. Additionally, you teach the family and patient how to use PMR with imagery. After 3 days, the patient's persistent pain level has decreased to 2 to 4 out of 10, breakthrough pain level has decreased to 1 to 3 out of 10, nausea has decreased to 3 to 4 out of 10, and he is taking lorazepam only once per day for anxiety. Additionally, the patient is using PMR and imagery with the help of his family three times per day, and his family decides to take him home.

NURSING IMPLICATIONS

Based on the current lack of literature on palliative care for symptoms such as nausea and vomiting,[1] it is vital that nurses in all settings (e.g., administrators, clinicians, educators, and researchers) lead the way in learning how to manage these symptoms appropriately for terminally ill patients. From a clinical perspective, nurses need to provide initial and ongoing assessment of the patient's symptom experience, implement appropriate drug and nondrug interventions, evaluate all interventions, and provide patient and family education. Administrators play a key role in providing the resources necessary for clinical nurses to give quality, but cost-effective palliative care in all settings (hospitals, inpatient hospice units, hospice houses, homes, and outpatient/ambulatory units).

Educators must begin to incorporate end-of-life issues and symptom management for terminally ill patients into the nursing curriculum and into textbooks. Educators can work collaboratively with clinicians to develop educational tools for patients and families (pamphlets, videos, and audiotapes). Additional research is desperately needed regarding appropriate antiemetic regimens, nonpharmacological interventions, appropriate self-care activities, and QOL issues for patients receiving palliative care. Nurse researchers can be actively involved in this research and in the dissemination of the results to clinicians and educators. Nurse researchers should design studies using prospective, longitudinal models, adequate sample sizes, and appropriate control groups. Findings should be reported in terms of clinical and statistical significance. Through collaborative efforts nurse administrators, clinicians, educators, and researchers can help to decrease the incidence of nausea and vomiting and improve the QOL of terminally ill patients.

CONCLUSION

A major goal of palliative care is to improve QOL by decreasing undue suffering. This can be achieved through symptom management, such as adequate treatment of nausea and vomiting in terminally ill cancer patients. It is often difficult for nurses to meet the challenge of providing palliative care when there is a limited amount of research or literature to guide interventions for symptom management. This body of research and literature is growing but significantly less than the information available related to symptom management for patients receiving active cancer treatment. Nurses in all settings (e.g., administrators, clinicians, educators, and researchers) need to help increase our knowledge base and skills in the areas of symptom management and QOL issues for patients receiving end-of-life care. Vigilant assessment, appropriate use and evaluation of pharmacological and nonpharmacological interventions, appropriate patient and family education and support, and further research can accomplish this. Nausea and vomiting profoundly affect all aspects (physical well-being, psychological well-being, social well-being, and spiritual well-being) of an individual's QOL, even at the end of life. It is essential that nurses meet the challenge to improve QOL for patients with advanced disease by decreasing or abolishing nausea and vomiting.

REFERENCES

1. Ferrell B, Virani R, Grant M. Analysis of end-of-life-content in nursing textbooks. Oncol Nurs Forum 1999;26:869–876.

2. Baines MJ. ABC of palliative care: nausea, vomiting and intestinal obstruction. BMJ 1997; 315:1148–1150.

3. Rueben DB, Mor V. Nausea and vomiting in terminal cancer patients. Arch Intern Med 1986;146:2021–2023.

4. Dunlop GM. A study of the relative frequency and importance of gastrointestinal symptoms and weakness in patients with far advanced cancer. Palliat Med 1989;4:37–43.

5. Mannix KA. Gastrointestinal symptoms. In: Doyle D, Hanks GWC, MacDonald N, eds. Oxford Textbook of Palliative Med. Oxford: Oxford University Press, 1998:489–571.

6. Ferrell B, Grant M, Padilla G, Vemuri S, Rhiner M. The experience of pain and perceptions of quality of life: validation of a conceptual model. Hospice J 1991;7:9–24.

7. Grant M. Nausea and vomiting, quality of life and the oncology nurse. Oncol Nurs Forum 1997;24:5–7.

8. Rhodes VA. Criteria for assessment of nausea, vomiting and retching. Oncol Nurs Forum 1997;24:13–19.

9. McCorkle R, Young K. Development of a symptom distress scale. Cancer Nurs 1978;1:373–378.

10. Rhodes VA, Watson PM, Johnson MH, Madsen RW, Beck NC. Patterns of nausea and vomiting and distress in patients receiving antineoplastic drug protocols. Oncol Nurs Forum 1987;14:35–44.

11. Hogan CM, Grant M. Physiologic mech-

anisms of nausea and vomiting in patients with cancer. Oncol Nurs Forum 1997;24:8–12.

12. Woodruff R. Symptom Control in Advanced Cancer. Melbourne: Asperula, 1997.

13. Fallon BG. Nausea and vomiting unrelated to cancer treatment. In: Berger A, Portenoy RK, Weissman DE, eds. Principles and Practice of Supportive Oncology. Lippincott Williams-Wilkins: Philadelphia, 1998:179–189.

14. Ladd LA. Nausea in palliative care. J Hospice Palliat Nurs 1999;1:67–70.

15. Andrews PRL, Davis CJ. The mechanism of induced anticancer therapies. In: Andrews PRL, Sanger GJ, eds. Emesis in Anticancer Therapy: Mechanisms and Treatment. New York: Chapman and Hall, 1993:113–161.

16. Enck RE. The Medical Care of Terminally Ill Patients. Baltimore: John Hopkins University Press, 1994.

17. Ventrafridda VM, Tamruini A, Caraceni F, DeConno, Naldi F. A validation study of the WHO method for cancer pain relief. Cancer 1987;59:850–856.

18. Goodman M. Risk factors and antiemetic management of chemotherapy-induced nausea and vomiting. Oncol Nurs Forum 1997;26:20–32.

19. Kaye P. Notes on Symptom Control in Hospice and Palliative Care. Essex, CT: Hospice Education Institute, 1995.

20. Cotanch P. Relaxation training for the control of nausea and vomiting in patients receiving chemotherapy. Cancer Nurs 1983;6:277–283.

21. Del Fauvero A, Tonato M, Roila F. Issues in the measurement of nausea. Br J Cancer 66(Suppl 19):S69–S71.

22. McDaniel RW, Rhodes VA. Symptom experience. Semin Oncol Nurs 1995;11:232–234.

23. Morrow G. Assessment of nausea and vomiting. Past problems, current issues and suggestions for future research. Cancer 1984;53:2267.

24. Hogan CM. Advances in the management of nausea and vomiting. Nurs Clin North Am 1990;25:475–497.

25. Gonzalez-Rosales F, Walsh D. Intractable nausea and vomiting due to gastrointestinal mucosal metastases relieved by tetrhydrocannabinol (dronabinol). J Pain Symptom Manage 1997;14:311–314.

26. Levy MH and Catalano RB Control of common physical symptoms other than pain in patients with terminal disease. Semin Oncol 1985; 12:411–430.

27. Kris MG, Grall RJ, Clark RA. Antiemetic control and prevention of side effects of anticancer therapy with lorazepam or diphenhydramine when used in combination with metoclopramide plus dexamethasone. Cancer 1987;60: 2816–2822.

28. Fox SM, Einhorn LH, Cox E, Powell N, Abdy A. Ondansetron versus ondansetron, dexamethasone and chlorpromazine in the prevention of nausea and vomiting associated with multiple-day cisplatin chemotherapy. J Clin Oncol 1993;11: 2391–2395.

29. Roila F, Tonato M, Cognetti F, et al. (1991). Prevention of cisplatin-induced emesis: a double-blind multicenter randomized crossover study comparing ondansetron and ondansetron plus dexamethasone. J Clin Oncol 1991;9:675–678.

30. Joss RA, Bacchi M, Buser K. Ondansetron plus dexamethasone is superior to ondansetron alone in the prevention of emesis in chemotherapy naïve and previously treated patients. Ann Oncol 1994;5:253–258.

31. Malik IA, Khan WA. Clinical efficacy of lorazepam prophylaxis of anticipatory, acute and delayed nausea and vomiting induced by high doses of cisplatin. Am J Clin Oncol 1995;18: 170–175.

32. Ettinger DS. Preventing chemotherapy induced nausea and vomiting: an update and review of emesis. Semin Oncol 1995;22:6–18.

33. King CR. Nonpharmacologic management of chemotherapy-induced nausea and vomiting. Oncol Nurs Forum 1997;24 (Suppl):41–48.

34. Yasko JM. Holistic management of nausea and vomiting caused by chemotherapy. Top Clin Nurs 1985;7:26–38.

35. Burish TG, Tope DM. Psychological techniques for controlling the adverse side effects of cancer chemotherapy: findings from a decade of research. J Pain Symptom Manage 1992;7:287–301.

36. Fallowfield LJ. Behavioral interventions and psychological aspects of care during chemotherapy. Eur J Cancer 1992;28A (Suppl 1): S39–S41.

37. Cotanch P, Hockenberry M, Herman S. Self-hypnosis as an antiemetic therapy in children receiving chemotherapy. Oncol Nurs Forum 1985;12:41–46.

38. LaBaw W, Holton C, Tewell K, Eccle D. The use of self-hypnosis by children with cancer. Am J Clin Hypn 1975;17:233–238

39. Morrow GR, Hickok JT. Behavioral treatment of chemotherapy-induced nausea and vomiting. Oncology 1993;7:83–89.

40. Redd WH, Andresen GV, Minagawa RY. Hypnotic control of anticipatory emesis in patients receiving chemotherapy. J Consult Clin Psychol 1982;50:14–19.

41. Zeltzer LK, LeBaron S, Zeltzer P. The effectiveness of behavioral interventions for reducing nausea and vomiting in children receiving chemotherapy. J Clin Oncol 1984;2:683–690.

42. Burish TG, Carey MP, Krozely MG, Greco A. Conditioned side effects induced by cancer chemotherapy. Prevention through behavioral treatment. J Consult Clin Psychol 1987;55:42–48.

43. Burish TG, Lyles JN. Effectiveness of relaxation training in reducing the aversiveness of chemotherapy in the treatment of cancer. J Behav Ther Exp Psychiatry 1979;10:357–361.

44. Burish TG, Snyder SL, Jenkins RA. Preparing patients for cancer chemotherapy. Prevention through behavioral treatment. J Consult Clin Psychol 1991;59:518–525.

45. Lyles JN, Burish TG, Krozely MG, Oldham RK. Efficacy of relaxation training and guided imagery in reducing the aversiveness of cancer chemotherapy. J Consult Clin Oncol 1982; 50:509–526.

46. Burish TG, Vasterling JJ, Carey MP, Matt D, Krozely MG. Posttreatment use of relaxation training by cancer patients. Hospice J 1988; 4:1–8.

47. Morrow GR. Effectiveness of behavioral treatments for chemotherapy side effects administered by nurses and oncologists compared with behavioral psychologists. Proc Am Soc Clin Oncol 1989;8:314. Abstract no. 1221.

48. Burish TG, Jenkins RA. Effectiveness of biofeedback and relaxation training in reducing the side effects of cancer chemotherapy. Health Psychol 1992;11:17–23.

49. Morrow GR, Angel C, DuBeshter B. Autonomic changes during cancer chemotherapy induced nausea and emesis. Br J Cancer 1992;66 (Suppl 19):S42–S45.

50. Achterberg, J, Lawlis F. Imagery and health intervention. Top Clin Nurs 1982;3:55–60.

51. Frank JM. The effects of music therapy and guided visual imagery on chemotherapy induced nausea and vomiting. Oncol Nurs Forum 1985;12:47–52.

52. Greene R, Reyher J. Pain intolerance in hypnotic analgesia and imagination states. J Abnorm Psychol 1972;79:29–38.

53. Troesch LM, Rodehaver CB, Delaney EA, Yanes B. The influence of guided imagery on chemotherapy-related nausea and vomiting. Oncol Nurs Forum 1993;20:1179–1185.

54. Redd WH, Jacobsen PB, Die-Trill M, Dermatis H, McEvoy M, Holland J. Cognitive–attentional distraction in the control of conditioned nausea in pediatric cancer patients receiving chemotherapy. J Consult Clin Psychol 1987;55:391–395.

55. Kolko DJ, Rickard-Figueroa JL. Effects of video games in the adverse corollaries of chemotherapy in pediatric oncology patients: a single case analysis. J Consult Clin Psychol 1985;53: 223–225.

56. Vasterling J, Jenkins RW, Tope DM. Cognitive distraction and relaxation training for the control of side effects due to cancer chemotherapy. J Behav Med 1993;16:65–80.

57. Morrow GR, Asbury R, Hammon S, et al. Comparing the effectiveness of behavioral treatment for chemotherapy-induced nausea and vomiting when administered by oncologists, oncology nurses, and clinical psychologists. Health Psychol 1992;11:250–256.

58. Morrow GR, Dobkin PL. Anticipatory nausea and vomiting in cancer patients undergoing chemotherapy treatment. Prevalence, etiology, and behavioral interventions. Clin Psychol Rev 1988;8:517–556.

59. Redd WH. Behavioral intervention for cancer treatment side effects. Acta Oncol 1994; 33:113–117.

60. Hailey BJ, White JG. Systematic desensitization for anticipatory nausea associated with chemotherapy. Psychosomatics 1983;24:287–291.

61. Hoffman ML. Hypnotic desensitization for the management of anticipatory emesis in chemotherapy. Am J Clin Hypn 1983;25:173–176.

62. Morrow GR. Effect of the cognitive hierarchy in the systematic desensitization treatment of anticipatory nausea in cancer patients: a component comparison with relaxation only, counseling, and no treatment. Cogn Ther Res 1986;10:421–466.

63. Hare ML. Shiatsu acupressure in nursing practice. Holistic Nurs Pract 1988;2:68–74.

64. Dundee JW, Ghaly RG, Fitzpatrick KTJ. Randomized comparison of the antiemetic effects of metoclopramide and electroacupuncture in cancer chemotherapy. Br J Clin Pharmacol 1988;25:678P–679P.

65. Dundee JW, Ghaly RG, Fitzpatrick KTJ, Abram WP, Lynch GA. Acupuncture prophylaxis of cancer chemotherapy-induced sickness. J R Soc Med 1989;82:268–271.

66. Dundee JW, Yang J. Acupressure prolongs the antiemetic action of P6 acupuncture. Br J Clin Pharmacol 1990;29:644P–645P.

67. Dundee JW, Yang J. Prolongation of the antiemetic action of P6 acupuncture by acupressure in patients having cancer chemotherapy. J R Soc Med 1990;83:360–362.

68. Dundee JW, Yang J, Macmillan C. Noninvasive stimulation of the P(6) (Neiguan) antiemetic acupuncture point in cancer chemotherapy. J R Soc Med 1991;84:210–212.

69. Aglietti L, Roila F, Tonato M, et al. A pilot study of metoclopramide, dexamethasone, diphenhydramine and acupuncture in women treated with cisplatin. Cancer Chemother Pharmacol 1990;26:239–240.

70. Brown S, North D, Marvel, MK, Fons R. Acupressure wrist bands to relieve nausea and vomiting in hospice patients. Do they work? Am J Hospice Palliat Care 1992;9:26–29.

71. Dossey BM. Psychophysiologic self-regulation interventions. In: Dossey B, ed. Essentials of Critical Care Nursing: Body, Mind, Spirit. Philadelphia: Lippincott, 1990:42–54.

72. Standley JM. Clinical applications of music and chemotherapy; the effects on nausea and emesis. Music Ther Perspect 1992;10:27–35.

73. Ezzone S, Baker C, Rosselet R, Terepka E. Music as an adjunct to antiemetic therapy. Oncol Nurs Forum 1998;25:1551–1556.

74. Pervan V. Practical aspects of dealing with cancer therapy induced nausea and vomiting. Semin Oncol Nurs 1990;6 (Suppl):3–5.

75. Weitzner MA, Moody LN, McMillan SC. Symptom management issues in hospice care. Am J Hospice Palliat Care 1997;14:190–195.

10 Dysphagia, Dry Mouth, and Hiccups

CONSTANCE M. DAHLIN and TESSA GOLDSMITH

I like to eat small bits. Sometimes I just start coughing and gagging. I try to drink water to help my dry mouth, but then I get these belch-like spasms. They hit me so suddenly. Nothing helps, but after awhile, they subside. I am left utterly exhausted.

—D.C., 64-year-old man with metastatic lung cancer

Dysphagia and dry mouth are disturbing symptoms that occur frequently in progressive terminal illness. Hiccups, while less frequent, can be as distressing, adversely affecting quality of life. More importantly, these problems impact the pleasure of food, communication, and social interaction, as well as nutrition.

In a culture where food is the essence of life, lack of interest in food and lack of the ability to eat can cause distress for both patients and family. Thus, care for patients with terminal illnesses who are experiencing dysphagia, hiccups, or dry mouth should focus on the following principles: *(1)* the patient and family are the unit of care, *(2)* relief of suffering is the primary goal, and *(3)* care is best delivered with the underlying aspect of the life-threatening disease reflected in the plan.[1]

DYSPHAGIA

Case Study: J.D., a Patient with ALS

J.D. was a 67-year-old woman with advanced bulbar-onset amyotrophic lateral sclerosis (ALS). Since her diagnosis 3 years earlier, J.D. had experienced progressive decline in her oral motor function, to the point where she was unable to move her tongue or close her mouth. Her speech was extremely unintelligible and swallowing was laborious, accompanied by frequent choking episodes that frightened her and her husband. Meal times were exhausting and time-consuming, lasting up to 2 hours. The result was limited nutritional intake and significant weight loss. J.D. repeatedly resisted the recommendation of a gastrostomy feeding tube, fearing capitulation to the disease. She preferred instead to compensate for her swallowing dysfunction by implementing some of the strategies suggested in the comprehensive speech language pathology evaluation. These suggestions included thickening fluids, postural modifications, small and frequent meals with high-calorie supplements, and careful mouth care to clear oral secretions and food/liquid debris after eating. The increased risks of aspiration and pneumonia secondary to decreased cough and respiratory function were explained to the patient. In spite of the extreme effort of eating, the patient's autonomy regarding eating by mouth was respected. Unfortunately, the efficacy of these strategies was short-lived as the patient was hospitalized due to inability to breath unassisted.

A tracheotomy was performed, to provide mechanical ventilation. Through augmentative communication, the patient continued to refuse a gastrostomy tube but agreed to intravenous hydration. Nurses and family were instructed on optimal feeding strategies to minimize risks for aspiration. Special attention was given to mouth care and suctioning for control of oral secretions that were impossible for the patient to swallow. Medications were crushed and placed in applesauce or thickened liquids. Oral intake dwindled to a few teaspoons of pureed foods and thickened liquids per meal. Food and liquid were repeatedly suctioned from the tracheotomy tube in spite of an inflated cuff indicating recurrent aspiration. Inevitably, the patient succumbed to aspiration pneumonia. However, she maintained both autonomy with respect to eating by mouth and control in choosing how she died.

DEFINITION

Dysphagia is defined as difficulty in swallowing food or liquid. Typically, chronically difficult swallowing affects the efficiency and safety with which oral alimentation is maintained. Patients may complain of food getting caught along the upper digestive tract anywhere from the throat to the esophagus. In addition, diversion of food or liquid into the trachea may occur, causing aspiration, choking, and in severe cases asphyxiation. Chronically difficult swallowing can be frustrating as well as frightening for patients, resulting in generalized weakness and loss of appetite and weight. Malnutrition is an outcome in severe cases. Pneumonia, secondary to aspiration, may result, causing fevers, malaise, shortness of breath, and sometimes death. The psychological impact of dysphagia is an individual's increased isolation from family and friends since so many social interactions center around consumption of food.

PHYSIOLOGY OF SWALLOWING

Swallowing involves the passage of food or liquid from the oral cavity through the esophagus and into the stomach, where the process of digestion begins. Swallowing is an extremely complex physiological act, and its correct execution demands exquisite timing and coordination of greater than 30 pairs of muscles under voluntary and involuntary nervous control. Given that humans swallow hundreds of times per day and are largely unaware of the activity, it is remarkable that difficulties do not occur more frequently.

The act of swallowing is divided into four stages. In reality, these stages occur simultaneously (Fig. 10–1). The act of swallowing takes no longer than 20 seconds from the moment of bolus propulsion into the pharynx until the bolus reaches the stomach. The longest phase comprises the transit of the bolus through the esophagus.

The first stage of swallowing, **the oral preparatory stage,** is responsible for readying the bolus for swallowing. Bolus preparation is under voluntary control and can be halted or changed at any point. Mastication of solid boluses and gathering and placement of semisoft and liquid boluses on the tongue are the primary activities. It is during this stage that we take pleasure from the flavor and texture of our food through the receptors of the tongue. The length of this stage is variable and depends on the viscosity or consistency of the material being prepared as well as individual styles in chewing.

During mastication, the tongue moves the bolus to the dental arches for grinding into smaller pieces. Opening of the jaw and rotary and lateral movements accomplish the masticatory process. Cohesive bolus formation of solids is dependent on several factors: the presence of enzyme-rich saliva to bind the material together, the ability of the tongue to gather particles from the sulci of the cheek and the mouth floor, and the prevention of food falling out of the oral cavity anteriorly and spilling into the pharynx prematurely.[2]

During **oral transit,** the second stage of swallowing, the prepared bolus, now positioned on the blade of the tongue, is propelled into the pharynx. The tongue contacts the hard palate laterally and the central incisors anteriorly. The soft palate elevates, permitting the bolus to enter the pharynx, and closes off the nasopharynx, preventing regurgitation of the bolus into the nose. The muscles of the floor of the mouth contract, and the base of the tongue depresses, forming a chute down which the bolus can flow. Through a series of contractions by the intrinsic tongue muscles pressed against the hard palate, the torpedo-shaped bolus is propelled in a rolling motion from anterior to posterior into the pharynx. Depending on the consistency of the bolus, this stage lasts approximately 1 second.

The **pharyngeal stage** of swallowing

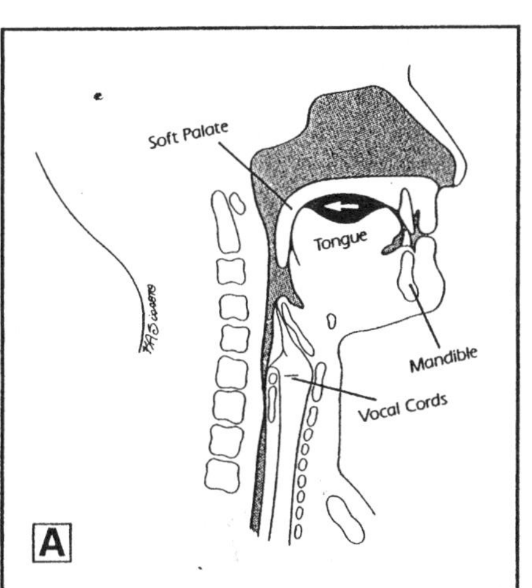

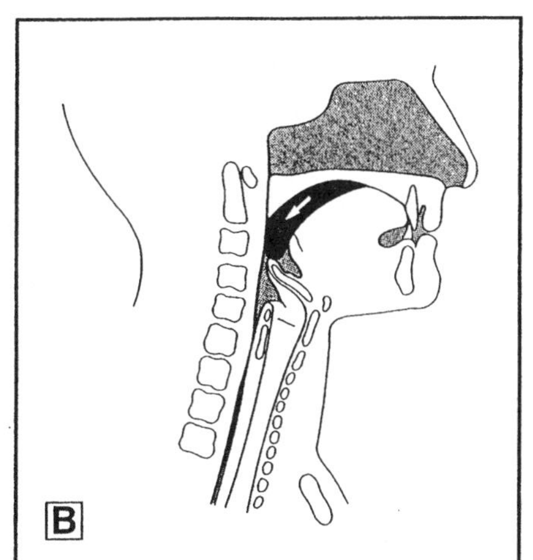

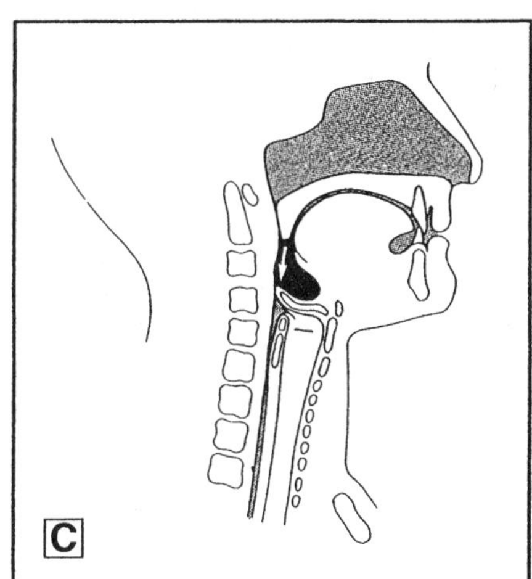

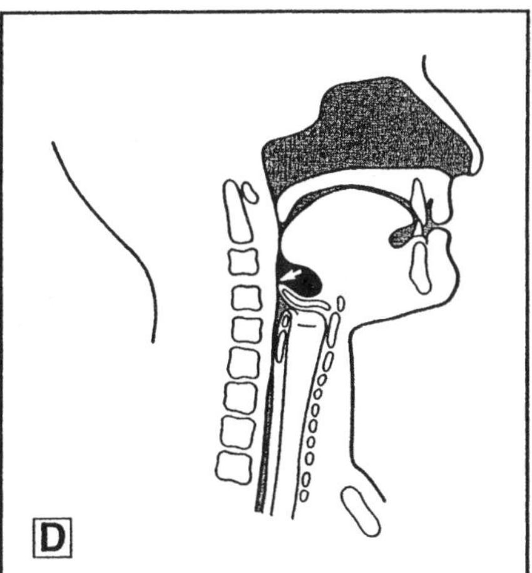

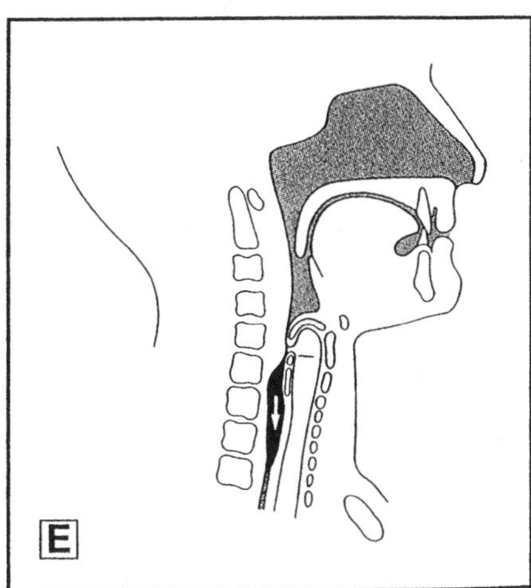

Fig. 10–1. Stages of swallowing, beginning with voluntary initiation of the swallow by the tongue *(A)*, oral transit *(B)*, pharyngeal stage of swallowing with airway protection *(C)* and *(D)*, and esophageal stage *(E)*. From Logemann (1998), reference 2.

is elicited as the posterior movement of the tongue and passage of the bolus stimulate the sensory impulses of the glossopharyngeal and vagus nerves, which travel to the afferent swallowing center located in the lower medulla of the brain stem and then to the cortex. The pharyngeal and oral transit stages are closely associated. The oral cavity and the pharynx become one continuous tube with the entrance to the larynx closed off.[2,3] The pharyngeal stage of swallowing is the most complex, requiring the most precise timing and coordination. It is during this stage that the airway is protected by the cessation of respiration. Simultaneously, the upper esophagus opens to accept the bolus.

The process of airway protection, that is, closure of the airway, is quite remarkable and complex. There are several levels of airway protection. Laryngeal closure occurs from inferior to superior so that if material is present in the laryngeal entrance, it will be extruded into the hypopharynx during the swallow. As the floor of the mouth/ tongue muscles contract to propel the bolus from the oral cavity, the larynx moves upward, closing the laryngeal vestibule. The vocal folds adduct simultaneously, and the epiglottis begins to invert over the entrance of the larynx, further protecting the airway. Cessation of respiration can last up to 2.5 seconds, but the average is 0.3 to 0.6 second for a single sip.[2,4] Swallows usually occur during the expiratory stage of the respiratory cycle, with expiration preceding and following the swallow. The superior–anterior movement of the larynx is responsible for opening the upper esophageal segment. The greater the excursion of the larynx, the larger the diameter of the opening of the upper esophagus.

As the bolus enters the pharynx, its tail is driven toward the hypopharynx and esophagus by the positive pressure generated from the base of the tongue contacting the pharyngeal walls. The pharyngeal constrictor muscles contract sequentially, and their topographic arrangement has the effect of stripping the bolus through the hypopharynx and clearing the pharyngeal recesses.

The duration of the pharyngeal stage of swallowing is approximately 1 second. The order of contraction of muscles is invariant, but the timing of contraction depends on the viscosity and size of the bolus.[5] The biomechanical events involved in this stage of swallowing are under involuntary control and carefully sequenced in a pattern by the central swallowing center in the lower medulla. In the medulla, sensory feedback continually modulates the motor response. For example, if the bolus is dense, the firing of a particular group of muscles of the tongue may be increased, or the opening of the upper esophagus may last longer with a large bolus volume. If the sensory feedback loop is disturbed, the onset of the pharyngeal stage of swallowing may be delayed or, in severe cases, absent.[5]

The **esophageal stage** of swallowing involves transport of the bolus from the upper esophageal segment, through the lower esophageal segment, and into the stomach, a distance of approximately 25 cm.[6] The esophageal stage is coordinated with the pharyngeal stage, with continued sequential contraction of muscles in the cervical esophagus. Like the pharyngeal phase of swallowing, the esophageal stage is under involuntary neuromuscular control. Unlike the pharyngeal stage, however, the speed of propagation of the bolus is much slower, with a rate of 3 to 4 cm/second compared to 12 cm/second in the pharynx.[7] The upper esophagus consists of approximately 8 cm of striated skeletal muscle beginning at the upper esophageal segment. The outer fibers of the cervical esophagus are arranged longitudinally, while the inner fibers are arranged in a circular configuration. As the bolus reaches the esophagus, the longitudinal muscles contract, followed by contraction of the circular fibers, constituting the primary peristaltic wave. The primary wave carries the bolus through the lower esophageal sphincter in a series of relaxation–contraction waves. The lower esophageal sphincter remains open until the peristaltic wave passes. A secondary peristaltic wave is generated, where the striated muscle meets the smooth muscle and clears the esophagus of residue. This wave is reflexive in nature and initiated by distention of the esophagus during the primary peristaltic wave.[8]

After passage of the bolus, the upper and lower esophageal sphincters contract to their baseline tonic posture. This contains the gastric contents within the stomach and prevents regurgitation of material into the hypopharynx and airway.[6]

Pressure Gradient Model of Swallowing

Difficulty swallowing can occur during any of the four stages described above, either within a stage or across stages depending on the underlying disease. Evaluation and treatment of dysphagia is dependent on a thorough understanding of the underlying aberrant anatomical and physiological components. It is helpful to conceptualize the process of bolus transfer through the oral cavity according to a piston–chamber model.[2,9] The oral cavity forms the chamber, and the tongue acts as the piston that creates pressure on the bolus to drive it into the esophagus. The ability of the oral cavity to fulfill its function as a closed chamber depends on the integrity of a number of muscular contractions, which form valves that open and close. Bolus flow and, hence, swallowing will be affected if there is dysfunction in the chamber or the piston. If the chamber leaks, this may result in residue, regurgitation, or aspiration. Inefficient bolus flow results from weakness in the tongue driving force on the bolus. The valves of the oral cavity are illustrated in Figure 10–2 and are described in detail below.

The oral cavity, or chamber, comprises the area extending from the lips anteriorly to the hard palate superiorly and the pharyngeal wall posteriorly, bounded by the floor of the mouth inferiorly.

Lips. The lips form the most anterior seal of the oral cavity and together with the jaw muscles are responsible for opening the oral cavity to accept bites of

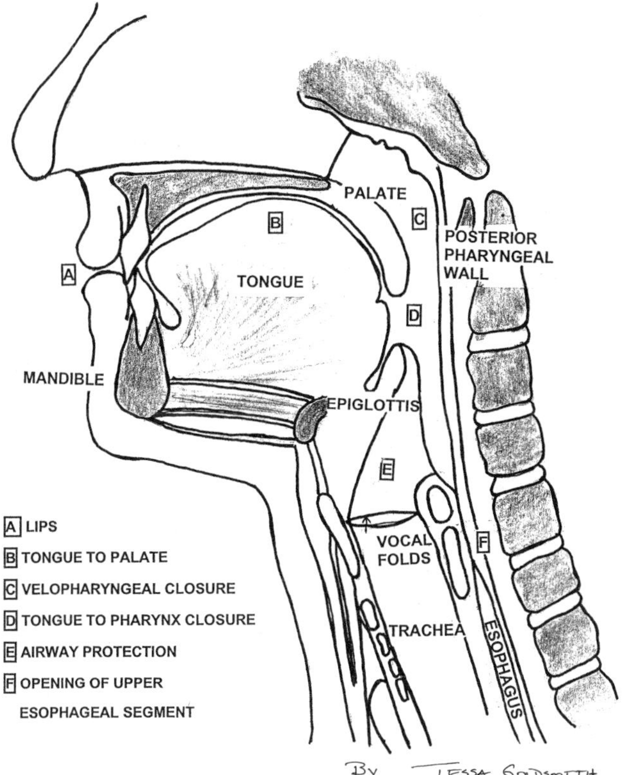

Fig. 10–2. Valves of the oral cavity illustrating twin function.

different sizes from a variety of utensils: cup, spoon, fork, straw, etc. The lips close during manipulation of the food or liquid, to prevent leakage anteriorly. Patients with muscle weakness due to stroke, degenerative neuromuscular disease, or neoplastic lesions involving motor and sensory function of the lips may experience difficulty containing the bolus in the oral cavity, and drooling may result. Patients with severe dementia may not be aware of the food in their mouth and may fail to close their lips.

Buccal or Cheek Seal. During chewing and formation of the bolus, contraction of the buccal muscles helps to maintain the bolus on the tongue blade. Where facial weakness is present, for example, in patients with Parkinson's disease or ALS, the boluses may pocket in the lateral buccal sulci and be difficult to retrieve. In cases where sensation is reduced, pocketed food may remain in the oral cavity for several hours, which would increase the risk of aspiration.

Tongue to Palate Seal. During bolus formation, especially of liquids and semisolids, approximation of the tongue to the soft palate prevents the bolus from spilling prematurely into the pharynx and airway. As the swallow is triggered, the palate elevates, allowing the tongue to propel the material into the pharynx.

Velopharyngeal Closure. The port connecting the oral with the nasal cavity (velopharyngeal port) is closed by elevation of the soft palate and its approximation with the lateral and posterior pharyngeal walls. This action prevents regurgitation of solids, particularly through the nose during swallowing. Nasal regurgitation of liquids is common in patients with cancer of the palate or pharynx.

Tongue to Pharynx Closure. The force against the bolus is greatest at the base of the tongue.[2,9] As the bolus reaches the back of the tongue, the tongue base exerts a strong driving force behind the bolus and contacts the pharyngeal walls, ensuring that the bolus, in its entirety, enters the hypopharynx. This posterior action of the tongue also assists in elevation of the larynx, initiating the first stages of deflection of the epiglottis over the laryngeal inlet. Weak driving force of the tongue results in a significant amount of residue in the pharyngeal recesses, loss of control over the bolus, or incomplete laryngeal closure, causing aspiration before, during, or after the swallow.

Airway Protection. The larynx comprises a vestibule or inlet and two sets of vocal folds that work synchronously for phonation, respiration, and airway protection during swallowing. Valving of the larynx during the swallow is important for prevention of aspiration into the tracheobronchial tree. During swallowing, complete laryngeal closure is necessary. This is accomplished by the following:

- Adduction of the true vocal folds, preventing airflow into the lower respiratory tract
- Adduction of the false vocal folds, preventing air escape from the lower respiratory tract
- Anterior and lateral rocking of the arytenoid cartilages to meet the base of the epiglottis
- Excursion of the hyoid and laryngeal muscle complex superiorly and anteriorly, resulting in complete inversion of the epiglottis over the laryngeal entrance[2,9,10]

Failure of the larynx to close due to timing or muscular incompetence can result in aspiration of liquids or solid materials. Reduced sensory function and weakened laryngeal musculature impair expectoration of aspirated material. Complete laryngeal valving is crucial during not only oropharyngeal swallowing but also periods of gastroesophageal reflux, regurgitation, or emesis.

Opening of the Upper Esophageal Segment. The final valve in the oropharyngeal swallow involves the cricopharyngeus muscle. This muscle is innervated by the vagus nerve and by sympathetic nervous system inputs, which help to maintain its tonic contraction. Opening of the upper esophageal segment is the result of traction of the cricoid lamina away from the posterior pharyngeal wall as a result of superior and anterior laryngeal movement. This movement creates a negative pressure in the esophagus, helping to propel the bolus toward the lower esophageal sphincter.[7,9,10]

ETIOLOGY OF DYSPHAGIA

A multitude of diseases can affect the "chamber–piston" relationship, causing dysphagia especially in patients receiving palliative care. These include degenerative neuromuscular diseases, progressive cognitive decline such as multiinfarct dementia, recurrent or fatal neoplastic lesions of the nervous system or aerodigestive tract, obstructive lesions from systemic diseases such as acquired immunodeficiency syndrome (AIDS), or pervasive debilitation from multisystem decline. In some cases, side effects of treatment, such as radiation therapy or chemotherapy, are the precipitating causative factor. In other cases, the progressive nature of a disease leads to unsafe and inefficient swallowing.

Understanding the physiological impact of the illness is critical in evaluation of the swallowing disorder and the method of management. For example, generalized weakness of the oropharyngeal musculature may be the overwhelming observation in two patients, one with a diagnosis of ALS who requires artificial ventilatory support and one who has undergone a second cycle of chemotherapy for extensive neck squamous cell carcinoma. Knowing that the weakness in the patient with ALS is likely to progress rapidly would deter one from suggesting effortful swallows as this may promote fatigue. On the other hand encouraging effortful swallows to preserve motor flexibility in the patient with neck cancer may assist this patient to take some food by mouth in the short term. Following is a description of some of the more commonly encountered etiological categories and their impact on swallowing.

Neoplasms

Tumors involving the nervous system as well as the head and neck and upper aerodigestive tract can interfere with swallowing.

Brain Tumors. Primary brain tumors are associated with oropharyngeal swallowing deficits as they affect the corticobulbar tracts involved in both the oral and pharyngeal stages of swallowing. Intrinsic brain stem neoplasms, such as gliomas, affect oropharyngeal swallowing because of the progressive invasion of the brain stem nuclei and tracts responsible for the coordination of sensory and motor inputs.[2]

Extrinsic tumors occurring around the brain stem, such as acoustic neuromas and meningiomas, as well as those originating in the skull base, such as glomus jugulare, glomus vagale tumors, and chordomas, may compress or invade the lower medulla and, hence, the cranial nerves and their nuclei that are critical for swallowing. The specifics of the swallowing impairment depend on which cranial nerves are affected. Compromise of the glossopharyngeal, vagus and hypoglossal cranial nerves singly or in combination results in the greatest swallowing dysfunction. Treatment approaches to neoplastic lesions of the brain comprise surgical excision, chemotherapy, and radiation treatment, all of which carry risks of morbidity and mortality. The relative inaccessibility of these tumors for treatment is associated with recurrence, which in turn can result in increased cranial nerve and swallowing impairment.[11,12]

Head and Neck Cancer. Oropharyngeal dysphagia is a common consequence of head and neck cancer and can result from tumors that invade structures and impair their functioning and from the obstructive effect of the tumor itself. Tumors of the head and neck are located in a variety of sites in the oral cavity, including the bony structures, the lips, floor of the mouth, tongue, palate, and tonsillar fossa, as well as the hypopharynx and larynx. Treatment of head and neck neoplasms varies according to cell type, location, and size of the tumor. In addition, treatment approaches vary among institutions and patient preferences. Some patients are treated with primary high-dose radiation and chemotherapy using "an organ preservation" approach.[2] Other facilities employ primary surgical excision followed by radiation therapy and/or chemotherapy as necessary. Prognosis and long-term survival rates vary with location of the tumor, distant metastases, and lymph node involvement.

Many patients with advanced head and neck cancer are unable to resume oral nutrition as a result of the surgical resection or from the sequelae of radiation treatment or chemotherapy. These side effects include mucositis in the acute stage and muscle fibrosis, scarring, and xerostomia (or dry mouth) even after the treatment phase is complete. Some patients manage to compensate for their dysphagia by utilizing changes in posture or diet consistencies suggested by speech language pathologists or nutritionists. Other patients rely on nutritional supplements delivered orally or via a gastrostomy tube. In any case, by the time the patient with advanced head and neck cancer reaches the terminal stage, he or she has already been fighting dysphagia and its very visible consequences for many months.

Malignant Esophageal Tumors. The incidence of malignant esophageal tumors is approximately 3 to 4 per 100,000.[13,14] Symptomatic presentation of dysphagia usually occurs late in the disease, and a diagnosis of advanced malignancy is commonly made. Esophageal carcinoma can arise either from squamous cells of the mucosa or as adenocarcinomas of the columnar lining of Barrett's epithelium.[13] Patients complain of weight loss and progressive dysphagia for solids more than for liquids. In some cases, an intractable cough may indicate extension of the tumor to the mediastinum or trachea. The presence of local extension to the aorta, trachea, or other mediastinal structures eliminates the possibility of surgical resection. Survival rates are reported to be between 10% and 20% at 5 years,[12,13] and thus, palliative care is the foundation of management of this disease.

If diagnosed early, esophagectomy or esophagogastrectomy may be the treatment of choice. However, in cases of advanced disease, symptomatic relief of dysphagia can be accomplished by radiation therapy,[13] esophageal dilation,[14] yttrium-argon-garnet laser electrocautery,[15] chemotherapy, or placement of an esophageal stent[16] to open the lumen of the esophagus. Each of these treatments is associated with considerable side effects, including esophagitis from radiation treatment and mucositis from chemotherapy. Perforation of the esophagus during laser surgery and dilation and migration of the esophageal stents are complications that may arise from some of the palliative procedures.[16] Frequently jejunostomy tubes must be placed as access for non-oral feeding.

Progressive Neuromuscular Diseases

Amyotrophic Lateral Sclerosis. Amyotrophic lateral sclerosis, or ALS, is encountered with unfortunate regularity in patients on a palliative care service. It is a rapidly progressive degenerative disease of unknown etiology that involves the motor neurons of the brain and spinal cord.[17,18] One-quarter of ALS patients present with difficulty swallowing as their initial complaint. The other patients begin with distal weakness that travels proximally to involve the bulbar musculature. Upper and lower motor neurons are involved as the disease progresses, and the respiratory system declines in the later stages. Respiratory failure is the usual cause of death in patients with ALS because of weakness in diaphragmatic, laryngeal, and lingual function.[18]

Typically, patients with ALS have a reduction in tongue mobility, affecting the ability to lateralize food for chewing and to control material in the mouth. As the disease progresses, heavier foods are difficult to manipulate, even those that are pureed. This results in significant residue in the oral cavity and hypopharynx. As oral musculature weakens further, there is nasal regurgitation of fluids; loss of control over liquids may result in aspiration and coughing before the swallow is triggered. Speech impairment parallels swallowing difficulty, affecting communication as well as alimentation. Diet modifications with calorie-dense foods and postural alterations are necessary if oral intake is to continue; however, many patients reach a point where the effort involved in eating is too great and the pleasure is lost. If the patient choses, a gastrostomy tube is placed percutaneously to provide nutrition, and sometimes supplemental oral intake for pleasure is possible.[2,18,19]

Parkinson's Disease. Parkinson's disease is a relatively common, slowly progressive disease of the central nervous system, marked by an inability to execute learned motor skills automatically.[17,18] A classic triad of symptoms, including resting tremor, bradykinesia, and rigidity, accompanies Parkinson's disease. An imbalance between dopamine-activated and acetylcholine-activated neural pathways in the basal ganglia causes the symptoms.[18,20] The largest etiological group is idiopathic, but Parkinson-like symptoms may occur as a result of medications, toxins, head trauma, or degenerative conditions.[17]

Dysphagia in Parkinson's disease is related to changes in striated muscles under dopaminergic control and in smooth muscles under autonomic control.[20] The oral stage is associated with rigidity of the lingual musculature rather than weakness. Small-amplitude, ineffective tongue-rolling movements are observed as patients attempt to propel the boluses into the pharynx. As a result, pharyngeal swallow responses are delayed and aspiration can occur before and during the swallow. Expectoration of aspirated material is weak because of rigidity of the laryngeal musculature. Incomplete opening of the upper esophageal sphincter and esophageal dysmotility are also commonly observed in patients with Parkinson's disease.[20]

In the early stages, antiparkinsonian medications such as L-dopa improve flexibility during swallowing. As the disease progresses, however, the medications are ineffective, and sometimes nonoral feeding is necessary.[19] Pneumonia is one of the most prevalent causes of death in patients with Parkinson's disease.

Multiple Sclerosis. Swallowing difficulty is uncommon in the early stages of multiple sclerosis.[18,19] The scattered inflammatory white matter lesions observed in the central nervous system result in varying combinations of motor, sensory, and cognitive deficits, which usually run a remitting-relapsing course.[2,18,19] Swallowing problems are less common in this disease, occurring in the end stages in approximately 10% to 33% of cases.[21] Difficulties arise with respect to the feeding process because of hand tremors and spasticity. Sclerosed plaques can be found in the cortex and the brain stem and can affect cranial nerves. Therefore, swallowing dysfunction will depend on the location of the lesions.

Sometimes the swallowing dysfunction is mild and goes unnoticed by the patients.[2] In patients who complain of dysphagia, the most commonly observed symptoms are delayed oropharyngeal swallowing initiation, reduced tongue strength, and weak pharyngeal contractions. These result in pharyngeal residue after the swallow and a sense of food getting caught in the throat.

A coexisting feature of multiple sclerosis in the later stages is cognitive decline and dementia.[18,21] Patients may be unaware of the act of eating and may be dependent on being fed. Family and caregivers require specific information to help patients compensate for reduced awareness.

Dementia

Dementia can result from several causes, including cumulative brain damage from multiple small cerebral infarcts in patients with hypertension and diabetes,

Alzheimer's disease, advanced stages of other diseases such as Parkinson's or Huntington's disease, or multiple sclerosis. In addition, patients can demonstrate cognitive decline from chronic metabolic derangement, sedating medications, and/or depression.[2,17,20] Patients with dementia frequently encounter pneumonia, particularly in the advanced stages of the disease.

Dementia causes fluctuating attention span, inactivity, agitation, confusion, and memory loss. These symptoms may necessitate medications to calm the wandering, agitation, and somnolence. Decreased consciousness predisposes patients to aspirate food and liquid.[20]

No single dysphagia profile exists for demented patients because of the variety of causes of the disease. However, common observations include inability to recognize food and accept it into the mouth, inability to feed self independently, slow or absent attempts at forming a bolus, delayed transit of boluses to the pharynx, and delayed pharyngeal swallow. Moreover, patients may exhibit distractible or agitated behavior, prolonging the feeding time and reducing the amount of nutrition and hydration received. Malnutrition and dehydration can produce medical complications that in turn exacerbate the cognitive decline even further.[2,19,20]

Systemic Dysphagia

The broadest category of causes of dysphagia includes inflammatory and infectious factors, which affect oral, pharyngeal, and esophageal stages of swallowing. Candida esophagitis can occur in an immunocompromised host, such as in patients with AIDS or patients who have undergone chemotherapy. Dysphagia for solids is greater than for liquids, and patients frequently complain of food getting caught. Heartburn, nausea, and vomiting are other common complaints.[12]

Autoimmune inflammatory disorders can affect swallowing in either specific organs or the immune system as a whole. This category of diseases includes polymyositis, scleroderma, and secondary autoimmune diseases. Sometimes intrinsic obstruction is observed, as in Wegener's granulomatosis; with other disorders, there is external compression, abnormal motility as in scleroderma, or inadequate lubrication as in Sjögren's syndrome. Pharyngeal and esophageal symptoms are common. Poor esophageal motility restricts patients to small meals of pureed or liquid substances. Patients report the sensation of solid foods getting caught in the esophagus. Weight loss is frequent. Gastroesophageal reflux results from poor esophageal peristalsis.[12,22]

General Deconditioning

Multisystem diseases, including the more frequently encountered progressive diseases such as end-stage chronic obstructive pulmonary disease, coronary artery disease, and chronic renal failure, cause insidious weakness. Weight loss in these patients is a common consequence because of reduced endurance for activities of daily living, including eating and swallowing. Patients with emphysema have difficulty coordinating swallowing and respiration and may be unable to tolerate the obligatory cessation of breathing required for airway protection during the swallow. General immobility impairs spontaneous pulmonary clearance, resulting in inability to expectorate material if it is aspirated. Patients are often discouraged and depressed by their loss of independence and declining health.

Medications can play a major role in causing dysphagia. The number of medications increases proportionally to the number of disorders to be treated, but their reaction may be exponential. Medications can affect lubrication of the oral cavity and pharynx, reduce coordination or motor function, and cause local mucosal toxicity.[23] The drugs that produce inhibitory effects, such as anticholinergics, tricyclic antidepressants, and calcium channel blockers, reduce esophageal peristalsis and decrease the tone in the lower esophageal sphincter.[23] Antipsychotic or neuroleptic medications can produce extrapyramidal motor disturbances, resulting in impaired function of the striated musculature of the oral cavity, pharynx, and esophagus. Medications such as haloperidol (Haldol), chlorpromazine (Thorazine), and thioridazine (Mellaril) can lead to dry mouth and nasal congestion. Long-term use of antipsychotics may result in tardive dyskinesias, with choreiform tongue movements affecting the coordination of swallowing. Delayed swallow initiation is a reported side effect of some neuroleptic medications.[24]

ASSESSMENT OF DYSPHAGIA

Approaching the evaluation of swallowing in the terminally ill patient demands a holistic view and reaches beyond the physiology of deglutition. While aspiration of food or liquid could realistically evolve into aspiration pneumonia, paradoxically, committing a patient to nonoral feeding or *non per os* (NPO) is also fraught with complications. It therefore behooves caregivers to consider very carefully the multiple parameters involved in making a decision about oral nutrition in the terminally ill patient. The matter is not a simple decision of "if the patient is aspirating food he or she should not receive nutrition orally."

In the terminally ill patient, the goals of the clinical swallowing evaluation are to *(1)* identify the underlying physiological nature of the disorder; *(2)* determine whether any short-range interventions can alleviate the dysphagia; and *(3)* together with the patient, family, and caregivers decide on the safest and most efficient method of providing nutrition and hydration.

Evaluation of dysphagia is best accomplished within a multidisciplinary framework. Nurses and family caregivers usually report that the patient has difficulty swallowing as the problems are witnessed regularly at meals and while administering medications. Speech language pathologists who are skilled at identifying causes of oropharyngeal swallowing and understand the complications of dysphagia can be consulted to evaluate the swallowing behavior and suggest compensatory management strategies to alleviate the dysphagia. In terminally ill patients, it may be possible to determine the least restrictive diet that will provide the patient with safe and efficient oral intake while at the same time preserving a modicum of the pleasures associated with eating by mouth. The assistance of a gastroenterologist may be required in cases requiring palliative dilation of the esophagus.

History

A comprehensive understanding of the difficulties involved in swallowing depends in large part on a detailed history from the patient and caregivers. Eliciting a description of the patient's complaints about swallowing is critical to building a picture of the physiological basis of the problem and to integrating these hypotheses with attitudes and wishes around eating and not eating. Details of the progression of the disease and the emotional and physiological impact it has created thus far on the patient and the family should also be appreciated, to gauge the intensity of the swallowing work-up and the treatment that can be undertaken.

The swallowing history may point to a mechanical obstruction as the etiology or to an underlying neuromuscular cause. Asking the patient which foods are easier and which are avoided, with special focus on liquids versus solids, provides clues about the location of the disorder. For example, patients who complain of solid food dysphagia and localize the area of difficulty to the throat may present with problems with bolus propulsion, whereas those who choke on liquids may have difficulty with airway protection. However, there is low diagnostic specificity regarding the patient's localization of the problem when compared with radiographic or endoscopic findings.[25] Sometimes a distal esophageal obstruction can give rise to a sensation of food getting caught in the cervical region or in the area of the retrosternal notch.

Information about the patient's current eating habits and diet should be obtained. Does the patient choke on all consistencies of solids foods and fluids? Can the patient feed himself or herself? How have meal times changed since the illness? Length of meal times and effort required are indicators of eating efficiency. Additional areas of concern include appetite, factors that appear to alleviate or exacerbate the problem, ability to swallow medication, and the presence of pain on swallowing.

The current complaints with respect to the physiology of swallowing are as important as the patient's prior attitudes toward eating. Was the act of eating important to this patient? Do the patient and caregivers understand the competing benefits and risks with regard to decisions around method of nutrition and the patient's preferences?

Table 10–1 lists frequently encountered complaints by patients regarding swallowing and their potential physiological counterparts.

Examination of Swallowing

Direct observation, by a perceptive clinician, of the patient while eating, drinking, or taking medications can yield valuable information about the underlying disorder. As discussed previously, the speech and language therapist is vigilant for indications of aspiration or obstruction. Warning signs associated with a swallowing disorder and aspiration risk relate to cognitive features, alterations in attitudes toward eating in general and mealtimes in particular, manifestations of oral and pharyngeal dysfunction, and specific patient complaints (Table 10–2).

Usually, the clinician assesses oral motor and sensory function, observes the patient partaking of a variety of liquid and solid foods (e.g., semisolid, soft solid, and—where appropriate—food requiring mastication), and assesses cognitive and communicative function. The speech and voice are analyzed, bearing in mind the chamber–piston model[9] described earlier, to determine the underlying physiology of the swallowing disorder. Since aspiration may be silent in up to 40% of patients with dysphagia, close attention is paid to occult signs of aspiration, including wet vocal quality or gurgliness, frequent throat clearing, delayed coughing, and oral/pharyngeal residue.[2]

Assessment of Oral Hygiene. The status of the oral mucosa and general oral hygiene reflect a patient's ability to manage secretions and swallowing. As mentioned earlier, xerostomia caused by radiation treatment, medications, oral candidiasis, mucositis, or poor oral hygiene may exacerbate, and in some cases even cause, difficulty swallowing. Patients who require supplemental oxygen delivered via a nasal cannula frequently

Table 10–1. Patient Complaints of Swallowing Difficulty and Their Possible Physiological Correlates

Patient's Complaint	Physiological Impairment
Choking on fluids	Poor tongue control for oral manipulation Impaired laryngeal closure Delayed onset of pharyngeal swallow
Protracted meal times	Weak chewing Diminished endurance
Nasal regurgitation of fluids	Incompetent velopharyngeal mechanism
Difficulty getting swallow started	Reduced oral and hypopharyngeal sensation
Dry mouth	Reduced or impaired saliva production
Solids caught in throat	Weak tongue driving force Impaired laryngeal excursion fails to open upper esophageal segment Weak pharyngeal contractions cause residue
Regurgitation or emesis after swallowing	Poor esophageal motility or esophageal obstruction
Sour taste in mouth after eating	Gastroesophageal reflux
Pain on swallowing	Esophagitis, mucositis, esophageal obstruction

Table 10–2. Indications of a Swallowing Disorder

Reduced alertness or cognitive impairment
- Coma, heavy sedation, dementia, delirium
- Impulsivity with regard to eating, playing with food, inattention during eating

Alterations in attitudes toward eating
- Refusal to eat in the presence of others
- Avoidance of particular foods or fluids
- Protracted meal times, incomplete meals, large amounts of fluids to flush solids
- Changes in posture or head movements during eating
- Laborious chewing, multiple swallows per small bites

Signs of oral–pharyngeal dysfunction
- Dysarthria or slurred, imprecise speech
- Dry mouth with thick secretions coating the tongue and palate
- Wet voice with "gurgly" quality
- Drooling or leakage from the lips
- Residual in the oral cavity after eating
- Frequent throat clearing
- Coughing or choking
- Nasal regurgitation

Specific patient complaints
- Sensation of food getting caught in the throat
- Coughing and choking while eating
- Regurgitation of solids after eating
- Pain on swallowing
- Food or fluid noted in tracheotomy tube
- Inability to manage secretions
- Drooling
- Shortness of breath while chewing or after meals
- Regurgitation of food or fluid through the nose
- Difficulty initiating the swallow
- Unexplained weight loss

experience dryness in the oral cavity. It is not uncommon to find dry secretions crusted along the tongue, palate, and pharynx in patients who have not eaten orally in some time. Dental caries and dentures that are not well cared for can also contribute to a state of poor oral hygiene as well as poor quality of life. Prior to giving the patient food or liquids, even for assessment purposes, it is vital to clear the oral cavity of extraneous secretions, using mouth swabs, tongue scrapers, toothbrushes, and oral suction if necessary. Dried oral secretions may loosen during trials of fluid and inadvertently obstruct the airway.

Evaluation of the Gag Reflex. A word of caution is needed regarding the gag reflex and oropharyngeal swallowing. Health care professionals routinely assess the gag reflex as a predictor of swallowing behavior. The gag reflex and the pattern of neuromuscular events comprising the swallow are very different, both in their innervation and in their execution. The gag reflex is a protective reflex that prevents noxious substances arising from the oral cavity or digestive tract from entering the airway. It involves simultaneous constriction of the pharyngeal and laryngeal muscles closing the airway and the pharyngeal lumen and results in anterior movement of the tongue.[26] A gag reflex is not elicited during the normal swallow.[27] Unlike the pattern of events in the swallow, the gag reflex can be extinguished or reduced by a nasogastric feeding tube, endotracheal intubation, or repeated stimulation. The pharyngeal swallow response, which closes the airway and opens the upper esophagus, cannot be extinguished once it begins, and it continues in a predetermined progression until the sequence of events is completed. These inherent differences highlight the need to examine the gag reflex and the swallow separately. Only evaluation of the biomechanical events of the swallow, not the gag reflex, can predict the safety of airway protection.

Assessment of Airway Protection. Functional airway protection is a critical predictor of safe swallowing and, thus, an important element of the clinical swallowing evaluation. Airway protection implies the speed and completeness of laryngeal closure during swallowing and the efficiency with which material is expectorated in response to aspiration. Patients who have weak voices and weak respiratory force for coughing and pulmonary clearance are at greater risk for pulmonary compromise than those whose cough is strong at the glottis. Patients whose cough on detection of aspiration is delayed may also be at increased risk of developing pulmonary complications. A functional cough is audible at the glottis, and the patient is able to expectorate secretions.

Compensatory Swallowing Strategies. If the clinical swallowing evaluation reveals signs of oropharyngeal or even esophageal dysphagia, the effectiveness of compensatory management strategies can be evaluated. These include alterations in head and neck posture, consistency of food, sensory awareness, and feeding behaviors.

1. *Postural changes:* Postural changes during swallowing often have the effect of diverting the food or liquid to prevent aspiration or obstruction but do not change the swallowing physiology.[2,28] Head rotation to the weak side in a patient with head and neck cancer may assist bolus flow down the intact side by obstructing the weak side and, hence, preventing residue or aspiration. Although it is not possible to detect the effectiveness of these strategies with complete certainty at the bedside, they may have empiric benefit that could be tested with an instrumental procedure if that is deemed necessary in the future.

   Table 10–3 lists some of the postural strategies that may be introduced during the bedside evaluation and their potential benefits on bolus flow.
2. *Changes in texture and consistency of food:* Underlying physiological constraints, such as reduced tongue control or strength, may affect the safety of swallowing certain solids or liquids. The patient with advanced ALS or Parkinson's

Table 10–3. Compensatory Postural Changes Which Improve Bolus Flow and Reduce Aspiration and Residue During Swallowing

Postural Strategy	Effects on Bolus Flow
Chin tuck	Closes laryngeal vestibule, pushes tongue closer to posterior pharyngeal wall, and promotes epiglottic deflection
Head back	Promotes posterior bolus movement with assistance of gravity
Head tilt to stronger side	Directs bolus down stronger side with assistance of gravity
Head turned to weaker side	Diverts bolus away from weaker side by obstruction of weaker pharyngeal channel, promotes opening of upper esophagus
Head tilt plus chin tuck	Directs bolus down stronger side while increasing closure of laryngeal vestibule
Head rotation plus chin tuck	Diverts bolus away from weaker side while facilitating closure of laryngeal vestibule and vocal folds

Source: Logemann (1998), reference 2.

disease with profound tongue weakness may show signs of aspiration on thin liquids but may have sufficient control to drink thickened liquids in small sips. Patients who are debilitated by chronic disease and who lack endurance to complete a meal may benefit from ground or pureed moist foods that require limited mastication. In certain circumstances, altered food consistency is the only way a patient can continue to eat orally, for example, in the patient with esophageal carcinoma or a severe esophageal motility disorder.

Changes in the consistency of food and liquid are frequently difficult for patients because they often lack appeal. Thus, this management strategy should be used as a last resort and reserved for patients who are unable to follow directions to use postural changes or for whom other compensatory strategies are not feasible.[2]

3. *Increased sensory awareness*: Sensory enhancement techniques include increasing downward pressure of a spoon against the tongue when presenting food in the mouth and presenting a sour bolus, a cold bolus, a bolus requiring chewing, or a large-volume bolus. These techniques may increase speed of elicitation of the pharyngeal swallow response while reducing the risk of aspiration. Some patients benefit from receiving food or liquid at a slower rate, while others are more efficient with smaller boluses delivered more rapidly. Patient responses to these behaviors can be evaluated at the bedside, and the findings can be easily communicated to the caregivers.[2]
4. *Secondary behaviors:* Attention is focused on the secondary behaviors that have an impact on the efficiency of swallowing. For example, the patient's attitude toward eating, endurance, efficiency of swallowing, and the length of time it takes to eat a meal influence the overall nutritional picture and, ultimately, quality of life.

Instrumental Evaluation

The clinical examination of swallowing is not conclusive with regard to location of the swallowing disorder or the underlying physiology. Radiographic or endoscopic evaluation of swallowing can provide valuable information for management.

Videofluorographic Evaluation of Swallowing. Radiographic swallowing studies are helpful in understanding the underlying physiology of swallowing. The modified barium swallow study examines oropharyngeal swallowing with the patient positioned upright and swallowing a variety of consistencies of barium-coated foods (liquids, semisolids, and solids) in controlled volumes. Speech pathologists and radiologists perform these studies together. The goal of this study is not only to determine the presence or absence of aspiration but also to evaluate the effectiveness of compensatory swallowing strategies, to decrease the risk of aspiration and increase swallowing efficiency. The test is not invasive, takes a short time to administer, and provides valuable information that can be used in managing the dysphagia.[2,6,28]

A barium swallow study examines esophageal function during swallowing. This test is conducted with the patient in a semireclined position and swallowing liquid barium. Mucosal abnormalities, esophageal strictures, esophageal motility, and gastroesophageal reflux are evaluated. If necessary, gastric emptying can also be assessed.[13]

Endoscopic examination of oropharyngeal swallowing can be performed at the bedside by a trained speech-language pathologist. The oropharynx can be visualized while the patient is swallowing. Endoscopic evaluation of the esophagus and stomach can confirm the presence of strictures and mucosal anomalies.[6]

MANAGEMENT OF DYSPHAGIA

Effortless, efficient, and safe swallowing are important criteria for continued oral nutrition. Experience has shown that most patients would like to continue to eat orally even if it means they do not receive sufficient nutrition. Patient autonomy in shared decision making is a critical ethical principle to respect but should be accompanied by a clear understanding of the risks involved in eating by mouth. In other words, families and patients should be informed about the risks and consequences of developing aspiration pneumonia and malnutrition so that they may make their decision. Health care professionals must present the information in as objective a manner as possible, taking the patient's wishes or the wishes of the surrogate decision maker into consideration. If the decision is to continue with oral intake, the safest diet should be suggested and aspiration precautions introduced using assessment of the swallowing problem as a guide.

The decision to pursue the option of nonoral nutritional support has significant ramifications for both the patient and the family. The family may feel that they have neglected their obligation to nourish their loved one safely and may be overwhelmed by the practical obligations demanded by the nonoral route, for example, frequent nocturnal feedings, monitoring of gastric residuals, etc. However, tube feeding may provide the patient with several more months of improved quality of life afforded by strength and endurance. Patients and families may also feel a sense of reduced pressure to eat by mouth because of the tube feeding.

Suggestions for Management of Dysphagia

Pharmacological Management. Candida esophagitis requires oral antifungal agents such as nystatin topical every 4 hours for 2 to 3 weeks. Other antifungal medications include ketoconazole, miconazole, fluconazole, and amphotericin B. Immunocompromised patients with candidiasis require potent systemic antifungal medications. Resistance can occur, however, in patients with long-term prophylaxis. Patients who fail the above regimen may be considered for anti-viral agents. The prokinetic agent or ranitidine may be prescribed for poor esophageal motility, and antireflux agents may be necessary (Prilosec, Zantac) for patients with gastroesophageal reflux disease.[29]

Dietary Changes. Evaluation results highlight the most appropriate nutritional method for the patient. If oral ingestion has been determined to be safe, the guiding principle for diet is to ingest the maximum amount of calories for the least amount of effort. Examples of modified diets are listed in Table 10–4. Nutritionists can provide individualized suggestions for calorie-dense foods depending on the patient's metabolic status. Patients with oropharyngeal dysphagia may require thickened liquids. Commercial thickening agents from modified food starch can be used to thicken liquids. These release the fluid in the gastrointestinal tract and provide water for hydration requirements.[30]

Feeding the Patient. While there is no cure for the swallowing disorder in the terminally ill patient, the continued ability to eat by mouth may be facilitated by careful feeding techniques and strategies employed by family and caregivers. These techniques will vary depending on the underlying swallowing/feeding difficulty. Compliance with feeding strategies is often related to understanding of the rationale. Family members are more likely to feed a patient a particular diet if they understand the physiological and psychological reasons for the recommendation and if they have been included in the decision making.[2]

Additional suggestions for feeding the patient include the following:

1. Removing distractions at mealtime. This is appropriate for patients who need to concentrate on swallowing to increase safety, such as patients with head and neck cancer who are using compensatory swallowing strategies, and for patients who easily lose their attention and need to be fed, such as patients with Alzheimer's dementia.[31]
2. Emphasize heightened awareness of sensory clues such as feeding patients larger boluses, increased downward pressure of the spoon on the tongue to alert the patient that food is in the mouth, or feeding patients cold or sour boluses or foods requiring some mastication.
3. Feeding utensils. Patients with multiple sclerosis who have feeding difficulties associated with hand tremors may be aided with devices such as weighted cuffs that reduce the intention tremor.[32] These may also be useful in patients with Parkinson's disease. Occupational therapists are often able to provide individualized assistive devices to patients.
4. Positioning the patient. Ensure optimal posture of the patient at meals; that is, reduce the tendency to slump forward, causing loss of food from the oral cavity, or head extension, making the airway vulnerable to aspiration.
5. Scheduling meal times. Some medications enhance swallowing function. For example, patients with Parkinson's disease may become more alert and flexible after their medications.[18] Thus, timing of meals to coincide with increased function may enhance swallowing efficiency and safety. In contrast, some medications, particularly sedatives such as haloperidol, may increase somnolence and produce bradykinesias, affecting the efficiency of swallowing. In such cases, withholding oral intake may reduce the risk of aspiration.

Nonoral Nutrition. Some patients require primary nonoral feeding, and gastrostomy or jejunostomy tubes are placed

Table 10–4. Diet Modifications for Patients with Dysphagia

Diet	Definition	Example	Indication
Pureed diet	Blenderized food with added liquid to form smooth consistency	Applesauce, yogurt, moist mashed potatoes, puddings	Reduced tongue function for chewing, impaired pharyngeal contraction, esophageal stricture
Mechanically altered diet	Ground, finely chopped foods that form a cohesive bolus with minimal chewing	Pasta, soft scrambled eggs, cottage cheese, ground meats	Some limited chewing possible but protracted due to impaired tongue control
Soft diet	Naturally soft foods requiring some chewing; food is cut in small pieces	Soft meats, canned fruits, baked fish; avoid raw vegetables, bread, and tough meats	Reduced endurance for prolonged meal due to tongue weakness for chewing, reduced attention span

endoscopically or in open surgical procedures. Some patients, such as those with esophageal cancer, head and neck cancer, or ALS, have had their feeding tubes in place for several months prior to the terminal period. For other patients, families and caregivers may have recently decided to pursue the nonoral feeding option. Irrespective of the scenario, the following should be considered:

1. The presence of a feeding tube does not imply NPO, or nothing by mouth. Some patients are able to take small amounts of food for their pleasure. Restrictions to reduce the risk of aspiration may apply during these "trials" of oral intake, such as texture of the food, postural requirements, and length of the trial.
2. Patients who are fed nonorally remain at risk for aspiration of either oral secretions or refluxed gastric contents, including tube feeding and aspiration pneumonia. A long-term study by Langmore and associates[33] examined the predictors of aspiration pneumonia in 189 elderly patients, including such factors as oropharyngeal and esophageal dysphagia, medical and dental status, feeding status, and functional status. They found that the dominant risk factor for aspiration pneumonia was dependence for feeding, that is, inability to feed oneself. This variable included those patients who were tube-fed as well as those who were fed orally by a caretaker. This study found that patients who were tube-fed had a significantly increased risk of developing aspiration pneumonia. The authors posited that oral hygiene is frequently neglected in tube-fed patients, promoting colonization of bacteria, and aspiration of these secretions can result in pneumonia.

Gastroesophageal Reflux Precautions. Poor esophageal motility or reduced tone of the lower esophageal sphincter can be managed either pharmacologically with the pro-motility agents described above or nonpharmacologically. Ideally, a combination approach is most efficacious. Gastroesophageal reflux precautions include elevation of the head of the bed to 45 degrees at night (blocks under the front feet of the bed are most effective); frequent small meals; upright posture for 45 to 60 minutes after eating; monitoring of gastric residuals in tube-fed patients, and avoidance of spicy foods, coffee, tea, chocolate, and alcohol.[34]

Administration of Medication. Oral medications can present enormous challenges to patients with dysphagia. Patients who take pills with fluid complain that they can swallow the water but the pills get caught in the throat. This phenomenon is explained by the differences in speed of transit of the fluid and the pill: the water travels more rapidly than the pill. Patients with delayed pharyngeal swallow initiation, reduced tongue strength, and/or pharyngeal contractions are unable to coordinate propulsion of the entire bolus. Crushing medications or burying them whole in a semisolid such as applesauce or ice cream creates a similar consistency and makes swallowing easier.

Tracheotomy Tubes and Oral Intake. The presence of a tracheotomy tube does not preclude oral intake. In fact, access to the upper respiratory tract improves pulmonary toilet in patients who have chosen to eat in spite of aspiration. Contrary to common thinking, an inflated tracheotomy cuff is not fully protective against aspiration.[2,34] The seal in the trachea is not complete, and material sitting above the cuff can be aspirated. Tracheal suctioning should be performed after meals in patients with dysphagia who have chosen to eat. Ideally, the cuff should be deflated and the patient encouraged to cough, to clear material that may have been aspirated.

DRY MOUTH (XEROSTOMIA)

Case Study: M.C., a Woman with Peripheral Vascular Disease

M.C. was a 73-year-old woman with peripheral vascular disease, atrial fibrillation, anxiety, foot pain, weakness, and fatigue. She had undergone surgery to her left foot for venous insufficiency. She was to undergo the same surgery to her right foot. However, preoperative diagnostics revealed a tumor in her left lung. Further diagnostic testing revealed stage IIIA lung cancer. M.C. decided to forego any treatment, including radiation and chemotherapy. Instead, she chose to go home with hospice care as she felt she had multiple medical problems in addition to her cancer. She started taking long-acting morphine for her foot and chest pain. M.C. said the pain "isn't too troublesome." Rather, she was frustrated by her constant dry mouth. Review of her medications showed she was receiving three that contributed to her problem: morphine, diuretics, and digitalis. She tried oral stimulants but had a bad reaction of anxiety. She did not like the taste of substitute saliva. This necessitated constant water drinking, which made her urinate frequently, exhausting her. However, given the alternatives, M.C. did not want to be on any more medications. So, she chose to continue to drink smaller sips of water, suck on ice chips, and keep lip balm by her side at all times.

DEFINITION

Xerostomia is the sensation of oral dryness, usually accompanied by decreased salivary secretions, and is commonly experienced by patients receiving palliative care.[35,36] It may be difficult to identify the exact underlying cause and contributing factors. However, treatment offers much comfort to patients.

PHYSIOLOGY

Although saliva is necessary for oral nutrition; it also facilitates chewing, swallowing, tasting, and talking. Additionally, saliva breaks down bacterial substances, offering immunoprotection for oral mucosa and dental structures. Saliva thereby inhibits dental caries and infections, while providing protection against extreme temperatures of food and drink.[37,38]

Saliva is comprised of several elements. It is largely composed of water and mucus, which provides the lubricative element. In addition, there are calcium bicarbonate ions and enzymes such as pytalin, antibodies, and other antimicrobial agents.[35,37,38]

The salivary glands and numerous glands in the oral pharynx produce saliva.[37–39] The average healthy adult produces up to 1.5 liters of saliva a day.

The parotid glands, the submandibular glands, and the sublingual glands produce 90% of saliva. Parotid glands produce a serous and watery saliva. Therefore, damage to the parotid gland will produce a thicker saliva. Submandibular glands secrete mostly serous saliva with some mucinous elements. Sublingual glands produce purely mucous saliva.[37,39] The overall viscosity of saliva is dependent on the functioning of the various glands.

Radiation to the head and neck can produce a 50% to 60% reduction of saliva within the first week of treatment because of inflammation. Usually, dry mouth sensations are worse at night. Salivary secretions may be further reduced due to the duration of radiation and/or greater radiation doses.[38] However, it eventually may become a more persistent issue the longer radiation continues or as disease progresses.[39]

Table 10–5. Assessment Questions for Xerostomia

Does oral dryness bother you?
Do you need to take increased fluids?
Is your mouth sore?
Do you experience altered taste sensations?
Is it difficult to speak?
Do you use tobacco? If so, what type and how much?
Do you drink alcohol or caffeine? If so, how much?
Are you on any medications, including over-the-counter preparations, prescriptions, or herbs?

Sources: Sreebny and Valdini (1987), reference 36; Cooke et al. (1996), reference 37.

ETIOLOGY

Xerostomia results from four causes. First, it may be the result of reduced salivary secretion. Common causes include surgery performed on head and neck areas, radiation aimed at head and neck regions, medication side effects, infections, hypothyroidism, autoimmune processes, and sarcoidosis. Second, xerostomia may be caused by buccal erosion. Potential factors are cancer and cancer treatment, particularly chemotherapy and radiation. Additionally, immunocompromised conditions such as AIDS, arthritis, or lupus may exacerbate dry mouth. Third, xerostomia may be induced by local or systemic dehydration. Factors contributing to dehydration include anorexia, vomiting, diarrhea, fever, drying oxygen therapies, mouth breathing, polyuria, diabetes, hemorrhage, and swallowing difficulties. Fourth, xerostomia can result from depression, coping reactions, anxiety, and pain.[35–37,40]

ASSESSMENT

Xerostomia may be accompanied by discomfort of the mucosa and the tongue such as burning, smarting, and soreness with or without the presence of ulcers. Additionally, there may be difficulty with mastication, swallowing, and speech. Taste alterations, difficulty with dentures, and an increase in dental caries may also be associated with xerostomia. Therefore, a thorough history should review these problem areas along with the subjective distress of xerostomia (Table 10–5).

The objective assessment begins with a thorough oral exam. Examination includes inspection of both mucosal and buccal dryness, noting whether the mouth is pale and dry, the presence of a dry and fissured tongue or cracked lips, the absence of salivary pooling, and the presence of oral ulcerations, gingivitis, or candidiasis.[36,37]

Two quick bedside tests are the cracker biscuit test and the tongue blade test. The cracker biscuit test involves giving a patient a dry cracker or biscuit. If she or he cannot eat it, xerostomia is present.[36] The tongue blade test is an extension of mouth inspection. After inspection is complete, the tongue blade is placed on the tongue. If it sticks, xerostomia is present.[37]

Another, more aggressive test is unstimulated or stimulated sialometric measurement of saliva. This test measures the amount of saliva collected by spitting into a container, swabbing the mouth with a cotton-tipped applicator, or salivating into a test container at a set time.[36,37]

To document the extent of xerostomia, it may be helpful to use the Oncology Nursing Society rating scale, specifically designed for this purpose. The scale, contained in Table 10–6, rates xerostomia in a four-point system.

MANAGEMENT OF XEROSTOMIA

Much of the treatment for xerostomia centers on patient and family education. A stepwise approach to treating xerostomia, as summarized in Table 10–7, would involve the following:

1. *Treat underlying infection or disease.* Candidiasis can cause xerostomia. Treating it with nystatin swish and swallow or with fluconazole 150 mg PO can improve xerostomia.[35,37,40]
2. *Review and, if necessary, alter current medications.* Anticholinergics, antihistamines, phenothiazines, antidepressants, opioids, beta-blockers, diuretics, anticonvulsants, sedatives, and tobacco may cause oral dryness. It is important to evaluate the necessity of specific xerostomia-inducing drugs. Decreasing the dosage may decrease dryness, or altering the schedule may assure that peak effect of medication does not coincide with peak time of xerostomia.[35–37,40,42–44]

Table 10–6. Oncology Nursing Society Documentation for Xerostomia

0	No dry mouth
1	Mild dryness, slightly thickened saliva; little change in taste
2	Moderate dryness, thick and sticky saliva, markedly altered taste
3	Complete dryness of mouth
4	Salivary necrosis

Source: Oncology Nursing Society (1994), reference 41.

Table 10–7. Stepwise Process for Managing Xerostomia

Treat underlying infections
Review and alter current medications
Stimulate salivary flow
Replace lost secretions with saliva substitutes
Protect teeth
Rehydrate
Modify diet

3. *Stimulate salivary flow.* Salivary stimulation can occur with both nonpharmacological and pharmacological interventions.

Nonpharmacological Interventions

Nonpharmacological use of gustatory stimulation includes simple measures. All of these interventions, except acupuncture, are inexpensive and may be as efficacious as medications for some patients, without side effects. However, relief is not long-lasting.[37,38]

- Peppermint water. The peppermint stimulates saliva. It can be taken as needed. However, do not use with metoclopramide as they have opposing actions.[45]
- Vitamin C. Use in lozenges or other forms as preferred. Although inexpensive, vitamin C may be irritating to the mouth, particularly if the patient has mouth sores.[40]
- Citric acids. Present in malic acid or in sweets. Again, similar to vitamin C, citric acids can cause a burning sensation.[40]
- Chewing gum, mints. Preferably sugarless, to prevent caries and infections, as an immunocompromised state can hasten cavities and infections. Most preferred by patients, cheap, no side effects.[39,40]
- Acupuncture. Effective with a variety of types of xerostomia. One study showed that 6 weeks of twice-weekly treatment increased salivation for up to 1 year.[46]

Pharmacological Interventions

- Pilocarpine. Pilocarpine is a parasympathetic agent that increases exocrine gland secretion and stimulates residual functioning tissue in damaged salivary gland. Saliva production is greatest after a dose and response lasts for about 4 hours. Dose is 2.5 mg PO tid and can be slowly titrated up to 10 mg PO tid. Response varies with severity of xerostomia. Side effects include mild to moderate sweating. May also cause nausea, rhinitis, chills, flushing dizziness, abdominal cramping, and asthenia. Should not be used in patients with chronic obstructive pulmonary disease or bowel obstruction.[37,40,47–49]
- Bethanechol. Bethanechol relieves anticholinergic side effects of tricyclic antidepressants. Few studies have been done with its solo use for xerostomia.[37,40]
- Methacholine. Methacholine is a parasympathomimetic compound that increases salivation. One side effect is hypotension. It is short-acting. Dose is 10 mg a day.[37,40]
- Yohimbine. Yohimbine blocks alpha$_2$-adrenorecpetors. Side effects include drowsiness, confusion, and atrial fibrillation, lasting up to 3 hours. Dose is 14 mg a day.[37,50]

4. *Replace lost secretions with saliva substitutes.*

- Water. Water is simple and inexpensive. It is usually well tolerated and easily accessible. Temperature is a personal choice.[37,40]
- Artificial saliva. Artificial saliva contains carboxymethylcellulose or mucin; dose 2 ml every 3 to 4 hours.[37,40,44]

5. *Protect teeth.* Oral hygiene, such as frequent brushing with soft brushes, water jet, denture cleaning, fluoride rinses, mouthwash, and flossing, stimulate salivation. Also, use of lip balm prevents cracked lips and use of saliva moistens lips. Care should be taken not to use products with alcohol since these can be very irritating.[39,41,51]
6. *Rehydrate.* Rehydrate by sipping water, spraying water, increasing humidity in the air.[39,43,51]
7. *Modify diet.* Education regarding the avoidance of sugars, spicy foods, sometimes salt, and dry or piquant foods is important. Patients may dip such foods in milk, tea, or water to assist in swallowing. In addition, instruct patients to take fluids with all meals and snacks. The use of gravies and juices with foods can add moisture to swallowing. Again, tastes may vary from one patient to the next in terms of preferred tastes of salt, sweet, and sour. For dry mouth without oral ulcerations, provide carbonated drinks such as ginger ale, cider, apple juice, or lemonade. Fresh fruits, papaya juice, or pineapple juice may be helpful.[39,50]

DECISION MAKING IN XEROSTOMIA MANAGEMENT

The degree of xerostomia varies from one patient to the next. Little research has focused on dry mouth; therefore, it has received scant attention. Clear evidence of one treatment over another has not been demonstrated, nor has one treatment been more efficacious. However, patients seem to prefer saliva stimulants to saliva substitutes.[40] If saliva substitutes are utilized, those based in mucin appear to be better tolorated than those derived from carboxymethylcellulose.[52] However, both preparations are better tolerated as an oral spray rather than a gel or rinse.[52] The issue of prophylactic antifungal therapy occasionally arises. The evidence thus far has not shown it to be beneficial. Finally, cost of therapy may be of concern for patients. Many patients choose nonpharmacological therapy since it is inexpensive and has fewer side effects.[40]

HICCUPS

Case Study: S.T., a Patient with AIDS

S.T. is a 60-year-old health care provider with end-stage AIDS, contracted 10 years ago secondary to a finger stick. She has undergone various treatments, including antiretroviral treatment and chemotherapy. S.T. has been fairly healthy in the past years, not requiring any hospitalizations, and was therefore able to maintain a busy lifestyle and schedule. In the last year, however, she became more confused. Work-up revealed central nervous system involvement of non-Hodgkin's lymphoma. She was finally admitted to the hospital for treatment of a viral infection. In addition to fevers, abdominal distress, and pain, S.T. developed long bouts of hiccups. They began suddenly, without warning or apparent trigger. They were intense and loud, lasting about 6 to 8 hours. The hiccups made her unable to eat and left her exhausted. Her husband felt hopeless and helpless during these episodes since they made S.T. so miserable and exhausted and increased her pain. Multiple regimens were attempted. Antiemetics and a nasogastric tube were used to decrease gastric distention. Phenothiazines were tried, to relax the phrenic muscle. Muscle relaxants were used to interrupt the hiccup cycle. With each one, S.T. experienced side effects worse than the hiccups themselves, including delirium, dystonic reactions, and altered blood counts. Eventually, morphine was chosen; it eased the pain as well as sedated her, which interrupted the hiccup cycle.

DEFINITION

Hiccups, or singulatus, are defined as sudden, involuntary contraction of one or both sides of the diaphragm, terminated by an abrupt closure of the glottis, producing a characteristic sound of "hic." [53–55] Hiccup frequency is usually 4 to 60 per minute.[56] Prolonged hiccups can produce fatigue and exhaustion if sleep is interrupted. Additionally, anxiety, depression, and frustration may arise as daily activities such as eating or sleeping are interrupted. Hiccups can also cause wasting because they can interfere with eating. Therefore, intractable hiccups affect the quality of life.[53,56–58]

PHYSIOLOGY

The precise pathophysiology of hiccups is unknown, as is their physiological function. The anatomical cause for hiccups is thought to be associated with the phrenic or vagus nerve.[56,57] There is thought to be a hiccup reflex arc located in the phrenic nerves, the vagal nerves, and T6–T12 sympathetic fibers, as well as a possible hiccup center in either the respiratory center, the brain stem, or the cervical cord between C3 and C5.[59] However, there is not a discrete hiccup center, such as the chemoreceptor trigger zone for nausea.[56,58,59]

Evidence suggests an inverse relationship between partial pressure of carbon dioxide (P_{CO2}) and hiccups; that is, an increased P_{CO2} decreases the frequency of hiccups and a decreased P_{CO2} increases frequency of hiccups.[43] Interestingly, hiccup strength or amplitude varies from patient to patient as well as among separate episodes.[55] Moreover, hiccups have a minimal effect on respiration.

ETIOLOGY

There are three types of hiccup. First are benign, self-limiting hiccups, which occur frequently. Such a bout of hiccups can last from several minutes to 2 days. Benign hiccups are primarily associated with gastric distention.[53,59,60] However, sudden changes in temperature, alcohol ingestion, excess smoking, and psychogenic causes may also induce benign hiccups.[53,55–57] Second are persistent, or chronic, hiccups. These continue for more than 48 hours but less than 1 month. Third and last are intractable hiccups, which persist longer than 1 month.[43,53,55] Intractable hiccups have over 100 different causes, varying from simple electrolyte imbalances to complex structural lesions of the central nervous system or infections.[43,53,55] The basis for these hiccups ranges from neurological processes to metabolic disturbances. Particular causes can be distilled into four conditions: structural, metabolic, inflammatory, and infectious disorders.[53] Specifically, these conditions affect the peripheral branches of the phrenic and vagus nerves, central nervous disorders, metabolic and drug-related disorders, infectious diseases, and psychogenic disorders.[55]

ASSESSMENT

Unlike primary care, where extensive work-up may be done, palliative care may choose not to perform a comprehensive work-up unless other measures have failed. Because the goal is comfort, work-up may be impractical and more uncomfortable than the hiccups themselves. Nonetheless, assessment should include both a subjective review of how much distress the hiccups cause the patient as well as physical examination of the patient's mouth.

Subjective assessment includes the history and duration of the current episode of hiccups; previous episodes; and interference with rest, eating, or daily routines. Inquiry into possible precipitates of the episodes may be helpful. In addition, a review of recent trauma, surgery, or acute illness and medication history is important to focus on potential causes of the hiccups.[43,57]

Physical observation includes inspection of the patient's general appearance, observing for signs of a toxic or septic process. More specifically, it includes evaluating for tenderness of the temporal artery, foreign bodies in the ear, infection of the throat, goiter in the neck, pneumonia or pericarditis of the chest, abdominal distention or ascites, and signs of stroke or delirium.[43]

Specific testing may be warranted to eliminate other causes. Chest x-ray may rule out pulmonary or mediastinal processes as well as phrenic/vagal irritation. Further, blood work including a complete blood count with differential electrolytes may rule out infection as well as electrolyte imbalances and other causes.[43,55,57]

MANAGEMENT

As when treating dysphagia or xerostomia, treatment for hiccups should be focused on underlying disease. If the etiology questionably includes simple causes such as gastric distention or temperature changes, "empiric" treatment should be initiated. Both nonpharmacological and pharmacological interventions may be utilized.[55–61]

Nonpharmacological Treatment

Nonpharmacological treatments can be divided into seven categories. First are simple respiratory maneuvers. These include breath holding, rebreathing in a bag, compression of the diaphragm, ice application in the mouth, and induction of sneeze or cough.[53,57] Second is nasal and pharyngeal stimulation. These techniques utilize pressure on the nose, inhalation of a stimulant, traction of the tongue, drinking from the far side of a glass, swallowing sugar, eating soft bread, or soft touch to the palate with a cotton-tipped applicator.[56] Third is miscellaneous vagal stimulation, which includes ocular compression, digital rectal massage, and carotid massage. Fourth are psychiatric treatments, which focus on behavioral therapy. Fifth is gastric distention relief, which encompasses fast-

Table 10–8. Pharmacological Treatment Suggestions for Hiccups

First-line treatment
Simethicone 15–30 cc PO q 4 h
Metoclopramide 10–20 mg PO q 4–6 h (do not use with peppermint water)
Baclofen 5–10 mg PO q 6–12 h
Second-line treatment
Chlorpromazine 10–25 mg PO/IM q 6 h
Haloperidol 1–5 mg PO/SQ every 12 h
Third-line treatment
Amitriptyline 25–90 mg PO q day
Valproic acid 5 mg/kg PO, then increase by 250 mg/week until hiccups stop
Nifedipine 10–80 mg PO q day
Mephenesin 1000 mg PO q day

Compiled from Launois, Walker, Watanbe, Bruera, 1998, Twycross, 1995, WHO
Sources: Launois et al. (1993), reference 57; Walker et al. (1998), reference 58; Twycross (1995), reference 60; World Health Organization (1998), reference 61.

ing, use of a nasogastric tube to decrease distention, lavage, and induction of vomiting.[53] Sixth is phrenic nerve disruption, such as an anesthetic injection.[53] Seventh are miscellaneous benign remedies, such as bilateral compression of radial arteries, peppermint water to relax the lower esophagus, use of distraction, or acupuncture.[45,53,56–58]

Pharmacological Treatment

Common pharmacological interventions are illustrated in Table 10–8. Initial therapy should attempt to decrease gastric distention, hasten gastric emptying, and relax the diaphragm. If ineffective, second-line therapy should focus on suppression of the hiccup reflex. Third-line therapy is the use of other drugs to disrupt diaphragmatic irritation or other possible causes of hiccups.

DECISION MAKING IN HICCUP MANAGEMENT

Although hiccups appear to be a simple reflex, their specific mechanism of action is unclear since myriad factors cause the response. Thus, the focus should be on comfort, with the goal of terminating the hiccups. The extent of aggressive treatment will depend on the degree of distress the hiccups impart on the patient's daily routine, particularly to what degree they are affecting sleep and nutrition.

Little research has been done because the mechanisms of hiccups are not well understood. Therefore, reports of therapy have been anecdotal, leading to lack of consensus on treatment. The result is that clinicians treat according to previous success with various medications rather than by a systematic approach based on research.

However, there are specific classes of medications to utilize. They include antacids, which decrease gas; antiemetics, which affect dopamine levels; and muscle relaxants, which affect the gamma-aminobutyric acid channels and skeletal muscle.[62] Persistence is necessary as patients may respond to different medications. If one class or type of medication fails, another class should be attempted until all possible medications have been utilized. If all of these medications fail to affect the hiccups, referral to a pain service or anesthesia service may be warranted as it may be appropriate for a patient to undergo a nerve block. However, as always, discussion with the patient should include their prognosis and the benefit and burden of any procedure.

CONCLUSION

Dysphagia, xerostomia, and hiccups are common problems that often receive little attention. Since they are considered trivial by many health care providers, these symptoms are probably underreported and underestimated.[37] However, nurses at the bedside, either in a facility or at home, may be the first to realize and witness the extent to which these symptoms cause discomfort and affect a patient's life. The mere act of a nurse listening to a patient's distress is an acknowledgment of his or her concerns. The patient feels she or he is taken seriously, as a unique individual. Moreover, the simple act of initiating treatment to manage these symptoms may promote psychological healing in itself because the patient feels respected about his or her concerns and experiences treatment as life-affirming.

Having established that the patient and family are the unit of care, the family should be brought into discussions concerning decision making. The nurse can elicit their concerns, promoting understanding and relief of anxiety and fears. Additionally, when death is imminent and aggressive treatment may not be warranted, specific discussion with the patient and family should focus on the individual circumstances that suggest comfort measures.

In summary, dysphagia, xerostomia, and hiccups are distressing symptoms that may affect nutrition, cause discomfort, and affect a person's sense of well-being. Left untreated, a patient may experience physical suffering and lose a sense of dignity. Because patients talk differently to physicians and nurses, nurses may be the first to identify these symptoms as well as evaluate the impact they have on a patient's daily routine. Therefore, nurses are in a pivotal role to address these symptoms and to initiate holistic management, providing relief, enhancing a patient's self-opinion, improving functional status, and promoting quality of life.

REFERENCES

1. Von Gunton C, Twaddle M. Terminal care in non-cancer patients. Clin Geriatr Med 1996; 12:349–358.
2. Logemann JA. Evaluation and Treatment of Swallowing Disorders, 2nd Ed. Austin, TX: Pro-Ed, 1998.
3. Perlman AL, Christensen J. Topography and functional anatomy of the swallowing structures. In: Perlman AL, Schulze-Delrieu K, eds. Deglutition and Its Disorders: Anatomy, Physiology, Clinical Diagnosis and Management. San Diego: Singular Publishing, 1997:15–42.
4. Selley WG, Ellis RE, Flack FC, Bayliss CR, Pearce VR. The synchronization of respiration and swallow sounds with videofluoroscopy during swallowing. Dysphagia 1994;9:162–167.
5. Miller AJ. The Neuroscientific Principles

of Swallowing and Dysphagia. San Diego: Singular Publishing, 1999.

6. Murray J. Manual of Dysphagia Assessment in Adults. San Diego: Singular Publishing, 1999.

7. Dantas RO, Kern MK, Massey BT, et al. Effect of swallowed bolus variables on the oral and pharyngeal phases of swallowing. Am J Physiol 1990;258:G675–G681.

8. Miller A, Bieger D, Conklin JL. Functional controls of deglutition. In: Perlman AL, Schulze-Delrieu K, eds. Deglutition and Its Disorders: Anatomy, Physiology, Clinical Diagnosis and Management. San Diego: Singular Publishing, 1997:43–98.

9. McConnel FM, Cerenko D, Mendelsohn MS. Manofluorographic analysis of swallowing. Otolaryngol Clin North Am 1988;21:625–635.

10. Cook IJ, Dodds WJ, Dantas RO, et al. Opening mechanism of the human upper esophageal sphincter. Am J Physiol 1989;257:G748–759.

11. Brin MF, Younger D. Neurologic disorders and aspiration. Otolaryngol Clin North Am 1988;21:691–699.

12. Schechter GL. Systemic causes of dysphagia in adults. Otolaryngol Clin North Am 1998;31:525–535

13. Murray JA, Rao SS, Schulze-Delrieu K. Esophageal diseases. In: Perlman AL, Schulze-Delrieu K, eds. Deglutition and Its Disorders: Anatomy, Physiology, Clinical Diagnosis and Management. San Diego: Singular Publishing, 1997:383–418.

14. Aste H, Munizzi F, Martines H, Pugliese V. Esophageal dilation in malignant dysphagia. Cancer 1992;56:2713–2715.

15. Nwokolo CU, Payne-James JJ, Silk DBA, Misiewicz JJ, Loft DE. Palliation of malignant dysphagia by ethanol induced tumor necrosis. Gut 1994;35:299–303.

16. Tietjen TG, Pasricha PJ, Kalloo AN. Management of malignant esophageal stricture with esophageal dilation and esophageal stents. Gastrointest Endosc Clin North Am 1994;4:851–862.

17. Buchholz DW, Robbins JA. Neurologic diseases affecting oropharyngeal swallowing. In: Perlman AL, Schulze-Delrieu K, eds. Deglutition and Its Disorders: Anatomy, Physiology, Clinical Diagnosis and Management. San Diego: Singular Publishing, 1997:319–342.

18. Yorkston KM, Miller RM, Strand EA. Management of Speech and Swallowing in Degenerative Diseases. Tucson: Communication Skill Builders, 1995.

19. Dray TD, Hillel AD, Miller RM. Dysphagia caused by neurologic deficits. Otolaryngol Clin North Am 1998;31:507–524.

20. Coyle JL, Rosenbek JC, Chignell KA. Pathophysiology of neurogenic oropharyngeal dysphagia. In: Carrau RL, Murry T, eds. Comprehensive Management of Swallowing Disorders. San Diego: Singular Publishing, 1999:93–108.

21. Hartelius L, Svensson P. Speech and swallowing symptoms associated with Parkinson's disease and multiple sclerosis. Folia Phoniatr Logop 1994;46:9–17.

22. Soliman AMS, Buchinsky FJ. Autoimmune disorders. In: Carrau RL, Murry T, eds. Comprehensive Management of Swallowing Disorders. San Diego: Singular Publishing, 1999: 199–209.

23. Alvi A. Iatrogenic swallowing disorders: medications. In: Carrau RL, Murry T, eds. Comprehensive Management of Swallowing Disorders. San Diego: Singular Publishing, 1999:119–124.

24. Stoschus B, Allescher HD. Drug-induced dysphagia. Dysphagia 1993;8:154–159.

25. Cooke IJ, Kahrilas PJ. AGA Technical Review on Management of Oropharyngeal Dysphagia. Gastroenterology 1999;116:455–478.

26. Leder SB. Gag reflex and dysphagia. Head Neck Surg 1996;18:138–141.

27. Leder SB. Videofluoroscopic evaluation of aspiration with visual examination of the gag reflex and velar movement. Dysphagia 1997;12: 21–23.

28. Rasley A, Logemann JA, Kahrilas PJ, Rademaker AW, Pauloski BR, Dodds WJ. Prevention of barium aspiration during videofluoroscopic swallowing studies: value of change of posture. Am J Roentgenol 1992;160:1005–1009.

29. Grandis JR. Infectious diseases. In: Carrau RL, Murry T, eds. Comprehensive Management of Swallowing Disorders. San Diego: Singular Publishing, 1999:229–233.

30. Lewis MM, Kidder JA. Nutrition Practice Guidelines for Dysphagia. Chicago: American Dietetic Association, 1996.

31. Groher ME, McKaig MT. Dysphagia and dietary levels in skilled nursing facilities. J Am Geriatr Soc 1995;43:528–532.

32. Broadhurst MJ, Stammers CW. Mechanical feeding aids for patients with ataxia. J Biomed Eng 1990;13:209–214.

33. Langmore SE, Terpenning MS, Schork A, et al. Predictors of aspiration pneumonia: how important is dysphagia? Dysphagia 1998;12: 69–81.

34. Leonard R, Kendall K, McKenzie S, Goodrich S. The treatment plan. In: Leonard R, Kendall K, eds. Dysphagia Assessment and Treatment Planning; A Team Approach. San Diego: Singular Publishing, 1999 pp. 181–218.

35. Speilman A, Ben Aryad H, Gutman D, Szargel R, Duetsch E. Xerostomia—diagnosis and treatment. Oral Med 1981;51:144–147.

36. Sreebny L, Valdini A. Xerostomia. Arch Intern Med 1987;147:1333–1337.

37. Cooke C, Admedzel S, Mayberry J. Xerostomia—a review. Palliat Med 1996;10:284–292.

38. Guchelaar H, Vermes A, Meerwaldt J. Radiation induced xerostomia: pathophysiology, clinical course, and supportive treatment. Support Cancer Care 1997;5:281–288.

39. Grant M, Ropka M. Alterations in oral status. In: Baird S, McCorkle R, Grant M, eds. Cancer Nursing: A Comprehensive Textbook. Philadelphia: WB Saunders, 1991:717–741.

40. Davies A. The management of xerostomia: a review. Eur J Cancer Care 1997;6:209–214.

41. Oncology Nursing Society. Radiation Therapy Patient Care Record: A Tool for Documenting Nursing Care. Pittsburgh: Oncology Nursing Society Press, 1994.

42. Ripamonti C, Sbanotto A, De Conno F. Oral complications of advanced cancer. In: Bruera E, Higginson I, eds. Cachexia–Anorexia in Cancer Patients. New York: Oxford University Press, 1996:38–56.

43. Waller A, Caroline N. Handbook of Palliative Care in Cancer. Boston: Butterworth-Heinemann, 1996.

44. Rust D. Anorexia and cachexia. In: Yasko J, ed. Nursing Management of Symptoms Associated with Chemotherapy. Bala Cynwyd: Menicus Health Care Communications, 1998: 38–56.

45. Kaye P. Notes on Symptom Control in Hospice and Palliative Care. Essex: Hospice Education Institute, 1989.

46. Blom M, Dawidson I, Angmar-Mansson B. The effect of acupuncture on buccal blood flow assessed by laser doppler flowmetry: a pilot study. Caries Res 1992;24:428.

47. Fox P, Atkinson J, Macynski A, et al. Pilocarpine treatment of salivary gland hypofuntion and dry mouth (xerostomia). Arch Intern Med 1991;151:1149–1152.

48. Rousseau P. Pilocarpine in radiation-induced xerostomia. Am J Hospice Palliat Care 1995; vol 12:38–39.

49. Oral pilocarpine for xerostomia. Med Lett 1994;36:76–77.

50. Chatelut E, Rispail Y, Berlan M, Montastruc J. Yohimbine increases human salivary secretion. Br J Clin Pharmacol 1989;28:366–368.

51. Oncology Nursing Society. Manual for Radiation Oncology Nursing Practice and Education. Pittsburgh: Oncology Nursing Press, 1998.

52. Sweeney M, Bagg J, Baxter W, Aitchison T. Clinical trial of mucin-containing oral spray for treatment of xerostomia in hospice patients. Palliat Med 1997;11:225–232.

53. Lewis J. Hiccups: causes and cures. J Clin Gastroenterol 1985;7:539–552.

54. Wilcock A, Twycross R. Midazolam for intractable hiccup. J Pain Symptom Manage 1996; 12:59–61.

55. Rousseau P. Hiccups in terminal disease. Am J Hospice Palliat Care 1994; vol 11 no 6:7–10.

56. Kolodzik P, Eilers M. Hiccups (singultus): review and approach to management. Ann Emerg Med 1991;20:565–573.

57. Launois S, Bizec J, Whitelaw W, Cabane J, Derenne J. Hiccups in adults: an overview. Eur Respir J. 1993;6:563–575.

58. Walker P, Watanabe S, Bruera E. Baclofen, a treatment for chronic hiccup. J Pain Symptom Manage 1998;16:125–132.

59. Pertel P, Till M. Intractable hiccups induced by the use of megestrol acetate. Arch Intern Med 1998;158:809–810.

60. Twycross R. Introducing Palliative Care. New York: Radcliffe Medical Press, 1995.

61. World Health Organization. Symptom Relief in Terminal Illness. Geneva: World Health Organization, 1998.

62. Friedman N. Hiccups: a treatment review. Pharmacotherapy 1996;16:986–995.

11 Bowel Management: Constipation, Diarrhea, Obstruction, and Ascites

DENICE CARACCIA ECONOMOU

Constipation is feeling stuffed all the time. Something's off, and my stomach feels tight. It puts an edge on everything. You worry because you haven't gone, but you are afraid to take too much laxative. It is like a double-edged sword.

—N.K., 45-year-old patient with advanced sarcoma

Constipation affects 10% of the general population, but the incidence may be as high as 20% to 50% in older or ill persons.[1] Constipation is a major problem in cancer patients, with as many as 78% of cancer patients having this distressing symptom.[2] The use of opioids for pain is a contributory factor to constipation, and this side effect is the principal reason for their discontinuation.[1,3]

PHYSIOLOGY OF CONSTIPATION

Understanding the normal functioning of the bowel can provide insight into the contributing factors that lead to constipation, diarrhea, and obstruction. *Constipation* is the infrequent passage of hard feces. Associated symptoms of constipation vary but may include excessive straining, a feeling of fullness or pressure in the rectum, the sensation of incomplete emptying, abdominal distention, and cramps.[4] The subjective experience of constipation may vary for different individuals. Connell and associates[5] observed that the definition of constipation varied greatly, with their study population reporting a normal frequency of bowel movement ranging from three times a day to three times a week. This variability underscores the importance of individualized patient assessment and management.

Normal bowel function includes three areas of control: small intestinal motility, colon motility, and defecation. Small intestinal activity is primarily the mixing of contents by bursts of propagated motor activity, which are associated with increased gastric, pancreatic, and biliary secretion. This motor activity occurs every 90 to 120 minutes but is altered when food is ingested. Contents are mixed to allow for digestion and absorption of nutrients. When the stomach has emptied, the small intestine returns to regular propagated motor activity.

The colon propels contents forward through peristaltic movements. The colon movement is much slower than that of the small intestine. Contents may remain in the colon for up to 2 to 3 days, whereas small intestinal transit is 1 to 2 hours. Motor activity in the large intestine occurs approximately six times per day, usually grouped in two peak bursts. The first is triggered by awakening and breakfast, and a smaller burst is triggered by the afternoon meal. Contractions are stimulated by ingestion of food, psychogenic factors, and somatic activity. Sykes[6] found that 50% of the constipated patients in a hospice setting had a transit time between 4 and 12 days.

The physiology of defecation involves coordinated interaction between the involuntary internal anal sphincter and the voluntary external anal sphincter. The residual intestinal contents distend the rectum and initiate expulsion. The longitudinal muscle of the rectum contracts, and with the voluntary external anal sphincter relaxed, defecation can occur. Additional coordinated muscle activity also occurs and includes contraction of the diaphragm against a closed glottis, tensing of the abdominal wall, and relaxation of the pelvic floor.

The enteric nervous system plays an important role in the movement of bowel contents through the gastrointestinal tract as well. Smooth muscles in the gastrointestinal tract has spontaneous electrical, rhythmic activity, resembling pacemakers in the stomach and small intestine, and communicating with the remainder of the bowel. There are both submucosal and myenteric plexuses of nerves. These nerves are connected to the central nervous system through sympathetic ganglia, splanchnic nerves, and parasympathetic fibers in the vagus nerve and the presacral plexus. Opioid medications affect the myenteric plexus, which coordinates peristalsis. Therefore, peristalsis is decreased and stool transit time is decreased, leading to harder, dryer, and less frequent stools, or constipation.[1,7]

Important factors that promote normal functioning of the bowel include the following:

1. *Fluid intake.* Nine liters of fluid (which includes 7 liter secreted from the salivary glands, stomach, pancreas, small bowel, and biliary system and the average oral intake of 2 liter) are reduced to 1.5 liter by the time they reach the colon. At this point, water and electrolytes continue to be absorbed and the end volume for waste is 150 ml. Therefore, decreased fluid in-

take can make a significant difference in the development of constipation.

2. *Adequate dietary fiber.* The presence of food in the stomach initiates the muscle contractions and secretions from the biliary, gastric, and pancreatic systems that lead to movement of the bowels. The amount of dietary fiber consumed is related to stool size and consistency.[8]
3. *Physical activity.* Colonic propulsion is related to intraluminal pressures in the colon. Lack of physical activity and reduced intraluminal pressures can significantly reduce propulsive activity.[9]
4. *Adequate time or privacy to defecate.* Changes in normal bowel routine, like morning coffee or reading the paper, can decrease peristalsis and lead to constipation. Emotional disturbances are also known to affect gut motility.[8]

PRIMARY, SECONDARY, AND IATROGENIC CONSTIPATION

Cimprich[8] offered three classifications of constipation:

1. Primary constipation is caused by reduced fluid and fiber intake, decreased activity, and lack of privacy.
2. Secondary constipation is related to pathologic changes. These changes may include tumor, partial intestinal obstruction, metabolic effects of hypercalcemia, hypothyroidism, hypokalemia, as well as spinal cord compression at the level of the cauda equina or sacral plexus.
3. Iatrogenically induced constipation is related to pharmacologic interventions. Opioids are the primary medications associated with constipation. In addition, vinca alkaloid chemotherapies (vincristine), anticholinergic medications (belladonna, antihistamines), tricyclic antidepressants (nortriptyline, amitriptyline), neuroleptics (haloperidol and chlorpromazine), antispasmodics, anticonvulsants (phenytoin and gabapentin), muscle relaxants, aluminum antacids, iron, diuretics (furosemide), and antiparkinsonian agents cause constipation.[1,7]

CONSTIPATION RELATED TO CANCER AND ITS TREATMENT

Multiple factors associated with cancer and its treatment cause constipation. When it involves the gastrointestinal system primarily or is anatomically associated with the bowel, cancer itself causes constipation. Pelvic cancers, including, ovarian, cervical, and uterine cancers, are highly associated with constipation and mechanical obstruction.[10] Malignant ascites, spinal cord compression, and paraneoplastic autonomic neuropathy also cause constipation. Cancer-related causes include surgical interruption of the gastrointestinal tract, decreased activity, reduced intake of both fluids and food, changes in the personal routines associated with moving the bowels, bedrest, confusion, and depression.[1,8,11]

OPIOID-RELATED CONSTIPATION

Opioids affect bowel function primarily by inhibiting propulsive peristalsis through the small bowel and colon.[1,11] McMillan and Williams[12] found that 100% of the patients in their study who had received at least 30 mg of morphine in the previous 24 hours developed constipation. Opioids bind with the receptors on the smooth muscles of the bowel, affecting the contraction of the circular and longitudinal muscle fibers that cause peristalsis or the movement of contents through the bowel.[13] Colonic transit time is lengthened, contributing to increased fluid and electrolyte absorption and dryer, harder stools.[14] Peristaltic changes occur 5 to 25 minutes after administration of the opioid and are dose-related. Patients do not develop tolerance to the constipation side effects even with long-term use of opioids.[3] The use of laxatives and stool softeners with opioids represents a rational, proactive approach to opioid-induced constipation.

ASSESSMENT OF CONSTIPATION

History

The measurement of constipation requires more than assessing the frequency of stools alone. Managing constipation requires a thorough history and physical examination. The use of a quantifying tool can be helpful in understanding what the patient is experiencing and how different that may be from the usual or baseline bowel habit. A tool developed in 1989 has been tested for validity and reliability and found to have a significant ability to measure constipation as well as its severity between moderate and severe constipation. It is a simple questionnaire that requires 2 minutes to complete. This Constipation Assessment Scale (CAS) includes eight symptoms associated with constipation.[12]

The CAS includes *(1)* abdominal distention or bloating, *(2)* change in amount of gas passed rectally, *(3)* less frequent bowel movements, *(4)* oozing liquid stool, *(5)* rectal fullness or pressure, *(6)* rectal pain with bowel movement, *(7)* small volume of stool, and *(8)* inability to pass stool.

These symptoms are rated as 0, not experienced; 1, some problem; or 2, severe problem. A score between 0 and 16 is calculated and can be used as an objective measurement of subjective symptoms for ongoing management (Fig. 11–1).

The CAS gives a good sense of bowel function.[12] Sykes[15] also outlines similar questions to use in taking a constipation history. It is important to start by asking patients when they moved their bowels last and following up by asking what their normal movement pattern is. Remember, what is considered constipated for one is not for someone else. What are the characteristics of their stools and did they note any blood or mucus? Were their bowels physically difficult to move? This is especially important if they have cancer in or near the intestines or rectal area that may contribute to physical obstruction. Ovarian cancer patients usually complain of feeling severely bloated. They may say things like "If you stick a pin in me, I know I will pop!" Evaluating the abdomen or asking patients if they feel bloated or pressure in the abdomen is important. Does the patient feel pain when moving the bowels? Is the patient oozing liquid stool? Does the patient feel that the volume of stool

Directions: Circle the appropriate number to indicate whether, during the past three days, you have had NO PROBLEM, SOME PROBLEM or a SEVERE PROBLEM with each of the items listed.

Item	No Problem	Some Problem	Severe Problem
1. Abdominal distension or bloating	0	1	2
2. Change in amount of gas passed rectally	0	1	2
3. Less frequent bowel movements	0	1	2
4. Oozing liquid stool	0	1	2
5. Rectal fullness or pressure	0	1	2
6. Rectal pain with bowel movement	0	1	2
7. Smaller stool size	0	1	2
8. Urge but inability to pass stool	0	1	2

Patient's Name Date

Fig. 11–1. Constipation Assessment Scale. (Reproduced with permission from McMillan et al. (1989), reference 12.)

passed is small? Many patients may experience unexplainable nausea.[16]

Medication- or Disease-Related History

The patient's medical status and anticipated disease process are important in providing insight into areas where early intervention could prevent severe constipation or even obstruction. Constipation may be anticipated with primary and secondary bowel cancer, as well as pelvic tumors, peritoneal mesothelioma or spinal cord compression, previous bowel surgery, or a history of vinca alkaloid chemotherapy. Changes in dietary habits related to the above medications or the addition of new medications may contribute to constipation.[1] Anticholinergic medications, antihistamines, tricyclic antidepressants, aluminum antacids, and diuretics can cause constipation. Hypercalcemia and hypokalemia contribute to constipation by slowing down motility.

Physical Examination

Begin the physical examination in the mouth, to ensure that the patient is able to chew foods and that there are no lesions or tumors in the mouth that could interfere with eating. Does the patient wear dentures? Patients who wear dentures and have lost a great deal of weight may have dentures that do not fit properly, which would make eating and drinking very difficult. Patients may choose to eat only what they are able to chew related to their dentures or other dental problems. Therefore, they may not be eating enough fiber and, thus, contributing to primary constipation.

Abdominal Examination

Inspect the abdomen initially for bloating, distention, or bulges. Distention may be associated with obesity, fluid, tumor, or gas. Remember, the patient should have emptied the bladder. Auscultation is important, to evaluate the presence or absence of bowel sounds. If no bowel sounds are heard initially, listen continuously for a minimum of 5 minutes. The absence of bowel sounds may indicate a paralytic ileus. If the bowel sounds are hyperactive, it could indicate diarrhea. Percussion of the bowel may result in tympany, which is related to gas in the bowel. A dull sound is heard over intestinal fluid and feces. Palpation of the abdomen should start lightly; look for muscular resistance and abdominal tenderness. This is usually associated with chronic constipation. If with coughing or light palpation rebound tenderness is detected, peritoneal inflammation should be considered. Deep palpation may reveal a "sausage-like" mass of stool in the left colon. Feeling stool in the colon indicates constipation.[11] Although Sykes[15] points out that the distinction between tumor and stool is hard to make, recognizing the underlying anatomy is helpful in distinguishing the stool along the line of the descending colon or more proximal colon, including the cecum. A digital examination of the rectum may reveal stool or possible tumor or rectocele. If the patient is experiencing incontinence of liquid stool, obstruction must be considered. Examining for hemorrhoids, ulcerations, or rectal fissures is important, especially in the neutropenic patient. Patients with a neutropenia can complain of rectal pain well before a rectal infection is obvious. Evaluating the patient for infection, ulceration, or rectal fissures is very important. Additionally, determine whether the patient has had previous intestinal surgery, alternating diarrhea and constipation, complaints of abdominal colic pain or nausea, and vomiting. Examining the stool for shape and consistency can also be useful. Stools that are hard and pellet-like suggest slow transit time, whereas stools that are ribbon-like suggest hemorrhoids. Blood or mucus in the stool suggests tumor, hemorrhoids, or possibly a preexisting colitis.[15] Elderly patients may experience urinary incontinence related to fecal impaction.[1,11,15] Abdominal pain may also be related to constipation. Patients will complain of colic pain related to the effort of colonic muscle to move hard stool. The history may be complicated by known abdominal tumors. Patients in pain should still be treated with opioids as needed.

MANAGEMENT OF CONSTIPATION

Preventing constipation whenever possible is the most important management strategy. Constipation can be extremely distressing to many patients and severely affects quality of life. The complicating factor remains the individuality of a patient's response to constipation therapy. Therefore, there is no set rule for the most effective way to manage constipation. Patients with primary bowel cancers, pelvic tumors like ovarian or uterine cancers, or metastatic tumors that press on colon structures will experience a difficult-to-manage constipation. It is not unusual for those patients to be admitted to the hospital, for constipation management and to rule out obstruction. To minimize those admissions whenever possible, as Dame Cicely Saunders, the founder of hospice recommends, "do not forget the bowels." Nurses are at the bedside most often and are the ones who see the cumulated number and types of medication a patient may be taking. Understanding which medications and disease processes put a patient at high risk for constipation is essential for good bowel management.

Assessing the patient's constipation as discussed earlier is the best place to start. The patient's problem list should reflect the risk for constipation and the need for aggressive constipation management. For example, diabetic patients who are taking opioids for pain are at extremely high risk for constipation. Diabetes damages the sensory fibers that are most important for temperature and pain sensation . The neuronal influence on intestinal motility is also affected through diabetes.[15,17]

In addition to assessing the extent of the patient's constipation, determining the methods the patient has used to manage the constipation in the past is essential. This can usually provide information regarding what medications the patient tolerates best and where to start with recommendations for management. According to Sykes[7], using radiography to evaluate whether constipation has advanced to obstruction may be useful if there is indecision, but in palliative medicine the use of x-ray procedures should be limited. He also suggests that blood work be limited to corrective studies. In constipation, if hypercalcemia or hyperkalemia can be reversed to improve constipation, such blood work may be useful.

Improving three important primary causes of constipation is essential. Encouraging fluid intake is a priority. Increasing or decreasing fluid intake by as little as 100 ml can contribute to constipation.[1,15] Increase dietary intake as much as possible. This is a difficult intervention for many patients. Focusing on food intake for some patients can increase their anxiety and discomfort. If a patient is feeling that bowel movements are less frequent, think about dietary intake. The Western diet is fiber-deficient.[1,7,8] Caution is needed for patients who use bulk laxatives like psyllium, especially if they also are taking other bowel medications (Table 11–1). Increasing the fiber intake for patients in general may be helpful, but in palliative care, high fiber in the diet can cause more discomfort and constipation. Fiber without fluid absorbs what little liquid the patient may have available in the bowel and makes the bowels more difficult to move.[1,7] For example, an elderly patient who experiences reduced appetite and decreased fluid intake related to chemotherapy or disease, and whose symptoms are nausea or vomiting with reduced activity, is at extreme risk for constipation. Encouraging activity, even in end-of-life care, whenever possible can be very helpful. Increased activity helps to stimulate peristalsis and to improve mood.[1,7] Physical therapy should be used as part of a multidisciplinary bowel management approach. Providing basic range of motion, either active or passive, can improve bowel management and patient satisfaction.[8,11]

Types of Laxative

Bulk Laxatives. Laxatives can be classified by their actions. Bulk laxatives do just that; they provide bulk to the intestines to increase mass, which stimulates the bowel to move. Increasing dietary fiber is considered a bulk laxative. Other bulk laxatives include bran, psyllium, carboxymethylcellulose, and methylcellulose. Bulk laxatives are more helpful for mild constipation. Because bulk laxatives work best when patients are able to increase their fluid intake, they may be inappropriate for end-stage patients. In palliative care, patients may not ingest enough fluid. It is recommended that the patient increase fluids by 200 to 300 ml when using bulk laxatives. Patients may have difficulty with the consistency of bulk laxatives and find this approach unacceptable. Patients using bulk laxatives without the additional fluid intake are at risk of developing a partial bowel obstruction or, if an impending one exists, may risk complete bowel obstruction. The benefits of bulk laxatives in severe constipation are questionable.

Additional complications include allergic reactions, fluid retention, and hyperglycemia.[1] Bulk laxatives produce gas as the indigestible or non-soluble fiber breaks down or ferments. The result can be uncomfortable bloating and gas.

The recommended dosage of bulk laxatives is to start with 8 g daily, then stabilize at 3 to 4 g for maintenance.

Table 11–1. Causes of Constipation in Cancer/Palliative Care Patients

Cancer-Related

Directly related to tumor site. Primary bowel cancers, secondary bowel cancers, pelvic cancers.
Hypercalcemia. Surgical interruption of bowel integrity.

Etiology
Intestinal obstruction related to tumor in the bowel wall or external compression by tumor. Damage to the lumbosacral spinal cord, cauda equina, or pelvic plexus. High spinal cord transection mainly stops the motility response to food. Low spinal cord or pelvic outflow lesions produce dilation of the colon and slow transit in the descending and distal transverse colon. Surgery in the abdomen can lead to adhesion development or direct changes in the bowel.

Hypercalcemia

Cholinergic control of secretions of the intestinal epithelium is mediated by changes in intracellular calcium concentrations. Hypercalcemia causes decreased absorption, leading to constipation, whereas hypocalcemia can lead to diarrhea.

Secondary Effects Related to the Disease
Decreased appetite, decreased fluid intake, low-fiber diet, weakness, inactivity, confusion, depression, change in normal toileting habits.

Etiology
Decreased fluid and food intake leads to dehydration and weakness. Decreased intake, ineffective voluntary elimination actions, as well as decreased normal defecation reflexes. Decreased peristalsis; increased colonic transit time leads to increased absorption of fluid and electrolytes and small, hard, dry stools. Inactivity, weakness, changes in normal toileting habits, daily bowel function reflexes, positioning affects ability to use abdominal wall musculature and relax pelvic floor for proper elimination. Psychological depression can increase constipation by slowing down motility.

Concurrent disease

Diabetes, hypothyroidism, hypokalemia, diverticular disease, hemorrhoids, colitis, chronic neurological diseases.

Etiology
Electrolytes and therefore water are transported via neuronal control. Like hypercalcemia, abnormal potassium can affect water absorption and contribute to constipation. Chronic neurological diseases affect the neurological stimulation of intestinal motility.

Medication-Related

Opioid medications
Anticholinergic effects (hydroscine, phenothiazines)
Tricyclic antidepressants
Antiparkinsonian drugs
Iron
Antihypertensives, antihistamines
Antacids
Diuretics
Vinka alkaloid chemotherapy

Etiology
Opioids in particular suppress forward peristalsis and increase sphincter tone. Opioids increase electrolyte and water absorption in both the large and small intestine; this leads to dehydration and hard, dry stools. Morphine causes insensitivity of the rectum to distention, decreasing the sensation of the need to defecate. Vinca alkaloid chemotherapy has a neurotoxic effect that causes damage to the myenteric plexus of the colon. This increases nonpropulsive contractions. Colonic transit time is increased, leading to constipation. Antidepressants slow large bowel motility. Antacids (bismuth, aluminum salts) cause hard stools.

Sources: Levy (1991), reference 1; Sykes (1996), reference 71.

Psyllium is recommended at 2 to 4 teaspoons daily as a bulk laxative. Action may take 2 to 3 days.

Lubricant Laxatives. Mineral oil is probably the most common lubricant laxative used. It can help by lubricating the stool surface and softening the stool by penetration, leading to an easier bowel movement. Overuse of mineral oil can cause seepage from the rectum and perineal irritation. It has also been shown with chronic use to lead to malabsorption of fat-soluble vitamins (vitamins A, D, E, and K). Levy[1] recommends caution when giving mineral oil at bedtime or to patients at risk for aspiration. Aspiration pneumonitis or lipoid pneumonia is common in the frail and elderly patient; caution should be used when giving mineral oil at bedtime, to prevent aspiration. A complication should be noted when mineral oil is given with docusate. If patients are on daily docusate (Colace) and are given mineral oil in addition, to assist with constipation, the absorption of mineral oil increases, leading to a risk of lipoid granuloma in the intestinal wall.[1]

The recommended dosage of mineral oil is 10 to 30 ml/day, and action may occur in 1 to 3 days.

Surfactant/Detergent Laxatives. Surfactant/detergent laxatives reduce surface tension, which increases absorption of water and fats into dry stools, leading to a softening effect. According to Levy[1] and Sykes,[7] medications like docusate exert a mucosal contact effect, which encourages secretion of water, sodium, and chloride in the jejunum and colon and decreases electrolyte and water reabsorption in the small and large intestine.[2] At higher doses, these laxatives may stimulate peristalsis. Docusate is used in a compounded or fixed combination with bowel stimulants like casanthranol (Peri-Colace) or senna (Senokot S). Castor oil also works like a detergent laxative by exerting a surface-wetting action on the stool and directly stimulates the colon, but Levy[17] discourages its use in cancer-related constipation because results are difficult to control.

The recommended dosage of surfactant/detergent laxatives includes docusate (Colace) starting at 300 mg daily and calcium salt (Surfak) at 240 mg daily to twice a day. (This may take 1 to 3 days to be effective.)

Combination Medications. Peri-Colace is a combination of a mild stimulant laxative, casanthranal, and the stool softener docusate (Colace).

The recommended dosage of Senokot S is two tablets daily to twice a day (see Senokot S flow chart in Table 11–2). Senokot is a combination of senna as a laxative and a stool softener for smoother and easier evacuation. Results occur in 6 to 12 hours. Flexibility of dosing allows individual needs to be met.

Table 11–2. Senokot S Laxative Recommendations for Cancer-Related Constipation

Day 0
- Senokot S 2 tablets at bedtime

If no BM on day 1
- Senokot S 2 tablets bid

If no BM on day 2
- Senokot S 3 or 4 tablets bid or tid

If no BM on day 3
- Dulcolax 2 or 3 tablets tid and/or hs
- If no BM, rule out impaction
- If impacted
  Lubricate rectum with oil retention enema
  Medicate with opioid and/or benzodiazepine
  Disimpact
  Give enemas until clear
  Increase daily laxative therapy per above
- If not impacted
  Give additional laxatives
  - Lactulose (45–60 ml PO)
  - Magnesium citrate (8 oz)
  - Dulcolax suppository (1 PR)
  - Fleet enema (1 PR)

At any step, if medication is effective, continue at that dose. If <1 BM per day, increase laxative therapy per steps. If >2 BM per day, decrease laxative therapy by 24% to 50%.

Source: Adapted from Levy (1991), reference 1.

Osmotic Laxatives. Osmotic laxatives are nonabsorbable sugars that exert an osmotic effect in both the small and, to a lesser extent, the large intestines. They have the additional effect of lowering ammonia levels. This is helpful in improving confusion, especially in hepatic failure patients. According to Levy,[1] 30 ml of lactulose can increase the colon volume by 400 to 600 ml within 1 to 3 hours. These laxatives can be very effective for chronic constipation, especially when related to opioid use. Drawbacks of these agents are that effectiveness is completely dose-related and, for some patients, the sweet taste is intolerable. The bloating and gas associated with higher doses may be too uncomfortable or distressing to tolerate. Lactulose or sorbitol can be put into juice or other liquid to lessen the taste. Patients may prefer hot tea or hot water to help reduce the sweet taste. Lactulose is more costly than sorbitol liquid. It can range from about $5.00 for 960 ml of sorbitol to between $30.00 and $50.00 for the same amount of lactulose. A study that compared the two medications found that there was no significant difference, except with regard to nausea, which increased with lactulose ($P < 0.05$).[18]

The recommended dosage of lactulose/sorbitol is 30 to 60 ml initially for severe constipation every 4 hours until a bowel movement occurs. Once a bowel movement occurs, calculate the amount of lactulose used to achieve that movement, then divide in one-half for recommended daily maintenance dose.[1] An example would be if it took 60 ml to have a bowel movement, then 30 ml daily should keep the bowels moving regularly. Action can occur within 4 hours, depending on the dose.

Osmotic rectal compounds include glycerine suppositories and sorbitol enemas. Glycerine suppositories soften stool by osmosis and act as a lubricant. In one study, bisacodyl (Dulcolax) suppositories were more effective for moving the bowel than glycerine suppositories in chronically ill and geriatric patients.[19]

Dulcolax acts directly on the mucous membrane of the large intestine, causing a reflex stimulation. Because it is not absorbed in the small intestine, it can pass through without side effects.

It can be especially helpful for bowel training or bedridden patients with dyschezia, or an incomplete reflex for defecation.

Suppositories should never be used in patients with severely reduced white cell or platelet counts due to the risk of bleeding or infection.

Saline Laxatives. Magnesium hydroxide (Milk of Magnesia) and magnesium citrate are the most commonly used saline laxatives. They increase gastric, pancreatic, and small intestinal secretion, as well as motor activity throughout the intestine. Aluminum salts in many of the antacid medications counteract the laxative effect of magnesium. Also, this laxative can cause severe cramping and discomfort. This medication is recommended for use only as a last resort in chronically ill patients. Opioid-related constipation requires the use of aggressive laxatives earlier than later, to prevent severe constipation, referred to as *obstipation*, which leads to obstruction.

The recommended dosage of Milk of Magnesia is 30 cc to initiate a bowel movement. For opioid-related constipation, 15 cc of Milk of Magnesia may be added to the baseline bowel medications either daily or every other day. Magnesium citrate comes in a 10-ounce bottle. For severe constipation, it is used as a one-time initial therapy. It can be titrated up or down, depending on patient's response. For patients with abdominal discomfort or pain, it is recommended that obstruction be ruled out prior to using this medication. If the patient were obstructed, even only partially, this would only increase the discomfort or lead to perforation.[15]

Bowel Stimulants. Bowel stimulants work directly on the colon to increase motility. These medications stimulate the myenteric plexus to induce peristalsis. They also reduce the amount of water and electrolytes in the colon. They are divided into two groups: the diphenylmethanes and the anthraquinones. The diphenylmethanes are commonly known as phenolphthalein (Ex-Lax, Fen-a-ment, Correctol, and Doxidan) and bisacodyl (Dulcolax). Phenolphthalein must be metabolized in the liver rather than in the colon. Levy[1] points out that because the effect is difficult to control and hepatic circulation is significant, this class of stimulants may not be appropriate for cancer-related constipation. The anthraquinones are bowel stimulants that include senna and cascara. They are activated in the large intestine by bacterial degradation into the large bowel, stimulating glycosides. The negative side of bisacodyl is its cramping side effect. This action causes a 6- to 12-hour delay when taken orally. Rectal absorption is much faster, at 15 to 60 minutes. It is recommended that bisacodyl be taken with food, milk, or antacids, to avoid gastric irritation. One Senokot S can counter the constipation caused by 120 mg of codeine.[13] Senna is available in a liquid form called X-Prep Liquid. This is used for bowel cleansing prior to radiology procedures; 72 ml of X-Prep is equivalent to ten Senokot tablets. Cascara, another anthraquinone, is commonly combined with Milk of Magnesia to make a mixture referred to as "Black and White." This is a mild combination that reduces colic pain. Casanthranol is derived from cascara and is used as the stimulant component in Peri-Colace.

Recommendations for use are senna 15 mg tablets used alone or as Senokot S. Starting dose is two tablets daily (Table 11–2). These stimulating laxatives are the most effective management for opioid-related constipation. Bisacodyl comes in 10 mg tablets or suppositories. It is used daily. The suppository medication has a faster onset, which is much appreciated in the uncomfortable, constipated patient.

Suppository Medications. As discussed above, bisacodyl (Dulcolax) comes in a suppository. Although the thought of rectal medications for many patients is unpleasant, their quick onset of action makes them more acceptable. Bisacodyl comes in 10 mg for adults and 5 mg as a pediatric dose.

Liquid rectal laxatives or lubricants should be used infrequently. In severely constipated patients, they may be necessary. Most commonly, saline enemas are used to loosen the stool and to stimulate rectal or distal colon peristalsis. Repeated use can cause hypocalcemia and hyperphosphatemia. In ill patients with a history of hemorrhoids, one study found that repeated use of phosphate enemas could produce gangrene.[20] It is important to use enemas cautiously. Enemas should never be considered part of a standing bowel regimen.

Oil retention enemas, however, are particularly helpful for severely constipated patients, for whom disimpaction may be necessary. They work best when used overnight, to allow softening. Overnight retention is effective only if the patient is able to retain it that long. The general rule is the longer the enema is retained, the better the results. Bisanz[22] recommends a milk and molasses enema for patients with low impaction, to ease stool evacuation in a nonirritating way. It is a low-volume enema of 300 cc and, therefore, thought to cause less cramping:

MILK AND MOLASSES ENEMA RECIPE

8 oz warm water
3 oz powdered milk
4.5 oz molasses

- Put water and powdered milk in a plastic jar. Close the jar and shake until the water and milk appear to be fully mixed.
- Add molasses, and shake the jar again until the mixture appears to have an even color throughout.
- Pour mixture into enema bag. Administer enema high by gently introducing tube about 12 inches. Do not push beyond resistance. Repeat every 6 hours until good results are achieved.[22]

Combining an enema with an oral saline-type cathartic (Lactulose, Cephylac) is helpful when a large amount of stool is present.[1,21] This may help to push the stool through the gastrointestinal tract.

If disimpaction is necessary, remember that it can be extremely painful and to premedicate the patient with either opioid and/or benzodiazepine anxiolytics, to reduce physical and emotional pain.[2,22]

There are few studies outlining the efficacy of one enema over another. The percentage of success for rectal enemas within 1 hour has been reported to include phosphate enemas (100%), mini-enemas (Micralax) (95%), bisacodyl suppositories (66%), and glycerine suppositories (38%).[15] If none of the above enemas is effective, Sykes[7] recommends rectal lavage with approximately 8 liters of warmed normal saline. It is important to remember that if a patient's constipation requires this invasive intervention, once this bowel crisis is resolved you must change the usual bowel regimen. For severe constipation associated with opioids, Levy[1] suggests four Senokot S and three Dulcolax tablets three times a day and 60 ml of lactulose, every other night, for a goal of a bowel movement every other day (Table 11–2).

New Approaches to Constipation Management

Oral naloxone has been studied for the treatment of opioid-related constipation resistant to other treatments. Culpepper-Morgan and colleagues[23] found that the majority of opioid effect on the human intestine is mediated peripherally rather than centrally. Naloxone, which is an opioid antagonist, has a less than 1% availability systemically when given orally, due to the first-pass effect in the liver. Therefore, the risk of causing a withdrawal response when using naloxone orally is small. Although the risk is small, patients who are opioid-dependent must be monitored closely for signs of withdrawal. It has been recommended that the dose start with 5 mg daily and be titrated as a percentage of the current morphine dose. A dose of approximately 20% of the daily morphine dose has been found to be most effective.[15,23] The cost of oral naloxone also prohibits its use beyond rare circumstances. Diarrhea associated with radiation can occur by the second or third week of treatment and continue after radiation has been discontinued.[15]

Oral erythromycin has been shown to cause diarrhea in 50% of patients who use it as an antibiotic.[15] Currently, researchers are investigating its use to promote diarrhea. There is also interest in identifying a medication that would increase colon transit time without being antibacterial.

Many herbal medicines have laxative properties. Some are mulberry and constituents of rhubarb, which are similar to senna. These herbs are being evaluated for use as laxatives. Patients have been known to develop rashes; in one patient, changes were found in warfarin (Coumadin) levels that were related to natural warfarin found in a laxative tea. Many patients prefer these options instead of pharmaceutical laxatives, but patients should be cautious about where they purchase any herbal product and alert to any unexplained side effects as their content is unregulated.

Important Points in Planning Laxative Therapy

Nurses should always be proactive in initiating laxative therapy. Bowel function requires continued evaluation to follow the trajectory of the disease and the changes that occur in normal activities that affect bowel function. Nurses should also be alert to medications that can increase the risk of constipation (Table 11–1). Some patients, especially those on long-term opioid therapy, sometimes need at least two different regimens that can be interchanged when one or the other loses its effectiveness for a time. Like opioids, over time, a standing laxative regimen may be less effective if tolerance develops.[1,15] It is also important to be aware of medication dosing changes as it is common to forget to increase anti-constipation therapy when there is an increase in opioid therapy. Patients generally have increased risk of constipation when opioids are increased. The importance of effective bowel management cannot be stressed enough. It remains the most distressing symptom in end-stage cancer patients.

DIARRHEA

Diarrhea is much less common than constipation in cancer patients.[2] It is a main symptom of 7% to 10% of hospice admissions.[15] Treating diarrhea requires a thorough assessment and therapy directed at the specific cause. Diarrhea is usually acute and short-lived, lasting only a few days, as opposed to chronic diarrhea, which lasts 3 weeks or more.[15] Diarrhea can be especially severe in human immunodeficiency virus (HIV)–infected patients. Forty-three percent of bone marrow transplant patients develop diarrhea related to radiation or graft-versus-host disease (GVHD).[24] Similar to constipation, this symptom can be very debilitating and severely affect quality of life.[25] Diarrhea can prevent patients from leaving their homes, increase weakness and dehydration, and contribute to feelings of lack of control and depression. Nurses can play a significant role in recognizing, educating, and managing diarrhea and its manifestations.

Definitions

Diarrhea is described as an increase in stool volume and liquidity resulting in three or more bowel movements per day.[1] Secondary effects related to diarrhea include abdominal cramps, anxiety, lethargy, weakness, dehydration, dizziness, loss of electrolytes, skin breakdown and associated pain, dry mouth, and weight loss.

Causes of Diarrhea

Cancer patients may have multiple causes of diarrhea. It may be due to infections or related to tumor type or its treatment. A common cause of diarrhea is overuse of laxative therapy or dietary fiber. Additional causes include malabsorption disorders, motility disturbances, stress, partial bowel obstruction, enterocolic fistula, villous adenoma, endocrine-induced hypersecretion of serotonin, gastrin calcitonin, and vasoactive intestinal protein prostaglandins.[1,26,27] Treatment-related causes include radiation and chemotherapy, which cause overgrowth of bacteria with endotoxin production that has a direct effect on the intestinal mucosa. Local inflammation and increased fluid and electrolyte secretion occur, resulting in interference with amino acid and electrolyte transport and a shift toward secretion by crypt cells with shortened villi.[28]

Diarrhea associated with radiation can occur by the second or third week of treatment and continue after radiation has been discontinued.[15] The risk is increased in acquired immunodeficiency syndrome (AIDS), GVHD, or HIV patients.[27,29] The end result could be a change in the intestinal mucosa that results in a limited ability to regenerate epithelium, which can lead to bleeding and ileus. The damaged mucosa leads to increased release of prostaglandins and malabsorption of bile salts, which increase peristaltic activity.[15]

Surgical patients who have had bowel-shortening procedures or gastrectomy related to cancer experience a "dumping syndrome," which causes severe diarrhea. This type of diarrhea is related to both osmotic and hypermotile mechanisms.[1] Patients may experience weakness, epigastric distention, and diarrhea shortly after eating.[32] The shortened bowel can result in a decreased absorption capacity and an imbalance in absorptive and secretory function of the intestine.

Mechanism of Diarrhea

Diarrhea can be grouped into four types, each with a different mechanism: osmotic diarrhea, secretory diarrhea, hypermotile diarrhea, and exudative diarrhea. Cancer patients rarely exhibit only one type. Understanding the mechanism of diarrhea permits more rational treatment strategies.[31]

Osmotic Diarrhea. Osmotic diarrhea is produced by intake of hyperosmolar preparations or non-absorbable solutions like enteral feeding solutions.[31] Enterocolic fistula can lead to both osmotic diarrhea from undigested food entering the colon and hypermotile diarrhea. Hemorrhage into the intestine can cause an osmotic-type diarrhea since intraluminal blood acts as an osmotic laxative. Osmotic diarrhea may result from insufficient lactase when dairy products are consumed.

Secretory Diarrhea. Secretory diarrhea is the most difficult to control. Villous adenoma is a local hypersecreting tumor. Malignant epithelial tumors that produce hormones that can cause diarrhea include metastatic carcinoid tumors, gastrinoma, and medullary thyroid cancer. The primary effect of secretory diarrhea is related to the hypersecretion stimulated by endogenous mediators that affect the intestinal transport of water and electrolytes. This results in accumulation of intestinal fluids.[32] Diarrhea associated with GVHD results from mucosal damage and can produce up to 6–8 liters of diarrhea in 24 hours.[33] Surgical shortening of the bowel leads to diarrhea due to decreased reabsorption by reducing intestinal mucosal contact and shortening colon transit time. Active treatment requires vigorous fluid and electrolyte repletion, antidiarrheal therapy, and specific anticancer therapy.[1]

The somatostatin analogue octreotide is used for severe diarrhea associated with GVHD. In a study done by Ippoliti and Neuman,[33] octreotide was given as 500 mcg IV three times daily for a median of 7 days, and 71% of the patients experienced complete resolution of their diarrhea.[33]

Hypermotile Diarrhea. Partial bowel obstruction from abdominal malignancies can cause a reflex hypermotility that may require bowel-quieting medications like loperamide.[32] Enterocolic fistula can lead to diarrhea from irritative hypermotility and osmotic influence of undigested food entering the colon. Biliary or pancreatic obstruction can cause incomplete digestion of fat in the small intestine, resulting in interference with fat and bile sale malabsorption, leading to hypermotile diarrhea, also called *steatorrhea*. Malabsorption is related to pancreatic cancer, gastrectomy, ileal resection or colectomy, rectal cancer, pancreatic islet cell tumors, or carcinoid tumors.

Chemotherapy-induced diarrhea is frequently seen with 5-fluorouracil or N-phosphonoacetyl-L-aspartate. High-dose cisplatin and irinotecan (Camptosar) cause severe hypermotility. Other chemotherapy drugs that cause diarrhea include cytosine arabinoside, nitrosourea, methotrexate, cyclophosphamide, doxorubicin, daunorubicin, hydroxyurea and biotherapy-2, interferon and topoisomerase inhibitors (CPT-II).

Exudative Diarrhea. Radiation therapy of the abdomen, pelvis, or lower thoracic or lumbar spine can cause acute exudative diarrhea.[28] The inflammation caused by radiation leads to the release of prostaglandins. Treatment using aspirin or ibuprofen was shown to reduce prostaglandin release and decrease diarrhea associated with radiation therapy.[34]

Bismuth subsalicylate (Pepto-Bismol) has also been shown to be helpful for diarrhea caused by radiotherapy.[21]

According to Sykes,[15] there are multiple causes of diarrhea in palliative medicine. Concurrent diseases such as diabetes mellitus, hyperthyroidism, inflammatory bowel disease, irritable bowel syndrome, and gastrointestinal infection (c-dif) can contribute to the development of diarrhea. Finally, the dietary influences of fruit, bran, hot spices, and alcohol as well as of over-the-counter nonsteroidal anti-inflammatory drugs (NSAIDs) and laxatives need to be included as sources of diarrhea.[15]

Diarrhea Assessment

Diarrhea assessment requires a careful history to detail the frequency and nature of the stools. The National Cancer Institute Scale of Severity of Diarrhea uses a grading system from 0 to 4. Stools are rated by (*1*) number of loose stools per day and (2) symptoms (Table 11–3). This scale permits an objective score to define the severity of diarrhea.

The initial goal of assessment is to identify and treat any reversible causes of diarrhea. If diarrhea occurs once or twice a day, it is probably related to anal incontinence. Large amounts of watery stools are characteristic of colonic diarrhea. Pale, fatty, malodorous stools, called steatorrhea, are indicative of malabsorption secondary to pancreatic or small intestinal causes. If a patient complains of sudden diarrhea with little warning and has been constipated, fecal

Table 11–3. National Cancer Institute Scale of Severity of Diarrhea

	National Cancer Institute Grade				
	0	1	2	3	4
Increased number of loose stools/day	Normal	2–3	4–6	7–9	>10
Symptoms		None	Nocturnal stools and/or moderate cramping	Incontinence and/or severe cramping	Grossly bloody diarrhea and/or need for parenteral support

impaction with overflow is the probable etiology.[15]

Evaluate medications that the patient may be taking now or in the recent past. Is the patient on laxatives? If the stools are associated with cramping and urgency, it may be the result of peristalsis-stimulating laxatives. If stools are associated with fecal leakage, it may be the result of overuse of stool-softening agents such as Colace.[15]

Depending on the aggressiveness of the treatment plan, additional assessment could include stool smears for pus, blood, fat, ova, or parasites. Stool samples for culture and sensitivity testing may be necessary to rule out additional sources of diarrhea through *Clostridium difficile* toxin, *Giardia lamblia*, or other types of gastrointestinal infection.[1] If patients experience diarrhea after 2 to 3 days of fasting, secretory diarrhea should be evaluated. Osmotic and secretory causes are considered first; if ruled out, then hypermotility is the suspected mechanism.

Management of Diarrhea

A combination of supportive care and medication may be appropriate for palliative management of diarrhea. If the patient is dehydrated, oral fluids are recommended over the intravenous route.[15] Oral fluids should contain electrolytes and a source of glucose to facilitate active electrolyte transport. Following diarrhea, the diet should start with clear liquids, flat lemonade, ginger ale, and toast or simple carbohydrates. It is recommended that the patient avoid milk if diarrhea is related to infection due to acute lactase deficiency. Protein and fats can be added to the diet slowly as diarrhea resolves.[15]

Recommended Medications. There are many nonspecific diarrhea medications that should be used unless infections are suspected as the cause. Diphenoxylate (Lomotil 2.5 mg with atropine 0.025 mg) is given as one or two tablets orally as needed for loose stools, maximum of eight/day. Diphenoxylate is derived from meperidine and binds to opioid receptors to reduce diarrhea. Atropine was added to this antidiarrheal to prevent abuse.[1] Diphenoxylate is not recommended for patients with advanced liver disease because it may precipitate hepatic coma in patients with cirrhosis. Loperamide (Imodium) has become the drug of choice for the treatment of nonspecific diarrhea. It is a long-acting opioid agonist.[2] The recommended dose is two 2 mg capsules orally as needed for loose bowel movements (maximum of eight/day). The 2 mg dose has the same antidiarrheal action as 5 mg, two tablets of diphenoxylate, or 45 mg of codeine.[1] The usual management of diarrhea begins with 4 mg of loperamide, with one capsule following each loose bowel movement. Most diarrhea is managed by loperamide 2 to 4 mg once to twice a day.[1] Neither diphenoxylate nor loperamide is recommended for use in children under 12 years old.[1] Codeine as an opioid for the reduction of diarrhea can be very helpful. It is also less expensive than some opioid medications. Most cancer-related diarrheas respond well to this drug. For specific mechanisms, other medications might be more beneficial. Anticholinergic drugs like atropine and scopolamine are useful to reduce gastric secretions and decrease peristalsis. Octreotide is also effective for secretory diarrhea that may result from endocrine tumors, AIDS, GVHD, or post gastrointestinal resection.[1,21] They may be helpful for patients who experience painful cramping.[1] Side effects to that class of drug can complicate their use: dry mouth, blurred vision, and urinary hesitancy.

Mucosal antiprostaglandin agents like aspirin, indomethacin, and bismuth subsalicylate (Pepto-Bismol) are useful for diarrhea related to enterotoxic bacteria, radiotherapy, and prostaglandin-secreting tumors. Octreotide (Sandostatin) is especially effective for secretory diarrhea but also for patients with AIDS, GVHD, diabetes, or gastrointestinal resection. Octreotide is administered subcutaneously at a dose of 50 to 200 mg, two or three times per day.[35] Ranitidine is a useful adjuvant to octreotide for patients with Zollinger-Ellison syndrome with gastrin-induced gastric hypersecretion.[1] Side effects include nausea and pain at injection site. Patients may also experience abdominal or headache pain.[1] Clonidine is effective at controlling watery diarrhea in patients with bronchogenic cancer. Clonidine effects an α_2-adrenergic stimulation of electrolyte absorption in the small intestine.[1] Streptozocin is used for watery diarrhea from pancreatic islet cell cancer because it decreases intestinal secretions. Hypermotile diarrhea involves problems with fat absorption. The recommended treatment is pancreatin before meals. Pancreatin is a combination of amylase, lipase, and protease that is available for pancreatic enzyme replacement. Lactaid may also be helpful for malabsorption-related diarrhea.

Managing diarrhea in the cancer patient is challenging at best. The nurse's role in helping the patient and caregivers talk about this difficult symptom is essential (Table 11–4). It is important to respect comfort levels about the topic

Table 11–4. Nursing Role in the Management of Diarrhea

Environmental assessment

- Assess the patient's and/or caregiver's ability to manage the level of care necessary.
- Evaluate home for medical equipment that may be helpful (bedpan or commode chair).

History

- Frequency of bowel movements in last 2 weeks
- Fluid intake (normal 2 quarts/day)
- Fiber intake (normal 30–40 g/day)
- Appetite and whether patient is nauseated or vomiting. Does diet include spicy foods?
- Does patient complain of pain or abdominal cramping?
- Assess for current medications the patient has taken that are associated with causing diarrhea (laxative use, chemotherapy, antibiotics, enteral nutritional supplements, nonsteroidal anti-inflammatory drugs).
- Surgical history that may contribute to diarrhea (gastrectomy, pancreatectomy, bypass or ileal resection)
- Recent radiotherapy to abdomen, pelvis, lower spine
- Cancer diagnosis associated with diarrhea includes abdominal malignancies, partial bowel obstruction; enterocolic fistulae; metastatic carcinoid tumors; gastrinomas; medullary thyroid cancer
- Immunosuppressed, susceptible to bacterial, protozoan, and viral diseases associated with diarrhea
- Concurrent diseases associated with diarrhea: gastroenteritis, inflammatory bowel disease, irritable bowel syndrome, diabetes mellitus, lactose deficiency, hyperthyroidism

Physical assessment

- Examine perineum or ostomy site for skin breakdown, fissures, or external hemorrhoids.
- Gentle digital rectal exam for impaction
- Abdominal exam for distention or palpable stool in large bowel
- Examine stools for signs of bleeding.
- Evaluate for signs of dehydration.

Interventions

- Treatment should be related to cause; i.e., if obstruction is cause of diarrhea, giving antidiarrheal medications would be inappropriate.
- Assist with correcting any obvious factors related to assessment, e.g., decreasing nutritional supplements, changing fiber intake, holding or substituting medications associated with diarrhea.
- If bacterial causes are suspected, notify physician and culture stools as instructed. *Clostridium difficile* is most common.
- Educate patient and family on importance of cleansing the perineum gently after each stool, to prevent skin breakdown. If patient has a colostomy, stomal area must also be watched closely and surrounding skin protected. Use skin barrier like Desitin ointment to protect the skin. Frequent sitz baths may be helpful.
- Instruct patient and family on signs and symptoms that should be reported to the nurse or physician: excessive thirst, dizziness, fever, palpitations, rectal spasms, excessive cramping, watery or bloody stools.

Dietary measures

- Eat small, frequent, bland meals
- Low residue diet—potassium-rich (bananas, rice, apples (peeled), dry toast
- Avoid intake of hyperosmotic supplements (e.g. Ensure, Sustacal)
- Increase fluids in diet. Approximately 3 liters of fluid a day if possible. Drinking elecrolyte fluids like Pedialyte may be helpful.
- Homeopathic treatments for diarrhea include: ginger tea, glutamine, and peeled apples

Pharmacologic management

- Opioids - Codiene, paregoric, dihenoxylate, loperamide, tincture of opium
- Absorbents - Pectin, aluminum hydroxide
- Adsorbents - Charcoal, kaolin
- Antisecretory - Aspirin, Bismuth subsalicylate, prednisone, Sandostatin, ranitidine hydrochloride, indomethacin,
- Anticholinergics-Scopolamine, atropine sulfate, belladonna
- A2 - adrenergic agonists - Clonidine

Report to nurse or physician if antidiarrheal medication seems ineffective

(continued)

Table 11–4. Nursing Role in the Management of Diarrhea (*Continued*)

Psychosocial interventions

- Provide support to patient and family. Recognize negative effects of diarrhea on quality of life.
- Fatigue
- Malnutrition
- Alteration in skin integrity
- Pain and discomfort
- Sleep disturbances
- Limited ability to travel
- Compromised role within the family
- Decreased sexual activity
- Caregiver burden

Source: Levy (1991), reference 1; Bisanz (1997), reference 21; Hogan (1998), reference 25.

between nurse, patient, and caregiver, to allow information sharing. Goals of diarrhea therapy should be to restore an optimal pattern of elimination, maintain fluid and electrolyte balance, preserve nutritional status, protect skin integrity, and patient's comfort and dignity.[21,32]

MALIGNANT OBSTRUCTION

Definition and Pathophysiology

Intestinal obstruction is occlusion of the lumen or absence of the normal propulsion which affects elimination from the gastrointestinal tract.[16] As primary tumors grow in the large intestine, they can lead to obstruction. Obstruction is related to the site of disease. Tumors in the splenic flexure obstruct 49% of the time but those in the rectum or rectosigmoid junction, only 6% of the time.[36] Obstruction can occur intraluminally related to primary tumors of the colon. Intramural obstruction is related to tumor in the muscular layers of the bowel wall. The bowel appears thickened, indurated, and contracted.[15] Extramural obstruction is related to mesenteric and omental masses and malignant adhesions. The common metastatic pattern in relation to primary disease in the pancreas or stomach in general goes to the duodenum, from the colon to the jejunum and ileum, and from the prostate or bladder to the rectum.[15]

Motility disruption, either impaired or absent, leads to a mechanical obstruction but without occlusion of the intestinal lumen. Mechanical obstruction results in the accumulation of fluids and gas proximal to the obstruction. Distention occurs as a result of intestinal gas, ingested fluids, and digestive secretions. It becomes a self-perpetuating phenomenon as when distention increases, intestinal secretion of water and electrolytes increases. A small bowel obstruction causes large amounts of diarrhea. The increased fluid in the bowel leads to increased peristalsis with large quantities of bacteria growing in the intestinal fluid of the small bowel.[37]

Obstruction is related to the surrounding mesentery or bowel muscle, such as in ovarian cancer. Lung cancer patients may experience a pseudo-obstruction as a result of paraneoplastic neuropathy.[38] Additional factors include multiple sites of obstruction along the intestine to constipating medications (Table 11–4), fecal impaction, fibrosis, or change in normal flora of the bowel. The goal of treatment is to prevent obstruction from happening whenever possible.

History of the Problem

Treatment of bowel obstruction in a patient with advanced cancer remains undetermined.[39–45] The difficulty is knowing which patients will truly benefit from surgical intervention. Jong and colleagues[45] found, in a retrospective study, that palliative surgery for bowel obstruction in advanced ovarian cancer achieved successful alleviation, defined as patient survival longer than 60 days after surgery, ability to return home, and relief of bowel obstruction for longer than 60 days. Past studies associated with ovarian or abdominal cancers found survival rates in general to be less than 6 months.[40,42,43] In patients for whom a definitive procedure could take place, such as a resection, bypass, colostomy, or ileostomy, the mean survival was 6 months. For these patients, who were not surgical candidates, the mean survival rate was 1.8 months. Progressive cancer was the cause of obstruction in 86% of patients.[42] There was a postoperative complication rate of 49%, which included wound infection, enterocutaneous fistulae, and other septic sequelae. Median postoperative survival was 140 days. In general, the operative mortality rate for this group was 12% to 25%.[42]

Further research needs to be done similar to that of Jong and colleagues,[45] who evaluated the effects of surgical intervention on quality as well as quantity of life. The result of unrelieved intestinal obstruction, for the patient and loved ones, on quality of life is devastating.

Assessment and Management

Patients may experience severe nausea, vomiting, and abdominal pain associated with a partial or complete bowel obstruction. General signs and symptoms associated with different sites of obstruction are listed in Table 11–5. Providing thoughtful and supportive interventions may be more appropriate than aggressive, invasive procedures. The

Table 11–5. Sites of Intestinal Obstruction and Related Side Effects

Site	Side Effects
Duodenum	Severe vomiting with large amounts of undigested food. Bowel sounds : succussion splash may be present. No pain or distension noted.
Small Intestine	Moderate to severe vomiting; usually hyperactive bowel sounds with borborygmi; pain in upper and central abdomen, colic in nature; moderate distension.
Large intestine	Vomiting is a late side effect. Borborygmi bowel sounds, severe distension. Pain central to lower abdomen, colic in nature.

Source: Baines (1998), reference 16.

signs and symptoms of obstruction may be acute with nausea, vomiting, and abdominal pain. A majority of the time, however, obstruction is a slow and insidious phenomenon, which may progress from partial to complete obstruction. Palliative care should allow for a thoughtful and realistic approach to management of obstruction within the goals of care. Radiologic examination should be limited unless surgery is being considered. Putting a patient through an x-ray of the abdomen may be helpful, to confirm the obstruction and identify where it is, but defining the goal of therapy is essential. When patients exhibit signs of obstruction, a physical exam may be helpful to assess the extent of the problem. Asking the patient for a bowel history, last bowel movement, and a description of consistency can be helpful. Does the patient complain of constipation? Physical examination should include gentle palpation of the abdomen for masses or distention. A careful rectal exam can identify the presence of stool in the rectum or a distended empty rectum. An empty, or "ballooned," rectum may be a symptom of high obstruction. It is also difficult to distinguish stool from malignant mass.[16,21] The ability to assess whether an impaction is low or high in the intestinal tract is important to help guide the intervention planning. As discussed above, lack of stool noted in the rectum during a digital exam is usually indicative of a high impaction. Stool has not or cannot move down into the rectum. The goal then would be to use careful assessment to be sure the obstruction is not a tumor and to concentrate on softening the stool and moving it through the gastrointestinal tract. Again, using a stimulant laxative for this type of patient would result in increasing discomfort and possible rupture of the intestinal wall.[16,21] Low impactions are uncomfortable, and patients may need more comforting measures. Patients may need to lay down to decrease pressure on the rectal area and avoid drinking hot liquids or eating big meals, which may increase peristalsis and discomfort until the impaction can be cleared.[21]

Radiological Examination. Barium enemas may be necessary to identify the cause of the obstruction. In patients whose prognosis is greater than 3 months, extensive testing for possible surgical intervention may be justified.[15]

Surgical Intervention. A percentage of cancer patients may experience nonmalignant obstruction.[41,44] Therefore, assuming the obstruction is related to worsening cancer may prevent the health care team from setting realistic treatment goals. A thorough assessment should be done, with attention to poor prognostic factors.[16,45] These factors historically include general medical condition or poor nutritional status, ascites, palpable abdominal masses or distant metastases, previous radiation to the abdomen or pelvis, combination chemotherapy, and multiple small bowel obstructions.[40,44,46]

A study on the palliative benefit of surgery for bowel obstruction in advanced ovarian cancer found that surgical intervention provided successful palliation in 51% of the patients studied.[45] Four prognostic factors for the probable success of palliative surgery were found: *(1)* absence of palpable abdominal or pelvic masses, *(2)* volume of ascites less than 3 liters, *(3)* unifocal obstruction, and *(4)* preoperative weight loss less than 9 kg. Sixty-eight percent of the patients survived longer than 60 days and recovered enough to be able to return home.[45]

Surgical interventions can involve resection and reanastomosis, decompression, either colostomy or ileostomy, gastroenterostomy or ileotransverse colostomy, or lysis of adhesions.[16] Prospective trials need to be done to further assess the success of surgical interventions and their effect on the quality as well as the quantity of life.[45]

Surgical intervention should be a decision made between patient and physician within the established goals of care. The patients' right to self-determine their paths is essential. As patient advocates, our role is to educate the patient and family. Helping them to understand physician recommendations as well as their personal desires and options in an effort to develop their treatment plan is essential. Surgical resection for obstructing cancers of the gastrointestinal tract, pancreatic, or biliary tracts was found to have a 3- to 7-month survival.[44] This study pointed out the importance of nutritional status at baseline and assessing performance status for its relationship to "reasonable quality of life."[44] The important conclusion of these studies was to leave the decision to operate with the patient. Mortality is possible. The need for additional surgeries remains high due to recurrence of the obstruction. Survival rates with each subsequent surgery lessen.[39]

Alternative Interventions. Nasogastric or nasointestinal tubes have been used to decompress the bowel and/or stomach. Use of these interventions, although uncomfortable for the patient, has been suggested for symptom relief while evaluating the possibility of surgery. Venting gastrostomy or jejunostomy can be a relatively easy alternative, which is especially effective for severe nausea and vomiting. It can be placed percutaneously with sedation and local anesthesia. Patients can then be fed a liquid diet with the tube clamped for as long as tolerated without nausea or vomiting.[16,47]

Symptom Therapy. Providing aggressive pharmacologic management of the distressing symptoms associated with malignant bowel obstruction (MBO) can prevent the need for surgical intervention.[15,37,48–50,53] The symptoms intestinal colic, vomiting, and diarrhea can be effectively controlled with medications for most patients.

Depending on the location of the obstruction, either high or low, symptom severity can be affected. As accumulation of secretions increase, abdominal pain also increases. Distention, vomiting, and prolonged constipation occur. With high obstruction, onset of vomiting is sooner and amounts are larger. Intermittent borborygmi and visible peristalsis may occur.[37] Patients may experience colic pain on top of continuous pain from a growing mass. In chronic bowel obstruction, colic pain subsides. As stated above, the goal of treatment is to prevent obstruction whenever possible. The use of subcutaneous (SQ) or intravenous (IV) analgesics, anticholinergic drugs, and antiemetic drugs can be effective for reducing the symptoms of inoperable and hard-to-manage obstruction.[49] Octreotide may be an option in early management to prevent partial obstructions from becoming complete.[37] Although octreotide is used for diarrhea because it decreases peristalsis, it also slows the irregular and ineffective peristaltic movements of obstruction, reducing the activity and balancing out the intestinal movement.[37] It reduces vomiting because it inhibits the secretion of gastrin, secretin, vasoactive intestinal peptide, pancreatic polypeptide, insulin, and glucagon. Octreotide directly blocks the secretion of gastric acid, pepsin, pancreatic enzyme, bicarbonate, intestinal epithelial electrolytes, and water.[49] It has been shown to be effective in 70% of patients for the control of vomiting.[15] Octreotide is administered by SQ infusion or SQ injection every 12 hours. A negative aspect of this drug is its cost. It is expensive and requires SQ injections or IV infusion over days to weeks. The recommended starting dose is 0.3 mg/day and may increase to 0.6 mg/day.[15] Hyoscine butylbromide is thought to be as effective as octreotide at reducing gastrointestinal secretions and motility. Hyoscine butylbromide is less sedating since it is thought to cross the blood–brain barrier less due to its low lipid solubility.[50] A recent study compared octreotide and scopolamine butylbromide for inoperable bowel obstruction with nasogastric tubes.[52] Both medications relieve colicky pain; both reduce the continuous abdominal pain and distention. Although this was a small study done over 3 days, they were able to remove the nasogastric tube in 3 of the 7 patients on the first dose of octreotide 0.3 mg/day subcutaneously; 3 more patients were able to have the nasogastric tube removed when the dose was doubled to 0.6 mg/day. Scopolamine was similar in results, but the octreotide arm was felt to be overall more effective. The negative effect is associated with the cost of drug; a definite consideration for overall quality of life. Scopolamine is less expensive at approximately $1.35US for 60 mg versus octreotide at $37.73US for 0.3 mg.

Analgesic Medication. Opioid medications have been used to relieve pain associated with obstruction.[15] Providing the opioid through SQ infusion via a patient-controlled analgesic (PCA) pump is beneficial for two reasons: patients may receive improved pain relief over the oral route due to improved absorption and giving access to a PCA pump allows patients some control over their pain management. Alternative routes of opioid administration, like rectal or transdermal, may also be effective but usually are inadequate if the pain is severe or unstable or there are frequent episodes of breakthrough pain.

Antiemetic Medications. Some antiemetic medications can be given SQ as well and combined with an opioid.[15] Haloperidol (Haldol) is the classic first-line antiemetic.[48] Phenothiazine, butyrophenone, and antihistamine antiemetics are the most helpful. Recent additions of the selective serotonin antagonists, the 5-hydroxytryptamine blockers (5-HT3), have made a significant difference in the treatment of nausea, especially when combined with corticosteroids for chemotherapy-induced nausea.[51] (See also Chapter 9.) Metoclopramide at 10 mg q 4 hours is the drug of choice for patients with incomplete bowel obstruction.[48] It stimulates the stomach to empty its contents into the reservoir of the bowel. Once complete obstruction is present, metoclopramide is discontinued and haloperidol or another antiemetic medication is started. Haloperidol is less sedating than other antiemetic or antihistamine medications.[16,48] The dose ranges from 5 to 15 mg/day, and at some institutions, it is combined with cyclizine.[16] Corticosteroids are particularly helpful antiemetics, especially when related to chemotherapy.[48]

In practice, it is recommended that morphine, haloperidol, and hyoscine butylbromide be given together by continuous SQ infusion. If pain or colic increases, the dose of morphine and hyoscine butylbromide should be increased; if emesis increases, increase the haloperidol dose.[16]

Fluid and nutrient intake should be maintained as tolerated. Usually, patients whose vomiting has improved will tolerate fluids with small, low-residue meals. Dry mouth is managed with ice chips, although this has been suspected to wash out saliva that is present in the mouth. The use of artificial saliva may be more beneficial.[16]

Corticosteroid Medications. Corticosteroids have been helpful as antiemetic medications. The recommended dose of dexamethasone is between 8 and 20 mg/day; the prednisolone dose starts at 50 mg/day (injection or SQ infusion).[16] Twycross and Lack[2] recommend starting with 4 mg bid for 5 days, then decreasing to 4 mg daily. One possible side effect to this medication is oral candidiasis.[48]

Antispasmodic Medications. Colic pain results from increased peristalsis against the resistance of a mechanical obstruction. Analgesics alone may not be effective. Hyoscine butylbromide has been used to relieve spasm-like pain and to reduce emesis.[16] Dosing starts at 60 mg/day and increases up to 380 mg/day given by SQ infusion.[50] Side effects are related to the anticholinergic effects, including tachycardia, dry mouth, sedation, and hypotension.[50]

Laxative Medications. Stimulant laxatives are contraindicated due to increased peristalsis against an obstruction. Stool-softening medications may be helpful if there is only a single obstruction in the colon or rectum. If the obstruction is in the small bowel, laxatives will not be of benefit.[16]

Antidiarrheal Medications. Patients who experience a subacute obstruction or a fecal fistula may complain of diarrhea. Antidiarrheal medicine, like codeine or loperamide, may be helpful. The benefit of these medications is that they may also help to relieve pain and colic.

Helping families cope with symptoms associated with obstruction is important. Historically, the management of obstruction involved aggressive surgical intervention or symptom management alone. The initial assessment should include: *(1)* evaluating constipation; *(2)* evaluating for surgery; *(3)* providing pain management; and *(4)* managing nausea with metoclopramide if incomplete obstruction, dexamethasone, haloperidol, dimenhydrinate, chlorpromazine, or hyoscine butylbromide.[48] The introduction of new medications, like octreotide, and newer antiemetics has made a difference in the quality of life a patient with a malignant bowel obstruction may experience. The important thing to remember is that the treatment plan must always be in agreement with the patient's wishes. Discussing the patient's understanding of the situation and the options available are essential to effective and thoughtful care of bowel obstruction in the palliative care patient.

ASCITES

Ascites associated with malignancy results from a combination of impaired fluid efflux and increased fluid influx.[54] Ascites may be divided into three different types. Central ascites is the result of tumor invading hepatic parenchyma, resulting in compression of the portal venous and/or the lymphatic system.[55] There is a decrease in oncotic pressure as a result of limited protein intake and the catabolic state associated with cancer.[55] Peripheral ascites is related to deposits of tumor cells found on the surface of the parietal or visceral peritoneum. The result is a mechanical interference with venous and/or lymphatic drainage.[55] There is blockage at the level of the peritoneal space rather than the liver parenchyma. Macrophages increase capillary permeability and contribute to greater ascites. Mixed-type ascites is a combination of central and peripheral ascites. Therefore, there is both compression of the portal venous and lymphatic systems, as well as tumor cells in the peritoneum. Chylous malignant ascites occurs when tumor infiltration of the retroperitoneal space causes obstruction of lymph flow through the lymph nodes and/or the pancreas.[55] Additional sources of ascites not related to malignancy include the following:

- Preexisting advanced liver disease with portal hypertension
- Portal venous thrombosis
- Congestive heart failure
- Nephrotic syndrome
- Pancreatitis
- Tuberculosis
- Hepatic venous obstruction
- Bowel perforation

Severe ascites is associated with poor prognosis (40% 1-year survival, less than 10% 3-year survival).[55] The pathological mechanisms of malignant ascites make the prevention or reduction of abdominal fluid accumulation difficult.[56] Invasive management of ascites is seen as appropriate whenever possible, in contrast to intestinal obstruction. Although survival is limited, the effects of ascites on the patient's quality of life warrant an aggressive approach.[56]

Tumor types most associated with ascites include ovarian, endometrial, breast, colon, gastric, and pancreatic cancers.[55,56] Less common sources of ascites include mesothelioma, non-Hodgkin's lymphoma, prostate cancer, multiple myeloma, and melanoma.[55]

Symptoms Associated With Ascites

Patients complain of abdominal bloating and pain. Initially, patients complain of feeling a need for larger-waisted clothing and notice an increase in belt size or weight. They may feel nauseated and have a decreased appetite. Many patients will complain of increased symptoms of reflux or heartburn. Pronounced ascites can cause dyspnea and orthopnea due to increased pressure on the diaphragm.[55,56]

Physical Examination

The physical examination may reveal abdominal or inguinal hernia, scrotal edema, and abdominal venous engorgement. Radiologic findings show a hazy picture, with distended and separate loops of the bowel. There is a poor definition of the abdominal organs and loss of the psoas muscle shadows. Ultrasound and computed tomographic scans may also be used to diagnose ascites.[55]

Treatment

Traditionally, treatment of ascites is palliative due to decreased prognosis.[55,57] Ovarian cancer is one of the few types where the presence of ascites does not necessarily correlate with a poor prognosis. In this case, survival rate can be improved through surgical intervention and adjuvant therapy.[56]

Medical Therapy. Advanced liver disease is associated with central ascites. There is an increase in renal sodium and water retention. Therefore, restricting sodium intake to 100 mmol/day or less along with fluid restriction for patients with moderate to severe hyponatremia (125 mmol/l) may be beneficial. Using potassium-sparing diuretics is also important. Spironolactone (100 to 400 mg/day) is the drug of choice.[55,58] Furosemide is also helpful at 40 to 80 mg/day to initiate diuresis. Over-diuresis must be avoided. Over-diuresis may precipitate electrolyte imbalance, hepatic encephalopathy, and prerenal failure. The above regimen of fluid and sodium reduction and diuretics may work for mixed-type ascites, which results from compression of vessels related to tumor and peripheral tumor cells of the parietal or visceral peritoneum as well. Because mixed-type ascites is associated with chylous fluid, adding changes to the diet, such as decreased fat intake and increased medium-chain triglycerides, may be important. Chylous ascites results from tumor infiltration of the retroperitoneal space, causing obstruction of lymphatic flow.[55]

Medium-chain triglyceride oil (Lipisorb) can be used as a calorie source in these patients. Because the lymph system is bypassed, the shorter fatty acid chains are easier to digest. For patients with refractory ascites and a shortened life expectancy, paracentesis may be the most appropriate therapy.[59]

Paracentesis. Paracentesis for tense ascites associated with cirrhosis or nonmalignant ascites has been shown to shorten hospitalization by 60%.[55] Multiple studies have found that removing 4–6 liters/day was a safe and effective treatment.[61–63] This treatment has been altered to include albumin infusions, which prevent hypovolemia and renal impairment, as well as hyponatremia.[55,63]

It is recommended that a maximum of 6 liters of ascites fluid be taken off. In a study examining the risks of paracentesis, a mean volume of 4.8 liters was removed without any sign of hypovolemia.[67] This can be a very safe and effective way to promptly relieve patients of discomfort associated with ascites and to improve quality of life.[54,55,64,65]

Peritoneovenous shunts (Denver or LeVeen shunt) can be helpful for the removal of ascites in 75% to 85% of patients.[55] These shunts are used primarily for nonmalignant ascites. The shunt removes fluid from the site, and the fluid is shunted up into the internal jugular vein.[55] This procedure is not done for malignant ascites because malignant cells can be dumped into the circulation, and malignant ascites has shown less improvement with such shunts.[66]

Past interventions for the relief of ascites have included surgery aimed at increasing absorption capacity. In one study, no patient survived beyond 30 postoperative days.[67] Pharmacological attempts to relieve ascites have also been disappointing. Radioactive isotopes were given to decrease production of ascitic fluid. Unfortunately, the side effects presented greater problems (nausea, pain, fever, and bone marrow suppression). The costs of those interventions were also prohibitive. A newer treatment is evolving using intraperitoneal α-interferon for malignant ascites.[68] Controlled research is in progress.

Ascites management involves understanding the mechanism initially, then using interventions appropriately. The reality of recurring ascites requiring repeated paracentesis is present. Acknowledging the risk/benefit ratio of repeated paracentesis is essential, especially in palliative care. Nurses need to remember good supportive care in addition to other resources, including skin care, to help prevent breakdown, and comfort interventions like pillow support, and loose clothing whenever possible. Educating the patient and caregivers on the rationale behind fluid and sodium restrictions when necessary can help understanding and compliance. The cycle of a patient who feels thirsty, receives IV fluids, and has more discomfort is difficult for the patient to understand. Careful explanations about why an intervention is or is not recommended can go a long way toward improving the quality of life for these patients.

REFERENCES

1. Levy MH. Constipation and diarrhea in cancer patients. Cancer Bull 1991;43:412–422.

2. Twycross RG, Lack SA. Diarrhea. In: Control of Alimentary Symptoms in Far Advanced Cancer. New York: Churchill Livingstone, 1986: 208–229.

3. Agency for Health Care Policy and Research. In: Management of Cancer Pain (AHCPR Guidelines), AHCPR Publication 94-0592. Washington DC: US Department of Health and Human Services, 1994.

4. Devroede G. Constipation. In: Sleisenger MH, Fordtran JS, eds. Gastrointestinal Disease. Philadelphia: WB Saunders, 1989:331–381.

5. Connell AM, Hilton C, Irvin EG, Lennard-Jones JE, Misiewicz JJ. Variation in bowel habit in two population samples. BMJ 1965;2:1095–1099.

6. Sykes NP. A clinical comparison of laxatives in a hospice. Palliat Med 1991;5:307–314.

7. Sykes NP. A volunteer model for the comparison of laxatives in opioid-related constipation. J Pain Symptom Manage 1996;11:363–369.

8. Cimprich B. Symptom management: constipation. Cancer Nurs 1985;8(Suppl 1):39–43.

9. Holdstock DJ, Misiewicz JJ, Smith T, Rowlands EN. Propulsion (mass movements) in the human colon and its relationship to meals and somatic activity. Gut 1970;11:91–99.

10. Kavanagh JJ, Copeland LJ, Gershenson DM. Continuous-infusion vinblastine in refractory carcinoma of the cervix: a phase II trial. Gynecol Oncol 1985;21:211–214.

11. McMillan SC. Assessing and managing narcotic-induced constipation in adults with cancer. Cancer Control. Moffitt Cancer Ctr 1999; 6:198–204.

12. McMillan SC, Williams FA. Validity and reliability of the constipation assessment scale. Cancer Nurs 1989;12:183–188.

13. Maguire LC, Yon JL, Miller E. Prevention of narcotic induced constipation. N Engl J Med 1981;305:1651–1652.

14. Adler HF, Atkinson AJ, Ivy AC. Effect of morphine and Dilaudid on the ileum and of morphine, Dilaudid and atropine on the colon of man. Arch Intern Med 1942;69:974–985.

15. Sykes NP. Constipation and diarrhea. In: Doyle D, Hanks GWC, MacDonald N, eds. Oxford Textbook of Palliative Medicine, Vol 2. New York: Oxford University Press, 1998:513–526.

16. Baines MJ. The pathophysiology and management of malignant intestinal obstruction. In: Doyle D, Hanks GWC, MacDonald N, eds. Oxford Textbook of Palliative Medicine, Vol 2. New York: Oxford University Press, 1998:526–534.

17. Levy MH. Pharmacologic treatment of cancer pain. N Engl J Med 1996;335:1124–1132.

18. Lederle FA, Busch DL, Mattox KM, West MJ, Aske DM. Cost-effective treatment of constipation in the elderly: a randomized double-blind comparison of sorbitol and lactulose. Am J Med 1990;89:597–601.

19. Mandel L, Silinsky J. Bisacodyl (Dulcolax) an evacuant suppository: a controlled therapeutic trial in chronically ill and geriatric patients. Can Med Assoc J 1960;83:384–387.

20. Sweeney WJ, Hewett R, Riddell P, Hoffman DC. Rectal gangrene: a complication of phosphate enema. Med J Austr 1986;144:374–375.

21. Bisanz A. Managing bowel elimination problems in patients with cancer. Oncol Nurs Forum 1997;24:679–688.

22. Walsh TD. Constipation. In: Walsh TD, ed. Symptom Control. Cambridge, MA: Blackwell Scientific, 1989:69–80.

23. Culpepper-Morgan JA, Inturrisi CE, Portenoy RK, et al. Treatment of opioid-induced constipation with oral naloxone: a pilot study. Clin Pharmacol Ther 1992;52:90–95.

24. Cox GJ, Matsui S, Kim RS, et al. Etiology and outcome of diarrhea after marrow transplantation: a prospective study. Gastroenterology 1994;107:1398–1407.

25. Hogan CM. The nurse's role in diarrhea management. Oncol Nurs Forum 1998;25:879–886.

26. Doughty D. Maintaining normal bowel function in the patient with cancer. J Enterostomal Nursing 1991;18:90–94.

27. Mercadante S. Diarrhea in terminally ill patients: pathophysiology and treatment. J Pain Symptom Manage 1995;10:298–308.

28. Cascinu S. Drug therapy in diarrheal diseases in oncology/hematology patients. Crit Rev Oncol Hematol 1995;18:37–50.

29. Cello JP, Grendell JH, Basuk P, et al. Effect of octreotide on refractory AIDS-associated diarrhea: a prospective, multicenter clinical trial. Ann Intern Med 1991;115:705–710.

30. Farthing MJG. Octreotide in dumping and short bowel syndromes. Digestion 1993;54 (Suppl 1):47–52.

31. Engelking C, Rutledge DN, Ipoliti C, Neumann J, Hogan CM. Cancer-related diarrhea: a neglected cause of cancer-related symptom distress. Oncol Nurs Forum 1998;25:859–860.

32. Rutledge DN, Engelking C. Cancer-related diarrhea: selected findings of a national survey of oncology nurse experiences. Oncol Nurs Forum 1998;25:861–872.

33. Ippoliti C, Neumann J. Octreotide in the management of diarrhea induced by graft versus host disease. Oncol Nurs Forum 1998;25:873–878.

34. Mennie AJ, Dalley V, Dinneen L, Collier H. Aspirin in radiation induced diarrhoea. Lancet 1973;1:1303–1311.

35. Gordon P, Comi RJ, Maton PN, Go VL. NIH conference: somatostatin analogue (SMS 201-995) in treatment of hormone-secreting tumors of the pituitary and gastrointestinal tract and non-neoplastic diseases of the gut. Ann Intern Med 1989;110:35–50.

36. Phillips RKS, Hittinger R, Fry JS, Fielding LP. Malignant large bowel obstruction. Br J Surg 1985;72:296–302.

37. Mercadante S, Kargar J, Nicolosi G. Octreotide may prevent definitive intestinal obstruction. J Pain Symptom Manage 1997;13:352–355.

38. Schuffler MD, Baird HW, Flemming CR. Intestinal pseudo-obstruction as the presenting manifestation of small-cell carcinoma of the lung. Ann Intern Med 1983;98:129–134.

39. Ketcham AS, Hoye RC, Pilch YH, Morton DL. Delayed intestinal obstruction following treatment for cancer. Cancer 1969;25:406–410.

40. Gallick HL, Weaver DW, Sachs RJ, Bouwman DL. Intestinal obstruction in cancer patients: an assessment of risk factors and outcome. Am Surg 1985;52:434–437.

41. Walsh HPJ, Schofield PF. Is laparotomy for small bowel obstruction justified in patients with previously treated malignancy. Br J Surg 1984;71:933–935.

42. Clarke-Pearson DL, Chin NO, DeLong ER, Rice R, Creasman WT. Surgical management of intestinal obstruction in ovarian cancer. Gynecol Oncol 1987;26:11–18.

43. Rubin SC, Hoskins WJ, Benjamin I, Lewis JL. Palliative surgery for intestinal obstruction in advanced ovarian cancer. Gynecol Oncol 1988;34:16–19.

44. Turnbull ADM, Guerra J, Starnes HF. Results of surgery for obstructing carcinomatosis of gastrointestinal, pancreatic, or biliary origin. J Clin Oncol 1989;7:381–386.

45. Jong P, Sturgeon J, Jamieson CG. Benefit of palliative surgery for bowel obstruction in advanced ovarian cancer. J Crit Care 1995;38(5): 454–457.

46. Krebs JB, Goplerud DR. Surgical management of bowel obstruction in advanced ovarian carcinoma. Obstet Gynecol 1983;61:327–330.

47. McCarthy D. Strategy for intestinal obstruction in peritoneal carcinomatosis. Arch Surg 1986;121:1081–1082.

48. Fainsinger RL, Spachynski K, Hanson J, Bruera E. Symptom control in terminally ill patients with malignant bowel obstruction. J Pain Symptom Manage 1994;9:12–18.

49. Mercadante S, Maddaloni S. Octreotide in the management of inoperable gastrointestinal obstruction in terminal cancer patients. J Pain Symptom Manage 1992;7:496–498.

50. DeConno F, Caraceni A, Zecca E, Spoldi E, Ventafridda V. Continuous subcutaneous infusion of hyoscine butylbromide reduces secretions in patients with gastrointestinal obstruction. J Pain Symptom Manage 1991;6:484–486.

51. Osoba D, MacDonald N. Principles governing the use of of cancer chemotherapy in palliative care: In *Oxford Textbook of Palliative Medicine*, Doyle D, Hanks G, MacDonald N, eds. Vol. 2. Oxford: Oxford University Press, 1998: 249–267.

52. Ripamont C, Mercadante S, Groff L, Zecca E, DeConno F, Casuccio A. Role of Octreotide, Scopolamine Butylbromide, and hydration in symptom control of patients with inoperable bowel obstruction and nasogastric tubes: A prospective randomization trial (2000). J Pain Symptom Manage 19(1):23–34.

53. Baines M, Carter RL, Oliver DJ. Medical management of intestinal obstruction in patients with advanced malignant disease. Lancet 1985;2: 990–993.

54. Lee CW, Bociek G, Faught W. A survey of practice in management of malignant ascites. J Pain Symptom Manage 1998;16:96–101.

55. Bain VG. Jaundice, ascites, and hepatic encephalopathy. In: Doyle D, Hanks GWC, MacDonald N, eds. Oxford Textbook of Palliative Medicine, Vol 2. Oxford: Oxford University Press, 1998:557–571.

56. Mercadante S, La Rosa S, Nicolosi G, Garofalo SL. Temporary drainage of symptomatic malignant ascites by a catheter inserted under computerized tomography. J Pain Symptom Manage 1998;15:374–378.

57. Garrison RN, Kaelin LD, Galloway RH, Heuser LS. Malignant ascites: clinical and experimental observations. Ann Surg 1986;203:644–651.

58. Pockros PJ, Esrason KT, Nguyen C, Duque J, Woods S. Mobilization of malignant ascites with diuretics is dependent on ascitic fluid characteristics. Gastroenterology 1992;103:1302–1306.

59. Abrahm J. Promoting symptom control in palliative care. Semin Oncol Nurs 1998;14:95–109.

60. Tito L, Gines P, Arroyo V, et al. Total paracentesis associated with intravenous albumin management of patients with cirrhosis and ascites. Gastroenterology 1990;98:146–151.

61. Runyon B. Paracentesis of ascitic fluid: a safe procedure. Arch Intern Med 1986;146:2259–2261.

62. Panos M, Moore K, Vlavianos P, et al. Single, total paracentesis for tense ascites: sequential hemodynamic changes and right atrial size. Hepatology 1990;11:662–667.

63. Gotlieb WH, Feldman B, Feldman-Moran O, et al. Intraperitoneal pressures and clinical parameters of total paracentesis for palliation of symptomatic ascites in ovarian cancer. Gynecol Oncol 1998;71:381–385.

64. Rose PG, Basile V. Palliative sclerosis of intra-abdominal cystic ovarian or peritoneal carcinoma. Gynecol Oncol 1999;72:256–260.

65. Gough IR, Balderson GA. Malignant ascites: a comparison of peritoneovenous shunting and non-operative management. Cancer 1993; 71:2377–2382.

66. Chu DZ, Lang NP, Thompson C, Osteen PK, Westbrook KC. Peritoneal carcinomatosis in nongynecologic malignancy. A prospective study of prognostic factors. Cancer 1989;63: 364–367.

67. Rath U, Kaufmann M, Schmid H, et al. Effect of intraperitoneal recombinant human tumor necrosis factor alpha on malignant ascites. Eur J Cancer 1991;27:121–125.

68. Sykes N. A Volunteer model for the comparison of laxatives in opioid-related constipation. J Pain Sympt Manage 1996;11:363–369.

12 Hydration, Thirst, and Nutrition

PAMELA KEDZIERA

How can I not give him food and water—you need food and water to live.

—Wife of a patient

Providing food and water is fundamental and basic for human existence. From birth, our growth is directly linked to nutrition. Socially, providing food is seen as an expression of caring, of meeting the needs of those for whom we care. Ethically, there is an obligation to feed the hungry and give drink to the thirsty. The imperative to provide nutrition and fluids for the dying individual who is unable and/or unwilling to eat and drink, however, is a controversial issue. There is no consensus among experts on whether it is physically, psychologically, socially, or ethically appropriate to provide artificial hydration and nutrition to a terminally ill person. Do these therapies improve the way an individual feels physically? Do they cause harm? Can an individual die comfortably without these interventions? Choices can be guided by careful assessment of the physical condition of the individual and exploring his or her personal belief system, as well as social, cultural, and psychological needs. These elements are illustrated in the following case report:

Case Report

Mrs. S. was a 70-year-old woman with advanced uterine cancer. She was a Holocaust survivor, as was her husband. Receiving and giving food were all-important to them both. Mrs S. was obstructed, had a draining percutaneous endoscopic gastrostomy tube and was unable to take food by mouth. Total parenteral nutrition (TPN), which had originally been started as nutritional support during intensive chemotherapy, became an expression of nurturing and life in both their minds, when the focus of care became directed toward end-of-life care. Although discontinuing chemotherapy had been a difficult transition for the patient and family, to discontinue TPN was inconceivable. This attitude continued until the end of life. The patient continued to receive TPN up until the time of her death.

The deep-seated, unimaginable horror of living through the Holocaust and the deprivation of food they had experienced strongly impacted on this patient and her family's unshakeable belief that food and water must be given up until death.

A contrasting situation is illustrated through a man in his 40s, dying of gastric cancer, who had received TPN for nutritional support during chemotherapy. Administration of TPN had repeatedly been associated with increased pain. The patient had been willing to tolerate the increased pain when the goal of care was for prolongation of life. When this goal was no longer possible, the patient associated the TPN with diminished quality of life and asked that it be discontinued. The meaning of food and water, and the meaning of discontinuing food and water, needs careful exploration and ongoing discussion of the benefits and burden for each individual. There are no absolutes.

HYDRATION

Water is an essential component of the human body. Complex cellular functions, like protein synthesis and metabolism of nutrients, are affected by hydration status. The maintenance of hydration is dependent on a balance between intake and output, which is regulated by neuroendocrine influences. Homeostasis is maintained through parallel neuroendocrine activity on excretion of fluid via the kidneys[1] and on intake via thirst. Increased osmotic pressure is the prime stimulus for thirst, stimulating the release of vasopressin. Renal excretion is mainly dependent on the action of vasopressin, which is secreted by the posterior pituitary gland. This hormone, known as antidiuretic hormone (ADH), increases water reabsorption in the collecting ducts of the kidneys.[2] Thirst stimuli include hypertonicity; depletion of the extracellular fluid compartment arising from vomiting, diarrhea, or hemorrhage; and renal failure, where plasma sodium is low but plasma renin levels are high.[(3)]

Dehydration is a loss of normal body water. There are several types of dehydration.[2,4] *Isotonic* dehydration results from a balanced loss of water and sodium. This occurs during a complete fast and during episodes of vomiting and diarrhea with the loss of water and electrolytes in the gastric contents. Billings[5] theorized that the terminally ill have this type of balanced decrease in food and fluid intake, causing *eunatremic* (sodium levels in normal range) dehydration, whereby there is simultaneous loss of salt and water. *Hypertonic* dehydration occurs if water losses are greater than sodium losses. Fever can cause this problem, by loss of water through the lungs and skin and a limited ability to take in oral fluids. *Hypotonic* dehydration occurs when sodium loss exceeds water loss. This generally occurs when water is consumed but food is not. Overuse of diuretics is a major factor. *Osmotic* diuresis (e.g., from hyperglycemia), salt-wasting renal conditions, third spacing (ascites), and adrenal insufficiency are other common etiologies of sodium loss.[6]

Table 12–1. Signs and Symptoms of Dehydration

Hyponatremic Dehydration	Hypernatremic Dehydration	Isotonic Dehydration
Volume depletion	Thirst	Morose
Anorexia, taste alteration, and weight loss	Fatigue	Aggression
Nausea and vomiting	Muscle weakness	Demoralized
Diminished skin turgor	Mental status changes	Apathetic
Dry mucous membranes	Fever	Uncoordinated
Reduced sweat		
Orthostatic hypotension		
Lethargy and restlessness		
Delirium		
Seizures (related to cerebral edema)		
Confusion, stupor and coma		
Psychosis (rare)		
Lab Results		
Azotemia	Increased sodium	Minor or no abnormalities
Disproportionate blood urea nitrogen compared to creatinine		
Hyponatremia		
Hemoconcentration		
Urine osmolarity with sodium concentration		

The methodology for assessing dehydration has not been well studied and tends to vary among practitioners. The clinical sensitivity of each method has not been determined. Clinical assessment should include mental status changes, thirst, oral/parenteral intake, urine output, and fluid loss. Physical findings, weight loss, dry mouth, dry tongue, reduced skin turgor, and postural hypotension should be noted. Laboratory tests, including increased hematocrit, elevated serum sodium, azotemia with a disproportionate rise in blood urea nitrogen in relation to creatinine, concentrated urine, and hyperosmolarity, are indicative of dehydration.

Physical findings (Table 12–1) are complicated to evaluate.[6] Comorbid conditions can be the cause of many of these symptoms in the chronically or terminally ill individual. Dry mouth, for example, can be associated with mouth breathing or anticholinergic medication. Skin turgor can be hard to evaluate in the cachexic individual and is unreliable. Obtaining weights may be impracticable, but a rapid weight loss of greater than 3% is indicative of dehydration.[4] Postural hypotension can be related to medications and cardiac pathology. Confusion is common in the advanced cancer patient relative to multiple etiologies, including the disease state itself. Thirst may be absent or mild in patients with hyponatremic dehydration, although marked volume loss may stimulate ADH and water craving.

There is evidence that elderly individuals do not perceive thirst in the same manner as healthy young adults.[3] In a study comparing the role of thirst sensation and drinking behavior in young versus older adults, water was restricted for 24 hours. Only the young healthy study group reported a dry, unpleasant mouth and a general sense of thirst; the healthy elders had a deficit in the awareness of thirst despite plasma osmolarity and sodium and vasopressin concentrations that were greater than those in the younger group. During the rehydration period, the younger group consumed enough fluid to correct their laboratory values. Elder subjects did not consume enough fluid to correct the laboratory values.[7] There is not, however, any evidence to support this observation in the terminally ill. In hypernatremia, thirst is a powerful stimulus and normally persons with access to water will take in sufficient amounts of fluid. Confused or somnolent individuals or those unable to drink are at risk because water may not be adequately replaced. Dehydrated, terminally ill patients generally present with mixed disorders of fluid and salt loss.

Dehydration causes confusion and restlessness in patients with nonterminal disease. These same symptoms are frequently reported in terminally ill persons and could be aggravated by dehydration.[8] Reduced intravascular volume caused by dehydration can result in renal failure. Opioid metabolite accumulation can result from renal failure and cause confusion, myoclonus, and seizures.[9] Dehydration has been associated with an increased risk of bedsores and constipation, particularly in the elderly. Discomfort, especially problems with xerostomia and thirst, may result from dehydration.[10]

Dehydration may improve physical care-giving for some patients. For example, less urine results in less incontinence and the subsequent need for physical care. Urinary catheters may be avoided if the frequency of urination decreases. The evidence regarding dehydration in palliative care patients, however, is very limited. With dehydration, there is less gastrointestinal fluid, with fewer bouts of vomiting, and a reduction in pulmonary secretions, with less coughing, choking, and the need for suctioning. It is often contended that terminal dehydration causes suffering, which should be relieved. This suffering includes thirst, dry mouth, fatigue, nausea, vomiting, confusion, muscle cramps, and perhaps the hastening of death.[11,12] Dehydration as a cause of renal failure has been well documented.[13,14] A study of terminally ill cancer patients, however, showed that the group receiving intravenous fluids at a rate of 1 to 2 l/day consistently had more abnormal laboratory values of serum sodium, urea, and osmolarity than the group who were not hydrated.[15] In a study of 82 patients in the last 2 days before death, analysis showed no statistically significant relationship between the level of hydration, respiratory tract secretions, dry mouth, and thirst.[16] The researchers concluded that artificial hydration to alleviate symptoms may be futile. This contrasts with a study of 100 palliative care patients receiving hypodermoclysis, in which researchers concluded that this therapy was useful for achieving better symptom control.[17] An anecdotal study of three patients being hydrated by hypodermoclysis reported that hydration may have contributed to improved cognitive function and allowed patients to deal with end-of-life issues.[18] Some experts suggest that hydration may relieve symptoms other than thirst, such as confusion and restlessness.[13] Still others who have looked at the issue of dehydration-related suffering have stressed the role of inappropriate medical interventions that cause their own problems. Hydrating a patient can involve repetitive needle sticks, decreased mobility, increased secretions, increased edema, and possibly congestive heart failure.[19,20] Improving the cognition of an individual in pain may make him or her more aware of pain, requiring more medication and then decreasing cognition with analgesics. Comatose patients may feel no symptoms; fluids may prolong dying, and dehydration may act as an anesthetic.[13] In the only descriptive research on symptoms of dehydration in the terminally ill, no association was found between fluid intake, serum sodium, osmolality, blood urea nitrogen, and symptom severity.[11] A survey of physicians found that there was no consensus with respect to the assessment of "suffering" from dehydration or thirst. The physicians who chose artificial hydration were more likely to perceive suffering and thirst as serious problems. Two-thirds of the doctors did not believe that artificial hydration was the best way to respond to terminal dehydration.[21]

The decision to use artificial means of hydration comes more from tradition than from science. To avoid unnecessary interventions in the course of the dying process, some practitioners have avoided artificial fluid replacement secondary to its perceived negative effects. Their conclusion, that artificial hydration may cause harm to some dying patients, keeps them from offering this therapy. Palliative care clinicians have noted that some individuals are more comfortable without artificial fluids, which may prolong the dying process. Unfortunately, most of these arguments are based on anecdotal reports, not research. Emotional issues are often involved in the decision to provide artificial hydration. The need to provide fluids may be directed by very strong cultural, religious, and/or moral convictions. For some patients, caregivers, and family members, "everything must be done," even if there is no certainty that the therapy does provide comfort.

Screening for dehydration in the palliative setting may include recording intake and output, examining skin turgor and mucous membranes, and monitoring mental status and blood pressure. Subjective reports of fatigue, muscle weakness, anorexia, and taste alteration are correlated with these signs and laboratory values (Table 12–1). The benefits and possible adverse effects of hydration should be discussed and the wishes of the patient explored. Each situation will have unique aspects that will affect choices and the outcome of therapy. Finally, there is a need for regular reassessment to allow for changes in therapy and frequent discussions with patients and families to provide opportunities to reevaluate decisions.

The treatment of dehydration starts with a review of medications and elimination, if possible, of any agents (diuretics) that may be contributing to the dehydration. Mouth care should be provided regularly. Intervening or treating dehydration may include various routes of administration. A standard goal for fluid intake is 1500 to 3000 ml, or eight to ten glasses, of water daily.[6] The least invasive approach to replacing fluids is to offer liquid orally at regular intervals. For those able to swallow, this approach can help the patient as well as promote the emotional well-being of the caregivers. Those who are very weak, depressed, confused, agitated, or demented may need significant assistance in getting the fluids in on a regular basis. Care must be taken to avoid overhydration by a well-meaning but misdirected aggressive approach, and the patient should be monitored for new orthopnea, shortness of breath, or change in mental status. If the ability to swallow is diminished, there is a risk of aspiration and causing more distress to the patient. Small, frequent sips of fluid or ice chips can be provided. Choice of fluids should be patient-driven. Some individuals find sports replacement fluids a good choice as they are easily absorbed by the stomach and can correct hypertonic dehydration.[4] Using a fine mist spray can also help to keep mucous membranes moist.[22] Hot, humid weather conditions can add to the risk of dehydration, so the use of air conditioning and fans should be considered.

If there are days or weeks of life expected, a more reliable route of fluid replacement may be chosen. Rehydration by proctoclysis is relatively risk-free and less expensive than parenteral means of administration.[23] Using a nasogastric tube placed rectally, tap water or saline is instilled, starting at about 100 cc/h. If there is no discomfort, leakage, or tenesmus (spasm of the anal sphincter), the rate can be increased to 400 cc/h. A liter of fluid can be instilled over 6 to 8 hours. Care must be taken, however, not to overhydrate. Side effects of this route of hydration can include pain, edema, rectal leakage of fluid, and pain during insertion of the tube. Researchers report that although effective, safe, and economical, most patients preferred hypodermoclysis.[23] It is possible to foresee cultural and social reluctance to accept the rectal mode of fluid administration. In an inpatient setting, clinical staff would administer the fluids, but in a home setting, it may be impractical to use professional staff daily for this treatment. Family caregivers or patients may be uncomfortable with relatives or friends having to assume this type of care.

Standard methods of replacement of fluids can be achieved by enteral feeding tubes and by parenteral methods, such as subcutaneously (hypodermoclysis) or intravenously. A feeding tube placed through the nose is often uncomfortable and may agitate the confused individual. Patients often extubate themselves when agitated. Endoscopic gastrostomy tubes have become more popular but are usually placed for decompression or feeding rather than for fluid replacement. If the individual has a feeding tube or a permanent intravenous access device (port or peripherally inserted central catheter), these may be used safely without any added burden for the patient. Placement of these devices, however, needs to be considered in the context of overall goals of therapy, cost, and feasibility. In addition, placement of these devices can be inconvenient and cause complications.

Hypodermoclysis, subcutaneous fluid administration, does not require special access devices. This method has the advantage over the intravenous route in people who have poor venous access. Using this method may prevent transfer to an acute setting for line placement. Hypodermoclysis can be started by any professional staff member who can give a subcutaneous injection. It does not require monitoring for clotting in the line, and there is no fear of letting the line "run dry." There can be local irritation at the site of infusion, however, as well as minor bleeding. Sloughing of tissue is possible with overinfusion and abscess formation may occur (Table 12–2). Hypotonic or isotonic solutions, with or without hyaluronidase or corticosteroids, are administered through needles inserted into the subcutaneous tissue of the abdomen or anterior or lateral thigh. Most individuals can tolerate 100 ml/h or more. Up to 1500 ml can be administered into a single site.[7,24] The following case report illustrates the use of hypodermoclysis:

Case Report

Mr. G was a 55-year-old man with advanced colon cancer. He was obstructed and unable to take oral food or water. His goal was to remain alert and interactive with his wife and children for as long as possible. Enteral feedings were not feasible, and venous access for fluids was complicated by recurrent port and line infections. Maintaining hydration, however, was felt to be important for achieving the patient's goals. Because of the complications associated with his venous access, hypodermoclysis was chosen as the most appropriate route for fluid administration. Subcutaneous fluids at 100 ml/h were continued for the last 4 months of his life. This subcutaneous access also provided a parenteral route for opioid administration. Mr. G remained alert and interactive up until the last day of life.

In this case, hypodermoclysis appeared to have been an appropriate use of technology and hydration in end-of-life care.

Replacement of fluids by the intravenous route is more technically complicated, and access to a competent vein must be available. Care must be taken not to overhydrate accidentally. In this era of technology, some individuals have permanent-access devices, placed for therapy earlier in their treatment, that are more than adequate for this type of administration. Others may wish to have a device placed. Using a regular intravenous line for ongoing hydration can be hard to maintain and may require frequent replacement. There is always the possibility of displacement, infiltration, or clotting of the line. Small, portable pumps are available for use in the inpatient or home setting, which can help to prevent run-away intravenous fluids. Some individuals choose to run fluids via the permanent-access devices only at night. This allows for more mobility during the daylight hours. There needs to be a competent caregiver to monitor the therapy, and because caregivers accept many duties, this can be overwhelming to some.

Consensus on volume or type of fluid replacement does not exist. Clinicians make choices based on their previous experience and knowledge of the patient's condition and wishes. Some practitioners allow the individual to have a liter a day despite the fact that it is inadequate replacement. Considerations also include safety and reality of the care burden on all caregivers. Providing a liter of fluid a day may only partially correct the patient's deficits but may relieve the emotional burden of needing to provide fluids. A liter a day can often be worked into the patient/family schedule better. If fluids are given only at night, the patient may be more mobile during the day. Fluid administration can be scheduled to accommodate the goals of living. More aggressive fluid replacement will require monitoring of serum electrolytes and blood counts by regular laboratory testing. This type of approach requires monitoring laboratory results and making adjustments every 24 to 48 hours.

Table 12–2. Potential Complications of Routes for Artificial Hydration [intravenous (IV), subcutaneous (SC)]

IV Peripheral	IV Central	SC Hypodermoclysis
Pain	Sepsis	Pain
Short duration of access	Hemothorax	Infection
Infection	Pneumothorax	Third spacing
Phlebitis	Central vein thrombosis	Tissue sloughing
	Catheter fragment thrombosis	Local bleeding
	Air embolus	
	Brachial plexus injury	
	Arterial laceration	

Patients and family members can be taught to manage hydration techniques at home. An assessment of their concerns should precede the instruction about the actual procedures. Adequate time must be allowed for education and return demonstration. Backup support should be provided, and repetitive sessions may be required. When possible, direct instruction to more than one caregiver should be provided, to allow them to help each other with the tasks required. Printed materials that are age- and reading level–appropriate should be given. In addition, if available, video instructions can be helpful. Follow-up visits or calls should be scheduled to assess level of functioning, to give support, and to reinforce teaching. These therapies may mean more home visits, to accommodate those who learn more slowly or are not able to master all or part of the procedure. Specific protocols will vary between institutions/agencies; however, written policies and procedures should guide practice.

Other symptoms related to dehydration can be assessed and treated. Thirst can be relieved by small amounts of fluid offered frequently. Immersion in cool water can also influence the sensation of thirst,[25] although this is frequently impractical. Dry mouth is treated with an intensive q 2-hour schedule of mouth care, including hygiene, lip lubrication, and ice chips or popsicles. Eliminating medications that cause dry mouth, such as tricyclic antidepressants and antihistamines, should be considered. Generally, however, the drugs that may contribute to these symptoms are being administered to palliate other symptoms. Mouth breathing can also cause dry mouth. Candida infection, a frequent etiology of dry mouth in the debilitated individual, can be treated. Agents such as pilocarpine (Salagen) can be used to increase salivation.

The controversy over providing hydration in terminally ill individuals stems from trying to balance the medical tradition of doing everything possible to heal and prolong life with the idea of allowing patients to die comfortably without unnecessary interventions. What is the role of medical intervention at the final stage of illness? Dehydration may aggravate or alleviate the discomfort of terminal disease (Table 12–3).[5] Current research does not clearly guide practice. Dehydration causes unpleasant symptoms, such as confusion and restlessness, in nonterminally ill patients. These problems are common in the dying. Dehydration can cause renal failure with an accompanying accumulation of opioid metabolites, which causes further symptoms, such as myoclonus and even seizures. Dehydration is also associated with constipation and increased risk of bedsores. Clinicians report that these symptoms are mild and easily treated without hydration and that some symptoms, like increased secretions, are actually made worse.[5,11,19] Hospice nurses have reported that the dehydrated patient is not uncomfortable.[26,27] There is concern that artificial hydration diminishes quality of life by adding tubes, which create a physical barrier that separates the terminally ill from their loved ones. There is often fear that hydration unnecessarily prolongs dying. Those who support the use of hydration point to the prevention or relief of some symptoms like delirium.[12,15] Fluids can be viewed as a symbol of life. To remove fluids may cause spiritual or emotional conflict for some individuals.

These issues are complex and involve not only physical, psychological, and social concerns but also ethical dilemmas. The prime goal of care of the dying should be the comfort of the patient and family. Whenever possible, the patient should have input into the decision making. Clinicians agree on the goal of comfort and the role of the patient in decisions regarding care. It is the absence of definitive research that makes guiding these decisions difficult.

Table 12–3. Hydration and Rehydration at the End of Life: Potential Effects

Body System	Effects of Dehydration	Effects of Rehydration
General appearance	Sunken eyes	Improved appearance
Mouth	Decreased saliva	Oral comfort
	Thirst	Relief of thirst
	Bad taste	Improved taste
	Dry, cracked lips	
Pulmonary	Dry airway, viscous secretions	Normal or increased secretions
	Reduced death rattle	
	Reduced secretions, cough	Facilitates productive cough
	Reduced congestion, wheezing, dyspnea, pleural effusions	Easier suctioning
Gastrointestinal tract	Constipation	More normal bowel function
	Decreased secretions	
	Less vomiting, diarrhea	
	Anorexia	
	Reduced ascites	Ascites
Urinary tract	Reduced renal function	Improved renal drug clearance
	Edema	Reduced toxic metabolites
	Possible drug accumulation	May need more drug administration

Source: Billings (1998), reference 6.

NUTRITION

Malnutrition is a common problem in chronic, advanced illnesses like acquired immune deficiency syndrome and cancer. *Anorexia*, a loss of appetite, occurs in most patients in the last weeks of life. Cancer cachexia refers to a complex syndrome characterized by loss of appetite, generalized tissue wasting, skeletal muscle atrophy, immune dysfunction, and a variety of metabolic alterations.[28,29] It is likely that *asthenia*, mental and physical fatigue coupled with generalized weakness, is directly related to malnutrition.[30–32] Administration of nutrition in the terminally ill is sometimes proposed as a medical intervention for nutrition-related symptoms or management of side effects, such as weight loss, weakness, constipation, pressure sores, intestinal obstruction, and dehydration. Nutritional intervention is also recommended to prevent further morbidity and maintain quality of life by controlling blood sugars or electrolyte imbalance. Lastly, nutritional therapy is offered to provide enough dietary intake to maintain energy. Enteral and parenteral feedings are, however, interventions with the potential for associated morbidity and increased suffering (Table 12–4).

Anorexia is influenced by alteration in taste, alterations in the gastrointestinal system, changes in metabolism, and effects of the tumor itself. In addition, psychological factors such as depression or anxiety can change eating habits. Pain, fatigue, and nausea may also decrease the desire for oral intake. Many aspects of the cancer experience decrease caloric intake. Taste changes may come from the tumor itself or result from various treatments like chemotherapy, surgery, radiation, or antibiotics.[33] These taste changes may in turn decrease digestive enzymes and delay digestion.[34] The gastrointestinal tract may be altered by tumor, opportunistic infections such as *Candida*, or ulcerations from chemotherapy or radiation that cause diarrhea. These can interfere with ingestion, digestion, and absorption. Nausea and vomiting may ensue. Abnormalities in glucose metabolism, increases in circulating amino acids or lactic acid, and increases in free fatty acids can cause early satiety.[35] Increased blood sugar and serotonin levels in the brain may also suppress appetite.[36] In addition, cytokines such as interluken 1 and tumor necrosis factor released from tumors may mediate anorexia and decrease gastric emptying.[37]

The advanced chronically ill patient may have increased caloric needs due to changes in metabolism. The basal metabolic rate can be increased by infection or malignancy. Age, nutritional status, temperature, hormones, and trauma can change the metabolic rate. Unlike the healthy person, there is no adaptation to a decrease in food intake; metabolism does not slow down. Cytokines increase resting energy expenditure and skeletal muscle wasting.[37] Nutrients which help to maintain immune function are decreased, and the resulting immunosuppression increases the risk of infection. Tumors invading the esophagus, stomach, or bowel can cause compression or obstruction and may limit oral intake. Surgery to remove tumors can remove all or part of the organs that produce digestive enzymes. This results in incomplete digestion. A shortened intestine reduces the number of villi available for absorption of nutrients.[35]

Table 12–4. Potential Complications of Enteral Support

Complication	Symptom	Etiology
Aspiration	Coughing Fever	Excess residual Large-bore tube
Diarrhea	Watery stool	Hyperosmotic solution Rapid infusion Lactose intolerance
Constipation	Hard, infrequent stools	Inadequate fluid Inadequate fiber
Dumping syndrome	Dizziness	High volume Hyperosmotic fluids

Nutritional assessment starts with a diet history. The history should include the individual's usual dietary habits, current eating habits, and disease symptoms. Food preferences and aversions should be explored as well as family support and the ability to obtain and prepare foods. The educational needs of the patient and caregivers should also be assessed. A food diary may be helpful in this situation, and dieticians recommend a 72-hour history followed by weekly documentation. A physical examination to screen for changes in oral mucosa and dentition should be performed.

Anthropometric measurements are part of nutritional assessment. These are often limited in scope at the end stages of disease. A history of weight loss of 20% or greater is indicative of increased morbidity and mortality.[38] In the patient with advanced disease, weight gain may indicate the presence of edema or ascites, whereas weight loss may indicate dehydration. Other anthropometric measurements, like skin-fold thickness and mid-arm circumference, are used to assess muscle and fat stores and can be used to monitor progress. Laboratory values are also used to estimate protein stores. These biochemical measurements are the mainstay for determining TPN. The appropriateness of each of these assessment parameters is controversial in the terminally ill.

Nutritional therapy is aimed at improving intake and managing cachexia. Increasing appetite is sometimes possible with pharmacological therapy. Steroids have been known to increase appetite, but long-term use can cause muscle weakness. High-dose megastrol acetate has been shown to increase appetite with subsequent weight gain.[39,40] Hydrazine sulfate did not improve appetite more than placebo.[41] Metoclopramide, tetrahydrocannabinol, and insulin have shown some improvement, but toxicities were problematic and the data often insufficient. Exercise has been shown to stimulate appetite; however, few end-stage patients are able to participate in the type of exercise necessary to increase appetite.

Nursing measures to promote oral intake include managing other symptoms, such as constipation, pain, and nausea, which negatively affect appetite. In addition, patients may require more seasoning than usual for food to taste good. Good oral care and unhurried meals should be encouraged. Suggesting that the patient allow others to cook may preserve energy for eating as well as decrease the negative effects of food odors. Wine or beer has been known to stimulate appetite but may be poorly tolerated in terminally ill patients or those receiving multiple medications with sedating properties.

Enteral feedings utilize the gastrointestinal tract for delivery of nutrients, and oral supplementation of nutrients can be tried in individuals who have the capacity to swallow. Care must be taken, however, to monitor the use of these supplements. Caregivers and patients sometimes feel a moral obligation to provide food and "push" the supplements at the risk of harm to the patient, such as aspiration pneumonia. Feedings may also be given through a nasogastric tube, an esophagostomy tube, a gastrostomy tube, or a jejunostomy tube. In addition to the possibility of aspiration with enteral feedings, there is the risk of dumping syndrome, diarrhea, constipation, skin irritation at tube site insertion, and clogging of feeding tubes. Finally, it is possible to provide nutrition parenterally. This approach may be useful to a small and carefully selected group of patients. However, TPN can be complicated by venous thrombosis, air embolism, infection, sepsis, hyperglycemia, hypoglycemia, and increased pain. Overall, enteral and parenteral nutritional support is an area of controversy in cancer therapy, not just at the end of life.

SUMMARY

We inherit beliefs that govern behavior. Among them are numerous contradictory notions which associate support with sustenance. The rites of family meals and celebrations provide bonding and sharing as well as food, fundamental components of personal and social life. The issues of hydration and nutrition at the end of life are complex and require a thoughtful, individualized approach.

REFERENCES

1. Rolls BJ, Phillips PA. Aging and disturbances of thirst and fluid balance. Nutr Rev 1990;48:137–144.
2. Smith SA. Patient-induced dehydration—can it ever be therapeutic? Oncol Nurs Forum 1995;22:1487–1491.
3. Rolls BJ, Wood RJ, Rolls ET. Thirst following water deprivation in humans. Am J Physiol 1980;8:R476–R482.
4. Weinberg AD, Minaker KL, Council on Scientific Affairs, American Medical Association. Dehydration evaluation and management in older adults. JAMA 1995;274:1552–1556.
5. Billings JA. Comfort measures for the terminally ill; is dehydration painful? J Am Geriatr Soc 1985;33:808–810.
6. Billings JA. Dehydration. In: Billings JA, Berger A, Portenoy R, Weissman D, eds. Principles and Practice of Supportive Oncology. Philadelphia: Lippincott-Raven, 1998:589–601.
7. Phillips PA, Rolls BJ, Ledingham JG, et al. Reduced thirst after water deprivation in healthy elderly men. N Engl J Med 1984;311:753–759.
8. MacDonald N. Ethical issues in dehydration and nutrition. In: Bruera E, Portenoy RK, eds. Topics in Palliative Care, Vol 2. New York: Oxford University Press, 1998:153–169.
9. Fassing R. Dehydration and palliative care. Palliat Care Letter 7 (1): insert 1.
10. Twycross R, Lichter I. The terminal phase. chapter 17 In: Doyle D, Hanks GWC, MacDonald N, eds. Oxford Textbook of Palliative Medicine, 2nd Ed. Oxford: Oxford University Press, 1998:977–994.
11. Burge FI. Dehydration symptoms of palliative care cancer patients. J Pain Symptom Manage 1993;8:454–464.
12. del Rosario B, Martin AS. Hydration for control of syncope in palliative care. J Pain Symptom Manage 1997;14:5–6.
13. Fainsinger RL, Bruera E. Hypodermoclysis for symptom control versus the Edmonton injector. J Palliat Care 1991;7:5–8.
14. Fainsinger R, Bruera E. The management of dehydration in terminally ill patients. J Palliat Care 1995;10:55–59.
15. Waller A, Hershkowitz M, Adunsky A. The effect of intravenous fluid infusion on blood and urine parameters of hydration and on state of consciousness in terminal cancer patients. Am J Hospice Palliat Care 1994;11:22–27.
16. Ellershaw JE, Sutcliffe JM, Saunders CM. Dehydration and the dying patient. J Pain Symptom Management 1995;10:192–197.
17. Fainsinger R, MacEachern T, Miller MJ, et al. The use of hypodermoclysis for rehydration in terminally ill cancer patients. J Pain Symptom Manage 1994;9:298–302.
18. Yan E, Bruera E. Parenteral hydration of the terminally ill. J Palliat Care 1991;7:40–43.
19. Zerwekh J. The dehydration question. Nursing 1983;13:47–51.
20. Printz LA. Is withholding hydration a valid comfort measure in the terminally ill? Geriatrics 1988;43:84–88.
21. Collard T, Rapin CH. Dehydration in dying patients: study with physicians in French-speaking Switzerland. J Pain Symptom Manage 1991;6:230–240.
22. Kemp C. Dehydration, fatigue and sleep. In: Kemp C, ed. Terminal Illness: A Guide to Nursing Care, 2nd Ed. Philadelphia, Lippincott, 1999:205–210.
23. Bruera E, Pruvost M, Schoeller T, Montejo G, Watanabe S. Proctoclysis for hydration of terminally ill cancer patients. J Pain Symptom Manage 1998;8:454–464.
24. Berger EY. Nutrition by hypodermoclysis. J Am Geriatr Soc 1984;32:199–203.
25. Sagawa S, Miki K, Tajima H, et al. Effect of dehydration on thirst and drinking during immersion in men. J Appl Physiol 1992;72:128–134.
26. Andrews M, Bell ER, Smith SA, Tischler JF, Veglia JM. Dehydration in terminally ill patients: is it appropriate palliative care? Postgrad Med 1993;93:201–208.
27. Andrews MR, Levine AM. Dehydration in the terminal patient: perception of hospice nurses. Am J Hospice Care 1989;1:31–34.
28. Rivadeneira DE, Envoy D, Fahey TJ, Lieberman MD, Daly JM. Nutritional support of the cancer patient. CA Cancer J Clin 1998; 48:69–80.
29. Costa G. Cachexia, the metabolic component of neoplastic diseases. Cancer Res 1977;37: 2327–2335.
30. Neuenschwander H, Bruera E. Asthenia. In: Doyle D, Hanks GWC, MacDonald N, eds. Oxford Textbook of Palliative Medicine, 2nd Ed. New York: Oxford University Press, 1998:573–581.
31. Bruera E. Clinical management of cachexia and anorexia in patients with advanced cancer. Oncology 1992;49 (Suppl 2):35–42.
32. Storey P. Symptom control in advanced cancer. Semin Oncol 1994;21:748–753.
33. Bender CM. Taste alterations. In: Yasko JM, ed. Nursing Management of Symptoms Associated with Chemotherapy, 3rd Ed. Columbus, OH: Adria Laboratories, 1993:67–74.
34. Kesner DL, DeWys WD. Anorexia and cachexia in malignant disease. In: Newell GR, Ellison NM, eds. Nutrition and Cancer: Etiology and Treatment. New York: Raven Press, 1981: 303–317.
35. Tait NS. Anorexia-cachexia syndrome. In: Groenwald SL, Frogge MH, Goodman M, Yarbro CH, eds. Cancer Symptom Management. Boston: Jones and Bartlett, 1997:171–185.
36. Grant M, Ropka ME. Alterations in nutrition. In: Baird S, McCorkle R, Grant M, eds.

Cancer Nursing: A Comprehensive Textbook. Philadelphia: WB Saunders, 1991:717–741.

37. Moldawer LL, Rogy MA, Lowry SF. The role of cytokines in cancer cachexia. J Parent Nutr 1992;16(Suppl):43s–49s.

38. Bernard M, Jacobs D, Rombeau J. Nutrient requirements. In: Bernard M, Jacobs J, Romeau D, eds. Nutritional and Metabolic Support of Hospitalized Patients. Philadelphia: WB Saunders, 1986:11–45.

39. Tchekmedyian NS, Hickman M, Siau J, et al. Megastrol acetate in cancer anorexia and weight loss. Cancer 1992;69:1269–1274.

40. Schmoll E, Wilke H, Thole R, Preusser P, Wildfang I, Schmoll HJ. Megastrol acetate in cancer cachexia. Semin Oncol 1991;18(Supp 2):32–34.

41. Loprinzi CL, Goldberg RM, Su JQ, et al. Placebo-controlled trial of hydrazine sulfate in patients with newly diagnosed non small-cell lung cancer. J Clin Oncol 1994;11:1126–1129.

13 Dyspnea, Death Rattle, and Cough

DEBORAH DUDGEON

I struggled to breathe, hoping that the attack would soon end. I was so scared. I thought I'd die!

—A patient

Dyspnea, an unpleasant awareness of breathing, is a very common symptom in people with advanced disease. Its prevalence varies according to the disease: chronic obstructive pulmonary disease (COPD), 95%; congestive heart failure, 61%; stroke, 37%;[1] amyotrophic lateral sclerosis, 47% to 50%; and dementia, 70%.[2] Approximately 50% of a general outpatient cancer population describe some breathlessness,[3] with this number rising to 45% to 70% in the terminal phases of the disease.[4–9] The prevalence of dyspnea is even more common in patients with lung cancer, almost 90% of whom complain of breathlessness just prior to death.[10]

In a study of late-stage cancer patients, Roberts and associates[11] used patient self-report surveys, chart audits of patients under the care of a hospice program, and interviews of patients and nurses in the home-care hospice program to examine the occurrence of dyspnea during the last weeks of life. They found that 62% of patients with dyspnea had been short of breath for a duration exceeding 3 months. Various activities intensified dyspnea for these patients: climbing stairs, 95.6%; walking slowly, 47.8%; getting dressed, 52.2%; talking or eating, 56.5%; and rest, 26.1%. The patients universally responded by decreasing their activity to whatever degree would relieve their shortness of breath. The majority of the patients had received no direct medical or nursing assistance with their dyspnea, leaving them to cope in isolation. Brown and colleagues[12] found that 97% of lung cancer patients studied had decreased their activities and 80% believed they had socially isolated themselves from friends and outside contacts to cope with their dyspnea.

Brown and colleagues[12] also found that dyspnea was typically chronic, with most patients experiencing episodes of acute shortness of breath. Acute shortness of breath can be a very frightening experience. One patient described it as feeling like she was "at the bottom of a swimming pool and unable to get up to catch her breath."

Dyspnea, like pain, is multidimensional in nature, with not only physical elements but also affective components, which are shaped by previous experience.[13,14] The neuropathways responsible for the sensation of dyspnea are poorly understood,[15] and no simple physiological mechanism or unique peripheral site can explain the varied circumstances that lead to the perception of breathlessness.[13,16] Stimulation of a number of different receptors (Fig. 13–1) and the conscious perception this invokes can alter ventilation and result in a sensation of breathlessness.

PATHOPHYSIOLOGY OF DYSPNEA

Management of dyspnea requires an understanding of its multidimensional nature and the pathophysiological mechanisms that cause this distressing symptom. Exertional dyspnea in cardiopulmonary disease (Table 13–1) is caused by *(1)* increased ventilatory demand, *(2)* impaired mechanical responses, or *(3)* a combination of the two.[17] The effects of abnormalities of these mechanisms can also be additive.

Increased Ventilatory Demand

Ventilatory demand is increased because of increased physiological dead space due to reduction in the vascular bed (from thromboemboli, tumor emboli, vascular obstruction, radiation, chemotherapy toxicity, or concomitant emphysema); hypoxemia and severe deconditioning with early metabolic acidosis (with excessive hydrogen ion stimulation); alterations in carbon dioxide output (V_{CO_2}) or in the arterial partial pressure of carbon dioxide (P_{CO_2}) set point; and non-metabolic sources, such as increased neural reflex activity, or psychological factors, such as anxiety and depression.

Impaired Mechanical Response/Ventilatory Pump Impairment

Impaired mechanical responses result in restrictive ventilatory deficits due to inspiratory muscle weakness,[18] pleural or parenchymal disease, reduced chest wall compliance, airway obstruction from coexistent asthma or COPD, or tumor obstruction. Patients may also have a mixed obstructive and restrictive disorder.

MULTIDIMENSIONAL ASSESSMENT OF DYSPNEA

Dyspnea, like pain, is a subjective experience that may not be evident to an observer. *Tachypnea*, a rapid respiratory rate, is not dyspnea. Medical personnel must learn to ask and accept the patient's assessments, often without measurable physical correlates. When patients say they are having discomfort with breath-

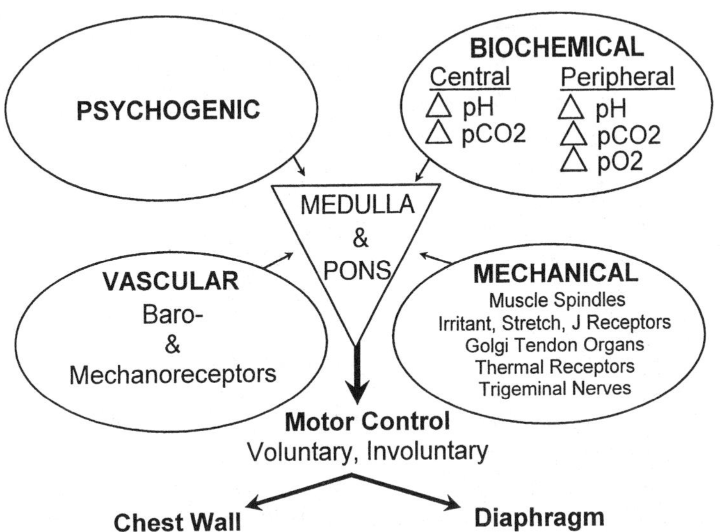

Fig. 13–1. Schematic diagram of the neuroanatomical elements involved in the control of ventilation. (From Portenoy and Bruera (2000), reference 115, with permission.)

Table 13–1. Pathophysiological Mechanisms of Dyspnea

Increased ventilatory demand
Increased physiological dead space
Thromboemboli
Tumor emboli
Vascular obstruction
Radiation therapy
Chemotherapy
Emphysema
Severe deconditioning
Hypoxemia
Change in V_{CO_2} or arterial P_{CO_2} set point
Psychological: anxiety, depression
Increased neural reflex activity
Impaired mechanical response/ventilatory pump impairment
Restrictive ventilatory deficit
Respiratory muscle weakness
Cachexia
Electrolyte imbalances
Peripheral muscle weakness
Neuromuscular abnormalities
Neurohumoral
Steroids
Pleural or parenchymal disease
Reduced chest wall compliance
Obstructive ventilatory deficit
Asthma
Chronic obstructive pulmonary disease
Tumor obstruction
Mixed obstructive/restrictive disorder (any combination of the above)

V_{CO_2} = carbon dioxide output; P_{CO_2} = partial pressure of carbon dioxide.

ing, we must believe that they are dyspneic.

To determine if dyspnea is present, it is important to ask more than "Are you short of breath?" Patients often respond in the negative to this simple question as they have limited their activities so that they will not become short of breath. It is therefore helpful to ask about shortness of breath in relation to activities such as "walking at the same speed as someone of your age," "stopping to catch your breath when walking upstairs," or "eating."

QUALITATIVE ASPECTS OF DYSPNEA

Dyspnea is also not a single sensation. Recent work suggests that the sensation of breathlessness encompasses several qualities.[16] Just as the descriptions "burning" and "numb" suggest neuropathic pain, phrases such as "chest tightness," "exhalation," and "deep" were among a cluster of words associated with asthma in the study of Simon and colleagues.[16] It is possible that dyspnea mediated by similar receptors evokes common word descriptors. From the research to date, it is not known whether qualitative assessments of dyspnea in breathless patients permits any discrimination among the various cardiopulmonary disorders. O'Donnell and coworkers[19–21] found that while descriptor choices were clearly different between health and disease states, they provided no discrimination, for example, between COPD, restrictive lung disease, and congestive heart failure.

CLINICAL ASSESSMENT OF DYSPNEA

Clinical assessments are usually directed at determining the underlying pathophysiology to decide appropriate treatment and evaluating response to therapy.

The clinical assessment of dyspnea should include a complete history of the symptom, including its temporal onset (acute or chronic), whether it is affected by positions, qualities, associated symptoms, precipitating, relieving events or activities, and response to medications. A past history of smoking, underlying lung or cardiac disease, concurrent medical conditions, allergy history, and details of previous medications or treatments should be elicited.[22,23]

Careful physical examination focused on possible underlying causes of dyspnea should be performed. Particular attention should be directed at signs associated with certain clinical syndromes that are common causes of dyspnea. An example of this would be an elevated jugular venous pressure, an audible third heart sound (S_3), and bilateral crackles audible on chest examination associated with congestive heart failure.[22,23]

Gift and co-workers[24] studied the physiological factors related to dyspnea in subjects with COPD with high, medium, and low levels of breathlessness. There were no significant differences in respiratory rate, depth of respiration, or peak expiratory flow rates at the three levels of dyspnea. There was, however, a significant difference in the use of accessory muscles between patients with high and low levels of dyspnea, suggesting that this is a physical finding which reflects the intensity of dyspnea.

Diagnostic tests helpful in determining the etiology of dyspnea include chest radiography; electrocardiography; pulmonary function tests; arterial blood gases; complete blood counts; serum potassium, magnesium, and phosphate levels; cardiopulmonary exercise testing; and tests specific for suspected underlying pathologies, such as echocardiogram for suspected pericardial effusion.[22] The choice of appropriate diagnostic tests should be guided by the stage of disease, the prognosis, the risk/benefit ratios of any proposed tests or interventions, and the desires of the patient and family.

Results of pulmonary function tests do not necessarily reflect the intensity of a person's dyspnea. Individuals with comparable degrees of functional lung impairment may experience considerable differences in the perceived intensity of dyspnea.[13]

DYSPNEA AND PSYCHOLOGICAL FACTORS

The person's perception of the intensity of his/her breathlessness is also affected by psychological factors. Anxious, obsessive, depressed, and dependent persons appear to experience dyspnea that is disproportionately severe relative to the extent of their pulmonary disease.[13] Burns and Howell[25] found that patients with disproportionately severe breathlessness were more likely to have a psychiatric disorder (commonly depression) and that their breathlessness resolved with the resolution of the psychiatric problem. Gift and colleagues[24] found that anxiety was higher during episodes of high or medium dyspnea levels when compared with low dyspnea. Others have found that anxiety and depression seem to perpetuate episodes of disproportionate breathlessness.[26] Kellner and associates[27] found that in multiple regression analyses depression was predictive of breathlessness. Studies in cancer patients by Dudgeon and Lertzman[18,28] and others[3,9,29] have also shown that anxiety is significantly correlated with the intensity of dyspnea. The correlations between dyspnea intensity and anxiety are often significant but low, explaining only 9% of the variance. These studies have been done on people with a chronic level of dyspnea, who have often adapted to the sensation. As stated earlier, however, patients often experience episodes of acute shortness of breath in which anxiety is a much more prominent factor.

MANAGEMENT OF DYSPNEA

The optimal treatment of dyspnea is to treat reversible causes. When this is no longer possible, both nonpharmacological and pharmacological methods are used (Table 13–2).

Nonpharmacological Interventions

Simple Techniques. Many patients obtain relief of dyspnea by leaning forward while sitting and supporting their upper arms on a table. This technique is effective for patients with emphysema,[30] probably because of an improved length–tension state of the diaphragm, which increases efficiency.[31]

Pursed-lip breathing slows the respiratory rate and increases intra-airway pressures, thus decreasing small airway collapse during periods of increased dyspnea.[32] Mueller and co-workers[33] found that pursed-lip breathing led to an increase in tidal volume and a decrease in respiratory rate at rest and during exercise, with seven of the 12 COPD patients experiencing an improvement in dyspnea. Pursed-lip breathing reduces dyspnea in about 50% of patients with COPD.[34]

People who are short of breath often obtain relief by sitting near an open window or in front of a fan. Cold directed against the cheek[35] and through the nose[36,37] can alter ventilation patterns and reduce the perception of breathlessness, perhaps by affecting receptors in the distribution of the trigeminal

Table 13–2. Management of Dyspnea

Sit upright, supported by pillows or leaning on overbed table
Fan ± oxygen
Relaxation techniques and other appropriate nonpharmacological measures
Identify and treat underlying diagnosis (if appropriate)
Pharmacologic management
- Chronic
  - Opioids
  - Add phenothiazine (chlorpromazine, promethazine)
- Acute
  - Opioids
  - Add anxiolytic

nerve that are responsive to both thermal and mechanical stimuli.[35,36]

Corner and colleagues[38] found that weekly sessions with a nurse research practitioner over 3 to 6 weeks using counseling, breathing retraining, relaxation, and coping and adaptation strategies significantly improved breathlessness and the ability to perform activities of daily living compared to the control group. Carrieri and Janson-Bjerklie[39] found that patients used self-taught relaxation to help control their breathlessness. Others have found that formal muscle-relaxation techniques decrease anxiety and breathlessness.[40] Guided imagery[41] and therapeutic touch[42] have resulted in significant improvements in quality of life and sense of well-being in COPD and terminal cancer patients, respectively, without any significant improvement in breathlessness.

In an open pilot study on 20 patients with cancer-related breathlessness, the safety and efficacy of acupuncture was tested.[43] Seventy percent of patients reported marked symptomatic benefit, with a significant reduction in visual analogue scale (VAS) scores of breathlessness and a significant reduction in respiratory rate.

Nursing actions which intubated patients thought helpful included friendly attitudes, empathy, providing physical support, staying at the bedside, being reminded or allowed to concentrate on changing their breathing pattern, and providing information about the possible cause of the breathlessness and possible interventions.[44]

Oxygen. The usefulness of oxygen for the terminally ill patient has been questioned.[45,46] Most authorities currently recommend oxygen for dyspneic hypoxic patients, even in the face of increasing hypercapnea, to achieve and maintain a (PAO_2) of 55 to 60 mm Hg and oxygen saturation of 88% to 90%.[47,48] Bruera and colleagues[49,50] have also demonstrated the benefit of oxygen therapy in 20 hypoxic patients with terminal cancer. Patients' ratings of dyspnea, respiratory rate, oxygen saturation, and respiratory effort improved with oxygen to a significantly greater degree than with air. In hypoxic patients with COPDs, oxygen supplementation improves survival, pulmonary hemodynamics, exercise capacity, and neuropsychological performance.[48] Guidelines for oxygen therapy are shown in Table 13–3.

Table 13–3. Guidelines for Oxygen Therapy

Continuous oxygen

- PAO_2 ≤55 mm Hg or oxygen saturation ≤88% at rest
- PAO_2 of 56 to 59 mm Hg or oxygen saturation of 89% in the presence of the following:
  - Dependent edema, suggesting congestive heart failure
  - Cor pulmonale
  - Polycythemia (hematocrit >56%)
  - Pulmonary hypertension

Noncontinuous oxygen during exercise:

- PAO_2 ≤55 mm Hg or oxygen saturation ≤88% with a low level of exertion or during sleep:
- PAO_2 of ≤55 mm Hg or oxygen saturation ≤88% associated with pulmonary hypertension, daytime somnolence, and cardiac arrhythmias

PAO_2 = partial pressure of oxygen in alveoli.
From Tarsy SP, and Celli BR: N Engl J Med 1995;333:710–714.

The role of oxygen in the treatment of nonhypoxic dyspneic patients is less clear. Woodcock and co-workers[51] studied the effect of oxygen on breathlessness in nonhypoxic patients with COPD. Oxygen not only reduced breathlessness but also increased the distance that patients were able to walk.

Pharmacological Interventions

Opioids. Since the late nineteenth century, opioids have been used to relieve breathlessness of patients with asthma, pneumothorax, and emphysema.[52] Although most trials have demonstrated the benefit of opioids in the treatment of dyspnea,[33,52–61] some have been negative[62–65] and/or produced undesirable side effects.[55,62]

In recent years, there has been tremendous interest in the use of nebulized opioids for the treatment of dyspnea. Opioid receptors are present on sensory nerve endings in the airways,[66] and therefore, it is hypothesized that if the receptors are interrupted directly, lower doses, with less systemic side effects, would be required to control breathlessness. There is only one randomized controlled trial that demonstrates a beneficial effect of nebulized opioids on shortness of breath,[67] but there are a number of anecdotal and uncontrolled reports.[68–72] Seven randomized controlled trials, however, did not find that nebulized opioids relieved breathlessness.[57,73–78] There was one report of acute respiratory depression as a complication of nebulized morphine.[79] It is recommended that patients with a history of poorly controlled asthma be excluded from receiving this treatment[80] and that all first administrations be observed as there is a risk for acute bronchoconstriction due to histamine release. The scientific evidence for the usefulness of nebulized opioids is very limited, and although nebulized opioids may help in certain clinical situations, these have yet to be identified.

Physicians have been reluctant to prescribe opioids for dyspnea since the potential for respiratory failure was recognized in the 1950s.[81] It is now known that whether clinically significant hypoventilation and respiratory depression develop from opioids depends on the rate of change of the dose, the history of previous exposure to opioids, and possibly the route of administration.[82] Early use of opioids improves quality of life and allows the utilization of lower doses while tolerance to the respiratory depressant effects develops.[83] Twycross[84] suggests that early use of morphine or another opioid, rather than hastening death in dyspneic patients, might actually prolong survival by reducing physical and psychological distress and exhaustion.

Sedatives and Tranquilizers. Chlorpromazine decreases breathlessness without affecting ventilation or producing sedation in healthy subjects.[85] Woodcock and colleagues[86] found that promethazine reduced dyspnea and improved exercise tolerance of patients with severe COPD. O'Neill and associates[85] did not find that promethazine improved breathlessness in healthy people, nor did Rice and co-workers[62] find it benefited patients with stable COPD. McIver and colleagues[87] found that chlorpromazine was effective for relief of dyspnea in advanced cancer.

Clinical trials to determine the effectiveness of anxiolytics for the treatment of breathlessness have also been quite variable. Two studies showed that diazepam was not effective at treating dyspnea,[86,88] and one showed a reduction in dyspnea.[89] Greene and colleagues[90] reported an improvement in dyspnea with alprazolam; however, a randomized, placebo-controlled, double-blind study did not find any relief of dyspnea with alprazolam.[91] Clorazepate was not effective for breathlessness.[92] Buspirone, a nonbenzodiazepine anxiolytic, had no effect on pulmonary function tests or arterial blood gases in patients with COPD but improved exercise tolerance and decreased dyspnea.[93] This drug warrants further study.

Combinations. In a double-blind, placebo-controlled, randomized trial, Light and colleagues[94] studied the effectiveness of morphine alone, morphine and promethazine, and morphine and prochlorperazine for the treatment of breathlessness in COPD patients. The combination of morphine and promethazine significantly improved exercise tolerance without worsening dyspnea compared to placebo, morphine alone, or the combination of morphine and prochlorperazine.[94] Ventafridda and colleagues[95] have also found the combination of morphine and chlorpromazine to be effective.

Other Medications. Indomethacin reduced exercise-induced breathlessness in a group of normal adults,[96] but no benefit was obtained in patients with diffuse parenchymal lung disease[97] or COPD.[98] Although inhaled bupivacaine reduced exercise-induced breathlessness in normal volunteers,[99] it failed to decrease the breathlessness of patients with interstitial lung disease.[100] Inhaled lidocaine did not improve dyspnea in six cancer patients.[101] Dextromethorphan did not improve breathlessness of patients with COPD.[102] None of these medications can be recommended for the treatment of dyspnea.

Patient and Family Teaching

Carrieri and Janson-Bjerklie[39] identified strategies patients used to manage acute shortness of breath. These strategies could be taught to patients and their families. Patients benefited from keeping still with positioning techniques, such as leaning forward on the edge of a chair with arms and upper body supported, and used some type of breathing strategy, such as pursed-lip or diaphragmatic breathing. Some of the patients distanced themselves from aggravating factors, and others used self-adjustment of medications. Several subjects isolated themselves from others to gain control of their breathing and diminish the social impact. Others used structured relaxation techniques, conscious attempts to calm down, and prayer and meditation. The study of Carrieri and Janson-Bjerklie[39] and another by Brown and colleagues[12] demonstrated that most subjects reported some changes in activities of living, such as changes in dressing and grooming, avoidance of bending or stooping, advanced planning of or reduction in activities, staying in a good frame of mind, avoidance of being alone, and acceptance of the situation.

Patients and families should be taught about the signs and symptoms of an impending exacerbation and how to manage the situation. They should learn problem-solving techniques to prevent panic, ways of conserving energy, how to prioritize activities, use of fans, and ways to maximize the effectiveness of their medications, such as using a spacer with inhaled drugs or taking an additional dose of an inhaled beta-agonist before exercise.[103] Patients should avoid activities where their arms are unsupported as these often increase breathlessness.[40]

Patients in distress should not be left alone. Social services, nursing, and family input will need to be increased as the patient's ability to care for himself or herself decreases.[104]

Case Study: Mr. D.S., a Patient with Dyspnea

You are called to the room of Mr. D.S. and find him sitting at the bedside gasping for breath. You know that Mr. D.S. is a 63–year-old man with a long history of COPD. He is receiving Ventolin and Atrovent by nebulizers every 4 hours and was recently started on a course of steroids. While getting an overbed table and pillow for him to rest on, you calmly instruct him to take slow, deep breaths and use the breathing technique that you previously had taught him. You note that he is cyanosed and institute oxygen and fan to help relieve his breathlessness. On further examination he exhibits no evidence of heart failure, but you note that there are very few breath sounds throughout his chest. With the institution of the oxygen, fan, and focused breathing, you note that he is slightly less distressed, but you ask his wife to stay with him while you prepare a prn dose of nebulized Ventolin. On your return 5 minutes later, his breathing has improved even more; but there is still little evidence of air entry, so you administer the Ventolin. His wife stays with him, and 15 minutes later, when you return, she has just helped him back into bed, where he is resting comfortably.

Summary

Dyspnea is a very common symptom in people with advanced disease. It is often unrecognized, and therefore, patients receive little assistance in managing their breathlessness. Interventions for the management of dyspnea need to be instituted early in the course of disease, to improve quality of life.

DEATH RATTLE

I can't stay in the room. It sounds like she's drowning to death!

—A family member

Noisy, moist breathing, commonly known as death rattle, occurs in 35% to 92% of patients in their last hours prior to death.[80,105,106] Studies have shown that there is an increased incidence of respiratory congestion in patients with primary lung cancer[80] or cerebral metastases.[107] In one study, the median time from onset of death rattle to death was 23 hours.[106] This noisy, moist breathing can be very distressing for the family and health care workers as it may appear that the person is drowning in his or her own secretions. Most commonly, this symptom occurs when the person is comatose, but if the person is alert, the respiratory secretions can cause him or her to feel very agitated and fearful of suffocating.

Pathophysiology

The primary defense mechanism for the lower respiratory tract is the mucociliary transport system. This system was developed as a protective device to prevent the entrance of viruses, bacteria, and other particulate matter into the body.[108–110] The surface of the respiratory tract is lined with a liquid sol phase near the epithelium and a superficial gel phase in contact with the air.[108] Ciliated epithelial cells, located at all levels of the respiratory tract except the alveoli and the nose and throat, are in constant movement to propel the mucus up the respiratory tract to be either subconsciously swallowed or coughed out. The mucus is produced by submucosal glands, which are under neural and humoral control. The submucosal glands are under parasympathetic, sympathetic, and noncholinergic nonadrenergic nervous control. Resting glands secrete approximately 9 ml/min, but mechanical, chemical, or pharmacological stimulation (via vagal pathways) of the airway epithelium can augment gland secretion. Surface goblet cells also produce mucous secretions, which can be increased with irritant stimuli, such as cigarette smoke. The secretory flow rate and amount, as well as the viscoelastic properties, of the mucus can be altered.[108] The audible breathing of the so-called death rattle is produced when turbulent air passes over or through pooled secretions in the oropharynx or bronchi. The amount of turbulence depends on the ventilatory rate and airway resistance.[107] Mechanisms of death rattle include excessive secretion of respiratory mucus, abnormal mucus secretions inhibiting normal clearance, dysfunction of the cilia, inability to swallow, decreased cough reflex due to weakness and fatigue, and the supine recumbent position. Factors that may contribute to respiratory congestion include infection or inflammation, pulmonary embolism producing infarction and fluid leakage from damaged cells, pulmonary edema or congestive heart failure,[110] dysphagia, and odynophagia. Although it has been suggested that a state of relative dehydration will decrease the incidence of problematic bronchial secretions,[111] Ellershaw and colleagues[80] found no statistically significant difference in the incidence of death rattle in a biochemically dehydrated group of patients versus a group of hydrated patients.

Bennett[107] has proposed two types of death rattle. Type 1 involves mainly salivary secretions, which accumulate in the last few hours of life when swallowing reflexes are inhibited. Type 2 is characterized by the accumulation of predominantly bronchial secretions over several days prior to death as the patient becomes too weak to cough effectively. This characterization has not been confirmed by research, but if true, it may prove useful for determining appropriate treatment.

Assessment

Assessment of death rattle includes a focused history and physical examination to determine potentially treatable underlying causes. If the onset is sudden and associated with acute shortness of breath and chest pain, it might suggest a pulmonary embolism or myocardial infarction. Physical findings consistent with congestive heart failure and fluid overload might support a trial of diuretic therapy; the presence of pneumonia indicates a trial of antibiotic therapy. The effectiveness of interventions should be included in the assessment. The patient's and family's understanding and emotional response to the situation should also be assessed so that appropriate interventions can be undertaken.

Patient and Family Teaching

The patient and/or family can be very distressed by this symptom. It is important to explain the process, to help them understand why there is a build-up of secretions and that there is something that can be done to help. The Victoria Hospice Society suggests using the term "respiratory congestion" as opposed to "death rattle," "suffocation," or "drowning in sputum" as these instill strong emotional reactions.[110] When explaining to families the changes that can occur prior to death, this is one of the symptoms that should be mentioned. If the person is being managed at home, the family should be instructed as to the measures available to relieve it and to notify their hospice/palliative care team if it occurs so that appropriate medications can be ordered.

Management

Nonpharmacological Interventions. There are times when the simple repositioning of the patient may help him or her to clear the secretions (Table 13–4). Suc-

Table 13–4. Management of Death Rattle

- Change position
- Reevaluate if receiving IV hydration
- Pharmacological management
  - Chronic
    - Glycopyrrolate or hyoscine hydrobromide patch
    - *If treatment fails:* subcutaneous hyoscine hydrobromide or subcutaneous atropine sulfate
  - Acute
    - Subcutaneous hyoscine hydrobromide or subcutaneous atropine sulfate

tioning is generally not recommended as it can be very uncomfortable for the patient and cause significant agitation and distress. Pharmacological measures are usually effective and prevent the need for suctioning. If the patient has copious secretions that can be easily reached in the oropharynx, then suctioning may be appropriate. In a study conducted at St. Christopher's Hospice, suctioning was required in only three of 82 patients to control the secretions.[80] In another study, 31% of patients required only nursing interventions with reassurance, change in position, and occasional suctioning to manage respiratory congestion in the last 48 hours of life.[112]

Pharmacological Interventions. Primary treatment should be focused on the underlying disorder if possible and/or appropriate to prognosis and the wishes of the patient and family. If this is not possible, then anticholinergics are the primary mode of treatment. Hyoscine hydrobromide (scopolamine), hyoscine butylbromide (Buscopan), and glycopyrrolate (Robinul) are the anticholinergics used to treat death rattle. Anticholinergic drugs can prevent vagally induced increased bronchial secretions but reduce basal secretions by only 39%.[108]

Hyoscine hydrobromide (Scopolamine) is the primary medication used for the treatment of death rattle. It inhibits the muscarinic receptors and causes anticholinergic actions such as decreased peristalsis, gastrointestinal secretions, sedation, urinary retention, and dilatation of the bronchial smooth muscle. It is administered subcutaneously, intermittently or by continuous infusion, or transdermally.[80,105,107,113] In one study,[112] hyoscine hydrobromide 0.4 mg subcutaneously was immediately effective and only 6% of the patients required repeated doses. In other studies, 22% to 65% of patients did not respond to hyoscine hydrobromide, with a recurrence of secretions occurring from 2 to 9 hours following the injection.[105] In a retrospective study of 100 consecutive deaths in a 22–bed hospice, 27% received an infusion of hyoscine hydrobromide with 5 of 17 requiring injections despite being on an infusion.

Atropine Sulfate is another anticholinergic drug, which is preferred by some centers for the treatment of respiratory congestion.[110] In a study of 995 doses of atropine, congestion was decreased in 30%, remained the same in 69%, and increased in 1%.[110] Atropine is the drug of choice of this group as it has less central nervous system depression, delirium, and restlessness and more bronchodilatory effect than hyoscine hydrobromide. There is, however, the risk of increased tachycardia with atropine sulfate when doses >1.0 mg are given.

Glycopyrrolate (Robinul) is also an anticholinergic agent. It has the advantages of producing less sedation and agitation and a longer duration of action than scopolamine. In the one study where its effectiveness was assessed, however, it was not as effective as scopolamine at controlling secretions.[105] Glycopyrrolate is available in an oral form and can be useful at an earlier stage of disease, when sedation is not desired.

Hyoscine butylbromide (Buscopan) is another anticholinergic drug, but it has not been evaluated for its effectiveness in this condition. It is available as an injection, suppository, and tablet.

Case Study: M.C., a 25-Year-Old Woman with an Inoperable Astrocytoma

Over the past 72 hours, M.C.'s condition has significantly deteriorated. She is no longer responsive to verbal stimuli. The decision had been made the day before by the team in consultation with the family to discontinue the intravenous hydration and continue only with the dexamethasone (Decadron) and other "comfort" measures. When you come on your shift, you notice that the mother is standing outside of the room, very distressed. The mother, in tears, says "I can't stay in the room. It sounds like she's drowning to death." When you enter the room, you notice that M.C. is very restless and has moist, gurgly respirations. You help to reposition M.C. on her side and explain to the mother and other family members why this is happening and that there is medication that can help dry up the secretions. You give her an injection of hyoscine hydrobromide subcutaneously, and within 20 minutes she has settled.

Summary

Although death rattle is a relatively common problem in people who are close to death, very few studies have evaluated the effectiveness of treatment. Anticholinergics are the drugs of choice at this time. This can be very distressing for family members at the bedside, and they need to receive good teaching and reassurance.

COUGH

I'm so exhausted; every time I fall asleep I start to cough.

—A patient

Cough is a natural defense of the body to prevent entry of foreign material into the respiratory tract. In people with advanced disease, it can be very debilitating, leading to sleepless nights, fatigue, pain, and at times pathological fractures. Cough is often present in people with advanced diseases such as bronchitis, congestive heart failure, uncontrolled asthma, human immunodeficiency virus, infection, and various cancers. In a study of 289 patients with non-small-cell lung cancer, cough was the most common (over 60%) and severe symptom at presentation.[10] Eighty percent of the group had cough prior to death. Over time, cough and breathlessness were much less well controlled than the other symptoms in this group of patients.

Pathophysiology

Cough is characterized by a violent expiration, with flow rates that are high enough to sheer mucous and foreign particles away from the larynx, trachea, and large bronchi. The cough reflex can be stimulated by irritant receptors in the larynx and pharynx or pulmonary stretch receptors, irritant receptors, or C-fiber stimulation in the tracheobronchial tree.[114] The vagus nerve carries sensory information from the lung that initiates the cough reflex. Infection may physically or functionally strip away epithelium, exposing sensory nerves and increasing the sensitivity of these to mechanical and chemical stimuli. It is also thought that inflammation produces prostaglandins, which further increase the sensitivity of these receptors, leading to bronchial hyperreactivity and cough. When cough is associated with increased sputum production, it probably results from excess secretion stimulating the irritant receptors.[114] Cough is associated with respiratory infection, bronchitis, rhinitis, postnasal drip, esophageal reflux, medications including angiotensin-converting enzyme inhibitors,[114] asthma, COPD, pulmonary fibrosis, congestive heart failure, pneumothorax, bronchiectasis, and cystic fibrosis.[46] In the person with cancer, cough may be caused by any of these things; however, direct tumor effects such as obstruction, indirect cancer effects such as pulmonary emboli, and cancer treatment effects such as radiation therapy could also be the cause.[115]

Assessment

In assessing someone with cough, it is important to do a thorough history and physical examination. This will help to determine the underlying etiology and appropriate treatment. Depending on the person's diagnosis, prognosis, and the patient and family wishes, it may be appropriate to do diagnostic tests, including chest or sinus x-rays, spirometry with pre- and postbronchodilator and histamine challenge, and in special circumstances in early-stage disease, upper gastrointestinal endoscopy and 24-hour esophageal pH monitoring. In the history and physical examination, one should look for a link between cough and the associated factors listed in the previous section, whether the cough is productive or not, the nature of the sputum, precipitating and relieving factors, and associated symptoms.

Management

It is important to base management decisions on the etiology and whether it is appropriate to treat the underlying diagnosis versus just suppressing the symptom. This decision is based on the diagnosis, prognosis, cost and possible benefits of the intervention, and wishes of the patient and family. Management strategies also depend on whether the cough is productive or not (Table 13–5). Theoretically, cough suppressants, by causing mucous retention, could be harmful in conditions with excess mucous production.[114]

Table 13–5 Treatment of Nonproductive Cough

Nonopioid antitussive (dextromethorphan, benzonatate)
Opioids
Inhaled anesthetic (lidocaine, bupivacaine)

Nonpharmacological Interventions. If cough is induced by a sensitive cough reflex, then the person should attempt to avoid the stimuli that produce this. If smoking, they should stop or cut down and avoid smoky rooms, cold air, exercise, and pungent chemicals. If medication is causing the cough, it should be decreased or stopped if possible; or if the etiology is esophageal reflux, then elevation of the head of the bed could be tried. Adequate hydration, humidification of the air, and chest physiotherapy may help the patient expectorate viscid sputum.[46] Radiation therapy to enlarged nodes, endoscopically placed esophageal stents for tracheoesophageal fistulas, or injection of polytef (Teflon) into a paralyzed vocal cord may improve cough.[46]

Pharmacological Interventions

Demulcents are a group of compounds that form aqueous solutions and help to alleviate irritation of abraded surfaces. They are often found in over-the-counter cough syrups. Their mode of action for controlling cough is unclear, but it is thought that the sugar content encourages saliva production and swallowing, which leads to a decrease in the cough reflex; stimulates the sensory nerve endings in the epipharynx and decreases the cough reflex by a "gating" process; or acts as a protective barrier by coating the sensory receptors.[114]

Opioids suppress cough, but the dose is higher than that contained in commercially available cough mixtures.[114] The exact mode of action is unclear, but it is thought that they inhibit the mu receptor peripherally in the lung; act centrally by suppressing the cough center in the medulla or the brain stem respiratory centers; or stimulate the mu receptor, thus decreasing mucous production or increasing mucous ciliary clearance.[114] Codeine is the most widely used opioid for cough, but it has no advantages over other opioids and provides no additional benefit to patients already receiving high doses of opioids for analgesia.[116]

Nonopioid Antitussive Agents More than 200 synthetic nonopioid antitussive agents are available; most are less effective than codeine.[117] Dextromethorphan, a dextro isomer of levorphanol, is an exception and is nearly equiantitussive to codeine. Dextromethorphan acts centrally through nonopioid receptors to increase the cough threshold.[116] Benzonatate is a nonopioid antitussive with a sustained cough-depressing action[118] that provided excellent symptomatic relief in a case report of three cancer patients with opioid-resistant cough.[119] Opioid and nonopioid antitussives may act synergistically,[116] but further studies are needed to confirm this hypothesis.

Inhaled anticholinergic **bronchodilators,** alone or in combination with beta$_2$-adrenergic agonists, effectively decrease cough in people with asthma and normal subjects.[120] It is thought that they decrease input from the stretch receptors, therefore decreasing cough reflex and changing mucociliary clearance.

The local anesthetic lidocaine is a potent suppressor of irritant-induced cough and has been used as a topical anesthetic for the airway when performing bronchoscopy. **Inhaled local anesthetics** such as lidocaine and bupivacaine delivered by nebulizer suppress some cases of chronic cough for as long as 9 weeks.[114,121–123] Higher doses can cause bronchoconstriction; therefore, it is wise to observe the first treatment. Patients must also be warned not to eat or drink anything for 1 hour after the treatment or until their cough reflex returns, to avoid choking or aspiration.

Productive Coughs

Interventions for productive coughs include chest physiotherapy, oxygen, humidity, and suctioning. In cases of increased sputum production, expectorants, mucolytics, and agents to decrease mucous production can be employed. Opioids, antihistamines, and anticholinergics decrease mucous production and thereby decrease the stimulus for cough.

Patient and Family Education

Education should include practical matters such as proper use of medications, avoidance of irritants, use of humidification, and ways to improve the effectiveness of cough. One such way is called "huffing." The person should lie on his or her side, support the abdomen with a pillow, blow out sharply three times, hold his or her breath, and then cough. This technique seems to improve the effectiveness of a cough and helps to expel sputum.

Case Example: P.B., a Patient with Small-Cell Carcinoma of the Lung

Mr. P.B. is a 58–year-old man with extensive small-cell carcinoma of the lung. He has known mediastinal and bone metastases, for which he has received maximum chemo- and radiotherapy. He has been admitted to the hospice for control of severe right-sided chest pain and was found on admission to have a pathological fracture of his right ninth rib. He is receiving morphine 40 mg PO every 4 hours for his pain and Ventolin and Atrovent every 6 hours for his underlying COPD. You note that he continues to have severe incident pain with coughing. He has had a trial of demulcents, dextromethorphan, and opioids for his cough, with little effect. He has no history of fever, postnasal drip, or esophageal reflux and is not on any medications known to produce cough. You note that his cough is nonproductive, with no evidence of pneumonia on physical examination. You suggest a trial of inhaled lidocaine and, after receiving the order, instruct Mr. P.B. not to eat or drink anything for 1 hour after the treatment, to avoid choking or aspiration. He receives the treatment and amazingly has no coughing episodes for 24 hours, when he receives his next prn inhalation.

Summary

Chronic cough can be a disabling symptom for patients. A thorough history and physical examination should be conducted to determine the underlying etiology, which should then be treated appropriately. Both nonpharmacological and pharmacological interventions can be helpful. When the underlying cause is unresponsive to treatment, suppression of the unproductive cough is the major therapeutic goal.

Dyspnea, death rattle, and cough are common symptoms in people with advanced disease. It is always important to do a thorough assessment to determine the underlying etiology so that appropriate pharmacological and nonpharmacological interventions can be used.

REFERENCES

1. Zeppetella G. The palliation of dyspnea in terminal disease. Am J Hospice Palliat Care 1998; 15:322–330.

2. Voltz R, Borasio GD. Palliative therapy in the terminal stage of neurological disease. J Neurol 1997;244(Suppl 4):S2–S10.

3. Dudgeon D, Kristjanson L, Sloan J, Lertzman M. Dyspnea in cancer patients: prevalence and associated factors. J Pain Symptom Manage 1999; in press.

4. Reuben DB, Mor V. Dyspnea in terminally ill cancer patients. Chest 1986;89:234–236.

5. Fainsinger R, MacEachern T, Hanson J, Miller MJ, Bruera E. Symptom control during the last week of life on a palliative care unit. J Palliat Care 1991;7:5–11.

6. Twycross RG, Lack SA. Respiratory symptoms. In: Twycross RG, Lack SA, ed. Therapeutics in Terminal Cancer, 2nd Ed. London: Churchill Livingston, 1990:123–136.

7. Curtis EB, Krech R, Walsh TD. Common symptoms in patients with advanced cancer. J Palliat Care 1991;7:25–29.

8. Heyse-Moore LH, Ross V, Mullee MA. How much of a problem is dyspnoea in advanced cancer? Palliat Med 1991;5:20–26.

9. Heyse-Moore LH. On Dyspnoea in Advanced Cancer. Southampton University, Southampton, UK., 1993. Dissertation.

10. Muers MF, Round CE. Palliation of symptoms in non-small cell lung cancer: a study by the Yorkshire Regional Cancer Organisation Thoracic Group. Thorax 1993;48:339–343.

11. Roberts DK, Thorne SE, Pearson C. The experience of dyspnea in late-stage cancer. Patients' and nurses' perspectives. Cancer Nurs 1993; 16:310–320.

12. Brown ML, Carrieri V, Janson-Bjerklie S, Dodd MJ. Lung cancer and dyspnea: the patient's perception. Oncol Nurs Forum 1986;13:19–24.

13. Cherniack NS, Altose MD. Mechanisms of dyspnea. Clin Chest Med 1987;8:207–214.

14. Tobin MJ. Dyspnea: pathophysiologic basis, clinical presentation, and management. Arch Intern Med 1990;150:1604–1613.

15. Manning HL, Schwartzstein RM. Mechanisms of dyspnea. In: Mahler D, ed. Dyspnea. New York: Marcel Dekker, 1998:63–95.

16. Simon PM, Schwartzstein RM, Weiss JW, Fencl V, Teghtsoonian M, Weinberger SE. Distinguishable types of dyspnea in patients with shortness of breath. Am Rev Respir Dis 1990; 142:1009–1014.

17. O'Donnell DE. Exertional breathlessness in chronic respiratory disease. In: Mahler D, ed. Dyspnea. New York: Marcel Dekker, 1998:97–147.

18. Dudgeon D, Lertzman M. Dyspnea in the advanced cancer patient. J Pain Symptom Manage 1998;16:212–219.

19. O'Donnell DE, Chau LL, Bertley J, Webb KA. Qualitative aspects of exertional breathlessness in CAL: pathophysiological mechanisms. Am J Respir Crit Care Med 1997;155:109–115.

20. O'Donnell DE, Chau LKL, Webb KA. Qualitative aspects of exertional dyspnea in interstitial lung disease. J Appl Physiol 1998;84:2000–2009.

21. D'Arsigny C, Raj S, Abdollah H, Webb KA, O'Donnell DE. Ventilatory assistance improves leg discomfort and exercise endurance in stable congestive heart failure (CHF). Am J Respir Crit Care Med 1998;157:A451.

22. Silvestri GA, Mahler DA. Evaluation of dyspnea in the elderly patient. Clin Chest Med 1993;14:393–404.

23. Ferrin MS, Tino G. Acute dyspnea. AACN Clin Issues 1997;8:398–410.

24. Gift AG, Plaut SM, Jacox A. Psychologic and physiologic factors related to dyspnea in subjects with chronic obstructive pulmonary disease. Heart Lung 1986;15:595–601.

25. Burns BH, Howell JBL. Disproportionately severe breathlessness in chronic bronchitis. Q J Med 1969;38:277–294.

26. Howell J. Behavioral breathlessness. In: Breathlessness. The Campbell Symposium May 16–19, 1991. Ingelheim: Boehringer-Ingelheim, 1992:149–155.

27. Kellner R, Samet J, Pathak D. Dyspnea, anxiety, and depression in chronic respiratory impairment. Gen Hosp Psychiatry 1992;14:20–28.

28. Dudgeon D, Lertzman M. Etiology of dyspnea in advanced cancer patients [abstract]. Proc Am Soc Clin Oncol 1996;15:165.

29. Bruera E, Schmitz B, Pither J, Neumann CM, Hanson J. The frequency and correlates of dyspnea in patients with advanced cancer. Personal communication, 1997.

30. Barach AL. Chronic obstructive lung disease: postural relief of dyspnea. Arch Phys Med Rehabil 1974;55:494–504.

31. Sharp JT, Drutz WS, Moisan T, Foster J, Machnach W. Postural relief of dyspnea in severe chronic obstructive pulmonary disease. Am Rev Respir Dis 1980;122:201–211.

32. Thoman RL, Stoker GL, Ross JC. The efficacy of pursed-lips breathing in patients with chronic obstructive pulmonary disease. Am Rev Respir Dis 1966;93:100–106.

33. Mueller RE, Petty TL, Filley GF. Ventilation and arterial blood gas changes induced by pursed lip breathing. J Appl Physiol 1970;28:784–789.

34. Make B. COPD: management and rehabilitation. Am Fam Physician 1991;43:1315–1324.

35. Schwartzstein RM, Lahive K, Pope A, Weinberger SE, Weiss JW. Cold facial stimulation reduces breathlessness induced in normal subjects. Am Rev Respir Dis 1987;136:58–61.

36. Burgess KR, Whitelaw WA. Effects of nasal cold receptors on pattern of breathing. J Appl Physiol 1988;64:371–376.

37. Burgess KR, Whitelaw WA. Reducing ventilatory response to carbon dioxide by breathing cold air. Am Rev Respir Dis 1984;129:687–690.

38. Corner J, Plant H, A'Hern R, Bailey C. Non-pharmacological intervention for breathlessness in lung cancer. Palliat Med 1996;10:299–305.

39. Carrieri VK, Janson-Bjerklie S. Strategies patients use to manage the sensation of dyspnea. West J Nurs Res 1986;8:284–305.

40. van den Berg R. Dyspnea: perception or reality. Canadian Association of Critical Care Nurses CACCN 1995;6:16–19.

41. Moody LE, Fraser M, Yarandi H. Effects of guided imagery in patients with chronic bronchitis and emphysema. Clin Nurs Res 1993;2: 478–486.

42. Giasson M, Bouchard L. Effect of therapeutic touch on the well-being of persons with terminal cancer. J Holist Nurs 1998;16:383–398.

43. Filshie J, Penn K, Ashley S, Davis CL. Acupuncture for the relief of cancer-related breathlessness. Palliat Med 1996;10:145–150.

44. Shih F, Chu S. Comparisons of American-Chinese and Taiwanese patients' perceptions of dyspnea and helpful nursing actions during the intensive care unit transition from cardiac surgery. Heart Lung 1999;28:41–54.

45. Shepard KV. Dyspnea in cancer patients. Palliat Care Lett 1990;2:6.

46. Cowcher K, Hanks GW. Long-term management of respiratory symptoms in advanced cancer. J Pain Symptom Manage 1990;5:320–330.

47. Kaplan JD. Acute respiratory failure. In: Woodley M, Whelan A, eds. Manual of Medical Therapeutics: The Washington Manual, 27th Ed. Boston: Little, Brown and Company, 1992:179–195.

48. Tarpy SP, Celli BR. Long-term oxygen therapy. N Engl J Med 1995;333:710–714.

49. Bruera E, de Stoutz N, Velasco-Leiva A, Schoeller T, Hanson J. Effects of oxygen on dyspnoea in hypoxaemic terminal-cancer patients. Lancet 1993;342:13–14.

50. Bruera E, Schoeller T, MacEachern T. Symptomatic benefit of supplemental oxygen in hypoxemic patients with terminal cancer: the use of the N of 1 randomized controlled trial. J Pain Symptom Manage 1992;7:365–368.

51. Woodcock AA, Gross ER, Geddes DM. Oxygen relieves breathlessness in "pink puffers." Lancet 1981:907–909.

52. Woodcock AA, Gross ER, Gellert A, Shah S, Johnson M, Geddes DM. Effects of dihydrocodeine, alcohol, and caffeine on breathlessness and exercise tolerance in patients with chronic obstructive lung disease and normal blood gases. N Engl J Med 1981;305:1611–1616.

53. Bruera E, Macmillan K, Pither J, MacDonald RN. Effects of morphine on the dyspnea of terminal cancer patients. J Pain Symptom Manage 1990;5:6:341–344.

54. Bruera E, MacEachern T, Ripamonti C, Hanson J. Subcutaneous morphine for dyspnea in cancer patients. Ann Intern Med 1993;119:906–907.

55. Cohen MH, Johnston Anderson A, Krasnow SH, et al. Continuous intravenous infusion of morphine for severe dyspnea. South Med J 1991;84:229–234.

56. Light RW, Muro JR, Sato RI, Stansbury DW, Fischer CE, Brown SE. Effects of oral morphine on breathlessness and exercise tolerance in patients with chronic obstructive pulmonary disease. Am Rev Respir Dis 1989;139:126–133.

57. Masood AR, Subhan MMF, Reed JW, Thomas SHL. Effects of inhaled nebulized morphine on ventilation and breathlessness during exercise in healthy man. Clin Sci (Colch) 1995;88: 447–452.

58. Robin ED, Burke CM. Single-patient randomized clinical trial: opiates for intractable dyspnea. Chest 1986;90:888–892.

59. Johnson MA, Woodcock AA, Geddes DM. Dihydrocodeine for breathlessness in "pink puffers." BMJ 1983;286:675–677.

60. Sackner MA. Effects of hydrocodone bitartrate on breathing pattern of patients with chronic obstructive pulmonary disease and restrictive lung disease. Mt Sinai J Med 1984;51: 222–226.

61. Timmis AD, Rothman MT, Henderson MA, Geal PW, Chamberlain DA. Haemodynamic effects of intravenous morphine in patients with acute myocardial infarction complicated by severe left ventricular failure. BMJ 1980;280:980–982.

62. Rice KL, Kronenberg RS, Hedemark LL, Niewoehner DE. Effects of chronic administration of codeine and promethazine on breathlessness and exercise tolerance in patients with chronic airflow obstruction. Br J Dis Chest 1987;81:287–292.

63. Eiser N, Denman WT, West C, Luce P. Oral diamorphine: lack of effect on dyspnoea and exercise tolerance in the "pink puffer" syndrome. Eur Respir J 1991;4:926–931.

64. Boyd KJ, Kelly M. Oral morphine as symptomatic treatment of dyspnoea in patients with advanced cancer. Palliat Med 1997;11:277–281.

65. Poole PJ, Veale AG, Black PN. The effect of sustained-release morphine on breathlessness and quality of life in severe chronic obstructive pulmonary disease. Am J Respir Crit Care Med 1998;157:1877–1880.

66. Belvisi MG, Chung KF, Jackson DM, Barnes PJ. Opioid modulation of non-cholinergic neural bronchoconstriction in guinea-pig in-vivo. Br J Pharmacol 1988;95:413–418.

67. Young IH, Daviskas E, Keena VA. Effect of low dose nebulised morphine on exercise endurance in patients with chronic lung disease. Thorax 1989;44:387–390.

68. Farncombe M, Chater S. Case studies outlining use of nebulized morphine for patients with end-stage chronic lung and cardiac disease. J Pain Symptom Manage 1993;8:221–225.

69. Farncombe M, Chater S, Gillin A. The use of nebulized opioids for breathlessness: a chart review. Palliat Med 1994;8:306–312.

70. MacLeod RD, King BJ, Potter M. Relieving breathlessness with nebulized morphine. Palliat Med 1995;9:169.

71. Tooms A, McKenzie A, Grey H. Nebulised morphine. Lancet 1993;342:1123–1124.

72. Zeppetella G. Nebulized morphine in the palliation of dyspnoea. Palliat Med 1997;11: 267–275.

73. Harris-Eze AO, Sridhar G, Clemens RE, Zintel TA, Gallagher CG, Marciniuk DD. Low-dose nebulized morphine does not improve exercise in interstitial lung disease. Am J Respir Crit Care Med 1995;152:1940–1945.

74. Masood AR, Reed JW, Thomas SHL. Lack of effect of inhaled morphine on exercise-induced breathlessness in chronic obstructive pulmonary disease. Thorax 1995;50:629–634.

75. Beauford W, Saylor TT, Stansbury DW, Avalos K, Light RW. Effects of nebulized morphine sulfate on the exercise tolerance of the ventilatory limited COPD patient. Chest 1993;104: 175–178.

76. Leung R, Hill P, Burdon JGW. Effect of inhaled morphine on the development of breathlessness during exercise in patients with chronic lung disease. Thorax 1996;51:596–600.

77. Davis CL, Hodder C, Love S, Shah R, Slevin M, Wedzicha J. Effect of nebulised morphine and morphine 6–glucuronide on exercise endurance in patients with chronic obstructive pulmonary disease. Thorax 1994;49:393P.

78. Noseda A, Carpiaux JP, Markstein C, Meyvaert A, de Maertelaer V. Disabling dyspnoea in patients with advanced disease: lack of effect of nebulized morphine. Eur Respir J 1997;10:1079–1083.

79. Lang E, Jedeikin R. Acute respiratory depression as a complication of nebulised morphine. Can J Anaesth 1998;45:60–62.

80. Ellershaw JE, Sutcliffe JM, Saunders CM. Dehydration and the dying patient. J Pain Symptom Manage 1995;10:192–197.

81. Wilson RH, Hoseth W, Dempsey ME. Respiratory acidosis: I. Effects of decreasing respiratory minute volume in patients with severe chronic pulmonary emphysema, with specific reference to oxygen, morphine and barbiturates. Am J Med 1954;17:464–470.

82. Dudgeon DJ, Rosenthal S. Management of dyspnea and cough in patients with cancer. Hematol Oncol Clin North Am 1996;10:157–171.

83. Dudgeon D. Dyspnea: Ethical Concerns. J Palliat Care 1994;10:48–51.

84. Twycross R. Morphine and dyspnoea. In: Pain Relief in Advanced Cancer. New York: Churchill Livingstone, 1994:383–399.

85. O'Neill PA, Morton PB, Stark RD. Chlorpromazine—a specific effect on breathlessness? Br J Clin Pharmacol 1985;19:793–797.

86. Woodcock AA, Gross ER, Geddes DM. Drug treatment of breathlessness: contrasting effects of diazepam and promethazine in pink puffers. BMJ 1981;283:343–346.

87. McIver B, Walsh D, Nelson K. The use of chlorpromazine for symptom control in dying cancer patients. J Pain Symptom Manage 1994;9: 341–345.

88. Sen D, Jones G, Leggat PO. The response of the breathless patient treated with diazepam. Bri J Clin Pract 1983;37:232–233.

89. Mitchell-Heggs P, Murphy K, Minty K, et al. Diazepam in the treatment of dyspnoea in the "pink puffer" syndrome. Q J Med 1980;49: 9–20.

90. Greene JG, Pucino F, Carlson JD, Storsved M, Strommen GL. Effects of alprazolam on respiratory drive, anxiety, and dyspnea in chronic airflow obstruction: a case study. Pharmacotherapy 1989;9:34–38.

91. Man GCW, Hsu K, Sproule BJ. Effect of alprazolam on exercise and dyspnea in patients with chronic obstructive pulmonary disease. Chest 1986;90:832–836.

92. Eimer M, Cable T, Gal P, Rothenberger LA, McCue JD. Effects of clorazepate on breathlessness and exercise tolerance in patients with chronic airflow obstruction. J Fam Pract 1985;21: 359–362.

93. Argyropoulou P, Patakas D, Koukou A, Vasiliadis P, Georgopoulos D. Buspirone effect on breathlessness and exercise performance in patients with chronic obstructive pulmonary disease. Respiration 1993;60:216–220.

94. Light RW, Stansbury DW, Webster JS. Effect of 30 mg of morphine alone or with promethazine or prochlorperazine on the exercise capacity of patients with COPD. Chest 1996;109: 975–981.

95. Ventafridda V, Spoldi E, De Conno F. Control of dyspnea in advanced cancer patients. Chest 1990;98:1544–1545.

96. O'Neill PA, Stark RD, Morton PB. Do prostaglandins have a role in breathlessness? Am Rev Respir Dis 1985;132:22–24.

97. O'Neill PA, Stretton TB, Stark RD, Ellis SH. The effect of indomethacin on breathlessness in patients with diffuse parenchymal disease of the lung. Br J Dis Chest 1986;80:72–79.

98. Schiffman GL, Stansbury DW, Fischer CE, Sato RI, Light RW, Brown SE. Indomethacin and perception of dyspnea in chronic airflow limitation. Am Rev Respir Dis 1988;137:1094–1098.

99. Winning AJ, Hamilton RD, Shea SA, Knott C, Guz A. The effect of airway anaesthesia on the control of breathing and the sensation of breathlessness in man. Clin Sci (Colch) 1985;68: 215–225.

100. Winning AJ, Hamilton RD, Guz A. Ventilation and breathlessness on maximal exercise in patients with interstitial lung disease after local anaesthetic aerosol inhalation. Clin Sci (Colch) 1988;74:275–281.

101. Wilcock A, Corcoran R, Tattersfield AE. Safety and efficacy of nebulized lignocaine in patients with cancer and breathlessness. Palliat Med 1994;8:35–38.

102. Giron AE, Stansbury DW, Fischer CE, Light RW. Lack of effect of dextromethorphan on breathlessness and exercise performance in patients with chronic obstructive pulmonary disease (COPD). Eur Respir J 1991;4:532–535.

103. Tiep BL. Inpatient pulmonary rehabilitation. A team approach to the more fragile patient. Postgrad Med 1989;86:141–150.

104. Grey A. The nursing management of dyspnoea in palliative care. Nurs Times 1995;91: 33–35.

105. Hughes AC, Wilcock A, Corcoran R. Management of death rattle. J Pain Symptom Manage 1996;12:271–272.

106. Morita T, Ichiki T, Tsunoda J, Inoue S, Chihara S. A prospective study on the dying process in terminally ill cancer patients. Am J Hospice Palliat Care 1998;15:217–222.

107. Bennett MI. Death rattle: an audit of hyoscine (scopolamine) use and review of management. J Pain Symptom Manage 1996;12:229–233.

108. Nadel JA. Regulation of airway secretions. Chest 1985;87:111S–113S.

109. Kaliner M, Shelhamer H, Borson B, Nadel JA, Patow C, Marom Z. Human respiratory mucus. Am Rev Respir Dis 1986;134:612–621.

110. Medical Care of the Dying, 3rd Ed. Victoria: Victoria Hospice Society, 1998.

111. Andrews MR, Levine AM. Dehydration in the terminal patient: perception of hospice nurses. Am J Hosp Care 1989;6:31–34.

112. Lichter I, Hunt E. The last 48 hours of life. J Palliat Care 1990;6:7–15.

113. Dawson HR. The use of transdermal scopolamine in the control of death rattle. J Palliat Care 1989;5:31–33.

114. Fuller RW, Jackson DM. Physiology and treatment of cough. Thorax 1990;45:425–430.

115. Dudgeon D, Rosenthal S. Pathophysiology and assessment of dyspnea in the patient with cancer. In: Portenoy RK, Bruera E, eds. Topics in Palliative Care. New York: Oxford University Press, 2000, p. 237–254.

116. Hagen NA. An approach to cough in cancer patients. J Pain Symptom Manage 1991;6: 257–262.

117. Eddy NB, Friebel H, Hahn KJ, Halbach H. Codeine and its alternatives for pain and cough relief. Potential alternatives for cough relief. Bull WHO 1969;40:639–719.

118. Eddy NB, Friebel H, Hahn KJ, Halbach H. Codeine and its alternatives for pain and cough relief. Discussion and summary. Bull WHO 1969; 40:721–730.

119. Doona M, Walsh D. Benzonatate for opioid-resistant cough in advanced cancer. Palliat Med 1997;12:55–58.

120. Lowry R, Wood A, Johnson T, Higenbottam T. Antitussive properties of inhaled bronchodilators on induced cough. Chest 1988;93: 1186–1189.

121. Louie K, Bertolino M, Fainsinger R. Management of intractable cough. J Palliat Care 1992;8:46–48.

122. Howard P, Cayton RM, Brennan SR, Anderson PB. Lignocaine aerosol and persistent cough. Br J Dis Chest 1977;71:19–24.

123. Sanders RV, Kirkpatrick MB. Prolonged suppression of cough after inhalation of lidocaine in a patient with sarcoid. JAMA 1984;252:2456–2457.

14 Urinary Tract Disorders

MIKEL GRAY and FERN G. CAMPBELL

Didi's end was painful, incontinent of urine and feces which caused so much pain. It was hard during the last month, giving her pills, narcotics, drugging her out, and yet having to give them because of the pain. And the indignity. It created such ambivalence.

—Family caregiver

The urinary system is frequently the cause of bothersome or deleterious symptoms that affect the patient receiving palliative care. A malignancy or systemic disease may affect voiding function and produce urinary incontinence (UI), urinary retention, or upper urinary tract obstruction. Typical lower urinary tract symptoms (LUTS) include intermittent or continuous urinary leakage, diurnal frequency, nocturia, urgency, feelings of incomplete bladder emptying, or the abrupt cessation of urination. Upper urinary tract symptoms include flank or abdominal pain and constitutional symptoms related to acute renal insufficiency or failure.

Urinary system disorders may be directly attributable to a malignancy, systemic disease, or a specific treatment such as radiation or chemotherapy. This chapter reviews urinary tract disorders commonly encountered when providing palliative care, including UI, bladder spasms, urinary stasis or retention, and hematuria.

LOWER URINARY TRACT DISORDERS

Lower Urinary Tract Physiology

The lower urinary tract comprises the bladder, urethra, and supportive structures within the pelvic floor. Together, these structures maintain *urinary continence*, which can be simply defined as control over bladder filling and storage and the act of micturition. Continence is modulated by three interrelated factors: *(1)* anatomic integrity of the urinary tract, *(2)* control of the detrusor muscle, and *(3)* competence of the urethral sphincter mechanism.[1,2] Each may be compromised in the patient receiving palliative care, leading to UI, urinary retention, or a combination of these disorders.

Anatomic Integrity. From a physiological perspective, the urinary system comprises a long tube originating in the glomerulus and terminating at the urethral meatus. When contemplating urinary continence, anatomic integrity of the urinary system is often assumed, particularly since extraurethral UI is uncommon. However, anatomic integrity may be lost in the patient receiving palliative care due to a fistula that bypasses the urethral sphincter. This epithelialized tract allows continuous urinary leakage, which varies from an ongoing dribble in a patient with otherwise normal urine elimination habits to total UI characterized by failure of bladder filling and micturition.[3]

Control of the Detrusor. In addition to a structurally intact urinary system, continence requires volitional control over detrusor contraction.[1,2] Control of this smooth muscle can be conceptualized on three levels. Multiple modulatory centers within the central nervous system modulate the detrusor reflex, allowing inhibition of detrusor activity until the person wishes to urinate. Detrusor control is also influenced by its histological characteristics. On a molecular level, detrusor control relies on neurotransmitters that stimulate or inhibit its tone.

The nervous control of the detrusor relies on input from multiple modulatory areas within the brain and spinal cord.[4] Bilateral detrusor motor areas are found within the lobes of the frontal cortex.[5] This modulatory center interacts with neurons in the thalamus,[6] hypothalamus,[7] basal ganglia,[8] and cerebellum[9] to modulate bladder filling and voiding. The net effect of these areas on continence is the maintenance of a stable detrusor that does not contract, even when provoked, until the person desires to urinate.[1,2]

While modulatory centers within the brain are essential for continence, the primary integration centers for bladder filling and micturition are found within the brain stem.[10] Specific areas within the brain stem control bladder filling and storage under the influence of higher brain regions, and a pontine micturition center initiates the detrusor contraction necessary for normal micturition while coordinating the reflexive response of the urethral sphincter mechanism. Recognition of the significance of the brain stem micturition center is particularly important when providing palliative care since a neurological lesion above the brain stem causes urge UI with a coordinated sphincter response, while lesions below this center affect bladder sensations and the coordination between the detrusor and the urethral sphincter.

The brain stem micturition center communicates with the bladder via spinal roots in the thoracolumbar and sacral segments.[4] Segments in the thoracolumbar spine (T10–L2) carry sympathetic nervous impulses that promote bladder filling and storage, while segments S2–S4 transmit parasympathetic impulses to the bladder wall, allowing micturition under the modulation of the brain and brain stem. These impulses are carried through several peripheral nerve plexus, including the pelvic and inferior hypogastric plexus.

Histological characteristics of the detrusor also contribute to its voluntary control.[11] Unlike the visceral smooth muscle of the bowel, stomach, or ureter, the detrusor muscle bundles are innervated on an almost one-to-one basis. They also lack the gap junctions, observed in other visceral organs, needed to propagate a contraction independent of nervous stimulation. These characteristics promote urinary continence since they discourage spontaneous contractions of the detrusor in response to the bladder filling characteristic of other visceral organs.

On a molecular level, specific chemical substances, commonly called neurotransmitters, exert local control over the detrusor muscle.[12] Several neurotransmitters are released from the axons of neurons within the bladder wall and act at specific receptors to produce smooth muscle contraction or relaxation. Norepinephrine acts through beta-adrenergic receptors, causing detrusor muscle relaxation, and acetylcholine acts through cholinergic receptors, leading to detrusor contraction and micturition. While it has long been known that the cholinergic receptors within the detrusor are muscarinic, physiological studies have identified at least five muscarinic receptor subtypes (M1 through M5).[13] Receptors M2 and M3 predominate within the bladder wall and are primarily responsible for the detrusor contraction that leads to micturition. Identification of these receptor subtypes is clinically relevant because it has facilitated the development of drugs that act upon the bladder but produce fewer side effects than the older (nonselective) drugs traditionally used to manage urge UI or bladder spasms.

Competence of the Urethral Sphincter Mechanism. The urethral sphincter comprises a combination of compressive and tension elements to form a watertight seal against urinary leakage, even when challenged by physical exertion or sudden increases in abdominal pressure caused by coughing, laughing, or sneezing.[1,2] The soft urethral mucosa interacts with mucosal secretions and the submucosal vascular cushion to ensure a watertight seal that rapidly conforms to changes. While the elements of compression provide a watertight seal for the urethra, striated and smooth muscle within the urethral wall and within the surrounding pelvic floor are necessary when sphincter closure is challenged by physical exertion. The muscular elements of the urethral sphincter comprise the smooth muscle of the bladder neck and proximal urethra (including the prostatic urethra in men), the rhabdosphincter, and the periurethral striated muscles. The efficiency of these muscles requires both neurological modulation from the brain and spinal cord and support from the endopelvic fascia and adjacent pelvic floor muscles to maintain continence.

Pathophysiology of Urinary Incontinence

Urinary incontinence is defined as the uncontrolled loss of urine of sufficient magnitude to create a problem.[14] It is initially characterized as acute or chronic, according to its presentation and underlying pathophysiology. Causes of acute UI may be classified according to the DIAPERS pneumonic (Table 14–1). Several conditions, including acute delirium, restricted mobility, stool impaction, and specific medications may occur in patients receiving palliative care and should be considered when assessing and managing UI.

Chronic UI is subdivided into types according to its presenting symptoms or underlying pathophysiology. For the purposes of this discussion, the pathophysiological system outlined by Gray and Dougherty[15] will be used to classify chronic UI. Stress UI occurs when physical stress (exertion) causes urine loss in the absence of a detrusor contraction. Two conditions lead to stress UI, urethral hypermobility and intrinsic sphincter deficiency. While urethral hypermobility is rarely the primary cause of significant stress UI in the patient re-

Table 14–1. Causes of Acute Urinary Incontinence (UI)

Delirium	Acute delirium may cause functional UI, which resolves when underlying disease and related delirium subside.
Infection	A urinary tract infection may cause or exacerbate UI.
Atrophic urethritis	Although atrophic urethritis has been associated with irritative voiding symptoms and stress UI, hormone replacement therapy has not been shown to alleviate associated UI.
Pharmacy	Multiple drugs may contribute to UI.
	Opioids, sedatives, antidepressants, antipsychotics, and antiparkinsonian drugs suppress detrusor contractility and increase the risk of urinary retention and overflow UI. Alpha-adrenergic blocking agents may cause stress UI in women. Alpha-adrenergic agonists increase smooth muscle tone in the male urethra and raise the risk of acute urinary retention.
Excessive urine production	Diabetes mellitus or insipidus causes polyuria and subsequent UI.
Restricted mobility	Restriction of mobility leads to UI when it prevents access to toileting facilities.
Stool impaction	Stool impaction increases the risk of UI, urinary retention, and urinary tract infection.

Table 14–2. Causes of Intrinsic Sphincter Deficiency in the Patient Receiving Palliative Care

Urethral surgery
Radical prostatectomy
Transurethral prostatectomy
Cryosurgery
Multiple urethral suspensions in women
Surgery indirectly affecting the urethra via local denervation
Abdominoperineal resection
Pelvic exenteration
Radical hysterectomy
Neurological lesions of the lower spine
Primary or metastatic tumors of the sacral spine
Pathological fracture of the sacral spinal column
Multiple sclerosis
Tertiary syphilis

ceiving palliative care, intrinsic sphincter deficiency may compromise sphincter closure and lead to severe urinary leakage. Intrinsic sphincter deficiency occurs when the nerves or muscles necessary for sphincter closure are denervated or damaged.[16] Table 14–2 lists conditions likely to cause intrinsic sphincter deficiency among patients receiving palliative care.

Instability UI occurs when unstable (overactive) detrusor contractions produce urinary leakage.[14] It can be subdivided into urge and reflex UI, based on the symptoms it produces and its underlying cause. Urge UI is characterized by a precipitous desire to urinate followed by urinary leakage unless the patient rapidly gains access to a toilet. In contrast, while reflex UI is also caused by overactive detrusor function, it produces little or no sensation of urgency, owing to denervation of afferent sensory pathways from the lower urinary tract. In addition, since reflex UI results from a neurological lesion below the brain stem micturition center, it also causes loss of coordination between the detrusor and sphincter muscles (detrusor-sphincter dyssynergia).

Functional UI occurs when deficits in mobility, dexterity, or cognition cause or contribute to urinary leakage.[17] A variety of conditions may produce functional UI in the patient receiving palliative care. For example, neurological deficits or pain may reduce the patient's ability to reach the toilet in a timely fashion. Cognitive deficits caused by malignancies or diseases of the brain may predispose the patient to functional UI. In addition, sedative or analgesic medications may reduce awareness of bladder fullness and the need to urinate, particularly in the patient who experiences nocturia.

Extraurethral UI occurs when a fistula creates an opening between the bladder and the vagina or skin, allowing urine to bypass the urethral sphincter. Within the context of the patient receiving palliative care, fistulae are usually caused by invasive pelvic or gynecological malignancies, extensive pelvic surgery, or radiation treatment.[3]

ASSESSMENT AND MANAGEMENT OF URINARY INCONTINENCE

The results of a focused history, physical assessment, urinalysis, and bladder log are essential to the evaluation of UI in the patient receiving palliative care. Urine culture and sensitivity testing, blood tests, urodynamic evaluation, or imaging studies also may be completed in specific cases.

The history focuses on the duration of the problem and the likely UI type. Acute UI is typically characterized by a sudden occurrence of symptoms or by an acute exacerbation of preexisting symptoms. These symptoms are typically similar to urge or stress UI. In contrast, chronic or established UI usually evolves over a period of time, typically weeks to months or possibly years.

The history can also be used to provide clues about the type of chronic UI. Stress UI is characterized by urine loss occurring with physical exertion or a sudden increase in abdominal pressure caused by coughing or sneezing. Urge UI is more difficult to diagnose when relying on reported symptoms.[18] It is typically present when the patient reports a combination of diurnal frequency (voids more often than every 2 hours while awake), nocturia (awakened two or more times per night by the need to urinate), and the symptom of urge UI (urinary leakage associated with a sudden desire to urinate). However, its presence cannot be accurately inferred from a report of the symptom of urge UI alone.

Reflex UI is suspected in the patient who experiences a paralyzing neurological lesion affecting spinal segments below the brain stem and above S2. The patient frequently reports periodic urination with little or no warning and little or no associated urgency. The urinary stream may be intermittent (stuttering), and the patient may perceive a sensation of incomplete bladder emptying or report additional urinary leakage soon after completing micturition.

Functional UI is suspected when a general evaluation of the patient reveals significant limitations in mobility, dexterity, or cognition. Continuous urinary leakage that is not associated with physical exertion raises the suspicion of extraurethral UI associated with a fistula, but it is also associated with severe stress UI caused by intrinsic sphincter deficiency.

A focused physical examination provides additional evidence concerning the UI type and its severity. A general examination is used to evaluate the presence of functional UI and to determine the influence of functional limitations on other types of UI. A pelvic examination is completed to assess perineal skin integrity, to identify the presence of obvious fistulae or severe sphincter incompetence, and to evaluate local neurological function. Altered skin integrity, particularly when accompanied by a monilial rash or chemical dermatitis, indicates high-volume (severe) urinary leakage. In certain cases, the source of severe leakage can be easily identified as a large fistula or massive intrinsic sphincter deficiency associated with a gaping (patulous) urethra. A local neurological examination, focusing on local sensations, pelvic floor muscle tone, and the presence of the bulbocavernosus reflex provides clues to underlying neurological problems leading to voiding dysfunction.

A bladder log (a written record of the timing of urination, volume, and timing of UI episodes and/or fluid intake) is useful because it allows a semiquantitative analysis of the patterns of urinary elimination, UI, and associated symptoms. A bladder log also may be used to assess fluid intake or the patient's response to prompted voiding. Ideally, a bladder log is maintained for 7 days, but data obtained from 1- to 3-day logs can be valuable.[19]

Urinalysis serves several useful purposes in the evaluation of the patient with UI. The presence of nitrites and leukocytes on dipstick analysis or bacteriuria and pyuria on microscopic analysis indicates a clinically relevant urinary tract infection. Blood in the urine may coexist with a urinary tract infection, or it may indicate significant hematuria demanding prompt management (see Hematuria, below). In the patient receiving palliative care, glucosuria may indicate poorly controlled diabetes mellitus causing osmotic diuresis and subsequent UI. In contrast, a low specific gravity may indicate diabetes mellitus or excessive fluid intake from oral or parenteral sources.

Other diagnostic tests are completed when indicated. For example, a urine culture and sensitivity are obtained when urinalysis reveals bacteriuria and pyuria, and an endoscopy is indicated when significant hematuria occurs without an obvious explanation. Urodynamic testing is indicated after acute UI is excluded and when simpler examinations fail to establish an accurate diagnosis leading to an effective plan for management.

The management of UI is based on its type, the desires of the patient and family, and the presence of complicating factors. Acute UI is managed by addressing its underlying cause.[20] A urinary tract infection should be treated with sensitivity-driven antibiotics. Similarly, medication regimens are altered as feasible when they produce or exacerbate UI. Atrophic urethritis may be managed with local hormone replacement when feasible. Alternatively, topical vitamin E preparations may offer some benefit when hormone replacement therapy is contraindicated. Fecal impaction must be relieved and constipation aggressively managed using a combination of fluids and fiber. Following disimpaction, a scheduled elimination program is frequently indicated. This program usually combines a peristaltic stimulant, such as a warm cup of coffee or tea or a suppository and a scheduled elimination program. In addition, stool softeners or laxatives may be used when simpler programs fail to alleviate constipation. Refer to Chapter 11 for a detailed discussion of bowel elimination problems.

A number of techniques are used to manage chronic or established UI. Every patient should be counseled about lifestyle alterations that may alleviate or occasionally relieve UI and associated LUTS.[21,22] Patients are advised to avoid routinely restricting fluid intake to reduce UI since this strategy only increases the risk of constipation and concentrates the urine irritating the bladder wall. Instead, they are counseled to obtain the recommended daily allowance for fluids (30 ml/kg or 0.5 oz/lb),[23] to sip fluids throughout the day, and to avoid intake of large volumes of fluids over a brief period of time. Patients may also be taught to reduce or avoid bladder irritants that increase urine production or stimulate detrusor muscle tone, including caffeine and alcohol, depending on the goals of care and short-term prognosis.

Containment devices may be used to provide protection while treatments designed to address underlying UI are undertaken, or they may be used for added protection if these interventions improve but fail to eradicate urine loss.[24] Women and men should be counseled about the disadvantages of using home products and feminine hygiene pads when attempting to contain urine. Specifically, they should be counseled that home products, such as tissues or paper towels, are not designed to contain urine and feminine hygiene products are designed to contain menstrual flow. As an alternative, patients should be advised about products specifically designed for UI, including disposable and reusable products, inserted pads, and containment undergarments.

Patients who experience primarily stress UI are initially managed with behavioral methods. Pelvic floor muscle training is strongly recommended for mild to moderate stress UI.[25] Ideally, visual biofeedback is used to assist the patient to identify, isolate, and contract the pelvic floor muscles. When visual biofeedback is not available, vaginal palpation may be used to assist the patient to identify and contract the pelvic muscles. This task may be supplemented by asking the patient to occasionally interrupt the urinary stream during micturition, but this maneuver should not be routinely employed since it interferes with the efficiency of bladder evacuation. After the patient demonstrates mastery of muscle identification, isolation, and contraction, he or she is taught the "knack" of pelvic muscle contractions in response to physical exertion.[26] This maneuver increases urethral closure and resistance to UI and relieves or sometimes corrects stress UI.

Medications also may be used to treat mild to moderate stress UI.[27] Alpha-adrenergic agonists, including pseudoephedrine and phenylpropanolamine, are available in over-the-counter preparations, such as Sudafed SA and Dexatrim without caffeine, respectively. Other medications are available via prescription, including the combination of quaifenesin and phenylpropanolamine (Entex LA) and imipramine. Imipramine is a tricyclic antidepressant with both alpha-adrenergic effects that increase urethral resistance and anticholinergic actions useful when patients experience mixed stress and urge UI. While these medications are often effective at alleviating stress UI, their potential benefits must be weighed carefully against their side effects. In addition to enhancing urethral sphincter closure, alpha-adrenergic agonists may cause tachycardia, restlessness, insomnia, and hypertension. Imipramine may produce these side effects as well as anticholinergic effects, including dry mouth, blurred vision, flushing, and heat intolerance. It also may affect the central nervous system, leading cognitive dysfunction, hallucinations, and nightmares. These side effects may be particularly significant in aged patients or persons with preexisting cognitive defects related to a primary disease or disorder.

An indwelling catheter may be indicated when intrinsic sphincter deficiency and subsequent stress UI are severe. Although not usually indicated, a larger catheter size may be required, to prevent urinary leakage (bypassing) around the catheter.[28] A detailed discussion on catheter management is provided below, see Managing the Indwelling Catheter.

Urge UI is also managed by behavioral and/or pharmacological modalities when possible.[29] In addition to the lifestyle and dietary factors discussed earlier, biofeedback methods are used to allow the patient to identify and contract the pelvic muscles. These skills are applied to a technique called urge suppression, which is used to inhibit specific episodes of urgency before UI occurs. When a sudden urge to urinate occurs, the patient is taught to stop, tighten the pelvic muscles in rapid succession using several "quick flick" contractions until the urge has subsided, and to proceed to the bathroom at a normal pace. The patient also may be taught relaxation or other distraction techniques to cope with specific urge episodes. Behavioral methods are particularly helpful for the patient who is at risk for falling and related injuries.

Anticholinergic or antispasmodic medications also may be used to manage urge UI. A variety of agents are available, although we prefer two relatively new drugs, tolterodine (Detrol) and extended-release oxybutynin (Ditropan XL) because they are associated with fewer side effects when compared to other medications used to manage urge UI.[30,31] Anticholinergic medications work by increasing the functional bladder capacity, inhibiting unstable detrusor contractions and reducing urinary frequency. The principal side effect is dry mouth, which can be severe and interfere with appetite and mastication.[27] Other side effects include blurred vision, constipation, flushing, heat intolerance, and cognitive effects such as nightmares or altered short-term memory. While antispasmodic medications are often viewed as an alternative to behavioral therapies, they are better viewed as complementary modalities. Specifically, all patients who wish to use anticholinergic medications for urge UI should be advised to void according to a timed schedule (usually every 2 to 3 hours, depending on the urinary frequency documented on a bladder log obtained during assessment) and taught urge-suppression skills. Similarly, patients whose urge UI is not managed adequately by behavioral methods should be counseled about anticholinergic medications before recommending placement of an indwelling catheter.

Intermittent catheterization or an indwelling catheter may be used in selected cases when urge UI is severe and the patient proves refractory to other treatments. It is also indicated when urge UI is complicated by clinically relevant urinary retention or when the patient is near death and immobile.

Because reflex UI is typically associated with diminished sensations of bladder filling, it is not typically responsive to behavioral treatments.[32] A minority of patients with reflex UI retain the ability to urinate spontaneously, but the majority must be managed with an alternative program. For men, a condom catheter may be used to contain urine. A condom that is latex-free is typically selected. In some patients, an alpha-adrenergic blocking agent such as terazosin, doxazosin, or Tamsulosin is administered, to minimize obstruction caused by detrusor-sphincter dyssynergia. Intermittent catheterization is encouraged whenever feasible. The patient and at least one significant other should be taught a clean intermittent catheterization technique. For the patient with reflex UI, an anticholinergic medication is usually required in addition to catheterization, to prevent UI. When intermittent catheterization is not feasible, an indwelling catheter may be used to manage reflex UI. While the indwelling catheter is associated with serious long-term complications and avoided in the spinal cord–injured patient with a significant life expectancy, it is a more attractive alternative for the patient receiving palliative care.

Functional UI is treated by minimizing barriers to toileting and the time required to prepare for urination.[33,34] Strategies designed to remove barriers to toileting are highly individualized and best designed using a multidisciplinary team, combining nursing with physical and occupational therapy as indicated. Strategies used to maximize mobility and access to the toilet include the use of assistive devices such as a walker or wheelchair, widening bathroom doors, adding support bars, or providing a bedside toilet or urinal. The time required for toileting may be reduced by selected alterations in the patient's clothing such as substituting tennis shoes with good traction for slippers or other footwear with slicker soles and substituting Velcro- or elastic-banded clothing for articles with multiple buttons, zippers, or snaps.

Patients with significant cognitive disorders contributing to functional UI are usually managed by a prompted voiding program.[35,36] Baseline evaluation includes a specialized bladder log, which is completed over a 48- to 72-hour period. The caregiver is taught to assist the patient to void on a fixed schedule, usually every 2 to 3 hours. The caregiver is taught to help the patient move to the toilet and prepare for urination; the caregiver also uses this opportunity to determine whether the pad incontinence brief reveals evidence of UI since the previous scheduled toileting. Patients who are successful (dry and able to urinate with prompting) during the majority of attempts completed during this trial period are considered good candidates for an ongoing prompted voiding regimen, while those who are unsuccessful are considered poor candidates and are managed using alternative methods, including indwelling catheterization in selected cases.

Because extraurethral UI is caused by a fistulous tract and produces continuous urinary leakage, it must be initially managed by containment devices and preventive skin care.[3] The type of containment device depends on the severity of the UI; an incontinent brief is frequently required. Preventive skin care consists of routine cleansing with water and an incontinence cleanser or mild soap, followed by thorough drying using a soft towel and hair dryer on the low (cool) setting. Additionally, a skin barrier may be applied when altered skin integrity is particularly likely.

In some cases, the fistula may be closed using conservative (nonsurgical) means. Initially, an indwelling catheter is inserted and the fistula allowed to heal spontaneously.[37] This intervention is most likely to work when repairing a traumatic (post-operative) fistula. Unfortunately, when a fistula is caused by an invasive tumor or following radiation therapy, it is not as likely to heal spontaneously. In this case, cauterization and a fibrin glue may be used to promote closure.[38] Alternatively, a suspension containing tetracycline or a related antibiotic may be prepared and used as a sclerosing agent. The adjacent skin is prepared by applying a skin barrier, such as a petrolatum-based ointment, to protect it from the sclerosing agent. A small volume of the agent, perhaps 5 to 10 ml, is then injected into the fistula by a physician and the fistula monitored for signs of scarring and closure. If UI persists for 15 days or longer, the procedure may be repeated under the physician's direction. For larger fistulae or those that fail to respond to conservative measures, surgical repair is undertaken when feasible.

URINARY STASIS OR RETENTION

A precipitous drop or sudden cessation of urinary outflow is a serious urinary system complication that may indicate oliguria or *anuria* (failure of the kidneys to filter the blood and produce urine), *urinary statis* (blockage of urine transport from the upper to lower urinary tracts), or *urinary retention* (failure of the bladder to evacuate itself of urine). This chapter reviews the pathophysiology and management of urinary stasis or acute postrenal failure caused by bilateral ureteral obstruction and urinary retention.

Obstruction of the Upper Urinary Tract

Upper urinary tract stasis in the patient receiving palliative care is usually caused by obstruction of one or both ureters.[39] The obstruction is typically attributable to a primary or metastatic tumor; most arise from the pelvic region. In men, prostatic cancer is the most common, while cervical cancers produce most ureteral obstructions in women. In addition to malignancies, retroperitoneal fibrosis secondary to inflammation or radiation may obstruct one or both ureters. Unless promptly relieved, bilateral ureteral obstruction leads to acute renal failure with uremia and elevated serum potassium, which will compromise cardiac function unless promptly managed.

When a single ureter is obstructed, the bladder will continue to fill with urine from the contralateral (unobstructed) kidney. In this case, urinary stasis will produce symptoms of ureteral or renal colic. Left untreated, the affected kidney is prone to acute failure and infection, and it may produce systemic hypertension because of increased renin secretion.

Urinary Retention

Urinary retention is the inability to empty the urinary bladder despite micturition.[40] Acute urinary retention is the sudden inability to void. Patients are almost always aware of acute urinary retention because of the increasing suprapubic discomfort produced by bladder filling and distension and the associated anxiety. Chronic urinary retention occurs when the patient is partly able to empty the bladder by voiding but a significant volume of urine remains behind. While no absolute cut-off point for chronic urinary retention can be defined, patients with a residual volume of 200 ml or more deserve further evaluation.

Urinary retention is caused by two disorders, bladder outlet obstruction or deficient detrusor contraction strength. Bladder outlet obstruction occurs when intrinsic or extrinsic factors compress the urethral outflow tract. For the patient receiving palliative care, malignant tumors of the prostate, urethra, or bladder may produce anatomic obstruction of the urethra, while lesions affecting spinal segments below the brain stem micturition center but above the sacral spine cause functional obstruction associated with detrusor-sphincter dyssynergia.[41] In addition, brachytherapy may cause inflammation and congestion of the prostate, producing a combination of urinary retention and urge UI.[42] In the patient receiving palliative care, deficient detrusor contraction strength usually occurs as a result of denervation or medication. Alternatively, it may result from histological damage to the detrusor muscle itself, usually owing to radiation therapy, or to detrusor decompensation following prolonged obstruction. Neurological lesions commonly associated with deficient detrusor contraction strength include primary or metastatic tumors affecting the sacral spine or spinal column, multiple sclerosis lesions, tertiary syphilis, and disease-causing peripheral polyneuropathies such as advanced-stage diabetes mellitus or alcoholism. Poor detrusor contractility also may occur as a result of unavoidable denervation from surgical resection of large abdominopelvic surgeries such as abdominoperineal resection or pelvic exenteration.

Assessment and Management of Upper Tract Obstruction and Urinary Retention

Accurate identification of the cause of a precipitous drop in urine output is essential since the management of upper urinary tract obstruction compared to urinary retention is different. Because both conditions cause a precipitous drop in urinary output, the LUTS reported by the patient may be similar. Both cause an inability to urinate and a dribbling, intermittent flow. However, upper urinary tract obstruction is more likely to produce flank pain, while acute urinary retention is more likely to produce discomfort localized to the suprapubic area. The flank pain associated with upper urinary tract obstruction is usually localized to one or both flanks, although it may radiate to the abdomen and even to the labia or testes if the lower ureter is obstructed. Its intensity varies from moderate to intense. It is typically not relieved by changes in position, and the patient is often restless. The discomfort associated with acute urinary retention is typically localized to the suprapubic area or the lower back. The patient with acute urinary retention also may feel restless, although this perception is usually attributable to the growing desire to urinate.

A focused physical examination should be completed. The patient with bilateral ureteral obstruction and acute renal failure may have systemic evidence of uremia, including nausea, vomiting, and hypertension. In some cases, obstruction may by complicated by pyelonephritis, causing a fever and chills. Abdominal assessment also should be completed. Physical assessment of the patient with upper urinary tract obstruction will reveal a nondistended bladder, while the bladder may be grossly distended and may extend above the umbilicus. Serum blood analysis will reveal an elevated serum creatinine, blood urea nitrogen, and potassium in the patient with bilateral ureteral obstruction; but these values are typically normal in the patient with urinary retention or unilateral ureteral obstruction.[39] Ultrasonography of the kidneys and bladder will reveal ureterohydronephrosis above the level of the obstruction or bladder distension in the patient with acute urinary retention.

In contrast to the patient with ureteral obstruction or acute urinary retention, the person with chronic retention may remain unaware of any problem, despite large residual volumes of 500 ml or more.[40] The LUTS vary and may include feelings of incomplete bladder emptying, a poor force of stream, or an intermittent urinary stream. Patients are also likely to note diurnal frequency and nocturia. While acute renal failure is uncommon in the patient with chronic urinary retention, serum creatinine may be elevated, indicating renal insufficiency attributable to lower urinary tract pathology.

Obstruction of the upper urinary tract is initially managed by reversal of fluid and electrolyte imbalances and prompt drainage.[39] Urinary outflow can be reestablished by insertion of a ureteral stent (drainage tube extending from the renal pelvis to the bladder). A ureteral stent is preferred because it avoids the need for a percutaneous puncture and a subsequent drainage bag. In the case of bilateral obstruction, a stent is placed in each ureter under ureteroscopic guidance, or a single stent is placed when unilateral obstruction is diagnosed. The patient is advised that the stent(s) will drain urine into the bladder. However, since the stents are potentially irritating, the patient is counseled to ensure adequate fluid intake while avoiding bladder irritants, including caffeine and alcohol. In certain cases, an anticholinergic medication may be administered to reduce irritative voiding symptoms associated with a ureteral stent.

If the ureter is significantly scarred because of radiation therapy or distorted because of a bulky tumor, placement of a ureteral stent may not be feasible and a nephrostomy tube may be substituted. The procedure may be done in an endoscopy suite or in an interventional radiographic suite under local and systemic sedation or anesthesia. Unlike the ureteral stent that drains into the bladder, the nephrostomy tube is drained via a collection bag. The patient and family are taught to monitor urinary output from the bag and to secure the bag to the flank or abdomen while avoiding kinking the tube. The success of placement of a ureteral stent or nephrostomy tube is measured as reduction in pain and serum creatinine and potassium, indicating reversal of acute renal insufficiency.

Acute urinary retention is managed by prompt placement of an indwelling urethral catheter.[40] The patient is closely monitored as the bladder is initially drained because of the small risk of transient hypotension and pallor. This risk may be further reduced by draining 500 ml, interrupted by a brief period where the catheter is clamped (approximately 5 minutes), and followed by further drainage until the retained urine is evacuated. The catheter is left in place for up to 1 month; this period allows the bladder to rest and recover from the overdistension typical of acute urinary retention. Following this period, the bladder may be filled with saline and the catheter removed.[43] The patient is allowed to urinate, and the voided volume is measured. This volume is compared to the volume infused, to estimate the residual volume, or a bladder ultrasound can be completed to assess the residual volume. If the patient is unable to evacuate the bladder successfully, the catheter is left out and the patient is taught to recognize and promptly manage acute urinary retention. If the patient is unable to urinate effectively, the catheter may be replaced or an intermittent catheterization program may be initiated, depending on the cause of the retention and the patient's ability to perform self-catheterization.

The patient with chronic urinary retention may be managed by behavioral techniques, intermittent catheterization, or an indwelling catheter.[40] Behavioral methods are preferred because they are noninvasive and not associated with any risk of adverse side effects. Scheduled toileting with double voiding may be used in the patient with low urinary residual volumes (approximately 200 to 400 ml). The patient is taught to attempt voiding every 3 hours while awake and to double void (urinate, wait for 3 to 5 minutes, and urinate again before leaving the bathroom). Those with higher urinary residual volumes and those with clinically relevant complications caused by urinary retention, including urinary tract infections or renal insufficiency, are usually managed by intermittent catheterization or an indwelling catheter.

Many factors enter into the choice between intermittent versus indwelling catheterization, including the desires of the patient and family, the presence of obstruction or low bladder wall compliance (a small or contracted bladder), and the prognosis. From a purely urological perspective, intermittent catheterization is preferable because it avoids long-term complications associated with an indwelling catheter, including chronic bacteriuria, calculi, urethral erosion, and catheter bypassing. However, an indwelling catheter may be preferable when the patient has a guarded prognosis, a urethra that is technically difficult to catheterize, a small capacity with low bladder wall compliance, or limited upper extremity dexterity.

MANAGING THE INDWELLING CATHETER

While the decision to insert a catheter may be directed by a physician or nurse practitioner, decisions concerning catheter size, material of construction, and drainage bag are usually made by the nurse.[28,44,45] A relatively small catheter is typically sufficient to drain urine from the bladder. In men, a 14-16 French catheter is adequate, and a 12-14 French catheter is usually adequate for women. Larger catheters (18-20 French) are reserved for patients with significant intrinsic sphincter deficiency, hematuria, or sediment in the urine. Silastic, Teflon-coated tubes are avoided when the catheter is expected to remain in place more than 2 to 3 days. Instead, a silicone- or lubricant-coated catheter is selected because of its reduced affinity for bacterial adherence and increased comfort.

In men, water-soluble lubricating jelly should be injected into the urethra prior to catheterization, and such jelly should be liberally applied to the urethral meatus and adjacent mucosa prior to catheterization in women. A lubricant containing 2% xylocaine is preferred because it reduces the discomfort associated with the procedure. The catheter is inserted to the bifurcation of the drainage port. A 5 ml balloon is filled with 10 ml, to fill the dead space in the port while ensuring proper inflation.

A drainage bag that provides adequate storage volume and reasonable concealment under clothing should be chosen. A bedside bag is preferred for bed-bound patients and for overnight use in ambulatory persons. The bedside bag should hold at least 2000 ml, contain an antireflux valve to prevent retrograde movement of urine from bag to bladder, and a drainage port that is easily manipulated by the patient or care provider. In contrast, a leg bag is preferred for ambulatory patients. It should hold at least 500 ml, be easily concealed under clothing, and attach to the leg using elastic straps or a cloth pocket rather than latex straps, which are likely to irritate the underlying skin.

The patient is taught to keep the drainage bag level or below the symphysis pubis and to secure the catheter so that unintentional traction against the thigh is avoided. Typically, the patient is encouraged to drink at least the recommended daily allowance of fluids and additional fluids when hematuria or sediment is present. However, these recommendations may be altered depending on the clinical setting and the patient's short-term prognosis. The catheter is routinely monitored for blockage caused by blood clots, sediment, or kinking of the drainage bag above the urinary bladder. The patient and family are also advised to monitor for signs and symptoms of clinically relevant infection, including fever, new hematuria, or urinary leakage around the catheter. They are also advised that bacteriuria is inevitable, even with the use of catheters containing a bacteriostatic coating, and that only clinically relevant (symptomatic) urinary tract infections should be treated.

BLADDER SPASM

Irritative LUTS, including a heightened sense of urgency and urethral discomfort, are common in patients managed with a long-term indwelling catheter. In certain cases, these irritative symptoms are accompanied by painful spasms. Bladder spasms are characterized by intermittent episodes of excruciating, painful cramping localized to the suprapubic region. They are caused by high-pressure, unstable detrusor contractions in response to a specific irritation.[39] Urine may bypass (leak around) the catheter. Painful bladder spasms may be the direct result of catheter occlusion from blood clots, sediment, or kinking or of a needlessly large catheter or improperly inflated retention balloon. Other risk factors include pelvic radiation therapy, chemotherapeutic agents (particularly cyclophosphamide), the presence of an intravesical tumor, urinary tract infections, and a bladder or lower ureteral calculus.

Bladder spasms are managed by altering modifiable factors or by administering anticholinergic medications when indicated (Table 14–3). Changing the urethral catheter may relieve bladder spasms. An indwelling catheter is usually changed every 4 weeks because of the risk of blockage and encrustation with precipitated salts, hardened urethral secretions, and bacteria.

In addition to changing the catheter, the nurse should consider altering the type of catheter. For example, a catheter with a smaller French size may be inserted if the catheter is larger than 16 French, unless the patient is experiencing a build-up of sediment causing catheter blockage. Similarly, a catheter with a smaller retention balloon (5 ml)

Table 14–3. Instability Urinary Incontinence (UI) in the Patient Receiving Palliative Care

Condition	UI Type
Neurological lesions above the brain stem micturition center Neurological lesions below the brain stem micturition center but above sacral spinal segments	Urge UI • Primary or metastatic tumors of the brain • Posterior fossa tumors causing increased intracranial pressure • Cerebrovascular accident (stroke) • Diseases affecting the brain, including multiple sclerosis, AIDS Reflex UI • primary or metastatic tumors of the spinal cord • Tumors causing spinal cord compression because of their effects on the spinal column • Systemic diseases directly affecting the spinal cord, including advanced-stage AIDS, transverse myelitis, Guillain-Barré syndrome
Inflammation of the bladder	Urge UI • Primary bladder tumors, including papillary tumors or carcinoma in situ • Bladder calculi (stones) • Radiation cystitis, including brachytherapy • Chemotherapy-induced cystitis
Bladder outlet obstruction	Urge UI • Prostatic carcinoma • Detrusor sphincter dyssynergia associated with reflex UI • Urethral cancers • Pelvic tumors causing urethral compression

may be substituted for a catheter with a larger balloon (30 ml), to reduce irritation of the trigone and bladder neck. Using a catheter that is constructed of hydrophilic polymers or latex-free silicone may relieve bladder spasms and diminish irritative LUTS because of their greater biocompatibility when compared to Teflon-coated catheters.

Instruction about the position of the catheter, drainage tubes, and bags is reinforced; and the drainage tubes and urine are assessed for the presence of sediment or clots likely to obstruct urinary drainage. In certain cases, a suprapubic indwelling catheter may be substituted for a urethral catheter, such as when the urethral catheter produces significant urethritis with purulent discharge from the urethra. A suprapubic catheter also may be placed in patients who tend to encrust the catheter, despite adequate fluid intake.

Bladder spasms also may indicate a clinically relevant urinary tract infection. The catheter change provides the best opportunity to obtain a urine specimen. This specimen should be obtained from the catheter and never the drainage bag. While bacteriuria is inevitable with the long-term indwelling catheter, cystitis associated with painful bladder spasms should be managed with sensitivity-guided antibiotic therapy.

The patient is taught to drink sufficient fluids to meet or exceed the recommended daily allowance of 0.5 oz/lb whenever feasible. A reduction of beverages or foods containing bladder irritants, such as caffeine or alcohol, also may reduce bladder spasms in some cases.

When conservative measures or catheter modification fails to relieve bladder spasms, an anticholinergic medication may be administered. These medications work by inhibiting the unstable contractions that lead to painful bladder spasms. Table 14–4 summarizes the dosage, administration, and nursing considerations of common anticholinergic medications used to manage bladder spasms, as well as urge or reflex UI.

HEMATURIA

Hematuria is defined as the presence of blood in the urine. It results from a variety of renal, urological, and systemic processes. When gross hematuria is present as an initial complaint or finding in an adult, further evaluation in one study revealed that 23% of patients had an underlying malignancy.[45] In the palliative care setting, hematuria occurs more commonly following pelvic irradiation, chemotherapy, or as the result of a major coagulation disorder or newly diagnosed or recurring malignancy.

Hematuria is divided into two subtypes according to its clinical manifestations. Microscopic hematuria is characterized by hemoglobin or myoglobin on dipstick analysis and more than three to five red blood cells per high-power field under microscopic urinalysis, but the presence of blood remains invisible to the unaided eye. Macroscopic (gross) hematuria is also characterized by dipstick and microscopic evidence of red blood cells in the urine, as well as a bright red or brownish discoloration that is apparent to the unaided eye.

In the context of the patient receiving palliative care, it can also be subdivided into three categories depending on its severity.[46] Mild hematuria is microscopic or gross blood in the urine that does not produce obstructing clots or cause a clinically relevant decline in hematocrit or hemoglobin. Moderate and severe hematuria are associated with more prolonged and high-volume blood loss; hematuria is classified as moderate when it requires six units or less to replace blood lost within the urine and as severe when more than six units are required. Both moderate and severe hema-

Table 14–4. Pharmacologic Management—Agents Used to Decrease Bladder Contractility

Drug	Action	Dosage	Adverse Effects	Nursing Considerations
Oxybutynin chloride, Ditropan 5 mg tablets 5 mg/5 ml syrup	Anticholinergic—inhibits muscarinic action of acetylcholine on smooth muscle Antispasmodic effect on detrusor smooth muscle Local anesthetic	Child <5 yr: Age in yr = ml/dose bid/tid Child >5 yr: 0.2 mg/kg bid/qid Adult: 5 mg tid-qid Geriatric: 5 mg qd	Dry mouth, flushing, decreased sweating, constipation, drowsiness, increased heart rate, behavioral changes, blurred vision.	Contraindicated in patients with narrow angle glaucoma. Drink plenty of fluids; avoid heat prostration
Ditropan XL extended release 5 mg, 10 mg tablets	Similar action to classic oxybutynin except for osmotic release vehicle	Single daily dose Recommended starting dose is 5 mg daily, up to 30 mg/day	Side-effect profile similar to oxybutynin but prevalence and severity of side-effects reduced.	Tablets to be swallowed whole; cannot be chewed, divided, or crushed
Propantheline Pro-Banthine 7.5 mg, 15 mg tablet	Anticholinergic—inhibits muscarinic action of acetylcholine on smooth muscle; direct antispasmodic effect of detrusor smooth muscle	Child: 0.5 mg/kg bid-qid Adult: 7.5 mg, up to 30 mg bid-qid	Same	
Hyoscyamine Levsin SL tabs 0.125 mg	Same	Child 2–12 yr: ½–1 tab q 4 hr. Child 12 yr and older: 1–2 tab q 4 hr Child 6 mo–2 yr: 5–10 mg tid–qid Child 2–12 yr: 10 mg tid–qid	Same	Also available in elixir, extended-release.
Dicyclomine hydrochloride Bentyl Caps 10 mg Tabs 20 mg Solution 10 mg/5 ml	Musculotropics/antimuscarinics, antispasmodics	Adult: 20–40 mg/qid	Same	

Flavoxate Urispas 100 mg tablets	Direct spasmolytic (papaverine-like) action on smooth muscle Local anesthetic effect	Adult >12 yr: 100–200 mg tid, qid	Dry mouth, nausea/vomiting, dizziness, headache, increased heart rate, hyperpyrexia, drowsiness	Contraindicated for GI obstruction or glaucoma
Belladonna and opium suppositories 16.2 mg belladonna 30 or 60 mg opium	Antimuscarinic/antispasmodic Analgesic	Adult: 1 suppository q 4–6 hr	Same Hallucinations	Child dose not known. Addictive
Tolterodine tartrate Detrol 1 mg tablets 2 mg tablets	Muscarinic receptor antagonist Antimuscarinic/antispasmodic	Adult: 1–2 mg twice daily	Same Less dry mouth	Caution: drug interaction with cytochrome P450 enzyme
Imipramine Tofranil	Tricyclic anti depressant with anticholinergic, direct musculotropic, adrenergic and anxiolytic properties. It has mild anesthetic and antihistaminic effects at nerve terminals. Used monthly for enuresis.	Adult: 25–75 mg. daily or twice daily Child <12 yr: 25–50 mg@HS	Weakness, sedation, lethargy, irritability, postural hypotension, nausea, abdominal distress. Lowers seizure threshold	Avoid using with MAO inhibitors. Check for h/o seizures

turia may produce obstructing clots that lead to acute urinary retention or obstruction of the upper urinary tracts.

Pathophysiology

Hematuria originates as a disruption of the endothelial–epithelial barrier somewhere within the urinary tract.[47] Inflammation of this barrier may lead to the production of cytokines, with subsequent damage to the basement membrane and passage of red blood cells into the urinary tract. Laceration of this barrier may be caused by an invasive tumor, iatrogenic or other trauma, vascular accident, or arteriovenous malformation. Hematuria that originates within the upper urinary tract is often associated with tubulointerstitial disease or an invasive tumor, while hematuria originating from the lower urinary tract is typically associated with trauma, an invasive tumor, or radiation- or chemotherapy-induced cystitis.

In the patient receiving palliative care, significant hematuria most commonly occurs as the result of a hemorrhagic cystitis related to cancer, infection (viral, bacterial, fungal, or parasitic), chemical toxins (primarily from oxazaphosphorine alkylating agents), radiation, anticoagulation therapy, or an idiopathic response to anabolic steroids or another agent.[46] Radiation and chemotherapeutic agents account for the majority of moderate to severe hematuria cases.

Radiation cystitis is typically associated with pelvic radiotherapy for cancer of the uterus, cervix, prostate, rectum, or lower urinary tract. Approximately 10% to 20% of patients treated with pelvic radiation will experience clinically relevant cystitis.[48,49] In certain cases, radiation cystitis is limited to LUTS, including diurnal urinary frequency, urgency, and dysuria with low bladder compliance and a small vesical capacity. However, friability of the bladder wall and hematuria occur in more severe cases. Radiation cystitis may occur during therapy or develop months to years after treatment. The acute effects of radiation on the bladder include mucosal edema, vascular telangiectasia, and submucosal hemorrhage. These effects may be followed by interstitial and smooth muscle fibrosis with lowered bladder compliance and a reduced capacity.[46] When severe, the fibrosis associated with radiotherapy can lead to moderate to severe hematuria, as well as upper urinary tract distress caused by chronically elevated intravesical pressures.

Chemotherapy-induced cystitis usually occurs after treatment with an oxazaphosphorine alkylating agent, such as cyclophosphamide or isophosphamide.[46] A urinary metabolite produced by these drugs, acrolein, is believed to be responsible. Hemorrhage usually occurs during or immediately following treatment, but delayed hemorrhage may occur in patients on long-term therapy. The effects on the bladder mucosa are similar to those described in radiation cystitis.

Assessment

Because bleeding may occur at any level in the urinary tract from the glomerulus to the meatus, a careful, detailed history is needed to identify the source of the bleeding and to initiate an appropriate treatment plan. The patient should be asked whether the hematuria represents a new, persistent or a recurrent problem. This distinction is often helpful since recurrent or persistent hematuria may represent a benign predisposing condition and a new or recent onset is more likely to result from conditions related to the need for palliative care. A review of prior urinalyses also may provide clues to the onset and history of microscopic hematuria in particular. The patient is queried about the relation of grossly visible hematuria to urinary stream. Bleeding limited to the initiation of the stream is often associated with a urethral source, bleeding during the entire act of voiding generally indicates a source in the bladder or upper urinary tract, and bleeding near the termination of the stream often indicates a source within the prostate or male reproductive system.

The patient with gross hematuria should also be asked about the color of the urine: a bright red hue indicates fresh blood, while a darker hue (often described as brownish or "Coke color") indicates older blood. Some patients with severe hematuria will also report the passage of blood clots; clots that are particularly long and thin, resembling a shoestring or fishhook, suggest an upper urinary tract source, while larger and bulkier clots suggest a lower urinary tract source.

The patient is asked about any pain related to the hematuria; this questioning should include the site and character of the pain and any radiation to the flank, lower abdomen, or groin. Flank pain usually indicates upper urinary tract problems, abdominal pain radiating to the groin usually indicates lower ureteral obstruction and bleeding, and suprapubic pain suggests obstruction or infection causing hematuria.

In addition to questions about the hematuria, the nurse should ask about specific risk factors, including a history of urinary tract infections; systemic symptoms suggesting infection or renal insufficiency including fever, weight loss, rash, and recent systemic infection; any history of primary or metastatic tumors of the genitourinary system; and chemotherapy or radiation therapy of the pelvic or lower abdominal region. A focused review of medications includes all chemotherapeutic agents used currently or in the past and the current or recent administration of anticoagulant medications, including warfarin, heparin, aspirin, nonsteroidal antiinflammatory drugs, or other anticoagulant agents.

Physical Examination. Physical examination also provides valuable clues to the source of hematuria. When completing this assessment, the nurse should particularly note any abdominal masses or tenderness, skin rashes, bruising, purpura (suggesting vasculitis, bleeding, or coagulation disorders), or telangiectasia (suggesting von Hippel-Lindau disease). Blood pressure should be assessed since a new onset or rapid exacerbation of hypertension may suggest a renal source for hematuria. The lower abdomen is examined for signs of bladder distension, and a rectal assessment is completed to evaluate apparent prostatic or rectal masses or induration.

Laboratory Testing. A dipstick and microscopic urinalysis is usually combined with microscopic examination when evaluating hematuria. This provides a semiquantitative assessment of the severity of hematuria (evaluated as the number of red blood cells per high-power microscopic field), and it excludes pseudohematuria (reddish urine caused by something other than red blood cells, such as ingestion of certain drugs, vegetable dyes or pigments).

Urinalysis provides further clues to the likely source of the bleeding.[50] Dysmorphic red blood cells, cellular casts, renal tubular cells, and proteinuria indicate upper urinary tract bleeding. In contrast, hematuria from the lower urinary tract is usually associated with a normal red blood cell morphology.

Additional evaluation is guided by clues from the history, physical examination, and urinalysis. For example, the presence of pyuria and bacteriuria suggests cystitis as the cause of hematuria and indicates the need for a culture and sensitivity testing. Random urine calcium:creatinine ratios should be assessed in patients with painful macroscopic hematuria, to evaluate the risk for stone formation, particularly in patients with hyperparathyroidism or prolonged immobility. Random urine protein:creatinine ratios and C3 component of complement are obtained in all patient with proteinuria or casts, to evaluate for glomerulopathy or interstitial renal disease. Further studies also may be completed, to evaluate the specific cause of hematuria and implement a treatment plan.

In selecting those who should undergo a more extensive evaluation, one should also consider the presence of other risk factors for urological cancer, such as age greater than 40 years, tobacco use, analgesic abuse, pelvic irradiation, cyclophosphamide use, and occupational exposure to rubber compounds and dyestuffs.[51]

Imaging Studies. Ultrasound is almost always indicated in the evaluation of hematuria in the patient receiving palliative care.[46] It is used to identify the size and location of cystic or solid masses that may act as the source of hematuria and to assess for obstruction, most stones, larger blood clots, and bladder-filling defects. An intravenous pyelogram also may be used to image the upper and lower urinary tracts, but its clinical use is limited by the risk of contrast allergy or nephropathy. Cystoscopy is performed when a bladder lesion is suspected, and ureteroscopy with retrograde pyelography may be completed if an upper urinary tract source of bleeding is suspected.

Management

The management of hematuria is guided by its severity and its source or cause. Preventive management for chemotherapy-induced hematuria begins with administering sodium 2-mercaptoethanesulfonate (Mesna) to patients receiving an alkylating agent for cancer.[52] This is given parenterally, and it oxidizes to a stable, inactive form within minutes of administration. It becomes active when it is excreted into the urine. Once there, it neutralizes acrolein (the metabolite postulated to cause chemotherapy-induced cystitis and hematuria) and slows the degradation of the 4-hydroxy metabolites produced by administration of alkylating drugs. It is given with cyclophosphamide (20 mg/kg at time 0 and every 4 hours for 2 or 3 doses). When combined with vigorous hydration, it has been shown to protect the bladder from subsequent damage and hematuria.

Mild urinary retention is managed by identifying and treating its underlying cause. For example, sensitivity-guided antibiotics are used to treat a bacterial hemorrhagic cystitis, and extracorporeal lithotripsy may be used to treat hematuria associated with a urinary stone. While hematuria persists, the patient is encouraged to drink more than the recommended daily allowance for fluids, to prevent clot formation and urinary retention. In addition, the patient is assisted in obtaining adequate nutritional intake to replace lost blood, and iron supplementation is provided if indicated.

In contrast to mild hematuria, moderate to severe cases often lead to the formation of blood clots, causing acute urinary retention and bladder pain. In these cases, complete evacuation of clots from the bladder is required before a definitive assessment and treatment strategy are implemented.[39] A large-bore urethral catheter is placed (24 or 26 French in the adult), and manual irrigation is performed with a Toomey syringe. The bladder is irrigated with saline until no further clots are obtained and the backflow is relatively clear.[39] A 22 or 24 French three-way indwelling catheter is then placed, to allow continuous bladder irrigation using cold or iced saline. Percutaneous insertion of a suprapubic catheter is not recommended because of limitations of size and the potential to "seed" the tract if a bladder malignancy is present.

Unsuccessful attempts to place a urethral catheter or recurrent obstruction of the irrigation catheter provide strong indications for endoscopic evaluation. Rigid cystoscopy is preferred because it allows optimal evacuation of bladder clots and further evaluation of sites of bleeding; retrograde pyelography or ureteroscopy may also be completed if upper urinary tract clots are suspected. Based on the findings of endoscopic evaluation, sites of particularly severe bleeding are cauterized or resected.

Following initial evacuation of obstructing clots, bladder irrigations or instillations may be completed when multiple sites of bleeding are observed or when the risk of recurrence is high, as in the case of radiation- or chemotherapy-induced hematuria. Table 14–5 summarizes agents used to stop moderate to severe hematuria and their route, administration, and principal nursing considerations. The following case report summarizes a case of recurring hemorrhagic cystitis following radiation therapy for endometrial cancer.

Case Study: D.Y., a Patient with Diabetes

D.Y. is a 69-year-old white woman with type 2 diabetes mellitus, hypertension, and idiopathic cirrhosis with a mild coagulopathy. She was diagnosed with endometrial

Table 14–5. Treatment Options for Hemorrhagic Cystitis

Agent	Action	Route of Administration/Dosage	Problems/Contraindications
Epsilon aminocaproic acid	Acts as an inhibitor of fibrinolysis by inhibiting plasminogen activation substances.	5 g loading dose orally or parenteral, followed by 1–1.25 g hourly to max of 30 g in 24 hr. Max response in 8–12 hr	Potential thromboembolic complications Increased risk of clot retention Contraindicated in patients with upper tract bleeding or vesicoureteral reflux Decreased blood pressure
Silver nitrate	Chemical cautery	Intravesical instillation 0.5%–1.0% solution in sterile H_2O instilled for 10–20 min followed by no irrigation. Multiple instillations may be required.	Reported as 68% effective Case report of renal failure in patient who precipitated silver salts in renal collecting system causing functional obstruction.
Alum. May use ammonium or potassium salt of aluminum.	Chemical cautery	Continuous bladder irrigation 1% solution in sterile H_2O pH 4.5 (salt precipitates at pH 7)	Requires average of 21 hr of treatment Thought to not be absorbed by bladder mucosa. However, case reports of aluminum toxicity in renal failure patients
Formalin. Aqueous solution of formaldehyde	Cross-links proteins; exists as monohydrate methylene glycol and as mixture of polymeric hydrates and polyoxyethylene glycols. Rapidly "fixes" the bladder mucosa.	Available as 37%–40% aqueous formaldehyde = 100% formalin diluted in sterile H_2O to desired concentration. 1% formalin = 0.37% formaldehyde Instillation = 50 cc for 4–10 min or endoscopic placement of 5% formalin-soaked pledgets onto bleeding site for 15 min and then removed.	Painful; requires anestheisa Vesicoureteral reflux (relative contraindication, patients placed in Trendelenburg position with low-grade reflux or ureteral occlusive balloons used with high-grade reflux). Extravasation causes fibrosis, papillary necrosis, fistula, peritonitis.

Phenol Carbonic acid	Destroys the urothelium but not the muscularis	Suprapubic cystostomy under general anesthesia, instill 30 cc 100% phenol with 30 cc glycerin for 1 min. Suctioning, instill 60 cc absolute 95% ethanol for 1 min, suction, follow with copious saline irrigation.	Reduced risk of bladder fibrosis as compared to formalin. 1 case report of failure to drain bladder in child led to death caused by methemoglobinemia.
Prostaglandins Prostaglandin E_2	These prostaglandins are naturally produced in bladder, synthesis is affected by multiple factors including distention, pH, osmolarity, carcinogens, PG synthesis and release in vitro are regulated partly by reduced glutathione, which is also involved in protection of membranes from lipid peroxidation	0.75 mg in 200 ml saline instilled into bladder left in situ for 4 hr. Repeat daily until bleeding stops.	Prostaglandin E_2 may cause severe bladder spasms. High cost, strict storage requirements
Prostaglandin F_2 Carboprost tromethamine		1.4 mg in 200 cc saline instilled as above.	
Hyperbaric oxygen	Found to enhance healing in a variety of of radiation-injured tissues. Animal models produced an 8-9 fold increase in vascular density in irradiated tissues raising transcutaneous O_2 levels to within 85% of normal. This angiogenesis appears to be mediated through tissue macrophages responding to the steep oxygen gradient.	100% oxygen in a hyperbaric chamber @ 2.0–2.4 atm absolute for 90 min, 5 days/week	Noninvasive Number of treatments average 40; good short-term results, questionable long-term results.

Source: References 33–61.

cancer at age 65 years and treated with external beam radiation therapy and interstitial radium seed implants. She began noting lower urinary tract symptoms, including frequency, urgency, and dysuria; and she developed gross hematuria with clots approximately 3 years after completing radiation therapy. She was initially treated with continuous bladder irrigation, intravesical alum, and prostaglandin instillations with minimal response. She underwent a cystoscopy for evacuation of blood clots. At that time, random bladder biopsies were obtained, which revealed chronic inflammation, hemorrhage, hemosiderin-laden macrophages, and vascular telangiectasia. There was no evidence of malignancy. Several areas of bleeding were cauterized. Hyperbaric oxygen therapy was attempted, but the patient did not tolerate the procedure well and refused further treatments. Over the next 3 months, she continued to have intermittent episodes of gross hematuria and progressive weakness.

D.Y. again sought assistance when she experienced a particularly severe episode of hematuria with clot retention and a hematocrit of 12%. She was admitted to hospital for transfusions and management of recurring hemorrhagic cystitis. A voiding cystourethrogram (VCUG) was obtained on admission, and she was treated with transfusions and continuous bladder irrigations until her sixth hospital day, when she was taken to the operating room for a cystoscopy, performed under anesthesia. Prior to cystoscopy, Vaseline gauze was placed on the perineal skin. Since left vesicoureteral reflux was noted on the VCUG, a Fogarty balloon was passed into the distal left ureter and inflated to occlude the ureter. The bladder was filled, and her capacity was determined to be 300 ml. One hundred and fifty milliliters of a 1% formalin solution was then slowly infused into the bladder and retained for 20 minutes. The bladder was then drained and irrigated with saline. A three-way indwelling catheter was placed, and continuous bladder irrigation was restarted. Her hematuria partially resolved, and she returned to the operating room 3 days later for instillation of 150 ml of a 3% formalin solution. Her hematuria resolved following this second instillation, and the continuous bladder irrigation was discontinued within 24 hours. At the time of discharge on the next day, she was voiding well and her urine remained free of hematuria. Postprocedure pain was managed by a combination of urinary analgesics, such as phenazopyridine (Pyridium), and an oral narcotic analgesic (oxycodone). Both medications were discontinued 1 week after the final instillation.

Unfortunately, she presented with recurrent dysuria, hematuria, and clots requiring transfusion and repeated cystoscopy with instillation of a 1% formalin solution. She responded to this treatment and was discharged 2 days following treatment.

This case demonstrates the risk of recurrent hemorrhagic cystitis following treatment with a combination of external beam and interstitial radiotherapy. In this case, the initial episode of hematuria occurred 3 years following therapy, and it recurred over a period of 22 months despite treatment with continuous bladder irrigation, cystoscopy with electrocauterization, hyperbaric oxygen, intravesical alum, and prostaglandin. Ultimately, she failed to respond to intravesical instillation of a 1% formalin solution, but she responded to a 3% solution. Nonetheless, she experienced a single recurrence within a period of 14 months, which responded to a single instillation of a 1% formalin solution. She remains symptom-free at 1 year.

Fortunately, life-threatening blood loss is a rare complication of hemorrhagic cystitis and bladder tumors. Treatment usually begins with bladder irrigation, evacuation of clots, and intravesical instillations such as alum or silver nitrate and progresses to therapy with intravesical prostaglandin and formalin. Alternatives include cystoscopy with electrical cauterization or laser coagulation of individual bleeding sites. Selective embolization or ligation of the hypogastric artery, palliative cystectomy, or radical nephrectomy may be required as a last resort.

SUMMARY

Patients receiving palliative care frequently experience urinary system disorders. A malignancy or systemic disease may affect voiding function and produce urinary incontinence, urinary retention, or upper urinary tract obstruction. In addition, upper acute renal insufficiency or renal failure may occur when the upper urinary tract becomes obstructed. These disorders may be directly attributable to a malignancy or systemic disease, or they may be caused by a specific treatment such as radiation, chemotherapy, or a related medication. Nursing management of patients with urinary system disorders is affected by the nature of the urological condition, the patient's general condition, and the nearness to death.

REFERENCES

1. Gray ML. Genitourinary Disorders. St. Louis: Mosby, 1992.
2. Gray ML. Physiology of voiding. In: Doughty DB, ed. Urinary and Fecal Incontinence: Nursing Management. St. Louis: Mosby, 2000: 1–27.
3. Gray M. UI Pathophysiology WOCN Continence Conference. January, 1999, Austin, TX.
4. deGroat WC. Central nervous system control of micturition. In: O'Donnell PD, ed. Urinary Incontinence. St. Louis: Mosby, 1997:33–47.
5. Langworthy OR, Kolb LC. The encephalic control of tone in the musculature of the urinary bladder. Brain 1933;56:371–375.
6. Bruggermann J, Shi T, Apkarian AV. Squirrel monkey lateral thalamus. II. Viscerosomatic convergent representation of urinary bladder, colon and esophagus. J Neurosci 1994;14: 6796–6814.
7. Sakakibara R, Hattori T, Yasuda K, Yamanishi T. Micturitional disturbance after hemispheric stroke: analysis of the lesion site by CT and MRI. J Neurol Sci 1996;137:47–56.
8. Fowler CJ. Neurological disorders of micturition and their treatment. Brain 1999;122: 1213–1231.
9. Kohama T. Neuroanatomical studies of pontine urine storage facilitatory areas in the cat brain. Jpn J Urol 1992;83:1478–1483.
10. De Groat WC. Innervation of the lower urinary tract: an overview. Presented at the 20th Annual Meeting of the Society for Urodynamics and Female Urology. Dallas, Texas, May 1, 1999.
11. Elbadawi A. Functional anatomy of the organs of micturition. Urol Clin North Am 1996; 23:177–210.
12. Chai TC, Steers WD. Neurophysiology of voiding. Urol Clin North Am 1996;23:221–236.
13. Eglen RM, Choppin A, Dillon MP, Hegde S. Muscarinic receptor ligands and their therapeutic potential. Curr Opin Chem Biol 1999;3:426–432.
14. Urinary Incontinence Guideline Panel. Acute and Chronic Incontinence. Rockville, MD: Department of Health and Human Services, publication 96-0682, 1996.
15. Gray ML, Dougherty MC. Urinary incontinence: pathophysiology and treatment. J Enterostomal Therapy Nurs 1987;14:152–162.
16. McGuire EJ, English SF. Periurethral collagen injection and female sphincteric incontinence: indications, techniques and result. World J Urol 1997;15:306–309.

17. Jirovec MM, Wells TJ. Urinary incontinence in nursing home residents with dementia: the mobility–cognition paradigm. Appl Nurs Res 1990;3:112–117.

18. Gray M, Marx RM, Peruggio M, Patrie J, Steers WD. A model for predicting motor urge urinary incontinence. Nurs Res 1999 (in press).

19. Robinson D, McClish DK, Wyman JF, Bump RC, Fantl JA. Comparison between urinary diaries with and without intensive patient instructions. Neurourol Urodyn 1996;15:143–148.

20. Peggs JF. Urinary incontinence in the elderly: pharmacologic therapies. Am Fam Physician 1992;46:1763–1769.

21. Tomlinson BU, Doughery MC, Pendergrast JF, Boyington AR, Coffman PA, Pickens SM. Dietary caffeine, fluid intake and urinary incontinence in older rural women. Int J Urogynecol Pelvic Floor Dysfunct 1999;10:22–28.

22. Gray ML. Altered patterns of urinary elimination. In: Ackley BJ, Ladwig GB, eds. Nursing Diagnosis Handbook. St. Louis: Mosby, 1999: 643–646.

23. National Academy of Sciences, Food and Nutrition Board. Recommended Daily Allowances, 9th Ed. Washington DC: National Academy of Sciences, 1980.

24. Brink CA. The value of absorbent and containment devices in the management of urinary incontinence. J Wound Ostomy Cont Nurs 1996;23:2–4.

25. Gray M, Marx R. Results of behavioral treatment for urinary incontinence in women. Curr Opin Urol 1998;8:279–282.

26. Miller JM, Ashton-Miller JA, Delancey JO. A pelvic muscle precontraction can reduce cough-related urine loss in selected women with mild SUI. J Am Geriatr Soc 1998;46:870–874.

27. Ghoneim GM, Hassouna M. Alternative for the pharmacologic management of stress urinary incontinence in the elderly. J Wound Ostomy Cont Nurs 1997;24:311–318.

28. Moore KN, Rayome RG. Problem solving and troubleshooting: the indwelling catheter. J Wound Ostomy Cont Nurs 1995;22:242–247.

29. Burgio KL, Locher JL, Goode PS, et al. Behavioral vs. drug treatment for urge urinary incontinence in older women: a randomized controlled trial. JAMA 1998;280:1995–2000.

30. Larsson G, Hallen B, Nilvebrant L. Tolterodine in the treatment of overactive bladder: analysis of pooled phase II efficacy and safety data. Urology 1999;53:990–998.

31. Gelason DM, Susset J, White C, Munoz DR, Sand PK. Evaluation of a new once daily formulation of oxybutynin for the treatment of urge incontinence. Ditropan XL study group. Urology 1999;54:420–423.

32. Smith DA. Devices for continence. Nurse Pract Forum 1994;5:186–189.

33. Anson C, Gray M. Secondary urologic complications of spinal injury. Urol Nurs 1993;13: 107–112.

34. Van Gool JD, Vijverberg MA, Messer AP, Elzinga-Plomp A, De Jong TP. Functional daytime incontinence: non-pharmacologic treatment. Scand J Urol Nephrol 1992;141:93–105.

35. Colling J, Ouslander J, Hadley BJ, Eisch J, Campbell E. The effects of patterned urge response toileting (PURT) on urinary incontinence among nursing home residents. J Am Geriatr Soc 1992;40:135–141.

36. Schnelle JF, Keeler E, Hays RD, Simmons S, Ouslander JG, Siu AL. A cost and value analysis of two interventions with incontinent nursing home residents. J Am Geriatr Soc 1995; 43:1112–1117.

37. Golomb J, Ben-Chaim J, Goldwasser B, Korach J, Mashiach S. Conservative treatment of a vesicocervical fistula resulting from Shirodkar cervical cerclage. J Urol 1993;149:833–834.

38. Tostain J. Conservative treatment of urogenital fistula following gynecological surgery: the value of fibrin glue. Acta Urol Belg 1992;60: 27–33.

39. Norman RW. Genitourinary disorders. In: Oxford Textbook of Palliative Medicine. Oxford: Oxford University Press, 1998:667–676.

40. Gray M. Urinary retention: management in the acute care setting. Am J Nurs 2000;15:42–60.

41. Gray M. Functional alterations: bladder. In: Gross J, Johnson BL, eds. Handbook of Oncology Nursing. Boston: Jones and Bartlett, 1998: 557–583.

42. Stock RG, Stone NN, DeWyngaert JK, Lavagnini P, Undger PD. Prostate specific antigen findings and biopsy results following interactive ultrasound guided transperineal brachytherapy for early stage prostate carcinoma. Cancer 1996;77: 2386–2392.

43. Thees K, Dreblow L. Trial of voiding: what's the verdict? Urol Nurs 1999;19:20–24.

44. Fiers S. Management of the long-term indwelling catheter in the home setting. J Wound Ostomy Cont Nurs 1995;22:140–144.

45. Copley JB. Asymptomatic hematuria in the adult. Am J Med Sci 1986;29:101–111.

46. DeVries CB, Fuad SF. Hemorrhagic cystitis: a review. J Urol 1990;143:1–7.

47. Herrin JT. General Urology: Workup of Hematuria and Tubular Disorders. In Gonzales, ET and Bauer SB (eds.) Pediatric Urology Practice. Philadelphia: Lippincott, Williams, and Wilkins, 1999:69–79.

48. Levenbach C, Eifel PJ, Burke TW, et al. Hemorrhagic cystitis following radio therapy for stage Ib cancer of the cervix. Gynecol Oncol 1994;55:206–210.

49. Dean RJ, Lytton B. Urologic complications of pelvic irradiation. J Urol 1978;119:64–67.

50. Stapleton FB. Morphology of urinary red blood cells: a simple guide in localizing the site of hematuria. Pediatr Clin North Am 1987;34: 561–563.

51. Catalona WJ. Urothelial tumors of the urinary tract. In: Walsh PC, Retik AB, Stamey T, Vaughan ED, eds. Campbell's Urology, 6th Ed. Philadelphia: WB Saunders. 1992:1094–1158.

52. Droller MJ, Saral R, Santos G. Prevention of cyclophosphamide-induced hemorrhagic cystitis. Urology 1982;20:256.

53. Lowe BA, Stamey TA. Endoscopic topical placement of formalin soaked pledgets to control localized hemorrhage due to radiation cystitis. J Urol 1997;158:528–529.

54. Praveen BV, Sankaranarayanam A, Vaibyanathan S. A comparative study of intravesical instillation of 15 (5) 15 Me alpha and alum in the management of persistent hematuria of vesical origin. Int J Clin Pharmacol Ther Toxicol 1992;30:7–12.

55. Shoskes DA, Radzinski CA, Struthers NW, et al. Aluminum toxicity and death following intravesical alum irrigation in a patient with renal impairment. J Urol 1992;147:697–699.

56. Perazella M, Brown E. Acute aluminum toxicity and alum bladder irrigation in patients with renal failure. Am J Kidney Dis 1993;21:44–46.

57. Norkool DM. Hyperbaric oxygen therapy for radiation-induced hemorrhagic cystitis. J Urol 1993;150:332–334.

58. DelPizzo JJ, Chew BH, Jacobs SC. Treatment of radiation induced hemorrhagic cystitis with hyperbaric oxygen: long-term follow-up. J Urol 1998;160:731–733.

59. Singh I, Laungani Gobinl B. Intravesical epsilon aminocaproic acid in management of intractable bladder hemorrhage. Urology 1992;40: 227–229.

60. Dewan AK, Mohan GM, Ravi R. Intravesical formalin for hemorrhagic cystitis following irradiation of cancer of the cervix. Int J Gynecol Obstet 1993;42:131–135.

15 Lymphedema

JEAN K. SMITH and ANNE ZOBEC

For many years I had enlarged legs which were not only cosmetically unattractive but extremely uncomfortable. After many years of devices and medications that proved unsuccessful, I skeptically tried CDT. At last I have ankles!

—A patient

I can manage the spread of my cancer, but the lymphedema is unbearable.

—A patient

The world prevalence of lymphedema has been estimated at some 150 million,[1] but is poorly documented.[2] The etiology of secondary lymphedema varies geographically depending on climate, prosperity, and sophistication of cancer treatment. In industrialized nations with sophisticated cancer treatment, a significant proportion of people with secondary lymphedema are cancer survivors.[3] Filariasis, a tropical disease, is the predominant cause of secondary lymphedema in third-world nations with hot and humid climates,[1] while the etiology of primary lymphedema is unknown.[4]

All lymphedemas have the potential to grow worse over time, and without proper management, varying levels of disability are likely to occur. Overall, lymphedema has been neglected in the United States, particularly during end-of-life care. Since lymphedema is incurable,[5] current management is palliative. This chapter provides a brief overview of lymphedema, followed by principles and practice strategies based on traditional goals of palliative care. The information is applicable to various clinical settings, including inpatient, acute care, home care, and hospice.

DEFINITION

Lymphedema is a chronic swelling of an organ or tissue due to reduced lymphatic transport capacity rather than an increase in capillary filtration. Excess fluids, proteins, immunological cells, and debris in affected tissues produce chronic inflammation and connective tissue proliferation, which often progresses to subcutaneous and dermal fibrosis and hardening.[4,6–9]

Numerous criteria and methods have been reported for quantifying lymphedema of the extremities. "No standard degree of enlargement constitutes lymphedema."[10] A 10% variation between opposite extremities has been suggested for qualifying a diagnosis.[6] It appears that a 50% to 100% increase in interstitial fluid volume is present in skin before edema becomes clinically detectable.[8]

For the purposes of nursing practices, lymphedema management is justified for high-risk patients who experience even a sensation of edema. Appropriate management often provides edema reduction, comfort, improved skin integrity, prevention of additional complications, a sense of disease control, and improved quality of life. Skillful end-of-life lymphedema management, rarely expensive or time- and labor-intensive, can significantly improve both the patient's and the surviving family's quality of life.[11]

CLASSIFICATION AND INCIDENCE

Worldwide, there are several lymphedema classifications.[12] Dynamic, or low-protein, edema has been contrasted with lymphedema, or high-protein edema.[13] Trauma of various sorts and conditions, such as congestive heart failure, leads to low-protein edemas that are directly related to increased capillary filtration. Unresolved low-protein edemas can transition to lymphedema (or a combination of high- and low-protein edemas) as a result of eventual damage to lymphatics and impaired transport capacity.

Three stages of lymphedema have also been described.[14,15] Stage I is reversible lymphedema. Stage II, spontaneously irreversible, is responsive to treatment but no longer decreases without assistance. Stage III, elephantiasis, is characterized by significantly increased size; local immunological changes resulting in proliferation of connective tissue; inflammation, scarring and fibrosis of dermal tissues; and often various troublesome skin conditions such as warts, papillomas, and deep folds (Fig. 15–1). This advanced stage of lymphedema should be avoided and is particularly problematic in patients with metastatic cancer whose lymphedemas have not been managed by skilled staff (Fig. 15–2).

Nurses are most familiar with the "pitting" classification of edema (0 to 4+ quantification of level of pitting from digital compression on an area with edema). This classification is subjective[6] and mainly applicable to low-protein edemas and stage I lymphedema.

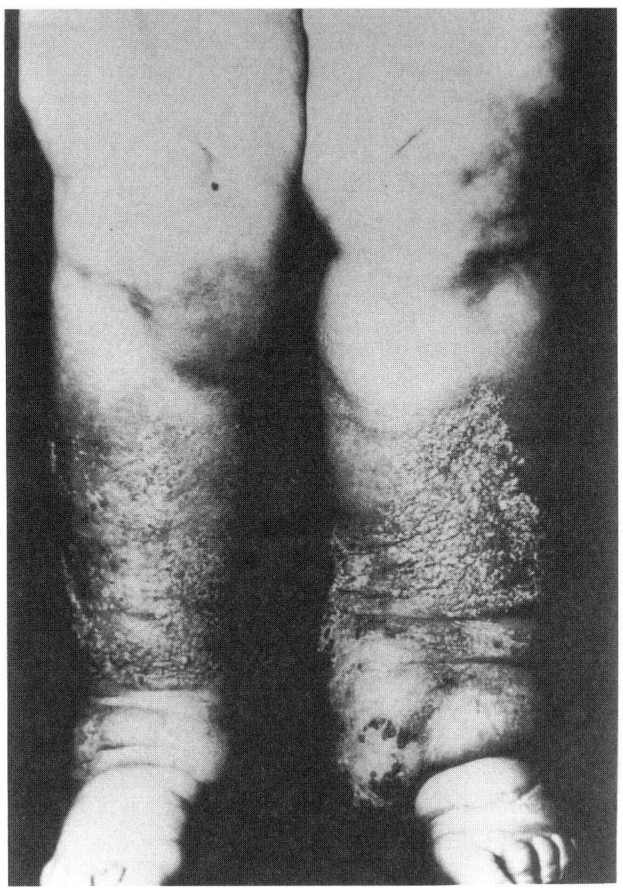

Fig. 15–1. Stage III Lymphedema (elephantiasis). (From Olzewski, 1991, reference 8, with permission.)

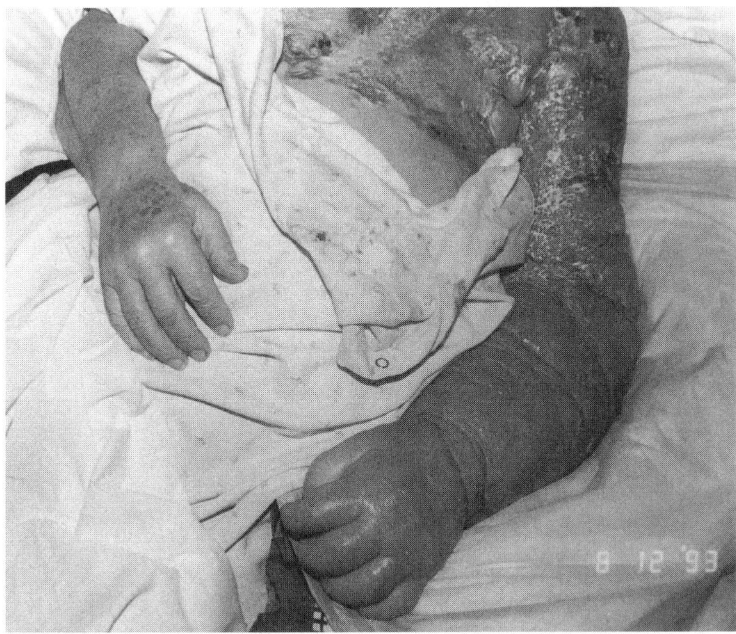

Fig. 15–2. Metastatic breast cancer patient with neglected lymphedema.

Lymphedemas of stages II and III involve tissue fibrosis, which is not addressed by the pitting classification.

Etiology is the basis for the most frequently used classification, primary and secondary lymphedemas. When the cause of the edema cannot be identified, the edema is called primary, idiopathic, or congenital.[8,16] Currently, etiology is attributed to embryonic developmental abnormalities, which may be sporadic or part of a syndrome due to either chromosomal abnormalities (i.e., Turner's syndrome) or inherited single-gene defects. Approximately 80% of primary lymphedemas develop well after birth, falling into two categories, either praecox (between adolescence and age 35) or tardia (after age 35).[8] The incidence of primary lymphedema has been reported to be 1:6000, with a male to female ratio of 1:3.[2] Potential abnormalities of lymphatic tissues in primary lymphedema include disorders of valves and vessel contractility, as well as lymphatic malformations such as hypoplasia, anaplasia, hypertrophy, and megalymphatics.

Secondary (acquired) lymphedema results from obstruction and/or obliteration of lymphatics.[16] Worldwide, filariasis causes the vast majority of noncancerous lymphedemas, with cases estimated at over 90 million. Trauma, surgery, childbirth, rheumatoid arthritis, and severe infections are also associated with noncancerous secondary lymphedema.[17] Cancer-related lymphedemas develop following surgical node dissection and/or radiation therapy to areas with concentrations of lymph nodes. These lymphedemas can also be secondary to invasion or compression of lymphatics from neoplasm.[7] Infection and thrombosis are known to precipitate lymphedema in patients treated for breast cancer.[18] Posttreatment weight gain,[19,20] repetitive and strenuous exercise/activity,[10] and sleep position on a high-risk limb[21] also appear to be associated with precipitation of lymphedema. Cancers commonly associated with lymphedema include breast, gynecological, prostate, sarcoma, melanoma, and lymphoma.

A wide range of lymphedema incidence has been reported for breast cancer survivors who have undergone axillary node dissection with or without radiation therapy. Ideally, incidence should be determined by quantitative measurement over many years following axillary node dissection[22] as lymphedema can occur 30 or more years after surgery.[23] Recent reports suggest a 25% incidence,[18,24] increasing to 38.3% when axillary radiation therapy is added.[25] For lymphedema of the lower extremity, an incidence range of 30% to 50% has been described.[26,27] Laparoscopic inguinal dissections are reported to reduce the incidence of lower-extremity lymphedema.[28,29] Sentinel biopsy also promises to reduce the incidence of secondary lymphedema in cancer patients undergoing node dissections.[30]

RELEVANT LYMPHEDEMA ANATOMY AND PHYSIOLOGY

The lymphatic system consists of interstitial space and fluid; lymph, lymph vessels, and nodes; lymphoid cells in the bone marrow, gut, spleen, and thymus gland; and free migrating lymphocytes. Functionally, this system regulates cellular environment in all tissues; removes cellular waste products, mutants and debris; eliminates non-self-antigens (organic and inorganic); and regulates local immune defense in the process of maintaining homeostasis.[31]

The lymphatic system is unidirectional, with vessels traversing from superficial to deep tissues, through 500 to 700 lymph nodes, to ultimately bring lymph to the right or left subclavian juncture (right or left terminus). Lymph nodes continually purify lymph, eliminating defective cells, toxins, and bacteria. Key nodal areas, consisting of concentrations of nodes, are located in the axillae, groin, neck, and gut (Fig. 15–3).

Increased tissue fluid causes tiny lymphatic capillaries (peripheral or initial lymphatics) to open and admit fluid and particles (Fig. 15–4). The presence of the fluid (officially lymph once it enters lymphatics) causes intrinsic pumping, further assisted by Starling's law of fluid balance. Transport advances to

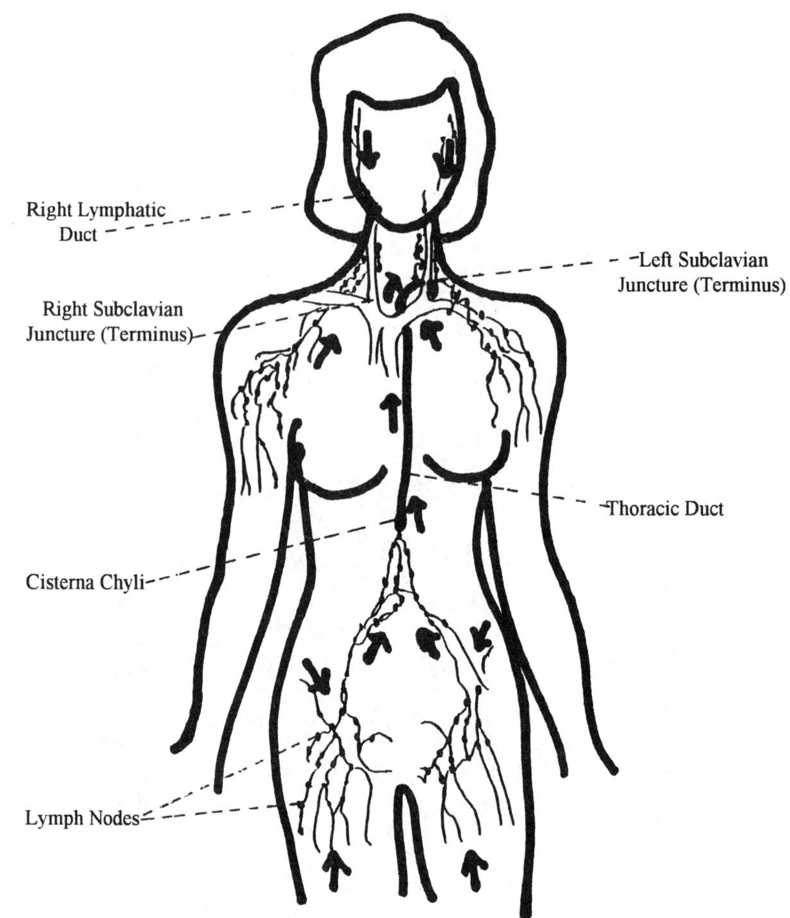

Fig. 15–3. Major components of lymphatic circulation. Large lymph vessels and key concentrations of lymph nodes are displayed. One-way directional flow causes all lymph to move to the subclavian junctures via either the thoracic duct or right lymphatic duct. The largest vessel, the thoracic duct, originates in the cisterna chyli.

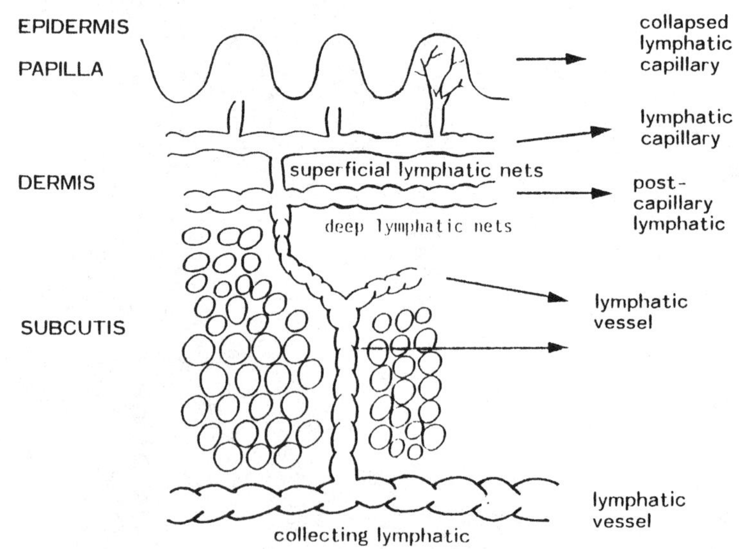

Fig. 15–4. Distribution of skin lymphatics. (Adapted from Olszewski, 1991, reference 8, with permission.)

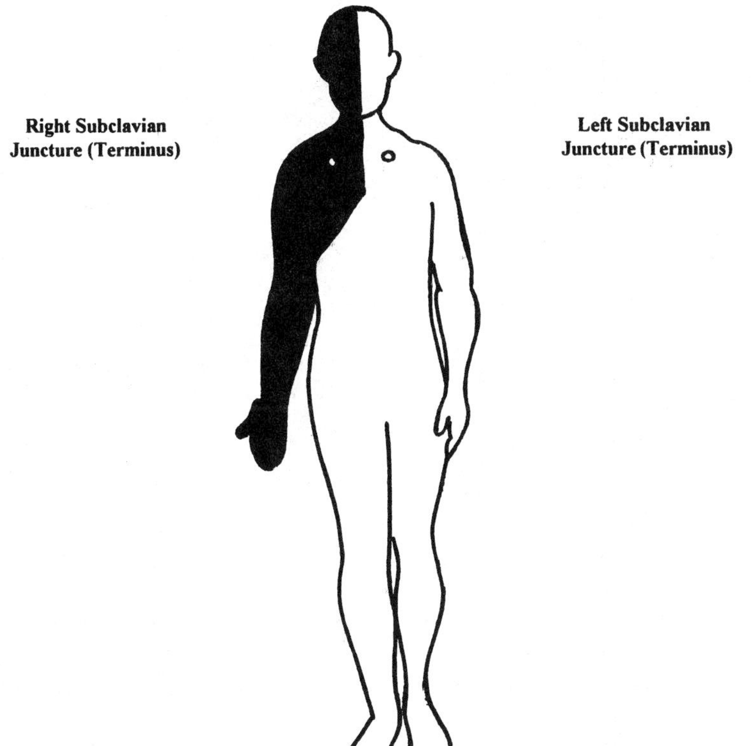

Fig. 15–5. Anatomical areas draining to the right and left subclavian junctures. Only the shaded area drains to the right. The rest of the body drains to the left subclavian juncture.

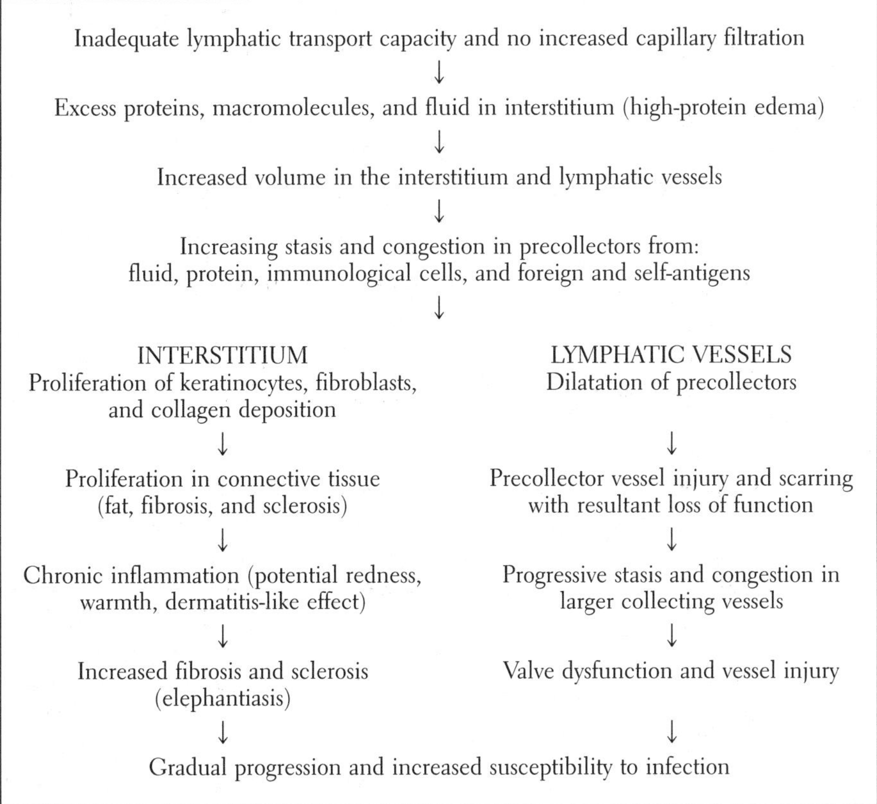

Figure 15–6. Basic lymphedema pathophysiology.

postcapillary vessels (precollectors), further to collecting lymphatics, to either the thoracic duct or the right lymphatic duct, and finally to the right or left subclavian juncture. Unequal distribution of drainage to these two circulatory entry sites is displayed in Figure 15–5. Respiration, as well as arterial and muscular contractions in the surrounding tissues, further stimulates lymphatic transport.

Lymphatic territories (also called lymphotomes or watersheds) have been described.[1,32] These anatomical regions of superficial lymphatics exhibit unidirectional flow of lymph on the journey to deeper lymphatics. Tiny collateral lymph vessels connect territories but provide minimal fluid transport. Knowledge of this directional flow and these collaterals is considered crucial to lymphatic fluid mobilization.

PATHOPHYSIOLOGY OF LYMPHEDEMA

Enlarging upon the definition provided earlier, Figure 15–6 summarizes the typical lymphedema pathophysiology. The common signs and symptoms of lymphedema, displayed in Table 15–1, reflect the results of this pathophysiology. Several researchers have reported decreased venous flow in limbs of cancer survivors with lymphedema[33,34] and increased arterial flow in limbs of breast cancer patients with lymphedema who have undergone axillary node dissection.[35,36] The significance of these findings is unclear, except to support the view that more remains to be learned about lymphedema pathophysiology.

DIAGNOSIS

A definitive diagnosis of lymphedema is often determined solely from a history and physical,[17,37] especially when conservative management is planned and symptomatology is not severe. A comprehensive history and physical exam substantiates the diagnosis and clarifies concomitant problems (i.e., infection, mobility, psychosocial issues). Components of a basic lymphedema assessment

Table 15–1. Lymphedema: Signs and Symptoms

Swelling and decreased skin mobility
Tightness, tingling, or bursting sensation
Decreased strength and mobility
Discomfort (ranging from aching to severe pain)
Changes in skin: color, texture, tone, temperature, and integrity

are listed in Table 15–2.[38,39] Undetected cancer, infection, thrombosis, as well as venous and arterial insufficiency must be ruled out or addressed during assessment. For example, assessment might reveal that a patient with suspected lymphedema actually has a low-protein edema related to mild congestive heart failure. Physical findings combined with a history revealing that the patient had replaced a cardiac medication with several "natural" supplements help to substantiate the diagnosis.

Imaging, such as lymphoscintigraphy, magnetic resonance imaging, or computed tomography, can be useful with unusual or severely problematic lymphedemas (i.e., chylus reflux or chylothorax).[40–42] In these situations, imaging might reveal additional problems and improve treatment decision making. Most experts recommend use of lymphoscintigraphy rather than lymphography when imaging is warranted. Lymphography/lymphangiography has been discouraged because of its potential to cause lymphatic injury.[16,43,44]

Two possible precipitators of lymphedema, neoplasms and thrombosis, require diagnostic evaluation. Venous ultrasound, rather than venography, offers safe evaluation for suspected thrombosis. Thrombotic precipitation of lymphedema, although uncommon, has been associated with breast cancer–related lymphedemas. Delayed or missed diagnosis can result in painful, large, and problematic lymphedema, especially in patients with metastatic disease. Anticoagulation is essential. Edema and symptom control generally improve with prompt attention.[11]

Table 15–2. Sequential Components of Lymphedema Assessment

Rule out or address immediate complications (i.e., infection, severe pain, cancer)
History and physical:
Past and current health status, including current medications and allergies
Current activities of daily living (job, home responsibilities, leisure activities)
Current psychological health
History of etiology, presentation, duration, and progression
Current signs and symptoms of lymphedema
Patient knowledge of lymphedema and interest in assistance
Support available to patient
Third-party payer status

LONG-TERM MANAGEMENT OF LYMPHEDEMA

In this text, "long-term management" is used to encompass all aspects of lifelong lymphedema management. The nine components of long-term management listed in Table 15–3 are the framework of this chapter and are applicable for nurses in all health care settings. In a climate of shrinking health care dollars, long-term management can produce better patient outcomes as well as save the time, anguish, and expense associated with complications.

Appropriate crisis management is the sequel to assessment, including referral of patients for multidisciplinary assistance. Infection, thrombosis, metastasis, or severe emotional distress must initially be addressed before launching into comprehensive management.[39] Occasionally, lymphedemas precipitated by thrombosis or metastasis resolve following the use of anticoagulant or antineoplastic crisis intervention therapy. In these situations, further nursing management simply requires instruction in lymphedema precautions (Table 15–4), and these patients will always have a high risk for developing lymphedema.

Table 15–3. Components of Long-Term Lymphedema Management

History, physical and ongoing assessment
Individualized and holistic care coordination
Multidiscipline referrals
Comprehensive patient instruction
Self-care (precautions and healthy lifestyle)
Psychosocial support
State-of-the-art treatment
Access and follow-up with knowledgeable health caregivers
Communication with health care providers
Management outcome measurement

TREATMENT OF LYMPHEDEMA

Lymphedema management and treatment decision making involve three essentials: knowledge of the principles of lymphedema and its management, individualized patient management, and critical thinking. For example, early-stage lymphedema is generally best managed by patient-directed self-care. Self-care typically includes adhering to precautions, weight management, exercise, a compression garment, optimal diet, and a healthy lifestyle. Allowing newly diagnosed patients an adjustment period before recommending a compression garment can improve overall patient self-care. Once patients see the lifelong nature of lymphedema and their need to be proactive, compliance to compression improves.

Complex Decongestive Physiotherapy (CDP, of the Foldi school) followed by Combined Decongestive Therapy (CDT, of the Vodder school) evolved in Europe.[45] These structured multimodality treatment approaches are considered "intensive therapy." Four modalities are included: skin care, exercise, external compression, and manual lymphatic therapy (a broad term used to describe manual fluid mobilization techniques based on *Dr. Vodder's Manual Lymph Drainage*[32]). Many titles are ascribed to variations of the four-component treatment strategy; all are referred to as "intensive therapy" here. Excellent results have been reported with intensive therapy, but a lack of standardized treatment, reliable and valid treatment outcome measures, compara-

Table 15–4. Lymphedema Precaution Activities

For the area with lymphedema
- Daily monitoring of skin
- Daily cleansing, drying, and lubrication
- Precaution against all irritation and breaks in the skin
- Immediately wash and treat any injuries or breaks in the skin
- Antibiotic therapy with any suspected or obvious infection

For an extremity
- Avoid heavy, strenuous, and repetitive activity
- Avoid limb dependence as much as possible
- Avoid restriction with tight shoes, clothing, jewelry, etc.
- Avoid venipuncture, all parenteral therapy, and blood pressure
- Avoid sleeping directly on the limb
- Use external compression during air travel

In general
- Healthy diet, high water intake, low sodium intake
- Maintain ideal weight
- Exercise to tolerance
- Regular medical follow-up
- Maintain all possible social and work activities
- Seek help for any problems

tive research, and third party payer reimbursement has hindered widespread use and acceptance. Since early detection and management often prevent the need for intensive therapy,[37,42] nurses' involvement in detection and prevention can significantly improve lymphedema control, reduce treatment expense, and help avoid the cancer metastasis complications depicted in Figure 15–2.

SKIN CARE

Standard lymphedema precautions emphasize meticulous care to protect skin health and integrity as well as to prevent cellulitis.[46] Lymphedema pathophysiology necessitates diabetic-like skin care. Bland, nonscented products are recommended for daily cleansing and moisturizing.[47] Emollients and moisturizers are essential for maintaining healthy skin. Water-based moisturizers (which absorb more readily) are less likely to damage compression products. Cotton clothing allows ventilation and is absorbent, helping skin to stay dry.

EXERCISE

While movement is essential in lymphedema management, no research has demonstrated the optimal exercise duration, intensity, activities, or precautions for people with lymphedema.[39] Restriction of strenuous and repetitive exercise has been encouraged based on practice results and anecdotal reports. Smith and Miller[39] have recommended establishing individual patient exercise tolerance through evaluation of patient response. Exercise tolerance can be determined through evaluation of edema volume, skin texture, and pain soon after exercise. Evaluation over time is also warranted. Since increased edema can occur slowly, very gradual increases in exercise will allow maximal safety in the exercise program.

Fitness is achieved by inclusion of aerobic, flexibility, and strengthening exercises. Physical, occupational, and exercise therapists who understand lymphedema pathophysiology are uniquely qualified to assist patients in establishing exercise programs. Weight-bearing exercise of the affected limb also requires gradual increases in intensity and careful limb evaluation. Higher levels of fitness should be possible for lymphedema patients through the use of external compressive support during exercise. Patient status and environment certainly affect the exercise program. The movement of the lymphatic flow is very important, and range-of-motion exercises (with caregiver assistance as needed) provide benefit for patients unable to carry out a more active program.

EXTERNAL COMPRESSION

External compression supports and protects skin and tissues as it reduces or controls edema. Without compression, the skin will stretch as much as necessary to accommodate fluid. Long-term benefits of compression include decreased accumulated protein, decreased arterial outflow into tissues, and improved valvular function.[48] Uneven compression, such as with blood pressure cuffs, tourniquets, watches, or elastic sleeves, is detrimental to lymphatic function.

Nonstretch (low-stretch or nonelastic) gradient external compression is paramount to lymphedema management. Gradient pressure refers to graduated pressure, which is greatest distally and slowly decreases proximally; gradient pressure enables physiological lymph flow. During exercise, muscle contractions stimulate lymphatic vessel contractions. Exercise combined with compression produces pressure above and below lymphatics to maximize lymphatic stimulation.[49]

Arterial disease, acute infection, or thrombosis in or near the area with edema usually precludes use of external compression.[50,51] Whenever compression causes pain or other neurological symptoms and/or discoloration or coolness of the fingers and toes, the compression should be removed. Readjustment of the compression product to avoid these problems or product replacement is necessary. The skin underneath external compression products often becomes dry and irritated; water-based moisturizers are recommended.[52] Commonly used products include compression garments (gloves, gauntlets, sleeves, and stockings), nonstretch bandages, and semirigid support. Manual Lymph Drainage and mechanical pumps are often classified as external compression. They also provide a more active component to fluid mobilization and are discussed individually.

Compression Garments

Compression garments maintain limb size[53] and are the least obtrusive form of compression. Since garments must have enough elasticity to allow application, their compression is inferior to nonstretch bandages.[54] Postoperative antiembolitic stockings are not appropriate substitutes for compression stockings because they do not provide either gradient pressure or a sufficient level of compression.

Contradictory instructions for the timing of garment usage are recommended by various manufacturers and experts. Both avoidance and inclusion of nighttime usage have been advocated.[21,48,54] Patient tolerance combined with effectiveness at edema control are crucial factors for establishing an individual patient's garment usage program. For example, if a patient finds daily edema greatest upon arising, nighttime garment use generally is helpful along with a change in the sleep position.

Since a variety of products exist, staff and patient persistence should result in patient satisfaction. Qualified, experienced fitters provide instruction in garment care, replacement, and wearing schedule. Long-term cost effectiveness (in the form of good lymphedema control) is enhanced by well-fitted garments that are used regularly. Use of rubber gloves while donning garments provides protection that increases garment life. Timely garment replacement is essential for good edema control. Garment life is 4 to 6 months,[48] depending on whether a patient uses one product or alternates between two. Acute home care and hospice settings generally require nurses to oversee garment replacement.

Bandaging

Nonstretch bandages (also called wrapping), not short stretch or Ace bandages, are used to reduce lymphedema volume, especially in combination with other treatments. These products (i.e., Comprilan, Rosidal) are more expensive than Ace bandages. Tubular gauze, followed by padding, is placed under bandages to improve effectiveness. The wrapping technique is very specific and somewhat labor-intensive. Bandages should be secured with tape rather than clips, to avoid skin abrasions. Since properly applied bandages provide adaptable compression for fluctuating limb size, bandages are essential during intensive therapy. Other indications for bandaging include gross edema, fragile or damaged skin, lymphorrhea, significant distortion in limb shape,[18] and as needed for patients at the end of life.

Semirigid Support

Several products have evolved that have been placed in a category of compression called semirigid support. Semirigid support provides nonstretch compression that is less time and labor intensive than nonstretch bandaging and more effective than traditional compression sleeves or stockings. These nonelastic products were initiated with the Unna boot, which utilized nonstretch compression combined with zinc oxide, calamine and glycerin gauze to assist in healing of foot ulcerations. The CircAid® semirigid product evolved next, designed and researched to address venous insufficiency complications.[55] Velcro was employed to attach segmental, nonstretch flaps/straps to encompass part or all of an extremity. CircAid advertises the provision of nonstretch compression that reduces the patient's need for manual dexterity, increases independent self care, and saves time and energy.

The Reid sleeve was designed by a medical oncologist to assist a patient with treatment-resistant lymphedema. This newer product has been substantiated by both manufacturer and nonaffiliated lymphedema treatment center research. Clear advantages of the Reid Sleeve include FDA approval, precisely gauged pressure, convoluted foam providing high/low pressure to improve peripheral and deep lymphatic transport, reduced tissue fibrosis, product longevity, and high patient compliance. Cost effectiveness has yet to be established, but since these products have the potential to significantly improve patient compliance and quality of life, future research is expected.

MANUAL LYMPHATIC THERAPIES

Manual lymph drainage (MLD) was developed by the Vodders in Europe.[56] Variations of this technique have evolved over time. For this chapter, all techniques following the principles of MLD are termed manual lymphatic therapy (MLT). These therapies are designed to alter tissue pressure, a necessary impetus for proper functioning of lymphatic capillaries and vessels.[39] A series of rhythmic skin-stretching movements using very light pressure stimulate lymphatics to improve lymphatic flow. In addition, MLT encourages lymphatic transport through collateral vessels and across lymphatic watersheds, creating new pathways for movement of fluid out of congested tissues. The trunk must initially be decongested during MLT, to stimulate systemic lymphatic transport as well as prepare for fluid input from the extremities. Deeper massage of fibrotic tissues is often provided.

CONTRAINDICATIONS TO LYMPHEDEMA TREATMENT

The Vodder school has delineated specific contraindications to MLT: untreated malignancy, acute generalized or local inflammation, thrombosis, and cardiac decompensation.[51] These recommendations are based on physiology, theory, and extensive experience and have been accepted by many experts.[45,50,57] Precautionary measures are advised for patients with treated cancer, precancerous lesions of the skin, chronic inflammation, bronchial asthma, functional disturbances of the thyroid, hypotonia, and autonomic dystonia. Precautionary measures related to MLT are also recommended for deep abdominal drainage and treatment of the neck.[51] Staff collaboration with physicians, in the face of any cardiac or respiratory problems, improves decision making as well as the local expert lymphedema knowledge base.

Acute infection generally precludes exercise and all forms of compression until signs and symptoms have resolved.

Compressive support should be avoided for 2 to 4 weeks after radiation therapy, to allow tissue healing. Following thrombosis, MLT and external compression are contraindicated until inflammation and embolism risk are no longer present.[51] CoWrap and CoBan Cohesive Bandages (made by Smith & Nephew and available over the counter) are self-adhering, nonadhesive wraps that provide gentle compression. Early use of one of these products has provided support and relief to patients with severe lymphedema soon after the presentation of thrombosis.[11] As with the use of all compression products, circulation must be monitored.

The Vodder and Foldi schools have traditionally precluded the use of MLT in the presence of cancer metastasis.[51] This viewpoint has been challenged by the International Society of Lymphology.[37] Current understanding of cancer metastasis demonstrates that lymphatic spread of cancer is only part of a complex process that is not yet fully understood. It is believed that metastasis may begin very early in the development of a primary tumor.[58] There are no data indicating that cancer can be spread through manipulation, especially for patients with suspected cancer or early metastatic cancer. In widely metastatic patients, with little hope of remission or cure, substantial comfort and quality of life can be achieved with combinations of treatments, including MLT. Appropriate decisions should be collaboratively made by the patient, treatment staff, and physician(s).

PNEUMATIC (MECHANICAL) PUMPS AND SURGICAL TREATMENTS

Robert Lerner's lymphedema treatment experience historically supports the superiority of intensive therapy over treatment by either compression pumps or surgery.[59] Lerner, a pioneer in American lymphedema treatment, has utilized all three modalities and concluded that intensive therapy is superior. Both Lerner and Foldi see no role for pumps and a minimal role for surgery in lymphedema management.[60,61] Some experts have concluded that pumps can assist in limb reduction by improving venous return, but pumps do not address tissue fibrosis.[1,39,62] No research currently substantiates the role of mechanical pumps in lymphedema management.

Other concerns are expressed. Unless MLT is combined with the use of pumps, mechanical compression can cause unwanted edema accumulations in the area just proximal to the compression sleeve (i.e., the trunk or genitalia).[60,61] In addition, pumps are confining, time-consuming, expensive, and potentially injurious to peripheral lymphatics and no research substantiates optimal treatment protocol.[48]

Multiple surgical interventions have been described for lymphedema, including both microsurgical anastamoses and debulking or reduction techniques. Surgical intervention is often described as a treatment of last resort[37] because cosmetic results and long-term effectiveness are not impressive. In Sweden, excellent reduction has been achieved with surgical liposuction.[63] Surgical intervention has also provided important benefits for patients with eyelid or genital edema.[5]

PHARMACOLOGICAL INTERVENTIONS

Medications commonly used in lymphedema management include antimicrobials, antifungals, antiinflammatories, anticoagulants, proteolytics (i.e., benzopyrones), and diuretics. Benzopyrones have been extensively researched by Casley-Smith and Casley-Smith.[64] Coumarin (5,6-benzo-[α]-pyrone) and flavonoids/bioflavonoids (y-benzopyrones) appear to increase both the number and activity of proteolytic cells (i.e., macrophages) in tissues, to help decrease interstitial protein accumulation.[65] These proteolytics were explored in order to address management of filariasis-related lymphedema for people in underdeveloped nations, where lymphedema treatment options were extremely limited. Liver toxicity, associated with the use of benzopyrone, resulted in the product's withdrawal from Australian medical practice. The Food and Drug Administration has never approved the use of benzopyrones for the treatment of lymphedema in the United States. Recently, the Mayo Clinic reported no edema reduction by coumarin/benzopyrone for breast cancer survivors with lymphedema.[66]

No data support the long-term use of diuretics in lymphedema management.[7] "Diuretics remain the most commonly used treatment because, to most doctors, edema is an indication for such drugs."[16] Diuretics contradict "the pathophysiology of edema and the pharmacology of diuretics."[61] Specifically, diuretics provide little benefit in lymphedema because they limit capillary filtration by reducing circulating systemic blood volumes.[16] Isotope lymphography has substantiated that removal of blood volume fluid in lymphedema patients decreases the rate of lymphatic drainage.[67]

The International Society of Lymphology concluded that diuretics offer marginal benefit to lymphedema patients and potentially complicate fluid and electrolyte disturbances.[34] Diuretics have been recommended by experts for lymphedema conditions that cause effusion of lymph into body cavities (i.e., abdomen or thorax) or lymphatic obstruction associated with malignancy.[34] Short-term use of diuretics following infection and thrombosis has been helpful for some patients.

UNUSUAL LYMPHEDEMAS

Nurses providing palliative care might be faced with unusual lymphedema of the breast, head, neck, trunk, or genitals. Such lymphedemas, in first-world nations, are generally secondary to malignancy or primary lymphedema. These conditions are more difficult to treat.[16] Manual lymphatic therapies, skin-softening techniques, and external compression (as possible) are recommended. External compression can be very challenging. Collars, vests, custom pants or tights, scrotal supports,[47] and spandex-type exercise apparel are examples of creative methods for providing compression. Expert seamstress skills might be required. Surgery has been recommended for some of these lymphedemas.[5] Consultation with one or more experts prior to surgery could be extremely beneficial.

PROBLEMS AND COMPLICATIONS OF LYMPHEDEMA

Many difficulties can arise following a lymphedema diagnosis, beginning with the presenting signs and symptoms (Table 15–1). Perhaps the most troublesome is the over-sized limb or body area, which makes an individual different from others. Society often does not accept those who are different, and as Ryan stated, "There is no disability worse than to be unwelcome." [68]

Early detection and management are the best strategies to prevent problems and complications.[69] Common problems of a lymphedema diagnosis are displayed in Table 15–5. The elderly, disabled, and patients with neglected lymphedemas, metastatic cancer, or other end-stage disease are most susceptible to difficulties. Limb circumference and/or volume is commonly used to quantify lymphedema status.[70] Use of additional "standard" outcome measures, such as incidence of infection, function, psychosocial status, and pain, could improve detection and management of lymphedema-related problems. Comprehensive, research-based outcome measures could also provide the basis for comparative treatment research.

Table 15–5. Lymphedema: Problems and Complications

Functional problems: range-of-motion limitations
Progressive gait problems
Limitations in activities of daily living
Various disabilities
Loss of self-sufficiency
Skin changes and pathologies
Weight gain
Discomfort/pain
Decreased self-esteem
Depression and anxiety
Decreased sexual activity
Increased risk of infectious disease
Lymphangiosarcoma

Functional problems are usually proportional to the extent of edema. Rehabilitation and social services enhance management. Weight gain is associated with increased risk and severity of lymphedema. Assisting patients in maintaining their ideal weight is therefore beneficial, though challenging. Dietitians as well as exercise and weight loss therapists/programs can be helpful.

Skin Complications

Complications of dermal integrity include pain, dermatitis, odor, hyperkeratosis, warts, papillomas, lymphorrhea, and both bacterial and fungal infections.[18] Prevention, through early lymphedema management, is the most effective strategy. When problems occur, referral for multidisciplined expertise is often appropriate. Dermatologists, wound clinics, and podiatrists specialize in skin problems.

Mild dermatitis and odor may respond to a combination of frequent cleansing; avoidance of moist, perspiring skin; and use of moisturizers (lubricants). Limb-reduction strategies are obviously most beneficial. Investigation of causes of the dermatitis might reveal allergy (occasionally to compression products) or eczema. Corticosteroid creams can be helpful. Dermatologist referrals are appropriate.[46] When dermatitis remains resistant to treatment, a biopsy will either identify or rule out malignancy.

Hyperkeratosis refers to thickening of the stratum corneum, causing excess hardened skin and scales.[46] Emollients should be massaged into the skin several times a day. Compression along with MLT are appropriate. The presence of warts and papillomas (benign epithelial tumors) and severe dermatitis are signs of neglected, long-standing lymphedema. Dermatology referral in combination with intensive therapy generally is appropriate. Lymphoceles (blisters) respond to external compression. Lymphorrhea describes leakage of lymph through a break in the skin. Immediate treatment of lymphorrhea is required to prevent infection. Paraffin gauze or a nonadhering dressing is recommended, followed by thick sterile pads and compression bandaging, which is changed as needed. Long-term compression is essential.[18]

Psychosocial Problems

Research suggests that breast cancer survivors who develop lymphedema have greater psychological, social, sexual, and functional morbidity than survivors without lymphedema. The most disability was reported for those who have poor social support, pain, lymphedema in the dominant hand, and/or passive or avoidant coping styles.[69] Spiritual distress, not addressed in the lymphedema literature, can also profoundly impact patient adjustment and quality of life. While cancer-related lymphedema complicates a patient's experience, many of these psychosocial issues should also be expected in patients with lymphedemas of other etiologies.

The concerned nurse can make significant improvements to a patient's quality of life by assessing for potential psychosocial problems. Referral avenues include counselors, chaplains, mentors, support groups, and nurses' caring strategies.[71] When the nurse takes time to explain the patient's diagnosis, etiology, and self-care activities, the patient frequently experiences a sense of empowerment. The knowledge and increased sense of control reduce the patient's fears. Other patients require additional support, repeated reinforcement of instruction, professional counseling, and/or referral to a support group. Patients with handicaps may have additional unique needs. One example is a breast cancer survivor who had a history of a head injury. She exhibited memory deficits that presented many challenges in her care.

Psychosocial problems can be minimized by the nurse who frequently follows up with the patient by offering support, reinforcing education, and assisting with garment replacement providers or services. Coordination of care and communication with physicians and other health care providers will significantly reduce stressors for the lymphedema patient.

Pain

The degree of pain associated with lymphedema is not known.[72] Foldi[73] reported that lymphedema is not associated with significant pain. He suggested that further exploration into the etiology is warranted in the face of pain. A 30% to 60% incidence of pain has been reported in breast cancer survivors with lymphedema.[72] Pain etiologies primarily included infection, postoperative changes in the axilla, postmastectomy pain syndrome, brachial plexopathy, and various arthritic conditions. Less common causes of pain included peripheral entrapment neuropathies, vascular compromise, and cancer recurrence.[72]

Sudden onset of pain always requires assessment for infection, thrombosis, or metastasis. Patients should be asked to quantify their pain level at regular intervals.[72] The 0 to 10 pain scale of Serlin and colleagues[74] has demonstrated effectiveness for the evaluation of pain.

Treatment of pain in patients with lymphedema uses the principles for treatment of chronic pain. The patient's self-report of pain must be believed. The most appropriate pain medications should be selected and other medications added as needed (i.e., antidepressants, antianxiety medications, nonsteroidal antiinflammatory drugs, etc.). Excellent patient teaching and communication about the pain management plan will assure the most beneficial outcome.

Infection

Infection, the most common lymphedema complication,[8] requires constant vigilance. Stasis, tissue congestion, and a protein-rich environment increase susceptibility for infection. Streptococci and/or staphylococci are frequent precipitators.[47,75] In addition to the normal signs and symptoms of infection, fever, lethargy, and nausea can be present.[72] Decreased local immune competence has also been documented.[76] Ample literature supports prompt antibiotic therapy.[16,77–80] Management is often improved by specialized wound care and infectious disease specialists. Intravenous antibiotic therapy is recommended for systemic signs of infection and/or insufficient response to oral antibiotics.[72] Once infection occurs, nurses contribute to management by assisting patients in obtaining prompt antibiotic therapy; encouraging high fluid intake; monitoring temperature, symptomatology, rest, and elevation of the affected limb; and avoiding use of external compression, MLT, or compression pumps.

The feet are especially susceptible to fungal infections in lower-extremity lymphedema. Peeling or scaly skin and toenail changes are frequent signs of fungal problems. Antifungal powders are recommended prophylactically. Antifungal creams should be used at the first sign of a fungal infection. Meticulous skin care, cotton socks, and well-fitting, sturdy shoes are also necessary.[46]

Prophylaxis has been recommended for patients who experience repeated serious infections.[5,31] Long-acting intramuscular benzathine penicillin (1,200,000 units every 3 weeks) has been effective.[31] Although injections are invasive, patients are spared taking a daily oral antibiotic and staff can monitor compliance. Penicillin V (phenoxymethyl penicillin) 500 mg daily has also been recommended.[16]

Lymphangiosarcoma

The most serious complication and the only potentially fatal one is lymphangiosarcoma, or Stewart-Treves syndrome. This malignancy is a form of sarcoma of the vascular endothelium[5] and occurs in patients with chronic lymphedema of any etiology. In postmastectomy patients, lymphangiosarcoma has been reported to occur 5 to 25 years after the presentation of lymphedema. Frequency has been described as between 0.07% and 0.45%. A single bruise or a cluster of bruises (*ecchymosis*) initially presents in or near the area with lymphedema. Lesions metastasize rapidly and profusely. Median survival has been reported as 1.3 years. Radical amputation, radiation therapy, and multimodality chemotherapy have provided cure or increased survival for some patients; but overall, prognosis is poor. Early recognition of skin lesions, followed by appropriate treatment interventions, could impact survival.[81,82]

CONCLUSION

The significance of nursing to lymphedema management began to emerge over the last decade.[10,39,46,83–89] Both the unique role of nursing and the nurse's immense patient access allow great opportunity to improve lymphedema management. This chapter has summarized the practice, literature, and research related to lymphedema management, to provide a broad knowledge base. It is hoped that this information will inspire additional nursing contributions to lymphedema care. At the very least, nursing can impact lymphedema prevention, access to care, and patient education and empowerment. Nurses providing lymphedema care can make significant contributions to developing standards, measuring treatment outcomes, and educating other health care providers. Nurses involved in end-of-life care of the lymphedema patient must ensure the cornerstones of palliative care, optimal symptom management and improved quality of life.

REFERENCES

1. Casley-Smith J. Modern treatment of lymphedema. Mod Med 1992;35:70–83.

2. Hafez H, Wolfe J. Lymphedema. Ann Vasc Surg 1996;10:88–95.

3. Witte C, Witte M. Advances in lymphatic imaging—implications for patients with lymphedema. Natl Lymphedema Netw Newslett 1992; 4:1–5.

4. Mortimer P. The pathophysiology of lymphedema. Cancer (Suppl) 1998;83:2798–2802.

5. Mortimer P. Therapy approaches for lymphedema. Angiology 1997;48:87–91.

6. Stanton A, Levick J, Mortimer P. Current puzzles presented by postmastectomy oedema (breast cancer related lymphoedema). Vasc Med 1996;1:214–215.

7. Brennan M, DePompolo R, Garden F. Postmastectomy lymphedema. Arch Phys Med Rehabil 1996;77(Suppl 3):S74–S80.

8. Olszewski W. Lymph Stasis: Pathophysiology, Diagnosis and Treatment. Boca Raton, FL: CRC Press, 1991:31, 187, 294–296, 348, 349.

9. Olszewski W. The world of lymphology—1995. Natl Lymphedema Netw Newslett 1995;7: 1–7.

10. Petrek J, Lerner R. Lymphedema. In: Harris JR, Morrow M, Lippman ME, Hellman S, eds. Diseases of the Breast. New York: Lippincott-Raven, 1996:896–903.

11. Smith J. Collaborative approach to treatment of lymphedema with breast cancer complications: a case study. Natl Lymphedema Netw Newslett 1997;9:1–7.

12. Browse N, Stewart G. Lymphedema: pathophysiology and classification. J Cardiovasc Surg 1985;26:91–106.

13. Foldi E, Foldi M, Clodius L. The lymphedema chaos: a lancet. Ann Plast Surg 1989;22: 505–506.

14. Foldi M, Foldi E. Lymphedema Methods for Treatment and Control: A Guide for Patients and Therapists. Malvern: Lymphoedema Association of Australia, 1993:48–49.

15. Klose G. Treatment choices for chronic extremity lymphedema. Phys Ther Forum 1991; X:6–7.

16. Mortimer P. Managing lymphoedema. Clin Exp Dermatol 1995;20:98–106.

17. Rockson S. Secondary lymphedema of the lower extremities. Natl Lymphedema Netw Newslett 1998;10:1–13.

18. Mortimer PS, Badger C, Hall JG. Lymphoedema. In: Doyle D, Hanks GW, MacDonald N, eds. Oxford Textbook of Palliative Medicine. Oxford. Oxford University Press, 1998:657–664.

19. Werner R, McCormick B, Petrek J, et al. Arm edema in conservatively managed breast cancer: obesity is a major predictive factor. Radiology 1991;180:177–184.

20. Bertelli G, Venturini M, Forno G, et al. An analysis of prognostic factors in response to conservative treatment of post-mastectomy lymphedema. Surg Gynecol Obstet 1992;175:455–460.

21. Casley-Smith J. Newsletter. Malvern: Lymphoedema Association of Australia, 1998.

22. Petrak J, Heelan M. Incidence of breast carcinoma-related lymphedema. Cancer (Suppl) 1998;83:2776–2781.

23. Brennan M, Weitz J. Lymphedema 30 years after radical mastectomy. Am J Phys Med Rehabil 1992;71:12–14.

24. Logan V. Incidence and prevalence of lymphoedema: a literature review. J Clin Nurs 1995;4:213–219.

25. Kissin M, della Rovere G, Easton D, et al. Risk of lymphoedema following the treatment of breast cancer. Br J Surg 1986;73:580–584.

26. Werngren-Elgstrom M, Lidman D. Lymphoedema of the lower extremities after surgery and radiotherapy for cancer of the cervix. Scand J Plast Reconstr Surg Hand Surg 1994;28:289–293.

27. James J. Lymphoedema following ilioinguinal lymph node dissection. Scand J Plast Reconstr Surg 1982;16:167–171.

28. Lang G, Ruckle H, Hadley H, et al. One hundred consecutive laparoscopic pelvic lymph node dissections: comparing complications of the first 50 cases to the second 50 cases. Urology 1994;44:221–225.

29. Kavoussi L, Sosa E, Chandhoke P, et al. Complications of laparoscopic pelvic lymph node dissection. J Urol 1993;149:322–325.

30. Giuliano A, Jones R, Brennan M, et al. Sentinal lymphadenectomy in breast cancer. J Clin Oncol 1997;15:2345–2350.

31. Olszewski W. What Is Lymphology? An Updated View, 1996. Paper presented at the International Society of Lymphology Conference, Madrid, Spain, September 1997.

32. Kasseroller R. Compendium of Dr. Vodder's Manual Lymph Drainage. Heidelberg: Karl F. Huag Verlag, 1998:58.

33. Svensson W, Mortimer P, Toho E, et al. Colour doppler demonstrates venous flow abnormalities in breast cancer patients with chronic arm swelling. Eur J Cancer 1994;30A:657–660.

34. Kim D, Huh S, Hwang J, Kim Y, Lee B. Venous dynamics in leg lymphedema. Lymphology 1999;32:11–14.

35. Martin KP, Foldi E. Are hemodynamic factors important in arm lymphedema after treatment of breast cancer? Lymphology 1996;29:155–157.

36. Svenson W, Mortimer P, Tohno E, et al. Increased arterial inflow demonstrated by doppler ultrasound in arm swelling following breast cancer treatment. Eur J Cancer 1994;30A:661–664.

37. International Society of Lymphology Executive Committee, Consensus Document. The diagnosis and treatment of peripheral lymphedema. Lymphology 1995;28:113–117.

38. Smith J. Oncology nursing in lymphedema management. Innov Breast Cancer Care 1998;3:82–87.

39. Smith J, Miller L. Management of patients with cancer-related lymphedema. Oncol Nurs Updates 1998;5:1–12.

40. Zelikovski A, Haddad M, Stelman E, et al. Primary long-standing chylous reflux into skin. Lymphology 1995;28:186–188.

41. Hillerdal G. Chylothorax and pseudochylothorax. Eur Respir J 1997;10:1157–1162.

42. Rockson S, Miller L, Senie R, et al. Workgroup III: Diagnosis and management of lymphedema. Cancer (Suppl) 1998;83:2883.

43. McNeill G, Witte M, Witte C, et al. Whole-body lymphangioscintigraphy: preferred method for initial assessment of the peripheral lymphatic system. Radiology 1989;172:495–502.

44. Weissleder H, Weissleder R. Lymphedema: evaluation of qualitative and quantitative lymphoscintigraphy in 238 patients. Radiology 1998;167:729–735.

45. Casley-Smith J, Boris M, Weindorf S, et al. Treatment for lymphedema of the arm—the Casley-Smith method. Cancer (Suppl) 1998;83: 2843.

46. Williams A, Venables B. Skin care in patients with uncomplicated lymphoedema. J Wound Care 1996;5:223–226.

47. Regnard C, Allport S, Stephenson L. ABC of palliative care: mouth care, skin care, and lymphoedema. BMJ 1997;315:1004–1005.

48. Rymal C. Compression modalities in lymphedema therapy. Innov Breast Cancer Care 1998;3:88–92.

49. Stemmer R, Marescaux J, Furderer C. Compression treatment of the lower extremities particularly with compression stockings. Dermatologist 1980;31:355–365.

50. Brennan M, Miller L. Overview of treatment options and review of the current role and use of compression garments, intermittent pumps, and exercise in the management of lymphedema. Cancer (Suppl) 1998;83:2821–2827.

51. Kurz I. III. Contraindications, side effects and precautionary measures with M.L.D. In: Harris RH, trans., ed. Textbook of Dr. Vodder's Manual Lymph Drainage. Treatment Manual, 3rd Ed. Brussels: Editions Haug International, 1996: 23–35.

52. Casley-Smith J, Casley-Smith J. Modern Treatment for Lymphoedema Malvern: Lymphoedema Association of Australia, 1997:159–160.

53. Yasuhara H, Shigematsu H, Muto T. A study of the advantages of elastic stockings for leg lymphedema. Int Angiol 1996;15:272–277.

54. Staudinger P. Compression bandaging for lymphedema. Natl Lymphedema Netw Newslett 1993;5:5–6.

55. Bergan J. Control of lower extremity L/e by semirigid support. Natl Lymphedema Netw Newslett 1994;6:1–6.

56. Connell M. Complete decongestive physiotherapy. Innov Breast Cancer Care 1998;3: 93.

57. Tunkel R, Lachmann E. Lymphedema of the limb—an overview of treatment options. Postgrad Med 1998;104:131–144.

58. LeMarbre P, Groenwald S. The metastatic sequence. In: Groenwald SL, Frogge MH, Goodman M, eds. Cancer Nursing: Principles and Practice, 4th Ed. Boston: Jones and Bartlett, 1997: 26–34.

59. Lerner R. Lymphedema: a 25 year perspective. Natl Lymphedema Netw Newslett 1997; 9:1–11.

60. Lerner R. Complete decongestive physiotherapy and the Lerner Lymphedema Services Academy of Lymphatic Studies. Cancer (Suppl) 1998;83:2861–2863.

61. Foldi M, Foldi E. Conservative treatment of lymphedema. In: Olszewski W, ed. Lymph Stasis: Pathophysiology, Diagnosis and Treatment. Boca Raton, FL: CRC Press, 1991:473–474.

62. Leduc O, Leduc A, Bourgeois P, et al. The physical treatment of upper limb edema. Cancer (Suppl) 1998;83:2836.

63. Brorson H, Svenson H, Norrgren K, et al. Liposuction reduces arm lymphedema without significantly altering the already impaired lymph transport. Lymphology 1998;31:156–172.

64. Casley-Smith J, Casley-Smith J. The pathophysiology of lymphedema and the action of benzo-pyrones in reducing it. Lymphology 1988; 21:190–194.

65. Casley-Smith J, Morgan R, Piller N. Treatment of lymphedema of the arms and legs with 5,6-benzo-*(a)*-pyrone. N Engl J Med 1993; 329:1158–1163.

66. Loprinzi C, Kugler J, Sloan J, et al. Lack of effect of coumarin in women with lymphedema after treatment for breast cancer. N Engl J Med 1999;340:346–350.

67. Tiedjen K. Isotopenlymphographische Untrusting (Technetium-Zinn-II-Schwefelkolloid) oberer Extremitäten beg Zustand nach Mam-

maamputation und Bestrahlung. Phlebol Proktol 1983;12:196.

68. Ryan T. Skin failure and lymphedema. Natl Lymphedema Netw Newslett 1996;8:1–5.

69. Passik S, McDonald M. Psychosocial aspects of upper extremity lymphedema in women treated for breast carcinoma. Cancer (Suppl) 1998;83:2817–2820.

70. Gerber L. A review of measures of lymphedema. Cancer (Suppl) 1998;83:2803–2804.

71. Mast ME. Nurse case managers bring element of caring to cost-contained care. Oncol Nurs Soc News 1999;13:1–5.

72. Brennan M. The complexity of pain in post breast cancer lymphedema. Natl Lymphedema Netw Newslett 1999;11:1–8.

73. Foldi E. The treatment of lymphedema. Cancer (Suppl) 1998;83:2833–2834.

74. Serlin R, Mendoza T, Nakamura Y, et al. When is cancer pain mild, moderate or severe? Grading pain severity by its interference with function. Pain 1995;61:277–284.

75. Tierney LM, Messina LM. Blood vessels and lymphatics/diseases of the lymphatic channels. In: Tierney LM, McPhee SJ, Papadakis MA, eds. Current Medical Diagnosis and Treatment, 37th Ed. Stamford, CT: Appleton & Lange, 1998: 473–474.

76. Mallon E, Powell S, Mortimer P, Ryan T. Evidence for altered cell-mediated immunity in postmastectomy lymphoedema. Br J Dermatol 1997;137:928–933.

77. Simon M, Cody R. Cellulitis after axillary lymph node dissection for carcinoma of the breast. Am J Med 1992;93:543–548.

78. Britton R, Nelson P. Causes and treatment of postmastectomy lymphedema of the arm. JAMA 1962;180:95–102.

79. Olszewski W. Episodic dermatolymphangioadenitis (DLA) in patients with lymphedema of the lower extremities before and after administration of benzathine penicillin: a preliminary study. Lymphology 1996;29:126–131.

80. Hughes L, Styblo T, Thomas W, et al. Cellulitis of the breast as a complication of breast-conserving surgery and irradiation. Am J Clin Oncol 1997;20:338–341.

81. Morton D, Antman K, Tepper J. Soft tissue sarcomas. In: Hollan JF, Morton DL, Frei E, Kufe DW, Weichselbaum RR, eds. Cancer Medicine, 4th Ed. Baltimore: Williams & Wilkins, 1997:2566.

82. Haskell C. Adjuvant treatment of breast cancer. In: Haskell C, ed. Cancer Treatment, 4th Ed. Philadelphia: WB Saunders, 1990:381–566.

83. Badger C. A problem for nurses—lymphedema. Surg Nurse 1988;1:14–19.

84. Thiadens S. Advances in the management of lymphedema. Perspect Plast Surg 1990; 4:181–182.

85. Woods M. Developing a service for the management of lymphedema. Nurs Stand 1991;5: 10–12.

86. Smith J. Lymphedema prevention: a systematic approach. ONS Spec Interest Group Newslett Lymphedema Manage 1992;2:1–3.

87. Jeffs E. Management of lymphoedema: putting treatment into context. J Tissue Viabil 1992;2:127–128.

88. Kirshbaum M. The development, implementation and evaluation of guidelines for the management of breast cancer related lymphoedema. Eur J Cancer Care 1996;5:246–251.

89. Knobf TM. Lymphedema management. Innov Breast Cancer Care 1998;3:81–116.

16 Skin Disorders

BARBARA M. BATES-JENSEN, LYNNE EARLY, and SUSIE SEAMAN

Palliative care for skin disorders is a broad area, encompassing prevention and care for pressure ulcers, management of tumor necrosis and fistulae, and management of stomas. The goals of treatment are often to reduce discomfort, manage odor and drainage, and provide for optimal functional capacity. In each area, involvement of the caregiver and family in the plan of care is important. Management of skin disorders involves significant physical care as well as attention to psychological and social care. To meet the needs of the patient and family, access to the multidisciplinary care team is crucial and consultation by an Enterostomal Therapy or certified Wound, Ostomy, Continence nurse is highly desirable.

Pressure ulcers are areas of local tissue trauma, usually developing where soft tissues are compressed between bony prominences and external surfaces for prolonged periods. Mechanical injury to the skin and tissues causes hypoxia and ischemia, leading to tissue necrosis. Caring for the patient with a pressure ulcer can be frustrating for clinicians because of the chronic nature of the wound and because additional time and resources are often invested in the management of these wounds. Pressure ulcer care is costly, and treatment costs increase as the severity of the wound increases. Additionally, not all pressure ulcers heal, and many heal slowly, causing a continual drain on caregiver and financial resources. The chronic nature of a pressure ulcer challenges the health care provider to design more effective treatment plans.

Once a pressure ulcer develops, the usual goal is to manage the wound, to support healing. However, some patients will benefit most from a palliative care approach. Palliative wound care means that the goals are comfort and limiting the extent or impact of the wound but without the intent of healing. Palliative care for chronic wounds such as pressure ulcers is appropriate for a wide variety of patient populations. Palliative care is often indicated for terminally ill patients such as those with end-stage cancer or in the terminal stages of other diseases. Institutionalized older adults with multiple comorbidities or older adults with severe functional decline may also benefit from palliative care. Sometimes individuals with longstanding wounds and other expectations for life benefit from a palliative care approach for a specified duration of time. For example, a wheelchair-bound young adult or teenager with a sacral pressure ulcer may choose (hopefully a fully informed choice) to continue to be up in a wheelchair to attend school even though the expectation for wound healing will be severely diminished. The health care professional may decide jointly with the patient to treat the wound palliatively during this time frame.

The foundation for designing a care plan for the patient with a pressure ulcer is a comprehensive assessment. This is true even if the goals of care are palliation. Comprehensive assessment includes assessment of wound severity, wound status, and the total patient. Generally, management of the wound is best accomplished within the context of the whole person, particularly when palliation is the outcome. Thus, assessment is the first step in maintaining and evaluating a therapeutic plan of care. Without adequate baseline wound and patient assessment and valid interpretation of the assessment data, the plan of care for the wound may be inappropriate or ineffective. At the least, the plan of care may be disjointed and fragmented from poor communication. An inadequate plan of care may lead to impaired or delayed healing, miscommunication regarding the goals of care (healing vs. palliation), and complications such as infection.

PATHOPHYSIOLOGY OF PRESSURE ULCER DEVELOPMENT

Pressure ulcers are the result of mechanical injury to the skin and underlying tissues. The primary forces involved are pressure and shear.[1–5] *Pressure* is the perpendicular force or load exerted on a specific area, causing ischemia and hypoxia of the tissues. High-pressure areas in the supine position are the occiput, sacrum, and heels. In the sitting position, the ischial tuberosities exert the highest pressure, and the trochanters are affected in the side-lying position.[2,6]

As the amount of soft tissue available for compression decreases, the pressure gradient increases. Likewise, as the tissue available for compression increases, the pressure gradient decreases; thus, most pressure ulcers occur over bony prominences, where there is less tissue for compression.[6] This relationship is important to understand for palliative care because most of the patients who are likely candidates for palliative care will have experienced significant changes in nutritional status and body weight with diminished soft tissue available for compression and a more prominent bony structure. This more prominent bony structure is more susceptible to skin breakdown from external forces as the soft tissue that is normally used to deflect physical forces (such as pressure or shear) is absent. Thus, the tissues are less tolerant of external forces and the pressure gradient within the vascular network is altered.[6]

Alterations in the vascular network allow an increase in the interstitial fluid pressure, which exceeds the venous flow. This results in an additional increase in the pressure and impedes arteriolar circulation. The capillary vessels collapse, and thrombosis occurs. Increased capillary arteriolar pressure leads to fluid loss through the capillaries, tissue edema, and subsequent autolysis. Lymphatic flow is decreased, allowing further tissue edema and contributing to the tissue necrosis.[3,5,7–9]

Pressure, over time, occludes blood and lymphatic circulation, causing deficient tissue nutrition and build-up of waste products due to ischemia. If pressure is relieved before a critical time period is reached, a normal compensatory mechanism, reactive hyperemia, restores tissue nutrition and compensates for compromised circulation. If pressure is not relieved before the critical time period, the blood vessels collapse and thrombose, causing tissue deprivation of oxygen, nutrients, and waste removal. In the absence of oxygen, cells utilize anaerobic pathways for metabolism and produce toxic by-products. The toxic by-products lead to tissue acidosis, increased cell membrane permeability, edema, and eventually cell death.[3,7]

Tissue damage may also be due to reperfusion and reoxygenation of the ischemic tissues or postischemic injury.[10] Oxygen is reintroduced into tissues during reperfusion following ischemia. This triggers oxygen-free radicals known as superoxide anion, hydroxyl radicals, and hydrogen peroxide, which induce endothelial damage and decrease microvascular integrity. Ischemia and hypoxia of body tissues are produced when capillary blood flow is obstructed by localized pressure. How much pressure and what amount of time is necessary for ulceration to occur has been a subject of study for many years. In 1930, Landis,[11] using single-capillary microinjection techniques, determined normal hydrostatic pressure to be 32 mm Hg at the arteriolar end and 15 mm Hg at the venular end. His work has been the criterion for measuring occlusion of capillary blood flow. Generally, a range from 25 to 32 mm Hg is considered normal and used as the marker for adequate relief of pressure on the tissues. In severely compromised patients, even this level of pressure may be too high.

Pressure is the greatest at the bony prominence and soft tissue interface and gradually lessens in a cone-shaped gradient to the periphery.[2,12,13] Thus, although tissue damage apparent on the skin surface may be minimal, the damage to deeper structures can be severe. In addition, subcutaneous fat and muscle are more sensitive than the skin to ischemia. Muscle and fat tissues are more metabolically active and, thus, more vulnerable to hypoxia with increased susceptibility to pressure damage. The vulnerability of muscle and fat tissues to pressure forces explains pressure ulcers, where large areas of muscle and fat tissue are damaged with undermining due to necrosis yet the skin opening is relatively small.[8] In patients with severe malnutrition and weight loss, there is less tissue between the bony prominence and the surface of the skin, so the potential for large ulcers with extensive undermining is much higher.

There is a relationship between intensity and duration of pressure in pressure ulcer development. Low pressures over a long period of time are as capable of producing tissue damage as high pressures for shorter periods of time.[2] Tissues can tolerate higher cyclic pressures versus constant pressure.[14] Pressures differ in various body positions. Pressures are highest (70 mm Hg) on the buttocks in the lying position and in the sitting position can be as high as 300 mm Hg over the ischial tuberosities.[2,6] These levels are well above the normal capillary closing pressure and capable of causing tissue ischemia. When tissues have been compressed for prolonged periods of time, tissue damage continues to occur even after the pressure is relieved.[12] This continued tissue damage relates to changes at the cellular level that lead to difficulties with restoration of perfusion. Initial skin breakdown can occur in 6 to 12 hours in healthy individuals and more quickly (less than 2 hours) in those who are debilitated.

More than 95% of all pressure ulcers develop over five classic locations: sacral/coccygeal area, greater trochanter, ischial tuberosity, heel, and lateral malleolus.[4] Correct anatomical terminology is important when identifying the true location of the pressure ulcer. For example, many clinicians often document pressure ulcers as being located on the patient's hip. The hip, or iliac crest, is actually an uncommon location for pressure ulceration. The iliac crest, located on the front of the body, is rarely subject to pressure forces. The area most clinicians are referring to is correctly termed the greater trochanter. The greater trochanter is the bony prominence located on the side of the body, just above the proximal, lateral aspect of the thigh, or "saddlebag" area. The majority of pressure ulcers occur on the lower half of the body. The location of the pressure ulcer may impact clinical interventions. For example, the patient with a pressure ulcer on the sacral/coccygeal area with concomitant urinary incontinence will require treatments that address the incontinence problem. Ulcers in the sacral/coccygeal area are also more at risk for friction and shearing damage due to the location of the wound. Figure 16–1 shows the correct anatomical terminology for pressure

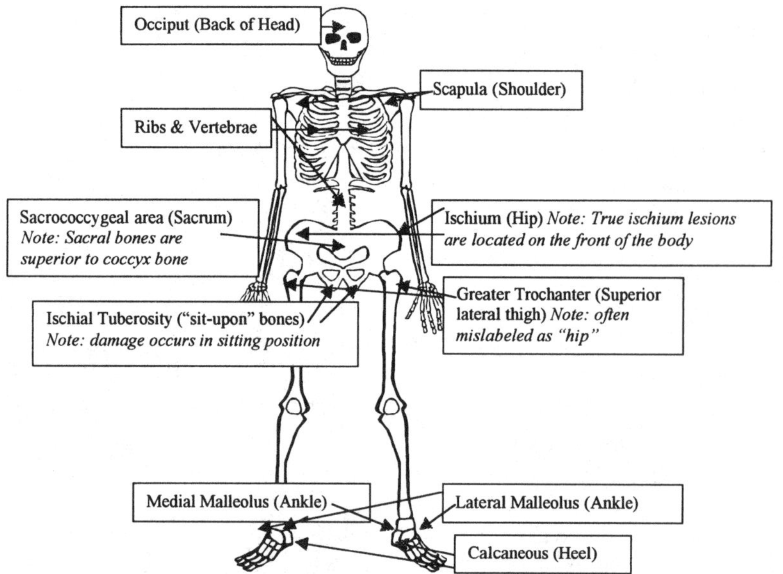

Fig. 16–1. Common anatomical location of pressure sores.

ulcer locations. Typical pressure ulcer locations for palliative care patients are the sacral/coccygeal area, trochanters, and heels. Patients with contractures are at special risk for pressure ulcer development due to the internal pressure of the bony prominence and the abnormal alignment of the body and its extremities. Institutionalized older adults with severe functional decline are particularly susceptible to contractures due to immobilization for extended perioods of time in conjunction with limited efforts for maintenance of range of motion.

RISK FACTORS FOR PRESSURE ULCERS

Pressure ulcers are physical evidence of multiple causative influences. Factors that contribute to pressure ulcer development can be thought of as those that affect the pressure force over the bony prominence and those that affect the tolerance of the tissues to pressure.

Mobility, sensory loss, and activity level are related to the concept of increasing pressure. Extrinsic factors including shear, friction, and moisture as well as intrinsic factors such as, nutrition, age, and arteriolar pressure relate to the concept of tissue tolerance.[15] Several additional areas may influence pressure ulcer development, including emotional stress, temperature, smoking, and interstitial fluid flow.[16]

Mobility

Immobility, inactivity, and decreased sensory perception affect the duration and intensity of the pressure over the bony prominence. Immobility or severely restricted mobility is the most important risk factor for all populations and a necessary condition for the development of pressure ulcers. *Mobility* is the state of being movable. Thus, the immobile patient cannot move, and facility or ease of movement is impaired. Closely related to immobility is limited activity.

Activity

Activity is the production of energy or motion and implies an action. Activity is often clinically described by the ability of the individual to ambulate and move about. Those persons who are bed- or chair-bound, and thus inactive, are more at risk for pressure ulcer development.[17,18] A sudden change in activity level may signal significant change in health status and increased potential for pressure ulcer development.

Sensory Loss

Sensory loss places patients at risk for compression of tissues and pressure ulcer development because the normal mechanism for translating pain messages from the tissues is dysfunctional.[19] Patients with intact nervous system pathways feel continuous local pressure, become uncomfortable, and change their position before tissue ischemia occurs. Spinal cord–injured patients have a higher incidence and prevalence of pressure ulcers.[20,21] Patients with paraplegia or quadriplegia are unable to sense increased pressure, and if their body weight is not shifted, pressure ulceration develops. Likewise, patients with changes in mental status functioning are at increased risk for pressure ulcer formation. They may not feel the discomfort from pressure, not be alert enough to move spontaneously, not remember to move, be too confused to respond to commands to move, or be physically unable to move.[19] This risk factor is particularly evident in the palliative care population, where individuals may be at the end of life, may not be alert enough to move spontaneously, or may be physically unable to move.

Shear

Extrinsic risk factors are those forces that make the tissues less tolerant of pressure. Extrinsic forces include shear, friction, and moisture. Whereas pressure acts perpendicularly to cause ischemia, shear causes ischemia by displacing blood vessels laterally and, thus, impeding blood flow to tissues.[22–24] Shear is caused by the interplay of gravity and friction. Shear is a parallel force that stretches and twists tissues and blood vessels at the bony tissue interface, and as such, affects the deep blood vessels and deeper tissue structures. The most common example of shear is the bed patient in a semisitting position with knees flexed and supported by pillows on the bed or by head-of-bed elevation. The patient's skeleton slides down toward the foot of the bed, but the sacral skin stays in place (with the help of friction against the bed linen). This produces stretching, pinching, and occlusion of the underlying vessels, resulting in ulcers with large areas of internal tissue damage and less damage at the skin surface.

Friction

Friction and moisture, although not direct factors in pressure ulcer development, have been identified as contributing to the problem by reducing tolerance of tissues to pressure.[24] Friction occurs when two surfaces move across one another. Friction acts on tissue tolerance to pressure by abrading and damaging the epidermal and upper dermal layers of the skin. Additionally, friction acts with gravity to cause shear. Friction abrades the epidermis, which may lead to pressure ulcer development by increasing the skin's susceptibility to pressure injury. Pressure combined with friction produces ulcerations at lower pressures than does pressure alone.[24] Friction acts in conjunction with shear to contribute to the development of sacral/coccyxgeal pressure ulcers on patients in the semi-Fowler position.

Moisture

Moisture contributes to pressure ulcer development by removing oils on the skin, making it more friable, as well as interacting with body support surface friction. Constant moisture on the skin leads to maceration of the tissues. The waterlogged tissues lead to softening of the skin's connective tissues. Macerated tissues are more prone to erosion, and once the epidermis is eroded, there is increased likelihood of further tissue breakdown.[25] Moisture alters the resiliency of the epidermis to external forces. Both shearing force and friction increase in the presence of mild to moderate moisture. Excess moisture may be due to wound drainage, diaphoresis, and fecal or urinary incontinence.

Incontinence

Urinary and fecal incontinence are common risk factors associated with pressure ulcer development. Incontinence contributes to pressure ulcer formation by creating excess moisture on the skin and by chemical damage to the skin. Fecal incontinence has the added detrimental effect of bacteria in the stool, which can contribute to infection as well as skin breakdown. Fecal incontinence is more significant as a risk factor for pressure ulceration because of the bacteria and enzymes in stool and the subsequent effects on the skin.[19,26] Inadequately managed incontinence poses a significant risk factor for pressure ulcer development, and fecal incontinence is highly correlated with pressure ulcer development.[17,27]

Nutrition

There is some disagreement on the major intrinsic risk factors affecting tissue tolerance to pressure. However, most studies identify nutritional status as playing a role in pressure ulcer development. Hypoalbuminemia, weight loss, cachexia, and malnutrition are commonly identified as risk factors predisposing patients to pressure ulcer development.[28–31] Individuals with low serum albumin levels are associated with both having a pressure ulcer and developing a pressure ulcer.

Age

Age itself may be a risk factor for pressure ulcer development, with age-related changes in the skin and wound healing increasing the risk of pressure ulcer development.[32] The skin and support structures undergo changes in the aging process. There is a loss of muscle, a decrease in serum albumin levels, diminished inflammatory response, decreased elasticity, and reduced cohesion between the dermis and epidermis.[32,33] These changes combine with other changes related to aging to make the skin less tolerant of pressure forces, shear, and friction.

Medical Conditions and Psychological Factors

Certain medical conditions or disease states are also associated with pressure ulcer development. Orthopedic injuries, altered mental status, and spinal cord injury are such conditions.[20,21,31,34,35] Others have examined psychological factors that may affect risk for pressure ulcer development.[36–38] Self-concept, depression, and chronic emotional stress have been cited as factors in pressure ulcer development; and the emerging role of cortisol levels in pressure ulcer development bears monitoring.

Environmental Resources

Environmental resources include socioeconomic, psychosocial, health care system, and therapy resources. These factors are less understood than other risk factors; however, several of them play an important role in determining risk for pressure ulcer development and course of pressure ulcer care in the patient receiving palliative care. Socioeconomic resources that may influence pressure ulcer development and healing are cost of therapy, type of payor (insurance type), and access to health care. In palliative care, cost of therapy becomes an important issue, particularly in long-term care facilities, where financial resources are limited and cost of therapy may hinder access to treatment.

Health care system resources are the type of health care setting and the experience, education level, and discipline of health care professionals. Patients receiving palliative care are often in long-term care facilities and dependent on the direct care practices of nurse aides with minimal education in health care, nursing, and especially the needs of the palliative care patient. Therapy resources include topical treatments for wounds and systemic treatments. Palliative care patients often receive concomitant therapy that impairs mobility or sensory perception, such as pain medication, or normal healing mechanisms, such as steroids.

Psychosocial resources include adherence to the therapy plan, cultural values and beliefs, social support network (family and caregiver support), spirituality support, and alternative medicine use. Social support network is a key factor for palliative care. Patients receiving palliative care are often cared for in the home or in a long-term care facility. Home caregivers may be family members of the patient and are often the spouse or significant other. When the patient is older and frail, it is typical to find that the caregiver is also older and frail yet responsible for providing direct care 24 hours a day with minimal respite or support. Many times the nurse is dealing with two patients, the patient receiving palliative care and the patient's caregiver, who may also be frail and in need of services. The family member may be physically unable to reposition the patient or to provide other care services. In long-term care facilities, the problem may not be physical inability to perform the tasks but lack of time or motivation. The availability of nurse attendants in the long-term care facility may be such that turning and repositioning the palliative care patient are not high-priority tasks. As is evident, environmental resources are not all well defined and typically are not included in formal risk-assessment tools for development of pressure ulcers; however, the importance of environmental resources in both the development and healing of pressure ulcers is clinically relevant in palliative care.

Use of Risk-Assessment Scales

For practitioners to intervene in a cost-effective way, a method of screening for risk factors is necessary. There are several risk-assessment instruments available to clinicians. Screening tools assist in prevention by distinguishing those persons who are at risk for pressure ulcer development from those who are not. The only purpose in identifying patients at risk for pressure ulcer development is to allow for appropriate use of resources for prevention. The use of a risk-assessment tool allows for targeting of interventions to specific risk factors for individual patients. The risk-assessment instrument selected is based on its reliability for the intended raters, its predictive validity for the population, its sensitivity and specificity under consideration, and its ease of use and the time required to complete. The most common risk-assessment tools are Braden's Scale for Predicting Pressure Sore Risk and Norton's Scale. There is minimal information on use of either instrument in palliative care patients, but both tools have been used in long-term care facilities, where many patients are assumed to be palliative care. This is an area where further study is warranted.

Norton's Scale. The Norton tool is the oldest risk-assessment instrument. Developed in 1961, it consists of five subscales: physical condition, mental state, activity, mobility, and incontinence.[39] Each parameter is rated on a scale of 1 to 4, with the sum of the ratings for all five parameters yielding a total score ranging from 5 to 20. Lower scores indicate increased risk, with a score of or below 16 indicating "onset of risk" and scores 12 and below indicating high risk for pressure ulcer formation.[40]

Braden Scale for Predicting Pressure Sores. The Braden Scale was developed in 1987 and is composed of six subscales that conceptually reflect degrees of sensory perception, moisture, activity, nutrition, friction and shear, and mobility.[15,16] All subscales are rated from 1 to 4, except for friction and shear, which is rated from 1 to 3. The subscales may be summed for a total score ranging from 6 to 23.

Lower scores indicate lower function and higher risk for developing a pressure ulcer. The cut-off score for hospitalized adults is considered to be 16, with scores of 16 and below indicating at-risk status.[16] In older patients, some have found cut-off scores of 17 or 18 to be better predictors of risk status.[15,30] Levels of risk are based on the predictive value of a positive test. Scores of 15 to 16 indicate mild risk, with a 50% to 60% chance of developing a stage I pressure ulcer; scores of 12 to 14 indicate moderate risk, with 65% to 90% chance of developing a stage I or II lesion; and scores below 12 indicate high risk, with 90% to 100% chance of developing a stage II or deeper pressure ulcer.[30,34] The Braden Scale has been tested in acute care and long-term care with several levels of nurse raters and demonstrates high interrater reliability with registered nurses.

Validity has been established by expert opinion, and predictive validity has been studied in several acute care settings, with good sensitivity and specificity demonstrated.[16,30] The Braden Scale is the model used in this chapter for prevention of pressure ulcers in patients requiring palliative care.

Regardless of the instrument chosen to evaluate risk status, the clinical relevance is threefold. First, assessment for risk status must occur at frequent intervals. Monitor assessment at admission to the health care organization (within 24 hours), at predetermined intervals (usually weekly), and whenever a significant change occurs in the patient's general health and status. The second clinical implication is the targeting of specific prevention strategies to identified risk factors. The final clinical implication is for those patients in whom prevention is not successful. For patients with an actual pressure ulcer, the continued monitoring of risk status may prevent further tissue trauma at the wound site and development of additional wound sites.

PREVENTION OF PRESSURE ULCERS

Prevention strategies are targeted at reducing risk factors and can be focused on eliminating specific risk factors. Thus, early intervention for pressure ulcers is risk factor–specific and prophylactic in nature. The prevention strategies are presented by risk factors, beginning with general information and ending with specific strategies to eliminate particular risk factors. Prevention is a key element for palliative care. If pressure ulcers can be prevented, the patient is spared tiresome, sometimes painful, and often overwhelming treatment. The Braden Scale is the basis for these prevention interventions. Prevention interventions that are appropriate to the patient's level of risk and specific to individual risk factors should be instituted.[18] For example, the risk factor of immobility is managed very differently for the comatose patient versus the patient with severe pain on movement or the patient who is still mobile even if bed-bound. The comatose patient requires caregiver education and caregiver-dependent repositioning. The patient with severe pain on movement requires special support surface intervention and minimal movement methods with a foam wedge, and the patient who is still mobile but bed-bound requires self-care education and may be able to perform self-repositioning. Thus, the intervention for the risk factor of immobility is very different for these patients.

Immobility, Inactivity, and Sensory Loss

Patients with impaired ability to reposition and who cannot independently change body positions must have local pressure alleviated by any of the following: passive repositioning by caregivers, pillow bridging, and pressure relief or reduction support surfaces for bed and chair.[18,19,34] In addition, measures to increase mobility and activity and to decrease friction and shear should be instituted.

Overhead bed frames with trapeze bars are helpful for patients with upper body strength and may increase mobility and independence with body repositioning. Wheelchair-bound patients with upper body strength can be taught and encouraged to do wheelchair pushups to relieve pressure and allow for reperfusion of the tissues in the ischial tuberosity region. For patients who are weak from prolonged inactivity, providing support and assistance for reconditioning and increasing strength and endurance will help prevent future debility.[19] Mobility plans for each patient should be individualized with the goal of attaining the highest level of mobility and activity possible. Mobility plans are the responsibility of nurses and physical therapists working together in all health care settings. It is essential that health care professionals train and observe home caregivers in the mobility plan and, in particular, passive repositioning techniques.

Caregivers in the home are often left to fend for themselves for prevention interventions and may be frail and have health problems themselves. A return demonstration of a repositioning procedure can be very informative to the nurse. The nurse may need to coach, improvise, and think of creative strategies for caregivers to use in the home setting to meet the patient's need for movement and tissue reperfusion.

Passive Repositioning by Caregiver

Turning schedules and passive repositioning by caregivers is the normal response for patients with immobility risk factors. Typically, turning schedules are based on time or event. If time-based, turning schedules are usually every 2 hours for full-body change of position and more often for small shifts in position. Event-based schedules relate to typical events during the day, for example, turning the patient after each meal. Full-body change of position involves turning the patient to a new lying position, for example, turning the patient from the right side-lying position to the left side-lying position or the supine position. When the side-lying position is used in bed, avoidance of direct pressure on the trochanter is essential. To avoid placing pressure on the trochanter, place the patient in a 30-degree, laterally inclined position instead of the commonly used 90-degree side-lying position, which increases tissue compression over the trochanter. The 30-degree, laterally inclined position allows for distribution of pressure over a greater area.

Small shifts in position involve moving the patient but keeping the same lying position, for example, changing the angle of the right side-lying position or changing lower-extremity position in the right side-lying position. Both strategies are helpful in achieving reperfusion of compressed tissues, but only full-body change of position completely relieves pressure. A foam wedge is very useful in positioning for frail caregivers and patients with severe pain on movement. The foam wedge should be a 30-degree angle when fully inserted behind the patient, usually extending from the shoulders to the hips/buttocks. Once in place, even the most frail of caregivers can easily pull the wedge out slightly every hour, providing for small shifts in position and tissue reperfusion. Even patients with pain on movement find the slight movement from the foam wedge tolerable. There are other techniques to make turning patients easier and less time-consuming. Turning sheets, draw sheets, and pillows are essential for passive movement of patients in bed. Turning sheets are useful in repositioning the patient to a side-lying position. Draw sheets are used for pulling patients up in bed and help prevent dragging the patient's skin over the bed surface. The recommended time interval for full change of position turning is every 2 hours, depending on the individual patient profile.

Similar approaches are useful for patients in chairs. Full-body change of position involves standing the patient and resitting the patient in a chair. Small shifts in position for those in chairs might be changing lower-extremity position or insertion of a small foam pillow or wedge. For the chair-bound patient, it is also helpful to use a foot stool to help reduce the pressure on the ischial tuberosities and to distribute the pressure over a wider surface. Attention to proper alignment and posture is essential. Individuals at risk for pressure ulcer development should avoid uninterrupted sitting in chairs and should be repositioned every hour. The rationale behind the shorter time frame is the extremely high pressures generated on the ischial tuberosities in the seated position.[42] Those patients with upper-body strength should be taught to shift weight every 15 minutes, to allow for tissue reperfusion. Again, pillows may be used to help position the patient in proper body alignment. Physical therapy and occupational therapy can assist in body-alignment strategies with even the most contracted patient. In many instances, patients receiving palliative care at home spend much of their time up in recliner chairs. The ability of recliner chairs to provide a pressure-reduction support surface is not known. Individual recliner chairs probably have various levels of pressure-reducing capability; thus, it is still prudent to institute a repositioning schedule for those using recliner chairs. Repositioning patients in recliner chairs is more difficult due to the physical properties of the chair and requires some creativity. The repositioning schedule should mimic the schedule for those in wheelchairs.

Pillow Bridging

Pillow bridging involves the use of pillows to position patients with minimal tissue compression. The use of pillows can help prevent pressure ulcers from occurring on the medial knees, the medial malleolus, and the heels. Pillows should be placed between the knees, between the ankles, and under the heels.

Pillow use is especially important for reducing risk of development of heel ulcers regardless of the support surface in use.[18] The best prevention strategy for eliminating pressure ulcers on the heels is to keep the heels off the surface of the bed. Use of pillows under the lower extremities will keep the heel from making contact with the support surface of the bed. Pillows help to redistribute the pressure over a larger area, thus reducing high pressures in one specific area. The pillows should extend and support the leg from the groin/perineal area to the ankle. Use of donut-type or ring cushion devices is contraindicated. Donut ring cushions cause venous congestion and edema and actually increase pressure to the area of concern.[18]

Use of Pressure Relief and Pressure-Reduction Support Surfaces

There are specific guidelines for the use of support surfaces to prevent and manage pressure ulcers.[42–44] Regardless of the type of support surface in use with the patient, the need for written repositioning and turning schedules remains essential. Support surfaces serve as adjuncts to strategies for positioning and careful monitoring of patients. The type of support surface chosen is based on a multitude of factors, including clinical condition of the patient, type of care setting, ease of use, maintenance, cost, and characteristics of the support surface. The primary concern should be the therapeutic benefit associated with the surface. Table 16–1 categorizes the types of support surface available and general performance characteristics.[42]

Pressure-Reducing Support Surfaces. Pressure-reduction devices lower tissue interface pressures but do not consistently maintain interface pressures below capillary closing pressures in all positions on all body locations. Pressure-reducing support surfaces are indicated for patients at risk for pressure ulcer development, who can be turned, and who have skin breakdown involving only one sleep surface.[18,19] Patients with an existing pressure ulcer who are still at risk for development of further skin breakdown should be managed on a pressure-reducing support surface.

Pressure-reduction devices can be classified as static or dynamic. Static devices do not move, they reduce pressure by spreading the load over a larger area. A simple definition of a static support surface is one that does not require electricity to function, usually a mattress overlay (lays on top of the standard hospital mattress). Examples of static devices are foam, air, or gel mattress overlays and water-filled mattresses. Foam devices have difficulties with retaining moisture and heat and not reducing shear. Air and water static devices also have difficulties associated with retaining moisture and heat. Dynamic support surfaces move. A simple definition of a dynamic support surface is one that requires a motor or pump and electricity to operate. One example is the alternating-pressure air mattress. Most of these devices use an electric pump to alternately inflate and deflate air cells or air columns, thus the term "alternating-pressure air mattress." The key to determining effectiveness is the length of time that cycles of inflation and deflation occur. Dynamic support surfaces may also have difficulties with moisture retention and heat accumulation.[42] Dynamic devices may be preferable for palliative care patients, especially those with significant pain on movement as the device may help with tissue reperfusion when patients cannot be turned because of pain. When using pressure-reduction devices, the caregiver must assure that the device is functioning properly and that the patient is receiving pressure reduction.

One concern when using mattress overlays, whether they are static or dynamic, is the bottoming out phenome-

Table 16–1. Selected Characteristics for Classes of Support Surface

Performance Characteristics	High Air Loss (Air Fluidized)	Low Air Loss	Alternating Air (Dynamic)	Static Flotation (Air or Water)	Foam	Standard Hospital Mattress
Increased support area	Yes	Yes	Yes	Yes	Yes	No
Low moisture retention	Yes	Yes	No	No	No	No
Reduced heat accumulation	Yes	Yes	No	No	No	No
Shear reduction	Yes	?	Yes	Yes	No	No
Pressure reduction	Yes	Yes	Yes	Yes	Yes	No
Dynamic	Yes	Yes	Yes	No	No	No
Cost per day	High	High	Moderate	Low	Low	Low

Source: Bergstrom et al. (1994), reference 42.

non. Bottoming out occurs when the patient's body sinks down, the support surface is compressed beyond function, and the patient's body lies directly on the hospital mattress. When bottoming out occurs, there is no pressure reduction for the bony prominence of concern. Bottoming out typically happens when the patient is placed on a static air mattress overlay that is not appropriately filled with air or when the patient has been on a foam mattress for extended periods of time. The nurse can monitor for bottoming out by inserting a flat, outstretched hand between the overlay and the patient's body part at risk. If the caregiver feels less than an inch of support material, the patient has bottomed out. It is important to check for bottoming out when the patient is in various body positions and to check at various body sites. For example, when the patient is lying supine, check the sacral/coccyxgeal area and the heels; and when the patient is side-lying, check the trochanter and lateral malleolus.[42]

Pressure-Relieving Support Surfaces. Pressure-relief devices consistently reduce tissue interface pressures to a level below capillary closing pressure in any position and in most body locations. Pressure-relief devices are indicated for patients at high risk for pressure ulcer development and who cannot turn independently or have skin breakdown involving more than one body surface. Most commonly, pressure-relief devices are grouped into low-air loss therapy, fluidized air, or high-air loss and kinetic therapy. These devices often assist with pain control as well as relieving pressure.

Low air-loss therapy uses a bed frame with a series of connected air-filled pillows with surface fabrics of low-friction material. The amount of pressure in each pillow can be controlled and calibrated to provide maximal pressure relief for the individual patient. They provide pressure relief in any position, and most models have built-in scales. There are newer models of low air-loss therapy devices that lay on top of standard hospital mattresses. These models may be of particular benefit for palliative care patients.

Fluidized air or high air-loss therapy consists of a bed frame containing silicone-coated glass beads and incorporates both air and fluid support. The beads become fluid when air is pumped through, making them behave like a liquid. High air-loss therapy has bactericidal properties due to the alkalinity of the beads (pH 10), the temperature, and entrapment of microorganisms by the beads. High air-loss therapy relieves pressure and reduces friction, shear, and moisture (due to the drying effect of the bed). These devices are difficult when transferring patients due to the bed frame. There is increased airflow, which can increase evaporative fluid loss, leading to dehydration. Finally, if the patient is able to sit up, a foam wedge may be required, thus limiting the beneficial effects of the bed on the upper back. In palliative care cases, use of high air-loss therapy is typically not indicated for pressure ulcers alone but may be indicated for patients with significant pain as well as pressure ulcers.

Support Surface Selection. Determining which support surface is best for individual patients can be confusing. The primary concern must always be the effectiveness of the surface for the individual patient's needs. The Agency for Health Care Policy and Research (AHCPR) recommends the following criteria as guidelines for determining how to manage tissue loading and support surface selection.[18]

1. Assess all patients with existing pressure ulcers to determine their risk for developing additional pressure ulcers. If the patient remains at risk, use a pressure-reducing surface.
2. Use a static support surface if the patient can assume a variety of positions without bearing weight on an existing pressure ulcer and without "bottoming out."
3. Use a dynamic support surface if the patient cannot assume a variety of positions without bearing weight on an existing pressure ulcer, if the patient fully compresses the static support surface, or if the pressure ulcer does not show evidence of healing.
4. If a patient has large stage III or stage IV pressure ulcers on multiple turning surfaces, a low air-loss bed or a fluidized air (high air-loss) bed may be indicated.
5. When excess moisture on intact skin is a potential source of maceration and skin breakdown, a support surface that provides airflow can be important in drying the skin and preventing additional pressure ulcers.
6. Any individual at risk for developing pressure ulcers should be placed on a static or dynamic pressure-reducing support surface.

There are additional concerns when choosing a support surface. Criteria for choosing support surfaces can be classified as intrinsic and extrinsic. Intrinsic criteria include wound burden (tissue history, such as previous ulcers, surgical repair, stress, duration of pressure ulcer, number of pressure ulcers present), body build (obese, thin, contractures present), and the magnitude and distribution of interface pressures (location of highest pressures, etc).[44] The following case examples illustrate how intrinsic criteria are used to determine a support surface. Patients who undergo specific surgical operative repair of the pressure ulcer may need to be placed on high air-loss or fluidized air therapy postoperatively. Patients with multiple ulcers involving more than one turning surface also need to be placed on pressure-relieving devices such as low air-loss therapy or high air-loss therapy. The patient with severe contractures may not require a support surface that has good heel pressure readings (with contraction of the legs, the heels do not reach the bottom of the mattress). If the bony prominence of concern is the greater trochanter, then the support surface must adequately reduce pressure over the trochanter. While algorithms are helpful tools used in many practice settings to aid in choosing a support surface, as these case examples illustrate, the clinician must also evaluate the individual patient's needs.

Evaluation of extrinsic criteria requires the clinician to review the goals for therapy. For example, the patient who uses the support surface only at night and spends most of the day up in a chair will require an aggressive approach to seating support surfaces, while a lesser support surface can be chosen for the bed. If the patient spends most of the day in bed, then the support surface chosen will be different. For agitated patients (particularly those with continual body motions), the support surface's ability to handle shearing and friction may be critical, and good choices may involve evaluation of the support surface covering. The external environment is also essential to include in choosing a support surface. If the patient is at home, with no air conditioning, incontinent of urine, and in a humid environment, the breathability of the support surface and the ability to handle moisture are essential to a positive outcome. Likewise, evaluation of the patient's prognosis is helpful in support surface choice. In palliative care, the patient is expected to decline in function, so choosing a support surface that will meet future as well as present skin care needs may be most prudent.

Seating Support Surfaces. Support surfaces for chairs and wheelchairs can be categorized as the support surfaces for beds. In general, providing adequate pressure relief for chair-bound or wheelchair-bound patients is critical as the patient at risk for pressure ulcer formation is at increased risk in the seated position because of the high pressures across the ischial tuberosities. Most pressure-reducing devices for chairs are static overlays, such as those made out of foam, gel, air, or some combination. Positioning chair- or wheelchair-bound individuals must include consideration of individual anatomy and body contours, postural alignment, distribution of weight, balance, and stability in addition to pressure relief.

Reducing Friction and Shear

Measures to reduce friction and shear relate to passive or active movement of the patient. To reduce friction, several interventions are appropriate. Providing topical preparations to eliminate or reduce the surface tension between the skin and the bed linen or support surface will assist in reducing friction-related injury. Use of appropriate techniques when moving patients so that skin is never dragged across linens will lessen friction-induced skin breakdown. Patients who exhibit voluntary or involuntary repetitive body movements (particularly the heels or elbows) require stronger interventions. Use of a protective film such as a transparent film dressing or a skin sealant, a protective dressing such as a thin hydrocolloid, or protective padding will help to eliminate the surface contact of the area and decrease the friction between the skin and the linens.[19] Even though heel, ankle, and elbow protectors do nothing to reduce or relieve pressure, they can be effective aids against friction.

Most shear injury can be eliminated by proper positioning, such as avoidance of the semi-Fowler position and limiting use of the upright position (positions over 30 degrees inclined). Avoidance of positions greater than 30 degrees inclined may prevent sliding- and shear-related injury. Use of foot boards and knee gatch (or pillows under the lower leg) to prevent sliding and to maintain position are also helpful in reducing shear effects on the skin when in bed. Observation of the patient when sitting is also important as the patient who slides out of the chair is at equally high risk for shear injury. Use of footstools and the foot pedals on wheelchairs and appropriate 90-degree flexion of the hip (may be achieved with pillows, special seat cushions, or orthotic devices) can help in preventing chair sliding.

Nutrition

Nutrition is an important element in maintaining healthy skin and tissues. There is a strong relationship between nutrition and pressure ulcer development.[28] The severity of pressure ulceration is also correlated with severity of nutritional deficits, especially low protein intake or low serum albumin levels.[28,30,31] Nutritional assessment is key in determining the appropriate interventions for the patient. A short nutritional assessment should be performed at routine intervals on all patients determined to be at risk for pressure ulcer formation.

Malnutrition can be diagnosed if serum albumin levels are below 3.5 mg/dl, total lymphocyte count is less than 1800 mm^3, or body weight decreases by more than 15%.[42] Malnutrition impairs the immune system, and total lymphocyte counts are a reflection of immune competence. If the patient is diagnosed as malnourished, nutritional supplementation should be instituted to help achieve a positive nitrogen balance. Examples of oral supplements are assisted oral feedings, dietary supplements, or tube feedings. Oral assisted feedings and dietary supplements are the first option for intervention, and tube feedings would be tried after other methods have failed. The goal of care is to provide approximately 30 to 35 calories per kilogram of weight per day and 1.25 to 1.5 g of protein per kilogram of weight per day.[42] It may be difficult for a pressure ulcer patient or an at-risk patient to ingest enough protein and calories necessary to maintain skin and tissue health. Oral supplements can be very helpful in boosting calorie and protein intake, but they are designed only to be an adjunct to regular oral intake. Monitoring of nutritional indices is helpful to determine the effectiveness of the care plan. Serum albumin, protein markers, body weight, and nutritional assessment should be performed every 3 months to monitor for changes in nutritional status if appropriate.

In palliative care, nutrition may be one of the biggest risk factors for pressure ulcer development. Nutritional supplementation may not be possible in all cases; however, if the patient can tolerate supplements, this should be encouraged. Involvement of a dietician during the early assessment of the patient is important to the overall success of the plan. Maintenance of adequate nutrition to prevent pressure ulcer development and to repair existing pressure ulcers is fraught with differing opinions in the palliative care patient. The issue is how to balance nutritional needs for skin care without providing artificial nutrition. One of the problems in this area is the limited research available. The inadequate evidence base leaves clinicians to rely on expert opinion and their own clinical experience. Perhaps the best advice is to look at the whole clinical picture rather than getting "caught up" and focused only on the wound. Viewing the pressure ulcer as a part of the whole, within the contextual circumstances of the patient, should provide some assistance in determining how aggressive to be in providing nutrition. The overriding concern in palliative care is to provide for comfort and to minimize symptoms. If providing supplemental nutrition aids in providing comfort to the patient and is mutually agreed upon by the patient, family caregivers, and health care provider, then supplemental nutrition (in any form) is very appropriate for palliative wound care. If the patient's condition is such that to provide supplemental nutrition (in any form) increases discomfort and the prognosis is expected to be poor and rapid, then providing supplemental nutrition should not be a concern and is not appropriate for palliative wound care. It is important to remember that little evidence for either of these viewpoints exists, yet expert opinions on the topic abound.

Managing Moisture

The preventive interventions related to moisture include general skin care, accurate diagnosis of incontinence type, and appropriate incontinence management.

General Skin Care. General skin care involves routine skin assessment, incontinence assessment and management, skin hygiene interventions, and measures to maintain skin health. Routine skin assessment involves observation of the patient's skin, with particular attention to bony prominences. Reddened areas should not be massaged. Massage can further impair the perfusion to the tissues.

Incontinence Management. Management of incontinence is a huge topic, and volumes have been written about various management techniques. This discussion is meant to serve as a stepping stone to those resources available to clinicians concerning management of the incontinent patient. The discussion will, therefore, by necessity be noninclusive of all management strategies and only briefly mention several strategies most pertinent to the palliative care patient at high risk of developing a pressure ulcer. Management of incontinence is dependent on assessment and diagnosis of the problem (see chapter 14).

Incontinence Assessment. Assessment of incontinence should include history of the incontinence, including patterns of elimination, characteristics of the urinary stream/fecal mass, and sensation of bladder/rectal filling. The physical examination is designed to gather specific information related to bladder/rectal functioning and, thus, is limited in scope. A limited neurological examination should provide data on the mental status and motivation of the patient/caregiver, specific motor skills, and back and lower extremities. The genitalia and perineal skin are assessed for signs of perineal skin lesions and perineal sensation.

The environmental assessment should include inspection of the patient's home or nursing home facility to evaluate for the presence of environmental barriers to continence. A voiding/defecation diary is very helpful in planning the treatment and management of incontinence. In cognitively impaired patients, the caregiver may complete the diary and management strategies, again, can be identified from the baseline data.

Incontinence Management Strategies. Palliative care patients at risk for pressure ulcer development are not candidates for all methods of behavioral management. The most successful behavioral management strategy for palliative care patients typically at risk of pressure ulcer development is a scheduled toileting program. Scheduled toileting is caregiver-dependent and requires a motivated caregiver to be successful. Scheduled intake of fluid is an important underlying factor for both strategies.

Scheduled toileting or habit training is toileting on a planned basis. The goal is to keep the person dry by assisting him or her to void at regular intervals. There can be attempts to match the interval to the individual patient's natural voiding schedule. There is no systematic effort to motivate patients to delay voiding or to resist the urge to void. Scheduled toileting may be based on the clock (toilet the patient every 2 hours) or based on activities (toilet the patient after meals and before transferring to bed).

Underpads and briefs may be used to protect the skin of patients who are incontinent of urine or stool. These products are designed to absorb moisture, wick the wetness away from the skin, and maintain a quick-drying interface with the skin. Studies with both infants and adults demonstrate that products designed to present a quick-drying surface to the skin and to absorb moisture do keep the skin drier and are associated with a lower incidence of dermatitis.[45] The critical feature is the ability to absorb moisture and present a quick-drying surface, not whether the product is disposable or reusable. Regardless of the product chosen, containment strategies imply the need for a check and change schedule for the incontinent patient so that wet linens and pads may be removed in a timely manner. Underpads are not as tight or constricting as briefs. Kemp[25] suggests alternating the use of underpads and briefs if the skin irritation is thought to be related to the occlusive nature of the brief. His recommendations echo the early work of Willis[46] on warm water immersion syndrome, who found that the effects of water on the skin could be reversed and tempered by simply allowing the skin to dry out between wet periods. Use of briefs when the patient is up in a chair, ambulating, or visiting and use of underpads when the patient is in bed is one suggestion for combining the strengths of both products.[25]

External collection devices may be more effective with male patients. External catheters or condom catheters are devices applied to the shaft of the penis to direct the urine away from the body to a collection device. Newer models of external catheters are self-adhesive and easy to apply. For patients with a retracted penis, a special pouching system, similar to an ostomy pouch, is available, the retracted penis pouch. A key concern with use of external collection devices is routine removal of the product and inspection and hygiene of the skin.

There are special containment devices for fecal incontinence as well. Fecal incontinence collectors consist of a self-adhesive skin barrier attached to a drainable pouch. Application of the device is somewhat dependent on the skill of the clinician, and the patient should be put on a routine for changing the pouch prior to leakage, to facilitate success. The skin barrier provides a physical obstacle on the skin to the stool and helps to prevent dermatitis and associated skin problems. In fact, skin barrier wafers without an attached pouch can be useful in protecting the skin from feces or urine.

The AHCPR recommends use of moisturizers for dry skin and use of lubricants for reduction in friction injuries.[18] They also discuss the use of moisture barriers to protect the skin from the effects of moisture. Although products that provide a moisture barrier are recommended, the reader is cautioned that the recommendation is derived from usual practice and professional standards and is not research-based. The success of the particular product is linked to how it is formulated and the hydrophobic properties of the product.[25] Generally, pastes are thicker and more repellent of moisture than ointments. A quick evaluation is the ease with which the product can be removed with water during routine cleansing: if the product comes off the skin with just routine cleansing, it probably is not an effective barrier to moisture. Use of mineral oil for cleansing some of the heavier barrier products, like zinc oxide paste, will ease removal from the skin.

PRESSURE ULCER ASSESSMENT

The foundation for designing a palliative care plan for the patient with a pressure ulcer is a comprehensive assessment. Comprehensive assessment includes assessment of wound severity, wound status, and the total patient.

Wound Severity

Assessment of wound severity refers to the use of a classification system for diagnosing the severity of tissue trauma by determining the tissue layers involved in the wound. Classification systems such as staging pressure ulcers provide communication regarding wound severity and the tissue layers involved in the injury.

Pressure ulcers are commonly classified according to grading or staging systems based on the depth of tissue destruction. The National Pressure Ulcer Advisory Panel (NPUAP) and the AHCPR recommend use of a universal four-stage classification system to describe depth of tissue damage. Staging systems measure only one characteristic of the wound and should not be viewed as a complete assessment independent of other indicators. Staging systems are best used as a diagnostic tool for indicating wound severity. Table 16–2 presents the pressure ulcer staging criteria according to the NPUAP and the AHCPR.

Wound Status

Pressure ulcer assessment is the base for maintaining and evaluating the therapeutic plan of care. Assessment of wound status involves evaluation of multiple wound characteristics. Initial assessment and follow-up assessments at regular intervals to monitor progress or deterioration of the sore are necessary to determine the effectiveness of the treatment plan. Adequate assessment is important even when the goal of care is comfort, not healing. The assessment data enable clinicians to communicate clearly about a patient's pressure ulcer, provide for continuity in the plan of care, and allow evaluation of treatment modalities. Assessment of wound status should be performed weekly and whenever a significant change is noted in the wound. Assessment should not be confused with monitoring the wound at each dressing change. Monitoring the wound can be performed by less skilled caregivers; however, assessment should be performed on a routine basis by health care practitioners. Use of a systematic approach with a comprehensive assessment tool is helpful.

There are few tools available that

Table 16–2. Pressure Ulcer Staging Criteria

Pressure Ulcer Stage	Definition
Stage I	A stage I pressure ulcer is an observable pressure-related alteration of intact skin whose indicators as compared to the adjacent or opposite area on the body may include changes in one or more of the following: • skin temperature (warmth or coolness) • tissue consistency (firm or boggy feel) • sensation (pain, itching) The ulcer appears as a defined area of persistent redness in lightly pigmented skin, whereas in darker skin tones, the ulcer may appear with persistent red, blue, or purple hues.
Stage II	Partial-thickness skin loss involving epidermis or dermis or both. The ulcer is superficial and presents clinically as an abrasion, blister, or shallow crater.
Stage III	Full-thickness skin loss involving damage or necrosis of subcutaneous tissue, which may extend down to, but not through, underlying fascia. The ulcer presents clinically as a deep crater with or without undermining of adjacent tissue.
Stage IV	Full-thickness skin loss with extensive destruction, tissue necrosis, or damage to muscle bone or supporting structures (such as tendon, joint capsule).

Source: National Pressure Ulcer Advisory Panel (1995), reference 47.

encompass multiple wound characteristics to evaluate overall wound status and healing. Two available tools are the Pressure Ulcer Scale for Healing (PUSH)[48] and the Pressure Sore Status Tool (PSST).[49]

The PUSH tool incorporates surface area measurements, exudate amount, and surface appearance. These wound characteristics were chosen based on principal component analysis to define the best model of healing.[48] The clinician measures the size of the wound, using length and width to calculate surface area (length × width), and chooses the appropriate size category on the tool (there are ten size categories, from 0 to 10). Exudate is evaluated as none (0), light (1), moderate (2), and heavy (3). Tissue type choices include closed (0), epithelial tissue (1), granulation tissue (2), slough (3), and necrotic tissue (4). The three subscores are then summed for a total score.[48]

Reliability testing of the tool with a large sample is under way.[48] The PUSH tool may offer a quick assessment to predict healing outcomes. The PUSH tool is best used as a method of prediction of wound healing and, therefore, may not be the best tool for palliative care patients since healing is not an expected outcome of care. Assessment of additional wound characteristics may still be needed, to develop a treatment plan for the pressure ulcer. The PSST includes additional wound characteristics that may be helpful in designing a plan of care for the wound.

The PSST (Figure 16–2), developed in 1990 by Bates-Jensen,[50] evaluates 13 wound characteristics with a numerical rating scale and rates them from best to worst possible. The PSST is recommended for use as a method of assessment and monitoring of pressure ulcers. It is a pencil-and-paper instrument comprised of 15 items: location, shape, size, depth, edges, undermining or pockets, necrotic tissue type, necrotic tissue amount, exudate type, exudate amount, surrounding skin color, peripheral tissue edema, peripheral tissue induration, granulation tissue, and epithelialization. Two items are nonscored, location and shape. The remaining 13 are scored items, and each appears with characteristic descriptors rated on a scale (1 = best for that characteristic and 5 = worst attribute of the characteristic). It is recommended that the pressure ulcer be scored initially for a baseline assessment and at regular intervals to evaluate therapy. Once a lesion has been assessed for each item on the PSST, the 13 item scores can be added to obtain a total score for the wound. The total score can then be monitored to "see at a glance" healing or degeneration of the wound. Total scores range from 13 (skin intact but always at risk for further damage) to 65 (profound tissue degeneration).

Reliability of the PSST has been evaluated in an acute care setting with enterostomal therapy (ET) nurses (nurses with additional training in wound care)[51] and in long-term care using a variety of health care professionals and one ET nurse expert in wound assessment.[52] Interrater reliability ranged from $r = 0.915$ ($P = 0.0001$) for the ET nurses[51] to 0.78% agreement for the variety of health care professionals.[52] The PSST is the most widely used of the instruments available.

Wound Characteristics

Adequate initial wound assessment should encompass a composite of wound characteristics as this forms a base for differential diagnosis, therapeutic intervention, and future reassessment comparisons.[53] The indices for wound assessment include all of the following: location, size of the ulcer, depth of tissue involvement, stage or classification, condition of the wound edges, presence of undermining or tunneling, necrotic tissue characteristics, exudate characteristics, surrounding tissue conditions, and wound healing characteristics of granulation tissue and epithelialization.[54–58] Wound characteristics of concern for the palliative care patient include wound edges, undermining and tunneling, necrotic tissue characteristics, exudate characteristics, and surrounding tissue conditions. These five characteristics as well as healing attributes of granulation tissue and epithelialization are discussed below.

Edges or Margins. Wound edge, or margin, includes characteristics of distinctness, degree of attachment to the wound base, color, and thickness. In pressure ulcers, as tissues degenerate, broad and indistinct areas, where the wound edge is diffuse and difficult to observe, become shallow lesions with more distinct, thin, separate edges. As tissue trauma from pressure progresses, the reaction intensifies, with a thickening and rolling inward of the epidermis so that the edge is well defined and sharply outlines the ulcer with little or no evidence of new tissue growth. In long-standing pressure ulcers, fibrosis and scarring result from repeated injury and repair, with the edges hyperpigmented, indurated, and firm[59] and possible impairment in the migratory ability of epithelial cells.[60] Pressure ulcers in palliative care may present with signficant tissue damage, and the edges may indicate areas of full-thickness tissue loss with other areas of partial-thickness damage. In palliative care, pressure ulcers may be present for prolonged periods of time with no change in the wound; thus, the wound edges will often exhibit hemosiderin staining or hyperpigmentation in conjunction with the rolled-under and thickened appearance.

When assessing edges, look for how clear and distinct the wound outline appears. If the edges are indistinct and diffuse, there are areas where the normal tissues blend into the wound bed and the edges are not clearly visible. Edges that are even with the skin surface and the wound base are attached to the base of the wound. This means the wound is flat, with no appreciable depth. Well-defined edges are clear and distinct and can be outlined easily on a transparent piece of plastic. Edges that are not attached to the base of the wound imply a wound with some depth of tissue involvement. A crater or bowl/boat shape indicates a wound with edges that are not attached to the wound base. The wound has walls or sides. There is depth to the wound.

PRESSURE SORE STATUS TOOL NAME ______________________________

Complete the rating sheet to assess pressure sore status. Evaluate each item by picking the response that best describes the wound and entering the score in the item score column for the appropriate date.

Location: Anatomic site. Circle, identify right **(R)** or left **(L)** and use **"X"** to mark site on body diagrams:

____ Sacrum & coccyx ____ Lateral ankle
____ Trochanter ____ Medial ankle
____ Ischial tuberosity ____ Heel ____Other Site

Shape: Overall wound pattern; assess by observing perimeter and depth.
Circle and <u>date</u> appropriate description:

____ Irregular ____ Linear or elongated
____ Round/oval ____ Bowl/boat
____ Square/rectangle ____ Butterfly ____ Other Shape

Item	Assessment	Date Score	Date Score	Date Score
1. Size	1 = Length x width < 4 sq cm 2 = Length x width 4 -16 sq cm 3 = Length x width 16.1 - 36 sq cm 4 = Length x width 36.1 - 80 sq cm 5 = Length x width > 80 sq cm			
2. Depth	1 = Non-blanchable erythema on intact skin 2 = Partial thickness skin loss involving epidermis &/or dermis 3 = Full thickness skin loss involving damage or necrosis of subcutaneous tissue; may extend down to but not through underlying fascia; &/or mixed partial & full thickness &/or tissue layers obscured by granulation tissue 4 = Obscured by necrosis 5 = Full thickness skin loss with extensive destruction, tissue necrosis or damage to muscle, bone or supporting structures			
3. Edges	1 = Indistinct, diffuse, none clearly visible 2 = Distinct, outline clearly visible, attached, even with wound base 3 = Well-defined, not attached to wound base 4 = Well-defined, not attached to base, rolled under, thickened 5 = Well-defined, fibrotic, scarred or hyperkeratotic			
4. Under-mining	1 = Undermining < 2 cm in any area 2 = Undermining 2-4 cm involving < 50% wound margins 3 = Undermining 2-4 cm involving > 50% wound margins 4 = Undermining > 4 cm in any area 5 = Tunneling &/or sinus tract formation			
5. Necrotic Tissue Type	1 = None visible 2 = White/grey non-viable tissue &/or non-adherent yellow slough 3 = Loosely adherent yellow slough 4 = Adherent, soft, black eschar 5 = Firmly adherent, hard, black eschar			
6. Necrotic Tissue Amount	1 = None visible 2 = < 25% of wound bed covered 3 = 25% to 50% of wound covered 4 = > 50% and < 75% of wound covered 5 = 75% to 100% of wound covered			

Fig. 16–2. Pressure Sore Status Tool (PSST). See Appendix 16–A for instructions in its use.

Item	Assessment	Date Score	Date Score	Date Score
7. Exudate Type	1 = None or bloody 2 = Serosanguineous: thin, watery, pale red/pink 3 = Serous: thin, watery, clear 4 = Purulent: thin or thick, opaque, tan/yellow 5 = Foul purulent: thick, opaque, yellow/green with odor			
8. Exudate Amount	1 = None 2 = Scant 3 = Small 4 = Moderate 5 = Large			
9. Skin Color Sur-rounding Wound	1 = Pink or normal for ethnic group 2 = Bright red &/or blanches to touch 3 = White or grey pallor or hypopigmented 4 = Dark red or purple &/or non-blanchable 5 = Black or hyperpigmented			
10. Periph-eral Tissue Edema	1 = Minimal swelling around wound 2 = Non-pitting edema extends < 4 cm around wound 3 = Non-pitting edema extends ≥ 4 cm around wound 4 = Pitting edema extends < 4 cm around wound 5 = Crepitus &/or pitting edema extends ≥ 4 cm			
11. Periph-eral Tissue Indura-tion	1 = Minimal firmness around wound 2 = Induration < 2 cm around wound 3 = Induration 2-4 cm extending < 50% around wound 4 = Induration 2-4 cm extending ≥ 50% around wound 5 = Induration > 4 cm in any area			
12. Granu-lation Tissue	1 = Skin intact or partial thickness wound 2 = Bright, beefy red; 75% to 100% of wound filled &/or tissue overgrowth 3 = Bright, beefy red; < 75% & > 25% of wound filled 4 = Pink, &/or dull, dusky red &/or fills ≤ 25% of wound 5 = No granulation tissue present			
13. Epithe-lializa-tion	1 = 100% wound covered, surface intact 2 = 75% to <100% wound covered &/or epithelial tissue extends >0.5cm into wound bed 3 = 50% to <75% wound covered &/or epithelial tissue extends to <0.5cm into wound bed 4 = 25% to < 50% wound covered 5 = < 25% wound covered			
	TOTAL SCORE			
	SIGNATURE			

PRESSURE SORE STATUS CONTINUUM

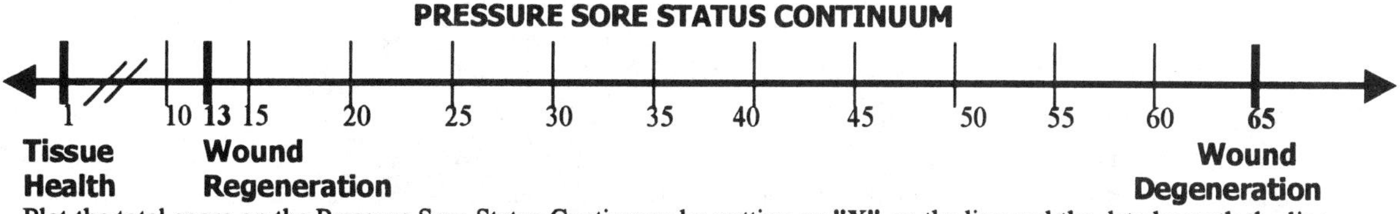

Plot the total score on the Pressure Sore Status Continuum by putting an "X" on the line and the date beneath the line. Plot multiple scores with their dates to see-at-a-glance regeneration or degeneration of the wound.

Fig. 16–2. *(Continued)*

As the wound ages, the edges become rolled under and thickened to palpation. The edge achieves a unique hyperpigmented coloring due to hemosiderin staining. The pigment turns a gray or brown color in both dark- and light-skinned persons. Wounds of long duration may continue to thicken, with scar tissue and fibrosis developing in the wound edge, causing the edge to feel hard, rigid, and indurated. Evaluate the wound edges by visual inspection and palpation.

Undermining and Tunneling. Undermining and tunneling are the loss of tissue underneath an intact skin surface. Undermining, or wound pockets, usually involve a greater percentage of the wound margins with more shallow length than tunneling. Undermining usually involves subcutaneous tissues and follows the fascial planes next to the wound.

Wounds with undermining have more aerobic and anaerobic bacteria than wounds in the process of healing with no undermining.[61] The degree and amount of undermining indicate the severity of tissue necrosis. As subcutaneous fat necroses, the skin undermines. Initially, deep fascia limits the depth of penetration, encouraging more internal undermining spread. Once the fascia is penetrated, undermining of deeper tissues may proceed rapidly.[59] Internal wound dimensions of undermining are commonly measured using cotton-tipped applicators and gently probing the wound. There are also premeasured devices that can be inserted under the wound edge and advanced into the deeper tissues to aid in determination of the extent of undermining.

Assess for undermining and wound pockets by inserting a cotton-tipped applicator under the wound edge; advance it as far as it will go without using undue force; raise the tip of the applicator so that it may be seen or felt on the surface of the skin; mark the surface with a pen; measure the distance from the mark on the skin to the edge of the wound. Continue this process all around the wound. Then use a transparent metric measuring guide with concentric circles divided into quadrants to help determine the percentage of the wound involved. Another noninvasive method of assessment of wound pockets is to use ultrasound to evaluate the undermined tissues. Ultrasound provides a visual picture of the impaired tissues and can be monitored for improvement.

Necrotic Tissue Type and Amount. Necrotic tissue characteristics of color, consistency, adherence, and amount present in the wound must be incorporated into wound assessment. As tissues die during wound development, they change in color, consistency, and adherence to the wound bed. The level and type of tissue death influence the clinical appearance of the necrotic tissue. For example, as subcutaneous fat tissues die, a collection of stringy, yellow slough is formed. As muscle tissues degenerate, the dead tissue may be more thick or tenacious.

The characteristic "necrotic tissue type" is a qualitative variable, with most clinicians using descriptions of clinical observations of a composite of factors as a method of assessment. The characteristics of color, consistency, and adherence are most often used to describe the type of necrosis. Color varies as necrosis worsens, from white/gray nonviable tissue to yellow slough and finally black eschar. Consistency refers to the cohesiveness of debris (i.e., is it thin or thick? stringy or clumpy?). Consistency also varies on a continuum as necrosis deepens and becomes more dehydrated.

The terms "slough" and "eschar" refer to different levels of necrosis and are described according to color and consistency. The term "slough" is described as yellow (or tan) and either thin, mucinous, or stringy, whereas eschar is described as black, soft or hard, and representing full-thickness tissue destruction. Adherence refers to the adhesiveness of the debris to the wound bed and the ease with which the two are separated. Necrotic tissue tends to become more adherent to the wound bed as the level of damage increases. Clinically, eschar is more firmly adherent than yellow slough.

Assess necrotic tissue for color, consistency, and adherence to the wound bed. Choose the predominant characteristic present in the wound. Necrotic tissue type changes as it ages in the wound, as debridement occurs, and as further tissue trauma causes increased cellular death. Slough usually is nonadherent or loosely adherent to the healthy tissues of the wound bed. Nonadherent is defined as appearing scattered throughout the wound; it looks like the tissue could be easily removed with gauze. Loosely adherent refers to tissue that is attached to the wound bed; it is thick and stringy and may appear as clumps of debris attached to wound tissue.

Eschar signifies deeper tissue damage. Eschar may be black, gray, or brown in color. It is usually adherent or firmly adherent to the wound tissues and may be soggy, soft or hard, and leathery in texture. A soft, soggy eschar is usually strongly attached to the base of the wound but may be lifting from (and loose from) the edges of the wound. A hard, crusty eschar is strongly attached to the base and the edges of the wound. Hard eschars are often mistaken for scabs. Sometimes nonviable tissue appears prior to a wound. This can be seen as a white or gray area on the surface of the skin. The area usually demarcates within a couple of days, and the wound appears and interrupts the skin surface.

The amount of necrotic tissue retards wound healing because it is a medium for bacterial growth and a physical obstacle to epidermal resurfacing, wound contraction, and granulation. The more necrotic tissue present in the wound bed, the more severe the insult to the tissue and the longer the time required to heal the wound. The amount of necrotic tissue usually affects the amount of exudate from the wound and causes wound odor, both of which are distressing to the patient and caregiver. In the process of treating the necrotic wound, the amount of necrotic tissue present leads to modification of treatment and debridement techniques. Depth of the wound cannot be assessed in the presence of necrosis that blocks visualization of the total wound.

The amount of necrotic tissue present in the wound is one of the easier characteristics to assess. Use a transparent measuring guide with concentric circles divided into quadrants, and lay this over the wound. Look at each quadrant, and judge how much necrosis is present. Add up the total percentage from judgments of each quadrant; this determines the percentage of the wound involved. The length and width of the necrotic tissue can also be measured to determine the surface area involved in the necrosis.

Exudate Type and Amount. Wound exudate (also known as wound fluid, wound drainage) is an important assessment feature because the characteristics of the exudate help the clinician to diagnose signs of wound infection, to evaluate appropriateness of topical therapy, and to monitor wound healing. Wound infection retards wound healing and must be treated aggressively. Proper assessment of wound exudate is also important because it affirms the body's brief, normal inflammatory response to tissue injury. Thus, accurate assessment and diagnosis of wound exudate and infection are critical components of effective wound management. One of the main goals of palliative wound care is to prevent infection and to control exudate as these conditions lead to discomfort from the wound.

The healthy wound normally has some evidence of moisture on its surface. Healthy wound fluid contains enzymes and growth factors, which may play a role in promoting reepithelialization of the wound and provide needed growth factors for all phases of wound repair. The moist environment produced by wound exudate allows efficient migration of epidermal cells and prevents wound desiccation and further injury.[62,63]

In pressure ulcers, increased exudate is a response to the inflammatory process or infection. Increased capillary permeability causes leakage of fluids and substrates into the injured tissue. When a wound is present, the tissue fluid leaks out of the open tissue. This fluid normally is serous or serosanguineous.

In the infected wound, the exudate may thicken, become purulent in nature, and continue to be present in moderate to large amounts. Examples of exudate character changes in infected wounds are the presence of *Pseudomonas,* which produces a thick, malodorously sweet-smelling, green drainage,[64] or *Proteus* infection, which may have an ammonia-like odor. Wounds with foul-smelling drainage are generally infected or filled with necrotic debris, and healing time is prolonged as tissue destruction progresses.[61] Wounds with significant amounts of necrotic debris will often have a thick, tenacious, opaque, purulent malodorous drainage in moderate to copious amounts. True wound exudate must be differentiated from necrotic tissue sloughing off the wound secondary to debridement efforts. Exudate from sloughing necrotic tissue is commonly attached to or connected with the necrotic debris; however, frequently, the only method of differentiation is adequate debridement of necrotic tissue from the wound site. Liquefied necrotic tissue occurs most often as a result of enzymatic or autolytic debridement. Often, removal of the necrotic tissue reduces the amount and changes the character of wound exudate.

Exudate should be assessed for the amount and type of drainage that occurs. The type and color of wound exudate vary depending on the degree of moisture in the wound and the organisms present. Characteristics used to examine exudate are color, consistency, adherence, distribution in the wound, and presence of odor.

Estimating the amount of exudate in the wound is difficult due to wound size variability and topical dressing types. One problem with assessment of exudate amount is the size of the wound. What might be considered a large amount of drainage for the smaller wound may be considered a small amount for the larger wound, making clinically meaningful assessment of exudate difficult.

Certain dressing types interact with or trap wound fluid to create or mimic certain characteristics of exudate, such as color and consistency of purulent drainage. For example, both hydrocolloid and alginate dressings mimic a purulent drainage upon removal of the dressing. Preparation of the wound site for appropriate assessment involves removal of the wound dressing and cleansing with normal saline to remove dressing debris in the wound bed, followed by evaluation of the wound for true exudate.

Although not a part of exudate assessment, evaluation of the wound dressing provides the clinician with valuable data about the effectiveness of treatment. Evaluation of the percentage of the wound dressing involved with wound drainage during a specific time frame is helpful for clinical management that includes dressings beyond traditional gauze. In estimating the percentage of the dressing involved with the wound exudate, clinical judgment is quantified as the clinician must put a number to visual assessment of the dressing. For example, the clinician might determine that 50% percent of the hydrocolloid dressing was involved with wound drainage over a 4-day wearing period. Based on the above data, the clinician might quantify judgment for this type of dressing, length of dressing wear time, and wound etiology as a "minimal" amount of exudate. Clinical judgment of amount of wound drainage requires some experience with expected wound exudate output in relation to phase of wound healing and type of wound, as well as knowledge of absorptive capacity and normal wear time of topical dressings.

Certain characteristics of exudate indicate wound degeneration and infection. If signs of cellulitis (erythema or skin discoloration, edema, pain, induration, and purulent drainage) present at the wound site the exudate amount may be copious and seropurulent or purulent in character. The amount of exudate remains high or increases in amount, and the character may change to frank purulence with further wound degeneration. Wound infection must be considered in these cases.

Pressure ulcers present with a variety of wound exudate types and amounts. In partial-thickness pressure ulcers, the wound exudate is most likely to be serous or serosanguineous in nature and presents in minimal to moderate amounts. In clean full-thickness pressure ulcers, the wound exudate is similar, with minimal to moderate amounts of serous to serosanguineous exudate. As healing progresses in the clean full-thickness pressure ulcer, the character of the exudate changes and may become bloody if the fragile capillary bed is disrupted and lessens in amount.

For full-thickness pressure ulcers with necrotic debris, wound exudate is dependent on the presence or absence of infection and the type of therapy instituted. Exudate may appear moderate to large but, in fact, be related to the amount of necrotic tissue present and liquefaction of the debris in the wound. Typically, the necrotic full-thickness pressure ulcer presents with serous to seropurulent wound exudate in moderate to large amounts. With appropriate treatment, the wound exudate amount may also temporarily increase, although the character gradually assumes a serous nature.

Surrounding Tissue Condition. The tissues surrounding the wound should be assessed for color, induration, and edema. The tissues surrounding the wound are often the first indication of impending further tissue damage and are a key gauge of successful prevention strategies. Color of the surrounding skin may indicate further injury from pressure, friction, or shearing. Assess the tissues within 4 cm of the wound edge. Dark-skinned persons show the colors "bright red" and "dark red" as a deepening of normal skin color or a purple or blacker hue. As healing occurs in dark-skinned persons, the new skin is pink and may never darken. In both light- and dark-skinned patients, new epithelium must be differentiated from tissues that are erythematous. To assess for blanchability, press firmly on the skin with a finger, lift the finger, and look for "blanching," or sudden whitening, of the tissues followed by prompt return of color to the area. Nonblanchable erythema signals more severe tissue damage.

Edema in the surrounding tissues will delay wound healing in the pressure ulcer. It is difficult for *neoangiogenesis,* or the growth of new blood vessels into the wound, to occur in edematous tissues. Again, assess tissues within 4 cm of the wound edge. Nonpitting edema appears as skin that is shiny and taut, almost glistening. Identify pitting edema by firmly pressing a finger down into the tissues and waiting for 5 seconds; on release of pressure, tissues fail to resume their previous position and an indentation appears. *Crepitus* is accumulation of air or gas in tissues. Measure how far edema extends beyond the wound edges.

Induration is a sign of impending damage to the tissues. Along with skin-color changes, induration is an omen of further pressure-induced tissue trauma. Assess tissues within 4 cm of the wound edge. *Induration* is an abnormal firmness of tissues with margins. Palpate where the induration starts and where it ends by gently pinching the tissues. Induration results in an inability to pinch the tissues. Palpate from healthy tissue, moving toward the wound margins. It is usual to feel slight firmness at the wound edge itself. Normal tissues feel soft and spongy; induration feels hard and firm to the touch.

Granulation Tissue and Epithelialization. Granulation and epithelial tissues are markers of wound health. They signal the proliferative phase of wound healing and usually foretell wound closure. Granulation tissue is the growth of small blood vessels and connective tissue into the wound cavity. It is more observable in full-thickness wounds because of the tissue defect that occurs in such wounds. In partial-thickness wounds, granulation tissue may occur so quickly and in concert with epithelialization, or skin resurfacing, so as to make it unobservable in most cases. The granulation tissue is healthy when bright, beefy red; shiny; and granular with a velvety appearance. The tissue looks "bumpy" and may bleed easily. Unhealthy granulation tissue due to poor vascular supply appears as pale pink or blanched to a dull, dusky red. Usually, the first layer of granulation tissue to be laid down in the wound is pale pink and as the granulation tissue deepens and thickens, the color becomes bright, beefy red.

The percent of the wound filled with granulation tissue and the color of the tissue are characteristics indicative of the health of the wound. Judge what percent of the wound has been filled with granulation tissue. This is much easier if there is some past history with the wound. If the wound has been followed by the same person over multiple observations, it is simple to judge the amount of granulation tissue present. If the initial observation was done by a different observer or if the data are not available, simply use best judgment to determine the amount of tissue present.

Partial-thickness wounds heal by epidermal resurfacing and regeneration. Epithelialization happens from lateral migration at the wound edges and the base of hair follicles as epithelial cells proliferate and resurface the wound. Full-thickness wounds heal using scar formation: the tissue defect fills with granulation tissue, edges contract, and the wound is resurfaced by epithelialization. So epithelialization may occur throughout the wound bed in partial-thickness wounds but only from the wound edges in full-thickness wounds.

Epithelialization can be assessed by evaluating the amount of the wound that is surrounded by new tissue and the distance new tissue extends into the wound base. Epithelialization appears as pink or red skin. Visualizing the new epithelium takes practice. Use a transparent measuring guide to help determine the percentage of the wound involved and to measure the distance the epithelial tissue extends into the wound.

Monitoring the Wound. In palliative care, monitoring of the wound is important, to continue to meet the goals of comfort and reduction in wound pain. Evaluation of wound characteristics at scheduled intervals will allow the nurse to revise the treatment plan as appropriate and often provides an indication of the overall health of the patient. In many cases, the pressure ulcer may worsen as death approaches and as the patient's condition worsens. The skin may be the first organ to actually "fail," with other systems following the downward trend. Progressive monitoring is also important to determine if the treatment is effectively controlling odor, managing exudate, preventing infection, and minimizing pain (the main goals of wound care for palliative care).

Total Patient Assessment

Comprehensive assessment includes assessment of the total patient as well as of wound severity and wound status. Generally, diagnosis and management of the wound are best accomplished within the context of the whole person. Comprehensive assessment includes a focused history and physical examination, attention to specific laboratory and diagnostic tests, and a pain assessment.

It is important to obtain a focused history and physical examination as part of the initial assessment. The patient history determines which relevant systems reviews are needed in the physical examination. The goals for treatment and the direction of care (e.g., curative with a goal of wound closure or palliative with a goal of reduced wound pain) can be best determined with a minimum of the following patient history information: reason for admission to care facility/agency; expectations and perceptions about wound healing; psychological, social, cultural, and economic history; presence of medical comorbidities; current wound status; and previous management strategies.

The systems review portion of the patient history and physical examination provides information on comorbidities that may impair wound healing. Specific comorbidities, such as diabetes,[65–68] vascular disease,[69,70] and immunocompromise,[71–73] have been related to impaired healing. The individual's capacity to heal may be limited by specific disease effects on tissue integrity and perfusion, patient mobility, nutrition, and risk for wound infection. Thus, throughout the patient history, systems review, and physical examination, the clinician considers host factors that affect wound healing.

Specific laboratory and diagnostic tests in a comprehensive assessment include data on nutrition, glucose management, and tissue oxygenation and perfusion. Nutritional parameters typically include evaluation of serum albumin. Serum albumin is a measure of protein available for healing; a normal level is greater than 3.5 mg/dl. Clinicians should evaluate laboratory values such as arterial blood gases to assess tissue perfusion and oxygenation abilities. Review of laboratory values is prudent to determine level of diabetic control. Normal glucose levels are 80 mg/dl. Levels of 180 to 250 mg/dl or greater indicate that glucose levels are out of control. Look specifically for a fasting blood glucose of less than 140 mg/dl, and a glycosylated hemoglobin (HgbA1C) of less than 7%. The HgbA1C helps to determine the level of glucose control the patient has had over the last 2 to 3 months.

The final aspect of the comprehensive assessment is pain assessment. Pain is thought to be an important factor in healing. Until recently, chronic wound pain has been largely ignored as a cofactor in healing. Krasner[74] proposed a chronic wound pain experience model and described the typical pain experiences for persons with chronic wounds as noncyclic acute wound pain (as with sharp debridement), cyclic acute wound pain (as with daily dressings or repositioning), and chronic wound pain (as persistent pain with no wound manipulation). Krasner[74] suggests that the model is best used as a guide for assessment, intervention, and evaluation.

Evaluate wound pain by having the patient rate the pain on a scale from 0 to 10, with 0 equal to no pain and 10 equal to the worst pain ever felt, or by use of a visual analogue scale. For patients who are nonverbal, observe for withdrawal, grimacing, crying out, or other nonverbal signs of pain. Pain assessments should be done prior to and during wound procedures, such as dressing changes or debridement, as well as when the dressing is intact and no procedures are in progress. Encourage the patient or caregiver to keep a pain diary as the data may be valuable in evaluating changes in wound pain over time. The focused history, physical examination, evaluation of laboratory and diagnostic data, and pain assessment provide the context for the wound itself and, along with wound severity and wound status assessment, the basis for pressure ulcer treatment. Total patient assessment should also encompass evaluation of treatment appropriateness in light of the overall condition of the patient and the goals of palliative care. Table 16–3 presents an overview of assessment for the patient with a pressure ulcer.

PRESSURE ULCER MANAGEMENT

Pressure ulcer management can be based on published guidelines. Existing guidelines are helpful in developing a palliative care plan. The existing guidelines are broad-based and general and, as such, form a good basis for wound care when the goal is comfort as well as when the goal is healing.

Agency for Health Care Policy and Research Guidelines for Pressure Ulcer Treatment

In the United States, most pressure ulcer care is based on the AHCPR algorithms for treatment.[42] The AHCPR guidelines present a general approach to use in developing a care plan for the patient with a pressure ulcer. The AHCPR guidelines base pressure ulcer care on three main areas of concern: nutritional assessment and support, management of tissue loads, and ulcer care, including management of bacterial colonization

Table 16–3. Pressure Ulcer Assessment Overview

Assessment Parameter	Assessment Methods	Notes & Considerations	Frequency
Wound severity	Pressure ulcer staging classification Partial vs. full thickness classification	Provides diagnosis of severity of tissue insult	• Baseline, initial observation of wound • Reassess if wound deteriorates • Does not change over time
Wound status	Evaluate wound characteristics (location, size, shape, depth, edges, undermining, and tunneling), necrotic tissue characteristics, exudate characteristics, surrounding skin characteristics, granulation tissue and epithelialization	Use of standardized tool is easiest: Pressure Sore Status Tool	• Baseline or initially • Weekly • Whenever significant change in wound status noted
Total patient: history	Interview or patient questionnaire. Include review of systems and specific questions: • Goals for care? • Reason for admission to facility? • Expectations about wound progress? • Psychosocial, cultural, economic history? • Presence of medical comorbidities? • Previous wound treatments?	Look for relevant systems to then include in physical exam	• Baseline data
Total patient: physical exam	Physical examination should focus on items identified during patient history	Focus on areas that would impact wound healing, such as disease effects on tissue perfusion, tissue integrity, mobility, nutrition, and risk for infection	• Baseline data
Total patient: labs and diagnostic tests	Nutritional parameters: serum albumin Tissue perfusion: arterial blood gases, hemoglobin and hematacrit, blood glucose levels, glycosylated hemoglobin	Specific tests depend on individual patient	• Baseline or initially • Every 3 months for nutritional markers, tissue perfusion markers • If performing self-blood glucose monitoring, daily levels are helpful
Total patient: pain	Assess for wound pain prior to and during procedures and when no procedure is occurring	Use 0–10 point scale, with 0 = no pain and 10 = worst pain ever, and have patient state level of pain. For non-verbal patients, observe for grimacing, pulling away, crying out, or withdrawal	• Baseline or initially • Every day as needed • Prior to and during procedures such as dressing changes, debridement, or repositioning

and infection.[42] These general guidelines are also appropriate for palliative care.

Nutritional Support. Because many studies have linked malnutrition with pressure ulcers, adequate nutritional support is an important part of pressure ulcer management. Figure 16–3 presents the nutritional assessment and support algorithm for pressure ulcer management from the AHCPR guidelines. The clinician must ensure that dietary intake is adequate in the patient with a pressure ulcer. Prevention of malnutrition will reduce the patient's risk for further tissue trauma related to pressure or impaired wound healing. As noted in the prevention discussion, maintenance of adequate nutrition in the palliative care patient may not be possible.

Management of Tissue Loads. Management of tissue loads refers to care related

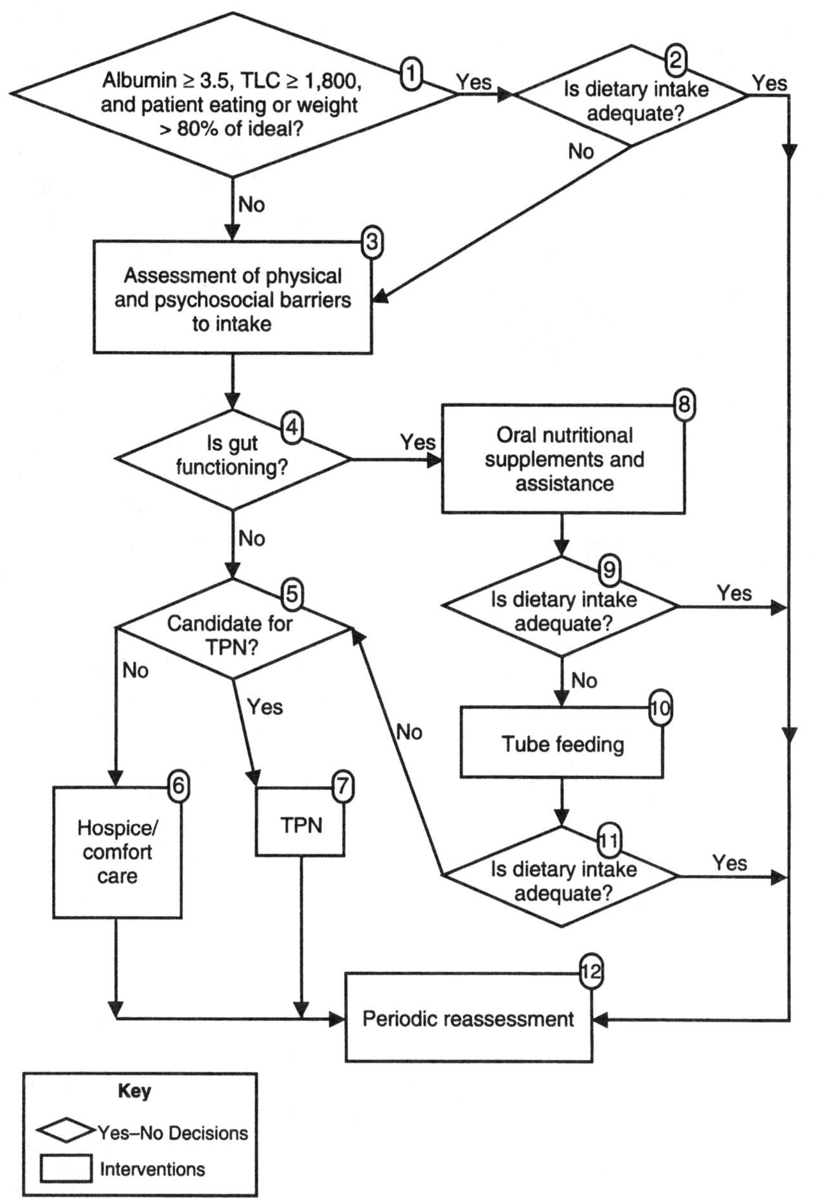

Fig. 16–3. Nutritional assessment and support algorithm from the United States Agency for Health Care Policy and Research (AHCPR). (From Bergstrom et al. (1994), reference 42, with permission.)

to those with pressure ulcers who are at risk of developing additional pressure ulcers. Figure 16–4 presents the AHCPR algorithm for management of tissue loads with support surfaces. This is an important part of pressure ulcer treatment as many individuals with a pressure ulcer are at risk for further pressure-induced tissue trauma. More information on support surfaces and management of tissue loads can be found under Prevention of Pressure Ulcers, above. It is important to understand that the goal of managing tissue loads in the palliative care patient is to ease suffering and discomfort from the wound. Use of pressure-reduction devices, such as alternating air mattresses, is particularly appropriate for palliative care.

Ulcer Care: Debridement. Direct-pressure ulcer care involves adequate debridement of necrotic material, management of bacterial colonization and infection, wound cleansing, and selection of topical dressings. Figure 16–5 presents an algorithm for ulcer care from the AHCPR guidelines.

Adequate debridement of necrotic tissue is necessary for wound healing. Necrotic debris in the wound bed forms an obstacle to healing and provides a medium for bacterial growth. The patient's condition and the goals of care determine the method of debridement. Sharp, mechanical, enzymatic, or autolytic debridement techniques may be used when there is no urgent need for drainage or removal of devitalized material from the wound. In the presence of advancing cellulitis, sepsis, or large and adherent amounts of necrotic debris, sharp debridement should be performed. In palliative care, debridement is still important as the removal of nonviable material decreases wound odor. In the case of the black eschar that forms on heels, debridement may not be necessary. Observation of the black heel with attention to the development of pathological signs such as erythema, drainage, odor, or bogginess to the tissues is necessary. If signs of erythema, drainage, odor, or bogginess to the tissues appear, then the heel eschar must be debrided.

Mechanical debridement includes the use of wet-to-dry dressings at specific intervals, hydrotherapy, or wound irrigation. Of these three methods, wound irrigation is the most favorable for wound healing. Wet-to-dry dressings are not favorable due to the time and labor involved in performing the dressing technique correctly and the potential for pain. Wet-to-dry dressings are not recommended for palliative care due to the frequency of dressing changes and the increased potential for wound pain. Hydrotherapy or whirlpool may be helpful for wounds with large amounts of necrotic debris adherent to healthy tissues. In these cases, hydrotherapy helps to loosen the material from the wound bed for easier removal with sharp debridement.

Enzymatic debridement is per-

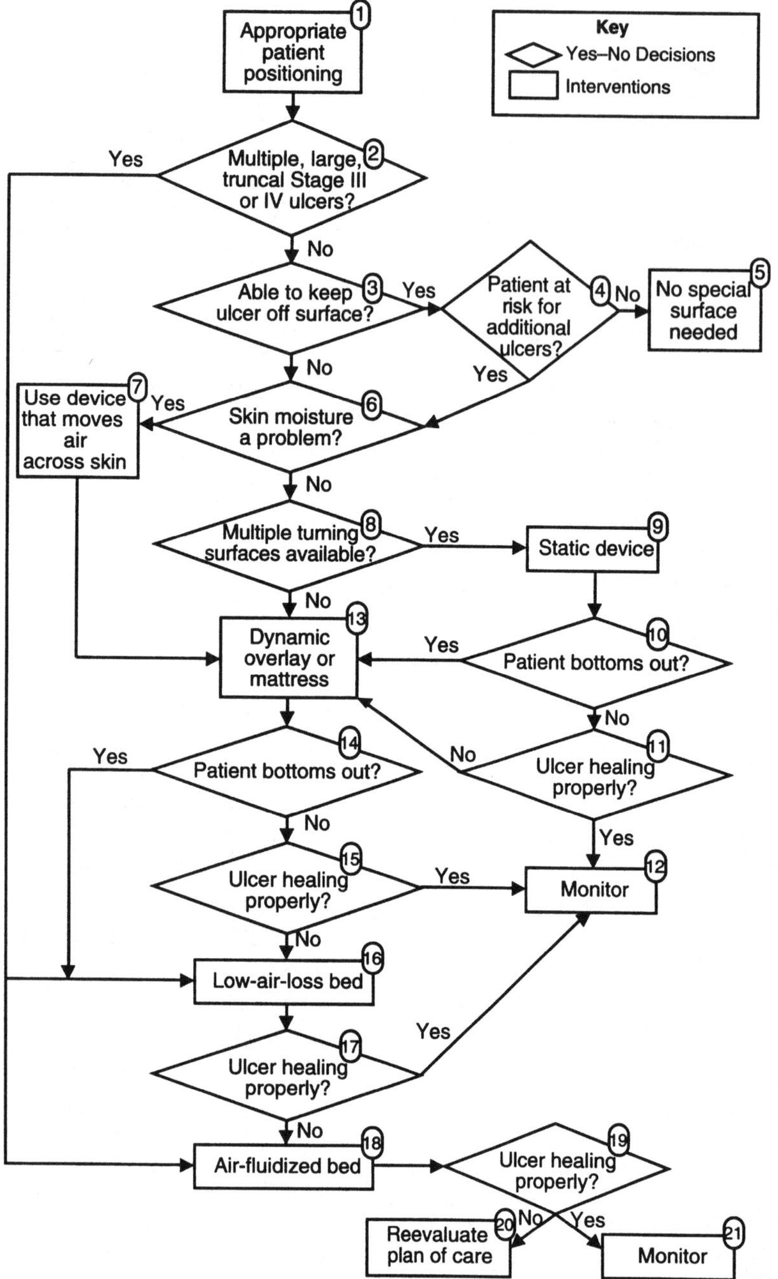

Fig. 16–4. Management of tissue loads algorithm from the United States Agency for Health Care Policy and Research (AHCPR). (From Bergstrom et al. (1994), reference 42, with permission.)

formed by applying a topical agent containing an enzyme that destroys necrotic tissue. Enzymatic debridement should be considered when an individual is not a candidate for sharp debridement or for those in long-term care or home care. Enzymes can be used alone or in conjunction with other debridement techniques. Enzymatic debridement may be an appropriate method for palliative care as the frequency of dressing changes is usually once a day and the method is easy to use in conjunction with periodic sharp debridement.

Autolytic debridement involves the use of moisture-retentive dressings to cover the wound and allow necrotic tissue to self-digest from enzymes normally found in wound fluid or exudate. Autolytic debridement may take longer than other methods and can be used in conjunction with other debridement methods such as intermittent sharp debridement or wound irrigation. Again, autolytic debridement may be particularly effective for palliative care. Autolytic debridement has the added benefit of decreased frequency of dressing changes (typically every 2 to 4 days), so the suffering associated with dressing changes is diminished.

Ulcer Care: Bacterial Colonization and Infection. Open pressure ulcers are typically colonized with bacteria. In most cases, adequate debridement and wound cleansing will prevent the bacterial colonization from proceeding to the point of clinical infection. Figure 16–6 presents a preferred pathway for management of bacterial colonization and infection according to the AHCPR guidelines. Wound healing can be enhanced in pressure ulcers by attention to debridement of necrotic debris and adequate wound cleansing. These two steps alone are often sufficient to prevent wound infection in pressure ulcers as they remove the debris that supports bacterial growth.[42] Prevention of infection is an important goal for the palliative care patient. Routine swab cultures should not be used to identify infection in most pressure ulcers. Swab cultures will simply reflect the bacterial contamination on the surface of the wound and, thus, may not truly reflect the organism(s) causing tissue infection. The recommended technique for diagnosing tissue infection in pressure ulcers is needle aspiration or tissue biopsy.[42] An alternative method involves use of surface swabs. After cleansing the wound with normal saline to remove any dressing debris, swab a 1 cm square area of the wound bed with the surface swab for 5 seconds until tissue fluid is apparent on the swab, then send directly to the laboratory. This technique may better reflect actual bacterial invasion of the wound tissues than standard swab methods.

There are cases where pressure ulcers appear clean and healthy, yet wound healing does not progress. The

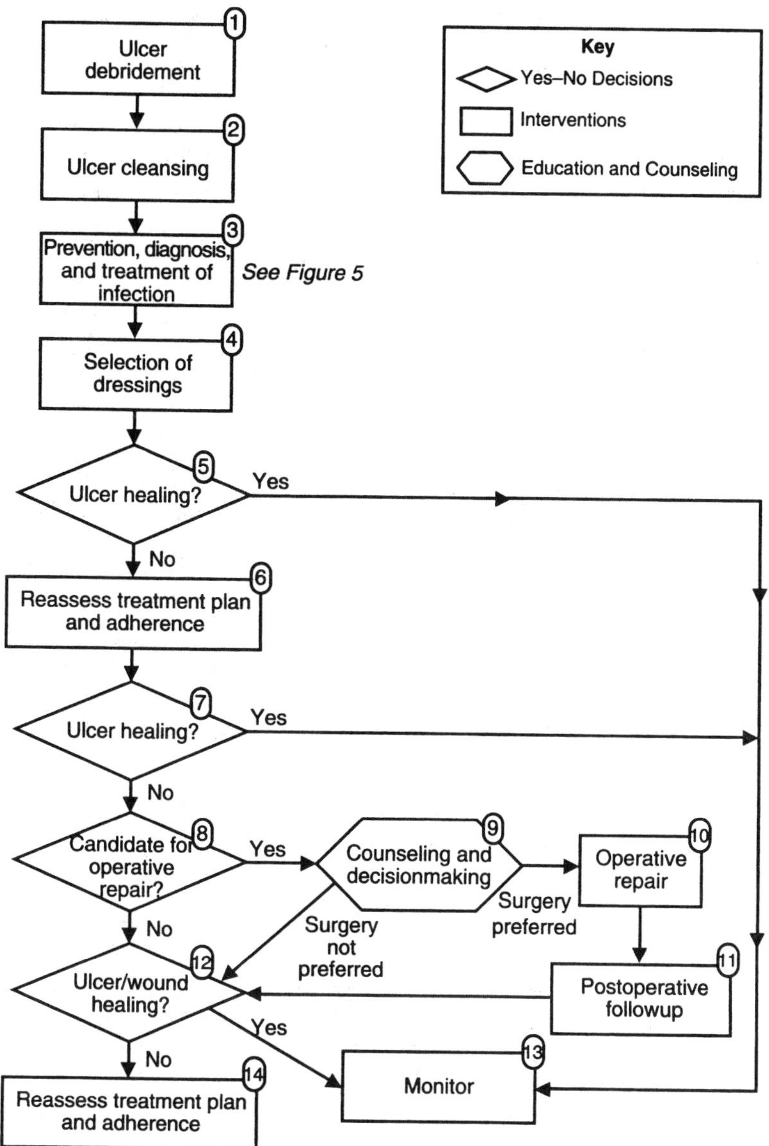

Fig. 16–5. Ulcer care algorithm from the United States Agency for Health Care Policy and Research (AHCPR). (From Bergstrom et al. (1994), reference 42, with permission.)

case of the nonhealing clean pressure ulcer may be handled by instituting a 2-week trial of topical antibiotics such as silver sulfadiazine or triple antibiotic. The topical antibiotic reduces the surface bacterial contaminants that may have impaired normal healing.

Use of topical antimicrobial solutions is not indicated for clean pressure ulcers. Indeed, most topical antimicrobial solutions are toxic to the fibroblast, which is the cell responsible for wound healing. Topical antiseptics, such as povidone iodine, iodophor, sodium hypochlorite, hydrogen peroxide, and acetic acid, do not significantly reduce the bacteria in wound tissue; however, they do harm the healing wound tissues.[42] As such, these substances usually have no place in the treatment of clean pressure ulcers. In necrotic debris-filled wounds, antiseptic/antimicrobial solutions may be used for a short course of therapy (typically 2 weeks) and then evaluated for further use.

Ulcer Care: Wound Cleansing. Cleansing a wound assists by removing necrotic tissue, excess wound exudate, and metabolic wastes from the wound bed. Wound healing is optimized and the potential for wound infection decreased when wound cleansing is a part of the treatment plan for pressure ulcers. Wound cleansing involves the selection of a solution for cleansing and a method of delivering the solution to the wound. Routine wound cleansing should be accomplished with minimal trauma to the wound bed. Wounds should be cleansed initially and at each dressing change. Minimal force should be applied when using gauze, sponges, or cloth to clean the wound bed. Skin cleansers and antimicrobial solutions are not indicated as solutions for cleaning pressure ulcers because they destroy the healthy wound tissues and are toxic to the fibroblast cell.[42] Normal saline is the preferred solution because it is physiological and will not harm healing tissues.

When using wound irrigation to cleanse wounds, the irrigation pressure should fall within the range of 4 to 15 pounds per square inch (psi). Higher pressures may drive bacteria deeper into wound tissues or cause additional wound trauma. A 35 ml syringe with a 19-gauge angiocatheter delivers saline at 8 psi and is an effective method of removing bacteria from the wound bed.

Ulcer Care: Dressings. In general, moisture-retentive wound dressings are the most appropriate for pressure ulcers. For palliative care, they are the dressings of choice because of the decreased frequency of required changes (typically every 2 to 4 days). The goal of the wound dressing is to provide an environment that keeps the wound bed tissue moist and the surrounding intact skin dry. Use of moist wound healing dressings supports a better rate of healing than use of dry gauze dressings,[42] but more importantly in palliative care, moist wound healing dressings contain odor, absorb exudate, and minimize dressing change discomfort. Clinical judgment is needed to determine the best dressing for the wound. The appropriate dressing should keep the surrounding intact skin dry while controlling wound exudate. The clinician must be aware of the absorptive capacity of the major dressing types. In general, thin film dressings have no

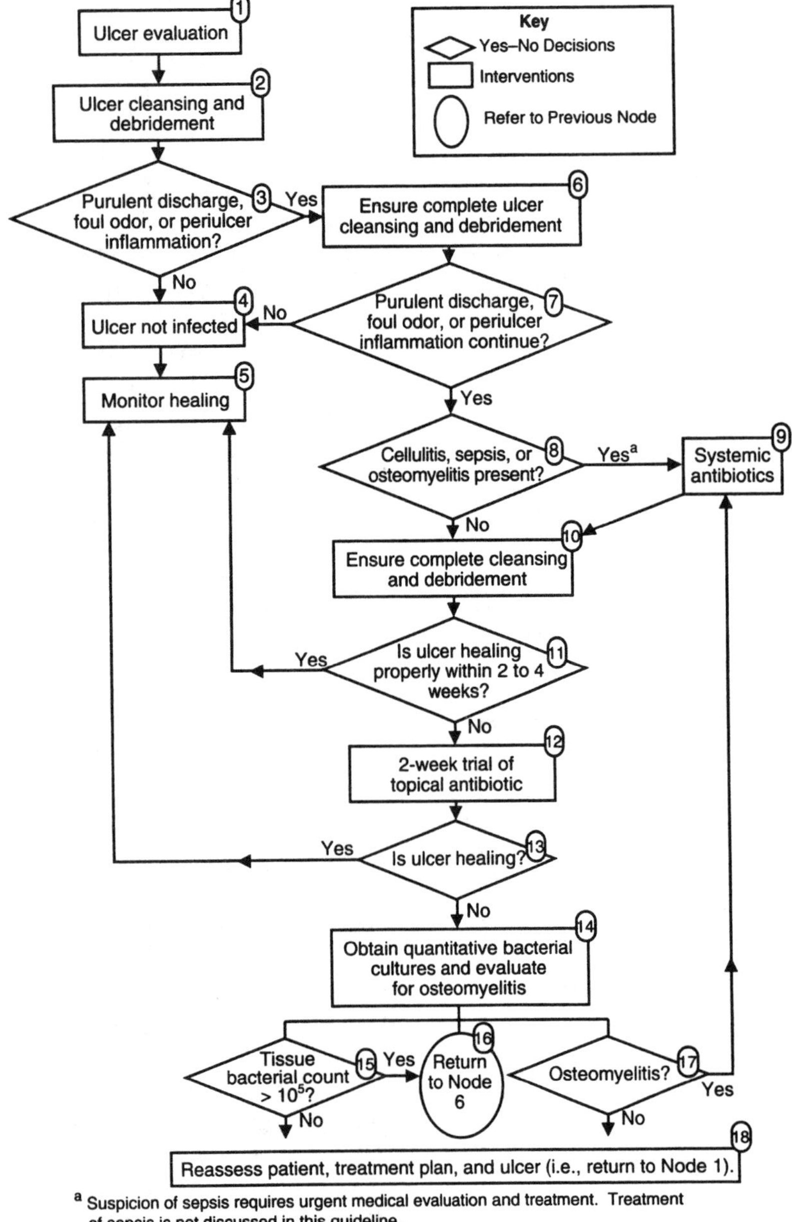

Fig. 16–6. Managing bacterial colonization and infection algorithm from the United States Agency for Health Care Policy and Research (AHCPR). (From Bergstrom et al. (1994), reference 42, with permission.)

absorptive capacity. Hydrocolloids, hydrogels, and foam dressings typically have a minimal to moderate absorptive capacity. Calcium alginates, alginate collagen dressings, and exudate absorbing beads, flakes, pastes, or powders absorb large amounts of drainage.

Wounds with small or minimal amounts of exudate will benefit from a variety of dressings, including hydrocolloids, hydrogels, thin film dressings, and foam dressings. Wounds with moderate amounts of exudate may require dressings with a higher absorptive capacity, such as hydrocolloids, foam dressings, hydrogel sheet dressings, or composite dressings (dressings with a combination of products included, such as a thin film with a foam island in the center). Wounds with a large amount of drainage will require dressings that are capable of absorbing large amounts, such as calcium alginates, alginate collagen combinations, or specific beads, pastes, or powders designed to handle large amounts of drainage. Wounds with significant odor benefit from dressings formulated with charcoal, such as charcoal foam and dressings with a charcoal filter overlay.

When a wound presents with a significant loss of tissue or when undermining or pockets are present, the wound cavities should be loosely filled with dressing to eliminate the potential for abscess formation. Eliminating the dead space will help to prevent premature wound closure with resulting abscess formation. Dressings such as calcium alginates, impregnated hydrogel gauze strips, or wound cavity fillers are useful for eliminating the dead space. Loosely filling the undermined areas also assists with exudate management as these wounds tend to have large amounts of exudate.

Wounds in the sacral area require additional protection from stool or urine contamination. Dressings near the anus may be difficult to maintain, and thus, the clinician must monitor dressings in this area more frequently. Some newer hydrocolloid dressings have been designed with specific shapes to improve their ability to stay in place over sacral/coccygeal wounds.

As evidenced by the above discussion, attention to multiple wound characteristics helps to determine the most appropriate wound dressing. Evaluation of wound characteristics in follow-up assessments provides the basis for changes in topical dressings. For example, a wound that is heavily exudative may be treated topically with a calcium alginate dressing for several weeks and as the amount of wound exudate decreases, the wound dressing may appear dry at dressing changes. This indicates that use of a dressing with high absorptive capacity may not be needed any longer and the wound dressing can be changed to one with minimal to moderate absorptive capacity, such as a hydrocolloid dressing. As the wound continues to heal and wound exudate becomes minimal or nonexistent, a thin film dressing may be used to provide protection from the environment.

PATIENT AND CAREGIVER TEACHING GUIDELINES

Patient and caregiver instruction in self-care must be individualized to specific pressure ulcer development risk factors, to individual learning styles and coping mechanisms, and to the ability of the patient or caregiver to perform procedures. In teaching prevention guidelines to caregivers, it is particularly important to use return demonstration to evaluate learning. Observing the caregiver perform turning manuevers, repositioning, managing incontinence, and providing general skin care can be enlightening and provide a context in which the clinician supports and follows up education. In palliative care, it is important to include the reasons for specific actions, such as the continuation of some level of turning and repositioning to prevent further tissue damage and lessen discomfort from additional wounds.

TUMOR NECROSIS

Tumor necrosis, also known in the literature as fungating wounds, ulcerating malignant wounds, or malignant cutaneous wounds, presents both a physical and an emotional challenge for the patient and even the experienced clinician. In dealing with tumor necrosis, the goals of care are symptom palliation. Treatments are directed at alleviation of the distressing symptoms associated with these lesions, with attention focused on minimizing pain and infection, management of exudate and odor, and control of bleeding. By far the most objectionable symptom for both patients and caregivers is the malodor that is often associated with tumor necrosis. Fungating or ulcerating wounds are often unsightly, malodorous, and painful. These wounds are a blow to self-esteem and may cause social isolation just when the patient needs more time with family and friends.

As pointed out in a literature review by Ivetic and Lyne,[75] there is a scarcity of information on tumor necrosis, with extremely limited data on the prevalence and incidence of malignant ulcerating wounds and even less on treatment methods. Tumor necrosis occurs in an estimated 8% of all patients with advanced cancer and is reported most frequently with breast cancer.[76] When tumor necrosis occurs as a result of primary malignancy metastasis, breast cancer accounts for 25% of cases, with the usual site of skin metastasis being the chest wall or scalp.[76]

Pathophysiology of Tumor Necrosis

Tumor necrosis may occur by infiltration of the epidermis by primary or metastatic tumor. Cutaneous infiltration occurs via the lymphatics or bloodstream or as a result of direct invasion from a primary lesion. Local invasion may initially manifest as inflammation with induration, redness, heat, and/or tenderness. The skin may have a *peau d'orange* appearance, and the area may be fixed to underlying tissue. As the tumor infiltrates the skin, ulcerating and fungating wounds develop. Initially, the tumor may present as an ulcerating wound and then progress to a necrotic wound with time. As the cancerous lesion infiltrates the epithelium, a fungating mass or an ulceration develops. There is uncertainty as to which develops first and whether one is a precursor to the other.

Once the fungating or ulcerating wound develops, perfusion of the tissues is altered such that as the mass expands, the center of the tumor becomes hypoxic and the result is tumor necrosis. Vascular permeability is altered in tumors such that it persists to provide a constant source of nutrition and oxygen to the tumor for unregulated tissue growth. Additionally, tumor cells secrete growth factors and have platelet-type functions that continually support the growth of new blood vessels and collagen, which enhance tumor growth. As the tumor grows larger, it is unable to sustain sufficient vasculature growth to support the entire mass; this results in fragile capillaries, poor perfusion, altered collagen synthesis, and resultant tissue ischemia and necrosis.[77] Additionally, tumor cells invade the vascular basement membrane, resulting in degeneration of the basement membrane by tumor cells through secretion of protease and other hydrolytic enzymes and formation of a hard fibrous mass.[78] The resulting lesion may be fungating, in which the tumor mass extends above the skin surface with a fungus or cauliflower-like appearance, or it may be erosive and ulcerative. The wound bed may be pale to pink with very friable tissue, completely necrotic, or a combination of both. The surrounding skin may be erythematous, fragile, and exceedingly tender to touch. The skin may also be macerated in the presence of excessive wound exudate. The ulceration itself results in local infection, offensive odor, and fragile capillaries with subsequent bleeding. There are often large amounts of necrotic material in these wounds, and the necrosis may account for much of the odor.

The odor of the wounds is also related to bacterial infection. Typical organisms that infiltrate tumor wounds include *Escherichia coli*, *Pseudomonas aeruginosa*, and strains of *Staphylococcus*, *Proteus*, and *Klebsiella*.[77,78] Odor may be due to anaerobic organisms, in most cases *Bacteroides*,[77] and the necrotic material in the wound provides an excellent medium for bacterial proliferation. Tumor necrosis, while mostly associated with breast cancer, can occur with any type of cancer and in any location. Indeed, many times the challenge in treating tumor necrosis is the location of the lesion, with wounds located in the head and neck area, labia and perineal area, rectal area, abdomen, and chest wall.

Tumor Necrosis Assessment

Assessment of tumor necrosis is inclusive of wound assessment with two caveats: assessment of potential complications and assessment of treatment appropriateness. Wound assessment for tumor necrosis is not intended only to document healing but as a precursor to determining treatment needs and treatment appropriateness. In particular, size of the lesion, necrotic tissue characteristics, exudate characteristics, and surrounding skin condition are important wound characteristics to consider in planning for topical dressing application. Table 16–4 presents assessment highlights for tumor necrosis or cutaneous lesions. Haisfield-Wolfe and Baxendale-Cox[78] have proposed a staging classification system for assessment of malignant cutaneous wounds. Use of wound classification may increase the effectiveness of communication among health care practitioners and make evaluation of treatment effectiveness consistent. In a pilot study with 13 wounds, they proposed a staging classification system that evaluates the wound depth with clinical descriptors, predominant color of the wound, hydration status of the wound, drainage, pain, odor, and presence of tunneling or undermining.[78] Use of this system provides a basis for a standard set of descriptors that nurses can use to both understand and assess tumor necrosis wounds.

Tumor necrosis and ulcerating wounds are expected to increase in size over time and to change in appearance. Tumor necrosis may occur singly or in groups, and nodules may enlarge and remit spontaneously.[79] While chemotherapy may bring about regression of lesions from breast cancer and radiation therapy may achieve healing of fungating lesions from breast cancer,[76] usual treatment is only symptomatic. Radiation therapy is used to destroy tumor cells and shrink the lesion. Reduction in the size of the lesion may result in decreased exudate and pain in addition to decreasing bleeding from lesions.[79]

Assessment of potential complications involves evaluation of the risk for

Table 16–4. Assessment of Cutaneous Malignancy

Assessment	Rationale
Wound Location	
• Is mobility impaired?	• Consider occupational therapy referral to facilitate activities of daily living
• Is the lesion easily covered from public view?	• Impacts dressing selection
• Located near wrinkled or flat skin?	• Impacts dressing fixation
Wound Appearance	
• Size: length, width, depth, undermining, deep structure exposure	• Impacts dressing selection, provides info on deterioration or response to palliative treatment
• Fungating or ulcerative	• Impacts dressing selection and fixation
• Percentage of viable vs. necrotic tissue	• Need for cleansing/debridement
• Tissue friability and bleeding	• Need for nonadherent dressings and other measures to control bleeding
• Presence of odor	• Need for odor-reducing strategies
• Presence of fistula	• Possible need for pouching
• Exudate amount	• Impacts dressing selection
• Wound colonized or clinically infected	• Need for local vs. systemic care
Surrounding Skin	
• Erythematous	• Infection or tumor extension
• Fragile or denuded	• Impacts dressing type and fixation
• Nodular	• Tumor extension/metastasis
• Macerated	• Need for improved exudate management
• Radiation-related skin damage	• Need for topical care of skin, impacts dressing fixation
Symptoms	
• Deep pain: aching, stabbing, continuous	• Need to adjust systemic analgesia
• Superficial pain: burning, stinging, may be only associated with dressing changes	• Need for topical analgesia and rapid-onset, short-acting analgesics
• Pruritis	• Related to dressings? If not, may need systemic antipruritic medications
Potential for Serious Complications	
• Lesion is near major blood vessels: potential for hemorrhage	• Need for education of patient/family about palliative management of severe bleeding
• Lesion is near major blood vessels: Potential for vessel compression/obstruction	• Need for education of patient/family about palliative management of severe swelling and pain, possible tissue necrosis
• Lesion is near airway: potential for obstruction	• Need for education of patient/family about palliative management of airway obstruction

infection and bleeding. In particular, bleeding can be a significant problem with tumor necrosis. Use of extreme care in dressing removal and attention to bleeding preparedness are essential. Infection risk increases with capillary fragility and bleeding. Decreasing the amount of necrosis present in the wound will decrease the risk for infection as well. The presence of infection increases wound odor and exudate. Treatment appropriateness must be assessed frequently. Because the prognosis with tumor necrosis is one of increasing degeneration of the wound site, the treatment may need to be changed more frequently than in other wound types. Dressing change frequency is often increased as the wound worsens, and additional products to contain exudate or control odor may be needed over time. Pain assessment is critical as these wounds are often severely painful. Analgesia is typically needed prior to dressing changes. Following assessment, the plan of treatment is developed and implemented.

Tumor Necrosis Management

Infection control, management of exudate, odor control, controlling bleeding, and minimizing pain are the cornerstones of nursing management for tumor necrosis. In determining the appropriate treatment regimen, the abilities of the caregiver must also be considered. The limited information on treatment effectiveness reflects the absence of evidence-based care in this area and the extreme need for further research and dissemination of findings. Many articles are based on expert opinion and the personal experience of practitioners knowledgeable in palliative and hospice care. Although research-based treatment is the gold standard of care, anecdotal reports on the successful treatment of patients with these challenging wounds is helpful to individual nurses striving to provide the best care.

Infection Control: Wound Cleansing and Debridement. Infection control is managed by focusing on wound cleansing and wound debridement. Because malignant cutaneous lesions are frequently associated with necrotic tissue and odor, wound cleansing is essential to remove necrotic debris, decrease bacterial counts, and thus reduce odor. If the lesion is not very friable, the patient may be able to get in the shower. This not only provides for local cleansing but also gives the added psychological benefit of helping the patient to feel clean. The patient should be instructed to allow the shower water to hit the skin above the wound and then to allow the water to run over the wound. If there is friable tissue (tissue that bleeds easily with minimal trauma) or the patient is not able to shower, the nurse/caregiver should gently irrigate the wound with normal saline or a commercial wound cleanser. Skin cleansers should generally be avoided because they tend to cause burning; however, they can be used to cleanse surrounding skin. Wound cleansing should be carried out using low-pressure irrigation with normal saline for those not able to shower and those requiring more aggressive cleansing. Saline has the advantage of not disturbing any tissues that might be healthy. Collinson[80] suggests using warmed saline, and Cormier and colleagues[81] have suggested use of a handheld shower head and tepid water with liquid soap. Use of antimicrobial solutions such as povidone iodine, sodium hypochlorite solution (Dakin's solution), chlorhexidine and hydrogen peroxide are not recommended by some,[75] but sodium hypochlorite solution and chlorhexidine are recommended by others.[77] The best approach may be short-term use of sodium hypochlorite solution or chlorhexidine for 2 weeks and then reevaluation of effectiveness. The rationale for antimicrobial solution use is the decrease of bacterial burden on the surface of the wound. However, the antimicrobial solutions do not inhibit further bacterial proliferation as they are inactivated by body fluids, blood, pus, and slough (all of which are found in abundance in tumor necrosis).[76,82,83] Cleansing of the wound is followed by adequate debridement of necrotic tissue at the wound site.

Necrotic tissue in tumor necrosis is typically dry, encrusted material, slough, or black eschar. Debridement of dry, encrusted material and black eschar may be best accomplished with the protocol described by Collinson.[80] After cleansing with warm normal saline, the wound is covered with an amorphous hydrogel dressing as the primary dressing and then with a thin film dressing as the secondary one. The dressing is changed daily at first and less frequently as debridement occurs. Collinson[80] describes initiation of liquefaction of necrotic tissue within 24 hours of starting the dressing. The hydrogel dressing allows for rehydration of the necrotic tissue and manages drainage associated with autolytic debridement. Procedures for sloughy, wet necrotic tissue differ. Collinson[80] advocates use of calcium alginate as a primary dressing and covering with either a thin film dresssing or a foam dressing. Use of the calcium alginate dressing has the additional advantage of controlling bleeding at the wound site. This procedure adequately debrides soft, sloughy necrotic tissue while protecting surrounding tissues from maceration by controlling exudate. Debridement is best done by autolytic methods and gentle mechanical methods (such as low-pressure irrigation) as opposed to wet-to-dry dressings, which are traumatic and can cause significant bleeding upon removal. If eschar on the tumor is extensive and thickly adherent to the tissues, surgical debridement may be indicated to allow for infection prevention, odor control, and exudate management. Frank wound infection, as evidenced by wound cultures of 10^5 organisms on wound culture, may be effectively treated with topical antibiotic preparations. This is in direct contrast to other wound types. The topical preparation may work better in tumor necrosis due to the decreased perfusion and vasculature throughout the tumor, which impede systemic antibiotic dissemination.

Management of Exudate and Odor Control. Management of exudate in tumor necrosis is similar to that in pressure ulcers and other wound types. The goal is to provide a moist wound environment to support epithelial cell migration across any healthy tissue, prevent trauma from drying and fissuring, and enhance tumor angiogenesis, which makes the tumor more susceptible to the effects of radiation or chemotherapy. While a moist wound environment is to be encouraged, a wet wound is to be avoided. Dressings should be chosen to conceal and collect exudate and odor. It is essential to use dressings that contain the exudate as a patient who experiences unexpected drainage on clothing or bedding may experience significant feelings of distress and loss of control. Specialty dressings, such as foams, alginates, or starch copolymers, are notably more expensive than gauze pads or cotton-based absorbent pads. However, if these dressings reduce the overall cost by reducing the need for frequent dressing changes, they may be cost-effective. Table 16–5 summarizes tumor necrosis dressing considerations. Nonadherent dressings are best for the primary contact layer as they minimize the trauma to the wound associated with dressing changes.

Seaman[84] suggests nonadherent contact layers, such as vaseline gauze, for the primary dressing on the wound bed covered with soft, absorbent dressings, such as gauze and ABDs, for secondary dressings to contain drainage, changing the dressing one to two times daily. When drainage increases, Seaman[84] recommends use of calcium alginate dressings to decrease the frequency of dressing changes. Grocott[85] also recommends use of calcium alginate dressings and discusses the use of hydrocolloids for less exudative wounds. Hydrocolloids may be difficult to apply to tumor necrosis because of the uneven wound surface and gel dressings may be easier for caregivers to manage. Protection of the surrounding skin and tissues is another goal of exudate management.

Use of skin barriers on the skin surrounding the wound and then taping dressings to the skin barriers (changing every 5 to 7 days) is one method of protecting surrounding skin from both excess drainage and tape and the resultant skin stripping with dressing changes. Another method of protecting the surrounding skin is use of a barrier ointment on the skin surrounding the ulcer. The barrier protects the fragile tissue from maceration and the caustic effects of the drainage on the skin. Dressings can then be held in place with Montgomery straps or tape affixed to a skin barrier placed on healthy skin, flexible netting, tube dressings, sports bras, panties, and the like.

Odor control is by far the most difficult management aspect of tumor necrosis. The literature supports use of metronidazole topically and systemically for controlling wound odor. For example, application of Metrogel (a 0.8% topical antibiotic wound deodorizing gel) to the wound results in a decrease in wound odor in 2 to 3 days even in the presence of resistant odor.[76,84,86,87] Typically, dressings are changed twice daily,

Table 16–5. Dressing Choices for Tumor Necrosis or Malignant Cutaneous Lesions

Type of Wound/Goals of Care	Dressing Choice
Low Exudate	

• Maintain moist environment
• Prevent dressing adherence and bleeding
	• Nonadherent contact layers
	  • Adaptic (Johnson & Johnson)
	• Dermanet (DeRoyal)
	  • Mepitel (MöInlycke)
	  • Petrolatum gauze (numerous manufacturers)
	  • Tegapore (3M Health Care)
	• Amorphous hydrogels
	• Sheet hydrogels
	• Hydrocolloids: contraindicated with fragile surrounding skin, may increase odor
	• Semipermeable films: contraindicated with fragile surrounding skin

High Exudate	
• Absorb and contain exudate • Prevent dressing adherence in areas of lesion with decreased exudate	• Alginates • Foams • Starch copolymers • Gauze • Soft cotton pads • Menstrual pads (excessive exudate)
Malodorous Wounds	
• Wound cleansing (see text) • Reduce or eliminate odor	• Charcoal dressings • Topical metronidazole (see text) • Iodosorb Gel (Healthpoint): iodine-based,may cause burning • Puri-Clens Wound Deodorizer (Coloplast Corporation): may cause burning

and the topical gel may be supplemented with irrigant solution and/or systemic metronidazole administration. Topical therapy is available by crushing metronidazole tablets in sterile water and creating either a 0.5% solution (5 mg/cc) or a 1% solution (10 mg/cc). Additionally, as an irrigant solution, 500 mg metronidazole in 100 ml normal saline intravenous (IV) solution can be used to irrigate the wound and may be used as a wet-to-moist gauze dressing (may be very effective for packing undermined or tunneled areas of the wound).[88,89] Metronidazole may also be given systemically to supplement the topical application. The usual dose for oral administration is 200 to 400 mg orally three times a day.[76] Systemic metronidazole 500 mg two to four times a day may also be administered orally, rectally, vaginally, or IV for wound odor management; but caution should be used because of the adverse gastrointestinal effects that may occur.[90]

Seaman[84] recommends that Puri-Clens, a gel wound deodorizer, be tried prior to instituting use of metronidazole. Puri-Clens gel contains benzethonium chloride, a cytotoxic antimicrobial compound that is effective against odor-causing bacteria. Seaman[84] notes that some patients may complain of burning despite use of topical anesthesia, and this may contraindicate further use.

Another topical antimicrobial agent is Iodosorb gel, an iodine complexed in a starch copolymer (cadexomer iodine). This product contains slow-release iodine and has been shown to decrease bacterial counts in wounds without cytotoxicity. Seaman[84] has had clinical experience with this product reducing odor associated with venous ulcers. Cadexomer iodine is available in a 40 g tube and is applied to the wound in a one-eighth inch layer. An advantage of this product is exudate absorption in that each gram absorbs 6 ml of fluid. Disadvantages include cost (comparable to metronidazole 0.75% gel) and possible burning on application.

Less conventional methods of odor management are also available. Topical use of yogurt or buttermilk has been reported to be successful at eliminating some tumor necrosis odors.[91,92] The yogurt or buttermilk is applied topically to the wound after cleansing. These may work by decreasing the wound pH, thus stunting bacterial proliferation and the resultant odor. It is theorized that the low pH of the lactobacilli present in the yogurt and buttermilk is responsible for the alteration in wound pH. There are limited studies supporting the use of yogurt or buttermilk, and none has addressed specific limitations or contraindications for use. Use of peppermint oil or other aromatherapy products in the environment around the patient may also help to eliminate wound odor.

Use of charcoal dressings may also be helpful in odor management. Many charcoal dressings are expensive and less flexible, so their use must be individualized as appropriate. Charcoal dressings typically are applied after the primary and secondary dressings have been applied and may be reused with each dressing change unless strike-through of wound drainage has occurred. Charcoal absorbs the odor from the wound. A basket of charcoal under the bed or table may also help in ridding the environment of wound odor for the home care patient.[81]

Controlling Bleeding. Wound bleeding is common in tumor necrosis. Prevention is the best therapy for controlling bleeding. Prevention involves use of a gentle hand in dressing removal and thoughtful attention to use of nonadherent dressings or moist wound dressings. On wounds with low exudate, the use of hydrogel sheets, or amorphous hydrogels under a nonadherent contact layer, may keep the wound moist and prevent dressing adherence. Even highly exudating wounds may require a nonadherent contact layer to allow for atraumatic dressing removal. When dressings stick to the wound on removal, they should be soaked away with normal saline to lessen the trauma to the wound bed. Even with use of nonadherent or moist wound dressings, bleeding may occur in tumor necrosis. Applying direct pressure to visible bleeding vessels for 10 to 15 minutes is the first intervention. If pressure alone is ineffective, several other options exist. Haisfield-Wolfe and Rund[79] suggest use of calcium alginate or collagen dressings as both have hemostatic properties. Waller and Caroline[76] advise use of gauze soaked in 1:1000 epinephrine over the bleeding point or application of sucralfate paste (crush a 1 g sucralfate table in 2 to 3ml of water-soluble gel) over widespread oozing. As an alternative, use of a topical absorbable hemostatic sponge or foam, such as Gelfoam, may be appropriate. Small bleeding points can be controlled with silver nitrate sticks. If bleeding continues, radiation therapy may be useful to stop it. Uncontrolled bleeding, as with capillary oozing, can result in acute and chronic anemia.

Minimizing Pain. There are several types of pain associated with tumor necrosis: deep pain, burning sensations, and superficial pain related to procedures. Deep pain should be managed by premedicating patients prior to dressing changes. Opioids for preprocedural medication may be needed, and rapid-onset, short-acting analgesics may be especially useful for those already receiving other opioid medication. Waller and Caroline[76] suggest use of nonsteroidal antiinflammatory agents. For management of superficial pain related to procedures, Seaman[84] recommends use of Hurricaine Topical Anesthetic Aerosol Spray, which is a reasonably priced, over-the-counter aerosol of benzocaine 20%. The onset of action is 15 to 30 seconds, and the spray is applied after removing the dressing prior to wound cleansing and again after wound cleansing for residual action. If the spray is applied to the chest wall or head/neck wounds, the patient's face should be covered, to prevent mouth and throat numbness if inhaled. Seaman[84] also suggests the use of ice packs over tender areas for pain relief. Maalox or a similar antacid applied directly to the wound area and allowed to dry may provide temporary relief of burning and superficial pain. Hurricaine Spray may also alleviate burning pain in these wounds.

Another emerging option for topical analgesia is the use of topical opioids, which bind to peripheral opioid receptors.[93–95] Back and Finlay[94] reported the use of diamorphine 10 mg added to an amorphous hydrogel and applied to the wounds of three patients on a daily basis. Two of the patients had painful pressure ulcers and the third had a painful malignant ulceration. All three were on systemic opioids. The patients noted improved pain control on the first day of treatment. Krajnik and Zbigniew[95] reported the case of a 76-year-old woman with metastatic lesions on her scalp that caused severe tension pain. Ibuprofen 400 mg tid was ineffective, and because the pain was in a limited area, the authors applied morphine gel 0.08% (3.2 mg morphine in 4 g of amorphous hydrogel). The patient's pain decreased from 7 on a 10-point visual analogue scale to 1 within 2 hours of gel application. Pain increased back to 6 at 25.5 hours postapplication. Therefore, the gel was reapplied daily and maintained pain control with no side effects. Nurses should discuss this new option for topical pain relief with the patient and physician. Since wound care is performed frequently in these patients, topical opioids may be an excellent adjunct to the pain management plan.

Patient and Caregiver Education

The same education provided to the patient and caregiver about basic wound care should be provided to those with tumor necrosis. Frequency and procedures for dressing changes, including time of premedication for pain management and alternatives for odor control, should be presented and reinforced. Patient and caregiver education must also focus on the psychosocial aspects of tumor necrosis. Patients are often unable to separate themselves from the wound and may feel as though their body is rotting away. Indeed, patients are often unable to view the wound, may become nauseous or retch when dressing changes are performed, or provide other signs of low self-esteem related to the wound. The nurse can facilitate a trusting relationship with the patient by reviewing the goals of care and by openly discussing issues that the patient may not have talked about with other providers. For example, it is helpful to acknowledge odor openly and then discuss how the odor will be managed. Attention to the cosmetic appearance of the wound with the dressing in place can assist the patient in dealing with body image disturbances. Use of flexible dressings (such as foam or thin film dressings) and dressings that can fill a defect (such as pastes or calcium alginates) may be appropriate to restore symmetry and provide adequate cosmesis for the patient.[79]

Isolation may result from embarrassment, shame, or guilt. Family caregivers may be overcome by the appearance of the wound or the other associated characteristics, such as odor. Assisting the patient and the caregiver to deal with the distressing symptoms of the tumor necrosis such that odor is managed, pain is alleviated, and exudate contained will allow for time to deal with the psychosocial issues related to body image disturbance. Improving the cosmetic appearance of the wound, eliminating odor, and containing exudate will help to achieve the goal of satisfactory psychological well-being.

Education must include realistic goals for the wound. Both the patient and the caregiver must understand the realistic goals of care. In tumor necrosis, the goal of complete wound healing is seldom achievable, but through attention to exudate, odor, and pain, quality of life can be maintained even as the tumor necrosis wound degenerates. Determination of priority goals in palliation may be the first step in patient and caregiver education. For example, if the patient is most disturbed by odor, measures to address wound odor should be foremost in the treatment plan. Continual education and evaluation of the effectiveness of the treatment plan are essential to maintaining quality of life for those suffering from tumor necrosis.

FISTULAS

A *fistula* is an abnormal passage or opening between two or more body organs or spaces. The most frequently involved organs are the skin and either the bladder or the digestive tract, although fistulas can occur between many other body organs/spaces. Often, the organs involved and the location of the fistula influence management methods and complicate care. For example, fistulas involving the small bowel and the vaginal vault and those involving the esophagus and skin create extreme challenges in care related to both the location and the organs involved in the fistula. While spontaneous closure occurs in at least 50% of all enteric or small bowel fistulas, the time required to achieve closure is from 4 to 7 weeks long, thus requiring long-term treatment plans for all patients with fistulas. Of those that will close spontaneously, 90% will do so within the 4- to 7-week time frame. So, if the fistula has not spontaneously closed with adequate medical treatment within 7 weeks, the goal of care may change to palliation, particularly when chances of closure are limited by other factors inhibiting closure. Factors that inhibit fistula closure include complete disruption of bowel continuity, distal obstruction, presence of a foreign body in the fistula tract, an epithelium-lined tract contiguous with the skin, presence of cancer, previous radiation, and Crohn's disease. The presence of any of these factors can be deleterious for spontaneous closure of a fistula. The goals of management for fistula care involve containment of effluent, management of odor, comfort, and protection of the surrounding skin and tissues.

Pathophysiology of Fistula Development

In cancer care, those with gastrointestinal cancers and those who have received irradiation to pelvic organs are at highest risk of fistula development. Fistula development occurs in 1% of patients with advanced malignancy.[76] In most cases of advanced malignancy, the fistula develops in relation to either obstruction from the malignancy or irradiation side effects. Radiation therapy damages vasculature and underlying structures. In cancer-related fistula development, management is almost always palliative. However, fistula development is not limited to those with cancer.

In addition to cancer or those who have received radiation therapy, postsurgical adhesions, inflammatory bowel disease (Crohn's disease), and small bowel obstruction place an individual at high risk for fistula development. The number one cause of fistula development is postsurgical adhesions. Adhesions are scar tissues that cause fistula development by providing an obstructive process within the normal passageway. Those with inflammatory bowel disease, Crohn's disease in particular, are prone to fistula development by virtue of the effects of the disease process on the bowel itself. Crohn's disease often involves the perianal area, with fissures and fistulas being common findings. Because Crohn's disease is a transmural disease, or involves all layers of the bowel wall, patients are prone to fistula development. Crohn's disease can occur anywhere along the entire gastrointestinal tract, and there is no known cure. Initially, the disease is managed medically with steroids, immunotherapy, and metronidazole for perianal disease. If medical management fails, the patient may be treated with surgical creation of a colostomy, to remove the bowel affected with the disease. In later stages of disease, if medical and surgical management has failed, multiple fistulas may present clinically and the goal for care becomes living with the fistula and palliation of symptoms.

Other factors contributing to fistula development include the presence of a foreign body next to a suture line, tension on a suture line, improper suturing technique, distal obstruction, hematoma/abscess formation, tumor or additional disease in anastomotic sites, and inadequate blood supply. Each of these can contribute to fistula formation by promoting an abnormal passage between two body organs. Typically, the contributing factor provides a tract for easier evacuation of stool or urine along the tract rather than through the normal route. Such is the case with a foreign body next to the suture line and hematoma or abscess formation. In some cases, the normal passageway is blocked, as with tumor growth or obstructive processes. Finally, in many cases, the pathology relates to inadequate tissue perfusion, as with tension on the suture line, improper suturing, and inadequate blood supply.

Fistula Assessment

Assessment of the fistula involves assessment of the source, surrounding skin, output, and fluid and electrolyte status. Evaluation of the fistula source may involve diagnostic tests such as radiographs to determine exact structures involved in the fistula tract. Assessment of the fistula source involves evaluation of fistula output, or effluent, for odor, color, consistency, pH, and amount. These provide clues to the origin. Fistulas with highly odorous output likely originate in the colon or may be related to cancerous lesions. Fistula output with less odor may have a small bowel origin. Color of fistula output also provides clues to the source: clear or white output is typical of esophageal fistulas, green output is usual of fistulas originating from the gastric area, light brown or tan output may indicate small bowel sources. Small bowel output is typically thin and watery to thick and pasty in consistency, while colonic fistulas have output with a pasty to a soft consistency. The volume of output is often an indication of the source. For small bowel fistulas, output is typically high, with volumes from 500 ml over 24 hours for low-output fistulas to 3000 ml over 24 hours for high-output fistulas. Esophageal fistula output may be as high as 1000 ml over 24 hours. Fistulas can be classified according to output, with less than 500 ml over 24 hours classified as low output and greater than 500 ml over 24 hours classified as high output.[96]

The anatomical orifice location, proximity of the orifice to bony prominences, regularity and stability of the surrounding skin, number of fistula openings, and level at which the fistula orifice exits onto the skin influence treatment options. Fistulas may be classified according to the organs involved and the location of the opening of the fistula orifice. Fistulas with openings from one internal body organ to another (such as from small bowel to bladder or bladder to vagina) are internal fistulas while those with cutaneous involvement (such as small bowel to skin) are external fistulas.[96]

The location of the fistula often impedes containment of output. Skin integrity should be assessed for erythema, ulceration, maceration, or denudation from fistula output. Typically, the more caustic the fistula output, the more impaired the surrounding skin integrity. Multiple fistula tracts may also impede containment efforts.

Assessment of fluid and electrolyte balance is essential due to the risk of imbalance in both. In particular, the patient with a small bowel fistula is at high risk for fluid volume deficit or dehydration and metabolic acidosis due to the loss of large volumes of alkaline small bowel contents. Significant losses of sodium and potassium are common with small bowel fistulas. Laboratory values should be monitored frequently. Evaluation for signs of fluid volume deficit is also recommended.

Fistula Management

Wherever anatomically possible, the fistula should be managed with an ostomy pouching technique. The surrounding skin should be cleansed with warm water without soap or antiseptics; skin barrier paste should be used to fill uneven skin surfaces so that a flat surface is created to apply the pouch. Pediatric pouches are often smaller and more flexible and may be useful for hard-to-pouch areas where flexibility is needed, such as the neck for esophageal fistulas. Pouch type should be chosen based on the output of the fistula. For example, if the fistula output is watery and thin, choose a pouch with a narrow spigot or tube for closure; in contrast, a fistula with a thick, pasty output would be better managed with a pouch with an open end and a closure clamp. Pouches must be emptied frequently, at least when one-third to one-half full. There are several wound drainage pouching systems on the market that allow for visualization and direct access to the fistula through a valve or door that can be opened and closed. These wound management pouches are available in large sizes and often work well for abdominal fistulas.[97] Pouching the fistula allows for odor control (many fistulas are quite malodorous), containment of output, and protection of the surrounding skin from damage. Gauze dressings with or without charcoal filters may be used when the output from the fistula is less than 250 ml over 24 hours and is not severely offensive in odor.[96] Colostomy caps (small closed-end pouches) may be very useful for low-output fistulas that continue to be odorous.

There are specific pouching techniques that are useful in complex fistula management, including troughing, saddlebagging, and bridging.[96] These techniques are particularly helpful when dealing with fistulas that occur in wounds, most commonly the small bowel fistula that develops in the open abdominal wound. Troughing is useful for fistulas that occur in the posterior aspect of large abdominal wounds.[98] Line the skin surrounding the wound and fistula with a skin barrier wafer and seal the edge nearest the wound with skin barrier paste. Then, apply thin film dressings over the top or anterior aspect of the wound down to the fistula orifice and the posterior aspect of the wound. Lastly, use a cut-to-fit ostomy pouch to pouch the opening in the thin film dressing at the fistula orifice. Wound exudate drains from the anterior portion of the wound (under the thin film dressing) to the posterior portion of the wound and out into the ostomy pouch along with fistula output. The trough technique does not prevent fistula output from contaminating the wound site.

The bridging technique prevents fistula output from contaminating the wound site and allows for a unique wound dressing to be applied to the wound site. Bridging is appropriate for fistulas that occur in the posterior aspect of large abdominal wounds, where it is important to contain fistula output away from the wound site. Using small pieces of skin barrier wafers, a bridge is built by consecutively layering the skin barriers together until the skin barrier has the appearance of a wedge or bridge and is the same height as the depth of the wound.[96] Using skin barrier paste, the skin barrier wedge is adhered to the wound bed (it will not harm the healthy tissues of the wound bed) next to the fistula opening. An ostomy pouch is then cut to fit the fistula opening, using the wedge or bridge as a portion of intact surrounding skin to adhere the pouch.[96] The anterior aspect of the wound may then be dressed with the dressing of choice.

Saddlebagging is used for multiple fistulas, where it is important to keep the output from each fistula separated and the fistula orifices are close together. Using two (or more for more fistulas) cut-to-fit ostomy pouches, the fistula openings are cut on the back of the pouch off-center or as far to the side as possible and the second pouch is cut to fit the next fistula and off-center as far to the other side as possible. The skin is cleansed with warm water, and skin barrier paste is applied around the orifices. Ostomy pouches are applied, and where they contact each other (down the middle) they are affixed/adhered to each other in a "saddlebag" fashion. Multiple fistulas can also be managed with one ostomy pouching system accommodating the multiple openings. Consultation with the ET nurse or ostomy nurse is extremely advantageous in these cases.

Another method of managing fistulas is by a closed suction wound drainage system. Jeter and colleagues[99] describe the use of a Jackson-Pratt drain and continuous low suction in fistula management. After cleansing the wound with normal saline, the fenestrated Jackson-Pratt drain is placed in the wound on top of a moistened gauze opened up to line the wound bed (primary contact layer), a second fluffed wet gauze is placed over the drain, and the surrounding skin is prepared with a skin sealant. Next, the entire site is covered with a thin film dressing, crimping the dressing around the tube of the drain where it exits the wound. The tube exit site is filled with skin barrier paste, and the drain is connected to low continuous wall suction; the connection site may have to be adjusted and may require use of a small "christmas tree" connector or device and tape to secure it. Jeter and colleagues[99] advise changing the system every 3 to 5 days. Others have used a similar set-up for pharyngocutaneous fistulas.[100] A vacuum-assisted closure device uses negative pressure and offers additional options for fistula management.

Pouching to contain the fistula output will usually involve odor as well. If odor continues to be problematic with an intact pouching system, internal body deodorants may be helpful, such as bismuth subgallete, charcoal compositions, or peppermint oil.[101] Taking care to change the pouch in a well-ventilated room will also help with odor. If odor is due to anaerobic bacteria, Waller and Caroline[76] suggest 400 mg metronidazole orally three times a day. Management of high-output fistulas may be improved with administration of octreotide 300 μg subcutaneously over 24 hours.[76]

Nutrition management and fluid and electrolyte maintenance are essential for adequate fistula care. Fluid and nutritional requirements may be greatly increased with fistulas, and there are difficulties with gastrointestinal system fistulas. As a general guideline, the intestinal system should be used whenever possible for nutritional support. If nutrition can bypass the fistula site, absorption and tolerance are better with use of the intestinal tract. For small bowel fistulas, bypassing the fistula orifice is not always feasible. If the small bowel fistula is located distally, there may be enough of the intestinal tract available to adequately absorb nutrients prior to the fistula orifice. If the fistula is located more proximally, there may not be enough intestinal tract available for nutrient absorption prior to the fistula orifice. Many of these patients must be managed with IV hyperalimentation during the early stages of fistula management. The specific goals of fluid and electrolyte and nutritional support for fistula management must be discussed with the patient and family in view of the palliative nature of the overall care plan.

Patient and Caregiver Education

Patient and caregiver teaching first involves adequate assessment of self-care ability and of the caregiver's abilities. The patient and caregiver must be taught the management method for the fistula, including pouching techniques, how to empty the pouch, odor-control methods, and strategies for increasing fluid and nutritional intake. Many of the pouching techniques used to manage fistulas are complicated and may require continual surveillance by an expert such as an ET nurse or ostomy nurse.

PALLIATIVE STOMA CARE

The significance of palliative care for an individual with a stoma is to improve the individual's well-being during this critical time and to attain the best quality of life possible. In regards to the stoma, palliative care is achieved by restoring the most efficient management plan and providing optimal function capacity. It is essential to involve the family in the plan of care and to provide care to the extent of the patient's wishes.

Management of the ostomy includes physical care as well as psychological and social care. To meet the needs of the patient and family, access to the multidisciplinary care team is crucial and may include the ET nurse, physicians such as the surgeon and oncologist, nutritionist, and social services. The urinary or fecal stoma can be managed (by the ET nurse) while incorporating the needs and goals of both the patient and the caregiver and providing the highest quality of life possible.

Pathophysiology

A *stoma* is an artificial opening in the abdominal wall surgically created to allow urine or stool to be eliminated by an alternative route. The most common indications for the creation of a stoma are as follows:

1. cancer which interferes with the normal function of the urinary or gastrointestinal system
2. inflammatory bowel diseases such as Crohn's or ulcerative colitis
3. congenital diseases such as Hirschsprung's disease or familial adenomatous polyposis,
4. trauma

In planning the care of an individual with a stoma, it is necessary to understand the type of ostomy that was created, including the contents which will be eliminated.

Types of Diversion

The three types of diversion created with a stoma as the outlet for urine or stool include the ileoconduit (urinary), the ileostomy (fecal) and the colostomy (fecal). Construction of any of these diversions requires the person to wear an external appliance to collect the output.

Ileoconduit. Since the early 1950s, the Bricker ileoconduit has been the cornerstone of diverting urinary flow in the absence of bladder function. This procedure involves isolation of a section of the terminal ileum. The proximal end is closed and the distal end brought out through an opening in the abdominal wall at a site selected prior to surgery. The ileal segment is sutured to the skin, creating a stoma. The ureters are implanted into the ileal segment, urine flows into the conduit, and peristalsis propels the urine out through the stoma. An external appliance is worn to collect the urine and emptied when the pouch is one-third to one-half full, or approximately every 4 hours.

Ileostomy. The ileostomy is created to divert stool away from the large intestine, generally utilizing the terminal ileum. Bringing the distal end of the ileum through an opening surgically created in the abdominal wall and suturing to the skin creates the stoma. The output is usually a soft, unformed to semi-formed stool. Approximately 600 to 800 cc per day are eliminated.[102] An external appliance is worn to collect the fecal material and emptied when the bag is one-third to one-half full, usually four to six times per day.

An ileostomy may be temporary or permanent. A temporary ileostomy is usually created when the colon needs time to heal or rest, such as after colon surgery or a colon obstruction. A permanent ileostomy is necessary when the entire colon, rectum, and anus have been surgically removed, such as in colorectal cancer or Crohn's disease.[103]

Colostomy. The colostomy is created proximal to the affected segment of the colon and/or rectum. A colostomy may be temporary or permanent. There are three sections of the colon: the ascending, transverse, and descending colon. The section of colon utilized to create the stoma determines in part the location and the consistency of output that may affect the nutritional and hydration status of the individual at critical times. The ascending colon stoma is generally created on the right mid-quadrant, and the output is a semiformed stool. The transverse stoma is created in the upper quadrants and is the largest stoma created; the output is usually a semiformed to formed stool. The descending colon stoma most closely mirrors the activity of normal bowel function. The stoma is generally located in the lower left quadrant.[103]

Bringing the distal end of the colon through an opening surgically created in the abdominal wall and suturing to the skin creates the stoma. An external appliance is worn to collect the fecal material and emptied when the bag is one-third to one-half full, usually one or two times per day. A second option for management is irrigation, to regulate the bowel. The patient is taught to instill 600 to 1000 cc of lukewarm tap water through the stoma utilizing a cone-shaped irrigation apparatus. This creates bowel distention, stimulating peristaltic activity and therefore elimination within 30 to 45 minutes. Repeating this process over time induces bowel dependence on the stimulus, reducing the spillage of stool between irrigations. The elimination process after initial evacuation is suppressed for 24 to 48 hours.[103]

Assessment

Stoma characteristics. Viability of the stoma is assessed by its color. This should be checked regularly, especially in the early postoperative period. Normal color of the stoma is deep pink to deep red. The intestinal stomal tissue can be compared with the mucosal lining of the mouth. The stoma may bleed when rubbed because of the capillaries at the surface. Bleeding that occurs spontaneously or excessively from stoma trauma can usually be managed by applying pressure. Bleeding that persists or that originates from the bowel requires prompt investigation, with the management plan based on the cause of the bleeding and the overall status of the individual.[104]

A stoma with a dusky appearance ranging from purple to black, or necrotic, indicates impairment of circulation and should be reported to the surgeon. A necrotic stoma may develop from abdominal distention causing tension on the mesentery, from twisting of the intestine at the time of surgery, or from arterial or venous insufficiency. Necrotic tissue below the level of the fascia indicates infarction and potential intraabdominal urine or stool leak. Prompt recognition and surgical reexploration are necessary.

Stoma edema is normal in the early postoperative period as a result of surgical manipulation. This should not interfere with stoma functioning, but a larger opening will need to be cut in the appliance to prevent pressure or constriction of the stoma. Most stomas decrease in size 4 to 6 weeks following surgery, with minor changes over 1 year. Teaching the individual to continue to measure the stoma with each change of appliance should alleviate the problem of the person wearing an appliance with an aperture too large for the stoma. The stoma needs only a space one-eighth of an inch in diameter to allow for expansion during peristalsis.

Stoma herniation is the process of the bowel moving through the muscle defect created at the time of the stoma formation and into the subcutaneous tissue. The hernia usually reduces spontaneously when lying in a supine position due to the decrease in intraabdominal pressure. Problems associated with the formation of a peristomal hernia are increased difficulty with ostomy pouch adherence and possible bowel strangulation and obstruction. The peristomal hernia can be managed conservatively using a peristomal hernia belt to maintain a reduction of the hernia. The belt is an abdominal binder with an opening to allow for the stoma and pouch. The belt is applied with the patient in a supine position, while the hernia is reduced, creating an external pressure that will maintain the bowel in a reduced position. Aggressive treatment includes surgical intervention for the correction of the peristomal hernia. However, this is usually reserved for emergency situations, such as obstruction or strangulation of the bowel. Colostomy patients who irrigate should be taught to irrigate with the hernia in a reduced position, to prevent perforation of the bowel.

Stoma prolapse occurs due to a weakened abdominal wall as a result of abdominal distention, formation of a loop stoma, or a large aperture in the abdominal wall. The prolapse is a telescoping of the intestine through the stoma. Stoma prolapse may be managed by conservative or surgical intervention. Surgical intervention is required if there is bowel ischemia, bowel obstruction, or prolapse of excessive length and unreducible. Conservative management includes reducing the stoma while in a supine position to decrease the intraabdominal pressure, then applying continuous gentle pressure at the distal portion of the prolapse until the stoma returns to skin level. If the stoma is edematous, apply cold soaks or hypertonic solution such as salt or sugar to reduce the edema before stoma reduction is attempted. Once the stoma is reduced, apply a support binder to prevent recurrence. In most cases, it is necessary to alter the pouching system by including a two-piece appliance and cutting the barrier size opening larger to accommodate changes in stoma size.

Retraction of the stoma below skin level can occur in the early postoperative period due to tension on the bowel or mesentery or related to breakdown at the mucocutaneous junction. Late retraction usually occurs as a result of tension on the bowel from abdominal distention, most likely as a result of intraperitoneal tumor growth or ascites. Stomal retraction is managed by modification of the pouching system, for example, using a convex appliance, to accommodate changes in skin contour. Stomas that retract below the fascia level require prompt surgical intervention.

Stenosis of the stoma can occur at the skin level or at the level of the fascia. Stenosis that interferes with normal bowel elimination requires intervention. Signs and symptoms of stenosis include change in bowel habits, such as decreased output or thin-caliber stools; abdominal cramping; abdominal distention; flank pain from urinary stomas; or nausea and/or vomiting. The stenotic area may be managed conservatively by dilatation or may require surgical intervention by local excision or lapotomy.[103,104] Many of the above stoma problems can occur from simple stretching and displacement of normal organs due to bulky tumors, as might occur in the end stages of some disease states.

Peristomal Skin Problems. Peristomal skin complications commonly include mechanical breakdown, chemical breakdown, rash, and allergic reaction. Mechanical breakdown is caused by trauma to the epidermal skin layer. This is most often related to frequent appliance changes, causing shearing or tearing to the epidermal skin. The result is denuded skin or erythematous, raw, moist, and painful skin. The use of pectin-based powder with or without a light coating of skin sealant will aid in healing and protecting the skin from further damage while allowing appliance adherence.

Chemical breakdown is caused by prolonged contact of urine or fecal effluent with the peristomal skin. Inappropriate use of adhesive skin solvents may also result in skin breakdown. The result of chemical breakdown is denudation of the peristomal skin that has been exposed to the caustic effects of the stool, urine, or adhesive solvents. Prompt recognition and management are essential. Modification of the pouching system, such as using a convex wafer instead of a flat wafer and/or adding protective skin products such as paste, can be utilized to correct the underlying problem. Instructing patients and caregivers to thoroughly cleanse the skin with plain water after using the skin solvent can eliminate the problem of denuded skin. Treatment of denuded skin is the same as described previously.

A peristomal fungal rash can occur as a result of excessive moisture or antibiotic administration which results in overgrowth of yeast in the bowel or at the skin level due to perspiration under a pouch or leakage of urine or stool under the barrier. The rash is characterized as having a macular, red border with a moist, red to yellow center; it is usually pruritic. Applying antifungal powder, such as nystatin powder, to the affected areas usually provides a prompt response. Blotting the powder with skin prep or sealant may allow the pouching system to adhere more effectively.

Allergic reactions are most often a result of the barrier and tape used for the pouching system. Erythematous vesicles and pruritis characterize the area involved. Management includes removal of the offending agent. The distribution of the reaction can usually aid in defining the allergen. It may be necessary to perform skin testing if the causative agent is not clear. Patients with sensitive skin and those who use multiple products may respond to simple pouching techniques such as the use of water to clean the skin, patting skin dry, and applying the wafer and pouch without the use of skin preparations. Changing manufacturers of products may also eliminate allergen. A nonadhesive pouching system, can be utilized temporarily for patients with severe blistering and hypersensitivity, to allow healing and prevent further peristomal skin damage. Patients with severe blistering and pruritis may also require temporarily systemic or topical administration of antihistamines or corticosteriods.[103,104]

Principles and Products for Pouching a Stoma. The continuous outflow of urine or stool from the stoma requires the individual to wear an external appliance at all times. Ideally, the stoma protrudes one-half to three-fourths of an inch above the skin surface to allow the urine or stool to drain efficiently into a pouch.[105] The objective of stoma management is to protect the peristomal skin, contain output, and control odor.

The skin around the stoma should be cleaned and thoroughly dried before positioning the appliance over the stoma. Although not always possible, an effective pouch should adhere for at least 3 days. If no leakage occurs, the same pouch can remain adhered to the skin for up to 10 days. It should then be changed for hygienic reasons and to observe the peristomal area. Today, there is a constant and ever-changing supply of new appliances. Materials and design are being updated rapidly to provide the consumer with the best protection and easiest care.[102] Factors to consider when choosing a pouch include consistency and type of effluent, contour of abdomen, and stoma size, shape, and extent of protrusion, as a well as patient preferences. Pouching systems are available as one-piece or two-piece systems. The one-piece system is constructed with the odor-proof pouch joined to a barrier ring that adheres to the skin. The barrier can be precut to the size of the stoma or it can be customized with a cut-to-fit barrier. A two-piece system usually consists of an individual barrier with a flange ring and an odor-proof pouch that attach (snap) together by matching the ring size of the barrier and pouch. The pouch barrier may be flat or convex and is chosen based on the contour of the abdomen and the extent of stoma protrusion. The colostomy pouch may be closed-ended or open-ended with a clip for closure. Some individuals may choose to clean the pouch daily. The pouch of the one-piece system can be cleaned by instilling water into the pouch (with a syringe or turkey baster) and rinsing while preventing the water from reaching the stoma area. The pouch of the two-piece system can be cleaned daily by detaching and washing it in the sink with soap and water and drying it before reattaching to the barrier. The urinary pouch has a spout opening to allow for controlled emptying of the pouch. This end may also be attached to a bedside bag or bottle to collect urine and usually holds up to 2000 ml of urine. The urinary system can be easily disassembled and cleaned with soap and water. After cleaning, a vinegar-and-water solution should be rinsed through the tubing and bag/bottle to prevent urine crystallization.

Skin barriers, skin sealants, powders such as stomahesive powder or karaya powder, and pastes such as stomahesive paste or karaya paste are available to protect the peristomal skin from the caustic affects of urine or stool. These products may also be used to aid in the healing of peristomal skin problems.

Belts and binders are available to assist in maintaining pouch adherence and for management of certain stoma problems.[105] Table 16–6 presents an overview of pouching options for patients with fecal or urinary diversions.

Interventions

Prevention of Complications. Stoma surgery performed as a palliative measure is not intended to provide a cure but rather to alleviate difficulties such as obstruction, pain, or severe incontinence. Unfortunately, at a difficult time in patients' and families' lives, the created stoma disrupts normal physical appearance, normal elimination of urine or stool, control of elimination, possible loss of body

Table 16–6. Pouch Options

Type	Barrier	Odor-Proof Pouch
1-piece	Flat	Open end with clip (ileostomy or colostomy)
2-piece	Convex	Closed end (colostomy)
	Cut-to-fit	Spout opening (urostomy)
	Precut	

parts, and sexual function. The patient then has to learn to care for the stoma or allow someone else to care for them. Physically and psychologically, the patient has to come to terms with the presence of the stoma, its function, and care. This takes time and energy to cope emotionally, physically, and socially.[103,104]

Educating the patient and family regarding management issues related to ostomy care and palliation could assist in the physical and psychological adaptation to the ostomy. Additional therapies that may be required for treatment of the underlying disease or a new disease process, such as progressed or recurrent cancer, may affect the activity of the stoma and/or the peristomal skin. Additional therapies may include chemotherapy, radiation therapy, or analgesics for pain management.

Chemotherapy and radiation therapy may affect a fecal stoma by causing diarrhea. Associated symptoms include abdominal discomfort, larger quantities of loose or liquid stool produced per day, and potential dehydration and loss of appetite with prolonged diarrhea. The ostomy bag will require more frequent emptying, and the ostomy pouch seal will need to be monitored more closely for leakage. In addition, radiation therapy that includes the stoma in the radiation field may cause peristomal skin irritation, particularly redness and maceration. The effects on the peristomal skin may be exacerbated by leakage of urine or stool as described above.[104]

Analgesic use may result in constipation and ultimately bowel obstruction. It is necessary to co-administer stool softeners or laxatives for the prevention of constipation. Irrigation of the colostomy may also assist in treating constipation. The patient and family need to be instructed regarding these measures so that they can be utilized to treat and prevent constipation. The patient and family need to be aware that adequate pain relief and prevention of constipation can be achieved.[103,104]

The patient may become very tired or experience anxiety, nausea, or pain as a result of the condition and palliative management. Patients often want to remain as independent as possible but may allow assistance from family and staff. For example, the patient may want to perform the actual pouch change but allow someone else to gather and prepare the supplies. This allows for conservation of energy during part of the task to be accomplished. The patient may also choose the time of day to perform such tasks, when they have the most energy and maximal pain and nausea control.[106]

Nutrition and Hydration

Anorexia and dehydration can be major problems for the patient and family in advancing disease and/or disease-related treatments such as chemotherapy and radiation therapy. Compromised ingestion, digestion, and absorption can have major influences on nutritional and hydration status.

Anorexia is the loss of appetite resulting from changes in gastrointestinal function, including change in taste, changes in metabolism, psychological behaviors, and the effects of disease and treatment. Decreased oral intake and changes in metabolism, including decreased protein and fat metabolism, increased energy expenditure, and increased carbohydrate consumption, result in loss of muscle mass, loss of fat stores, and fatigue, leading to weight loss and malnutrition.[107]

Managing the underlying cause of poor nutritional and hydration status, such as controlling the cancer or disease, treating an infection, or slowing down the high-volume ileostomy output, can improve the nutritional state. However, despite effective treatment, other assistance may be necessary, such as small and more frequent meals, nutritional liquid supplements, appetite stimulants such as megestrol acetate, corticosteroids, and/or parenteral or enteral support.[108] Foods and drinks need to be appealing to the patient. Strong odors and large-portion meals may result in appetite suppression. Promoting comfort prior to meals may also increase appetite, such as administering antiemetics or analgesics, oral care, or resting for 30 minutes prior to mealtime.[107]

Management Issues. Controlling odor, reducing gas, and/or preventing or managing diarrhea or constipation are management issues related to patients with a colostomy. Odor can be controlled by ensuring that the pouch seal is tight, using odor-proof pouches, and maintaining a clean pouch opening. In addition, deodorants such as bismuth subgallate or chlorophyllin copper complex, can be taken orally. Gas can be reduced by decreasing intake of gas-producing foods such as broccoli, cabbage, beans, and beer. Peppermint or chamomile tea may be effective in gas reduction.[103,104]

Diarrhea can be managed as in a patient with an intact rectum and anus. Diarrhea may be a result of viral illness or a chemotherapeutic agent. Management includes increasing fluid intake, a low-fiber and low-fat diet, and administration of antidiarrhea medications such as loperamide (Imodium), Pepto-Bismol, or Lomotil (diphenoxylate plus atropine) by prescription.[105,109] If the patient irrigates, it will be necessary to hold irrigation until formed stools return. Constipation more commonly occurs in patients with advanced malignancies due to the affects of analgesic use, reduced activity level, and reduced dietary fiber intake. Management of constipation includes administration of laxatives such as milk of magnesia, mineral oil, or lactalose, and initiation of a plan for prevention of constipation with use of stool softeners and laxatives as needed. Cleansing irrigation may be necessary for patients who normally do not irrigate. Cleansing irrigation is performed as described previously for individuals with a colostomy who irrigate for control of bowel movements.[105]

Skin protection, fluid and electrolyte maintenance, prevention of blockage, and modification of medications are management issues related to an ileostomy. Due to the high-volume liquid loose stools, protecting the skin from this effluent is critical. Leakage of effluent can cause chemical skin breakdown and pain from the irritated skin. The ET nurse can work with the patient and family to determine the cause of the effluent leak. It may be necessary to modify the pouching system, to ensure a proper fit. The peristomal skin may need to be treated with a powder and/or skin sealant to aid in healing. The transit time of food and wastes through the gastrointestinal system and out through the ileostomy is rapid and potentially contributes to dehydration and fluid and electrolyte imbalance. Ensuring adequate fluid and electrolyte intake is essential and may be accomplished by ingestion of sports drinks or nutrition shakes. Patients with an ileostomy are instructed to include fiber in their diet, to bulk stools and promote absorption of nutrition and medications. Food blockage occurs when undigested food particles and/or medications partially or completely obstruct the stoma outlet at the fascia level. It is necessary to instruct the patient and family about the signs of a blockage, including malodorous, high-volume liquid output or no output accompanied by abdominal cramping, distention, and/or nausea and vomiting. These symptoms should be reported as soon as they occur. Blockage is resolved by lavage or mini-irrigation performed by the physician or ET nurse. A catheter is gently inserted into the stoma until the blockage is reached, 30 to 60 cc of normal saline are instilled, and the catheter is removed to allow for the return. This process is repeated until the blockage has resolved. Reinforce teaching with the patient regarding the need to chew food well before swallowing, to prevent food blockage. Time-release tablets and enteric-coated medications should be avoided due to inadequate or unpredictable absorption. Medications often come in various forms, including liquid, noncoated, patch, rectal suppository, subcutaneous or IV administration. Choosing the most appropriate route that will provide the greatest efficacy for the individual is essential, such as utilizing a transdermal patch for analgesia instead of a time-released pain tablet. Patients who have an intact rectum that is no longer in continuity with the proximal bowel can effectively have medications administered rectally.[109]

Management issues for an individual with an ileoconduit include prevention of a urinary tract infection, stone formation, peristomal skin protection, and odor control. Each of these issues is preventable by the maintenance of dilute and acidic urine by adequate fluid intake (1800 to 2400 cc per day). Vitamin C (500 to 1000 mg per day) and citrus fruits and drinks may assist in accomplishing acidic urine. Alkaline urine can cause encrustations on the stoma and peristomal skin damage with prolonged exposure. Applying acetic acid soaks three or four times per day can treat the encrustations until they dissolve. Adjustments in the pouching system may be necessary to prevent leakage of urine onto the skin as well as the temporary addition of powder, paste, and/or skin sealant to aid in healing of the affected skin.[105]

Case Report: Mr A., a Patient with Colorectal Cancer

Mr. A is a 69-year-old patient diagnosed with colorectal cancer 1 year ago. Since diagnosis he has undergone abdominal perineal resection with a permanent sigmoid colostomy and has completed a course of adjuvant chemotherapy and radiation therapy. He presents as a thin, Caucasian male with dry and scaling skin, weakness, and fatigue. He has a left lower quadrant colostomy with the pouch seal intact. He is being cared for by his wife in his home. The goals of care have changed from life prolonging active treatment to palliative care within the last 3 to 4 months as his condition has progressively deteriorated. Currently, he is inactive and requires assistance for mobility. He spends most of the day up in a recliner chair in the family room. His wife has taken over most of the colostomy care and is concerned with difficulty in getting the irrigation procedure performed and stool leakage between procedures. Prior to Mr. A's change in status, he was irrigating his colostomy every other day and just wearing a small patch or closed-end pouch over the stoma. As a side effect of adjuvant therapy (and probably related to progressive disease), his stooling pattern has changed and he now has loose to thickened colostomy output. He is no longer able to irrigate the colostomy independently, so his wife has been performing the procedure and applying a closed-end pouch every other day. Unfortunately, because of the stool leakage, she has often had to change the pouch two or three times a day.

Mr. A has developed a clean, shallow, full-thickness stage III pressure ulcer over the sacral/coccygeal area. The pressure ulcer has a moderate amount of exudate, no necrotic tissue, and intact surrounding skin and tissues. There is no evidence of undermining or tunneling, and the wound bed exhibits pink granulation tissue filling 50% of the wound. There is minimal epithelialization. The total Pressure Sore Status Tool score is 35. The wound has deteriorated from a stage II partial-thickness injury to the current state over the last 2 weeks. Wound management involves cleansing with povidone iodine and daily application of a wet-to-dry saline gauze dressing. The patient rates pain from the ulcer as a 6 on a 10-point scale and rates procedural pain during dressing changes as a 7 on a 10-point scale.

The patient is still able to ingest food and fluids orally, and the patient and family have decided to refuse tube feedings for the future. They understand the consequences of the minimally nourished and dehydrated condition. His last serum albumin was 2.9 mg/dl, and he has lost 10 lb in the last 2 months. He has been taking oral supplements between meals.

In this case, palliative and prevention treatment is indicated. The wound can be kept clean and dressed to control drainage and odor. The patient is also a candidate for a pressure-relief support surface to prevent further skin breakdown with attention directed at the recliner chair. A turning schedule and techniques for repositioning while in the recliner chair are part of the prevention intervention plan with attention directed at training the caregiver. The wound-management system has failed to demonstrate improvement in the wound over the last 2 weeks and is burdensome and distressing to the patient and wife. The wound-management care plan now includes cleansing the wound with normal saline and applying a hydrocolloid dressing, which is changed every 3 to 4 days. The wife is instructed to administer the general pain medication about 20 to 30 minutes prior to dressing changes, to decrease pain. Colostomy care is changed as well. The irrigation procedure is discontinued because of stool leakage between procedures and because of the quality of the stool. The colostomy is recalibrated by the ET nurse, and a new drainable pouch is suggested. The wife is taught how to empty the pouch and how to change the pouch every 5 to 7 days. The changes in the care plan for this patient reflect care practices that are better suited to palliative care. The new wound dressing will limit the number of dressing changes and resulting discomfort and the changes in the management of the colostomy are also directed at management of the symptoms while easing some of the care burden and the patient's discomfort.

SUMMARY

Skin disorders are both emotionally and physically challenging for the patient and caregivers. Cutaneous symptoms may be the result of disease progression such as tumor necrosis or fistula development, complications associated with end-stage disease or the end of life such as pressure ulcers, or simple changes in function of urinary or fecal diversions. All cutaneous symptoms require attention to basic care issues, creativity in management strategies, and thoughtful attention to the psychosocial implications of cutaneous manifestations. Palliative care intervention strategies for skin disorders reflect an approach similar to nonpalliative care. Goals of care, while not to cure the condition, are always to alleviate the distressing symptomology and to improve quality of life. The most distressing symptoms associated with skin disorders are odor, exudate, and pain. The importance of attention to skin disorders for palliative care is related to the major effect of these conditions on the quality of life and general psychological well-being of the patient.

REFERENCES

1. Daniel RK, Priest DL, Wheatley DC. Etiologic factors in pressure sores: an experimental model. Arch Phys Med Rehabil 1981;62:492–498.

2. Kosiak M. Etiology and pathology of ischemic ulcers. Arch Phys Med Rehabil 1959;40: 62–69.

3. Reuler JB, Cooney TG. The pressure sore: pathophysiology and principles of management. Ann Intern Med 1981;94:661.

4. Seiler WD, Stahelin HB. Recent findings on decubitus ulcer pathology: implications for care. Geriatrics 1986;41:47–60.

5. Witkowski JA, Parish, LC. Histopathology of the decubitus ulcer. J Am Acad Dermatol 1982; 6:1014–1021.

6. Lindan O, Greenway RM, Piazza JM. Pressure distributor on the surface of the human body. Arch Phys Med Rehabil 1965;46:378.

7. Scales JT. Pressure on the patient. In: Kenedi RM, Cowden JM, eds. Bedsore Biomechanics. London: University Park Press, 1976.

8. Parish LC, Witkowski JA, Crissey JT. The Decubitus Ulcer. New York: Masson, 1983.

9. Slater H. Pressure Ulcers in the Elderly. Pittsburgh: Synapse, 1985.

10. Parish LC, Witkowski JA, Crissey JT. The Decubitus Ulcer in Clinical Practice. Berlin: Springer, 1997.

11. Landis EM. Micro-injection studies of capillary blood pressure in human skin. Heart 1930;15:209.

12. Husain T. An experimental study of some pressure effects on tissues, with reference to the bedsore problem. J Pathol Bacteriol 1953;66: 347–358.

13. Salcido R, Donofrio JC, Fisher SB, LeGrand EK, et al. Histopathology of decubitus ulcers as a result of sequential pressure sessions in a computer-controlled fuzzy rat model. Adv Wound Care 1994;7(5):40.

14. Kosiak M, Kubicek WG, Olsen ME. Evaluation of pressure as a factor in the production of ischial ulcers. Arch Phys Med Rehabil 1958;39:623.

15. Braden BJ, Bergstrom N. A conceptual schema for the study of etiology of pressure sores. Rehabil Nurs 1987;12:8–12.

16. Bergstrom N, Demuth PJ, Braden BJ. A clinical trial of the Braden Scale for Predicting Pressure Sore Risk. Nurs Clin North Am 1987; 22:417–428.

17. Allman RM, Goode PS, Patrick MM, Burst N, Bartolucci AA. Pressure ulcer risk factors among hospitalized patients with activity limitations. JAMA 1995;273:865–870.

18. Panel for the Prediction and Prevention of Pressure Ulcers in Adults. Pressure Ulcers in Adults: Prediction and Prevention. Clinical Practice Guideline Number 3. Rockville, MD: Agency for Health Care Policy and Research, US Department of Health and Human Services Publication AHCPR 92–0047, 1992.

19. Maklebust J, Sieggreen MY. Pressure Ulcers: Guidelines for Prevention and Nursing Management, 2nd Ed. Springhouse, PA Springhouse, 1996.

20. Curry K, Casady L. The relationship between extended periods of immobility and decubitus ulcer formation in the acutely spinal cord injured individual. J Neurosci Nurs 1992;24:185–189.

21. Hammond MC, Bozzacco VA, Stiens SA, Buhrer R, Lyman P. Pressure ulcer incidence on a spinal cord injury unit. Adv Wound Care 1994;7:57–60.

22. Reichel SM. Shearing force as a factor in decubitus ulcers in paraplegics. JAMA 1958;166: 762–763.

23. Bennett L, Kavner D, Lee BY, Trainor FS, Lewis JM. Skin stress and blood flow in sitting paraplegic patients. Arch Phys Med Rehabil 1969; 65:186–190.

24. Dinsdale SM. Decubitus ulcers: role of pressure and friction in causation. Arch Phys Med Rehabil 1974;55:147–152.

25. Kemp MG. Protecting the skin from moisture and associated irritants. J Gerontol Nurs 1994;20:8–14.

26. Bates-Jensen B. Incontinence management. In: Parish LC, Witkowski JA, Crissey JT, eds. The Decubitus Ulcer in Clinical Practice. Berlin: Springer, 1997:189–199.

27. Maklebust J, Magnan MA. Risk factors associated with having a pressure ulcer: a secondary analysis. Adv Wound Care 1994;7:25–42.

28. Pinchcovsky-Devin G, Kaminsky MV Jr. Correlation of pressure sores and nutritional status. J Am Geriatr Soc 1986;34:435–440.

29. Bobel LM. Nutritional implications in the patient with pressure sores. Nurs Clin North Am 1987;22:379–390.

30. Bergstrom N, Braden B. A prospective study of pressure sore risk among institutionalized elderly. J Am Geriatr Soc 1992;40:747–758.

31. Allman RM, Laprade CA, Noel LB, et al. Pressure sores among hospitalized patients. Ann Intern Med 1986;105:337–342.

32. Jones PL, Millman A. Wound healing and the aged patient. Nurs Clin North Am 1990; 25:263–277.

33. Eaglestein WH. Wound healing and aging. Clin Geriatr Med 1989;5:183.

34. Bergstrom N, Braden BJ, Boynton P, Bruch S. Using a research-based assessment scale in clinical practice. Nurs Clin North Am 1995; 30:539.

35. Versluysen M. Pressure sores in elderly patients. The epidemiology related to hip operations. J Bone Joint Surg Br 1985;67:10–13.

36. Shannon ML. Pressure sores. In: Norris CM, ed. Concept Clarification in Nursing. Rockville, MD: Aspen, 1982.

37. Anderson TP, Andberg MM. Psychosocial factors associated with pressure sores. Arch Phys Med Rehabil 1979;60:341–346.

38. Vidal J, Sarrias M. An analysis of the diverse factors concerned with the development of pressure sores in spinal cord patients. Paraplegia 1991;29:261–267.

39. Norton D, McLaren R, Exton-Smith NA. An Investigation of Geriatric Nursing Problems in Hospitals. London: National Corporation for the Care of Old People, 1962.

40. Norton D. Calculating the risk: reflections on the Norton scale. Decubitus 1989;2: 24–31.

41. Braden B, Bergstrom N. Clinical utility of the Braden scale for predicting pressure sore risk. Decubitus 1989;2:44–51.

42. Bergstrom N, Bennett MA, Carlson CE, et al. Treatment of Pressure Ulcers. Clinical Practice Guideline Number 15. Rockville, MD: Agency for Health Care Policy and Research, US Department of Health and Human Services Publication AHCPR 95-0652, 1994.

43. McLean J. Pressure reduction or pressure relief: making the right choice. J ET Nurs 1993; 20:211–215.

44. Krouskop TA, Garber SL, Cullen BB. Factors to consider in selecting a support surface. In: Krasner D, ed. Chronic Wound Care. King of Prussia, PA: Health Management Publications, 1990;135–141.

45. Zimmerer RE, Lawson KD, Calvert CJ. The effects of wearing diapers on skin. Pediatr Dermatol 1986;3:95–101.

46. Willis I. The effects of prolonged water exposure on human skin. J Invest Dermatol 1973; 60:166–171.

47. National Pressure Ulcer Advisory Panel. Consensus statement. Adv Wound Care 1995;8: 32–33.

48. Thomas DR, Rodeheaver GT, Bartolucci AA, et al. Pressure Ulcer Scale for Healing: derivation and validation of the PUSH tool. Adv Wound Care 1997;10:96–101.

49. Bates-Jensen BM, Vredevoe DL, Brecht ML. Validity and reliability of the Pressure Sore Status Tool. Decubitus 1992;5:20–28.

50. Bates-Jensen B. New pressure ulcer status tool. Decubitus 1990;3:14–15.

51. Bates-Jensen BM, Vredevoe DL, Brecht ML. Validity and reliability of the Pressure Sore Status Tool. Decubitus 1992;5:20–28.

52. Bates-Jensen BM, McNees P. Toward an intelligent wound assessment system. Ostomy Wound Manage 1995;41(Suppl 7A):80–87.

53. Bates-Jensen B. The Pressure Sore Status Tool: an outcome measure for pressure sores. Top Geriatr Rehabil 1994;9:17–34.

54. Bates-Jensen BM. The Pressure Sore Status Tool a few thousand assessments later. Adv Wound Care 1997;10:65–73.

55. Cooper DM. Indices to include in wound assessment. Adv Wound Care 1995;8:28-15–28-18.

56. Lazarus GS, Cooper DM, Knighton DR, et al. Definitions and guidelines for assessment of wounds and evaluation of healing. Arch Dermatol 1994;130:489–493.

57. Van Rijswijk L. Wound assessment and documentation. In: Kane DP, Krasner D, eds. Chronic Wound Care: A Clinical Sourcebook for Healthcare Professionals, 2nd Edition. Wayne, PA: Health Management Publications, 1997:16–28.

58. Yarkony GM, Kirk PM, Carlson C, et al. Classification of pressure ulcers. Arch Dermatol 1990;126:1218–1219.

59. Shea JD. Pressure sores: classification and management. Clin Orthop Rel Res 1975; 112:89–100.

60. Seiler WD, Stahelin HB. Identification of factors that impair wound healing: a possible approach to wound healing research. Wounds 1995;6:101–106.

61. Sapico FL, Ginunas VJ, Thornhill-Hoynes M, et al. Quantitative microbiology of pressure sores in different stages of healing. Diagn Biol Infect Dis 1986;5:31–38.

62. Winter GD. Formation of the scab and the rate of reepithelialization of superficial wounds in the skin of the young domestic pig. Nature 1965;193:293–294.

63. Kerstein MD. Moist wound healing: the clinical perspective. Ostomy Wound Manage 1995;41(Suppl 7A):37S–44S.

64. Stotts NA. Impaired wound healing. In: Carrieri-Kohlman VK, Lindsay AM, West, CM, eds. Pathophysiological Phenomena in Nursing, 2nd edition, Philadelphia: WB Saunders, 1993: 343–366.

65. Bagdade JD, Root RK, Bulger RJ. Impaired leukocyte function in patients with poorly controlled diabetes. Diabetes 1974;23:9–15.

66. Pecoraro RE, Ahroni JH, Boyko EJ, Stensel VL. Chronology and determinants of tissue repair in diabetic lower extremity ulcers. Diabetes 1991;40:1305–1313.

67. Goodson 3d WH, Hunt TK. Studies of wound healing in experimental diabetes mellitus. J Surg Res 1977;22:221–227.

68. Yue DK, McLennan S, Marsh M, et al. Effects of experimental diabetes, uremia, and malnutrition on wound healing. Diabetes 1987;36: 295–299.

69. Coleridge Smith PD, Thomas P, Scurr JH, Dormandy JA. Causes of venous ulceration: a new hypothesis. BMJ 1998;296:1726–1727.

70. Falanga V. Growth factors and wound healing. Dermatol Clin 1993;11:667–674.

71. Barbul A, Lazarou SA, Efron DT, Wasserkrug HL, Efron, G. Arginine enhances wound healing and lymphocyte immune responses in humans. Surgery 1990;108:331–336.

72. Kagan RJ, Bratescu A, Jonasson O, Matsuda T, Teodorescu M. The relationship between the percentage of circulating B cells, corticosteroid levels, and other immunologic parameters in thermally injured patients. J Trauma 1989;29:208–213.

73. Mosiello GC, Tufaro A, Kerstein M. Wound healing and complications in the immunosuppressed patient. Wounds 1994;6:83–87.

74. Krasner D. The chronic wound pain experience: a conceptual model. Ostomy Wound Management 1995;41:20–27.

75. Ivetic O, Lyne PA. Fungating and ulcerating malignant lesions: a review of the literature. J Adv Nurs 1990;15:83–88.

76. Waller A, Caroline NL. Smelly tumors. In: Waller A, Caroline NL, eds. Handbook of Palliative Care in Cancer. Boston: Butterworth-Heinemann, 1996:69–73.

77. Goodman M, Hilderley LJ, Purl S. Integumentary and mucous membrane alterations. In: Groenwald SL, Hansen Frogge M, Goodman M, Yarbro CH, eds. Cancer Nursing, Principles and Practice. Boston: Jones and Bartlett, 1997: 768–821.

78. Haisfield-Wolfe ME, Baxendale-Cox LM. Staging of malignant cutaneous wounds: a pilot study. Oncol Nurs Forum 1999;26:1055–1064.

79. Haisfield-Wolfe ME, Rund C. Malignant cutaneous wounds: a management protocol. Ostomy Wound Manage 1997;43:56–66.

80. Collinson G. Improving quality of life in patients with malignant fungating wounds In: Harding KG, Cherry G, Deale C, Turner TD, eds. Proceedings of the 2nd European Conference on Advances in Wound Management. Harrogate, October 20–23, 1992:59–63.

81. Cormier AC, McCann E, McKeithan L. Reducing odor caused by metastatic breast cancer skin lesions. Oncol Nurs Forum 1995;22:988–999.

82. Butler GA. Desloughing agents at work. Nurs Mirror 1985;160:29.

83. Leaper D. Antiseptics and their effect on healing tissue. Nurs Mirror 1986;82:45–47.

84. Seaman S. Home care for pain, odor, and drainage in tumor-associated wounds. Oncol Nurs Forum 1995;22:987.

85. Grocott P. Application of the principles of modern wound management for complex wounds in palliative care. In: Harding KG, Leaper DL, Turner TD, eds. Proceedings of the 1st European Conference on Advances in Wound Management. Cardiff, September 4–6, 1991:88–91.

86. Newman V, Allwood M, Oakes RA. The use of metronidazole gel to control the smell of malodorous lesions. Palliat Med 1989;3:303–305.

87. Rice T. Metronidazole use in malodorous skin lesions. Rehabil Nurs 1990;17:244–245.

88. Ashford RFU, Plant GT, Maher J, Teares L. Double-blind trial of metronidazole in malodorous ulcerating tumours. Lancet 1984;1:1232–1233.

89. McMullen D. Topical metronidazole use in malodorous ulcerating skin lesions. Presented at the 22nd Annual Meeting of the International Association of Enterostomal Therapists, Los Angeles, CA, June 1990.

90. Forman WB, Sheehan DC. Symptom management. In: Sheehan DC, Forman WB, eds. Hospice and Palliative Care. Boston: Jones and Bartlett, 1996:83–97.

91. Welch LB. Simple new remedy for the odour of open lesions. RN 1981;44:42–43.

92. Schulte MJ. Yogurt helps to control wound odor. Oncol Nurs Forum 1993;20:1262.

93. Stein C. The control of pain in peripheral tissue by opioids. N Engl J Med 1995;332: 1685–1690.

94. Back IN, Finlay I. Analgesic effect of topical opioids on painful skin ulcers. J Pain Symptom Manage 1995;10:493.

95. Krajnik M, Zbigniew Z. Topical morphine for cutaneous cancer pain. Palliat Med 1997;11:325.

96. Bryant RA. Management of drain sites and fistula. In: Bryant RA, ed. Acute and Chronic Wounds: Nursing Management. St. Louis: Mosby Year Book, 1992:248–287.

97. Schaffner A, Hocevar BJ, Erwin-Toth P. Small bowel fistulas complicating midline surgical wounds. J Wound Ostomy Cont Nurs 1994; 21:161–165.

98. Wiltshire BL. Challenging enterocutaneous fistula: a case presentation. J Wound Ostomy Cont Nurs 1996;23:297–301.

99. Jeter KF, Tintle TE, Chariker M. Man-

aging draining wounds and fistula: new and established methods. In: Krasner D, ed. Chronic Wound Care. King of Prussia, PA: Health Management Publications, 1990:240–246.

100. Harris A, Komray RR. Cost-effective management of pharyngocutaneous fistulas following laryngectomy. Ostomy Wound Manage 1993;39:36–44.

101. McKenzie J, Gallacher M. A sweet smelling success. Nurs Times 1989;85:48–49.

102. Anonymous. The 1998 ostomy/wound management buyers guide. Ostomy/Wound Manage 1998;44:4.

103. Breckman B. Rehabilitation in palliative care: stoma management. In: Doyle D, Hanks G, MacDonald N, eds. Oxford Textbook of Palliative Medicine. New York: Oxford University Press, 1994:543–549.

104. Doughty D. Principles of fistula and stoma management. In: Berger A, Portenoy R, Weissman D, eds. Principles and Practice of Supportive Oncology. New York: Lippincott-Raven, 1998:285–294.

105. Erwin-Toth P, Doughty DB. Principles and procedures of stomal management. In: Hampton BG, Bryant RA, eds. Ostomies and Continent Diversions: Nursing Management. Philadelphia: Mosby Year Book, 1992:29–94.

106. Dodd M. Self-care and patient/ family teaching. In: Yarbro C, Frogge M, Goodman M, eds. Cancer Symptom Management. Boston: Jones and Bartlett, 1999:20–32.

107. Tait N. Anorexia–cachexia syndrome. In: Yarbro C, Frogge M, Goodman M, eds. Cancer Symptom Management. Boston: Jones and Bartlett, 1999:183–208.

108. Bruera E. ABC of palliative care: anorexia, cachexia, and nutrition. BMJ 1997;315:1219–1222.

109. Martz C. Diarrhea. In: Yarbro C, Frogge M, Goodman M, eds. Cancer Symptom Management, Boston: Jones and Bartlett, 1999:522–545.

APPENDIX 16–A. Instructions for Use of the Pressure Sore Status Tool

General Guidelines:

Fill out the attached rating sheet to assess a pressure sore's status after reading the definitions and methods of assessment described below. Evaluate once a week and whenever a change occurs in the wound. Rate according to each item by picking the response that best describes the wound and entering that score in the item score column for the appropriate date. When you have rated the pressure sore on all items, determine the total score by adding together the 13-item scores. The HIGHER the total score, the more severe the pressure sore status. Plot total score on the Pressure Sore Status Continuum to determine progress.

Specific Instructions:

1. **Size**: Use ruler to measure the longest and widest aspect of the wound surface in centimeters; multiply length x width.

2. **Depth**: Pick the depth, thickness, most appropriate to the wound using these additional descriptions:
   - 1 = tissues damaged but no break in skin surface.
   - 2 = superficial, abrasion, blister or shallow crater. Even with, &/or elevated above skin surface (e.g., hyperplasia).
   - 3 = deep crater with or without undermining of adjacent tissue.
   - 4 = visualization of tissue layers not possible due to necrosis.
   - 5 = supporting structures include tendon, joint capsule.

3. **Edges**: Use this guide:
   - Indistinct, diffuse = unable to clearly distinguish wound outline.
   - Attached = even or flush with wound base, no sides or walls present; flat.
   - Not attached = sides or walls are present; floor or base of wound is deeper than edge.
   - Rolled under, thickened = soft to firm and flexible to touch.
   - Hyperkeratosis = callous-like tissue formation around wound & at edges.
   - Fibrotic, scarred = hard, rigid to touch.

4. **Undermining**: Assess by inserting a cotton tipped applicator under the wound edge; advance it as far as it will go without using undue force; raise the tip of the applicator so it may be seen or felt on the surface of the skin; mark the surface with a pen; measure the distance from the mark on the skin to the edge of the wound. Continue process around the wound. Then use a transparent metric measuring guide with concentric circles divided into 4 (25%) pie-shaped quadrants to help determine percent of wound involved.

5. **Necrotic Tissue Type**: Pick the type of necrotic tissue that is predominant in the wound according to color, consistency and adherence using this guide:
   - White/gray non-viable tissue = may appear prior to wound opening; skin surface is white or gray.
   - Non-adherent, yellow slough = thin, mucinous substance; scattered throughout wound bed; easily separated from wound tissue.
   - Loosely adherent, yellow slough = thick, stringy, clumps of debris; attached to wound tissue.
   - Adherent, soft, black eschar = soggy tissue; strongly attached to tissue in center or base of wound.
   - Firmly adherent, hard/black eschar = firm, crusty tissue; strongly attached to wound base and edges (like a hard scab).

(continued)

6. **Necrotic Tissue Amount**: Use a transparent metric measuring guide with concentric circles divided into 4 (25%) pie-shaped quadrants to help determine percent of wound involved.

7. **Exudate Type**: Some dressings interact with wound drainage to produce a gel or trap liquid. Before assessing exudate type, gently cleanse wound with normal saline or water. Pick the exudate type that is <u>predominant</u> in the wound according to color and consistency, using this guide:

Bloody	=	thin, bright red
Serosanguineous	=	thin, watery pale red to pink
Serous	=	thin, watery, clear
Purulent	=	thin or thick, opaque tan to yellow
Foul purulent	=	thick, opaque yellow to green with offensive odor

8. **Exudate Amount**: Use a transparent metric measuring guide with concentric circles divided into 4 (25%) pie-shaped quadrants to determine percent of dressing involved with exudate. Use this guide:

None	=	wound tissues dry.
Scant	=	wound tissues moist; no measurable exudate.
Small	=	wound tissues wet; moisture evenly distributed in wound; drainage involves ≤ 25% dressing.
Moderate	=	wound tissues saturated; drainage may or may not be evenly distributed in wound; drainage involves > 25% to ≤ 75% dressing.
Large	=	wound tissues bathed in fluid; drainage freely expressed; may or may not be evenly distributed in wound; drainage involves > 75% of dressing.

9. **Skin Color Surrounding Wound**: Assess tissues within 4cm of wound edge. Dark-skinned persons show the colors "bright red" and "dark red" as a deepening of normal ethnic skin color or a purple hue. As healing occurs in dark-skinned persons, the new skin is pink and may never darken.

10. **Peripheral Tissue Edema**: Assess tissues within 4cm of wound edge. Non-pitting edema appears as skin that is shiny and taut. Identify pitting edema by firmly pressing a finger down into the tissues and waiting for 5 seconds, on release of pressure, tissues fail to resume previous position and an indentation appears. Crepitus is accumulation of air or gas in tissues. Use a transparent metric measuring guide to determine how far edema extends beyond wound.

11. **Peripheral Tissue Induration**: Assess tissues within 4cm of wound edge. Induration is abnormal firmness of tissues with margins. Assess by gently pinching the tissues. Induration results in an inability to pinch the tissues. Use a transparent metric measuring guide with concentric circles divided into 4 (25%) pie-shaped quadrants to determine percent of wound and area involved.

12. **Granulation Tissue**: Granulation tissue is the growth of small blood vessels and connective tissue to fill in full thickness wounds. Tissue is healthy when bright, beefy red, shiny and granular with a velvety appearance. Poor vascular supply appears as pale pink or blanched to dull, dusky red color.

13. **Epithelialization**: Epithelialization is the process of epidermal resurfacing and appears as pink or red skin. In partial thickness wounds it can occur throughout the wound bed as well as from the wound edges. In full thickness wounds it occurs from the edges only. Use a transparent metric measuring guide with concentric circles divided into 4 (25%) pie-shaped quadrants to help determine percent of wound involved and to measure the distance the epithelial tissue extends into the wound.

17 Pruritus, Fever, and Sweats

MICHELLE RHINER and NEAL E. SLATKIN

It's not just the pain; pain is bad, but that's not the only thing. It's all the other things that go along, like the constant itching, itching, itching . . . it drove us crazy. The itch, the sweats, the nausea—they're all part of the pain.

—Family caregiver

Pruritus, derived from the Latin word *prurire*, which means "to itch," is a common and poorly understood symptom of both localized and systemic disorders (Table 17–1). The difficulties of defining the clinical characteristics of pruritus are in part related to the ambiguities of the available terminology and difficulties in quantitating this subjective disorder. "Itch," while describing the actual experience of sensory discomfort, is sometimes confused with the response used to relieve the discomfort, scratching. The literature is also less than clear on the distinction between itching and pruritus.[1,2] "Itch" is probably best reserved to describe the actual sensory discomfort that may arise in response to a fleeting stimulus or a pathological disorder.[3] The term "pruritus," is generally used to refer to a pathological condition in which the sensations of itch are intense and often generalized and trigger repeated scratching in an attempt to relieve the discomfort. Quantification of itch intensity, which is necessary for both clinical management and interventional studies, usually relies on the same 0 to 10 scale used to rate pain and other subjective symptoms. An assessment can also be made of "itch behaviors," such as rubbing and scratching, or the physical manifestations of these behaviors, such as the severity and distribution of scratch-induced excoriation.

PRURITUS

Although itching is not normally considered a "pain state," its neurotransmission parallels that of pain and the discomfort it causes can be just as distressing as conditions ordinarily considered painful. Words used to describe pruritus include "intense itch," "stinging," "burning," "pins and needles," "tickle," "a creeping or crawling sensation," and "pain." The particular descriptor used often depends on whether the cause of the itch is primarily cutaneous or neuropathic and, in the case of cutaneous conditions, which inflammatory mediators have been activated. Like persistent pain, persistent itch, especially when generalized, can cause considerable distress, including alterations in mood and loss of sleep. Moreover, persistent scratching can cause skin excoriations and cutaneous infection, which can also be painful and contribute to the vicious cycle of itching.[4]

Skin Anatomy

The skin is the body's first line of defense and its largest organ system. It consists of two layers, the *epidermis* (outer layer) and the *dermis* (inner layer), with a basement membrane zone dividing the two. Subcutaneous tissue, consisting primarily of fat and connective tissue, lends support to the neural and vascular systems that supply the skin and contains *eccrine* glands (ordinary sweat glands) and deep hair follicles.

The cells of the epidermis produce *keratin* (a fibrous protein), which imparts durability to the skin and protection against real-world frictions, and *melanin*, which protects against ultraviolet radiation. There are five layers of the epidermis: stratum corneum, stratum lucidum, stratum granulosum, stratum spinosum, and stratum germinativum (the single layer of basal cells attached to the basal membrane). Within these layers are found four major cell types: *keratinocytes* (which produce keratin), *melanocytes* (pigment-synthesizing cells), *Langerhans' cells* (derived from bone marrow cells, assist in cutaneous immune responses and produce prostaglandins), and *Merkel's cells* (mechanoreceptors).[5]

The dermis separates the epidermis from the subcutaneous tissues and is well vascularized, providing nutrients to the more superficial layers of skin. The two layers of the dermis are the *papillary dermis* (which contains capillary venules, lymph vessels, and nerve fibers) and the *reticular dermis* (the thicker layer of the dermis, consisting of collagen bundles interlaced by elastic fibers and ground substance). The cell types found in the dermis include *fibroblasts* (which secrete enzymes necessary to remodel the connective tissue matrix), *macrophages* (which synthesize enzymes that enhance or suppress lymphocytic activity and express inflammatory mediators), *lymphocytes*, and *mast cells* (which contain among other substances the pruitogenic mediator histamine).

Pathophysiology

Neural innervation of the skin is complex. As the barrier that functionally separates the self from the nonself, the skin's sensory innervation must allow for all manner of touch, temperature, and pain

Table 17–1. Differential Diagnoses for Pruritus

Systemic Causes

- Endocrine/metabolic
  - Hyper- and hypothyroidism
  - Hyper- and hypoparathyroidism
  - Diabetes mellitus
  - Zinc deficiency
  - Pyridoxine (vitamin B_6) and niacin deficiency
  - Chronic renal insufficiency and failure
  - Dialysis dermatosis
- Hepatic
  - Cholestasis, e.g., primary biliary cirrhosis, drug-induced
  - Extrahepatic biliary obstruction
  - Hepatitis
- Connective tissue disrders
  - Sjögren syndrome
  - Systemic lupus erythematosus
  - Chronic graft-versus-host disease
- Infectious
  - Syphilis
  - Human immunodeficiency virus
  - Parasitic, e.g., onchocerciasis, filariasis
- Neurological disorders
  - Stroke, brain tumor, brain injury (hemipruritus)
  - Multiple sclerosis (hemipruritus or paroxsymal pruritus)
  - Peripheral neuropathy (usually small-fiber neuropathy)
  - Post-herpes zoster
  - Tabes dorsalis
  - Notalgia paresthetica
- Other
  - Sarcoid
  - Pregnancy
- Psychological/psychiatric
  - Psychosis, psychogenic causes
- Malignancies
  - Polycythemia rubra vera
  - Carcinoid syndrome
  - Cutaneous T-cell lymphomas (mycosis fungoides, Sézary syndrome)
  - Other lymphomas and Hodgkin's disease
  - Plasma cell dyscrasias (e.g., multiple myeloma) with paraproteinemias
  - Other solid tumors
- Hematologic
  - Iron deficiency anemia
  - Systemic mastocystosis

Drug-Induced Causes

- Release of endogenous mediators
  - Opioids
  - Amphetamines
  - Cocaine
- Hypersensitivity
  - Acetylsalicylic acid (aspirin)
  - Quinidine
  - Niacinamide
  - Etretinate
  - Other medications

Dermatologic Causes

- Infections
  - Dermatophytosis
  - Folliculitis
- Infestations
  - Pediculosis (lice)
  - Scabies
- Inflammatory
  - Atopic dermatitis
  - Contact dermatitis
  - Drug hypersensitivity
  - Eczema
  - Psoriasis
  - Urticaria
- Miscellaneous
  - Insect bites
  - Systemic mastocytosis
  - Pregnanacy-associatred
  - Xerosis (dry skin)
  - Sunburn

Source: Lowitt and Bernhard (1992), reference 12.

sensitivity while at the same time responding to changes in environmental conditions. Receptors for pain, heat, cold, touch, pressure, and pleasure are distributed widely within the skin. These receptors are in turn innervated by a variety of afferent nerve types, including well-myelinated A fibers (which relay sharp pain, proprioception, direction of movement along the skin), myelinated D fibers, and unmyelinated C fibers. Afferent C fibers comprise 70% of all peripheral neurons transmitting to the central nervous system and are of three types: C mechanoreceptors, cold thermoreceptors, and C polymodal nociceptors. Maintenance of the skin's function as a protective barrier and temperature-regulating organ also requires a motor, or efferent, nerve supply. The ongoing turnover and replacement of epidermal cells, which maintains the skin's function as a protective barrier, requires a rich vascular supply. This vascular supply is in part regulated by sympathetic efferent fibers. The skin's function as a temperature-regulating system also depends on changes in cutaneous vascularity as well as the function of sweat glands and erector pili muscles (pilomotor muscles are responsible for "goosebumps"). Thermoregulatory sympathetic nerves help to modulate body temperature by either vasodilatation or vasoconstriction and by controlling the function of the sweat glands.

The sensation of itch can arise from either exogenous or endogenous stimuli. Regardless of the origin, evidence suggests that the sensation is transmitted by otherwise inactive nonmyelinated C nerve fibers. Such cutaneous sensory nerves can be activated by a variety of chemical or physical stimuli and serve as the final common sensory pathway for transmission of the itch stimulus. The ultimate sensation of itch, therefore, often provides little information about the etiology or provoking factors of itch. Chemical stimuli include caustic and abrasive substances, which cause skin injury, as well as a variety of potential topical allergens, including additives in perfumes and cleaning products. Physical stimuli that can cause pruritus include sunburn, negative pressure, moving suddenly from cold to heat in the presence of moisture, low-voltage electrical stimulation, and the epicutaneous application of caustic substances. Through uncertain mechanisms, repeated scratching itself can promote itch. Scratching causes *lichenification*, or thickening of the epidermis, which may decrease the sensitivity of large nerve fibers that may "gate" the perception of itch.[6] The exact mechanisms by which chemical and physical stimuli cause itch are in some instances stimulus-dependent, generally acting either directly on the free nerve endings or indirectly through the release of histamine (from dermal mast cells) or other inflammatory mediators.

As discussed above, the neurotransmission of itch typically begins with activation of the free, or penicillate, nerve endings of unmyelinated polymodal C nociceptive fibers, which lie at the epidermal–dermal junction. The terminal ends of these fibers form a rich arborization throughout the granular layers of the epidermis and dermis. Why some signals carried by these fibers are interpreted as itch and others as burning pain appears to depend on the pattern of neural firing and/or of coactivation of other nerve fibers.[7,8] Activated C polymodal nociceptive fibers transmit their signals back to their nerve cells in the dorsal root ganglia and then to the spinal cord to synapse in the substantia gelatinosa of the dorsal horn. After interacting with interneurons within the dorsal horn, fibers ascend in the anterolateral pathways (including the spinothalamic tract) to terminate within the brain stem and thalamus. The role played by the cerebral cortex in the mediation of itch remains undetermined but, as will be indicated below, appears to at least in part inhibitory. In both the laboratory and the clinic, brain injury can result in clinical itching.[9–11]

The neurochemical mediation of itch begins with activation of the polymodal nociceptive C fibers. These contain neuropeptides such as substance P, neurokinin A, vasoactive intestinal peptide, and calcitonin gene–related peptide.[3,12] Of these, substance P is the best studied and most abundant; it acts as the major puritogenic peptide. Its local release in response to neural activation may secondarily activate release of histamine from dermal mast cells, as well as other inflammatory mediators. These mediators may include prostaglandins, interleukins, serotonin, and neuropeptides such as endogenous opiates.[1,3,4] Capsaicin, an alkaloid from the chili pepper plant, typically evokes pain when applied to the mucous membranes or skin, due to release of substance P. When applied at very low concentrations, however, the sensation of itch rather than pain may occur. When chronically applied, capsaicin depletes substance P and, therefore, can block transmission of both itch and pain. Prostaglandins can lower the threshold to chemically induced itch, though prostaglandin antagonists do not typically have antipruritic effects except in certain hematologic disorders such as polycythemia vera.[13] Other mediators that produce itch are the endopeptidases. These include such enzymes as trypsin, chymotrypsin, bradykinin, kallikrein, and papain, which have been demonstrated to cause pruritus when injected into the skin even in the absence of dermal histamine. Itching powder, or cowhage, which is derived from the legume *Mucuna pruriens*, contains endopeptidases that cause the sensation of itch.[6] One mechanism by which microorganisms, such as bacteria, fungi, and parasites, may cause itching is the release of endopeptidases and other inflammatory mediators.

Serotonin is also an important mediator of pruritus, as revealed by the response of various pruritic states to antiserotonergic therapy. 5-Hydroxytryptamine-3 (5-HT3) antagonists (e.g., ondansetron, granisetron) have been used to palliate pruritus associated with uremia and cholestasis.[14,15] The temperature-dependent pruritus seen with polycythemia and lymphoreticular malignancies may also respond to antiserotonergic therapies.

Etiology

Pruritus, like pain, is multifactorial in origin and can be a symptom of diverse pathophysiologies. Like pain, pruritus can at times serve as a warning sign of external or internal threats to the organism or exist only as a discomforting and unwelcome symptom. Management of pruritus must begin with a thorough assessment of the various etiologic causes. Several different classification systems for pruritus have been proposed and are useful in conceptualizing its causes. When no cause can be found, even after a meticulous evaluation, it is referred to as primary, or idiopathic, pruritus. When symptoms are severe and generalized, the patient should remain under continued surveillance for the development of a possible malignancy.[16–18] Secondary pruritus can arise from either dermatologic or nondermatologic causes, and the distribution can be localized or systemic.

Secondary Pruritus. Secondary pruritus can be related to either exogenous agents, such as scabies, insect bites, and fungi, or endogenous factors, for example, atopic dermatitis, psoriasis, and biliary obstruction. Pruritus caused by a specific disease may require medical or surgical intervention. As noted above, itch can arise from a variety of exogenous physical and chemical stimuli, as well as from a large number of endogenous causes. Other endogenous causes for pruritus are not as well understood. In metabolic disorders, malignancies, and conditions of organ failure, pruritus may be due to hormonal imbalance, excessive production of cytokines, or buildup of metabolic by-products.

Various Common Clinical Situations

• Atopic Dermatitis. Pruritus in atopic dermatitis (AD) arises from the release of proinflammatory cytokines from mast cells and keratinocytes.[19] It is postulated that there is a dysfunction of bone marrow–derived cells migrating to the skin rather than an intrinsic cutaneous defect. Lymphocytic infiltrates of AD consist of T-helper cells. Both the Langerhans' cells and macrophages found in AD lesions have surface-bound immunoglobulin E (IgE). The patterns of cytokine production are also distinctive, due to the presence of interleukin-4 (IL-4) with the acute inflammatory phase and IL-5 and eosinophil infiltration with chronic inflammation.[19]

• Cholestatic Jaundice. In cholestatic liver disease, the accumulation of bile salts is presumed to be a causative factor in pruritus, though an association with bile levels in the skin and blood has not been consistently demonstrated.[20,21] Moreover, the response of pruritus to a variety of agents, each with differing mechanisms of action (e.g., ondansetron, rifampin, opiate antagonists, propofol, cholestyramine, norethandrolone, etc.) renders the primary causative factor even more obscure.[22–26] More recent evidence points to the accumulation of pruritogenic endogenous opiates. [27–29]

• Opioid-Induced Pruritus. Opioids can cause pruritus whether administered by the systemic, intraspinal, or intracisternal route. Clinically, itching is most commonly seen after intrathecal administration; then, typically, it is initially localized and most severely experienced in and about the face. Epidural administration, due to the higher systemic levels of opiate achieved with this route, tends to cause more generalized itching. Among opioid-naive cesarean section patients, as many as 60%–80% receiving epidural morphine report pruritus, with more than half of these requiring treatment.[30,31] The occurrence among palliative care patients, most of whom are not opiate-naive at the time of epidural placement, is considerably less, suggesting that tolerance to the pruritogenic effects of opiates develops with continued opioid exposure. The mechanisms for opioid induced pruritus are several. Opioids are known to trigger mast cell degranulation with histamine release, which probably accounts for the pruritus seen with systemic opioid administration. Opioid antagonists can attenuate histamine-induced itch unrelated to opioid administration, suggesting that endogenous opioids play an intermediary role in some forms of chemically induced pruritus.[32] Morphine, which appears to cause greater histamine release than fentanyl, meperidine, and oxymorphone, is most frequently implicated in opioid-induced pruritus; and changing to an alternative opioid (opioid rotation) may be a successful management strategy.[33–37] The fact that pruritus can be caused by either intrathecal or intracisternal opioid administration also speaks to a direct pruritogenic effect of opioids on the central nervous system.

• Pruritus Associated with Lesions of the Central Nervous System. Pruritus may also arise from disorders of the central nervous system (e.g., cerebrovascular accident pruritus).[10] Cases of hemipruritus have been described following stroke and with multiple sclerosis (MS). Phantom itch can occur in the amputated limb.[38] Paroxysmal itching may also result from nerve root demyelination in MS.[39,40]

• Anorectal Pruritus (Pruritus ani). While sometimes mistakenly viewed as a discrete diagnosis, anorectal pruritus is a common symptom of a large number of disorders affecting the lower colorectal area. Common etiologies include hemorrhoids, pinworms and other parasites, fungal infection, rectal irritation and dryness from detergent soaps, rectal seepage, and cryptitis from undigested food particles. Premalignant conditions, such as Bowen's disease and Paget's disease, may also present with these symptoms. In one reported series, 16% of 109 patients evaluated for pruritus ani were found to have a neoplastic lesion in the anorectal area.[41,42]

• Uremia. Pruritus can be a disabling symptom of end-stage renal disease and is not relieved by dialysis. Between 80% and 90% of patients undergoing hemodialysis suffer from this symptom.[43] As with many systemic causes of pruritus, the pathogenesis is poorly understood. Recent studies have shown affected patients to have high plasma histamine levels. These levels, as well as clinical pruritus, were significantly reduced by therapy with recombinant erythropoietin, the treatment reaching its maximal efficacy after 3–4 weeks. [44] Other potential causes of pruritus include secondary hyperparathyroidism, uremic and other forms of polyneuropathy, xerosis, and hypervitaminosis A.

Evaluation of the Patient with Pruritus

Evaluation of pruritus should be thorough and systematic, applying the same principles used when assessing pain. Quantify as much as possible any physical findings as well as subjective responses to the pruritus (e.g., distress associated with the itch based on a scale of 0–10, with 0 being "no distress" and 10 representing "severe distress").

Location. It is important to recognize whether the itch reported by the patient is generalized throughout the body, focal to a single region, or more widespread but in a particular pattern. Itching around skin creases of the wrists, axilla, and intertriginous areas, as well as the umbilicus and nipples, suggests scabies mite infestation. Anogenital itching may be due to contact dermatitis (e.g., from menstrual or continent pads, deodorants, washing products), *Candida* or other fungal infection, other infestations, or potentially psychogenic causes. Localized dermatitis, for instance, with a dermatomal distribution, may indicate prior herpes zoster infection or other segmental neurologic abnormality. Generalized pruritus may arise from a large number of causes, including organ failure, endocrinopathy, or dry skin.

Presence or Absence of Rash. Pruritus resulting from systemic disease is seldom characterized by a rash, though with histamine and serotonin release a mild flush may be present. It is important to distinguish between a true rash and the stigmata of frequent scratching, including excoriations and dermatographia. Focal rash may indicate contact sensitivity, evolving skin infection, or dryness of skin with associated flaking.

Quality of Symptoms. The common itch consists of an irresistible and persistent tickling sensation, which is usually at least transiently relieved with scratching. In addition to bearing the tickling sensation common to the itch experience, itch from irritant dermatitis and herpes zoster typically has a burning quality. Actual pain may coexist with itch in herpes zoster and other neuropathic lesions or arise from the trauma of repeated scratching.

Aggravating and Alleviating Factors. Topical application of heat often worsens itching, whereas cold diminishes the sensation. Worsening of pruritus after a hot shower is typical of Hodgkin's disease, myeloid metaplasia, and polycythemia vera. Consumption of alcohol may also induce itching in these conditions.

Treatment/ Management of Pruritus

Local Dermatologic Measures

• Topical treatment. Dry skin (xerosis) is common in patients who have undergone chemotherapy or radiation therapy. Xerosis arises either as a direct effect of therapy or as a manifestation of anorexia, dehydration, impaired nutrition, and weight loss, the skin becoming more vulnerable under these conditions to everyday traumas.[45]

Xerosis is also a common cause of pruritus in the aged. Other causes are related to reduced activity of the sebaceous and sweat glands, thinning of the skin, decreased subcutaneous tissue padding, and alterations in skin elasticity. Hydration of the skin is essential and can be accomplished by soaking in a warm bath for 15–20 minutes. The area should be patted dry, followed by application of an occlusive or moisturizer (Table 17–2). This is referred to by Nicol and Boguniewicz[19] as the "soak and seal" method and can relieve dryness by trapping moisture in the skin. Vaseline

Table 17–2. Medications Used to Treat Pruritus in Selective Conditions

Allergic/Autoimmune

Drug rotation or discontinuation[1]
Avoidance of offending allergen
5-HT_3 antagonists[13]
Antihistamines (e.g., diphenhydramine, cyproheptadine)
Corticosteroids
  Topical
  Systemic
Other immunosuppressive therapy

Opioid-Induced Pruritis

Opiate rotation (e.g., from morphine to alternative opiate, such as fentanyl)
Low-dose naloxone infusion
Low-dose nalbuphine infusion
Propofol[23]

Cholestatic Disorders

Acute palliative effects
  Propofol
  Naloxone and other opioid antagonists or agonist-antagonists
  Ondansetron
  External biliary drainage

Chronic palliative effects
  Cholestyramine
  Androgenic steroids
  Phototherapy
  Plasmapheresis
  Rifampicin (enhances hepatic microsomal function)
  Ursodeoxycholic acid
  Barbiturates
  Intravenous heparin
  Charcoal

Neuropathic Disorders

Local anesthetics, e.g., lidocaine, mexiletine, topical EMLA cream or lidoderm patch
Anticonvulsant agents, e.g., for paroxysmal symptoms of multiple sclerosis
Capsaicin[13]

Dermatoses

Skin cooling: increases the itch threshold, can break vicious cycle

Uremia

5-HT3 antagonists[14,15]
Ultraviolet B phototherapy
Erythropoietin
Parathyroidectomy
Thalidomide
Lidocaine

Polycythemia vera

Nonsteroidal antiinflammatory agents
Alpha-interferon

is considered an occlusive but must be used after hydration as it does not contain moisture. Moisturizers can be classified as lotions, creams, or ointments. Lotions can potentially be more drying to the skin since they contain more water and evaporate more quickly. There are a number of moisturizers (among them, Eucerin, Aquaphor, Vanicream, Moisturel, and Cetaphil) available in large containers that are alcohol- and fragrance-free. Among patients for whom cost is a treatment-limiting factor, a cooking shortening, such as Crisco, can be an inexpensive, alternative moisturizer. Moisturizers and occlusives should be applied several times per day.

For patients with pruritus, skin cleansing is important, especially if there are skin excoriations due to scratching. Many patients additionally seek relief by bathing or skin washing. The skin cleaners used in these situations should have a neutral pH and minimal defatting activity. Examples of such products include Dove, Oil of Olay, Basis, and Aveeno. Oatmeal baths and cold packs can be used to dry vesicles and relieve itch. Other topical agents such as calamine and topical Benadryl contain an antihistamine, which soothes and dries vesicles and decreases scratching. Camphor, phenol, and pramoxine may have local anesthetic properties; and menthol, a counterirritant, gives the impression of a cooling effect to the skin.[46]

A morphine- and lidocaine–based cream has been used in our clinical practice for pruritus described as burning and painful. Topical applications have been used for bullous pemphigoid lesions associated with graft-versus-host disease, cutaneous skin lesions associated with chest wall recurrence of breast cancer, and macerated rectal skin from persistent seepage. The preparation, when applied three times a day over affected areas, was highly effective at decreasing pain and pruritus. Creams compounded with antidepressants, such as doxepin (Zonalon), may decrease itch by local inhibition of H_1 and H_2 receptors, as well as through antiserotonergic effects.[4,19]

Topically applied corticosteroids can reduce inflammation and itching associated with urticaria and other acute conditions but are generally not indicated for chronic use. Key considerations when prescribing topical steroids are the potency of the product (high to low potency), the vehicle used (lotion, cream, ointment, solution, gel), and the area of application. Examples of high-potency steroids include betamethasone dipropionate (Diprolene 0.05%) ointment/cream and desoximethasone (Topicort 0.25%) ointment/cream; mid-range preparations include triamcinolone (Kenalog 0.1%) ointment/cream and betamethasone valerate (Valisone 0.1%) ointment; hydrocortisone (Hytone 2.5%) and 1% ointment/cream/lotion represent low-potency preparations.[19] The side effects from prolonged use may include thinning and hypopigmentation of the skin, secondary skin infections, acne, and striae. If high-potency topical steroids are used under occlusive dressings, greater skin and systemic absorption can occur, which increases the likelihood of localized atrophy and systemic side effects (e.g., Cushing's disease, cataracts, hyperglycemia, and avascular necrosis).[19,47,48] In the same manner, ointments are more occlusive than other vehicles and, therefore, may be associated with a higher skin penetration as well as a greater likelihood of side effects upon prolonged use. In hot, humid conditions, ointments may also cause folliculitis, thereby increasing pruritus. Under these conditions, creams may be a better option. Topical steroids should generally not be applied more often than twice per day. Hydration of the skin prior to each application will promote absorption through the stratum corneum, thereby improving local absorption and efficacy.[48] It is typical to start with a high-potency preparation and to move to a lower-potency agent as the dermatitis/pruritus improves.[47]

• Anti-Fungal Treatment. The most frequent superficial fungal infection of the skin is *Candida albicans*. Typical areas of infection involve the inframammary areas, inguinal folds, and vulvovaginal areas, with pruritus being a common manifestation. Patients predisposed to candidiasis include those who are obese and have overlapping skin folds, those who are immunosuppressed, are on broad-spectrum antibiotics, are receiving corticosteroids, or have diabetes. Skin involvement in the inframammary or inguinal folds often appears as a creamy white layer, but gentle removal of this layer may reveal an erythematous base, with areas of maceration and even papules and pustules. Vulvovaginal infections will have a cheesy vaginal discharge with itching and excoriation of the vulva.

Topical antifungal agents in use fall into three classifications: the polyene group (nystatin), the azole group (ketoconazole, fluconazole, itraconazole), and the allylamine/benzylamine group (ciclopiroxolamine, terbinafine).[49] The allylamine/benzalamine group is the newest generation of antifungals. They have greater bioavailability and a high cure rate with a shorter duration of treatment. To prevent recurrence, antifungal treatment should continue for 5–7 days after signs of infection have resolved. Ketoconazole should not be used in individuals with sulfite sensitivity. Some antifungals are prepared with corticosteroids; however, these should be avoided to prevent side effects from the corticosteroids.

Fungal infections not responsive to topical therapy will require systemic treatment. Systemic antifungals include griseofulvin, the azoles, and the allylamines. Gastrointestinal distress, headaches, exanthema, and liver toxicity (griseofulvin and fluconazole) are common side effects.

Tar preparations may reduce inflammation and limit the use of topical steroids in chronic pruritus/dermatitis. They may be used at night and washed off in the morning. Tar products are less costly; however, the smell and staining that occur with these products make them less than desirable.

Phototherapy with ultraviolet A may be an option for some individuals. Initially, treatments are given three or four times per week and, after several weeks, may progress to weekly. An oral preparation of psoralen prior to phototherapy may also be used for a wide range of disorders from AD to renal disease.[4] Side effects include sunburn and an increased risk of skin cancer.[19]

Systemic Measures

• Opioid antagonists. Naloxone hydrochloride (Narcan) is effective for relieving pruritus related to systemic and intraspinal opiates.[32,50,51] Infusion of naloxone at an hourly dose of 0.25 μg/kg was successful at relieving pruritus in patients receiving a continuous morphine infusion and appeared to enhance rather than diminish postoperative analgesia.[50] Nalbuphine, an agonist–antagonist analgesic, has also shown efficacy under similar conditions.[52] Naltrexone and nalmephene are oral agents, with a longer half-life than naloxone, that have been used in the treatment of pruritus associated with cholestasis, uremia, AD, and urticaria.[28,53] It is not known whether all centrally acting opioid antagonists are equal in their antipruritic effects. When naltrexone was used for pruritus in a patient with mycosis fungoides after initial success with subcutaneous naloxone, it was found to actually exacerbate itching[54] (Table 17–3). Because of the potential of opiate antagonists to induce a withdrawal syndrome, neither pure antagnoists nor agonist–antagonists should be prescribed for the treatment of pruritus, except by those experienced in their use.

• Systemic corticosteroids. Systemic corticosteroids can be highly effective in patients with pruritus related to inflammatory conditions, neoplasms, and certain dysmetabolic states. The presumed mechanism of action is inhibition of inflammatory and pruritogenic factors. Long-term use of these agents is limited by the well-known sequelae of chronic steroid use, including increases in skin friability, hyperglycemia, and the risks of fungal and other opportunistic infections. All of these can worsen preexisting pruritus. Other side effects may include avascular necrosis, hypertension, proximal muscle weakness, fluid retention, and osteoporosis.[55]

Table 17–3. Occlusives and Moisturizers

Vaseline (Chesebrough Ponds, Greenwich, CT)
Aquaphor ointment (Allscrips, Vernon Hills, IL)
Eucerin cream (Allscrips)
Vanicream (Pharm Spec, Rochester, MN)
Cetaphil cream (Galderma, Fort Worth, TX)
Moisturel cream (Westwood/Squibb, Buffalo, NY)
Crisco (Procter and Gamble, Cincinnati, OH)

• Antihistamines. H_1-specific antihistamines are useful primarily for histamine-mediated pruritus, such as that associated with hives; but these agents often fail to provide meaningful relief in other conditions. A trial of the more sedating histamines is often recommended in initial treatment, but many patients find that negative side effects outweigh the minimal benefit achieved. A trial of the nonsedating antihistamines (fexofenadine, cetirizine, and loratidine) may be a more reasonable first step in the treatment of nonspecific itch since these agents are well tolerated. The more sedating antihistamines, such as diphenhydramine, chlorpheniramine, clemastine, hydroxyzine, and cyproheptadine, can be useful at night when itch interferes with sleep. In addition to its antihistaminic effects, cyproheptadine has antiserotonergic activity, which may provide increased relief in some patients.

• Local anesthetics. Mexiletine (Mexitil) is similar in its chemical properties to lidocaine and has been used in patients with intractable pruritus. Other anesthetic agents given IV, intradermally, or intraarterially can block sensory transmission, including pruritus.[1,56] Side effects include lightheadedness, dizziness, tremors, and nervousness. Interferon-α has been reported to be effective in relieving pruritus refractory to antihistamines and steroids in B-cell chronic lymphocytic leukemia and in non-Hodgkin's lymphoma. It is thought to inhibit the proliferation of eosinophil differentiation.[57,58] Dermatomyositis-induced pruritus has been treated with high-dose human immunoglobulin.[59]

• Antidepressants. Doxepin, amitriptyline, nortriptyline, and imipramine have been used in the treatment of numerous neuropathic pain states. Pruritus is frequently a comorbid feature of neuropathic pain, and anecdotal reports suggest that the same tricyclic antidepressants that are efficacious in certain forms of neuropathic pain may also be beneficial in treating pruritus.[60–62] As the most antihistaminic of the group, doxepin may be the most effective. Mirtazapine also has potent H_1 antagonism, as well as antiserotonergic effects at both the 5-HT2 and 5-HT3 receptors. Since antagonism at each of these individual receptor types has been associated with antipruritic effects, mirtazepine may possess a theoretical advantage in pruritus treatment.

• Propofol. Subhypnotic doses of propofol have been successfully used in the treatment of pruritus resulting from neuraxial administration of opioids and cholestasis from pancreatic neoplasm, hepatic and bile duct metastasis, and primary biliary cirrhosis. Patients achieved rapid symptomatic control following both single injections and continuous low-dose infusion.[22,23,64] While the mechanism of action is unclear, the effect was unrelated to sedation.[22,23,64]

• Anticonvulsants. In general, anticonvulsant agents have not been investigated for utility in the treatment of pruritus. Several anticonvulsant agents, such as carbamezepine and gabapentin, are of established clinical efficacy in the treatment of a variety of neuropathic pain syndromes. When pruritus complicates a known neuropathic disorder (e.g., postherpetic neuralgia), a therapeutic trial of one of these agents should be considered.

• Other agents. Ondansetron, a 5-HT3 antagonist, has been used in cholestatic, uremic, and opioid-induced pruritus.[15,65,66] Benzodiazepines, such as lorazepam and alprazolam, may be helpful in relieving itch if anxiety is also present.[67] Benzodiazepines are not suggested for long-term use.

Sensory modulation can be accomplished through counterirritants, heat or cold, and transcutaneous electrical nerve stimulation (TENS). The Roman physician Scribonius Largus used the voltages of certain fish (electric rays and torpedo fish) in A.D. 47 for treatment of gout and headaches.[68] With the advent of the battery, TENS units that provided a more reliable source of current were developed. When applied directly over the pruritic area, surrounding area, or acupressure points, TENS may block transmission of polymodal nociceptive C fibers, thereby blocking pain and pruritus.[69,70]

Capsaicin depletes substance P when applied repeatedly to the mucous membrane or skin, decreasing both pain and itch sensations. When given in low concentrations, the stinging, burning itch may initially be exacerbated.[2]

The gate control theory of pain states that impulses carried by noxious stimuli to the spinal cord via thin myelinated and unmyelinated fibers are blocked at the dorsal horn by stimulation of larger-diameter myelinated nerve fibers by pressure, vibration, or a TENS unit.[69] Thick nerve fibers have a lower threshold than thin fibers and adapt more readily. No adaptation takes place in the large fibers when scratching or vibration occurs. This may explain why scratching or rubbing the affected part sometimes relieves mild to moderate pain.[69]

Case Study: An Elderly Woman with Pruritus

Ms. S is a 75-year-old woman with a history of non-Hodgkin's lymphoma, cervical cancer, breast cancer, chronic renal failure, hypothyroidism, hypertension, and seizure disorder. She was treated for a disseminated herpes zoster infection that involved several dermatomes (T2–L2) diagnosed 3 months earlier. Ms. S was seen in clinic for complaints of pruritus in the right posterior chest that had been present for 3 months that was thought to be a postherpetic neuralgia. The patient described the pruritus as a burning, unrelenting itch and stated she was "ready to give up." The following medications were prescribed and reported to be ineffective: amitriptyline (Elavil) 20 mg q hs, hydroxyzine (Atarax) 25 mg tid, diphenhydramine (Benadryl) 25 mg tid po, and doxepin cream 5% to the affected area qid. Nondrug interventions included ice pack to the back for 20 min tid. Famotidine (Pepcid) 20 mg bid, prednisone 20 mg bid, and triamcinolone acetonide (Kenalog) cream 0.025 topically applied tid were also used, again without relief. The patient was admitted to the hospital for cellulitus in the right arm, presumably a secondary bacterial infection resulting from the scratching, and was given cefazolin (Ancef) IV.

The patient denied any contact with pets; no new or changed soap/detergents, cosmetics, body lotions/creams, medications; no exposure to scabies or to new foliage. She denied pruritus in any area other than her back.

Clinical evaluation: a frail, elderly woman who appeared uncomfortable and at times restrained herself from scratching. No vesicular eruptions were noted. Numerous scratch marks and dry blood are present over the posterior thorax. Three raised erythematous areas were noted, in the right scapular, lower thorax, and lumbar areas. Skin turgor was good. There was no allodynia, and no lymphadenopathy in the head/neck, supraclavicular area, or axilla. There was no evidence of a rash, infection, or tracks. Blood urea nitrogen and creatinine were stable, and thyroid function tests were within normal limits.

The impression was that this woman with a history of herpes zoster infection had developed post-herpetic neuralgia.

Ms. S's pruritus was treated as a postherpetic neuralgia, and a prescription for mexiletine (Mexitil) 150 mg bid was given with instructions to take with food to minimize gastrointestinal side effects. Ms. S was asked to titrate by one pill (150 mg) every 5 days to a total of 300 mg tid. Amitriptyline (Elavil) 10 mg was prescribed with instructions to take every evening at 8:00. By taking this medication earlier in the evening, the patient was less likely to feel "hungover" in the morning.

The patient reported improvement in the "itchiness and discomfort" in her back once the mexiletine was started; however, she developed a tremor that she noted while in church. The patient became frightened and stopped the medication. Ms. S was evaluated in an urgent care clinic by an on-call physician. Upon examination, an essential tremor was diagnosed and the patient was advised to restart the mexiletine at 150 mg tid for 24 hours and then to increase to 300 mg tid. Ms. S. was reevaluated later that week and reported "dizziness" when taking mexiletine 300 mg tid. She stopped the amitriptyline at night and continued to report relief of the pruritus with the use of this drug. The patient was asked to decrease the mexiletine to 150 mg tid and to restart the amitriptyline 10 mg q hs. The patient called several days later to report that the pruritus was not controlled at this dose and that was afraid to increase the dose because of side effects (i.e., tremor). The patient was seen in clinic, and it was decided that since the mexiletine was the only medication that provided any relief of her symptoms, the dose would be adjusted again to 150 mg in the morning and evening and 300 mg at hs; propranolol (Inderal) 10 mg tid was added to decrease the tremor.

Nursing Implications

Assessment

1. Describe and document the color, characteristics, and size of any lesions.
2. Obtain a thorough history of any new products (detergents, lotions, soaps), exposure to new pets, recent travel and outdoor exposure, or any new medications.
3. Obtain a thorough patient and family history of allergies (e.g., food or seasonal), treatments previously used and their success, travel, hikes, and any exposure to known infectious agents/insect bites. Do other members of the family or others with whom the patient has had social contact have pruritus?
5. What has been the general health of the patient over the several weeks preceding the development of pruritus?
6. A skin biopsy may be required to determine the etiology of the pruritus.

Management

1. Teach safety measures with use of sedating antihistamines, such as not driving or operating potentially dangerous equipment until tolerance to the sedating effects of these medications has been established.
2. Psychological support is needed for any new diagnosis of malignancy.
3. Educate patients concerning the proper use of topical medications and the potential side effects.
4. Frequently assess the skin in pruritic areas for the presence of any secondary infections.

FEVER

Fever is defined as a rise in normal body temperature (above 37° ± 1°C), as a temperature ≥38°C for three consecutive readings performed 1 hour apart, or as one reading ≥38.5°C.[71] Fevers can be a result of inflammation (including malignancy), infection, immunologic disorders, hypermetabolic states (e.g., thyrotoxicosis), hyperthermia, heat stroke, or uncommonly, disorders of the central nervous system (e.g., cerebral stroke). Febrile illnesses have been recorded in the medical literature as far back as Hippocrates (5th century B.C.E.), though it was not possible to actually measure body temperature until the development of the thermometer in the mid-nineteenth century.[72,73] Determining the etiology of a fever is often essential to providing the most appropriate treatment of this symptom as well as of its underlying causes. Deciding when to treat the actual symptom of fever depends to a great extent on the symptoms associated with it (e.g., tachypnea, tachycardia, hyperhydrosis, feeling of dissipation, fatigue), age, general medical condition, any co-morbid conditions or diseases, and the goals of care relative to the patient's stage of illness. For example, the treatment of fever and associated tachycardia in an older patient with a known history of advanced coronary artery disease but few other co-morbid illnesses may itself be life-saving. Treating fever usually provides improved patient comfort. However, treating fever may at times have the unintended effect of inhibiting immunologic responses mounted as a means of defense against infectious pyrogens.[73] To what extent such inhibitory responses are of clinical significance is largely unknown.

In the setting of palliative care, decisions on treating an infectious etiology of fever can at times trigger controversy since doing so may prolong the dying process. How aggressively infection should be treated at the end of life depends on the factors listed above and the plan of care agreed upon by the patient, family, and health care professionals.

Pathophysiology of Fever

The body's thermoregulatory system is controlled by the preoptic region of the anterior hypothalamus. Under ordinary circumstances, the hypothalamus maintains the core body temperature by establishing a thermal set-point. This set-point, analogous to a thermostatic control, may be affected by the presence of various *pyrogens*, or fever-causing substances. Pyrogens may be produced by and released directly from infectious pathogens (bacteria, viruses, or fungi). These are typically called "exogenous" pyrogens. Pathogenic agents may also stimulate the release of endogenous pyrogens from the immune system. The four best recognized endogenous pyrogens are IL-1, IL-6, tumor necrosis factor-α (TNF-α), and interferon (IFN). Systemic release of either exogenous or endogenous pyrogens can trigger the fever response by elevating the hypothalamic set-point so that compensatory temperate lowering mechanisms are not activated until higher than normal temperatures are reached. At this time, it is not known if peripherally released cytokines cross the blood–brain barrier to directly influence the hypothalamic set point or whether this process occurs through other cytokine mediators or even neural means. At the hypothalamic level, prostaglandins, especially prostaglandin E_2, appear to play an important role in establishing the hypothalamic set-point. It is presumably through these inhibiting prostaglandin mediators that aspirin and certain other antipyretic agents work. Regardless of the actual mechanism, the hypothalamus continues to regulate body temperature, though this regulation is now around a higher set-point. When an antipyretic is given or the pyrogen level is decreased, the hypothalamic temperature is reset back to normal.[71,73,74] Temperatures above 41°C suggest that the source of fever may be either abnormal heat production (as in malignant hyperthermia) or problems with heat dissipation (as in heat stroke).

Phases of Fevers

There are often three stages of a fever. The "cold stage" occurs when there is a physiological discrepancy between the hypothalamic set-point, now at a higher level, and the existing body temperature. In response, hypothalamic mechanisms signal for peripheral vasoconstriction to occur, which diminishes cutaneous heat loss, and for shivering, which generates heat through increased muscle activity. The "hot stage," or febrile phase, occurs when body heat is maintained at a higher than normal level due to the higher set-point of hypothalamic thermoregulaton. During the febrile stage, symptoms often include flushing of the skin, increased sense of thirst, sensation of increased body warmth, lethargy, and restlessness or irritability. Less commonly seen central nervous system manifestations include hallucinations and seizures, though the latter are seen almost exclusively in young children. During febrile states, the basal metabolic rate is increased as tissue metabolism and oxygen requirements increase by 10% to 13% for each 1°C increase in body temperature. Associated physiologic changes include tachycardia with an increase in cardiac output and workload.[74,75] Decreases in the level of pyrogen produced or administration of an antipyretic at least temporarily resets the hypothalamic set-point. During the defervescence stage, or stage 3, heat dissipation is increased due to vasodilatation and sweating, causing an increase in evaporative skin cooling.[75,76] Heat-generating mechanisms (e.g., shivering) are inhibited, and the body temperature falls back within the normal range.[77,78]

Various Clinical Situations

Immunologic Responses. Blood products and certain medications, as well as allergic reactions and connective tissue disorders, liberate substances which in turn activate release of endogenous pyrogens, the three best recognized being IL-1, IL-6, TNF, and IFN. A variety of secondary immune reactions may trigger the release of pyrogens, including anaphylactic reactions (e.g., asthma), cytotoxic reactions (e.g., blood-transfusion reactions), immune complex—mediated reactions (e.g., serum sickness), and delayed hypersensitivity reactions (e.g., contact dermatitis and allograft rejection). Primary immune disorders that may be associated with a fever include systemic lupus erythematosus, giant cell arteritis, and rheumatoid arthritis.

Infections. Infectious pathogens elaborate pyrogens, such as bacterial lipopolysaccharides, which in turn promote the release of endogenous pyrogenic cytokines by stimulating the body's immune and other defensive reactions. The principal origins of these cytokines are activated monocytes, macrophages, and lymphocytes, which are recruited to respond to the infection. Endogenous pyrogens can also be produced by endothelial cells and fibroblasts.

Of pathogens found in new fevers, 85%–90% are of bacterial origin. Common origins of bacterial infections in cancer and immunosuppressed patients include the breakdown of skin integrity and mucosal barriers due to multiple venipunctures and lines or catheters, other invasive procedures, decubitus ulcers, cutaneous infections including herpes zoster, and mucositis. Bacteria, as well as other pathogens, induce the production of endogenous pyrogens in macrophages and monocytes. These pyrogens include TNF-α and IL-1β. Release of these substances into the inflammatory soup in turn stimulates the cascade of other cytokines, including IL-1, IL-6, and the prostaglandins.[71]

Increasing body temperature can itself increase phagocytic activity and affect the type and amount of pyrogenic cytokine released.[75] Although fever may contribute in this fashion to stimulation of the immune system, the tachycardia and hypermetabolism caused by the fever can prove fatal in an individual who is immunocompromised, in advanced cancer patients, and in those with acquired immunodeficiency syndrome (AIDS).[74,77,78]

Inflammation. Inflammation occurs with cellular damage due to cytotoxic agents, trauma (including surgery), radiation therapy, or exposure to heat. Fibroblasts and endothelial cells, as well as macrophages, release endogenous pyrogens, such as IL-1, IL-6, and TNF.[71,72,75] Postoperative fluid collections and large internal hematomas are therefore common causes of fever in the surgical patient. Although circumscribed superficial inflammation rarely causes significant fever, inflammation can predispose to secondary infection and a febrile state.[74,77,78] Radiation therapy, for example, can cause fevers through several mechanisms. First, immunocytes and endothelial cells damaged by radiation may release endogenous pyrogens. Second, radiation therapy may alter skin integrity (dry and moist desquamation) and damage mucosal barriers, thereby increasing the patient's predisposition to infection. Infection may also be associated with radiation-related myelosuppression when the radiation field includes the primary sites of blood cell production, such as the sternum, long bones, and iliac crests.[79–81] Finally, cranial radiation may cause temporary perturbations in the hypothalamic set-point.

Vascular causes of fever may include thrombophlebitis with or without pulmonary emboli, and regional or systemic tumor-associated vasculitis. The cause of fevers in these settings is thought to be release of pyrogens from phagocytic and endothelial cells. Several cancers, especially lymphomas and gastrointestinal malignancies, are associated with a higher than expected risk for developing deep vein thrombosis. It is not uncommon, in fact, for fever to be the earliest sign of thrombophlebitis. In one study of pulmonary emboli, approximately 18% of the patients had malignancies, 54% had a fever >37.5°C, and 19.6% had a fever >38°C.[82]

Even in the absence of vascular inflammation, fever may be the presenting symptom of many malignancies, including Hodgkin's lymphoma, bronchogenic carcinoma, breast cancer, non-Hodgkin's lymphoma, and multiple myeloma. Fevers related to tumors may be associated with the release of pyrogens, such as TNF-α and IL-6, either directly from the tumor or from tumor-reactive hypersensitivity reactions.[71,74,75] Pulsatile release of tumor pyrogens can cause a waxing and waning of fever, which correlates with disease activity.[71,74,83–85] The naproxen test has been used as a diagnostic tool to differentiate between a neoplastic fever and a fever associated with an infection. Chang and Gross[86] reported complete response of neoplastic fevers to naproxen within 24 hours of starting the drug, whereas no patient with an infectious fever showed any improvement.[71,79] It was postulated that the fever suppression was related to the interference/suppression or release of humoral factor(s).[86] The specificity of this test is uncertain, and the possibility of infection should not be dismissed on the basis of this test alone. Other noninfectious etiologies, such as allergic reaction, drug toxicity, and adrenal insufficiency, also need to be considered.[71]

Blood Transfusions. Allergic responses to white blood cells in blood products may be avoided by using irradiated blood products, removing white blood cells from blood (leukapheresis), or premedicating with antihistamines, hydrocortisone, and/or antipyretics.[76]

Medications Associated with Fevers. Certain medications may be antigenic; that is, they are interpreted by the body as a foreign substance, thereby initiating an allergic or immune response with accompanying fever. The categories of drug most often associated with a febrile response include antibiotics, cytotoxic agents, cardiovascular drugs, and biological therapies such as the interferons and interleukins.[78] The classes of antibiotic most commonly associated with fevers are the penicillins, cephalosporins, and certain antifungals, such as amphotericin.[71] Cytotoxic drugs such as bleomycin trigger a fever in 25% of individuals, and anaphylaxis results in 1% of cases.[71]

Hemorrhage. Gastrointestinal bleeding may result in fever within 24 hours, which may last a few days to a few weeks.[71,72] Although this has been mentioned in the literature, no clear explanation has been offered, but fever may be related to the release of IL-1 from the damaged gastrointestinal mucosa.[72]

Neutropenia. Neutropenia is defined as a polymorphonuclear neutrophil count of 500/μl or less, which may arise from decreased production of white blood cells (myelosuppression from chemotherapy or radiation therapy or tumor infiltration of bone marrow with inhibition of white blood cell production) or increased loss of white blood cells (usually through an autoimmune process). Of patients with neutropenia, 50% to 70% experiencing a fever will die within 48 hours if left untreated because of rapidly progressive sepsis.[76,78,87]

Miscellaneous Factors. Several general medical problems can be identified as contributing to fever (Table 17–4). Dehydration limits the body's compensatory response of heat loss through sweating. Severe obstipation has been associated with fever, due possibly to associated dehydration or ischemia of the bowel, causing a local inflammatory response. Hospitalization itself is a frequent cause of infection and fever, probably because of the frequency of procedures, such as venipuncture and the placement of intravenous catheters, which violate the integrity of skin defense mechanisms. Nosocomial infections account for more than 80% of infections in cancer patients.[88]

Opioids. Opioids have been found to cause a flush (vasodilatation) and sweating, especially involving the face, but have not been associated with fever.[89] Meperidine hydrochloride (pethidine hydrochloride) in combination with a monoamine oxidase inhibitor can cause hyperpyrexia, muscle rigidity, central nervous system excitability, or depression that can be severe or fatal.[71,90] Abrupt opioid cessation results in withdrawal symptoms, which include restlessness, rhinitis, abdominal pain, and fever. Withdrawal from benzodiazepines may also cause a fever.[71]

Clinical Evaluation

Patient History. A thorough history must be obtained to determine if there are coexisting symptoms suggestive of a urinary tract infection, upper respiratory infection, or any exposure to a person with infection or who has had a live-virus vaccination. A bowel history should be conducted to rule out constipation. If the patient has cancer, when was the last surgery? When was the last course of chemotherapy or immunotherapy? When was the last course of radiation therapy? Is there any history of blood transfusion within the preceding 6 months? It is important to determine the pattern of the patient's fevers, the time of day they occur, and the number of temperature peaks over 24 hours. In patients receiving end-of-life care, the focus of the treatment plan is palliation of symptoms. Determining the source of

Table 17–4. Common Causes of Fevers

Tumor
- Hodgkin's and non-Hodgkin's lymphoma (cell-mediated immune deficiency)
- Hypernephroma
- Carcinoma metastatic to the liver
- Leukemia
- Multiple myeloma (altered humoral immunity)
- Ewing's sarcoma
- Tumors that become necrotic, with secondary infections
- Adrenal carcinoma/pheochromocytoma
- Primary or metastatic tumors of the thermoregulatory areas of the brain
- Obstructive solid tumors of the gastrointestinal, genitourinary, or respiratory system

Cancer and treatment
- Changes in the body's natural defenses
- Foreign bodies (catheters, venous access devices)
- Degree and duration of neutropenia
- Immunosuppression
- Chemotherapeutic agents (e.g., bleomycin)
- Blood products
- Splenectomy

Inflammatory processess
- Thrombophlebitis
- Radiation
- Heat
- Trauma
- Surgery
- Cell necrosis (ischemic)
- Pulmonary embolism
- Regional enteritis
- Granulomatous disease of the colon
- Ulcerative colitis

Autoimmune and allergic processess
- Connective tissue disorders (systemic lupus)
- Anaphylactoid reactions
- Rheumatoid arthritis
- Polymyalgia rheumatica
- Acquired immunodeficiency syndrome
- Medications, e.g., antibiotics

Infections
- Bacteria, fungi, viruses, and parasites
- Tuberculosis
- Infective endocarditis
- Liver abscess/subphrenic abscess
- Anicteric hepatitis
- Nosocomial infection

Environmental
- Microbial flora that colonize in the nasopharynx, small and large bowel, and skin
- Travel to third-world countries; Central, North, and South America; tropics and subtropics
- Exposure to microorganisms from farm animals
- Allergic response to environmental allergens

Foods (immunocompromised patients)
- Fresh fruits and vegetables
- Fresh flowers
- Spices
- Tobacco

Others
- Constipation
- Dehydration

the fever will guide the clinician as to the appropriate intervention. If the patient is severely constipated, laxative-induced evacuation may not only reduce the fever but also improve nutritional status and eliminate or reduce nausea, if present. Treating a urinary infection may also improve comfort, promote rest, and improve cognition. Use of oral antibiotics to treat a urinary tract or upper respiratory infections may be appropriate to palliate symptoms, such as the distress that may accompany tachypnea, tachycardia, or shaking chills. Antibiotics are used in this manner to palliate symptoms due to infection rather than to eradicate the infection proper. If antibiotic therapy causes increased physical distress in the form of pruritus, drug-induced fevers, or nausea and vomiting, the role of antibiotic treatment needs to be reevaluated, to keep the focus of care on quality-of-life issues. As with all palliative treatments, it is important to routinely re-assess goals with the patient and family to be certain that everyone is in agreement.

Physical Examination. Since common sites of infection include the skin, respiratory tract, urinary system, perianal region, oral cavity, and sinuses, a comprehensive evaluation for infection should not overlook any of these sites. In chronically ill and emaciated patients, special attention should be paid to the skin overlying bony prominences as well as the perineal and perianal regions, evaluating for decubitus lesions and other areas of skin breakdown, necrotic tumors, and/or infection. If the patient has a intravenous line, central catheter, or other central venous access device (e.g., Porta-Cath), these need to be carefully evaluated for signs of infection. Decisions on the appropriateness of blood and sputum cultures and radiographic tests need to be made on a case-by-case basis, depending on the patient's status and the likelihood that test results will lead to a meaningful therapeutic intervention. This said, performance of a urinalysis is noninvasive and inexpensive and can provide information leading to straightforward therapies offering symptom relief.

Management of Common Sources of Skin Infection in End-of-Life Care

There are several interventions nurses can initiate to manage skin infections based on the location, characteristics of the affected area, and organism(s) involved. Dakin's solution is composed of bleach, sodium bicarbonate, and sterile water. It can be prepared as a 0.25%, 0.5%, 0.75%, or full-strength solution, depending on the contamination of the wound, and may be used to irrigate or pack wounds contaminated with *Pseudomonas.* Clean, healthy skin should not come in contact with Dakin's solution as it is very irritating.

Hypertonic saline gels (Panafil) can debride thick, necrotic eschar on a decubitus without surgical intervention. Morphine (powder or concentrated solution) is added to commercially prepared ointments and substances used for wound healing, such as Silvadene and lidocaine, and to Duoderm powder to pack inside wounds. These mixtures may be helpful in reducing secondary skin infections as well as promoting comfort and can be used to pack a venous stasis ulcer, decubitus, or fungating lesion. Fungal infections, generally characterized by a foul odor, maceration of the skin, and occasionally superficial bleeding, are commonly seen in the intertriginous areas (inframammary and inguinal folds). Daily cleansing with soap and water, thorough drying of the affected area, and use of antifungal powder or lotion (nystatin, clotrimazole) can be applied bid or tid until healed.

Treatment of Fever

Comfort should be the primary goal for the dying patient with a fever. Treatment should be initiated with antipyretics, such as acetaminophen, aspirin, or ibuprofen, which are the only drugs approved by the Food and Drug Administration for this purpose.

Acetaminophen can be administered in tablet, liquid, or suppository form. For tumor-related fever, a nonsteroidal anti-inflammatory drug (NSAID) may be especially beneficial. The presence of thrombocytopenia may be a limiting factor in the selection of NSAIDs. The specific cyclo-oxygenase-2 (COX-2)–inhibiting antiinflammatory agents, such as celecoxib (Celebrex) and rofecoxib (Vioxx), may in certain instances be preferred in this setting.

Cooling measures, such as a tepid cloth to the patient's forehead may be comforting, otherwise, cooling measures (such as as ice bags and cool cloths) should be avoided as they cause shivering, which is heat-generating. Oral fluids and/or ice chips should be encouraged, but the benefit of using parenteral or enteral fluids is highly debated, and it remains undetermined whether hydration improves cognition, especially in individuals using opioids.[91,92] Oral care with soft applicators should be offered frequently by the family caregiver; aside from promoting the patient's comfort, this allows the caregiver to participate in the loved one's care. A salt and soda solution can be used instead of mouthwash. A solution can be made by boiling one quart of water and adding one teaspoon of salt and one teaspoon of baking soda. Chill the solution and use several times a day as desired. Discard any unused solution after 1 week. Vaseline or other lubricants should be placed on the patient's lips to prevent dryness and cracking. Special attention to skin is essential; clothing and linens should be changed frequently and special attention given to skinfolds. Aquaphor, Eucerin, aloe vera, or Vaseline Intensive Care can be applied to maintain skin integrity. Lymphedema patients using a Jobst and Sigvarus compression garment should be instructed to avoid products that contain petroleum because they break down the rubber in the garment. Avoid skin products that contain alcohol as they may actually increase dryness and cause chemical irritation.

A bowel history should be obtained and a laxative or suppository given if constipation is present. An enema or disimpaction may be required. Corticosteroids are effective as antipyretics and can reduce inflammation and pain but are potentially dangerous insofar as immune function is hampered and an infectious process may be masked.[75] The risk:benefit ratio with respect to goals of care must always be considered. In a palliative care setting, neuroleptic agents can be used for centrally mediated fevers. Chlorpromazine (Thorazine) has been used primarily in this setting, probably because among the neuroleptics it is most likely to cause vasodilatation.[93]

Palliative radiation may be needed if the fever is tumor-related, as indicated by the tumor type and general condition of the patient.

Case Study: Fever

Mr. D was an 80-year-old retired pediatrician with a recent history of fever of unknown origin, leukocytosis, elevated erythrocyte sedimentation rate (ESR), anemia, and myalgias. The patient had been in good health until his return from Mexico, 2 months earlier, when he developed chills, myalgias, nonproductive cough, and fevers. Antibiotics were prescribed when a chest x-ray showed a left lower lobe infiltrate. Myalgias continued, especially in the triceps muscles and shoulder girdle muscles. The myalgias were partially relieved by NSAIDs. Throughout the 2 months, he had intermittent spikes of fever with episodes of profuse diaphoresis, generalized malaise, anorexia, and a 15 lb weight loss. He was admitted to a local hospital, where he underwent extensive testing.

The past medical history included Guillain-Barré syndrome in 1945, right bundle branch block, transurethral prostatectomy in 1988, and prostate cancer without evidence of metastatic disease. There was no history of rheumatic fever or heart murmur.

Clinical Evaluation revealed the patient as an alert, oriented man with intact cognitive functions. Funduscopic examination was impeded by cataract formation, but no Roth spots or areas of hemorrhage were visible. There was slight focal tenderness of the proximal superficial temporal artery, barely notable on the right and mild on the left. There was no nodularity or induration along the course of either of these arteries. Carotid bruits were absent and extracranial artery pulsations, normal. There was no nuchal rigidity. Motor examination was normal for age, without muscle masses or tenderness, except in the calves. He was, however, unable to rise from a chair without the use of his arms and was unsteady on his feet. Gait was wide-based and waddling, with some unsteadiness. Sensation was intact to all modalities, though Romberg's sign was positive for postural imbalance and tandem gait was slightly abnormal. Radial pulses were equal, and pedal pulses were present bilaterally. No cutaneous stigmata of infection or vasculitis was appreciated. Heart sounds were normal without murmur. There was no hepatomegaly or abdominal tenderness. Areas of bone tenderness were absent.

The impressions were (1) fever of unknown origin, (2) rule out temporal arteritis.

The diagnostic data were as follows: lumbar puncture was negative, carotid ultrasound showed moderate amount of plaque formation in both common carotid arteries with no significant stenosis, and temporal artery biopsy showed giant cell arteritis.

The patient was treated with prednisone 20 mg tid with regular monitoring of ESR.

The patient enjoyed complete relief of fevers, night sweats, and myalgias. He was encouraged to exercise, and bone density studies and blood sugar levels were monitored during the time he was on prednisone. His ESR returned to normal, and prednisone was gradually tapered.

SWEATING

The sweat glands of the skin, the piloerector muscles, and the vascular skin blood vessels are controlled, at least in part, by the sympathetic nervous system and are intimately involved in temperature regulation. Vasodilatation and sweating allow for evaporative heat loss to lower body temperature in a hot environment, with fevers, or during exercise. Approximately 5% of cancer patients experience sweating as a direct result of malignant disease.[94–96]

Pathophysiology

The hypothalamus interprets signals from the central and peripheral thermoreceptors. There are two types of thermosensitive neuron, warm-sensitive and cold-sensitive, both of which are located in the preoptic anterior hypothalamus. The more abundant warm-sensitive neurons respond to a rise in temperature in the periphery, whereas the cold-sensitive neurons are triggered by a decrease in body temperature in the periphery.[1] Body temperature is read at various thermoreceptors in the skin, spinal cord, and brain stem. Hypercapnia, plasma osmolality, intravascular blood volume changes, and dehydration can affect body temperature and set-point.[1]

The autonomic nervous system both transmits the thermoregulatory adjustments to the central nervous system and has a measure of thermoregulatory control independent of the central nervous system. Postganglionic sympathetic axons innervate sweat glands, blood vessels, and piloerector muscles. Through adjustments in adrenergic vasoconstrictor nerve fibers, cutaneous blood flow is increased or decreased depending on the need to dissipate or conserve heat. Cholinergic fibers innervate the eccrine glands. Thermal sweating occurs when the hypothalamic set-point is exceeded. Signals are transmitted from the hypothalamus by the autonomic nervous system to the effector sweat glands and cutaneous vasculature. Generalized diaphoresis ensues, which lowers body temperature. Emotional sweating is controlled primarily by the limbic system, rather than the hypothalamus, and may affect areas of the body differentially. Whereas sweating may be either depressed or increased over the trunk and proximal limbs, sweating always increases in the palms of the hands and soles of the feet. Under given circumstances, the quantity of sweating in response either to temperature elevation or emotion is often dependent on age, gender, exercise, hydration, ambient temperature, and sweat gland blood flow. Disorders of sweating include *hyperhidrosis* (excessive sweating), *anhidrosis* (absent or decreased sweating), and *gustatory sweating* (primarily of the face, associated with diabetes). Each of these disorders can arise from dysfunction of either the neural innervation or the sweat glands themselves or both.

Etiology

Anhydrotic ectodermal hypoplasia is an inherited condition in which heat loss through perspiration may be inadequate to lower body temperature. Other cooling methods must be used for thermoregulation (e.g., submersion in cool water, exposure to cool ambient temperatures, cool cloths) to lower temperature.

Hyperhidrosis may be a compensatory mechanism for anhidrosis of other body areas. Thermoregulatory sweat testing can be conducted to assess the peripheral and central sympathetic pathways. Reduced or absent sweating patterns can be identified and the pathology identified as either pre- or post-ganglionic abnormalities or abnormalities of the sweat glands. Abnormalities of sweating, either excessively dry or wet skin, accompanied by trophic skin changes and thin shiny skin are signs of a peripheral neuropathic disorder. When seen in the setting of limb pain, they typically indicate that the pain is arising, at least in part, on a neuropathic basis.

Generalized hyperhydrosis can occur with various endocrine disorders, such as estrogen deficiency due to menopause (related either to the climacteric medical treatment), hyperthyroidism, or hypoglycemia, as well as with various neuroendocrine tumors, such as carcinoid and pheochromocytoma. Hyperhidrosis may also be a sign of chronic infection, such as tuberculosis, or of inflammatory illnesses (e.g., lupus, vasculitis, regional enteritis) even in the absence of fevers. Various malignancies, most notably lymphomas, cause drenching sweats, especially at night. Such night sweats may be an early sign of tumor recurrence. Hyperhidrosis may announce many abstinence syndromes, such as from barbiturates, opioids, or ethanol.[1] With opioids, both agonists, such as morphine and methadone, and mixed agonists–antagonists, such as butorphanol and pentazocine, have been associated with excessive sweating, probably due to cutaneous vasodilatation. An opioid rotation may be beneficial in reducing this symptom.[1]

It is important to evaluate all reported regional disturbances of sweating. Patients with an area of anhidrosis (e.g., related to a Pancoast tumor as a component of Horner's syndrome) may not notice a decrease in sweating on the affected area but, instead, report hyperhidrosis on the unaffected side.

Nocturnal hyperhidrosis, or night sweats, can be associated with decreased estrogen production such as from menopause, other endocrine disorders, and malignancies. Hormonal therapy for breast and prostate cancers is often associated with troublesome hot flashes, which interfere with sleep patterns. Seventy-five percent of men receiving hormonal therapy experience hot flashes, although the symptom is often overlooked.

Clinical Evaluation/Treatment Options for Hot Flashes

Hot flashes occur as a result of estrogen depletion related to surgery, adjuvant chemotherapy, and hormonal therapy [such as tamoxifen, leuprolide (Lupron), and flutamide (Eulexin)]. Estrogen replacement therapy generally is not given to women with a history of breast cancer in the United States. Such women are predisposed not only to hot flashes but also to other problems associated with estrogen deficiency, such as osteoporosis and heart disease. In the nonhormonal treatment of hot flashes, such agents as ergotamine tartrate plus phenobarbital (Bellergal), methydopa, and clonidine have been tried, but often with limited success. Other purported remedies include moderate doses of vitamin E, certain antidepressant agents such as paroxetine (Paxil), venlafaxine Hcl (Effexor),[99] and anticholinergic agents such as oxybutynin chloride (Ditropan).[98] Oxybutynin is an antispasmodic, anticholinergic agent indicated for the treatment of urge incontinence and bladder hyperactivity disorders; it often effectively reduces sweating. It is now available in a sustained-release form, which minimizes the side effects of sleepiness and dry mouth. Patients living in hot climates must be cautioned against overactivity in the heat as diminished sweating can lead to heat stroke when taking anticholinergic agents. Adequate hydration is important if confusion and hyperthermia are to be avoided. In clinical practice, propranolol hydrochloride (Inderal) has been found to decrease the sympathetic symptoms of hot flashes and night sweats in a variety of illnesses, such as Parkinson's disease. Thalidomide has been reported to decrease TNF-α production and sweating in patients with tuberculosis, leprosy, rheumatoid arthritis, graft-versus-host disease, and mesothelioma (where TNF-α levels were elevated).[94] There are numerous references in the professional and lay literature regarding use of evening primrose oil and phytoestrogens for menopausal symptoms. Phytoestrogens are found in over 300 plants (coumestans: bean sprouts, red clover, and sunflower seeds; lignans: rye wheat, sesame seeds, linseed). Constituent isoflavones are reportedly similar in efficacy to endogenous estrogen at minimizing the symptoms of menopause (hot flashes) and pre-menstrual syndrome. A recent study evaluating soy phystoestrogens for treatment of hot flashes in breast cancer survivors concluded the soy product did not alleviate hot flashes.[97] Black cohosh (*Cimicifuga racemosa*) is a perennial herb that has emerged as a treatment for hot flashes, but there is no good evidence from controlled trials to support its use.[100,101]

Case Study: A 60-Year-Old Breast Cancer Survivor

Mrs. M is a 60-year-old woman with a prior history of oophorectomy, who in 1994 was diagnosed with breast cancer. Treatment included a lumpectomy, followed by a segmental resection with axillary node dissection and external radiation therapy. Since her diagnosis, she has taken tamoxifen 10 mg bid as a prophylactic measure. Hot flashes were reported as her most distressing symptom. Sleep was interrupted due to frequent linen changes (two or three per night), and frequent changes of nightwear were required. The patient described these episodes as being "drenched," and they impacted negatively on her quality of life. Past medical history included mitral valve prolapse, type II diabetes, hypertension, hypercholesterolemia, stress incontinence (status post bladder suspension), and oophorectomy.

Mrs. M is a very pleasant, well-developed,

well-nourished woman in no distress. Vital signs: T :35.9, P: 95. Her blood pressure was 162/92, she weighed 84 kg. The physical examination was unremarkable except for the area of the right breast, where a well-healed surgical deficit was present. There was increased density in the tissue of the right breast. There was no erythema and no palpable mass. There was no lymphadenopathy in the supraclavicular region or axillae. There was no nipple discharge.

Diagnostic data included fasting blood sugar 115. The impression is hot flashes related to tamoxifen use.

The patient was given a prescription for a clonidine TTS-1 patch, to be worn weekly as a means of blocking the symptoms of excessive sympathetic outflow that caused her hot flashes and sweats and as a means of treating her hypertension. The clonidine was tried for 1 month, but after this, the patient discontinued the patch, feeling it was ineffective and reporting symptoms of orthostatic hypotension. Hyosphen (Bellergal), which contains phenobarbital, ergotamine, and belladonna, was prescribed, twice a day. This agent was tried for several days, and while it had some efficacy, the patient found its sedating properties to be unacceptable. Oxybutynin chloride (Ditropan), an anticholinergic and antispasmodic agent, was prescribed. At the starting dose of 5 mg bid, the patient reported that the frequency and intensity of her hot flashes were considerably reduced and that her urinary urgency was also better controlled.

The patient's quality of life reportedly improved when she was able to sleep through the night without experiencing the hot flashes or nocturia. She was able to decrease the dose of oxybutynin to 5 mg once a day at sleep.

CONCLUSION

Pruritus, fever, and sweats are frequently seen in end-of-life care but are still not well managed. New pharmacologic therapies have evolved in the palliation of these symptoms, and the physiological processes are better understood. Symptoms of pruritus, fever, and sweats should be assessed and recognized as being distressing to the patient and negatively impacting on the patient's quality of life. In the palliative care setting, treatment of the underlying disease process may be limited but comfort should be a priority.

REFERENCES

1. Pittelkow MR, Loprinzi CL. Pruritus and wweating. In: Doyle D, Hanks G, MacDonald N, eds. Oxford Textbook of Palliative Medicine, 2nd Ed. Oxford: Oxford University Press, 1998:627–642.
2. Fleischer AB Jr, Michaels JR. Pruritus. In: Berger A, Portenoy RK, Weissman DE, Principles and Practice of Supportive Oncology. Philadelphia: Lippincott-Raven, 1998: 245–250.
3. Denman ST. A review of pruritus. J Am Acad Dermatol 1986;14:375–392.
4. Fleischer AB, Michaels JR. Pruritus. In: Berger A, Portenoy RK, Weissman DE, Principles and Practice of Supportive Oncology. Philadelphia: Lippincott-Raven, 1998:245–250.
5. Simandl G. Alterations in skin function and integrity. In: Porth CM, ed. Pathophysiology Concepts of Altered Health States 3rd Ed. Philadelphia: JB Lippincott, 1990:106–143.
6. Herndon JH Jr. Itching: the pathophysiology of pruritus. Int J Dermatol 1975;14:465.
7. Tuckett RP, Denman ST, Chapman CR, et al. Pruritus, cutaneous pain, and eccrine gland and sweating disorders. J Am Acad Dermatol 1985; 5:1000–1006.
8. Handwerker HO, Forster HC, Kirchhoff C. Discharge patterns of human C-fibers induced by itching and burning stimuli. J Neurophysiol 1991;66:307–315.
9. Bradford FK. Ablations of frontal cortex in cats with special reference to enhancement of the scratch reflex. J Neurophysiol 1939;2:192–201.
10. King CA, Huff FJ, Jorizzo JL. Unilated neurogenic pruritus: paroxysmal itching associated with central nervous system lesions. Ann Intern Med 1982;97:222–223.
11. Massey EW. Unilateral neurogenic pruritus following stroke. Stroke 1984;15:901–903.
12. Lowitt MH, Bernhard JD. Quantitation of itch and scratch. Semin Neurol 1992;12:374–384.
13. Lovell CR, Burton PA, Duncan EHL, Burton JL. Prostaglandins and pruritus. Br J Dermatol 1976;94:273.
14. Schworer H, Ramadori G. Treatment of pruritus: a new indication for serotonin type 3 receptor antagonists. Clin Invest 1993;71:659–662.
15. Raderer M, Muller C, Scheithauer W. Ondansetron for pruritus due to cholestasis. N Engl J Med 1994;330:1540.
16. Radossi P, Tison T, Vianello F, Dazzi F. Intractable pruritus in non Hodgkins lymphoma/CLL: rapid response to IFN α. Br J Haematol 1996;94:579–583.
17. Cooper DL, Gilliam AC, Perez MI. Hyperprolactinemic galactorrhea in a patient with Hodgkin's disease and intense pruritus. South Med J 1993;86:829–830.
18. Apel RL, Fernandes BJ. Malignant lymphoma presenting with an elevated serum CA-125 level. Arch Pathol Lab Med 1995;119:373–376.
19. Nicol NH, Boguniewicz M. Understanding and treating atopic dermatitis. Nurse Pract Forum 1999;10:48–55.
20. Malet KM. Pruritus associated with cholestasis. A review of pathogenesis and management. Dig Dis Sci 1994;39:1–8.
21. Losowsky T Jr. Opioid peptides and primary biliary cirrhosis. BMJ 1988;297:1501–1504.
22. Borgeat A, Savioz D, Mentha G, Giostra E, Suter PM. Intractable cholestatic pruritus after liver transplantation–management with propofol. Transplantation 1994;58:727–730.
23. Borgeat A, Wilder-Smith OHG, Saiah M, Rifat K. Subhypnotic doses of propofol relieve pruritus induced by epidural and intrathecal morphine. Anesthesiology 1992;76:510–512.
24. Bachs L. Rifampin more effectively relieves pruritus in patients with primary biliary cirrhosis, compared with phenobarbital. Lancet 1989; 1:574–576.
25. Jones EA, Bergasa NV. The pruritus of cholestasis: from bile acids to opiate agonists. Hepatology 1990;11:884–887.
26. Abboud TK, Lee K, Zhu J, et al. Prophylactic oral naltrexone with intrathecal morphine for cesarean section: effects on adverse reactions and analgesia. Anesth Analg 1990;71: 367–70.
27. Thornton JR, Losowsky MS. Opioid peptides and primary biliary cirrhosis. BMJ 1988;297: 1501–1504.
28. Bergasa NV, Alling DW, Talbot TL, et al. Effects of naloxone infusions in patients with the pruritus of cholestasis. A double-blind, randomized, controlled trial. Ann Intern Med 1995;123: 161–167.
29. Khandelwal M, Malet PF. Pruritus associated with cholestasis: a review of pathogenesis and management. Dig Dis Sci 1994;39:1–7.
30. Fuller JG, McMorland GH, Douglas MJ. Epidural morphine for analgesia after caesarean section: a report of 4880 cases. Can J Anaesth 1990;37:636–640.
31. Cohen SE, Ratner EF, Kreitzman TR, et al. Nalbuphine is better than naloxone for treatment of side effects after epidural morphine. Anesth Analg 1992;75:747–752.
32. Bertnstein JE, Swift RM, Soltani K, Lorincz A. Anti-pruritic effect of an opiate antagonist, naloxone hydrochloride. J Invest Dermatol 1982; 78:82–83.
33. Ackerman W, Juneja M, Kaczorowski D, Colclough G. A comparison of the incidence of pruritus following epidural opioid administration in the patient. Can J Anaesth 1989;36:388–391.
34. Hermens JM, Ebertz JM, Hanifin JM, Hirshman CA. Comparison of histamine release in human skin mast cells induced by morphine, fentanyl, and oxymorphone. Anesthesiology 1985; 62:124–129.
35. Sinatra RS, Lodge K, Sibert K, et al. A comparison of morphine, meperidine, and oxymorphone as utilized in patient-controlled analgesia following cesarean delivery. Anesthesiology 1989;70:585–590.
36. Woodhouse A, Hobbes AFT, Mather LE, Gibson M. A comparison of morphine, pethidine and fentanyl in the postsurgical patient-controlled analgesia environment. Pain 1996;64:115–121.

37. Bergasa NV, Talbot TL, Alling DW, et al. A controlled trial of naloxone infusions for the pruritus of chronic cholestasis. Gastroenterology 1992;102:544–549.

38. Bernhard JD. Phantom itch, pseudophantom itch and senile pruritus. Int J Dermatol 1992;33:856–857.

39. Yamamoto M, Yabuki S, Hayabara T, Otsuki S. Paroxysmal itching in multiple sclerosis: a report of three cases. J Neurol Neurosurg Psychiatry 1981;44:19–22.

40. Osterman PO. Paroxysmal itching in multiple sclerosis. Br J Dermatol 1976;95:555.

41. Daniel GL, Longa WE, Vernava AM III. Pruritus ani: causes and concerns. Dis Colon Rectum 1994;37:670–674.

42. Hejna M, Valencak J, Raderer M. Anal pruritus after cancer chemotherapy with gemcitabine. N Engl J Med 1999;340:655–656.

43. Gilchrest BA. Pruritus: pathogenesis, therapy and significance in systemic disease states. Arch Intern Med 1982;142:101–105.

44. De Marchi SD, Cecchin E, Villalta D, Sepiacci G, Santini G, Bartoli E. Relief of pruritus and decreases in plasma histamine concentrations during erythropoietin therapy in patients with uremia. N Engl J Med 1992;326:15.

45. Hunnuksela A, Kinnunen T. Moisturizers prevent irritant dermatitis. Acta Derm Venereol 1992;72:42–44.

46. Gatti S, Serri F. Pruritus in Clinical Medicine. New York: McGraw Hill, 1991.

47. Nicol NH, Baumeister LL. Topical corticosteroid therapy: Considerations for prescribing and use. Prim Care 1997;1:62–69.

48. Chaffman MO. Topical corticosteroids: a review of properties and principles in therapeutic use. Nurse Pract Forum 1999;10:95–105.

49. Jantzi Rudy S. Superficial fungal infections in children and adolescents. Nurse Pract Forum 1999;10:56–66.

50. Gan TJ, Ginsberg B, Glass PSA, Fortney J, Jhaveri R, Perno R. Opioid-sparing effects of a low-dose infusion of naloxone in patient-administered morphine sulfate. Anesthesiology 1997;87: 1075–1081.

51. Sullivan JR, Watson A. Naltrexone: a case report of pruritus from an antipruritic. Australas J Dermatol 1997;38:196–198.

52. Kendrick WD, Woods AM, Daly MY, Birch RF, DiFazio C. Naloxone versus nalbuphine infusion for prophylaxis of epidural morphine-induced pruritus. Anesth Analg 1996;82:641–647.

53. Monroe EW. Efficacy and safety of nalmefene in patients with severe pruritus caused by chronic urticaria and atopic dermatitis. J Am Acad Dermatol 1989;21:135–136.

54. Sullivan JR, Watson A. Naltrexone: a case report of pruritus from an antipruritic. Australas J Dermatol 1997;38:196–198.

55. Howser RL. What you need to know about corticosteroid therapy. Am J Nurs 1995: 95;44–48.

56. Fishman S, Stojanovic MP, Borsook D. Intravenous lidocaine for treatment-resistant pruritus. Am J Med 1997;102:584–585.

57. Radossi P, Tison T, Vianello F, Dazzi F. Intractable pruritus in non-Hodgkin lymphoma/cll: rapid response to ifn cx. Br J Haematol 1996; 94:579–583.

58. Neuber K, Berg-Drewniock B, Volkenandt M, Neumaier M, Gross G, Ring J. B cell chronic lymphocytic leukemia associated with high serum IGE levels and pruriginous skin lesions: successful therapy with IFN α after failure on IFNγ. Dermatology 1996;192:110–115.

59. Kikuchi-Numagami K, Sato M, Tagami H. Successful treatment of a therapy resistant severely pruritic skin eruption of malignancy associated dermatomyositis with high dose intravenous immunoglobulin. J Dermatol 1996;23:340–343.

60. Freilich RJ, Seidman AD. Pruritus caused by 3-hour infusion of high-dose paclitaxel and improvement with tricyclic antidepressants. J Natl Cancer Inst 1995;87:933–934.

61. Liddell K. Post-herpetic pruritus. BMJ 1974;4:165.

62. Procacci P, Maresca M. Case report. Pain 1991;45:307–308.

63. Zylicz Z, Smits C, Krajnik M. Paroxetine for pruritus in advanced cancer. J Pain Symptom Manage 1998;16:121–124.

64. Saiah M, Borgeat A, Wilder-Smith HG, Rifat K, Suter PM. Epidural morphine-induced pruritus: propofol versus naloxone. Anesth Analg 1994;78:1110–1113.

65. Wilde MI, Markham A. Ondansetron: a review of its pharmacology and preliminary clinical findings in novel applications. Drugs 1996;52: 773–794.

66. Larijani GE, Goldberg ME, Rogers KH. Treatment of opioid induced pruritus with ondansetron: report of four patients. Pharmacotherapy 1996;16:958–960.

67. Fried RG. Evaluation and treatment of psychogenic pruritus and self excoriation. J Am Acad Dermatol 1994;30:993–999.

68. Ostrowski MJ. Pain control in advanced malignant disease using transcutaneous nerve stimulation. Br J Clin Pract 1979;33:157–162.

69. Ostrowski MJ, Dodd A. Transcutaneous nerve stimulation for relief of pain in advanced malignant disease. Nurs Times 1977;11:1233–1238.

70. Carlsson CA, Augustinsson LE, Lund S, Roupe G. Electrical transcutaneous nerve stimulation for relief of itch. Experientia 1975;31:191.

71. Cleary J. Fever and sweats: including the immunocompromised hosts. In: Berger A, Portenoy RK, Weissman DE, Principles and Practice of Supportive Oncology. Philadelphia: Lippincott-Raven, 1998:119–131.

72. Porth CM, Curtis RL. Alteration in temperature regulation. In: Porth CM, ed. Pathophysiology Concepts of Altered Health States, 3rd Ed. Philadelphia: JB Lippincott, 1990:95–105.

73. Styrt B, Sugarman B. Antipyresis and fever. Arch Intern Med 1990;150:1591–1597.

74. Carpenter R. Fever. In: Chernecky CC, Berger BJ, eds. Advanced and Critical Care Oncology Nursing: Managing Primary Complications. Philadelphia: WB Saunders, 1998:156–171.

75. Bruce JL, Grove SK. Fever: pathology and treatment. Crit Care Nurse 1992;12:40–49.

76. Chernecky CC, Berger BJ. Fever. In: Chernecky CC, Berger BJ, eds. Advanced and Critical Care Oncology Nursing: Managing Primary Complications. Philadelphia: WB Saunders 1998:156–171.

77. Pizzo PA. Management of fever in patients with cancer and treatment induced neutropenia. N Engl J Med 1993;328:1323–1332.

78. Pizzo PA. Fever in immunocompromised patients. N Engl J Med 1999;341:893–897.

79. Wujcik D. Infection control in oncology patients. Nurs Clin North Am 1993;20:639–650.

80. Lokkevik E, Skovlund E, Reitan JB, Hannidsdal E, Tanum G. Skin treatment with bepanthen cream versus no cream during radiotherapy. Acta Oncol 1996;35:8.

81. Omand M, Meredith C. A study of acute side-effects related to palliative radiotherapy treatment of lung cancer. Eur J Cancer Care 1994; 3:149–152.

82. Manganelli D, Palla A, Donnamaria V, Giuntini C. Clinical features of pulmonary embolus. Doubts and certainties. Chest 1995;107: S25–S32.

83. Pitz CCM, Lokhorst HM, Hoekstra JBL. Fever as a presenting symptom of multiple myeloma. Neth J Med 1998;53:256–259.

84. Scully RE, Mark EJ, McNeely WF, Ebeling SH. Case presentation. N Engl J Med 1996; 335:1514–1521.

85. Gucalp R. Management of the febrile neutropenic patient with cancer. Oncology 1991; 5:137–144.

86. Chang JC, Gross HM. Neoplastic fever responds to adequate dose of naproxen. J Clin Oncol 1985;3:552–558.

87. Burke MB, Wilkes GM, Berg DB, Bean CK, Ingwersen K. Cancer Chemotherapy: A Nursing Process Approach. Boston: Jones and Bartlett, 1991.

88. Finkbiner KL, Ernst TF. Drug therapy management of the febrile neutropenic cancer patient. Cancer Pract 1993;1:295–304.

89. Rogers AG. Considering histamine release in prescribing opioid analgesics. J Pain Symptom Manage 1991;6:44.

90. Coyle N, Cherny N, Portenoy R. Pharmacologic management of cancer pain. In: McGuire DB, Henke Yarbro C, Ferrell B, eds. Cancer Pain Management, 2nd ed. Boston: Jones and Bartlett, 1995:89–130.

91. Waller A, Hershkowitz M, Adunsky A. The effect of intravenous fluid infusion on blood and urine parameters of hydration and on state of consciousness in terminal cancer patients. Am J Hospice Palliat Care 1994;11:22–37.

92. Fainsinger RL. Rehydration in palliative care. Palliat Med 1996;10:165–166.

93. Takata Y, Kurihara J, Suzuki S, Okubo Y,

Kato H. A rabbit model for evaluation of chlorpromazine-induced orthostatic hypotension. Biol Pharm Bull 1999;22:457–462.

94. Gates LK, Cameron AJ, Nagorney DM, Goellner JR, Farley DR. Primary leiomyosarcoma of the liver mimicking liver abscess. Am J Gastroenterol 1995;90:649–652.

95. Tuckett RP, Wei JY. Response to an itch-producing substance in cat. II. Cutaneous receptor populations with unmyelinated axons. Brain Res 1987;413:95–103.

96. Deaner P. Thalidomide for distressing night sweats in advanced malignant disease. Palliat Med 1998;12:208–209.

97. Quella SK, Loprinzi CL, Barton DL, Knost JA, Sloan JA, LaVasseur BI, Swan D, Krupp KR, Miller KD, Notovny PJ. Evaluation of soy phytoestrogens for the treatment of hot flashes in breast cancer survivors: A North Central Cancer Group Trial. J Clin Oncol 2000;18(5):1068–1074.

98. Stearns V, Isaacs C, Rowland J, Crawford J, Ellis MJ, Kramer R, Lawrence W, Hanfelt JJ, Haynes DF. A pilot trial assessing the efficacy of paroxetine hydrochloride (Paxil) in controlling hot flashes in breast cancer survivors. Ann Oncol 2000;11(1):17–22.

99. Loprinzi CL, Pisansky TM, Fonseca R, Sloan JA, et al. Pilot evaluation of venlafaxine hydrochloride for the therapy of hot flashes in cancer survivors. J Clin Oncol 1998;16(7):2377–2381.

100. Petit J. Alternative medicine. Black cohosh. Clin Rev 2000;10(4):117–121.

101. Lisle E. Therapeutic efficacy and safety of *Cimicifuga racemosa* for gynecologic disorders. Adv Ther 1998;15(1):45–53.

18 Neurological Disturbances

JUDITH A. PAICE

Four days before he died, he had seizures, 3 days of hell, didn't rest for 3 days and nights. I feel badly about the end, it wasn't handled well. He died in the hospital.

—A spouse

Myoclonus and spasms are frequently seen in palliative care settings. Seizures, although seen less frequently, can also occur. Astute palliative care clinicians can prevent some of these disorders and treat those that cannot be prevented. Patient and family involvement is mandatory since comfort and safety issues are prevalent with all three syndromes.

SEIZURES

Of the many neurological disorders that occur in advanced disease, seizures are the most frightening. This fear exists for the patient and for their caregivers. Furthermore, seizures can be exhausting for the patient, eliminating the few energy reserves that might be better spent on quality activities. Therefore, seizures must be prevented whenever possible. When prevention is not feasible, all attempts should be made to limit the extent of the seizure and ensure safety measures to prevent trauma during these episodes.

Seizures occur when a large number of neurons discharge abnormally.[1] This abnormal discharge produces involuntary paroxysmal behavioral changes. There are two types of seizure, including primary (also called generalized) and focal (also called partial). Primary seizures involve large parts of the brain and include both grand mal and petit mal types. Focal seizures are isolated to specific regions of the brain, and symptoms reflect the area of disturbance.[1] For example, Jacksonian motor seizures result from abnormal discharge in the motor cortex. These patients may have involuntary twitching of muscle groups, usually on the contralateral side of the body. If the tumor is located in the left motor cortex (anterior to the central sulcus), the activity is seen on the right side of the body. Often, activity begins in one area and spreads throughout that side of the body as abnormal discharge spreads to nearby cortical neurons. Patients generally remain conscious unless the abnormal cortical discharge spreads to the opposite hemisphere. In the palliative care setting, there are many potential causes of seizure activity.

Causes of Seizures

Careful consideration of the many causes of seizure activity must be included in the assessment of patients at the end of life, whether the patient has demonstrated seizure activity or not. This allows prevention whenever possible. Primary or metastatic neoplasms to the brain are common causes of seizures in palliative care, as are pre-existing seizure disorders.[1] Medications, including phenothiazines, butyrophenones, and tricyclic antidepressants, can lower the seizure threshold. Other medication-related causes of seizures include metabolites (e.g., normeperidine), preservatives within these compounds (e.g., sodium bisulfite), or the abrupt discontinuation of certain drugs (e.g., benzodiazepines).[2–5] Additional causes of seizures at the end of life include metabolic disorders, infection, stroke, hemorrhage, oxygen deprivation, and some very rare paraneoplastic syndromes (Table 18–1).[1,6]

Primary or Metastatic Brain Tumors. Brain tumors can result in either primary generalized or focal seizures. Seizures occur in approximately 25% of those with brain metastases.[7] Patients with malignancies known to metastasize to the brain, such as breast, lung, hypernephroma, and melanoma, should be considered at risk for seizures. Leukemias and lymphomas are also known to produce infiltrates in the brain. Multiple metastases or brain and leptomeningeal disease are more commonly associated with seizures.[7] The tumor location, size, and histology dictate whether seizures may result and the resulting symptoms associated with the seizure.

Medications. Medications can lead to seizures in the palliative care setting through several mechanisms. Medications such as the phenothiazines, butyrophenones, and tricyclic antidepressants can place patients at risk by lowering the seizure threshold. These agents should be used cautiously in patients with intracranial tumors or infection. There are reports of patients developing seizures due to fluoroquinolones, including ofloxacin and ifosfamide (more likely if serum creatinine is elevated and the patient has had prior treatment with cisplatin), as well as cephalosporins and monobactams.[8]

In very high doses, any opioid can lead to seizures. Several opioids are associated with much higher risk due to their metabolites that cause seizures. Meperidine is converted to normeperidine during metabolism. Individuals with renal dysfunction cannot excrete normeperidine efficiently; the metabolite then accumulates in the blood-

Table 18–1. Causes of Seizures in Palliative Care

Primary or metastatic neoplasm to the brain
Preexisting seizure disorder
Medications
Lower seizure threshold
Metabolites
Preservatives, antioxidants, or other additives
Abstinence
Metabolic disorders
Infection
Trauma
Strokes and hemorrhage
Paraneoplastic syndromes

stream and leads to seizures.[5] Therefore, the clinical practice guidelines developed by the Agency for Health Care Policy and Research for cancer pain strongly discourage the use of meperidine in any patient, a practice long known to those in palliative care.[4] These guidelines also discourage the use of propoxyphene (the weak opioid in Darvon) in persons with cancer due to the metabolite norpropoxyphene.[4]

More recently, morphine has been found to be metabolized to morphine-3-glucuronide and morphine-6-glucuronide. Morphine-3-glucuronide may produce adverse effects, including hyperalgesia (elevated pain intensity) and seizure in patients unable to excrete it efficiently.[9–11] Clinically, patients respond acceptably to morphine for the first day or two, then develop symptoms after the metabolite has accumulated. Morphine-6-glucuronide is a potent analgesic. Another opioid, tramadol, has been associated with seizure risk, especially when taken with other drugs that lower the seizure threshold.

Compounds added to medications to preserve the drug or prevent its breakdown (such as sodium bisulfite) are normally present in extremely small amounts. However, when high doses of a drug, usually opioids, are needed to treat severe pain, the concomitant dose of these additives increases. In this setting, there have been rare reports of seizures.[2] Using preservative-free solutions when administering high doses of any agent may prevent this activity. Hagen and Swanson[3] report a syndrome of opioid hyperexcitability that progressed to seizures in five patients with high-dose infusions. Parenteral midazolam infusion was used to treat the seizures, the patients were rotated to alternative opioids (including levorphanol and methadone), and aggressive supportive care was provided during the episodes.

Rapid cessation of various drugs can lead to seizure activity in the palliative care setting. Often, this occurs when staff are unaware that a patient uses certain medications and, as a result, these drugs are not provided when patients are hospitalized or unable to independently dispense their own drugs. Benzodiazepines, barbiturates, and baclofen are the most common drugs associated with seizures during abstinence.[1] This also can occur when the patient abuses these compounds or alcohol and the staff or family is unaware. Alcohol abuse often is underrecognized in the palliative care setting.[12]

Other Causes of Seizures in Palliative Care. Infection within the brain, as may be seen in persons with human immunodeficiency virus (HIV) or acquired immunodeficiency syndrome (AIDS), can lead to seizure activity.[6] The syndrome of inappropriate antidiuretic hormone, associated with lung cancer and other malignancies, can result in increased water and sodium content within the cells.[7] The resultant swelling of neuronal cells within the brain causes increased intracranial pressure (ICP). Anoxia deprives the brain of needed nutrients, resulting in an inability to drive sodium out of neuronal tissue. Water follows into the cells, creating increased ICP. Hyponatremia (<130 mEq/l) can also lead to mental status changes and seizures, especially when of rapid onset.

Assessment

Conduct a thorough history from the patient and caregiver to ascertain any symptoms existing with the onset of the seizure, the specific type of seizure activity, and whether there was any aura immediately prior to the seizure.[1] Headache, nausea, and projectile vomiting are associated with increased ICP and can occur immediately prior to seizure activity.[7] The family may relate a staring-type behavior, where the patient does not respond to stimuli for a brief moment.

The past medical history might reveal a seizure disorder. Review all drugs recently added to the plan of care for agents that might lower the seizure threshold or produce metabolites. Question whether the patient recently discontinued a drug, including recreational drugs. If the patient is currently taking anticonvulsants or corticosteroids for seizures and increased ICP, determine if there might be reasons that the drugs were not ingested or absorbed. These might include compliance issues or nausea and vomiting.

Often, the clinician may not witness the seizure and must rely on the observation and memory of family members and caregivers. Assist family members in differentiating between seizures and myoclonus (see following section) or altered level of consciousness due to other etiologies. A thorough exam is indicated, with attention to bruises and other signs of trauma. If these occur, additional teaching for family and caregivers regarding safety measures is warranted.

Measuring serum levels of anticonvulsants may be indicated to insure that the drug is adequately absorbed.[1] Dose adjustments may be done empirically based on the patient's condition. Electroencephalography may be used to identify the site of abnormal discharge. Brain lesions may be scanned using computed tomography or magnetic resonance imaging.

Treatment

Anticonvulsants are used when patients have demonstrated seizures (Table 18–2). The prophylactic use of anticonvulsants in patients who have not had a seizure is controversial. Only in the case of brain metastases from melanoma has prophylactic anticonvulsant therapy demonstrated benefit. The potential benefits must be weighed against the side effects associated with these agents.

Table 18–2. Prophylactic Pharmacological Management of Seizures

Drug	Adult Dose	Adverse Effects	Comments
Phenytoin (Dilantin) Tablets Capsules Suspension Parenteral	Loading dose: 5 mg/kg po q 3 h × 3 doses (loading dose not to be used in patients with renal or hepatic disease) Maintenance: 5 mg/kg po	Nystagmus, ataxia, slurred speech, mental confusion, Stevens-Johnson syndrome Too rapid IV injection (>50 mg/min) can result in cardiac toxicity	Usual serum level 10–20 mcg/ml (or 10–20 mg/l or 40–80 μmol/l)
Carbamazepine (Tegretol) Tablets Suspension	400 mg/day: Tablet: 200 mg bid Suspension: 1 teaspoon qid Maximum dose: 1600 mg/24 h	Aplastic anemia, agranulocytosis Patients with known sensitivity to tricyclic antidepressants may be hypersensitive to carbamazepine.	Periodic blood counts and liver function tests indicated Therapeutic plasma levels 4–12 mcg/ml
Valproic acid (Depakene) Capsules Syrup	15 mg kg daily, increasing weekly in 5–10 mg increments Syrup can be given rectally by a red rubber catheter 250–500 mg tid	Hepatic failure, coagulopathies, nausea, vomiting, sedation Chewing may produce irritation of the mouth and throat.	Therapeutic plasma levels 50–100 mcg/ml
Divalproex sodium (Depakote) Capsules Sprinkles Tablets	Same dosing for valproic acid and divalproex, although peaks and troughs may differ		
Phenobarbital Tablets Elixir Parenteral	Oral: 60–200 mg/day Parenteral: 3–4 mg/kg q 24 h continuous SQ infusion	Sedation, paradoxical excitation	—
Midazolam (Versed) Parenteral	1–3 mg/h continuous SQ or IV infusion	Sedation, respiratory depression if overdose	Antagonist, flumazenil, can result in seizures. Use same extreme caution as when giving naloxone for suspected opioid overdose.

SQ = subcutaneous; IV = intravenous.

Table 18–3. Acute Treatment of Seizures

Drug	Dose
Diazepam (Valium)	5–10 mg slow IV push (stop other infusions to prevent incompatibility problems) or 5–10 mg IM every 5–10 min if no IV access, can also use diazepam (Diastat) rectal gel, usually 10 mg per rectum
Fosphenytoin (Cerebyx)	15–20 mg phenytoin equivalents/kg IV loading dose
Lorazepam (Ativan)	1 mg/min up to 5 mg
Midazolam (Versed)	0.02–0.10 mg/kg continuous hourly infusion
Phenobarbital	20 mg/kg IV at a rate of 100 mg/min
Phenytoin (Dilantin)	Acute treatment: 20 mg/kg IV infusion over 20–30 min. An additional 5–10 mg/kg can be given if seizures persist. However, IV injections can cause severe local reactions, including edema, pain, and discoloration.

IV = intravenous; IM = intramuscular.

The most common anticonvulsants used in the United States to prevent seizures are phenytoin, carbamazepine, valproate, and phenobarbital (Table 18–2).[13] Newer anticonvulsants, such as gabapentin, vigabatrin, and lamotrigine, have not been studied in the palliative care setting.[7] Agents used during a seizure include diazepam, lorazepam, midazolam, phenytoin, and phenobarbital (Table 18–3).[13]

A particular challenge in palliative care is the administration of these drugs when the patient is unable to take oral medications. The intramuscular route can be used for some (diazepam and phenobarbitol), but since this route is painful and absorption is unpredictable, its use should be reserved for situations when no other access is practical or possible. Diazepam is available in a rectal gel. Doses are 200 mcg/kg body weight, rounded down to the next available unit dose (10 mg, 15 mg, and 20 mg unit doses for adults) in debilitated patients.[14] Pentobarbital (used more commonly in Canada and Europe) is available in rectal formulations. Intravenous phenytoin can lead to the purple glove syndrome, a potentially serious local complication including edema, discoloration, and pain distal to the injection site.[15] Fosphenytoin is a newer compound that has an advantage in palliative care as it can be given subcutaneously (by either intermittent injection or infusion) for prevention or treatment of seizures.[14] Dosing is based on phenytoin equivalents, generally 5 to 10 mg phenytoin equivalent/kg. Little research has compared the efficacy of these agents, particularly in the palliative care setting. The choice of agent is often based on the availability of the drug, comfort level of the practitioner, ability to use nonoral routes, and other factors. Because most medications are administered by nonprofessional caregivers in the home, often elderly spouses of aged patients, it is best to keep the drug regimen simple.[16]

Many patients with seizure disorders will also be taking dexamethasone. Dexamethasone is technically not an anticonvulsant, yet this compound is critical when intracranial lesions that might increase ICP are present.[7] Although most texts suggest qid dosing, the long half-life of dexamethasone allows daily dosing with adequate serum levels maintained throughout the 24-hour period.[13] Of additional concern is the interaction between phenytoin and dexamethasone. Phenytoin can decrease the bioavailability of dexamethasone by as much as 20%. Additionally, dexamethasone inhibits the metabolism of phenytoin, reducing the anticonvulsant effect of this drug. Thus, extreme care must be exercised when adding or titrating either drug when using combinations.[13] Phenytoin can alter plasma levels of several drugs (Table 18–4). In the palliative care settng, if a patient decides to stop all corticosteroids, the professional must evaluate the likelihood of developing seizures. Prophylactic therapy must be considered.

Status epilepticus is a seizure that persists longer than 5 minutes or repeated seizures without a return to consciousness between each episode.[1] This is considered a neuro-oncological emergency. Clear the airway, ensure adequate perfusion, give glucose (usually 50 ml of a 50% solution), evaluate electrolytes, and administer intravenous benzodiazepine (such as diazepam or lorazepam), followed by a loading dose of intravenous phenytoin. The Veterans Administration Cooperative Trial of Status Epilepticus revealed response rates during first-line treatment as follows: lorazepam 64.9%, phenobarbitol 58.2%, diazepam plus phenytoin 55.8%, and phenytoin alone 43.6%.[17] These results suggest that lorazepam should be the first drug of choice. If the seizure is not relieved in 5 to 7 minutes, add phenytoin or fosphenytoin. If recurrent, continuous infusion of phenobarbital or diazepam is indicated. In extreme cases, barbiturate anesthesia, neuromuscular blockade, and propofol may be indicated.

Table 18–4. Drugs that Interact with Phenytoin

Drugs that may increase phenytoin serum levels
Alcohol, amiodarone, choramphenicol, chlordiazepoxide, diazepam, dicumarol, disulfiram, estrogens, H_2 antagonists, halothane, isoniazide, methylphenidate, phenothiazines, phenylbutazone, salicylates, succinimides, sulfonamides, tolbutamide, trazodone
Drugs that may decrease phenytoin serum levels
Carbamazepine, chronic alcohol abuse, reserpine, sucralfate, antacids with calcium (should not be taken with phenytoin but at a different time)
Drugs that may have reduced efficacy due to phenytoin
Corticosteroids (including dexamethasone), coumarin anticoagulants, digitoxin, doxycycline, estrogens, furosemide, oral contraceptives, quinidine, rifampin, theophylline, vitamin D

Patient and Family Education

Witnessing a seizure can be extremely frightening for family members and caregivers. Preparation is critical. Explain that restraining the patient or attempting to place objects in the mouth can lead to significant harm. Educate family members to move items out of the way that might cause trauma and to get the patient to lay on one side if possible. Caregivers may be given information regarding the jaw lift technique if the airway is compromised. Pillows placed around the bed, between the patient and the siderails (if a hospital-style bed is in use), and around the room can be quickly positioned to prevent trauma. Caution family members to refrain from feeding or providing fluids until the patient is fully alert and able to swallow. However, if the patient has grossly unstable blood sugar levels and is prone to developing hypoglycemia, candy, glucose, juice, or other sources of glucose can be given only if the patient is able to swallow. Glucagon can also be given subcutaneously. Inform family members that loss of continence is common during a seizure and does not imply that the patient is not able to control these functions at other times. Encourage them to assist the patient while considering the patient's ability and dignity.

To help recovery after a seizure, the patient may benefit from reduced stimulation. Lower the lights, reduce the sound of televisions or radios, and speak softly and reassuringly. Assess for pain and treat accordingly. Relaxation exercises also may be helpful. Often, patients will sleep for several hours after the seizure.

Case Report: Complexities of Seizure Management

A 30-year-old man with HIV/AIDS and cryptosporidium in the brain. Despite aggressive anticonvulsant therapy, the patient experienced frequent seizures, which resulted in severe headache. The baseline headache was generally well controlled with transdermal fentanyl. The pain after seizures was controlled by oral liquid morphine; however, the patient was requesting large amounts of morphine. During assessment by the hospice nurse and social worker at the patient's home, it became clear that the seizures were associated with cocaine use by the patient. In an objective, nonjudgmental manner, they described the risk of lowered seizure threshold with cocaine and the need to be compliant with anticonvulsant therapies. They engaged the assistance of siblings and friends living nearby to limit exposure to recreational drugs and provide distraction. They also described strategies to help provide safety and comfort during a seizure and discouraged calls to 911 (this had created significant chaos). The patient lived just a few more weeks with reduced, although not completely eliminated, use of cocaine and episodes of seizures.

MYOCLONUS

Myoclonus consists of sudden, uncontrollable, nonrhythmic jerking, usually of the extremities.[1] Frequently seen in the palliative care setting, myoclonus can be exhausting and can progress to more severe neurological dysfunction. Early identification and rapid treatment are critical.

Causes of Myoclonus

In the palliative care setting, myoclonus is most often associated with opioids. The prevalence of opioid-induced myoclonus ranges greatly, from 2.7% to 87%.[18] Nocturnal myoclonus is common and often precedes opioid-induced myoclonus.[1,19] The precise cause of opioid-induced myoclonus is unknown; however, several mechanisms have been proposed.[3] High doses of opioids result in the formation of neuroexcitatory metabolites. The best characterized are morphine-3-glucuronide and morphine-6-glucouronide. Serum and cerebrospinal fluid levels as well as the ratios of these metabolites are elevated in patients receiving morphine for cancer and nonmalignant pain.[9] Hyperalgesia is particularly associated with morphine-3-glucuronide, although other opioids with no known metabolites have also been shown to produce myoclonus.[11]

Opioids given in high doses may result in myoclonus. Bruera and Pereira[20] reported the development of acute confusion, restlessness, myoclonus, hallucinations, and hyperalgesia due to a high dose of 5000 mcg subcutaneous fentanyl.[20] These symptoms were successfully treated with 0.2 mg intravenous naloxone.

Other reported causes of myoclonus include surgery to the brain,[21] placement of an intrathecal catheter,[22] AIDS dementia,[6] hypoxia,[23] chlorambucil,[24] and a paraneoplastic syndrome.[25] This paraneoplastic syndrome is rare, occurring in fewer than 1% of people with cancer. The etiology of the paraneoplastic syndrome can also be viral and is believed to be immunologically mediated. Symptoms of this paraneoplastic (also called opsoclonus-myoclonus) syndrome include myoclonus, opsoclonus, ataxia, and encephalopathic features.[26] Treatment of the underlying tumor or infection and immunosuppression are possible treatments.[25,26]

Assessment

An accurate history from the patient and family is essential. An analogy to help patients describe the symptoms is to compare the jerking to the feeling that often happens when one is close to falling asleep (a common condition called *nocturnal myoclonus*). The difference is that myoclonus is usually continuous. Physical exam will reveal jerking of the extremities, which is uncontrolled by movement or other activities. Jerking can be induced by single or repeated tapping of a muscle group.

Treatment

Opioid rotation is the primary treatment of myoclonus, particularly if the patient is receiving morphine and has renal dysfunction.[18] Different opioids have different side effect profiles, which may produce less risk of myoclonus. In addition, cross-tolerance is not complete. Therefore, lower doses may be used. Methadone has been used as an alternative agent with success,[27] although other opioids may be easier to titrate. Strategies, such as adding adjuvant analgesics, that reduce the necessary amount of opioid could reduce or eliminate myoclonus.

Little research is available regarding agents used to reduce myoclonic jerking. Benzodiazepines, including clonazepam, diazepam, and midazolam, have been recommended.[18,28] Muscle relaxants, such as dantrolene 50 to 100 mg/day, have also been reported to be successful.[29] This reduces spasticity but also reduces muscle strength. Therefore, dantrolene is not recommended in ambulatory patients. Furthermore, dantrolene can cause hepatotoxicity.[30] The antispasmodic baclofen has been used to treat myoclonus due to intraspinal opioid administration.[31]

Patient and Family Education

Safety measures are essential, as are interventions designed to reduce fatigue during myoclonus. Use padding around bed rails and assistive devices if the patient is ambulatory. Provide a calm, relaxing environment. Pain assessment is critical as opioids are rotated since equianalgesic conversions are approximations and wide variability exists. Therefore, patients and family members are encouraged to track pain intensity as opioids are titrated to provide optimal relief.

SPASTICITY

Spasticity is a movement disorder that results in a partial or complete loss of supraspinal control of spinal cord function. Patients may exhibit involuntary movement, abnormal posture, rigidity, and exaggerated reflexes. Spasticity may interfere with all aspects of life by limiting mobility, disturbing sleep, and causing pain.[30] Spasticity is often associated with advanced multiple sclerosis, spinal cord trauma, tumors of the spinal cord, meningitis, and other infections. In a study of 2104 patients with non-traumatic spasticity seen in a regional neuroscience center in the United Kingdom, 17.8% had multiple sclerosis, 16.4% had neoplasm, and 4.1% had motor neuron disease.[32]

Assessment

Patients will describe a gradual onset of loss of muscle tone, followed by resistance and jerking when muscles are flexed. A recent history of urinary tract infection, decubitus ulcer, constipation, or pain may immediately predate the onset, or increased episodes, of spasticity.

Physical exam will yield resistance and spasticity when doing passive limb movement.[30] The faster the passive movement, the more pronounced the effect. Reflexes may be hyperactive, particularly in the affected area. Bruises are common as patients inadvertently and uncontrollably move their limbs, resulting in trauma.

Management

The standard therapies for reducing spasticity include oral baclofen, a gamma-aminobutyric acid-B agonist. Baclofen is generally started with lower doses, 5 to 10 mg/day, and titrated upward gradually using tid or qid dosing. Although effective for some patients, higher doses are often necessary, frequently resulting in cognitive changes and dizziness. For this reason, intrathecal baclofen has been administered with good results.[30] Those in palliative care must weigh the benefits of intrathecal baclofen therapy given the patient's prognosis, the availability of skilled clinicians to administer the therapy, cost, and other factors.

Dantrolene diminishes the force of the contraction. Start at 25 mg daily and increase by 25 mg increments in divided doses every 4 to 7 days.[14] The contents can be mixed with liquids if the patient is unable to swallow capsules. Marijuana, and its active ingredient delta-9-tetrahydrocannabinol (THC), has been described by patients as useful in the relief of spinal cord spasticity.[33–35] Although not approved for this purpose, there is general agreement within the medical community that the treatment of spasticity is a legitimate use of THC. However, despite data supporting its safety and the availability of a commercially prepared product (Marinol), some patients, family members, and health care professionals continue to feel uneasy regarding the use of this compound.

Patient and Family Education

Patients and their caregivers should be educated about factors that may worsen spasticity, including constipation, urinary tract infection, pressure ulcers, fatigue, and psychosocial concerns.[30] Strategies to prevent and relieve these conditions should be clearly communicated, and early communication regarding their onset should be encouraged. When spasticity occurs, the patient and family members must understand the rationale for drug therapy. Nonpharmacological therapy also may be helpful. Family members may be encouraged to gently massage the affected extremities, although this may produce increased spasticity in some patients. Repositioning, heat, and range-of-motion exercises have been described by patients as being helpful. As with other neurological disorders, safety measures are imperative. Padding wheelchairs, bed rails, and any other furniture that might come in contact with spastic extremities will reduce trauma.

CONCLUSION

Neurological disorders, including seizures, myoclonus, and spasticity, create fear, reduce energy levels, increase pain, and can complicate the course of a patient's illness. The goal in palliative care is prevention whenever possible. When not possible, early diagnosis and treatment are critical. Knowledge of pharmacotherapy is essential, including agents that might precipitate these disorders, drugs used to treat these syndromes, as well as drug interactions that might occur in the palliative care setting. As with all aspects of palliative care, the patient and family are the center of care. Empowering them through education and support is extremely important. The interdisciplinary approach exemplified by palliative care is key.

REFERENCES

1. Gilroy J. Basic Neurology. New York: Pergamon Press, 1990.
2. Gregory RE, Grossman S, Sheidler VR. Grand mal seizures associated with high-dose intravenous morphine infusions: incidence and possible etiology. Pain 1992;51:255–258.
3. Hagen N, Swanson R. Strychnine-like multifocal myoclonus and seizures in extremely high-dose opioid administration: treatment strategies. J Pain Symptom Manage 1997;14:51–58.
4. Jacox A, Carr DB, Payne R, et al. Management of Cancer Pain. Clinical Practice Guideline 9. AHCPR Publication 94-0592. Rockville, MD: Agency for Health Care Policy and Research, US Department of Health and Human Services, Public Health Service.
5. Kaiko RF, Foley KM, Gralinski PY, et al. Central nervous system excitatory effects of meperidine in cancer patients. Ann Neurol 1983; 13:180–185.
6. Maher J, Choudhri S, Halliday W, Power C, Nath A. AIDS dementia complex with generalized myoclonus. Mov Disord 1997;12:593–597.
7. Ziai W, Hagen NA. Headache and other manifestations of intracranial pathology. In: Berger A, Portenoy RK, Weissman DE, et al. eds. Principles and Practice of Supportive Oncology. Philadelphia: Lippincott-Raven, 1998:435–447.
8. Walton GD, Hon JK, Mulpur TG. Ofloxacin-induced seizures. Ann Pharmacother 1997;31:1475–1477.
9. Sjogren P, Thunedborg LP, Christrup L, Hansen SH, Franks J. Is development of hyperalgesia, allodynia and myoclonus related to morphine metabolism during long-term administration? Six case histories. Acta Anaesthesiol Scand 1998;42:1070–1075.
10. Tiseo PJ, Thaler HT, Lapin J, Inturrisi CE, Portenoy RK, Foley KM. Morphine-6-glucuronide concentrations and opioid-related side effects: a survey in cancer patients. Pain 1995;61: 47–54.
11. Gong QL, Hedner J, Bjorkman R, Hedner T. Morphine-3-glucuronide may functionally antagonize morphine-6-glucuronide induced antinociception and ventilatory depression in the rat. Pain 1992;48:249–255.
12. Bruera E, Moyano J, Siefert L, Fainsinger RL, Hanson J, Suarez-Almazor M. The frequency of alcoholism among patients with pain due to terminal cancer. J Pain Symptom Manage 1995; 10:599–603.
13. Stringer JL. Drugs for seizure disorders (epilepsies). In: Brody TM, Larner J, Minneman KP, Neu HC, eds. Human Pharmacology: Molecular to Clinical. St. Louis: Mosby, 1994:351–361.
14. United States Pharmacopeial Convention. Drug Information for the Health Care Professional, Vol I. Englewood, CO. Micromedix, 1999.
15. O'Brien TJ, Cascino GD, So EL, Hanna DR. Incidence and clinical consequence of the purple glove syndrome in patients receiving intravenous phenytoin. Neurology 1998;51:1034–1039.
16. Ferrell BR. Home care. In: Berger A, Portenoy RK, Weissman DE, eds. Principles and Practice of Supportive Oncology. Philadelphia: Lippincott-Raven, 1998:709–715.
17. Bleck TP. Management approaches to prolonged seizures and status epilepticus. Epilepsia 1999;40 (Suppl):59–63.
18. Mercadante S. Pathophysiology and treatment of opioid-related myoclonus in cancer patients. Pain 1998;74:5–9.
19. Nunez-Olarte JM. Opioid-induced myoclonus. Eur J Palliat Care 1995;2:146–150.
20. Bruera E, Pereira J. Acute neuropsychiatric findings in a patient receiving fentanyl for cancer pain. Pain 1997;69:199–201.
21. Nishigaya K, Kaneko M, Nagaseki Y, Nukui H. Palatal myoclonus induced by extirpation of a cerebellar astrocytoma. Case report. J Neurosurg 1998;88:1107–1110.
22. Ford B, Pullman SL, Khandji A, Goodman R. Spinal myoclonus induced by an intrathecal catheter. Mov Disord 1997;12:1042–1045.
23. Werhann KJ, Brown P, Thompson PD, Marsden CD. The clinical features and prognosis of chronic posthypoxic myoclonus. Mov Disord 1997;12:216–220.
24. Wyllie AR, Bayliff CD, Kovacs MJ. Myoclonus due to chlorambucil in two adults with lymphoma. Ann Pharmacother 1997;31:171–174.
25. Pranzatelli MR. The immunopharmacology of the opsoclonus-myoclonus syndrome. Clin Neuropharmacol 1996;19:1–47.
26. Batchelor TT, Platten M, Hochberg FH. Immunoadsorption therapy for paraneoplastic syndromes. J Neurooncol 1998;40:131–136.
27. Sjogren P. Clinical implications of morphine metabolites. In: Portenoy RK, Bruera E, eds. Topics in Palliative Care, Vol 1. New York: Oxford University Press. 1997:163–176.
28. Eisele JH, Grisby EJ, Dea G. Clonazepam treatment of myoclonic contractions associated with high-dose opioids: case report. Pain 1992;49:213–222.
29. Mercadante S. Dantrolene treatment of opioid-induced myoclonus. Anesth Analg 1995;81: 1307–1308.
30. Gianino JM, York MM, Paice JA. Intrathecal Drug Therapy for Spasticity and Pain. New York: Springer, 1996.
31. Krames E, Lyons A, Taylor P, Gershow J, Kenefick T, Glassberg A. Continuous infusion of spinally administered narcotics for the relief of pain due to malignant disorders. Cancer 1985;56: 696–702.
32. Moore AP, Blumhardt LD. A prospective survey of the causes of non-traumatic spastic paraparesis and tetraparesis in 585 patients. Spinal Cord 1997;35:361–367.
33. Voth EA, Schwartz RH. Medicinal applications of delta-9-tetrahydrocannabinol and marijuana. Ann Intern Med 1997;126:791–798.
34. Taylor HG. Analysis of the medical use of marijuana and its societal implications. J Am Pharm Assoc (Washington) 1998;38:220–227.
35. Consroe P, Musty R, Rein J, Tillery W, Pertwee R. The perceived effects of smoked cannabis on patients with multiple sclerosis. Eur Neurol 1997;38:44–48.

19 Anxiety and Depression

JEANNIE V. PASACRETA, PAMELA A. MINARIK, and LESLIE NIELD-ANDERSON

My mother was diagnosed with breast cancer when I was 13; she was 40 years old, and she died 2 years later. I have lived in fear that I would go through the same experience, and sure enough, here I am, 42 years old and in a similar situation. I am so fearful of going through what she did that I can't sleep at night. . . . I am anxious and afraid to even think about dying, yet that is all I can think about at times.

—A patient

To palliate can be defined as the process of alleviating symptoms without curing; therefore, palliative care is not reserved for the period of terminal care as is often believed. Palliative care is active and compassionate care, which is directed primarily toward symptom management and improving the quality of life for the patient and family. Any chronic medical condition, particularly when the outcome of cure is not possible, often carries a large burden of emotional consequences. Involvement with a complicated and fragmented health care delivery system, the need for episodic treatment, remissions and exacerbations of acute and uncomfortable symptoms, family separation, financial burden, functional limitations, and role disruptions are but a few of the issues that characterize the lives of many patients with chronic and progressive illnesses.

The goal of this chapter is to provide information regarding the assessment and treatment of anxiety and depression among individuals who are faced with chronic illness and to delineate psychosocial interventions that are effective at minimizing these troubling symptoms. Practical guidelines regarding patient management and identifying patients who may require formal psychiatric consultation are offered. As psychiatric consultation liaison nurses who work primarily in nonpsychiatric settings, the authors have been consistently impressed by the lack of knowledge held by nursing and medical staff regarding key signs and symptoms that characterize depression and anxiety in the medically ill. Often, young patients with particularly poor prognoses, who elicit anxiety and sadness from staff, rather than their objectively depressed or anxious counterparts, are referred for psychiatric evaluation. Among depressed and/or anxious patients who are referred for evaluation, the decision to intervene with psychotherapy or pharmacological agents is often based largely on the style, philosophy, educational background, and past experience of individual clinicians. Often, a diagnosis of clinical anxiety or depression is ruled out if the symptoms seem reactive and appropriate to the situation or are viewed as organic in nature. Patients who exhibit depressive or anxious symptoms not considered severe enough to classify for "psychiatric" status are often not offered psychotherapeutic services, and the natural history of their symptoms is rarely monitored over time. The lack of attention to assessment and treatment of depression and anxiety among the medically ill may lead to ongoing dysphoria, family conflict, noncompliance with treatment, increased length of hospitalization, persistent worry, and suicidal ideation, to name just a few risks. Because depression and anxiety are common among individuals with chronic illness, and particularly because they are often responsive to treatment, recognition of those afflicted is of unquestionable clinical relevance.

Patients, family, and professional caregivers need to be informed of the factors that affect psychological adjustment, the wide range of psychological responses that accompany chronic and progressive disease, and the efficacy of various modes of intervention at minimizing psychological distress and thus promoting adaptation.

CLINICAL COURSE OF ILLNESS

Acute stress has been described as a usual response to the diagnosis of a life-threatening chronic illness that occurs at transitional points in the disease process (beginning treatment, recurrence, treatment failure, disease progression).[1] The response is characterized by shock, disbelief, anxiety, depression, sleep and appetite disturbance, and difficulty performing activities of daily living. Under favorable circumstances, these psychological symptoms should resolve within a short period.[1,2] The time period is quite variable, but the general consensus is that once the crisis has passed and individuals know what to expect in terms of a treatment plan, psychological symptoms diminish.[1,3]

The stage of disease at the time of diagnosis and its clinical course, including medical treatments, recurrence, and prominent symptoms, impact the psychosocial profiles of individuals. To a large extent, these factors will determine the emotional issues that are most pressing at any given point. Patients who are diagnosed with late-stage disease or have aggressive illnesses with no hope for cure are often most vulnerable to psychological distress, particularly anxiety, depression, family problems, and physical discomfort.

Diagnostic Phase

The period from time of diagnosis through initiation of a treatment plan is characterized by medical evaluation, the development of new relationships with unfamiliar medical personnel, and the need to integrate a barrage of information that, at best, is frightening and confusing. Patients and families experience heightened responsibility, concern, and isolation during this period. They are particularly anxious and fearful when receiving initial information regarding diagnosis and treatment. Consequently, care should be taken by professionals to repeat information over several sessions and to inquire about patients' and families' understanding of facts and options.

Weisman and colleagues[2] described the first 100 days following a cancer diagnosis as the period of "existential plight."[2] Psychological distress varied according to patient diagnosis. Individuals with lung cancer who had predominantly late-stage disease were more distressed than individuals with early-stage disease, supporting the need for palliative care services directed toward psychological symptoms. During the diagnostic period, patient concerns focus on existential issues of life and death more than on concerns related to health, work, finances, religion, self, or relationships with family and friends. While it is unusual to observe extreme and sustained emotional reactions as the first response to diagnosis, it is important to assess the nature of early reactions as they are often predictive of later adaptation.[4,5] Early assessment by clinicians can help to identify individuals at risk for later adjustment problems or psychiatric disorders who are in the greatest need of ongoing psychosocial support.[2,6] The initial response to diagnosis may be profoundly influenced by a person's prior association with a particular disease.[7] Those with memories of close relatives with the same illness often demonstrate heightened distress, particularly if the relative died or had negative treatment experiences. During the diagnostic period, patients may search for explanations or causes for their disease and may struggle to give personal meaning to their experience. Since many clinicians are guarded about disclosing information until a firm diagnosis is established, patients may develop highly personal explanations, which can be inaccurate and provoke intensely negative emotions. Ongoing involvement and accurate information will minimize uncertainty and the development of maladaptive coping strategies based on erroneous beliefs.

While the literature substantiates the devastating emotional impact of a life-threatening chronic illness, it also is well documented that many individuals cope effectively. Positive coping strategies, such as taking action and finding favorable characteristics in the situation, have been reported to be effective.[8] Contrary to the beliefs of many clinicians, denial also has been found to assist patients in coping effectively,[9] unless sustained and used excessively to a point that it interferes with appropriate treatment.

Health care practitioners play an important role in monitoring and supporting psychosocial adjustment. With an awareness of the unique meaning the individual associates with the diagnosis, it is vital that practitioners keep patients informed and involved in their care. Even though patients may not be offered hope for cure, assisting them in maintaining comfort and control promotes adaptation and improved quality of life.

Recurrence and Progressive Disease

Development of a recurrence after a disease-free interval can be especially devastating for patients and those close to them. The point of recurrence often signals a shift into a period of disease progression and is clearly a time when palliative care services aimed at alleviating psychological symptoms are indicated. The medical workup is often difficult and anxiety-provoking;[10] psychosocial problems experienced at the time of diagnosis frequently resurface, often with greater intensity.[11,12] Shock and depression often accompany relapse and require individuals and their families to reevaluate the future. This period is a difficult one, during which patients may also experience pessimism, renewed preoccupation with death and dying, and feelings of helplessness and disenchantment with the medical system. Patients tend to be more guarded and cautious at this time and feel as if they are in limbo.[12] Silverfarb and colleagues[13] examined emotional distress in a cross-sectional study of 146 women with breast cancer at three points in the clinical course (diagnosis, recurrence, stage of disease progression). The point of recurrence was found to be the most distressing time, with an increase in depression, anxiety, and suicidal ideation. As a disease progresses, the person often reports an upsetting scenario that includes frequent pain, disability, increased dependence on others, and diminished functional ability, which often potentiates psychological symptoms.[11] Investigators studying quality of life in cancer patients have demonstrated a clear relationship between an individuals' perception of quality of life and the presence of discomfort.[14] As uncomfortable symptoms increase, perceived quality of life diminishes. Thus, an important goal in the psychosocial treatment of patients with advanced chronic illness focuses on symptom control.

An issue that repeatedly surfaces among patients, family members, and professional care providers deals with the use of aggressive treatment protocols in the presence of progressive disease. Often, patients and families request to participate in experimental protocols even when there is little likelihood of extending survival. Controversy continues about the efficacy of such therapies and the role health professionals can play in facilitating patients' choices about participating. These issues become even more important as changes in the health care system may limit payment for costly and highly technical treatments, such as bone marrow transplants. Structured dialogue with patients, family members, and care providers regarding treatment goals and expectations is essential for health care professionals to establish. Despite the existence of progressive illness, certain individuals may respond to investigational treatment with increased hope. Efforts to separate and clarify values, thoughts, and emotional reactions of care providers, patients, and families to these delicate issues is important if individualized care with attention to psychological symptoms is to be provided. Use of resources such as psychiatric consultation-liaison nurses, psychiatrists, social workers, and chaplains can be invaluable in assisting patients, family members, and staff to grapple with these issues in a meaningful and productive manner.

Terminal Disease and Dying

Once the terminal period has begun, it is usually not the fact of dying but the quality of dying that seems to be the overwhelming issue confronting the patient and family.[15,16] Continued palliative care into the terminal stage of cancer relieves physical and psychological symptoms, promotes comfort, and increases well-being. Often, patients and families who have received such services along the illness trajectory will be more open and accepting of palliative efforts in the final stage of life. In addition, it is important that nurses caring for the terminally ill recognize the emotional impact on themselves and attend to self-care.

Patients living in the final phase of any advanced chronic illness experience fears and anxiety related to uncertain future events, such as unrelieved pain, separation from loved ones, burden on family, and loss of control. Psychological maladjustment is more likely in persons confronting diminished life span, physical debilitation associated with functional limitation, and/or symptoms associated with toxic therapies for which there are not effective interventions.[14,17] Therapeutic interventions should be directed toward increasing patients' sense of control and self-efficacy within the context of functional decline and increased dependence. In addition, if patients so desire, it is often therapeutic to let them know that there is help available to discuss the existential concerns that often accompany terminal illness.

Personal values and beliefs, socioeconomic and cultural background, and religious belief systems influence patients' expectations about quality of life and palliative care. Cultural affiliation has a significant influence on perception to pain; for example, the findings of Bates and colleagues[18] indicate that the best predictors of pain intensity are ethnic group affiliation and locus of control style. For example, an individual's stoic attitude, which serves to minimize or negate discomfort, may be related to a cultural value learned and reinforced through years of family experiences. Similarly, an individual's highly emotional response to routine events may become exaggerated during the terminal phase of illness and not necessarily signal maladjustment but, rather, a cultural norm. Awareness of the family system's cultural, religious, ethnic, and socioeconomic background is important to the understanding of their beliefs, attitudes, practices, and behaviors related to illness and death. Cultural patterns play a significant role in determining how individuals and families cope with illness and death.[19,20]

Delirium, depression, suicidal ideation, and severe anxiety are among the most common psychiatric complications encountered in terminally ill cancer patients.[21] When severe, these problems require urgent and aggressive assessment and treatment by psychiatric personnel who can initiate pharmacological and psychotherapeutic treatment strategies. Psychiatric emergencies require the same rapid intervention as distressing physical symptoms and medical crises. In spite of the seemingly overwhelming nature of psychosocial responses along the chronic illness trajectory, most patients do indeed cope effectively. Periods of intense emotions, such as anxiety and depression, are not necessarily the same as maladaptive coping.

FACTORS THAT AFFECT PSYCHOLOGICAL ADJUSTMENT

Psychological responses to chronic illness vary widely and are influenced by many individual factors. A review of the literature points to key factors that may impact psychological adjustment and the occurrence and expression of anxiety and depression. Three of the most important factors are previous coping strategies and emotional stability, social support, and symptom distress. In addition, there are common medical conditions, treatments, and substances that may cause or intensify symptoms of anxiety and depression (Tables 19–1, 19–2).

Previous Coping Strategies and Emotional Stability

One of the most important predictors of psychological adjustment to chronic illness is the emotional stability and coping strategies used by the person prior to diagnosis. Individuals with a history of poor psychological adjustment and of clinically significant anxiety or depression are at highest risk for emotional decompensation[23] and should be monitored closely throughout all phases of treatment. This is particularly true for people with a history of major psychiatric syndromes and/or psychiatric hospitalization.[24]

Social Support

Social support has consistently been found to influence a person's psychosocial adjustment to chronic illness.[25] The ability and availability of significant others in dealing with diagnosis and treatment can significantly affect the patient's view of him- or herself and potentially the patient's survival.[26]

Individuals diagnosed with all types of life-threatening chronic disorder experience a heightened need for interpersonal support. Individuals who are able to maintain close connections with family and friends during the course of illness are more likely to cope effectively

Table 19–1. Common Medical Conditions Associated with Anxiety and Depression

Anxiety

- Endocrine disorders: hyper- and hypothyroidism, hyper- and hypoglycemia, Cushing's disease, carcinoid syndrome, pheochromocytoma
- Cardiovascular conditions: myocardial infarction, paroxysmal atrial tachycardia, angina pectoris, congestive heart failure, mitral valve prolapse, hypovolemia
- Metabolic conditions: hyperkalemia, hypertemia, hypogycemia, hyperthermia, anemia, hyponatremia
- Respiratory conditions: asthma, chronic obstructive pulmonary disease, pneumonia, pulmonary edema, pulmonary embolus, respiratory dependence, hypoxia
- Neoplasms: islet cell adenomas, pheochromocytoma
- Neurological conditions: akathisia, encephalopathy, seizure disorder,vertigo, mass lesion, postconcussion syndrome

Depression

- Cardiovascular: cardiovascular disease, congestive heart failure, myocardial infarct, cardiac arrhythmias
- Central nervous system: cerebrovascular accident, cerebral anoxia, Huntington's disease, subdural hematoma, Alzheimer's disease, human immunodeficiency virus (HIV), infection, dementia, carotid stenosis, dementia, temporal lobe epilepsy, multiple sclerosis, postconcussion, myasthenia gravis, narcolepsy, subarachnoid hemorrhage
- Autoimmune: rhematoid arthritis, polyarteritis nodosa
- Endocrine: hyperparathyroidism, hypothyroidism, diabetes mellitus, Cushing's disease, Addison's disease
- Other: alcoholism, anemia, systemic lupus erythematosus, Epstein-Barr virus, hepatitis, HIV infection, malignancies, pulmonary insufficiency, pancreatic and liver disease, syphilis, encephalitis, malnutrition

Source: Stoudemire (1996), reference 22; Fernandez et al. (1995), reference 44; Kurlowicz (1994), reference 45; Wise & Taylor (1990), reference 23.

with the disease than those who are not able to maintain such relationships.[27] This is especially true during the palliative care period.

Symptom Distress

The effects of treatment for a variety of chronic diseases as well as the impact of progressive illness can inflict transient and/or permanent physical changes, physical symptom distress, and functional impairments in patients. It is a well known clinical fact supported by research[28] that excessive psychological distress can exacerbate the side effects of cancer-treatment agents. Conversely, treatment side effects can have a dramatic impact on the psychological profiles of patients.[29]

The potential for psychological distress, particularly anxiety and depression, appears to increase in patients with advanced illness,[30–33] especially when cure is not viable and palliation of symptoms is the issue. In a study that elicited information from oncology nurses regarding psychiatric symptoms present in their patients, almost twice as many patients with metastatic disease were reported to be depressed in contrast to those with localized cancers.[34] Investigators studying quality of life in cancer patients have demonstrated a clear rela-

Table 19–2. Common Medications and Substances Associated with Anxiety and Depression

Anxiety

- Alcohol and nicotine withdrawal
- Stimulants including caffeine
- Thyroid replacement
- Neuroleptics
- Corticosteroids
- Sedative-hypnotic withdrawal or paradoxical reaction
- Bronchodilators and decongestants
- Cocaine
- Epinepherine
- Benzodiazepines and their withdrawal
- Digitalis toxicity
- Cannabis
- Antihypertensives
- Antihistamines
- Antiparkinsonian medications
- Oral contraceptives
- Anticholinergics
- Anesthetics and analgesics
- Toxins

Depression

- Antihypertensives
- Analgesics
- Antiparkinsonian agents
- Hypoglycemic agents
- Steroids
- Chemotherapeutic agents
- Estrogen and progesterone
- Antimicrobials
- L-Dopa
- Benzodiazepines
- Barbiturates
- Alcohol
- Phenothiazines
- Amphetamines
- Lithium carbonate
- Heavy metals
- Cimetidine

Sources: Stoudemire (1996), reference 22; Fernandez et al. (1995), reference 44; Kurlowicz (1994), reference 45; Wise & Taylor (1990), reference 23.

tionship between an individuals' perception of quality of life and the presence of discomfort.[14] As uncomfortable symptoms increase, perceived quality of life diminishes and psychiatric symptoms often worsen. The presence of increased physical discomfort combined with a lack of control and predictability regarding the occurrence of symptoms often amplifies anxiety, depression, and organic mental symptoms in patients with advanced disease.

DIFFERENTIATING PSYCHIATRIC COMPLICATIONS FROM EXPECTED PSYCHOLOGICAL RESPONSES

Differentiating between symptoms related to a medical illness and symptoms related to an underlying psychiatric disorder is particularly challenging to health care practitioners. Anxiety and depression are normal responses to life events and illness and occur throughout the palliative care trajectory. It is the intensity, duration, and extent to which symptomatology affects functioning that distinguishes an anxiety or depressive disorder from symptoms that individuals generally experience in the progression of an illness.

Symptoms following stressful events (employment difficulties, retirement, death of a family member, loss of a job, diagnosis of a medical illness/life-threatening illness) in a person's life are expected to dissipate as an individual copes with reassurance and validation from family and friends and adapts to the situation. When responses predominantly include excessive nervousness, worry, and fear, diagnosis of an adjustment disorder with anxiety is applied; if an individual responds with tearfulness and feelings of hopelessness, he or she is characterized as experiencing an adjustment disorder with depressed mood; an adjustment disorder with mixed anxiety and depressed mood is characterized by a combination of both anxiety and depression.[35] Referrals from primary care providers for psychiatric assistance with psychopharmacological treatment are indicated when symptoms continue, intensify, or disrupt an individual's life beyond a 6-month period or when symptoms do not respond to conventional reassurance and validation by the primary care provider and support from an individual's social network. Most patients develop transient psychological symptoms that are responsive to support, reassurance, and information about what to expect regarding a disease course and its treatment. There are some individuals, however, who require more aggressive psychotherapeutic intervention such as pharmacotherapy and ongoing psychotherapy. Following are guidelines to assist clinicians to identify patients who exhibit behavior suggesting the presence of a psychiatric syndrome.

If the patient's problems become severe in that supportive measures are insufficient to control emotional distress, referral to a psychiatric clinician is indicated. Factors that may predict major psychiatric problems along the chronic illness trajectory include past psychiatric hospitalization; history of significant depression, manic-depressive illness, schizophrenia, organic mental conditions, or personality disorders; lack of social support; inadequate control of physical discomfort; history of or current alcohol and/or drug abuse; and currently prescribed psychotropic medication.

The need for psychiatric referral among patients receiving psychotropic medication deserves specific mention as it is often overlooked in clinical practice. Standard therapies used to treat major chronic diseases, such as surgery and chemotherapy, and/or disease progression itself can significantly change dosage requirements for medications used to treat major psychiatric syndromes such as anxiety, depression, and bipolar disorder. For example, dosage requirements for lithium carbonate, commonly used to treat the manic episodes associated with bipolar disorder and the depressive episodes associated with recurrent depressive disorder, can change significantly over the course of treatment for a number of chronic diseases. Therapeutic blood levels of lithium are closely tied to sodium and water balance. Additionally, lithium has a narrow therapeutic window, and life-threatening toxicity can develop rapidly. Treatment side effects such as diarrhea, fever, vomiting, and resulting dehydration warrant scrupulous monitoring of dosage and side effects. Careful monitoring is also indicated during pre- and postoperative periods. Another common problem among patients treated with psychotropic medication is that medications may be discontinued at specific points in the treatment process, such as the time of surgery, and not restarted. This may produce an avoidable recurrence of emotionally disabling psychiatric symptoms when the stress of a life-threatening chronic disease and its treatment is burden enough.

For a proportion of patients, psychological distress does not subside with the usual supportive interventions. Unfortunately, clinically relevant and severe psychiatric syndromes are often unrecognized by nonpsychiatric care providers.[36] Particularly as a chronic illness progresses, anxiety and depression may occur in greater numbers of patients and with greater intensity.[37] One of the reasons that it may be difficult to detect serious anxiety and depression in patients is that several of the diagnostic criteria used to evaluate their presence, such as lack of appetite, insomnia, decreased sexual interest, psychomotor agitation, and diminished energy, may overlap with usual disease and treatment effects.[38] Additionally, health care providers may confuse their own fears about chronic illness with the emotional reactions of their patients (e.g., "I too would be extremely depressed if I were in a similar situation").

The Coexisting Nature of Psychiatric and Medical Symptoms: Models of Interaction

Depression and anxiety are appropriate to the stress of having a serious illness, and the boundary between normal and abnormal symptoms is often unclear. Even when diagnostic criteria are met for a major depressive episode or anxiety disorder, there is disagreement regarding the need for psychiatric treatment as psychiatric symptoms may improve upon initiation of medical treatment. Another major source of confusion is the overlap of somatic symptoms associated with several chronic illnesses and their treatments and those pathognomic to depression and anxiety themselves (e.g., fatigue, loss of appetite, weakness, weight loss, restlessness, agitation). Separating out whether a symptom is due to depression, anxiety, the medical illness and its treatment, or a combination of factors is often exceedingly difficult. Nield-Anderson, the third author, extended and clarified the four models or modes of interaction between anxiety and depression and primary medical conditions that were identified by Derogatis and Wise[39]: anxiety or depression with a medical or pharmacological etiology; anxiety or depression with somatic preeminence; anxiety or depression precipitated by the experience of a medical disorder; anxiety or depression concomitant with a medical disorder. The models of interaction between anxiety and depression and primary medical disorders are examined as they relate to the three phases of palliative care identified earlier: diagnostic phase, recurrence and progressive disease phase, and terminal disease and dying phase.

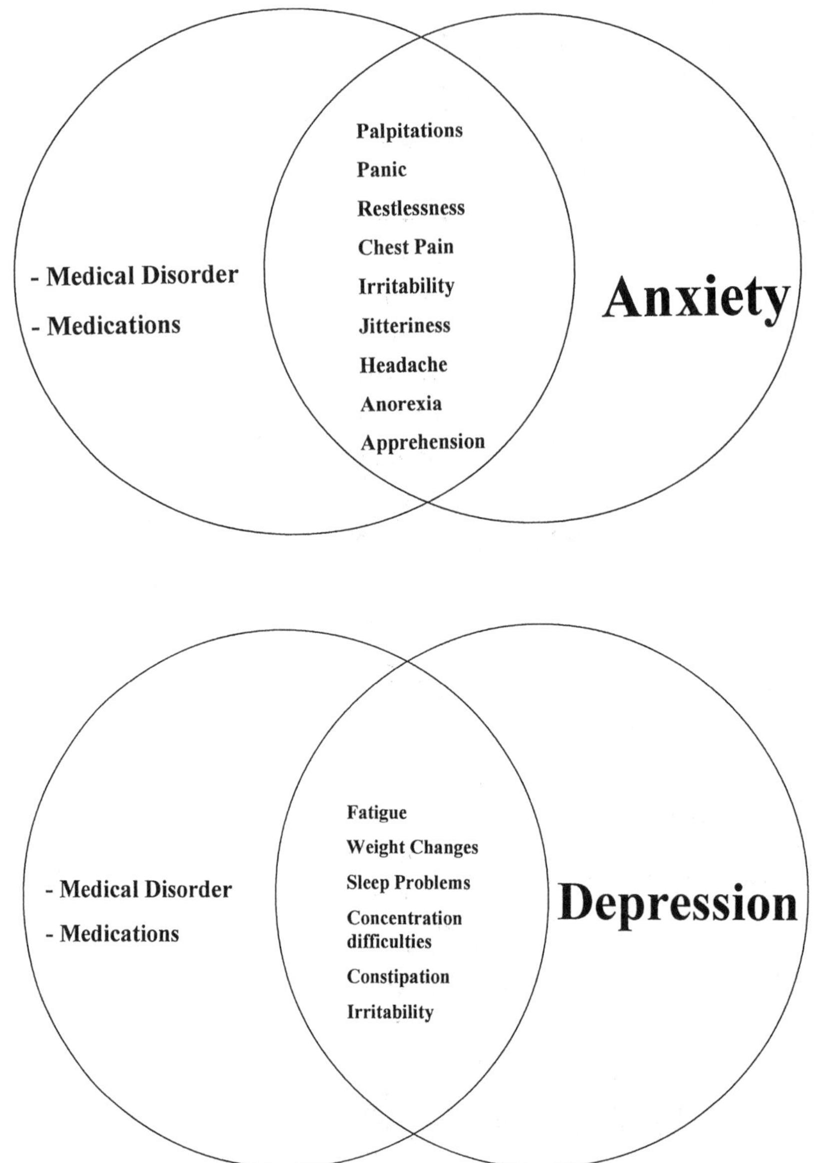

Fig. 19–1. Model 1. Symptoms of depression and anxiety with medical etiologies. Sources: Leslie Nield-Anderson, unpublished and adapted from Derogatis & Wise.[39]

Anxiety or Depression with a Medical or Pharmacological Etiology. Figure 19–1 diagrams the overlap between a medical condition or pharmacological intervention and the clinical manifestation of anxiety or depression. The symptoms of anxiety or depression are intrinsic to the medical disorder or induced by certain pharmacological agents. Symptoms cease when the medical disorder is treated or the medication is discontinued or decreased.

The interaction patterns denoted in Figure 19–1 are more likely to apply to the diagnostic phase and recurrence and progressive disease phase of palliative care treatment. If the medical condition is the primary source for psychiatric symptomatology, treatment of the medical condition results in symptom alleviation. However, pharmacological agents used in treatment may precipitate psychiatric symptomatology as well. During the recurrence and progressive disease phase, a time of relapse, the intrinsic symptoms of anxiety or depression caused by the medical condition or treating agents may recur. Data from a diagnostic assessment, preferably prior to the diagnostic phase, that includes a history and physical, medication history, mental status exam that includes neurological status, psychosocial and psychiatric histories (see Table 19–3 for screening instruments), electrocardiogram, comprehensive laboratory tests including a toxicology screening, and relevant information gathered from family members regarding an individual's lifestyle and functioning patterns allow for close monitoring throughout the palliative care trajectory, assisting health care providers to more accurately diagnose the etiology of anxiety or depression.

Anxiety or Depression with Somatic Preeminence. Model 2, shown in Figure 19–2, illustrates an interaction between a primary psychiatric disorder and pre-

Table 19–3. Brief Screening Measures for Cognitive Functioning, Anxiety, and Depression

Folstein Mini-Mental Exam
Beck Depression Inventory
Center for Epidemiological Studies of Depression Scale
Geriatric Depression Scale
Hamilton Depression Scale
Hamilton Rating Scale for Anxiety
Hospital Anxiety and Depression Scale
Zung Self-Rating Depression Scale
Zung Self-Rating Anxiety Scale
State-Trait Anxiety Inventory

senting somatic symptomotology. This pattern is frequently found in primary care settings and across the illness trajectory. During the diagnostic phase, fear and anxiety are expected reactions to the diagnosis of a life-threatening or potentially life-threatening disease. Heightened apprehension coincides with the anticipated course of treatment, uncertainty, and concerns about the potential impact on lifestyle. These initial responses usually resolve in a few weeks with the support of family and friends, use of personal resources, provision of professional care, and hope.[40] Lingering reports of feeling weak, dizzy, worried, or tense and of difficulty concentrating often are misleading to a provider and may mask an anxiety disorder. When accurately diagnosed and treated, somatic complaints fade. If symptoms, however, are not alleviated, practitioners must rule out a worsening medical condition.[39,41]

Depression occurs frequently during the recurrence and progressive disease phase. An illness course marked with recurrences engenders anxiety and fear with each relapse, as well as feelings of desperation. Individuals experiencing depression do not always present with a dysphoric affect or report distressing feelings of hopelessness and helplessness. They may instead present with somatic complaints such as dizziness, headaches, excessive fatigue, sleep disturbances, or irritability. An accurate diagnosis, appropriate use of antidepressants, and, depending on the willingness of the individual, psychotherapy and education regarding nonpharmacological interventions and cognitive behavioral therapy usually alleviate the original complaints as the underlying depressive disorder is treated.

Disturbances in appetite, sleep, energy, and concentration are hallmark symptoms in the diagnosis of depression. However, in the medically ill, these symptoms are frequently caused by the medical illness.[42] Symptoms such as fearfulness or depressed appearance, social withdrawal, brooding, self-pity, pessimism, a sense of punishment, and mood that cannot be changed (such as cannot be cheered up, not smiling, does not respond to good news) are considered to be more reliable. It has been recommended that assessment of these areas be included for a more accurate diagnosis of a major depression in a medically ill individual.[42–45] Tables 19–4 and 19–5 list general criteria to diagnosis an anxiety and depressive disorder in the medically ill.[35,44,46] Whenever symptoms are unremitting or intensify and do not respond to conventional professional and family support, psychiatric evaluations for psychopharmacological and psychotherapeutic interventions are essential. Untreated or undertreated psychiatric disorders are further disabling. Baseline data and use of the screening instruments listed in Table 19–3 can assist health care providers in assessing presenting symptoms.

The degree of anxiety and depression experienced by an individual during the terminal disease and dying phase will be dependent on the degree to which the individual and his or her family has been prepared for this stage, the speed and extent of physical devastation experienced, the presence of intractable pain, or an individual's prior history of psychiatric illness.[40] Fear, anxiety, and depression are to be expected as difficult decisions are made regarding comfort measures and diagnostic procedures and advanced technological treatments are withdrawn. Feelings of despair regarding separation from family and friends, bur-

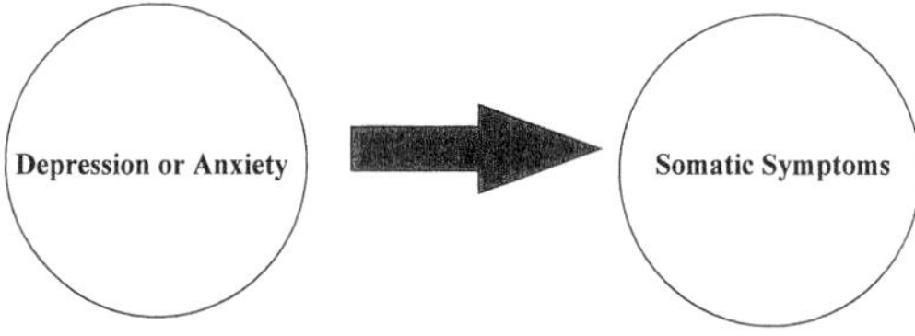

Fig. 19–2. Model 2: depression or anxiety with somatic preeminence. Source: Leslie Nield-Anderson, unpublished, based on Derogatis & Wise.[39]

Table 19–4. Symptoms Indicating an Anxiety Disorder in the Medically Ill

Chronic apprehension, worry, inability to relax not related to illness or treatment
Difficulty concentrating
Irritability or outbursts of anger
Difficulty falling asleep or staying asleep not explained by illness or treatment
Trembling or shaking not explained by illness or treatment
Exaggerated startle response
Perspiring for no apparent reason
Chest pain or tightness in the chest
Fear of places, events, certain activities
Unrealistic fear of dying
Fear of "going crazy"
Recurrent and persistent ideas, thoughts, or impulses
Repetitive behaviors to prevent discomfort

Sources: Barraclough (1997), reference 46; Fernandez et al. (1995), reference 44; American Psychiatric Association (1994), reference 35.

Table 19–5. Symptoms Related to Depressive Disorder in the Medically Ill

Enduring depressed or sad mood, tearful
Marked disinterest or lack of pleasure in social activities, family, and friends
Feelings of worthlessness and hopelessness
Excessive enduring guilt that illness is a punishment
Significant weight loss or gain not explained by dieting, illness, or treatments
Hopeless about the future
Enduring fatigue
Increase or decrease in sleep not explained by illness or treatment
Recurring thoughts of death or suicidal thoughts or acts
Diminished ability to think and make decisions

Sources: American Psychiatric Association (1994), reference 35; Cassem (1995), reference 42; Cavanaugh (1995), reference 43; Kurlowicz (1994), reference 45.

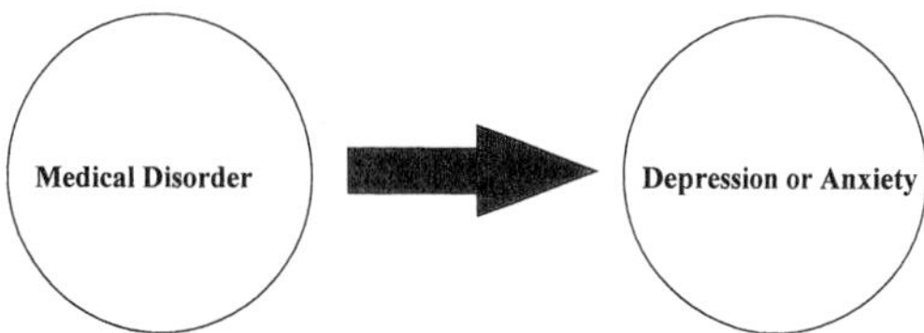

Fig. 19–3. Model 3: symptoms of depression or anxiety precipitated by medical disorder. Source: Leslie Nield Anderson, unpublished, based on Derogatis & Wise.[39]

dens of care, decisions regarding location for an individual's final stage of care, and living in existential uncertainty confront individuals and their family members during this phase. Severe distress with thoughts of suicide, panic episodes, or questions regarding assisted suicide may occur, in spite of health care providers and family members attempts at supportive interventions. These responses require immediate attention and intervention. Suicide and assisted suicide are discussed below.

Anxiety or Depression Precipitated by a Medical Disorder. Model 3 (Fig. 19–3) demonstrates an interaction between a primary medical disorder and an anxiety or depressive disorder. This interaction is associated more commonly with the recurrence and progressive disease phase and can extend into the terminal phase. In this model, the psychiatric disorder occurs secondary to the medical condition. The stressors of the medical illness induce anxiety or depression. Often, symptoms of anxiety or depression diminish when the individual progresses and progress renews hope. When an individual, however, experiences recurrences that lead to increasing physical dependence on others and prolonged pain with increasing loss of function and immobility, anxiety and depression can be heightened and sustained. Disease progression affects body image, self-esteem, social relationships, employment, and family roles. The extent of, and speed at which, these changes occur tax coping and adjustment skills. An individual's thoughts about death and dying and feelings of hopelessness can divert practitioners' attention from a disabling anxiety to presenting symptoms of depression; thus, the anxiety disorder remains undiagnosed or untreated.

Anxiety and depression often occur simultaneously. This is not to imply that they develop at the same time. Anxiety generally precedes depression, and depression is more likely to persevere in individuals who also have an anxiety disorder. When anxiety and depression coexist, assessment is more difficult and treatment generally must be more aggressive and extensive.

A common mistake by providers is to assume that the distress from a medical condition is natural and understandable, particularly when a cure is not available, significant losses are incurred, there is a quickened decrease in functioning, or prognosis is graver than foreseen. Minimizing presenting symptoms potentially results in underdiagnosing and delayed treatment. Untreated anxiety and depression increase suffering and further impair quality of life.[46]

Receiving the diagnosis of a serious medical condition and undergoing invasive medical and surgical procedures is not customarily perceived by providers as a catalyst to a stress response in an individual. Providers' dominant concerns are with a person's treatment in pursuit of curing, improving prognosis, and relieving physical discomfort. Often, providers are desensitized to the intrusiveness of medical protocols and treating environments. The experiences along the palliative care process, in particular during the recurrence and progressive disease phase and the terminal disease and dying phase, involve actual and threatened death to self. Patients do not often address their extreme feelings of helplessness, fearfulness, and horror with health care providers and family members; instead, they avoid discussions in attempts to decrease the burden on their families, and there is discomfort discussing more intimate responses with primary providers. A posttraumatic stress disorder (PTSD) is difficult to diagnose in the medically ill. Providers are apt to identify avoidance and withdrawal behaviors as acceptance, adjustment, and understandable. It is common for providers to hear "I do not remember anything about the hospitalization; it is a blur; I feel like I am/was in a daze; ask my wife/husband: my memory isn't so great." Psychopharmacological agents only partially treat this disorder. It is best treated by skilled professionals with group, individual, and cognitive–behavioral therapy expertise. Psychiatric evaluations and follow-up across the palliative care trajectory help to reduce the underdiagnosing and treatment of posttraumatic stress disorder.[35]

Anxiety or Depression Concomitant with a Medical Disorder. Model 4 (Fig. 19–4) represents a coexisting psychiatric disorder and medical disorder. There is no connection between the conditions; the treatment of one does not influence the other, except with the potential relief in the reduction of the collective burden of illness. Frequently, providers erroneously relate the symptoms of the psychiatric disorder to demoralization about the impact of the medical condition on the individual's lifestyle and do not treat the psychiatric illness. Comprehensive physical and psychiatric histories generally provide the necessary

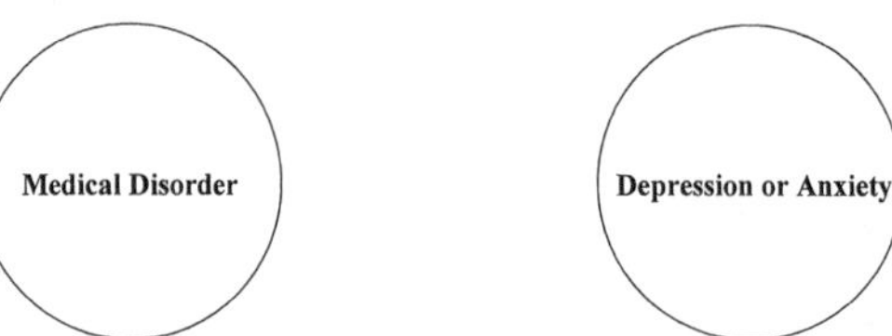

Fig. 19–4. Model 4: depression or anxiety concomitant with medical disorder. Source: Leslie Nield Anderson, unpublished, based on Derogatis & Wise.[39]

information for accurate and uninterrupted treatment of a psychiatric illness. In general, the pattern of interaction identified in Figure 19–4 is associated with the diagnostic phase of palliative care, prior to the initiation of treatment.

Teasing out anxiety and depressive disorders from an individual's unique responses to the diverse demands and intrusive nature of a medical illness is a challenge to health care practitioners. Comprehensive assessments and treatment enhance quality of life throughout the palliative care trajectory.

Recognition of Anxiety

The experience of anxiety is universal, especially when a person has a serious chronic illness. Anxiety is a vague, subjective feeling of apprehension, tension, insecurity, and uneasiness, usually without a known specific cause. Normally, anxiety serves as an alerting response that results from a real or perceived threat to a person's biological, psychological, or social integrity, as well as to self-esteem, identity, or status. This alert occurs in response to actual happenings, to thoughts about happenings, in the past, present, or future. The greater the perceived threat, the greater the anxiety response.[20]

A wide variety of signs and symptoms accompany anxiety along the continuum of mild, moderate, severe, and panic levels. Table 19–6 illustrates how anxiety affects attention, learning, and adaptation, all of which are essential to coping during the palliative care trajectory.[47] Anxiety responses can be adaptive, and anxiety can be a powerful motivating force for productive problem solving. Talking, crying, sleeping, exercising, deep breathing, imagery, and relaxation techniques are adaptive anxiety-relief strategies. Responses to anxiety also can be maladaptive and may indicate psychiatric disorder, but not all distressing symptoms of anxiety indicate a psychiatric disorder. Table 19–4 lists anxiety symptoms that indicate a psychiatric disorder and call for psychiatric assessment and treatment.

Skill in early recognition of anxiety is crucial so that care providers can intervene immediately to alleviate symptoms, to prevent escalation and loss of control, and to enable adjustment and coping. Anxiety is interpersonally contagious. As a result, therapeutic effectiveness can be severely compromised when care providers fail to recognize and manage their own anxiety.

Recognition of Depression

Often underrecognized and undertreated, depression has the potential to decrease immune response, decrease survival time, and impair quality of life.[48] The assessment of depression in any setting relies on the provider's awareness of risk factors associated with depression and the provider's ability to elicit from the patient key signs, symptoms, and history of illness. In addition to medical comorbidity, risk factors include prior episodes of depression, family history of depression, prior suicide attempts, female gender, age of onset under 40 years, postpartum period, lack of social support, stressful life events, personal history of sexual abuse, and current substance abuse.[49]

The experience of chronic and progressive disease may increase dependence, helplessness, and uncertainty and generate a negative, self-critical view. Cognitive distortions can easily develop, leading to interpretation of benign events as negative or catastrophic. Motivation to participate in care may be diminished, leading to withdrawal. Patients may see themselves as worthless and burdensome to family and friends. Family members may find themselves immobilized, impatient, or angry with the patient's lack of communication, cooperation, or motivation.[49]

Culture can influence depressive symptoms. In some cultures, depression may be expressed with somatic symptoms rather than with guilt or sadness.

Table 19–6. Symptoms of Anxiety and Effects on Attention, Learning, and Adaptation

Mild	Awareness, alert attention, skill in seeing relationships or connections available for use Notices more than previously, ability to observe improved If the person has well-developed learning and adaptive skills, will be able to use all steps in the learning process from observing and describing to analyzing, testing, and using what is learned
Moderate	Perceptual field is narrowed, ability to observe decreased, does not notice peripheral stimuli but can notice more if directed to do so (selective inattention) If the person has well-developed learning and adaptive skills, will be able to use all steps in the learning process from observing and describing to analyzing, testing, and using what is learned
Severe	Perceptual field is greatly reduced, focus on one detail or scattered details May be able to notice what is pointed out by another person, but as anxiety escalates will be unable to attend May dissociate to prevent panic, i.e., fail to notice what is happening in reference to self Even with well-developed learning and adaptive skill, behavior will orient to getting immediate relief Automatic (not requiring thought) behaviors used to reduce anxiety
Panic	Feelings of panic, awe, dread Previous foci of attention "blown up" or scatter of details increased Tendency to dissociate to prevent panic Inability to focus attention even when directed by another person Even with well-developed learning and adaptive skills, behavior will orient to getting immediate relief Automatic (not requiring thought) behaviors used to reduce anxiety

Source: Peplau (1963), reference 47.

Complaints of "nerves" and headaches (in Latino and Mediterranean cultures); of weakness, tiredness, or "imbalance" (in Chinese or Asian cultures); of problems of the "heart" (in Middle Eastern cultures), or of being "heartbroken" (among the Hopi) may be depressive equivalents. Cultures may differ in judgments about the seriousness of dysphoria; for example, irritability may be a greater concern than sadness or withdrawal. Experiences distinctive to certain cultures, such as fear of being hexed or vivid feelings of being visited by those who have died, must be differentiated from actual hallucinations or delusions that may be part of a major depressive episode with psychotic features. However, a symptom should not be dismissed because it is seen as characteristic of a particular culture (Table 19–5).[35,42,43,45]

The concept of depression has a variety of meanings; it has been used to describe a broad spectrum of human emotions and behaviors, ranging from expected, transient, and nonclinical sadness following upsetting life events to the clinically relevant extremes of suicidality and major depressive disorder. Depression is common among people with chronic illness. The term "depressive syndromes" refers to a specific constellation of symptoms that comprise a discrete psychiatric disorder, such as major depression, dysthymia, organic affective disorder, and adjustment disorder with depressed features. Depressive symptoms describe varying degrees of depressed feelings not necessarily associated with psychiatric illness.

Five major theoretical viewpoints have been used to understand and treat depression. In the psychodynamic view, depression represents the introjection of hostility subsequent to the loss of an ambivalently loved object. Cognitive views emphasize the mediating role that distorted and negative thinking plays in determining mood and behavior. In the sociological view, depression is a social phenomenon in which a breakdown of self-esteem involves the loss of possessions such as status, roles and relationships, and life meaning. Cultural and societal factors, including illness, increase vulnerability to depression. The biological view of depression emphasizes genetic vulnerability and biochemical alterations in neurotransmitters. In studies of medically ill patients, depression is often equated with a crisis response, in which demands on the individual exceed the ability to respond. These viewpoints influence the understanding and subsequent treatment of depression in those with chronic physical illness.

In many health care settings, nurses have the most patient contact and are likely to talk with individuals about their physical and emotional problems and to detect depression. Recognition begins with knowing that many people who experience depression seek treatment for related somatic symptoms in medical rather than mental health settings. Specific screening instruments, such as those listed in Table 19–3, may be used for assessment. In addition, direct questioning and clinical observation of mood, behavior, and thinking can be carried out concomitantly with physical care. Questions related to mood may include the following: How have your spirits been lately? How would you describe your mood now? Have you felt sad or blue? Questions about behavior relate to sleeping patterns, appetite, activity level, and changes in energy: How are you sleeping lately? How much energy do you have now compared with 1 month or 6 months ago? Have you experienced recent changes in your appetite? Have you lost or gained weight? What do you usually do to cope with stress (talk to someone? go to a movie? work? exercise? drugs? alcohol?). Questions related to cognition are as follows: What do you see in your future? What are the biggest problems facing you now? Are you as interested as usual in your family and friends, work, hobbies, etc.? Have you felt satisfied with yourself and with your life? Can you concentrate as well as you usually can? Do you have family or close friends readily available to help you? Do you feel able to call on them? As noted previously, disturbances in appetite, sleep, energy, and concentration may be caused by the illness and not necessarily indicative of depression.

SUICIDE

Suicide is the ninth leading cause of death in the United States. Five percent of suicides occur in patients with chronic medical illnesses, with spinal cord injuries, multiple sclerosis, cancer, and human immunodeficiency virus disease associated with increased suicide rates.[50] Because of underreporting, statistics underestimate the magnitude of suicide; intentional overdoses by the terminally ill and intentional car accidents are rarely labeled as suicides.[51] The strongest suicide predictor is the presence of a psychiatric illness, especially depression and alcohol abuse, although a chronic deteriorating medical illness with perceived poor health, recent diagnosis of a life-threatening illness, and recent conflict or loss of a significant relationship also are considered to be predictive.[50] Male gender, age over 45, and living alone and lacking a social support system are risk factors.[51] In one study, hopelessness was found to be more important than depression as a clinical marker of suicidal ideation in the terminally ill.[52] Individuals with progressive chronic illness, particularly during the terminal stages, are at increased risk for suicide.[51] Other cancer-related risk factors include oral, pharyngeal, or lung cancer; poor prognosis; confusion and delirium; inadequately controlled pain; and the presence of deficits, such as loss of mobility, loss of bowel or bladder control, amputation, sensory loss, inability to eat or swallow, and exhaustion.[48] The highest-risk patients are those with severe and rapidly progressive disease producing rapid functional decline, intractable pain, and/or history of depression, suicide attempts, or substance abuse.[53]

Physician-Assisted Suicide

Whereas suicide is the intentional ending of one's own life, physician-assisted suicide (PAS) refers to a physician acting to aid a person in the ending of his or her life.[54] Public demand for PAS has been fueled by burdensome, exhausting, and expensive dying in acute care settings.[16,55] It is highly controversial; the

American Medical Association, the American Nurses Association, and the National Hospice Organization have taken strong positions against it.[54,55] Implications for health care providers include the necessity of being knowledgeable about the legal and moral/ethical aspects of PAS; to do a personal evaluation and prepare responses for situations with patients where the topic may arise; to improve education about pain management, symptom control, and related issues in the care of dying and seriously ill patients; to conduct rigorous research on the attitudes and practices of health care professionals with respect to assisted suicide; and to develop effective mechanisms to address conflicts.[54,56]

There is an ongoing debate about the legalization of PAS. Only in Oregon have the voters approved legalization of PAS. The controversy potentially affects pain management in palliative care.[16] Current efforts to create a federal ban on PAS may have a "chilling" effect on the widely supported approach to pain management in terminal care of high doses of opiates, regardless of secondary effects on respiration and length of life.[16] Some fear that providing adequate pain relief might be seen as assisting the patient to die.[51] Although the Oregon law remains in dispute, the public dialogue in that state led to palliative care reform which significantly improved end-of-life care in Oregon.[16,55] Tilden[16] notes that economic hardship on the families of the seriously ill is common and that palliative care has the advantage of wise resource utilization. Events in Oregon highlight care as a priority and increase the understanding about the distinction between assisted suicide and honoring patient preferences for limiting life-sustaining treatment.[55] Patient concerns most often related to desire to suicide are unrelieved pain, poorly managed symptoms, depression, worries about loss of control, being a burden, being dependent on others for personal care, and loss of dignity.[51,53,54] Valente and Trainor[51] identified poor quality of life, failed requests for treatment withdrawal, and distressing treatments as typical reasons for suicide in the critically ill. Further, patient requests for PAS are not rare, and physicians do provide such services, even though they are not legal.[53] Requests to physicians may also be indirect, as in the reported case of a patient asking for pain relief with the unspoken intent to cause death.[57]

To further complicate the issue for health care providers, requests for suicide may be rational and not simply a symptom of depression.[51] Rationality has been defined as the capacity to deliberate, to communicate in relationships, and to reflect on and examine one's own values and purposes.[51] The accepted criteria for rational suicide among adults with terminal illness include the following:

- Rational considerations
- Understandable motives
- Careful planning
- Review of alternatives
- Absence of coercion
- Recognition of consequences.[51]

The patient's decisional capacity may be impaired by agitation, disorientation, major depression, poor reality orientation, grief and loss, medications, effects of illness, and ambivalence. Particularly in these circumstances, a formal psychiatric evaluation is warranted.[51]

Assessment of Suicide Risk

Assessment and treatment of depression, often overlooked in chronic illness treatment settings, is a key suicide-prevention strategy. In addition, symptom management, communication, and helping patients to maintain a sense of control are vitally important prevention strategies. An assessment of depression should always include direct questions about suicidal thinking, plans or attempts, despair or hopelessness, distress from poorly managed symptoms, and personal or family history of suicidal ideation, plans, or attempts.[51]

When any indicator of suicide risk is recognized, risk factors, clues, suicidal ideation, level of depression, hopelessness and despair, and symptom distress should be thoroughly evaluated to estimate individual lethality. The rationality of the suicidal request or intent must also be evaluated. Interview the patient and family members to find out why the patient is thinking about suicide now.[51] Find out what method the patient is considering and whether the means are available. Ask the patient what has prevented suicide before and if he or she wants help or hopes someone else will decide.[51] Most people are relieved to be asked about suicidal thoughts because it opens communication. Initial and periodic evaluation of suicidal potential is necessary for patients with history, thoughts, or risk factors of suicide.

Recognition of Clues. Suicidal persons usually give verbal and/or behavioral clues, such as isolated or withdrawn behavior or death wishes or death themes in art, writing, play, or conversation. Clues may be subtle or obvious, for example, joking about suicide, asking questions concerning death (e.g., "How many of these pills would it take to kill someone?"), comments with a theme of giving up, or statements that indicate hopelessness or helplessness. Resistance or refusal of treatments, food, or fluids may indicate suicidal ideation or intent and require further assessment.[49,51]

Ascertaining Lethality. Keys to determining lethality are suicide plan, method, intended outcome (e.g., death or rescue), and availability of resources and ability to communicate.[49,51] Lethal means include guns, knives, jumping from heights, drowning, or carbon monoxide poisoning. Other potentially lethal means include hanging or strangulation (using strong pieces of twine, rope, electric cords, sheets), taking high doses of aspirin or Tylenol, being in a car crash, or undergoing exposure to extreme cold. Low to moderately lethal methods are wrist cutting and mild aspirin overdose.

Suicide Interventions

Severely depressed and/or potentially suicidal patients must be identified as soon as possible to ensure a safe environment and appropriate treatment. Prompt action should be taken including provision of safety, supervision, and initiation of psychiatric evaluation. A patient with an immediate, lethal, and precise suicide plan needs strict safety precautions such as hospitalization and continuous or close supervision.[51] The low-risk patient should not be underestimated. If circumstances change, risk could change. In all cases, notify the primary provider, and document the patient's behavior and verbatim statements, suicide assessment, and rationale for decisions as well as the time and date the provider was notified.[51] If the provider is not responsive to the report of the patient's suicidal ideation, it is important to maintain observation and to pursue psychiatric consultation.

The motivation for suicide can be reduced through palliative care interventions such as improved pain and symptom management; referral and treatment for depression or other psychiatric disorders; discussion of alternative interventions to improve quality of life; referral to spiritual, social, and psychiatric resources; and education and accurate facts about options for terminal care or end-of-life decision making. Openness to talking about suffering, distress, death preferences, and decision making in a sensitive and understanding manner and advocacy to aid communication with others is helpful for patients and their families.[51]

MANAGEMENT OF ANXIETY AND DEPRESSION

Psychosocial interventions can exert an important effect on the overall adjustment of patients and their families to chronic illness and treatment.[58] Several studies document the beneficial effect of counseling on anxiety, feelings of personal control,[59] depression, and generalized psychological distress.[60] Increased length of survival from time of diagnosis has highlighted the need for psychopharmacological, psychotherapeutic, and behaviorally oriented interventions to reduce anxiety and depression and to improve quality of life for patients diagnosed with a chronic illness.

Pharmacological Interventions

Pharmacotherapy, as an adjunct to one or more of the psychotherapies, can be an important aid in bringing psychological symptoms under control.

Pharmacological Management of Anxiety. The prevalence of anxiety in medical illness is relatively high. As described in Figure 19–1, a variety of disorders have anxiety as a prominent symptom of the clinical presentation (Tables 19–1, 19–2), and many commonly used medications are associated with anxiety as a side effect. Studies have shown a high prevalence in cardiovascular, pulmonary, cerebrovascular, and gastrointestinal diseases, as well as cancer and diabetes. In addition, patients with a history of anxiety disorders have increased rates of diabetes, heart disease, arthritis, and physical handicaps compared to the general population. Pain, metabolic abnormalities, hypoxia, and drug withdrawal states can present as anxiety. Before instituting pharmacological treatment, any patient presenting with acute or chronic symptoms of anxiety should be thoroughly evaluated, including a review of medications to assess the contribution of medical condition and/or medication-related etiologies for their complaints.[22]

The following brief review of pharmacological treatment must be supplemented with other references concerning assessment, intervention, evaluation, and patient education (Table 19–7).

Benzodiazepines are the most frequently used medications for anxiety in both medical and psychiatric settings. When longer-acting benzodiazepines, such as diazepam, are used in the elderly or in the presence of liver disease, dosages should be decreased and dosing intervals increased. They may suppress respiratory drive. Consultation-liaison services often utilize lorazepam in medically ill patients because its elimination half-life is relatively unaffected by liver disease, age, or concurrent use of selective serotonin reuptake inhibitors (SSRIs) or nefazodone. Drawbacks include amnestic episodes and interdose anxiety caused by its short half-life. The latter can be remedied by more frequent dosing. If medically ill patients need a longer-acting benzodiazepine for panic disorder or generalized anxiety disorder, clonazepam is often used as it is not affected by concurrent use of SSRIs. Clonazepam may accumulate and result in oversedation and ataxia in the elderly; therefore, low doses are used. Temazepam is useful as a sedative-hypnotic.[22]

Buspirone, used primarily for generalized anxiety disorder, is attractive for anxiety in the medically ill because of its lack of sedation, lack of negative effects on cognition, insignificant effect of age on elimination half-life, and limited effect of liver disease on half-life. Buspirone has almost no clinically significant interactions with drugs commonly used in general medicine. It may stimulate the respiratory drive, which makes it useful in patients with pulmonary disease or sleep apnea.[22]

Cyclic antidepressants are well established as anxiolytic agents that are particularly effective in the treatment of panic disorder and in generalized anxiety disorder. If these drugs are used for anxiety in depressed medically ill patients or used because of their sedating properties in patients with major depression or panic disorder, the side effects must be carefully considered. Potentially deleterious side effects in the medically ill are sedative, anticholinergic, orthostatic hypotensive, and quinidine-like. Liver disease and renal disease may affect metabolism and excretion of the drug and, therefore, require careful dosage titration.[22]

Other drugs that may be used for anxiety include the beta-adrenergic blocking agents, antihistamines, monoamine oxidase inhibitors, and neuroleptics. Beta-adrenergic blocking agents may be used for milder forms of generalized anxiety, but there are cautions and contraindications in the presence of pulmonary disease, diabetes, and congestive heart failure. Antihistamines are sometimes used, although the effects are largely nonspecific and sedative. Side effects, such as sedation and dizziness, can be significant for medically ill patients. Monoamine oxidase inhibitors are rarely used in the medically ill because of the precautions that must be taken to prevent drug interactions. Neuroleptics, such as haloperidol in low doses, are

Table 19–7. Medications Appropriate for the Treatment of Anxiety in the Medically Ill

Benzodiazepines

Diazepam (Valium and others)
Flurazepam (Dalmane and others)
Helazepam (Paxipam)
Chlordiazepoxide (Librium and others)
Alprazolam (Xanax)
Triazolam (Halcion)
Clorazepate (Tranxene)
Prazepam (Centrax)
Midazolam (Versed, IM and IV only)
Quazepam (Doral)
Estazolam (ProSom)
Clonazepam (Klonopin)
Lorazepam (Ativan and others)
Temazepam (Restoril and others)
Oxazepam (Serax and others)

Azapirones

Buspirone (Buspar)

Cyclic Antidepressants

Amitriptyline (Elavil and others)
Imipramine (Tofranil and others)
Nortriptyline (Pamelor and others)
Protriptyline (Vivactil)
Trazodone (Desyrel and others)
Desipramine (Norpramin and others)
Amoxapine (Asendin)
Maprotiline (Ludiomil)
Doxepin (Sinequan and others)
Trimipramine (Surmontil)

Not Cyclic Antidepressants

Fluoxetine (Prozac, selective serotonin reuptake inhibitor)
Sertraline (Zoloft, selective serotonin reuptake inhibitor)
Paroxetine (Paxil, selective serotonin reuptake inhibitor)
Bupropion (Wellbutrin, dopamine reuptake blocker)
Nefazodone (Serzone, 5-HT2 receptor antagonist)
Venlafaxine (Effexor, serotonin/norepinephrine reuptake inhibitor)

Other Medications Selectively Used for Their Anxiolytic Effects

Beta-adrenergic blocking agents, such as propranolol
Monoamine oxidase inhibitors
Neuroleptics (antipsychotics), such as haloperidol

Source: Stoudemire (1996), reference 22.

used for anxiety associated with severe behavioral agitation or psychotic symptoms.[22]

When anxiety develops in the context of the terminal stages of cancer, it is often secondary to hypoxia and/or an untreated pain syndrome. Intravenous opiates and oxygen if hypoxia is present are usually an effective palliative treatment.[61]

Anxiolytics are most effective when doses are scheduled; if given on an as-needed basis, anxiety may increase in patients already frightened and anxious. Anxiolytic medications help patients gain control over agonizing anxiety. Use of these medications may also assist the patient in psychotherapy, which can aid control over symptoms.

All pharmacological treatments must be monitored for effectiveness and side effects. The effects of benzodiazepines are felt within hours, with a full response in days. Buspirone has no immediate effect, with a full response after 2 to 4 weeks. The sedating effects of benzodiazepines are associated with impaired motor performance and cognition. Benzodiazepines have dependence and abuse potential and the possibility of withdrawal symptoms when discontinued. Buspirone has no association with dependence or abuse.[62]

Pharmacological Management of Depression. Patients with chronic illness commonly exhibit transient depressive symptoms at various points in the disease trajectory, particularly during the palliative care period when a hope for cure is no longer possible. As explained previously (see The Coexisting Nature of Psychiatric and Medical Symptoms: Models of Interaction), depressive symptoms can be caused by the medical disorder itself, associated with medications used for treatment or symptom management, or caused or worsened by the stress related to coping with illness; also, depression can predate and recur with the medical illness. To further complicate matters, individuals with medical illness are often older with potentially greater risk of adverse effects from both psychotropic and nonpsychotropic medications. Medical illnesses and the medications required to treat or manage symptoms may impose significantly modified prescribing regimens on the use of antidepressants. Therefore, it is necessary to evaluate the possible role of existing medical conditions and medications that could cause the depressive symptoms. Other general guidelines include (*1*) use of the medication with the least potential for drug–drug interactions and for adverse effects based on the patient's drug regimen and physiological vulnerabilities and the greatest potential for improving the primary symptoms of the depression; (2) begin with low dosage, increase slowly, and establish the lowest effective dosage; (3) reassess dosage requirements regularly.[61]

In the past, antidepressant drug selection was limited by the nearly sole availability of tricyclic antidepressants, but new drugs, such as the SSRIs, bupropion, and venlafaxine, have vastly simplified the pharmacological treatment of depression in the medically ill.[62] No one medication is clearly more effective than another. The SSRIs have fewer long-term side effects than the tricyclic antidepressants, but they are more expensive.

Psychostimulants such as dextroamphetamine and methylphenidate have been useful in the treatment of depression in medically ill patients.[63–65] Advantages include rapid onset of action and rapid clearance if side effects occur.[66] They can also counteract opioid-induced sedation and improve pain control through a positive action on mood.[67] Common side effects of psychostimulants include insomnia, anorexia, tachycardia, and hypertension,[63] although incremental dosage increases allow adequate monitoring of therapeutic versus side effects. In patients with cardiac conduction problems, stimulants may be the treatment of choice. In medically ill patients, a 1- to 2-month trial can provide remission from depression even after discontinuation of the drug. Different studies have shown a 48% to 80% improvement in depressive symptoms,[67] and this class of medication is often quite effective but underutilized in medical settings (Table 19–8).

Certain medications and cancer treatment agents can produce severe depressive states. A diagnosis of major depression in medically ill patients relies heavily on the presence of affective symptoms, such as hopelessness, crying spells, guilt, preoccupation with death and/or suicide, diminished self-worth, and loss of pleasure in most activities such as being with friends and loved ones. The neurovegetative symptoms that usually characterize depression in physically healthy individuals are not good predictors of depression in the medically ill due to the fact that disease and treatment can also produce these symptoms. A combination of psychotherapy and antidepressant medication will often prove useful in treating major depression in medically ill patients.[68] Peak dosages of antidepressants irregardless of drug class are usually substantially lower than those tolerated by physically healthy individuals. Antidepressant medications may take 2 to 6 weeks to produce their desired effects. Patients may need ongoing support, reassurance, and monitoring prior to experiencing the antidepressant effects of medication. It is essential that patients are monitored closely during the initiation and modification of psychopharmacological regimens by a consistent provider. Patient education is essential in this area, to decrease the possibility of nonadherence to the medication regimen.[22]

Psychotherapeutic Modalities

According to Weisman, Worden and Sobel,[2] psychosocial interventions are defined as systematic efforts applied to influence coping behavior through educational or psychotherapeutic means. The goals of such interventions are to improve morale, self-esteem, coping ability, sense of control, and problem-solving abilities and to decrease emotional distress. The educational approach is directive, utilizing problem-solving and cognitive methods.[58] Clarifying medical information that may be missed due to fear and anxiety as well as misconceptions and/or misinformation regarding illness and treatment and normalizing emotional reactions throughout the illness trajectory are important components of the educational approach.

The psychotherapeutic approach utilizes psychodynamic and exploratory methods to help the individual understand aspects of the medical condition such as emotional responses and personal meaning of the disease. Psychotherapeutic interventions as opposed to educational interventions should be delivered by professionals with special training in both mental health and specific interventional modalities as applied to patients with chronic medical illnesses and palliative care needs.

Psychotherapy with a patient who has cancer should maintain a primary focus on the illness and its implications, utilizing a brief therapy and crisis-intervention model.[58] Expression of fears and concerns that may be too painful to reveal to family and friends is encouraged. Normalizing emotional distress, providing realistic reassurance and support, and bolstering existing strengths and coping skills are essential components of the therapeutic process. Gathering information about previous associations with the medical condition experienced through close relationships can also be instrumental in clarifying patients' fears and concerns and establishing boundaries for and differences from the current situation. Depending on the nature of the problem, the treatment modality may take the form of individual psychotherapy, support groups, family and marital therapy, or behaviorally oriented therapy such as progressive muscle relaxation and guided imagery.

A primary role for nurses is to facilitate a positive adjustment in patients under their care. Periodic emotional distress and coping problems can be expected during the palliative care trajectory and monitored routinely. Emotional display is not the same as maladaptive coping. Understanding an individual's unique circumstances can assist nurses in supporting the constructive coping abilities that seem to work best for a particular patient.[68]

Psychotherapeutic Interventions Targeted to Symptoms of Anxiety

Anxiety responses can be thought of as occurring along a continuum, from mild to moderate to severe to panic. Lazarus and Folkman's[69] differentiation of problem-focused coping and emotion-focused coping provides a framework for intervention strategies matched to the continuum of responses (Table 19–9).

As a person moves along the continuum to moderate, severe, and panic levels of anxiety, the problem causing distress is lost sight of and distress itself becomes the focus of attention. Both preventive and treatment strategies can be used with patients and family members in a variety of settings.

Before assuming that anxiety has a psychological basis, consider the models of interaction and review the patient's history for recent changes in medical condition and/or medications. Asking whether the patient was taking medications for "nerves," depression, or insomnia will help to determine whether drugs were inappropriately discontinued or whether anxiety symptoms predated the current illness. In addition, ask about over-the-counter medications, illegal drugs, alcohol intake, and smoking history. Documentation and communication of findings are essential to enhance teamwork among providers.

Table 19–8. Medications Appropriate for the Treatment of Depression in the Medically Ill

For Patients with Cardiovascular Disease

Selective serotonin reuptake inhibitors
- Sertraline (Zoloft)
- Paroxetine (Paxil)
- Fluoxetine (Prozac)
- Fluvoxamine (Luvox)
- Citalopram (Celexa)

Dopamine reuptake blocking compounds
- Bupropion (Wellbutrin, Zyban)

Serotonin/norepinephrine reuptake inhibitors
- Venlafaxine (Effexor)

5-HT2 receptor antagonist properties
- Nefazodone (Serzone)
- Trazodone (Desyrel)

For Patients with Gastrointestinal Disease

Tricyclic antidepressants
- Amitriptyline (Elavil)
- Amoxapine (Asendin)
- Clomipramine (Anafranil)
- Desipramine (Norpramin)
- Doxepin (Sinequan)
- Imipramine (Tofranil)
- Maprotiline (Ludiomil)
- Nortriptyline (Aventyl, Pamelor)
- Protriptyline (Vivactil)
- Trimipramine (Surmontil)

5-HT2 receptor antagonist properties
- Nefazodone (Serzone)
- Trazodone (Desyrel)

Dopamine reuptake blocking compounds
- Bupropion (Wellbutrin, Zyban)

For Patients with Renal Disease

Tricyclic antidepressants
- Amitriptyline (Elavil)
- Amoxapine (Asendin)
- Clomipramine (Anafranil)
- Desipramine (Norpramin)
- Doxepin (Sinequan)
- Imipramine (Tofranil)
- Maprotiline (Ludiomil)
- Nortriptyline (Aventyl, Pamelor)
- Protriptyline (Vivactil)
- Trimipramine (Surmontil)

Selective serotonin reuptake inhibitors
- Sertraline (Zoloft)
- Paroxetine (Paxil)
- Fluoxetine (Prozac)
- Fluvoxamine (Luvox)
- Citalopram (Celexa)

Serotonin/norepinephrine reuptake inhibitors
- Venlafaxine (Effexor)

Noradrenergic agonist
- Mirtazapine (Remeron)

For Patients with Hepatic Disease

Tricyclic Antidepressants
- Amitriptyline (Elavil)
- Amoxapine (Asendin)
- Clomipramine (Anafranil)
- Desipramine (Norpramin)
- Doxepin (Sinequan)
- Imipramine (Tofranil)
- Maprotiline (Ludiomil)
- Nortriptyline (Aventyl, Pamelor)
- Protriptyline (Vivactil)
- Trimipramine (Surmontil)

Serotonin/norepinephrine reuptake inhibitors
- Venlafaxine (Effexor)

Selective serotonin reuptake inhibitors
- Sertraline (Zoloft)
- Paroxetine (Paxil)
- Fluoxetine (Prozac)
- Fluvoxamine (Luvox)
- Citalopram (Celexa)

5-HT2 receptor antagonist properties
- Nefazodone (Serzone)
- Trazodone (Desyrel)

Noradrenergic agonist
- Mirtazapine (Remeron)

For Medically Ill Patients with Anergic Depression

Psychostimulants
- Dextroamphetamine (Dexedrine)
- Methylphenidate

Dopamine reuptake blocking compounds
- Bupropion (Wellbutrin, Zyban)

Sources: Beliles, K. & Stoudemire, A. (1998). Psychopharmacologic treatment of depression in the medically ill. *Psychosomatics* 39(3):52–19.

Frequently, patients can identify the factors causing their anxiety as well as coping skills effective in the past; when they do, their discomfort decreases. Anxiety may be greatly reduced by initiating a discussion of concerns which are painful, frightening, or shameful, such as being dependent or accepting help. Use open-ended questions, reflection, clarification, and/or empathic remarks, such as "You're afraid of being a burden?" Help the patient to identify previously effective coping strategies and integrate them with new ones, using statements such as "What has helped you get through difficult times like this before?" "How can we help you use those strategies now?" "How about talking about some new strategies that may work now?" Encourage the patient to identify supportive individuals who can help emotionally or with tasks.

Preventive Strategies. Preventive strategies can help to maintain a useful level of anxiety, one that enhances rather than interferes with problem solving. Effective preventive strategies that can be used by all providers involved with the patient follow.[20,70]

Table 19–9. Hierarchy of Anxiety Interventions

Anxiety Level	Interventions
Level 1	Prevention Strategies
Mild to moderate	Provide concrete objective information Ensure stressful event warning Increase opportunities for control Increase patient and family participation in care activities Acknowledge fears Explore near-miss events, past and/or present Control symptoms Structure uncertainty Limit sensory deprivation and isolation Encourage hope
Level 2	Treatment Strategies
Moderate to Severe	Use presence of support person as "emotional anchor" Support expression of feelings, doubts, and fears Explore near-miss events, past and/or present Provide accurate information for realistic restructuring of fearful ideas Teach anxiety-reduction strategies, such as focusing, breathing, relaxation, imagery techniques Use massage, touch, physical exercise Control symptoms Use antianxiety medications Delay procedures to promote patient control and readiness Consult psychiatric experts
Level 3	Treatment Strategies
Panic	Stay with the patient Maintain calm environment, reduce stimulation Use antianxiety medications, monitor carefully Control symptoms Use focusing and breathing techniques Use demonstration in addition to verbal direction Repeat realistic reassurances Communicate with repetition and simplicity Consult psychiatric experts

Sources: Minarik (1996), reference 20; Leavitt and Minarik (1989), reference 70.

1. Provide concrete objective information. Fear of the unknown, lack of recent prior experience, or misinterpretations about an illness, procedure, test, or medication, especially when coupled with a tendency to focus on emotional aspects of experiences, may be a source of anxiety. Help patients and families know what to expect, and focus attention by realistically describing the potentially threatening experience with concrete objective information.[71] Describe both the typical subjective (e.g., sensations and temporal features) and objective (e.g., timing, nature of environment) features of stressful health care events using concrete terminology. Avoid qualitative adjectives, such as "terrible." Also known as mental rehearsal and stress inoculation, concrete information increases the patient's understanding of the situation, allows for preparation under less emergent and more supportive conditions, and facilitates coping. Encourage the patient to ask questions, and then match the detail of the preparatory information to the request. Since anxiety hinders retention, use of understandable terms and repetition is helpful. Too much information at once may increase anxiety.
2. Ensure stressful event warning before the event. For example, a person may experience magnetic resonance imaging as entrapping or traumatic or the placement of a central line as painful and threatening. Giving time to anticipate and mentally rehearse coping with the experience helps the person to maintain a sense of control and endure the procedure.
3. Increase opportunities for control. Illness can seriously disrupt a person's sense of control and increase anxiety. Help the patient to make distinctions between what is controllable, partially controllable, or not controllable. Focus on what is controllable or partially controllable and create decision-making and choice opportunities that fit the patient's knowledge. Ask patients to make choices about scheduling the day of the visit and the readiness for and timing of procedures and interventions.
4. Increase patient and family participation in care. Participation in care helps directly in coping and can be taught to both the patient and family members. Participation may reduce helplessness and increase sense of control. Patients and family members may vary in their interest in participating and in their ability to do so. Often, female family members are more likely to be caregivers. Family roles such as spouse, parent, and sibling; quality of relationships; presence or absence of conflicts; and other commitments, such as work or other family roles, will influence the ability to participate. Cultures also vary in expectations and the duty or obligation about caregiving based on gender or family position. Participation may also help with the resolution of ineffective denial when a person's condition is deteriorating. Family members who are caring for a person may recognize and adjust to the deterioration.
5. Encourage self-monitoring and use of a stress diary. Self-monitoring of stress is a cognitive–behavioral intervention. Ask the patient to record the situations, thoughts, and feelings that elicit stress and anxiety. The patient may record incidences of treatment-related stress, illness-related stress, or other unrelated anxiety-provoking situations. Not only does this intervention provide assessment information, it enhances collaboration with the patient and helps the patient understand the relationship between situations, thoughts, and feelings.
6. Acknowledge fears. Encourage and listen to the expression of feelings. Avoid denying the existence of problems or reassuring anxious people that "everything will be fine." Structure your availability. Refrain from avoiding the anxious person or their fears. Avoidance is likely to increase vulnerability, isolation, helplessness, and anxiety. Early structured intervention is more economical of time and more effective.
7. Explore near-miss events. Past or current exposure to a near-miss event is a potent generator of extreme stress and anxiety,

with heightened vigilance. A near-miss is a harrowing experience that overwhelms the ability to cope. It may be a one-time experience, such as a person's own near-death experience, the cardiac arrest of another person in similar circumstances, or something faced repeatedly such as daily painful skin and wound care. Near-misses should be explored, fears acknowledged and realistically evaluated in view of the person's situation, and help given in developing coping strategies.

8. Symptom management. Managing symptoms such as pain, dyspnea, and fatigue is an essential part of promoting self-control. Symptoms such as pain signal threat and may lead to worries about the meaning of the symptom and whether necessary treatments will be worse or more frightening. Ensure pain control, especially prior to painful or frightening procedures. Severe anxiety may increase the perception of pain and increase the requirement for analgesia. Symptom management reduces distress and allows for rest.
9. Structure uncertainty. Even when there are many unknowns, the period of uncertainty can be framed with expected events, procedures, updates, meetings with providers, etc.
10. Reduce sensory deprivation. Sensory deprivation and isolation can heighten attention to various signals in the environment. Without the means to accurately interpret the signals, be reassured, and feel in control, the signals take on frightening meanings for the patient, such as abandonment and helplessness. Feeling isolated and helpless increases the sense of vulnerability and danger.
11. Build hope. Provide information about possible satisfactory outcomes and means to achieve them. Hope also may be built around coping ability, sustaining relationships, revised goals such as pain-free or peaceful death, and determination to endure.[72] Many additional suggestions are provided in Chapter 24.

Treatment Strategies. When it is evident that the person's anxiety level has escalated to the point of interfering with problem solving or comfort, the following strategies may be helpful:[20,70]

1. Presence of supportive persons. Familiar and supportive people, a family member, friend, or staff member can act as an "emotional anchor." Family and friends may need coaching to enable them to help in the situation without their own anxiety increasing.
2. Expression of feelings, doubts, and fears. Verbalizing feelings provides the opportunity to correct or restructure unrealistic misconceptions and automatic anxiety-provoking thoughts. Accurate information allows restructuring of perceptions and lends predictability to the situation. Aggressive confrontation of unrealistic perceptions may reinforce them and is to be avoided.
3. Use antianxiety medications. If medications are used, they should be given concurrently with other interventions and monitored. Use caution to avoid delirium from toxicity, especially in the aged person.
4. Promote patient control and readiness. If a patient is very frightened of a particular procedure, allow time for the patient to regain enough composure to make the decision to proceed. Forging ahead when a patient is panicked may appear to save time in the immediate situation, but it will increase the patient's sense of vulnerability and helplessness, possibly adding time over the long term.
5. Management of panic. When anxiety reaches panic, use presence and acknowledgment: "I know you are frightened. I will stay with you." Communicate with repetition and simplicity. Guide the person to a smaller, quieter area away from other people, and use quiet reassurance. Maintain a calm manner, and reduce all environmental stimulation. Help the patient to focus on a single object (see below), and guide the patient in recognizing the physical features of the object while breathing rhythmically. Consider using prescribed anxiolytic medication.
6. Massage, touch, and physical exercise. For those who respond well to touch, massage releases muscle tension and may elicit emotional release. Physical exercise is a constructive way of releasing energy when direct problem solving is impossible or ineffective as it reduces muscle tension and other physiological effects of anxiety.
7. Relaxation techniques. Relaxation techniques are likely to be effective for patients with mild to moderate anxiety who are able to concentrate and desire to use them. Some techniques require learning and/or regular practice for effectiveness. Environmental awareness is reduced by focusing inward, with deliberate concentration on breathing, a sound, or an image and suggestions of muscle relaxation. Progressive relaxation and autogenic relaxation are commonly used techniques which require approximately 15 minutes. Relaxation and guided imagery scripts are readily available for use by clinicians.[20,73]
8. Breathing techniques. Simple and easy to learn, breathing exercises emphasize slow, rhythmic, controlled breathing patterns that relax and distract the patient while slowing the heart rate, thus decreasing anxiety. Ask the patient to notice his or her normal breathing. Then, ask the patient to take a few slow, deep abdominal breaths and to think "Relax" or "I am calm" with each exhalation. Encourage practice during the day. Some patients are helped by seeing photographs and drawings of lungs and breathing, such as the images in *The Incredible Machine*,[74] to visualize their actions.
9. Focusing techniques. Useful for patients with episodes of severe to panic levels of anxiety, focusing repeatedly on one person or object in the room helps the patient to disengage from all other stimuli and promotes control. A combination of focusing with demonstration and coaching of slow, rhythmic breathing with a calm, low-pitched voice is helpful. These techniques enhance the patient's self-control, which is desirable when the stress reaction is excessive and the stressful event cannot be changed or avoided. Both focusing and deep breathing techniques can be used without prior practice and during extreme stress.
10. Music therapy. Soothing music or environmental sounds reduce anxiety by providing a tranquil environment and prompting recall of pleasant memories, which interrupt the stress response through distraction or direct sympathetic nervous system action.[75] Music most helpful for relaxation is primarily of string composition, low-pitched, with a simple and direct musical rhythm and a tempo of approximately 60 beats per minute,[75] although music with flute, a cappela voice, and synthesizer is also effective.
11. Imagery and visualization techniques. Imagery inhibits anxiety by invoking a calm, peaceful mental image, including memories, dreams, fantasies, and visions. Guided imagery is the deliberate, goal-directed use of the natural capacities of the imagination. Using all the

senses, imagery serves as a bridge for connecting body, mind, and spirit.[76] Imagery, especially when combined with relaxation, promotes coping with illness by anxiety reduction, enhanced self-control, feeling expression, symptom relief, healing promotion, and dealing with role changes. [20,49] Regular practice of imagery enhances success. Guided imagery for pain or anxiety reduction should not be attempted the first time in periods of extreme stress. Imagery in conversation is subtle and spontaneous. Often without awareness, health care providers' questions and statements to patients include imagery. Easily combined with routine activities, the deliberate use of conversational imagery involves listening to and positive use of the language, beliefs, and metaphors of the patient. Be aware of descriptors used for the effects of medications or treatments as they affect the patient's attitude and response. Health care providers can enhance hope and self-control if they give empowering, healing messages which emphasize how the treatment will help.[49]

Psychotherapeutic Interventions Targeted to Symptoms of Depression

Depression is inadequately treated in palliative care, although many patients experience depressive symptoms. Goals for the depressed patient are (*1*) to ensure a safe environment, (*2*) to assist the patient in reducing depressive symptoms and maladaptive coping responses, (*3*) to restore or increase the patient's functional level, (*4*) to improve quality of life if possible, and (*5*) to prevent future relapse and recurrence of depression.[49]

Crisis Intervention. Crisis intervention is appropriate treatment for a grief and loss reaction and when a patient feels overwhelmed. Effective strategies also include providing guidance on current problems, reinforcing coping resources and strengths, and enhancing social supports.[20,49]

Cognitive Interventions. Cognitive interventions (Table 19–10) are based on a view of depression as the result of faulty thinking. A person's reaction depends on how that person perceives and interprets the situation of chronic illness. Patterns of thinking associated with depression include self-condemnation, leading to feelings of inadequacy and guilt; hopelessness, which is often combined with helplessness; and self-pity, which comes from magnification or catastrophizing about one's problems. Cognitive approaches involve clarification of misconceptions and modification of faulty assumptions by identifying and correcting distorted, negative, and catastrophic thinking. Cognitive approaches are effective in treating forms of depression.[49] Therapy is usually brief, with the primary goal of reversing and decreasing the likelihood of recurrence of the symptoms of depression by modifying cognitions. It requires effort on the part of the patient. The effect is more powerful if homework and practice are included.

Cognitive restructuring is one of the strategies used in cognitive therapy. In this strategy, patients are aided in identifying and evaluating maladaptive attitudes, thoughts, and beliefs by self-monitoring and recording their automatic thoughts when they feel depressed. The patient is then helped to replace self-defeating patterns of thinking with more constructive patterns. For example, "The treatment is not working. I can't cope; nothing works for me." could be replaced with a rational response such as "I can cope. I have learned how to help myself and I can do it." New self-statements and their associated feeling responses can also be written on the self-monitoring form. Over time, the patient learns to modify thinking and learns a method for combating other automatic thoughts.[47a]

Imagery rehearsal is a strategy useful for helping patients to cope with situations in which they usually become depressed. The first step is to anticipate events that could be problematic, such as a magnetic resonance procedure. The patient is helped to develop constructive self-statements; then, imagery is used to provide an opportunity for the patient to mentally rehearse how to think, act, and feel in the situation. The combination of imagery with cognitive restructuring increases the effectiveness.[47a]

Interpersonal Interventions. Interpersonal interventions (Table 19–10) focus on improved self-esteem, the development of effective social skills, and dealing with interpersonal and relationship difficulties. Interpersonal difficulties that could be a focus include role disruptions or transitions, social isolation, delayed grief reaction, family conflict, or role enactment. Psychotherapies include individual, group, and support groups led by a trained professional. Patient-led support groups or self-help groups are effective for the general chronic illness population but less able to address the needs of depressed persons.[48]

Behavioral Interventions. Behavioral interventions (Table 19–10) are based on a functional analysis of behavior and on social learning theory. These interventions are often used in combination with cognitive interventions, such as self-monitoring and imagery rehearsal. The key to the behavioral approach is to avoid reinforcement of dependent or negative behaviors. Instead, provide a contingency relationship between positive reinforcement and independent behavior and positive interactions with the environment. This approach suggests that, by altering behavior, subsequent thoughts and feelings are positively influenced. It is helpful to structure this approach using the following self-care functional areas: behavior related to breathing, eating, and drinking; elimination patterns; personal hygiene behavior; rest and activity patterns; patterns of solitude and social interaction. The aim is to maintain involvement in activities associated with positive moods and, if possible, avoidance of situations that trigger depression.[77] This approach as been effective at helping family members of terminally ill patients to see and accept functional decline.

Alternative and Complementary Therapies. Complementary therapies may help reduce mild depressive symptoms, or they may be used as an adjunct to

Table 19–10. Nonpharmacological Interventions for Treatment of Depression

Cognitive Interventions
Review and reinforce realistic ideas and expectations
Help the patient test the accuracy of self-defeating assumptions
Help the patient identify and test negative automatic thoughts
Review and reinforce patient's strengths
Set realistic, achievable goals
Explain all actions and plans, seek feedback and participation in decision making
Provide choices, e.g., about the timing of an activity
Teach thought stopping or thought interruption to halt negative or self-defeating thoughts
Encourage exploration of feelings only for a specific purpose and only if the patient is not ruminating (constant repeating of failures, problems, etc.)
Direct the patient to activities with gentle reminders to focus as a way to discourage rumination
Listen and take appropriate action on physical complaints, then redirect and assist the patient to accomplish activities
Avoid denying the patient's sadness or depressed feelings or reason to feel that way
Avoid chastising the patient for feeling sad
Interpersonal Interventions
Educate the patient about the physical and biochemical causes of depression and good prognosis
Enhance social skills through modeling, role playing, rehearsal, feedback, and reinforcement
Build rapport with frequent, short visits
Engage in normal social conversation with the patient as often as possible
Give consistent attention even when the patient is uncommunicative, to show that the patient is worthwhile
Direct comments and questions to the patient rather than to significant others
Allow adequate time for the patient to prepare a response
Mobilize family and social support systems
Encourage the patient to maintain open communication and share feelings with significant others
Supportively involve family and friends and teach them how to help
Avoid sharing with the patient your personal reactions to the patient's dependent behavior
Avoid medical jargon, advice giving, sharing personal experiences, or making value judgments
Avoid false reassurance
Behavioral Interventions
Provide directed activities
Develop a hierarchy of behaviors with the patient and use a graded task assignment
Develop structured daily activity schedules
Encourage the at-home use of a diary or journal to monitor automatic thoughts, behaviors, and emotions; review this with the patient
Use systematic application of reinforcement
Encourage self-monitoring of predetermined behaviors, such as sleep pattern, diet, and physical exercise
Focus on goal attainment and preparation for future adaptive coping
Specific Behavioral Strategies
Observe the patient's self-care patterns, then negotiate with the patient to develop a structured, daily schedule
Develop realistic daily self-care goals with the patient to increase sense of control
Upgrade the goals gradually to provide increased opportunity for positive reinforcement and goal attainment
Utilize a chart for monitoring daily progress; gold stars may be utilized as reinforcement; a visible chart facilitates communication, consistency among caregivers, and meaningful reinforcement, i.e., praise and positive attention from others
Provide sufficient time and repetitive reassurance ("You can do it") to encourage patients to accomplish self-care actions
Positively reinforce even small achievements
Provide physical assistance with self-care activities, especially those related to appearance and hygiene, that the patient is unable to do
Adjust physical assistance, verbal direction, reminders, and teaching to the actual needs/abilities of the patient; avoid increasing unnecessary dependence by overdoing
Teach deep breathing or relaxation techniques for anxiety management
Complementary Therapies
Guided imagery and visualization
Art and music therapies
Humor
Aerobic exercise
Phototherapy
Aromatherapy and massage

Sources: Minarik (1996), reference 20; Leavitt and Minarik (1989), reference 70.

other therapies for more severe depressive symptoms.[48] Strategies described for anxiety, such as guided imagery and visualization, the use of drawings or photographs, and music therapy, also may be used for depression. Art therapy for creative self-expression, use of humor and laughter, aerobic exercise, and aromatherapy massage have been helpful for mild depressive symptoms.[48] *Phototherapy*, which is exposure to bright, wide-spectrum light, has shown promise in patients with cancer.[48]

CONCLUSION

The psychosocial issues in persons facing life-threatening illness are influenced by individual, sociocultural, medical, and family factors. Most patients receiving palliative treatment and their families experience expected periods of emotional turmoil that occur at transition points along the clinical course of cancer. Some patients experience anxiety and depressive disorders. This chapter has described the spectrum of anxiety and depressive symptoms during the palliative care trajectory, models of interaction useful for understanding the interaction of psychiatric and medical symptoms and for designing appropriate treatments, guidelines for referral to trained psychiatric clinicians, and a range of treatments for anxiety and depression. Supportive psychotherapeutic measures, such as those described in this chapter, should be used routinely as they minimize distress and enhance feelings of control and mastery over self and environment. Assessment and treatment of psychosocial problems including physical symptoms, psychological distress, caregiver burden, and psychiatric disorders can enhance quality of life throughout the palliative care trajectory.

Case Report

A 42-year-old housewife and the mother of two small children, Mrs. Brady, was referred for consultation following segmental resection for probable stage IV breast cancer with 15 positive nodes and one small area of questionable bone metastasis noted on her left hip. On being told that she required chemotherapy, she refused, saying "It is hopeless—why bother?" Her husband and oncologist together persuaded her to discuss her decision with a psychiatric consultation liaison nurse, and she reluctantly agreed. She was depressed and withdrawn, although moderately anxious. She wrung her hands throughout the interview, reported intrusive thoughts of death that kept her from sleeping at night, and stated that she preferred for her children to remember her as she was. An early death would be preferable to the lingering debilitation that she believed would be associated with chemotherapy. On further review, she described being 13 years old when her mother was diagnosed with breast cancer and that she had always feared that it would happen to her too. Her mother's mastectomy had been followed by painful bone metastasis despite chemotherapy. Mrs. Brady had distressing memories of her mother's suffering and had taken lengthy steps with her physicians to assure that mammograms and frequent breast exams would allow her to be diagnosed early should breast cancer develop. Several areas of calcification had been monitored for over a year. She now had anger toward her physician that her life was needlessly compromised by late diagnosis of something she had attempted to avoid for so long. The anger and hopelessness together were overwhelming, and she could not focus on anything else. Clarification that she would be receiving chemotherapy to halt disease progression and awareness that her reason for refusing was based on memories of her mother and, thus, assumptions about her own outcome led the patient to reconsider and accept treatment recommendations. A low-dose anxiolytic was suggested for use at bedtime, which the patient received on a short-term basis. Mrs. Brady was still well at the 1 year follow-up.

REFERENCES

1. Holland J. Clinical course of cancer. In: Holland JC, Rowland JH, eds. Handbook of Psychooncology: Psychological Care of the Patient with Cancer. New York: Oxford University Press, 1989:75–110.

2. Weisman AD, Worden JW, Sobel HJ. Psychosocial Screening and Intervention with Cancer Patients. Final report of the Omega Project (CA 19797). Bethesda, MD: National Cancer Institute.

3. Endicott J. Measurement of depression in patients with cancer. In: Proceedings of the Working Conference on Methodology in Behavioral and Psychosocial Cancer Research. American Cancer Society, April 21–23, 1983, St. Petersburg Beach, FL, pp. 2243–2247.

4. Graydon JE. Factors that predict patients' functioning following treatment for cancer. Int J Nurs Stud 1988;25:117–124.

5. Northouse L. The impact of cancer on the family: an overview. Int J Psychiatry Med 1984;14:215–242.

6. Worden JW. Psychosocial screening of cancer patients. J Psychosoc Oncol 1983;1:1–10.

7. Rowland JH, Massie MJ. Breast cancer. In: Holland JC, ed. Psycho-oncology. New York: Oxford University Press, 1989:380–401.

8. Gotay CC. Causal attributions and coping behaviors in early-stage cervical cancer. Presented at the Annual Meeting of the American Psychological Association, Los Angeles, CA, 1981.

9. Watson M, Greer S, Blake S, Sharpnell K. Reaction to a diagnosis of breast cancer: relationship between denial, delay, and rates of psychological morbidity. Cancer 1984;53:2008–2012.

10. Bope E. Follow-up of the cancer patient: surveillance for metastasis. Prim Care 1987;14:391–401.

11. Holland JC. Psychologic aspects of cancer. In: Holland JF, Frei, III E, eds. Cancer Medicine. Philadelphia: Lea and Febiger, 1982:1175–1184.

12. Weissman A. A model for psychosocial phasing in cancer. In: Moos RH, ed. Coping with Physical Illness, vol 2. New Perspectives. New York: Plenum, 1984:107–122.

13. Silverfarb PM, Maurer LH, Crouthamel CS. Psychosocial aspects of neoplastic disease: I. Functional status of breast cancer patients during different treatment regimens. Am J Psychiatry 1980;137:450–455.

14. McCorkle R, Benoliel JQ, Donaldson G, Georgiadou F, Moinpour C, Goodell B. A randomized clinical trial of home health nursing care for lung cancer patients. Cancer 1989;64:199–206.

15. Thomas SG. Breast cancer: the psychosocial issues. Cancer Nurs 1978;1:53–60.

16. Tilden VP. Ethics perspectives on end-of-life care. Nurs Outlook 1999;47:162–167.

17. Speigel D, Bloom JR, Kraemer HC. Effect of psychosocial treatment on survival of patients with metastatic breast cancer. Lancet 1989; 2:888–891.

18. Bates MS, Edwards WT, Anderson KO. Ethnocultural influences on variation in chronic pain perception. Pain 1993;52:101–112.

19. Pickett M. Cultural awareness in the context of terminal illness. Cancer Nurs 1993;16:102–106.

20. Minarik P. Psychosocial intervention with ineffective coping responses to physical illness: anxiety-related. In: Barry PD, ed. Psychosocial Nursing: Care of Physically Ill Patients and Their Families. New York: Lippincott-Raven, 1996: 301–322.

21. Roth AJ, Breitbart W. Psychiatric emergencies in terminally ill cancer patients. Hematol Oncol Clin North Am 1996;10:235–259.

22. Stoudemire A. Epidemiology and psychopharmacology of anxiety in medical patients. J Clin Psychiatry 1996;57 (Suppl 7):977–986.

23. Wise MG, Taylor SE. Anxiety and mood

disorders in medically ill patients. J Clin Psychiatry 1990;51 (Suppl 1):27–32.

24. Sinsheimer L, Holland JC. Psychosocial issues in breast cancer. Semin Oncol 1987;14: 75–82.

25. Penman DT, Bloom JR, Fotopoulou S, et al. The impact of mastectomy on self concept and ego function. A combined cross sectional and longitudinal study with comparison groups. Womens Health, 1986;11:3.

26. Bloom JR. Social support, accommodation to stress and adjustment to breast cancer. Soc Sci Med 1982;16:1329–1338.

27. Jamison KR, Wellisch DK, Pasnau RO. Psychosocial aspects of mastectomy: I. The woman's perspective. Am J Psychiatry 1978;135: 432–436.

28. Andrykowski MA, Redd WH, Hatfield AK. The development of anticipatory nausea: a prospective analysis. J Consult Clin Psychol 1985; 4:447–454.

29. Burish TG, Lyles JN. Effectiveness of relaxation training in reducing adverse reactions to cancer chemotherapy. J Behav Med 1981;4:65–78.

30. Sarna L, McCorkle R. Living with lung cancer: a prototype to describe the burden of care for patient, family and caregivers. Cancer Pract 1996;4:245–251.

31. Bukberg J, Penman D, Holland JC. Depression in hospitalized cancer patients. Psychosom Med 1984;46:199–212.

32. Derogatis LR, Morrow GR, Fetting J, et al. The prevalence of psychiatric disorders among cancer patients. JAMA 1983;249:751–757.

33. Massie MJ, Gagnon P, Holland JC. Depression and suicide in patients with cancer. J Pain Symptom Manage 1994;9:325–340.

34. Pasacreta JV, Massie MJ. Psychiatric complications in patients with cancer. Oncol Nurs Forum 1990;17:19–24.

35. American Psychiatric Association. Diagnostic and Statistical Manual of Mental Disorders (DSM IV), 4th Ed. Washington DC: APA, 1994.

36. Wells KB, Stewart A, Hays RD, et al. The functioning and well being of depressed patients: results from the medical outcomes study. JAMA 1989;262:914–919.

37. Breitbart W. Identifying patients at risk for and treatment of major psychiatric complications of cancer. Support Care Cancer 1995;3:45–60.

38. McDaniel JS, Messelman DL, Porter MR, Reed DA, Nemeroff CB. Depression in patients with cancer. Diagnosis, biology and treatment. Arch Gen Psychiatry 1995;52:89–99.

39. Derogatis LR, Wise TN. Anxiety and Depressive Disorders in the Medical Patient. Washington DC: American Psychiatric Press, 1989.

40. Pasacreta JV, Pickett M. Psychosocial aspects of palliative care. Semin Oncol Nurs 1998; 26:77–92.

41. Pasacreta JV, McCorkle R. Psychosocial aspects of cancer. McCorkle R, Grant M, Stromborg MF, Baird S, eds. Cancer Nursing: A Comprehensive textbook (2nd ed). Philadelphia: WB Saunders, pp. 1074–1090.

42. Cassem EH. Depressive disorders in the medically ill. Psychosomatics 1995;36:S2–S10.

43. Cavanaugh S. Depression in the medically ill. Psychosomatics 1995;36:48–59.

44. Fernandez R, Levy JK, Lachar BL, Small GW. The management of depression and anxiety in the elderly. J Clin Psychiatry 1995;56 (Suppl 2): 20–29.

45. Kurlowicz LH. Depression in hospitalized medically ill elders: evolution of the concept. Arch Psychiatric Nurs 1994;7:124–136.

46. Barraclough J. ABC of palliative care: depression, anxiety, and confusion. BMJ 1997;315: 1365–1368.

47. Peplau H. A working definition of anxiety. In: Burd SF, Marshall MA, eds. Some Clinical Approaches to Psychiatric Nursing. New York: Macmillan, 1963:323–327.

47a. Golden WL, Gersh WD, Robbins DM. Psychological Treatment of Cancer Patients: A Cognitive Behavioral Approach. New York: MacMillan, 1992.

48. Hurst M, Schulmeister L. Depression among patients with cancer. ONS Supplement. Am J Nurs 1999;99:24–27.

49. Minarik P. Psychosocial intervention with ineffective coping responses to physical illness: depression-related. In: Barry PD, ed. Psychosocial Nursing: Care of Physically Ill Patients and Their Families. New York: Lippincott-Raven, 1996:323–339.

50. Hall RCW, Platt DE. Suicide risk assessment: a review of risk factors for suicide in 100 patients who made severe suicide attempts: evaluation of suicide risk in a time of managed care. Psychosomatics 1999;40:18–27.

51. Valente SM, Trainor D. Rational suicide among patients who are terminally ill. AORN J 1998;68:252–264.

52. Chochinov HM, Wilson KG, Enns M, Lander S. Depression, hopelessness, and suicidal ideation in the terminally ill. Psychosomatics 1998;39:366–370.

53. Back AL, Wallace JI, Starks HE, Pearlman RA. Physician-assisted suicide and euthanasia in Washington State. Patient requests and physician responses. JAMA 1996;275:919–925.

54. Daley BJ, Berry D, Fitzpatrick JJ, Drew B, Montgomery K. Assisted suicide: implications for nurses and nursing. Nurs Outlook 1997;45: 209–214.

55. Tilden VP, Tolle SW, Lee MA, Nelson CA. Oregon's physician-assisted suicide vote: its effect on palliative care. Nurs Outlook 1996;44: 80–83.

56. Scanlon C. Euthanasia and nursing practice—right question, wrong answer. N Engl J Med 1996;344:1401–1402.

57. St John PD, Man-Son-Hing M. Physician-assisted suicide: the physician as an unwitting accomplice. J Palliat Care 1999;15:56–58.

58. Holland J, Massie MJ, Straker N. Psychotherapeutic interventions. In: Holland JC, Rowland JH, eds. Handbook of Psychooncology: Psychological Care of the Patient with Cancer. New York: Oxford University Press, 1989:455–469.

59. Bloom JR, Ross RD, Burnell G. The effect of social support on patient adjustment after breast surgery. Patient Counsel Health Educ 1978;1:50–59.

60. Linn MW, Linn BS, Harris R. Effects of counseling for late stage cancer patients. Cancer 1982;49:1048–1055.

61. Levenson J, Lesko LM. Psychiatric aspects of adult leukemia. Semin Oncol Nurs 1990;6:76–83.

62. Bailey K. Lippincott's Need-to-Know Psychotropic Drug Facts. Philadelphia: Lippincott, 1998.

63. Massie MJ, Lesko LM. Psychopharmacologic management In: Holland JC, Rowland JH, eds. Handbook of Psychooncology: Psychological Care of the Patient with Cancer. New York: Oxford University Press, 1989:470–492.

64. Woods SW, Tesar GE, Murray GB. Psychostimulant treatment of depressive disorders secondary to medical illness. J Clin Psychiatry 1986; 47:12–15.

65. Vigano A, Watanabe S, Bruera E. Methylphenidate for the management of somatization in terminal cancer patients. J Pain Symptom Manage 1995;10:167–170.

66. Shuster JL, Stern TA, Greenberg DB. Pros and cons of fluoxitine for the depressed cancer patient. Oncology 1992;11:45–55.

67. Eisendrath SJ. Psychiatric problems. In: Bongard FS, Sue DY, eds. Current Critical Care Diagnosis and Treatment. Norwalk, CT: Appleton and Lange, 1994:235–244.

68. Gellert GA, Maxwell RM, Siegel BS. Survival of breast cancer patients receiving adjuvant psychosocial support therapy: a 10 year follow up study. J Clin Oncol 1993;11:66–69.

69. Lazarus RS, Folkman S. Stress, Appraisal and Coping. New York: Springer, 1984.

70. Leavitt M, Minarik PA. The agitated, hypervigilant response. In: Riegel B, Ehrenreich D, eds. Psychological Aspects of Critical Care Nursing. Rockville, MD: Aspen, 1989:49–65.

71. Christman NJ, Kirchhoff KT, Oakley MG. Concrete objective information. In: Bulechek GM, McCloskey JC, eds. Nursing Interventions: Essential Nursing Treatments, 2nd Ed. Philadelphia: WB Saunders, 1992.

72. Morse JM, Doberneck B. Delineating the concept of hope. Image J Nurs Sch 1995;27:277–285.

73. Bulechek GM, McCloskey JC. Nursing Interventions: Essential Nursing Treatments, 2nd ed. Philadelphia: WB Saunders, 1992.

74. National Geographic Society. The Incredible Machine. Washington DC: National Geographic Society, 1986.

75. White JM. Music therapy: an intervention to reduce anxiety in the myocardial infarction patient. Clin Nurse Spec 1992;6:58.

76. Dossey BM. Imagery: awakening the inner healer. In: Dossey BM, Keegan L, Guzzetta CE, Kolkmeier LG, eds. Holistic Nursing: A Handbook for Practice. Rockville, MD: Aspen, 1988.

77. Tommassini N. The client with a mood disorder (depression). In: Antai-Otong D (ed.) Psychiatric Nursing: Biological and Behavioral Concepts. Philadelphia, PA: WB Saunders, 1995:178–179.

20 Delirium, Confusion, Agitation, and Restlessness

KIM K. KUEBLER, NANCY ENGLISH,
and DEBRA E. HEIDRICH

My grief became confused with anger at seeing this dignified, intelligent woman, my beloved aunt, laying naked in her bed, eyes wide and frightened, crying "Don't do this to me. . . . Get me out of here. I don't want to die." How can I respond? What could I do? The family expected me to know because I am the nurse who cares for the dying. I felt helpless.

The human "living" experience will eventually tread the path toward the inevitable physical decline that accompanies age and death. Yet each individual's dying experience is as unique as the life he or she has lived. Many of the common threads that often create fear in the dying process are similar and include the fear of pain, the fear of loss, and the fear of losing control over one's physical, emotional, and mental capacities. As nurses caring for the dying and their families, it is important that we understand how to empower both patients and families and how to reassure them that patients will receive the care and support necessary to control symptoms at life's end.

Unmanaged physical and psychiatric symptoms impact negatively on the quality of life for each person and his or her family.[1] Prompt recognition, assessment, and intervention of all symptoms become crucial for the well-being of the patient living with advanced disease. The patient with an advanced disease faces many stresses throughout the course of his or her illness, and the accompanying psychological distress is varied and dependent on personality, coping ability, social support, and medical factors.[1]

Cognitive disorders are frequently seen with dying patients. For example, in the advanced cancer patient, delirium has been found to be the main reason for cognitive failure.[1–3] This chapter specifically discusses the symptoms of delirium, confusion, agitation, and restlessness and provides a framework for approaching patients with cognitive disorders in the palliative care setting.

PREVALENCE

Many patients develop psychiatric symptoms during the terminal phase of illness, either alone or in combination with other physical symptoms. The varied psychiatric complications include anxiety, depression, and cognitive disorders.[4,5] A cognitive disorder is all too common in patients with advanced illness and has an impact on patient morbidity.[1,4,5] The American Psychiatric Association's *Diagnostic and Statistical Manual of Mental Disorders*, fourth edition (DSM-IV), categorizes cognitive disorders to include (*1*) delirium, dementia, amnesia, and other cognitive disorders; (2) mental disorders due to a general personality change as a result of an underlying medical condition; and (3) substance-related disorders.[6] Patients diagnosed with a terminal illness often have an escalation in the intensity of both the underlying medical condition and psychiatric syndromes.[4,7] The percentage and prevalence of cognitive disorders in the terminally ill cancer patient is higher than what was initially proposed.[8] Delirium is considered the most common cognitive disorder in the terminally ill.[4]

Delirium is found in 77% to 85% of terminally ill cancer patients[2,8–10] and in up to 57% of terminally ill acquired immunodeficiency syndrome (AIDS) patients.[11] Some clinicians may consider delirium to be the "hallmark" of dying, and its relevance to palliative care is evident. Delirium is also one of the most commonly encountered mental disorders in general hospital practice[5] and has been refered to as "everyman's psychosis," which can account for the fact that everybody is potentially susceptible.[5] While delirium can occur at any age, the high incidence in elderly patients is often overlooked. Delirium has also been referred to as the "reversible madness," which no clinician wants to overlook. Studies have indicated that 25% to 35% of episodes are reversible.[12,13] Early detection and assessment are likely to improve outcomes. Objective monitoring and a high level of clinical awareness and skill are necessary to detect and treat this syndrome in the palliative setting.

DEFINITION

Terminology of Cognitive Changes

Understanding the many symptoms, syndromes, and diagnoses associated with cognitive changes in persons with a terminal illness can be difficult at best, and the use of these definitions is often inconsistent in both clinical practice and the nursing and medical literature. "Confusion," for example, may at times be used to describe a symptom; at other times, "confusion" may be used to describe a syndrome. Terms such as "encephalopathy" and "acute confusional state" are often used to describe changes in mental status instead of using a psychiatric classification based on a set criteria from the DSM.[6,10,14] In addition, many of these are complex disorders having overlapping yet distinct etiologies and clinical characteristics. The use of imprecise terminology can lead to mislabeling of behaviors, miscommunication among health care professionals, and misdiagnoses of cognitive changes. The potential for the mismanagement of any cognitive change is, therefore, extremely high.

Symptoms Associated with Cognitive Changes

The various labels used to categorize cognitive changes are based on the observation and evaluation of symptoms and behaviors. A common language regarding these symptoms is essential for accurate communication among health care professionals.

Anxiety. Anxiety may be described as a fear of the unknown (not knowing what is expected) or fear of the known (knowing what to expect) and is considered a universal human experience. An anxious person experiences a vague, diffuse apprehension or uneasiness, often accompanied by feelings of uncertainty and helplessness.[15–17] Anxiety is a subjective experience and not directly observable. Its existence is either reported by the experiencing individual or inferred by observing overt behaviors. One can view anxiety as being on a continuum ranging from mild to extreme. Although mild anxiety can be beneficial, increased or sustained anxiety can be detrimental physiologically and psychologically.

The subjective experiences of the anxious person are often described as tension, nervousness, restlessness, headaches, and nausea. Observable signs of anxiety include holding a tense posture, fidgeting with fingers or clothing, sighing frequently, licking dry lips, sweating more than average, and trembling. The individual may be very quiet or speak more freely than usual. Physiologically, anxiety can be noted by an increase in heart rate, respiratory rate, and systolic blood pressure.[16]

Anxiety is a symptom that has many causes, including the physical, psychosocial, emotional, and spiritual. While anxiety is common in persons with terminal illness, it is neither helpful nor accurate to assume that a high level of anxiety is inevitable during the terminal phase of illness.[1] The various signs of anxiety must be used as cues to help assess the underlying causes and implement appropriate interventions.

Cognitive changes can lead to anxiety. Cognitive impairment, regardless of the underlying cause, can disrupt both the receiving and the processing of sensory information. This results in a diminished ability to handle stressful situations and creates the sensation of anxiety.[18] Thus, anxiety may be a symptom of a cognitive change. In addition, anxiety may be a cause of cognitive change. For example, Bowman[19] identified that unrelieved anxiety was associated with the development of postoperative delirium. Although there have been no studies looking at the association between anxiety and delirium in the terminally ill, it is prudent to view anxiety as a potential contributing factor to cognitive changes in this population of patients.

Confusion. Confusion is a very commonly used term to describe the behavior of patients at the end of life, yet it lacks both clarity and definition.[20] When used to describe a subjective experience, confusion is considered a symptom. When used to describe a patient's mental state, the term "confusion" is broad, indicating neither a symptom nor a diagnosis.[10] A number of different subjective experiences and objective or observational behaviors may be described as confusion. In one study, nurses identified certain behaviors that they believed to be indicative of confusion. Based on these observations, Williams and colleagues[21] operationally defined confusion as behaviors falling into one of the following four categories:

1. Disorientation to time, place, or persons in the environment
2. Inappropriate communication or communication unusual for the person, such as nonsensical speech, calling out, yelling, swearing, and/or silence
3. Inappropriate behavior, such as attempting to get out of bed, pulling at tubes, dressings, and/or picking at bedclothes
4. Illusions or hallucinations

Illusions are misinterpretations of real external stimuli. For example, a patient who misinterprets the pattern of the wallpaper to be snakes on the walls is experiencing an illusion. A *hallucination* is a subjective sensory perception in the absence of any relevant external stimuli. The individual experiencing the hallucination may or may not recognize that the experience is not real. Hallucinations may be auditory, visual, olfactory, gustatory, tactile, or somatic.[16]

Any decline in normal cognitive function may be labeled confusion. In the elderly, confusion is most likely a symptom of delirium or dementia but may also be associated with psychoses and/or major depression.[22] Because the term is not specific, it is best to describe the behaviors of patients and their self-reported experiences rather than identifying the patient as "confused."

Restlessness. Restlessness is defined in *Webster's New World Dictionary* as the inability to relax, being rarely quiet or still, or being active.[23] In the medical literature, restlessness has been described as being unable to keep still and being worried, uneasy, or anxious.[24] Again, this is a symptom with multiple etiologies and characteristics that often overlap with other symptoms, such as anxiety and agitation. Terminal restlessness, however, has frequently been described as a common occurrence within the last few hours of life. "Restlessness" and "agitation" are frequently used interchangeably.

Agitation. *Agitation* is another example of a symptom that does not have a clear definition. The term has been used to describe behaviors, syndromes, and outcomes of multiple psychiatric or medical problems.[14,18,25–27] Allen[18] has described agitation as being better understood as a group of symptoms that might characterize an underlying disorder.

Agitation includes many different behaviors, such as aimless wandering, pacing, cursing, screaming, calling out to a passerby, and arguing. In a factor analysis of agitated behaviors, Cohen-Mansfield and Billing[25] identified four types of agitation:

1. Physically aggressive behaviors: hitting, kicking, tearing, pushing, and cursing
2. Physically nonaggressive behaviors: pacing, inappropriate robing or disrobing, repetitious mannerism, and handling things inappropriately
3. Verbally agitated behaviors: constant request for attention, screaming, complaining, and negativism
4. Hiding/hoarding behaviors

These researchers further identified correlations between medical diagnoses and types of agitated behavior. They noted that nursing home residents who typically manifest agitation through physical behaviors usually suffer from dementia but are not otherwise generally ill. Verbal agitation was found to be prevalent in persons with a generally ill condition and in persons with unrelieved pain. However, verbal agitation was not associated with dementia. The researchers believed that the correlation of verbal agitation with disease and pain might be explained by the possibility that agitation is a form of expression of suffering from a medical disorder. This study[25] illustrates the importance of describing the agitated behavior and not simply describing a patient as being agitated.

Others have also noted a relationship between disease processes and agitated behaviors. Persons with dementia often exhibit agitation.[14,18] This probably results from alterations in the brain that cause impairments of memory, judgment, and impulse control. Agitation may be a person's attempt to express feelings and needs which cannot be verbalized, for instance, uncontrolled physical symptoms such as pain and dyspnea.[18]

Agitated behaviors have a negative impact on both patients and the families observing them. Persons who are agitated have a decreased sense of well-being, a poorer quality of life, and an increased likelihood of entering a long-term care facility. These behaviors may also lead to the overuse of physical restraints and the inappropriate use of antipsychotic medications.[18] In addition, studies have demonstrated that health care personnel are less likely to spend time with patients who are agitated and/or confused.[18,28]

Delirium. A variety of terms have been used to describe delirium, such as acute brain failure, acute confusional state, acute secondary psychosis, exogenous psychosis, sundown syndrome, and organic brain syndrome.[14] Based on the DSM-IV criteria, *delirium* may be defined as "an etiologically non-specific, global, cerebral dysfunction characterized by concurrent disturbances of level of consciousness, attention, thinking, perception, memory, psychomotor behavior, emotion, and the sleep–wake cycle."[1] It is often identified as a sudden and significant decline in a previous level of functioning and is conceptualized as a reversible process. Delirium can also affect sleep, psychomotor activity, and emotions.

Following are the DMS-IV criteria for delirium:[6]

1. Disturbance of consciousness with reduced ability to focus, sustain, or shift attention
2. A change in cognition (such as memory deficit, disorientation, language disturbance) or the development of a perceptual disturbance that is not better accounted for by preexisting, established, or evolving dementia
3. The disturbance develops over a short period of time (usually hours to days) and tends to fluctuate over the course of the day

Disturbance of Consciousness. To better understand this diagnosis, it may be helpful to discuss each of these criteria in more detail. Disturbance of consciousness with reduced clarity or awareness of the environment that does not reach the level of stupor or coma can manifest as delirium. A critical feature of this criterion is altered attention.[29] Attention is typically fluctuating and may present as a change in the level of consciousness, slowed or inadequate reactions to stimuli or the environment, and easy distractibility. Due to this distractibility, individuals may be unable to follow conversations or complete simple tasks.[10,30]

Change in Cognition. Memory deficits are a common indication of delirium, with short-term memory deficits being the most evident. This probably results from inattention or being easily distracted.[10,29] Persons who are easily distracted or simply cannot pay attention for more than a few minutes may not remember conversations, television shows, or verbal instructions. They may have no recollection of the conversation or remember only bits and pieces. For example, the person experiencing cognitive changes may remember the nurse visiting but not anything the nurse said or did.

Disorientation is a common, but not universal, feature of delirium[10] and usually manifests as disorientation to time or place, with time disorientation being the first to be affected. Disorientation to other persons occurs commonly, but disorientation to self is very rare.[30] Language disturbances associated with delirium include a lack of fluency and spontaneity. This may manifest itself in long pauses in the conversation or use of repetitious phrases by the patient. The person experiencing delirium may also have difficulty finding the correct word to use in conversation or naming objects (*anomia*). Chedru and Geschwind[31] noted that writing ability seems to be affected earlier in the advent of delirium and is more severe than other language-related skills.

Perceptual disturbances may include misinterpretations, illusions, or hallucinations. Visual misperceptions and hallucinations are most common; but auditory, tactile, gustatory, and olfactory misperceptions or hallucinations can also occur. The individual with delirium may have the delusional conviction that the hallucination is real and exhibit emotional and behavioral responses consistent with the hallucination's content.[30]

Additional Features of Delirium. Although not required for the diagnosis of delirium, other features are common, and it will be helpful to assess for these symptoms and monitor for any changes in these over time. Disturbance in sleep patterns is frequently observed in persons with delirium and was one of the criteria for delirium in the DSM-IIIR (third edition, revised) definition. However, this criteria was excluded from the DSM-IV definition of delirium because it lacked specificity.[32] It is all too common to observe daytime sleepiness, nighttime agitation, and disturbances in sleep continuity along with the other features of delirium.[30]

Persons with delirium may also exhibit disturbed psychomotor activity. This may be evident in a hyperactive or hypoactive form. Persons with the hyperactive variant of delirium more often experience hallucinations, delusions, agitation, and disorientation. Confusion and sedation are more commonly found in the hypoactive form of this condition.[30]

Persons with delirium may exhibit emotional disturbances. Anxiety, fear, depression, irritability, anger, euphoria, and apathy are common, with anxiety being the prevailing emotion. The delirious patient may be emotionally labile, rapidly and unpredictably shifting from one emotional state to another.[10,30]

Diagnosing Delirium. The diagnosis of delirium is primarily clinical, based on careful observation and awareness of its key features.[33] Because the signs and symptoms are nonspecific, the clinician must look for a constellation of findings (signs of a disturbance in consciousness and a change in cognition), identify the rapidity of onset, and assess for associated medical and environmental risks that lead to a definitive diagnosis. It is frequently unrecognized by clinicians[33] and misdiagnosed.[28] The fact that demented, depressed, and anxious patients may develop delirium makes the diagnosis difficult.[29] However, because of its prevalence in the hospitalized elderly and the terminally ill, any patient with a deterioration in mental status is best presumed to be delirious until it is proved otherwise.[8,22,33,34]

Clinicians expect delirium to present with agitation, hallucinations, and inappropriate behavior. Indeed, the hyperalert–hyperactive variant of delirium is most commonly recognized.[29,33] Characteristics of hyperactive–hyperalert delirium include plucking at bedclothes, wandering, verbal or physical aggression, increased alertness to stimuli, psychosis, and mood lability.[29]

In addition, hyperactive–hyperalert delirium may be more quickly identified due to the disruption of behavior associated with it. Verbal agitation, wandering, and mood swings can be very distressing to caregivers, leading to earlier reporting of symptoms. One study identified that the hyperactive–hyperalert variant of delirium is seen more frequently at the end of life. However, this may have been related to missing or misdiagnosing hypoactive delirium as some other cognitive disorder.[35]

Significantly, older patients with delirium often present with lethargy and decreased activity, that is, the hypoactive form of delirium.[33] As the majority of persons with terminal illness are older, one might anticipate this variant of delirium to be relatively common in the terminally ill. Hypoactive–hypoalert delirium is characterized by withdrawal from people and usual activities and decreased responsiveness to stimuli. The delirium in these patients is often overlooked.[12,33,35,36] Their symptoms may be attributed to dementia, depression, or senescence.[33,34,37] However, patients who lack alertness or have a clouded consciousness are more likely to have delirium than dementia.[22] A 6-month or longer duration of ongoing symptomatology is required for a definitive diagnosis of dementia.[34] The distinguishing characteristics among delirium, dementia, depression, and psychosis are outlined in Table 20–1.

Some patients experience the mixed type of delirium, fluctuating between hyperactive and hypoactive symptoms. A major concern in this population is that a change in behavior from hyperactive to hypoactive may be viewed as an improvement (less agitated) when, in actuality, the patient has gotten worse.[29] A complete assessment of all symptoms of delirium is required before a change in behavior can be labeled as an improvement.

Prodromal Signs of Delirium. Some patients manifest a subclinical delirium or prodromal symptoms such as restlessness, anxiety, irritability, distractibility, or sleep disturbance in the days before the onset of overt delirium. These may progress to full-blown delirium over 1 to 3 days.[30] Patients noted to be exhibiting one or more of the above symptoms or who report feeling "mixed up," having difficulty judging the passing of time, and having difficulty thinking or concentrating should be assessed for potentially reversible causes of delirium (such as dehydration, medications, and hypercalcemia), and appropriate interventions should be initiated.[29,38]

Delirium and Dementia. In addition to commonly shared symptoms, there appears to be an interrelationship or overlap between dementia and delirium.[33] It has been noted in the elderly that up to two-thirds of cases of delirium are superimposed on dementia. It has also been postulated that delirium may lead to chronic cognitive impairment. Many patients who have experienced delirium are slow to recover to their previous level of function.[32,34] Full recovery is less likely in the elderly versus younger patients and may not be possible in the terminally ill.

Cognitive Changes Specific to the Dying Patient

Terminal Restlessness. The symptom of restlessness is commonly observed in the

Table 20–1. Differentiating Delirium, Dementia, and Psychosis

Features	Delirium	Dementia	Psychosis
Consciousness	Clouded, reduced awareness of environment	Alert (unless delirium coexists)	Alert
Cognitive intellectual abilities	General loss	General loss	Variable
Attention	Reduced ability to focus, sustain, or shift attention	Relatively unaffected	Variable
Short-term memory	Impaired	Impaired	Intact, may be variable
Remote memory	Variable	Impaired	Intact, may be variable
Affect	Mood lability	Mood lability	Variable, mood lability
Orientation	Disorientation	May become impaired after months or years	May be impaired
Delusions	Common, usually transient and poorly organized	Sometimes	Common, usually bizarre and/or complicated
Hallucinations	Visual, tactile, olfactory	Uncommon	Auditory
Speech	Often incoherent, slow or rapid	Difficulty in finding words, preservation	Normal, slow or rapid
Personality change	Withdrawn irritability	Alteration or accentuation of premorbid traits	Variable
Psychomotor behavior	Variable: hypokinetic, hyperkinetic, mixed	Normal, may have apraxia	May be retarded or hyperactive, depends on type of psychosis
Sleep–wake cycle	Disturbed, may be reversed	Fragmented	Variable
Onset	Develops over short time period (hours–days)	Often slow and progressive, insidious	Variable
Course	Fluctuates over course of day, worse at night	Stable over course of day	Variable
Duration	Short days to weeks	Chronic	Variable

Sources: Haskell et al. (1997), reference 14; Trzepacz et al. (1999), reference 30; Milisen et al. (1998), reference 29; Foreman and Zane (1996), reference 82.

last hours of life.[38] Burke and associates[39] defined terminal restlessness as a specific form of delirium observed in patients in their last days or hours of life. Other names or descriptors used to identify this phenomenon include "agitated delirium"[39,40] and "the terrible agitation, the calling out, the can't-get-comfortable distress often experienced in the final days of life."[41] In 1997, the Hospice and Palliative Nurses Association published a clinical practice protocol on terminal restlessness in which terminal restlessness was defined as a common observable syndrome appearing in the last days of life. The observable indicators of terminal restlessness include frequent, nonpurposeful motor activity; inability to concentrate or relax; disturbances in sleep or rest patterns; fluctuating levels of consciousness, cognitive failure, and/or anxiety or potential progression to agitation.[20]

The causes of terminal restlessness are the same as those of delirium, but multiple causes often coexist. Although theoretically delirium can be reversed, it is important to recognize that terminal restlessness may be irreversible during the last 24 to 48 hours of life. This is due to the fact that irreversible processes such as multiple organ failure are occurring.[1] However, a reversible cause is always possible, and a thorough assessment is essential for quality symptom management. For example, hydrating a patient who has hypercalcemia or toxic accumulations of medications can clear cognition.

Terminal Anguish. Twycross and Lichter[38] defined *terminal anguish* as a tormented state of mind related to longstanding unresolved spiritual issues, emotional problems, interpersonal conflicts, and/or suppressed unpleasant memories. These are issues that have festered in the mind but have never been brought into the open. As persons with unresolved issues enter the dying process, their psychological defenses are no longer able to keep the unresolved issues away from conscious thought. Being weak and lacking the physical and psychosocial ability to address unresolved issues, these persons may experience the somatization of mental anguish. Restlessness, thrashing about, moaning, groaning, and even crying out are often observed in these patients. Inadequate sedation only makes this syndrome worse. Terminal sedation, either natural or induced, may be required. Terminal anguish should be suspected in the absence of cognitive failure, hallucinations, or delusion.[38] However, in reality, it may be very difficult to distinguish between a delirium with significant agitation symptoms and terminal anguish. It is important to utilize all disciplines (psychological and spiritual) in caring for the patient with terminal anguish.

DIFFERENTIATING DELIRIUM, DEMENTIA, DEPRESSION, AND PSYCHOSIS

Etiology

Despite the varied definitions of cognitive disorders, the predominant symptom of delirium represents a broad category of symptoms associated with the rapid onset of changes in the cognition. Although delirium and dementia often overlap, for the purposes of this chapter, the focus is on delirium. Delirium often represents a nonspecific syndrome due to widespread cerebral dysfunction as a direct result of many organic factors.[1,12,42]

The nonspecific etiology of delirium can be characterized as a universal cognitive disorder that impairs level of consciousness, gravely altering the ability to discern detail as well as affecting perception and memory and clouding consciousness. In addition, psychomotor abilities and the sleep–wake cycle are disturbed. Delirium will often present with an acute onset (hours to days) and has a fluctuating course; this clearly distinguishes delirium from dementia and can be easily noted on the patient's chart to reflect the sudden change in cognition. Often, the course of delirium is multifactorial, and occasionally no specific cause can be identified.[2,42–44] Bruera and colleagues[9] identified cognitive failure in 80% to 90% of 66 patients studied prior to death and a reversible cause of delirium in 44% of these patients.

The prognosis for the patient experiencing delirium is often poor, yet this should not deter the clinician from looking for the underlying cause since a significant number of cases are reversible.[2,12,43] Reversible delirium at the end of life makes a major difference in the quality of life for both patients and families. Providing sedation to comfort the delirious patient is a necessary part of palliative care but requires a thorough evaluation.[2,12,43] It is important that diagnostic work-up exclude any potentially reversible factors. Potentially reversible causes include medications, such as opioids, sedatives, anticholingerics, and steroids; hypoxia; dehydration; metabolic causes, such as hypercalcemia; and sepsis.[5,10,12] These potentially reversible causes can be identified in the following ways:

1. Simple physical examination
2. Thorough evaluation of medications
3. Complete blood count
4. Electrolytes, urea, creatine, and calcium levels
5. Pulse oximetry

Through a prospective study, Bruera and colleagues[9] identified that, in patients with reversible delirium, medications were the predominant source of cognitive impairment. Unfortunately, patients at the end of life may have multiple symptoms requiring multiple medications for management.[45] A careful reevaluation of the medication regimens on an ongoing basis is an important nursing aspect of the prevention and management of delirium.

Delirium is often referred to as the "hallmark" of dying. The person dying from a chronic progressive illness may experience a multisystem organ failure that ultimately affects the brain, leading to delirium, stupor, coma, and eventual death. Studies suggest that it is very rare for the dying to remain mentally clear throughout the final stages of illness.[8,9,12] Elizabeth Kubler-Ross identified the psychological stage of decathexis as the final emotional stage of dying that may result in cognitive functioning and precipitate the onset of delirium.[8]

Metabolic and cellular causes of delirium include, but are not limited to, hypoglycemia, ischemia, nutritional insufficiencies (thiamin, vitamin B_{12}), cachexia and the aging process, and specific diseases (such as Alzheimer's disease, cancer, paraneoplastic syndrome, AIDS, and end stage cardiac and renal diseases). Chronic social isolation may also result in delirium.[46–48]

Assessment

In the nursing process, assessment is the critical step toward understanding the complicated syndrome of delirium. Table 20–1 is a summary of characteristics to help distinguish these related symptoms. Standardized, reliable, and predictive methods of assessing patients in a palliative care environment can provide the nurse with tools to effectively communicate with other members of the interdisciplinary team and to discern the level of interventions required. Nurses utilizing assessment criteria for describing cognitive changes are able to identify risk factors often associated with delirium.

Mini-Mental State Examination

The Mini-Mental State Examination (MMSE) provides a systematic, scored method for evaluating cognitive function.[20,43,49] This scored examination can indicate early changes in cognition as it relates to the cortical function of the brain.[1] Orientation, attention, recall, and language are evaluated. Scores below 24 out of a maximum of 30 are indicative of cognitive changes.[43]

However, one of the ambiguities of this assessment instrument is that it is unable to provide the clinician with a definitive diagnosis for delirium. Also, it does not help to determine the differences between dementia, anxiety, and depression.[1,50,51] The MMSE relies heavily on patient cooperation and does not account for the abrupt changes that may occur in the patient's cognitive status during a 24-hour period. Other criticisms of the MMSE include that it does not account for the varied physical factors, such as pain and/or fatigue, and the frequency that these symptoms may contribute to the subjective score. Factors such as literacy, ethnicity, and language may have a significant influence on the resulting score and are not accounted for in the MMSE.[10,50,52]

The MMSE is intended to measure cognitive change over time and is easily administered in the palliative setting. Used over time, it is a consistent indicator of changes in cognition and can help direct clinicians to follow patients with a more predictive instrument that reflects the criteria outlined in both the DSM-III and the DSM-IV, to provide specific assessment of delirium.[6,43]

Predictive Model for Delirium

A simple predictive model for delirium based on risk factors was identified in two cohort studies of hospitalized elderly patients.[53] The Risk Assessment Model for Delirium consists of two parts: Predictive Risk Factors and Precipitating Risk Factors.

A study of 281 patients over the age of 70 admitted to a medical unit for varied reasons revealed that four predictive factors contributed to the emergence of delirium. The investigators excluded patients identified with an existing "severe" dementia. Patients experiencing a "mild cognitive impairment" (change in cognition of 6 months or less) were included. According to the researchers, there are significant risk factors for developing delirium that can be identified on admission to the acute care setting: vision impairment, severe illness, dehydration, and previous cognitive impairment.[53] One point was assigned for each risk factor present when patients were admitted to the inpatient setting. Accordingly, patients who scored a 0 were at very low risk, those scoring 1 or 2 had a moderate risk, and those scoring a 3 or 4 were considered at high risk for developing delirium during their hospitalization.[53]

Further investigations of this assessment instrument identified other factors that may precipitate the onset of delirium after hospitalization. Each event had occurred within 24 hours of the onset of a diagnosis of delirium and included the following factors: use of physical restraints, malnutrition, more than three medications added to the medication profile, and insertion of an indwelling catheter.[53] Each of these events was scored in a similar manner: low risk is 0 and high risk is 3 or more precipitating events. Subjects identified with a Predictable Risk Factor score of 0 on admission continued to be resistant to delirium even though they had 3 or more precipitating events during their hospitalization.[53]

The above two instruments are used predominantly as screening tools for cognitive impairment and are not recommended for the specific assessment of delirium. However, early identification of patients at risk for developing delirium can precipitate interventions that may reverse the delirious experience.

The following four instruments correlate with the criteria found in the DSM-III, DSM-IIIR, and DSM-IV for delirium. These instruments were selected for review because they distinguish delirium from dementia and assess the multiple features of delirium. Both the Delirium Rating Scale (DRS) and the Memorial Delirium Assessment Scale (MDAS) were found to be psychometrically valid and reliable in palliative care settings. The Confusion Assessment Method (CAM) and the Neecham Confusion Scale (NCS) were validated in the elderly patient population in an acute care setting.[53,54]

Memorial Delirium Assessment Scale

The MDAS is one of the most recent measurement scales specifically designed to quantify the presence of delirium identified from the DSM-IV criteria.[1,55,56] The MDAS (Fig. 20–1) has a high interrater reliability and internal consistency for each item.

The MDAS is a ten-item inventory, and each item is on a 0- to 3-point scale of none, mild, moderate, and severe; thus, scores range from 0 to 30. A score of 13 or above is considered positive for delirium. The MDAS was designed to quantify the severity or intensity of delirium in the medically ill. In addition, the MDAS takes into account physical factors such as fatigue and psychomotor abilities. Specific behaviors that can be assessed include disturbances in arousal and level of consciousness, psychomotor activity, memory, attention, orientation, and thinking. This rating scale requires about 10 minutes to administer and integrates both behavioral observations and operationalized descriptions of specific behaviors observed by the rater. The MDAS offers the nurse a standardized and reliable instrument to be utilized in the palliative care setting. It requires minimal training for use and is appropriate for both clinical practice and research.

Delirium Rating Scale

The DRS is the most widely used assessment instrument based on the DSM-III criteria.[50,57] The DRS has been validated predominantly in the psychiatric setting and has been found useful in the assessment of delirium in the terminally ill.[55] The DRS can discern between delirious and nondelirious patients. This ten-item scale, also rated from 0 to 3, utilizes information from patient and family interviews along with the medical history and nursing observations. A score of 12 or above (range 0–30) indicates the presence of delirium.[1,10] The ten items assessed in the DRS are as follows:

- Temporal onset of symptoms
- Perceptual disturbances
- Hallucination type
- Delusions
- Psychomotor behavior
- Cognitive status during formal testing
- Underlying physical disorder
- Sleep–wake cycle disturbance
- Lability of mood
- Variability of symptoms

The benefits of the DRS are clear as it takes into account many underlying causes of delirium, but limitations are that it lacks administrative ease for the clinician and is more appropriate for use in research environments.

Confusion Assessment Method

A nurse designed the CAM for use by a trained interviewer to assess cognitive functioning in patients on a daily scheduled basis.[58,59] The CAM contains ten domains, which are dependent on clinical observations along with patient interviews. The CAM is an algorithm of specific and abrupt onset of symptoms and reflects the patient's level of consciousness and clarity of thought changes from baseline data.

Despite its attempt to streamline a diagnosis, the CAM is a complex instrument that requires extensive instruction for the rater due to its subtleties. It specifies that the patient must have an abrupt onset of symptoms in congruence with his or her inattention and disorganized thinking. In addition, the patient's level of consciousness must reflect a change from baseline norms. The domains assessed on the CAM include:

- Acute onset
- Inattention
- Disorganized thinking
- Altered level of consciousness
- Orientation
- Memory
- Perceptual problems
- Psychomotor agitation
- Psychomotor retardation
- Altered sleep–wake cycle

INSTRUCTIONS: Rate the severity of the following symptoms of delirium based on current interaction with subject or assessment of his/her behavior or experience over past several hours (as indicated in each time.)

ITEM 1—REDUCED LEVEL OF CONSCIOUSNESS (AWARENESS): Rate the patient's current awareness of and interaction with the environment (interviewer, other people/objects in the room; for example, ask patients to describe their surroundings).

☐ 0: none (patient spontaneously fully aware of environment and interacts appropriately)
☐ 1: mild (patient is unaware of some elements in the environment, or not spontaneously interacting appropriately with the interviewer; becomes fully aware and appropriately interactive when prodded strongly; interview is prolonged but not seriously disrupted)
☐ 2: moderate (patient is unaware of some or all elements in the environment, or not spontaneously interacting with the interviewer; becomes incompletely aware and inappropriately interactive when prodded strongly; interview is prolonged but not seriously disrupted)
☐ 3: severe (patient is unaware of all elements in the environment with no spontaneous interaction or awareness of the interviewer, so that the interview is difficult-to-impossible, even with maximal prodding

ITEM 2—DISORIENTATION: Rate current state by asking the following 10 orientation items: date, month, day, year, season, floor, name of hospital, city state, and country.

☐ 0: none (patient knows 9–10 items)
☐ 1: mild (patient knows 7–8 items)
☐ 2: moderate (patient knows 5–6 items)
☐ 3: severe (patient knows no more than 4 items)

ITEM 3—SHORT-TERM MEMORY IMPAIRMENT: Rate current state by using repetition and delayed recall of 3 words [patient must immediately repeat and recall words 5 min later after an intervening task. Use alternate sets of 3 words for successive evaluations (for example, apple, table, tomorrow; sky, cigar, justice)].

☐ 0: none (all 3 words repeated and recalled)
☐ 1: mild (all 3 repeated, patient fails to recall 1)
☐ 2: moderate (all 3 repeated, patient fails to recall 2, 3)
☐ 3: severe (patient fails to repeat 1 or more words)

ITEM 4—IMPAIRED DIGIT SPAN: Rate current performance by asking subjects to repeat first 3, 4, then 5 digits forward and then 3, then 4 backwards; continue to the next step only if patient succeeds at the previous one.

☐ 0: none (patient can do at least 5 numbers forward and 4 backward)
☐ 1: mild (patient can do at least 5 numbers forward, 3 backward)
☐ 2: moderate (patient can do 4–5 numbers forward, cannot do 3 backward)
☐ 3: severe (patient can do no more than 3 numbers forward)

ITEM 5—REDUCED ABILITY TO MAINTAIN AND SHIFT ATTENTION: As indicated during the interview by questions needing to be rephrased and/or repeated because patient's attention wanders, patient loses track, patient is distracted by outside stimuli or over-absorbed in a task.

☐ 0: none (none of the above; patient maintains and shifts attention normally)
☐ 1: mild (above attentional problems occur once or twice without prolonging the interview)
☐ 2: moderate (above attentional problems occur often, prolonging the interview without seriously disrupting it)
☐ 3: severe (above attentional problems occur constantly, disrupting and making the interview difficult-to-impossible)

ITEM 6—DISORGANIZED THINKING: As indicated during the interview by rambling, irrelevant, or incoherent speech, or by tangential, circumstantial, or faulty reasoning. Ask patient a somewhat complex question (for example, "Describe your current medical condition.").

☐ 0: none (patient's speech is coherent and goal-directed)
☐ 1: mild (patient's speech is slightly difficult to follow; responses to questions are slightly off target but not so much as to prolong the interview)
☐ 2: moderate (disorganized thoughts or speech are clearly present, such that interview is prolonged but not disrupted)
☐ 3: severe (examination is very difficult or impossible due to disorganized thinking or speech)

(*continued*)

Fig. 20–1. Memorial Delirium Assessment Scale (MDAS). (Copyright ©1996 Memorial Sloan-Kettering Cancer Center. Reproduced with permission.)

ITEM 7—PERCEPTUAL DISTURBANCE: Misperceptions, illusions, hallucinations inferred from inappropriate behavior during the interview or admitted by subject, as well as those elicited from nurse/family/chart accounts of the past several hours or of the time since last examination:
☐ 0: none (no misperceptions, illusions, or hallucinations)
☐ 1: mild (misperceptions or illusions related to sleep, fleeting hallucinations on 1–2 occasions without inappropriate behavior)
☐ 2: moderate (hallucinations or frequent illusions on several occasions with minimal inappropriate behavior that does not disrupt the interview)
☐ 3: severe (frequent or intense illusions or hallucinations with persistent inappropriate behavior that disrupts the interview or interferes with medical care)

ITEM 8—DELUSIONS: Rate delusions inferred from inappropriate behavior during the interview or admitted by the patient, as well as delusions elicited from nurse/family/chart accounts of the past several hours or of the time since the previous examination.
☐ 0: none (no evidence of misinterpretations or delusions)
☐ 1: mild (misinterpretations or suspiciousness without clear delusional ideas or inappropriate behavior)
☐ 2: moderate (delusions admitted by the patient or evidenced by his/her behavior that do not or only marginally disrupt the interview or interfere with medical care)
☐ 3: severe (persistent and/or intense delusions resulting in inappropriate behavior, disrupting the interview or seriously interfering with medical care)

ITEM 9—DECREASED OR INCREASED PSYCHOMOTOR ACTIVITY: Rate activity over past several hours, as well as activity during interview, by circling (a) hypoactive, (b) hyperactive, or (c) elements of both present.
☐ 0: none (normal psychomotor activity)
☐ a b c 1: mild (Hypoactivity is barely noticeable, expressed as slightly slowing of movement. Hyperactivity is barely noticeable or appears as simple restlessness.)
☐ a b c 2: moderate (Hypoactivity is undeniable, with marked reduction in the number of movements or marked slowness of movement; subject rarely spontaneously moves or speaks. Hyperactivity is undeniable, subject moves almost constantly; in both cases, exam is prolonged as a consequence.)
☐ a b c 3: severe (Hypoactivity is severe; patient does not move or speak without prodding or is catatonic. Hyperactivity is severe; patient is constantly moving, overreacts to stimuli, requires surveillance and/or restraint; getting through the exam is difficult or impossible.)

ITEM 10—SLEEP-WAKE CYCLE DISTURBANCE (DISORDER OF AROUSAL): Rate patient's ability to either sleep or stay awake at the appropriate times. Utilize direct observation during the interview, as well as reports from nurses, family, patient, or charts describing sleep-wake cycle disturbance over the past several hours or since last examination. Use observations of the previous night for morning evaluations only.
☐ 0: none (at night, sleeps well; during the day, has no trouble staying awake)
☐ 1: mild (mild deviation from appropriate sleepfulness and wakefulness states: at night, difficulty falling asleep or transient night awakenings, needs medication to sleep well; during the day, reports periods of drowsiness or, during the interview, is drowsy but can easily fully awaken him/herself)
☐ 2: moderate (moderate deviations from appropriate sleepfulness and wakefulness states: at night, repeated and prolonged night awakening; during the day, reports of frequent and prolonged napping or, during the interview, can only be roused to complete wakefulness by strong stimuli)
☐ 3: severe (severe deviations from appropriate sleepfulness and wakefulness states: at night, sleeplessness; during the day, patient spends most of the time sleeping or, during the interview, cannot be roused to full wakefulness by any stimuli)

Fig. 20–1. *(Continued)*

Items 1 through 4 must be observed in order to confirm the diagnosis of delirium. Despite the attempt to streamline assessment and diagnosis of delirium, the Confusion Assessment Method is a very delicate and complex instrument and perhaps not particularly useful for use by a nurse at the bedside.

The Neecham Confusion Scale (NCS)

The NCS was developed by nurse researchers who recognized the prevalence of confusion in elderly hospitalized patients.[54] It was designed to be used by nurses in routine assessments of the elderly and takes approximately 8 to 10 minutes to administer.[36] The NCS has a high internal consistency and inter-rater and test–retest reliability. The NCS significantly correlates with the MMSE and the DSM-IIIR diagnostic criteria (Table 20–2).

The three scored subscales are designed to collect data regarding information processing and psychomotor behavior along with select vital functions. Subscale I evaluates attention and alertness, verbal and motor response, memory, and orientation. Each item has a weighted value and is scored from 0 to 14. Subscale II observes the patient's appearance, posture, sensorimotor performance, and verbal responses. Scores range from 0 to 6 and are given the least weight. Subscale III examines the possible etiology of an acute confessional episode. Physiological changes that may indicate existing or developing delirium include oxygen saturation, continence, and vital signs. The total maximum score for all three subscales is 27 to 30 and indicates a normal function. A score between 0 and 19 indicates moderate to severe confusion or delirium. Table 20–2 includes a summary of these assessment instruments.

Association Between Symptoms and Etiology

Clinical reports have identified that the presence of certain symptoms in delirium may give clues to the underlying etiological cause. The following associations have been noted:

- Nystagmus, ataxia, and extreme lethargy may accompany delirium due to medication intoxication.[29,30,59]
- Asterixis (sustained contraction of muscle groups, also called liver flap) may be observed with renal or hepatic insufficiency.[30,59]
- Restlessness, agitation, poor judgment, and inattentiveness are associated with hypoxia.[29,59a]
- Intermittent drowsiness, inattention, indifference to environment, forgetfulness, and difficulty following sequences of events are common with chronic obstructive pulmonary disease, probably due to carbon dioxide narcosis and hypoxia.[59]
- Hypoalert behaviors are associated with hepatic encephalopathy.[10]
- Hyperalert behaviors tend to be more closely associated with alcohol withdrawal.[10]

Interventions

Multiple medications are a frequent insult to cognitive functioning in the terminally ill patient. Changing an opioid is one useful intervention when delirium is thought to be a consequence of the accumulation of an opiate metabolite or the patient responds poorly to a particular opioid.[13,48] Accumulation of benzodiazepines and, to a lesser degree, antidepressants also contributes to delirium. A medication review will elicit what medications can be eliminated from the patient's regimen. Most palliative practices discontinue all medications that are not absolutely necessary.[12,46]

Liver failure that causes hepatic encephalopathy is more commonly encountered in the palliative care setting and should be considered when prescribing pharmaceuticals.[35] Benzodiazepines such as diazepam and alprazolam undergo oxidation in the liver into primary and secondary active metabolites, which can often exacerbate the symptom of cognitive failure.[35,45]

Hydration

Dehydration is a common condition, frequently assessed in the dying patient. As death approaches, patients often lose the ability to drink fluids. The lack of fluids precipitates fluid and electrolyte imbalances and leads to symptoms of headache, nausea, vomiting, cramps, thirst, and dry mouth.[59,60] It is possible that dehydration causes reabsorption of fluids or other processes that may negatively affect the patient's well-being.[61] Recent studies show that some clinicians believe that maintaining artificial hydration in dying patients alleviates many symptoms that gravely interfere with quality of life, not to mention relieving the distress experienced by patients, their families, and professional caregivers surrounding the symptom of dehydration.[62–64]

It has been established that dehydration exacerbates confusion, delirium, and restlessness; renal failure is often responsible for the accumulation of opioid metabolites, leading to confusion, myoclonus, and nausea. Dehydration can also increase the risk of bedsores as a result of circulatory insufficiency and decreased skin perfusion. Constipation, pyrexia, and electrolyte imbalance result from dehydration and can further contribute to disorientation, agitation, and neuromuscular irritability.[62–64]

There is an ongoing debate about the benefits of hydration, yet the ethical basis of most clinical decision making is assessment of the benefits and risks conferred by any particular intervention, as opposed to the burden it imposes on the patient and family. In the terminal phase of advanced diseases, length of life is limited and attention is directed to maintaining or improving quality of life. Symptom control and provision of comfort should be the primary goals of both medical and nursing care. Good symptom control or palliative care necessitates remedial treatment for conditions secondary to the illness.[64] The decision to administer artificial hydration should be based on individual patients and made in consensus with the patient's and family's wishes. One argument against parenteral hydration relates to the discomfort, cost, and complexity of maintaining this intervention. Hypodermoclysis or, occasionally, protoclysis is an inexpensive, comfortable method of replacing fluids.[62,63,65]

Pharmacological Interventions for Management of Delirium

When sequential trials of both pharmaceutical and complementary interventions used in tandem prove futile in treating the underlying cause of delirium, aggressive and skilled use of both the benzodiazepines and the neuroleptics should be considered.[35] Both complementary therapies and pharmaceuticals should be included in the plan of care.[10,66] Neuroleptics clear the sensorium and improve cognition in persons with delirium, while the benzodiazepines are most useful for the symptoms restlessness and agitation.[10,29] Brietbart and co-workers[1,56] suggest that benzodiazepines may increase the symptoms of agitation and restlessness in delirious patients. If sedation is required, the combination of a benzodiazepine with a neuroleptic is suggested. Pharmacological interventions used to treat the symptoms of delirium may be tapered over several days if the delirium has resolved.

Table 20–2. Overview of the Four Delirium Assessment Instruments

Description	Domains	Validation	Reference Standard	Reliability	Feasibility
Memorial Delirium Assessment Scale (MDAS)					
10-item, 4-point clinician-rated scale. Designed to quantify the severity of delirium. Establish diagnosis for delirium using DSM III-R and DSM IV.[50,56]	1. Level of awareness 2. Disorientation 3. Short-term memory impairment 4. Impaired digit span 5. Reduced ability to maintain and shift attention 6. Perceptual disturbance 7. Delusions 8/9. Psychomotor activity ↑ or ↓ 10. Sleep–wake cycle disturbances	Memorial Sloan-Kettering Cancer Center n = 33 study I n = 51 study II[56]	Psychiatrists interview based on DSM III-R and DSM IV Convergent agreement (MMSE, $P < 0.0001$) Global Accessibility Rating Delirium Rating Scale Distinguishes between delirium and non-delirious subject ($P < 0.0002$) Predictive score = 13, 92.3% positive Predictive accuracy = 75% Negative predictive power	Interrater correlation coefficient = 0.92 (psychiatrists) Internal consistency coefficient (−alpha = 0.91)	• Observer-rated • Time not specified • Requires minimal rater training
Delirium Rating Scale (DRS)					
10-item rating scale, with additive score 0–32, designed to be completed by a psychiatrist after complete psychiatric assessment.	1. Onset course 2. Cognitive status 3. Perceptual problems 4. Delusions 5. Hallucination types 6. Psychomotor behavior 7. Emotional liability 8. Sleep–wake cycle 9. Symptom variability 10. Physical disorder	Presbyterian Medical Center n = 20 Age 20–83 years mean = 58.8[57]	Psychiatrists interview based on DSM III Distinguishes between delirium and psychotic disorders: • Schizophrenia • Dementia (mild to moderately impaired) Predictive score >12 Range 0–32	Interrater: Intraclass correlation coefficient = 0.97	• Observer-rated based on lengthy interview and detailed assessment (time not specified) • Rater instruction required

Confusion Assessment Method (CAM)					
9 operationalized criteria from DSM III-R scored according to algorithm. Based on observations made during interview.	1. Onset/course 2. Attention 3. Organization of thought 4. Level of consciousness 5. Orientation 6. Memory 7. Perceptual problems 8. Psychomotor behavior 9. Sleep–wake cycle	Yale-New Haven General Medicine Units[59] University of Chicago n = 56 Age 65+ years MMSE κ = 0.64[59]	Gero-psychiatrists' diagnoses based on clinical judgment and DSM III-R criteria	Interrater: k = 1.0 overall	• Observer-rated • Extensive training manual required for raters
Neecham Confusion Scale (NCS)					
9 items organized in 3 domains, with an additive score of 30. Designed for nurses' use at bedside in hospitalized elderly. Establishes diagnosis using DMS III-R criteria. Assesses hypoactive delirium or "quiet confusion."[54]	1. Procesing • Attention/alertness (0–4) • Command of information (0–5) • Memory orientation (0–5) 2. Behavior • Appearances/posture control (0–2) • Sensory-motor performance (0–4) • Verbal manifestation (0–4) 3. Physiological control • Vital signs (0–2) • Oxygen stability (0–2) • Urinary continence (0–2)	General medical units n = 168 Age 65+ years n = 258 Age 65+ years Distinguishes between delirium and non-delirious subjects Predictive score <19 (0–30)[54]	Nurse researchers and staff nurses Convergent agreement (MMSE, r = 0.75) Apache II (Classifications Symptom Severity)	• Interrater reliability for staff nurses $r = 0.91$ • Interrater reliability for staff nurses/researchers [$\kappa = 0.65 < 91\%$) • Repeated 24-hour period correlation = −0.68 • Interitem correlation $P < 0.001$ • Internal consistency Cronbach's alpha coefficient = 0.90	• Observer-rated • 10-minute testing • Instruction required

DSM III-R = *Diagnostic and Statistical Manual of Mental Disorders,* 3rd edition revised (IV = 4th edition); MMSE = Mini-Mental State Examination; κ = kappa coefficient; n = number of subjects; r = Pearson coefficient; m = median.

Neuroleptics. The butyrophenones are the most frequently recommended medications for the management of delirium in cancer patients and the elderly.[10,12,30,35] Haloperidol is preferred by many clinicians as it has a short half-life, no active metabolites, and minimal anticholinergic and cardiovascular side effects.[1,12,32,35,66] It is less likely to cause sedation than the phenothiazine class of neuroleptics.[35] Haloperidol can be given orally, subcutaneously, intramuscularly, or intravenously, with the parenteral dose being roughly twice as potent as the oral route.[1,10] Subcutaneous or intravenous continuous infusions may eliminate frequent bolus dosing.

Dosage recommendations for haloperidol vary significantly. Liptzin[32] recommends haloperidol doses of 0.5 to 5 mg, given orally or parenterally every 4 hours up to a maximum of 20 mg/day depending on the patient's response. Jacobson[66] reported dosage schedules based on severity of symptoms: 0.5 mg for mild agitation, 1 mg for moderate agitation, and 2 mg for severe agitation. The dose may be repeated every 30 to 60 minutes until the patient is calm. Fainsinger and colleagues[12] discussed a protocol of 1 to 2 mg, orally or parenterally, every 6 hours plus an hourly PRN dose to be used for titration. There have been reports of using bolus doses as high as 50 mg, with total daily doses as high as 250 to 500 mg.[1,30] However, in the palliative care setting, it is recommended that if patient symptoms are not controlled by the time the dose has reached 20 to 30 mg/day, it is a sign to discontinue the haloperidol and begin a more sedating medication.[12,38]

Droperidol, another butyrophenone, has also been used to treat the symptoms of delirium. This medication is most often reserved for the critical care setting as it is more potent and more sedating than haloperidol.[66] Studies suggest that a more rapid response may be obtained with droperidol than with haloperidol.[30] However, there are no published data on the use of droperidol for delirium in the palliative care setting.

There is a risk of extrapyramidal side effects with the butyrophenones due to their dopamine-blocking properties. Parkinsonian symptoms have been noted in persons receiving high doses of haloperidol. However, this symptom can often be managed with benztropine.[10,12,35] Also, the extrapyramidal side effects may be less severe when these medications are given intravenously versus the oral route.[30]

The phenothiazines may be used when the patient is experiencing severe symptoms and sedation is required.[12,35] This class of medications is associated with sedation, anticholinergic effects, and alpha-adrenergic blocking effects, all of which may complicate delirium.[30] Methotrimeprazine, 10 mg every 8 hours with 10 mg every 1 hour PRN for breakthrough symptoms, or chlorpromazine, 25 mg every 8 hours with 25 mg every 1 hour PRN, are the most frequently used phenothiazines for delirium.[12] They can be very effective but very sedating.

One of the newer classes of neuroleptics, the thienobenzodiazepines, has also been reported to be effective at treating delirium in persons with cancer.[55] An advantage is that these medications cause less akithisia and fewer extrapyramidal effects than the butryophenones or phenothiazines. Passik and Cooper[44] reported successful use of olanzapine in the treatment of a patient with delirium who was profoundly sensitive to the side effects of other neuroleptics. However, there have not been any controlled clinical trials comparing these newer medications to the standard neuroleptics in the treatment of delirium at the end of life.

Although the neuroleptics are the preferred class of medications for delirium, Burke and co-workers[39] state that neuroleptics should be avoided in cases of terminal restlessness due to an increased risk of myoclonus, muscle twitching, and seizures due, in part, to the potential for these medications to lower the seizure threshold. As terminal restlessness is a variant of delirium, it is exceptionally difficult to determine the most appropriate course of action for delirium at the end of life. However, it is clear that restlessness without other symptoms of delirium should not be treated with neuroleptics. The benzodiazepines would be a more appropriate choice.

Benzodiazepines. Benzodiazepines are very helpful in treating anxiety and restlessness in persons with terminal illnesses.[1,24] However, their role in the treatment of delirium is not clear. The few studies evaluating the efficacy of the benzodiazepines as single therapy for delirium suggest that these medications alone are not effective.[30] Unlike the antipsychotics, the benzodiazepines do not clear sensorium or improve cognition in delirious patients.[10] However, they may be the medications of choice in the treatment of delirium if the patient has significant liver disease, if the delirium is related to alcohol or benzodiazepine withdrawal, or if the patient is refractory to monotherapy with antipsychotic medications.[10,30,38]

Clinical reports suggest that a combination of antipsychotics and benzodiazepines may increase clinical effectiveness while decreasing medication side effects. Benzodiazepines can be useful as they do not have anticholinergic or dopamine-blocking properties, decrease the anxiety associated with delirium, and do not lower the seizure threshold.[30,35]

Although used commonly, the benzodiazepines do have significant side effects, which need monitoring. These medications are associated with sedation, behavioral disinhibition, amnesia, ataxia, respiratory depression, physical dependence, rebound insomnia, withdrawal reactions, and delirium. Fainsinger and colleagues[12] noted that palliative care patients experiencing delirium are very sensitive to the sedative properties of the benzodiazepines. The elderly and children appear to be at greatest risk for adverse reactions.[30]

Concerns regarding potential adverse side effects should not prevent the clinician from using adequate doses of the benzodiazepines to control the symptoms of anxiety, restlessness, and agitation.[10] When used, short-acting medications with short-acting metabolites, for example, lorazepam or oxamepam, should be selected.[1,30] Lorazepam can be administered orally, sublingually, intramuscularly, or intravenously. The symptoms of restlessness and agitation may be treated with doses of 1 to 2 mg orally if mild or 0.25 to 2 mg parenterally if more severe, every 4 hours.[10,32] The dose may be repeated or doubled every 30 to 60 minutes, depending on the patient's level of sedation.[38] Liptzin[32] suggests a maximal dose of 8 mg/day. However, there have been clinical reports both of using higher doses effectively and of adverse effects at lower doses.

The disadvantage of the short-acting benzodiazepines is that patients may experience breakthrough anxiety or end-of-dose failure. These patients may benefit from switching to longer-acting medications, such as diazepam or clonazepam.[1] An additional advantage of clonazepam is that it appears to be particularly effective for myoclonus.[40] However, it is important to monitor for excessive sedation and depressive side effects when administering these longer-acting benzodiazepines.

Sedation. Terminal sedation is defined as the intentional use of pharmacological agents to induce sleep in the final days of life.[41] The most common indication for terminal sedation is in the presence of distressing symptoms that cannot be controlled by other means and usually after an exhaustive use of sequential trials of pharmacological, evidence-based interventions. Severe anxiety, disorientation, restlessness, agitation, hallucinations, illusions, and sleep disturbances associated with unresolved or unmanageable cognitive disorders can be extremely distressing and, thus, a legitimate reason to offer terminal sedation to a patient.[40] Syndromes that may produce these symptoms include hyeractive–hyperalert delirium, terminal restlessness, and terminal anguish.

Reversible causes of delirium at the end of life must be evaluated. In addition to a thorough physical assessment and review of medication, it is important to assess all potential causes of these cognitive changes, including the physical, psychosocial, emotional, and spiritual, with patient and family. The delirious patient is clearly distressed. In addition, the symptoms exhibited by the patient can lead to distress in family and health care providers. As a result, there may be pressure for quick results. Of concern is jumping to the use of sedative medications when a more thorough assessment would be of benefit.[62–64]

Delirium in the terminally ill is generally multifactorial. Some causes can be avoided, corrected, or modified; but this is not often feasible or appropriate in the terminal phase.[38] Delirium at the end of life may develop due to irreversible processes such as multiple organ failure.[1] When a cause cannot be determined or the delirium is irreversible, it is not feasible to treat it; conventional treatment of symptoms alone should be implemented. It is only in the presence of distress not responding to conventional therapy that terminal sedation is appropriate.

Medications should be chosen to accomplish the patient/family goal with the least morbidity. This includes administration via the route of choice, when possible.[41] As patients are often not able to take medications by mouth, frequently due to cognitive impairment, medications that can be given subcutaneously, sublingually, or rectally are preferred.[40]

When a neuroleptic medication, typically haloperidol, alone is not sufficient to address the distress experienced by an individual with delirium at the end of life, a medication with more sedative effects should be added. Droperidol is also a neuroleptic, but it is more sedating than haloperidol. It is effective for agitation symptoms, but no published data are available for its use in terminal sedation.[30]

Chlorpromazine is a phenothiazine neuroleptic often used for distressing delirium at the end of life.[40] One advantage of this medication is its availability in suppository form.[64] Because of its strong anticholinergic effects, there is potential for worsening delirium. It should, therefore, be used with caution in delirium. It may be very effective, however, for terminal anguish. When droperidol or chlorpromazine is used, it should replace haloperidol and not be used in addition to it.

The most commonly used classes of medication for sedation are the benzodiazepines and the barbiturates. The benzodiazepines are effective and safe medications for sedation in the person with unrelieved delirium. They are sedating, anxiolytic, and anticonvulsant.[40] The short-acting medications in this class, lorazepam and midazolam, are preferred, though diazepam has also been used for terminal sedation.

The benzodiazepine most frequently cited in the literature for terminal sedation is midazolam. Twycross and Lichter[38] suggest starting with 10 mg subcutaneously along with haloperidol. If further sedation is required, the dose can be increased to 60 mg in 24 hours; both the neuroleptic and the benzodiazepine can be titrated upward or downward as need, to a high of 100 mg midazolam and 30 to 40 mg haloperidol in 24 hours. If the patient still experiences distressing symptoms, a barbiturate can be added.

Phenobarbital is a suitable barbiturate for use in the patient with a terminal illness who is experiencing distressing delirium as it is anticonvulsant and sedative.[40] In acutely agitated and restless patients, the clinician might start 130 mg subcutaneously every 30 minutes until calm. Some patients have required doses greater than 1000 mg per day.[41] Pentobarbital may also be used for terminal sedation in the terminally ill. Pentobarbital is available in suppository form, which can be advantageous in the home care setting.[65,67] Another barbiturate, thiopental, is also available in suppository and intravenous forms.[64,68] Although both thiopental and methohexital are mentioned in reviews of terminal sedation,[41] they do not appear to have been used often in the clinical setting for terminal sedation.

Psychosocial, emotional, and spiritual support is essential for patients being treated with terminal sedation and for their families. Even when sedated, patients may be aware of the persons and sounds in the environment. All persons entering the rooms of sedated patients should introduce themselves, explain any procedures to be performed, and inform patients before touching them in any way. Patients and families often desire to hear an update of their condition as assessed by their nurses and physicians. This information should be shared with patients and families. Evaluate the need and desire for regular spiritual support from the patient/family's own clergy, the care facility's chaplain, or skilled volunteers.

Complementary Nursing Interventions

Historically, nurses have recognized how the environment influences a patient's mood, emotions, and well-being. A quiet, restful environment is a means of reducing the sensory stimuli, both internal and external, that often insult the patient's cortical brain; it has been recommended as a prudent intervention by experienced practitioners familiar with the course of delirium.[10,38,69]

Familiar sounds, smells, and textures convey warmth and caring for the agitated and restless patient. Patients who experience confusion as a result of a delirious episode may have a greater need to relate to the familiar voice of a significant caregiver or to the soft touch of a favorite pet. Since the visual field may present distorted images, sound, smell, and touch are avenues that nurses and caregivers can use to communicate understanding and reassurance for the cognitively impaired patient.

The significant caregiver may offer frequent reassurance, such as "You are going to be all right. I am here beside you." Often, family members can be reminded that the sound of a familiar voice is crucial, and caregivers can be offered reorienting scripts, such as "I know this must be frightening for you. The nurse is getting you medicine."[69] Repeating family names of children, grandchildren, or pets can also be of value. Reorienting to time is of minimal value in that time has little meaning to the patient. Television and extraneous noise should be avoided. It is through reducing the excess stimuli that pertinent relaxing sounds of music or a familiar voice can be received.[69]

The sound of familiar music can also quiet the restless mind. Assessing from the family or caregiver what the patient's favorite music has been in the past and encouraging its use not only includes the family but also promotes a soothing environment. When deemed appropriate by the professional support team, integrating the use of psalms and prayer may be of value to the family whose background is influenced by the Judeo-Christian religions. Knowledge of rituals utilized in various cultures, along with individual/family belief systems is essential. Professional caregivers cannot assume that the "Holy Bible" is regarded as a soothing sound. It may be the sound of drumming or chanting that creates the familiar in an individual patient's experience of confusion.

Complementary Interventions for Terminal Anguish

The final phase of a delirious episode is frequently referred to in the literature as terminal anguish.[38] The family may feel frightened and helpless as the patient's restlessness has evolved into distressed moans interspersed with crying. Nothing that caregivers offer seems to relieve the distress of the patient experiencing terminal anguish. Pharmacological intervention is often the medical remedy to such situations. Sedation is warranted when a patient's and/or family's safety is at risk or when families are unable to cope with the torment of watching the unrelieved discomfort of the dying patient.[8,38,40,69]

The importance of supportive interventions for the family and the patient should not be underestimated.[10,69,70] The experiences of seasoned nurses caring for the dying is recorded in *Final Gifts;* the authors discuss anecdotes of "nearing death awareness," when they were able to understand the confused words of their patients who speak of trips. These trips may be the symbolic expressions of the patient's own awareness that he or she is dying. A plea of "I want to go home" may be answered with "I know, it's time and you can go when you are ready," rather than with the more literal "You are home."[71]

Callahan and Kelly[71] emphasize the nurse's unique role in helping caregivers understand this symbolic communication. When the significant caregiver and nurse communicate compassionate understanding, the patient's restlessness is often subdued.[67,71,72] At times, caregivers can offer insight into the patient's troubled mind when the nurse queries the family on issues that may remain unresolved for the patient.[38] Many times, the pain and resentment within the family emerge when death is on the threshold. The chaplain or other spiritual caregiver in the palliative care setting can offer families solace and support.

In the final moments of dying, observers may regard confused and delirious patients as having visions or hallucinatory events as death approaches.[10,38,70,71] It is debatable whether or not this phenomenon is the normal process of dying or whether it is an authentic supernatural event.[70] One hypothesis is that such hallucinatory episodes may arise from a collective consciousness that treats icons like angels as real beings from another remote reality that are recognizable only as the gates of death stand ajar. Throughout the history of humankind, angels have symbolized unseen forces that aid in times of distress or visit at the time of death, hence the well-known image of the angel of death.

The phenomenon of angels extends beyond religious and/or cultural myths and pervades the core belief system of humankind. Matthew Fox, an Anglican priest, and Rupert Sheldrake, a renowned biologist, have explored the reality of angels.[73] Their conclusion, based on research of culture, arts, and religious traditions spanning from medieval times to the present, is that, indeed, "angels do accompany people from this life to the next." They cite, for example, soul guides, the winged creatures drawn with meticulous care over the Egyptian mummies that await the end as the promise of angels to take the person to another reality."

Acknowledging to the dying patient that his or her "hallucinations" of unseen helpers or guides may be real can dissipate the patient's anguish. The nurse's role should be to reach out to the family and patient during this time, reassuring the family through acknowledging that the dying patient's reality is valid and appropriate. This acknowledgment can lead to family discussions and help provide guidance on some of the misconceptions regarding death and dying This intervention can provide an opportunity for the family to enter into the sacred mystery of death and allow the dying patient to become the teacher of wisdom.

Use of Smell. The faint scent of freshly baked bread often conveys a sense of safety in one's remote memory. A pleasant scent is remembered as a time of joy, a safe and secure moment of love and caring. The sense of smell travels by way of the olfactory nerve to the central part of the brain, known as the limbic system. The limbic system is known as the "seat of emotion," where anxiety and fear are labeled as threatening to the self.[74]

In palliative care settings throughout England and Ireland, scents are used as an intervention in the form of essential oils. Essential oils are aromatic substances extracted from plants.[73,75] A minute drop of oil can be added to massage oil and applied to the skin in the form of a massage. Clinical studies have indicated a positive and prolonged effect in reducing anxiety when using scented oils in conjunction with massage.[74–75] A review of clinical studies of patients in the palliative care setting concluded that providing massage with essential oil is of therapeutic benefit.[75]

When patients experience the anxiety and fear associated with a delirious episode, a simple hand massage with lavender oil can help provide a calming and relaxing effect. The essential oil of lavender (*Lavandula angustifolia*) acts primarily on the central nervous system, resulting in a sedative effect. The relaxation effect is believed to be a direct result of the biochemical properties of lavender due to its high content of linalyl acetate (ester). In the home setting, scented candles can be placed in the room. The use of candles can also symbolize a sacred space of solitude and peace.

Use of Touch. Touch, with intent offered by the caregiver, nurse, or volunteer, may express caring and safety to the confused mind of the patient. The clinical experience of nurses using therapeutic touch has value in calming the patient who has reached the end of life's journey. Often the struggle between the physical body and the departing spirit is observed in the final tense moments before death. Therapeutic touch, a gentle and non-invasive expression by a nurse or caregiver, will relax the physical body, an effect that may be observed in the patient's facial expression and relaxation of muscles as the breath ceases. Cathleen Fanslow-Brunjes,[78] a nurse clinician who worked with Elisabeth Kübler-Ross and later at Calvary Hospital in the Bronx, pioneered the use of therapeutic touch while caring for the dying. She eloquently expressed that her clinical experience has shown that "therapeutic touch enables us to truly accompany the dying in a special way . . . it allows us to be truly present to the 'I' of the other person in their dying process."[77]

The hand–heart connection developed by Fanslow-Brunjes[78] is taught to nurses and caregivers as a relevant intervention for use in terminal restlessness and terminal anguish. Based on the principles of therapeutic touch[78] in conjunction with the ancient healing system of Tibetan Buddhism[79] and Ayurvedic medicine,[78] it encourages "letting go." This intervention is based on the belief that letting go of life occurs at the level of the heart. The heart is where the releasing emotions and relationships transpire. This is accomplished by holding the hand of the patient, which is symbolic of holding the heart. The caregiver or nurse sits at the left of the patient and holds the left hand with his or her own left hand. When the patient appears comfortable and relaxed, the caregiver places his or her right hand over the patient's left hand. Intuiting when to proceed, the right hand of the caregiver is placed over the heart area of the patient. The hands may remain in this position for 2 or 3 minutes. In closing the intervention, the right hand of the caregiver is momentarily placed on the left shoulder, then moved slowly down the arm, returning to the position of the left hand.[80] Those surrounding the deathbed can be taught this profoundly simple technique. This intervention may provide a sacred space in time for the dying to transition in peace and with the love of his or her family present.

Patient and Family Teaching. Patient and family education is the cornerstone of comprehensive end-of-life care. Through proper education and support, cognitive disorders may be avoided, recognized early, or shortened. When a cognitive disorder leads to distress, appropriate education and support can decrease the severity of symptoms by providing open and adequate communication to lessen the stimuli that exacerbate symptoms.[73]

Teaching activities associated with cognitive disorders at the end of life involve prevention, identification, intervention, and supportive care issues.

Preventing Terminal Anguish. As terminal anguish is related to unresolved issues, often involving guilt,[38] it is important to encourage the patient and family to identify and address unresolved issues. This sensitive topic can be introduced by telling the patient that many times people hold old grudges and hurts inside because they seem too painful or difficult to talk about. However, the common experience is that not talking about these concerns makes treating somatic symptoms even more emotional and difficult.

Preventing Delirium in the Terminally Ill. As medications are the most common reversible and preventable cause of delirium,[33] patients and families require education on the proper dosing and schedule of all medications. Delirium can be caused by both taking too much medication (leading to toxicity) or too little (causing discomfort or potential withdrawal). It is important for nurses who care for patients in home care and clinic settings to review all medications with the patient and primary caregiver. Ideally, patients or family caregivers will recognize both the generic and trade names of their medications. Patients and family caregivers need to know the schedule on which each medication is to be taken, the side effects of each to report to their clinicians, and what to do if they should lose or run out of a medication. Medication charts, pillboxes, and medication information cards or sheets may be useful tools.

Patients and family also need to understand that any discomfort that is not adequately addressed can lead to complications, such as feeling nervous, confused, or worse. Thus, education to manage symptoms such as pain, nausea, constipation, and insomnia is an important component of the teaching plan to prevent delirium.[29]

Knowing that sensory deprivation, sensory overload, and unfamiliar or threatening surroundings may contribute to the development of delirium, it becomes evident that patient and family education should include evaluating the patient's sensory environment and developing strategies to provide appropriate levels of sensory stimulation. For some patients, this may mean encouraging interactions with caregivers and others (e.g., hospice volunteers), having the television or radio at a level pleasing to the patient, being sure the patient can see out a window to sense day and night clues, encouraging touch (e.g., massage or range-of-motion exercises), and assuring that the patient uses any needed sensory aides, such as eyeglasses or hearing aides.

Conversely, the patient who is in an environment where sensory overload is a potential requires education on decreasing sensory stimuli. Acute care settings are well known for the potential for sensory overload. However, many times, the potential for sensory overload in the home is not assessed. The combination of noises from vacuums, mixers, dishwashers, televisions, radios, conversations, and patient equipment (e.g., oxygen concentrators) can be overwhelming. In the susceptible patient, it may be helpful to close room doors, to run dishwashers or other equipment at different times of the day, to turn off or turn down televisions and radios when conversing, or to unplug the telephone at certain times of the day.

Being in a strange or threatening environment can contribute to delirium. Should a patient need to be admitted to an acute care or extended care setting, it is important to make that environment as familiar as possible. Encourage the patient and family to bring in familiar photographs or objects, establish a plan for familiar persons to visit regularly, teach family to greet their loved one at eye level, and encourage the use of touch since this is very reassuring to the patient.

Early Identification of the Symptoms of Delirium. The prodromal symptoms of delirium may be easily overlooked. It is not uncommon for persons with advanced diseases to feel restless, anxious, depressed, irritable, angry, or emotionally labile. These symptoms may go unnoticed, only to be recalled later in family interviews.[10,30] Therefore, it is important to teach the patient and family to report any new feelings of uneasiness, anxiety, restlessness, or mood changes.

Lessening the Severity of the Symptoms of Delirium. The individual experiencing delirium may be very frightened regarding what is happening. Clinicians need to provide reassurance that delirium is usually temporary and that the symptoms are part of a medical condition.[30] This intervention may significantly decrease fear and anxiety. The purpose of all supportive measures needs to be explained to both the patient and the family. For example, discuss the purpose of any hydration ordered, the importance of adequate rest, and the rationale for orienting interactions on the part of nursing staff and family.[35]

The family should be informed regarding the fluctuating nature of delirium,[29] to prepare them for the changes in behavior and prevent them from misinterpreting these frequent changes. Reorienting the patient to time, place, and persons in the environment may assist him or her to stay oriented. Repetition is important to compensate for memory impairment.[38] Thus, the family should be taught to correct the patient's orientation errors gently and regularly. If, however, correcting orientation errors leads to increased distress in the patient, this strategy should be discontinued.[29]

The delirious patient is at risk for misinterpreting the environment. The family should be encouraged to evaluate the patient's environment for over- or undersensory stimulation. Interventions to correct the potential for sensory deprivation or overload, as mentioned above, may be appropriate.

Behaviors associated with delirium can be very distressing for family caregivers to observe and may lead to fears that their loved one has "gone crazy."[30,38] The family needs to hear that delirium is the result of a biological disorder and that the symptoms are generally temporary. The family should also be included in discussions of current, predicted, or resolving delirium in the patient. In addition, the family should be encouraged not to take behavior personally.[18]

Teaching Following an Episode of Delirium. Follow-up teaching will include a discussion with the patient about the apparent cause of delirium so that both the patient and family are aware of risk factors. The individual may or may not recall events during delirious episodes. Some individuals have frightening recollections of the delirious episode. Thus, it is important to assess the presence of any distressing memories. Extra psychotherapeutic support to work through the experience may be appropriate.[30]

CONCLUSION

The nurse is the bedside advocate in discerning changes in the patient's cognition. Early and prompt recognition of changes can initiate the appropriate interventions to discourage the progressive nature of delirium. Delirium is a broad category for many alterations in the cognitive realm of the person experiencing advanced disease. Becoming better acquainted with the assessment, etiology, and interventions to promote an improved quality of life is essential to help ease the transition of the dying patient.

REFERENCES

1. Breitbart W, Chochinov HM, Passik S. Psychiatric aspects of palliative care. In: Doyle D, Hanks GWC, MacDonald, N. eds. Oxford Textbook of Palliative Medicine, 2nd Ed. Oxford: Oxford University Press, 1998:933–954.
2. Pereira J, Bruera E. The Edmonton Aide to Palliative Care. Edmonton: Division of Palliative Care, University of Alberta, 1997.
3. Pereira J, Hanson J, Bruera E. The frequency and clinical course of cognitive impairment in patients with terminal cancer. Cancer 1997;79:835–842.
4. Brietbart W, Jacobson P. Psychiatric symptom management in terminal care. Clin Geriatr Med 1996;12:329–347.
5. Lipowski ZJ. Delirium in the elderly. N Engl J Med 1989;320:578–582.
6. American Psychiatric Association. Diagnostic and Statistical Manual of Mental Disorders, 4th Ed. Washington DC: American Psychiatric Association, 1994.
7. Minagawa H, Uchiltomi Y, Yamawaki S, Ishitani K. Psychiatric morbidity in terminally ill cancer patients: a prospective study. Manuscript presented at the 2nd International Congress of Psycho-Oncology. Kobe, Japan. October 20–22, 1995 and the 7th Scientific Meeting of the Pacific Rim College of Psychiatry. Fukuoka, Japan. October 25–27, 1995.
8. Massie MJ, Holland J, Glass E. Delirium in terminally ill cancer patients. Am J Psychiatry 1983;140:1048–1050.
9. Bruera E, Miller L, McCallion J, et al. Cognitive failure (CF) in patients with terminal cancer: a prospective study. J Pain Symptom Manage 1992;7:192–195.
10. Ingham J, Caraceni A. Delirium. In: Berger A, Portenoy R, Weissman D, eds. Principles and Practice of Supportive Oncology. Philadelphia: Lippincott-Raven, 1998:477–495.
11. Brietbart W. Suicide risk in cancer and AIDS patients. In: Chapman C, Foley K, eds. Current and Emerging Issues in Cancer Pain: Research and Practice. New York: Raven, 1993: 319–412.
12. Fainsinger R, Tapper M, Bruera E. A perspective on the management of delirium in terminally ill patients on a palliative care unit. J Palliat Care 1993;9:4–8.
13. Bruera E, Franco J, Maltoni M, Wantanabe S, Suarez-Almazor M. Changing patterns of agitated impaired mental status in patients with advanced cancer: association with cognitive monitoring, hydration and opioid rotation. J Pain Symptom Manage 1995;10:287–291.
14. Haskell R, Frankel H, Rotondo M. Agitation. AACN Clin Issues 1997;8:335–350.
15. Carpenito L. Handbook of Nursing Diagnosis. Philadelphia: JB Lippincott, 1989.
16. Thompson J, McFarland G, Hirsch J, et al. (eds.) Mosby's Manual of Clinical Nursing, 2nd Ed. St. Louis: Mosby, 1989.
17. Luckmann J. (ed.) Saunders Manual of Nursing Care. Philadelphia: WB Saunders, 1997.
18. Allen L. Treating agitation without drugs. Am J Nurs 1999;99:36–41.
19. Bowman AM. The relationship of anxiety to the development of postoperative delirium. J Gerontol Nurs 1992;18:24–30.
20. Kuebler KK. Hospice and Palliative Care Clinical Practice Protocol: Terminal Restlessness. Pittsburgh: Hospice and Palliative Nurses Association, 1997.
21. Williams M, Campbell E, Raynor W, et al. Predictors of acute confusional states in hospitalized elderly patients. Res Nurs Health 1985;8: 31–40.
22. Espino D, Jules-Bradley A, Johnston C, Mouton C. Diagnostic approach to the confused elderly patient. Am Fam Physician 1998;57: 1358–1366.
23. Neufeldt V. (ed.) Webster's New World Dictionary. New York: Warner Books, 1990.
24. Back I. Terminal restlessness in patients with advanced malignant disease. Palliat Med 1992;6:293–298.
25. Cohen-Mansfield J, Billing N. Agitated behaviors in the elderly. I. A conceptual review. J Am Geriatr Soc 1986;34:711–721.
26. Grossman S, Labedzki D, Butcher R, Dellea L. Definition and management of anxiety, agitation, and confusion in ICUs. Nurs Connect 1996;9(2):49–55.
27. Cohen-Mansfield J, Billing N, Lipson S, et al. Medical correlates of agitation in nursing home residents. Gerontology 1990;36:150–158.
28. Armstrong S, Cozza K, Watanabe K. The misdiagnosis of delirium. Psychosomatics 1997;38: 433–439.
29. Milisen K, Foreman MD, Godderis J, et al. Delirium in the hospitalized elderly: nursing assessment and management. Nurs Clin North Am 1998;33:417–439.
30. Trzepacz P, Breitbart W, Franklin J, et al. American Psychiatric Association practice guidelines: practice guidelines for the treatment of patients with delirium. Am J Psychiatry 1999; 156(Suppl 5):1–20
31. Chedru F, Geschwind N. Writing disturbances in acute confusional state. Neuropsychologia 1972;10:343–353.
32. Liptzin B. Delirium. Arch Fam Med 1995;4:453–458.
33. Inouye SK. The dilemma of delirium: clinical and research controversies regarding diagnosis and evaluation of delirium in hospitalized elderly medical patients. Am J Med 1994;97:278–288.
34. Chan D, Brennan N. Delirium: making the diagnosis, improving the prognosis. Geriatrics 1999;54:28–42.
35. Stiefel F, Fainsinger R, Bruera E. Acute confusional states in patients with advanced cancer. J Pain Symptom Manage 1992;7:94–98.
36. Csokasy J. Assessment of acute confusion: use of the NEECHAM Confusion Scale. Appl Nurs Res 1999;12:51–55.
37. Pereira J, Hanson J, Bruera E. The frequency and clinical course of cognitive impairment in patients with terminal cancer. Cancer 1997;79:835–842.
38. Twycross R, Lichter I. The terminal phase. In: Doyle D, Hanks G, MacDonald N, eds. Oxford Textbook of Palliative Medicine, 2nd Ed. Oxford: Oxford University Press, 1998:977–992.
39. Burke A, Diamond P, Hulbert J, et al. Terminal restlessness—its management and the role of midazolam. Med J Aust 1991;155:485–487.
40. Burke A. Palliative care: an update on terminal restlessness. Med J Aust 1997;166:39–42.
41. Storey P. Symptom control in dying. In: Berer A, Portenoy R, Weissman D, eds. Principles and Practice of Supportive Oncology. Philadelphia: Lippincott-Raven, 1998:741–748.
42. Neelon V, Champagne M, McConnell T, Calson J. The Neecham Confusional Scale. J Pain Symptom Manage 1996;13:128–135.
43. de Stoutz N, Tapper M, Fainsinger R. Reversible delirium in terminally ill patients. J Pain Symptom Manage 1995;10:249–253.
44. Passik S, Cooper M. Complicated delirium in a cancer patients successfully treated with olanzapine. J Pain Symptom Manage 1999;17:219–296.
45. Brietbart W, Rosenfeld B, Roth A, Smith M, Cohen K, Passik S. The Memorial Delirium Assessment Scale. J Pain Symptom Manage 1997; 13:128–135.
46. Inouye S. The dilemma of delirium: clinical and research controversies regarding diagnosis and evaluation of delirium in hospitalized elderly medical patients. Am J Med 1994;97:278–288.
47. Inouye S, van Dyck C, Alessi C, Balkin S, Siegal A, Horwitz R. Clarifying confusion: the confusion assessment method. Ann Intern Med 1990;113:941–948.
48. Sulkowski J, Judy K. Acute mental status changes. AACN Clin Issues 1997;8:319–334.
49. Folestein M, Folstein S, McHugh P. Mini-mental state: a practical method for grading the cognitive status of patients for the clinician. J Psychiatr Res 1975;12:189–193.
50. Armstrong-Esther C, Browne K. The influence of elderly patients' mental impairment on nurse–patient interactions. J Adv Nurs 1986;11: 379–387.
51. Inouye SK, Bogardus S, Charpentier P, et al. A multicomponent intervention to prevent delirium in hospitalized older patients. N Engl J Med 1999;340:669–439.
52. Mesulum M, Waxman S, Gerschwind N. Acute confusional state with right cerebral artery infarction. J Neurol Neurosurg Psychiatry 1976; 391:84–89.
53. Caraceni A. Delirium in palliative medicine. Eur J Palliat Care 1995;2:62–67.
54. Kemp C. Neurological problems and interventions. In: Terminal Illness Guide to Nursing Care. Philadelphia: JB Lippincott, 1995:149–153.
55. de Stoutz N, Stiefel F. Assessment and management of reversible delirium. In: Portenoy

R, Bruera E, eds. Topics in Palliative Care. New York: Oxford University Press, 1997:21–43.

56. Smith M, Brietbart W, Platt W. A critique of instruments and methods to detect, diagnose and rate delirium. J Pain Symptom Manage 1995; 10:35–70.

57. Kaasa T, Loomis J, Gills K, Bruera E, Hanson J. The Edmonton functional assessment tool: preliminary development and evaluation for use in palliative care. J Pain Symptom Manage 1997;13:10–17.

58. Trzepacz P. Cognitive Disturbances Basic Perspectives: Symptoms in Terminal Illness. Research Workshop. Baltimore: National Institutes of Health, 1997.

59. Inouye S, Viscoli C, Horwitz R, Hurst L, Tinetti M. A predictive model for delirium in hospitalized elderly medical patients and evaluation for use in palliative care. Ann Intern Med 1993; 119:474–481.

59a. Musgrave C, Bartal N, Opstad J. Intravenous hydration for terminal patients what are the attitudes of Israeli terminal patients, their families and their professional health professionals. J Pain Symptom Manage 1996;9:298–302.

59b. Ellershaw J, Sutcliffe J, Saunders C. Dehydration and the dying patient. J Pain Symptom Manage 1995;10:192–197.

60. Zerwekhi V. Do dying patients really need IV fluids? Am J Nurs 1997;3:26–30.

61. Fainsinger R, MacEachern T, Miller M. The use of hypodermoclysis for rehydration in terminally ill cancer patients. J Pain Symptom Manage 1994;9:298–302.

62. Fainsinger R, Bruera E. Hypodermoclysis (hdc) for symptom control vs. the Edmonton injector. J Palliat Care 1991;7:5–8.

63. Dunphy K, Finlay I, Rathbone G. Rehydration in palliative and terminal care: if not—why not? Palliat Med 1995;9:221–228.

64. Jones C. Electrolyte imbalances. In: Yarbo C, Frogge M, Goodman M, eds. Cancer Symptom Management, 2nd Ed. Boston: Jones and Bartlett, 1999:438–456.

65. Bruera E, Belizile M, Watanabi S, Fainsinger R. Volume of hydration in terminal cancer patients. Support Cancer Care 1996;4:147–150.

66. Jacobson S. Delirium in the elderly. Psychiatr Clin North Am 1997;20:91–110.

67. Skidmore-Roth L. Mosby's 1999 Nursing Drug Reference. St. Louis: Mosby, 1999.

68. Wrede-Seaman L. Symptom Management Algorithms for Palliative Care. Yakima, WA: Intellicard, 1996.

69. Boyle-McCaffery D, Abernathy G, Baker L, Wall A. End-of-life confusion in patients with cancer. Oncol Nurs Forum 1998;25:1335–1343.

70. Shuster J. Delirium, confusion and agitation at the end-of-life. J Palliat Med 1998;1: 177–185.

71. Callahan C, Kelly P. Final Gifts. New York: Poseidon Press, 1992.

72. Macleod A. The management of delirium in hospice practice. Eur J Palliat Care 1997; 4:116–120.

73. Fox M, Sheldrake R. The Physics of Angels: Exploring the Realm Where Science and Spirit Meet. San Francisco: Harper Collins, 1996.

74. Gannong W. Review of Medical Pathology, 13th Ed. Norwalk, CT: Appleton and Lange, 1987.

75. Vickers A. Complementary therapies in palliative care. Eur J Palliat Care 1996;3:150–153.

76. Wilkenson S. Aromatherapy and massage in palliative care. Int J Palliat Nurs 1995;1:21–30.

77. Versagi C. Hands of peace. Massage Mag 1999, pp. 68–77 Nov/Dec.

78. Fanslow-Brunjes C. Therapeutic touch: compassion for dying persons and their families. Lecture Presentation, Annual Conference of Nurse Healers–Professional Associates Annual Conference, Wichita, KS, October 15, 1988.

79. Foreman MD, Zane D. Nursing strategies for acute confusion in elders. Am J Nurs 1996; 96:44–51.

80. Inouye S, Schlesinger M, Lydon T. Delirium: a symptom of how hospital care is failing older persons and a window to improve quality of hospital care. Am J Med 1999;106:573.

21 Sexuality

MARGARET ANNE LAMB

As I gain the perspective of a dying person, I begin to realize what is and is not important in life. Paramount in my mind is the importance of my family. My wife of 45 years remains near and dear to my heart. I wish we could have some time alone together. The children, whom I also love dearly, have come home to be with me. Along with them arrived their respective spouses and my grandchildren. Add to that the nurses and other health care providers who stream through here on a daily basis and you can easily see why I long for just a little privacy. Just to lie in bed together and hold each other, maybe snuggle and kiss or even just fall asleep in each other's arms would mean the world to me.

—A patient with end-stage prostate cancer

Sexuality is a fundamental aspect of human life. It is a complex phenomenon, which, at its basis, comprises the greatest intimacy between two humans. The ability to give and receive physical love is very important for many individuals, even through the trajectory of an incurable illness. The ability to maintain close, sexual relations can be viewed as maintaining an essential part of one's "self." Sexuality can affirm love, relieve stress and anxiety, and distract one from the emotional and physical sequelae of an eventually terminal chronic illness. Health care providers, in all clinical settings in which palliative care is provided, can be pivotal in facilitating the expression of sexuality in the terminal stages of life. Holistic palliative care throughout the trajectory of an incurable illness should include aspects of promoting sexual expression and preventing or minimizing the untoward effects of the illness progression on a couple's intimacy.

IMPORTANCE OF PHYSICAL INTIMACY

The client and family are at the center of palliative care. A client's desire for and interest in maintaining sexual relations is highly variable. Some may find expression of physical love a very important aspect of their life right up to death, while others may relinquish their "sexual being" early in their end-of-life trajectory. Each individual's identity is influenced, in part, by his or her sexual identity. Roles between spouses or sexual partners are additionally defined by the sexual intimacy between them. Sexual integrity is altered and often compromised during the course of an incurable disease, and this may deleteriously affect both the identity and role fulfillment of the affected persons. Health care providers should not make assumptions about the level of interest or capacity a couple has for physical intimacy.

Sexuality is not merely "sexual intercourse." Sexuality may encompass physical touch of any kind as well as experiences of warmth, tenderness, and the expression of love. The importance of physical intimacy vacillates throughout a relationship and may be diminished or rekindled by a superimposed illness. Long-term palliative care providers may see sexual desire and expression ebb and flow between a couple throughout the course of care. The client may view sexual expression as an affirmation of life, a part of being human, a means to maintain role relationships, or the expression of passion in and for life itself. Some clients may view sexual expression an essential aspect of their being, while others may see it as ancillary or unimportant. Some clients may enter palliative care with an established sexual partner; some may lose a partner during this trajectory through separation, divorce, or widowhood; and others may begin a relationship during this period of time. Some clients may have several sexual partners; some couples may be gay or lesbian; while others, without a sexual partner, may gain pleasure by erotic thoughts and masturbation. All of these scenarios are within the realm of the palliative care provider's client base. Understanding the various forms of sexual expression and pleasure is paramount in providing comprehensive care.

A sexual partner's interest and ability to maintain sexual relations through the palliative care trajectory is also affected by many variables. Sexual expression may be impeded by the partner's mood state (anxiety, depression, grief, or guilt), exhaustion from caregiving and assuming multiple family roles, and misconceptions about sexual appropriateness during palliative care. Anxiety and depression have profound effects on sexual functioning. Decreases in libido and sexual activity result from depressive and anxious states.[1] A partner may feel that the client is "too ill" to engage in sexual activity. In turn, the partner may feel remorse or guilt for even thinking about their loved one in a sexual capacity during this time. Partners may fear that they may injure their loved one during sexual activity due to their perceived or actual weakened state or appearance. Furthermore, a partner may have difficulty adjusting to the altered physical appearance of the client (cachexia, alopecia, stomatitis, pallor, amputation, etc.) The role of caregiver may seem incompatible with that of sexual partner. As the ill partner's health deteriorates, the well partner may assume caretaking roles which may seem incompatible with those of a lover. Furthermore, the myriad of responsibilities sequentially assumed by the well partner may leave him or her exhausted. This can impede sexual interest and performance. Finally, the partner may harbor misconceptions about sexual relations with a terminally ill partner, including diminishing the patient's waning energy reserves or causing the illness to progress more rapidly.

Cultural issues may also play a part in the couple's willingness or interest in maintaining sexual intimacy during palliative care. In Part VIII of this book, the international perspective of palliative care is addressed. There exists tremendous diversity among cultural, religious, and spiritual beliefs in relation to sexual intimacy and death.[2] Culture often guides interactions between people, even the mores within sexual interactions. Culturally competent health care providers should take into consideration the effect of culture on sexual expression between a couple during palliative care. For example, does the couple possess the same cultural identity? If not, are their identities similar in respect to beliefs about intimacy? What are the couple's health, illness, and sexual beliefs and practices? What are their customs and beliefs around intimacy, illness, and death? Issues such as personal space, eye contact, touch, and permissible topics to discuss with health care providers and/or members of the opposite sex may influence one's ability to intercede within the realm of intimate relations. A cultural assessment is key to determining if these factors are an issue. Variations in sexual orientation must also be considered within the area of cultural competence. The beliefs, actions, and normative actions of homosexual and bisexual couples are important considerations when providing palliative care to a couple with alternate sexual expression.[3–6] Gay and lesbian couples may be offended by the assumption that they are heterosexual.

Case Study: Narrative Demonstrating the Need for Acknowledging and Respecting Individual Sexuality

A 45-year-old woman dying of ovarian cancer once stated that 'I have been gay all of my life. I have been with the same partner, Jane, for over 15 years. We are very close, emotionally, spiritually, and physically. We have been very forthright about our sexual orientation with our family and friends. However, when I come to the clinic for treatment, I feel very inhibited. It just seems that all the health care providers assume I am celibate or presently "uncoupled." I have Jane accompany me, but they see her as a friend who gives me rides. I know I should just come right out and explain the nature of my relationship; the problem is, I see so many different providers. I feel like I would have to keep going over this again and again. I don't want to be put in this position repeatedly.'

Developmental issues also take part in the client's ability to maintain intimacy during palliative care. Often, health care providers assume sexual abstinence in the elderly and, to some degree, in adolescents and unmarried young adults. However, intimacy may be a vital part of these individuals' lives. Chronological age may or may not be a determination of sexual activity. For underage clients, parental influence may interfere with the ability to express physical love; and likewise, the elderly may be inhibited by societal values and judgments they perceive about their sexuality. Maintaining an open, nonjudgmental approach to clients of all ages, sexual orientations, and marital status when inquiring about intimacy aspects will foster trust and communication.

PRIVACY

One of the main external obstacles of maintaining intimate relations during palliative care is the lack of privacy. In part VI of this book, the various settings in which end-of-life care may take place and the concomitant issues raised within each setting are addressed. In the acute care setting, privacy is often difficult to achieve. However, this obstacle can be removed or minimized by recognizing the need for intimacy and making arrangements to ensure quiet, uninterrupted time for couples. Private rooms are, of course, ideal; however, if this is not possible, arranging for roommates and visitors to leave for periods of time is necessary. Furthermore, a sign should be posted on the door which alerts health care providers, staff, and visitors that privacy is required. Finally, many rooms in the acute care setting have windows as opposed to walls. This requires the use of blinds and/or curtains to assure privacy. Such strategies should be offered by the nurse as opposed to expecting clients to suggest measures to obtain privacy.

Similar issues may arise in the long-term care environment. If privacy is a scarce commodity, assisting couples to maintain intimate relations as desired is crucial in providing holistic care. Nurses in long-term care can initiate strategies similar to those enumerated for the acute care setting. Furthermore, this issue may be even more paramount to the client since often the stay in long-term care is quite extended. In both the acute care and long term care settings, nurses can play a vital role in policy setting to allow for the expression of intimacy.

Home care may present an array of different obstacles for maintaining intimate relations. The ongoing presence of a health care provider other than the sexual partner is such an obstacle. Furthermore, the home setting is often interrupted by professional visits as well as visits from family, friends, and clergy. These visits may be unplanned or unannounced. The telephone itself may be an unwelcome interruption. Furthermore, the client may have moved from a more private, bedroom setting to a more convenient central location, such as a den or family room, to aid care giving and to maintain an integral role in family life. However, this move does not foster the privacy usually sought for intimate activity. There may not be a door to close. Alternately, proximity of the client's bed to the main rooms of the house may inhibit the couple's intimate activities. Negotiating for private time is often necessary. Scheduling "rest periods" when one will not be disturbed; turning the ringer on the phone off; asking health care providers, friends, and clergy to call before visiting; and having family members allow periods of uninterrupted time are necessary steps to maintaining sexual relations.

Case Study: A 26-year-old man with Acquired Immunodeficiency Syndrome

I've been in the hospital for over a week now. The nurses, doctors, and others come and go all day long, The patient in the next bed is in and out for tests, and I never know when he will be coming back to the room. I am too weak to go to the bathroom, so last night, when I thought he was asleep and the nurses were busy, I tried to masturbate. All of a sudden, the light went on and the curtain was pulled back. Come to find out my roommate heard the noise I was making and thought I was having a seizure. He had put on his call light for the nurse and was ready to help me. I was so embarrassed I wanted to die (just kidding). I really didn't want everyone to find out what I was doing, but they seemed to figure it out anyway. We were all embarrassed, but no one said anything. I'll never try that again.

SEXUAL ASSESSMENT

The promotion or restoration of sexual health begins with a sexual assessment. The assessment should include the client as well as his or her partner. Securing permission to include the sexual partner is necessary. For the nurse to perform this assessment, she or he must be comfortable with the topic of sexuality. Comfort with one's sexuality conveys comfort to others. Additionally, the nurse's values, beliefs, and attitudes regarding sexuality greatly influence the capacity to discuss these issues in a nonjudgmental way. Perceived insufficient knowledge on the part of the health care provider is often an obstacle to frank sexual discussions. Additional sexual education and consistent assessment and counseling approaches will allay this discomfort. Education can be gained informally via discussions with colleagues and through consultation with experts in the area of human sexuality. Formal training is gained through in-service education offerings, workshops, and sexual attitude reassessment programs. Knowledge can also be fostered by keeping abreast of new developments within the field by attending conferences and reviewing journals and professional information via the internet.

Assessment of sexuality begins with a sexual history and is then supplemented by data regarding the client and partner's physical health as it influences intimacy, psychological sequelae of the chronic illness, sociocultural influences, and possible environmental issues. Since sexual health is viewed as a relative matter, it is essential to determine if the couple is satisfied with their current level of sexual functioning. Celibacy, for example, may have been present in the relationship for years. However, the trajectory of palliative care may have forced celibacy on an otherwise sexually active couple. Determining the couple's need for interventions and assistance in this realm is key. The ability to prevent or minimize the untoward effects that palliative care may impose on intimacy is well within the realm of interventions on the part of the health care provider.

Obtaining a sexual history and performing a subsequent sexual assessment can be augmented using several communication techniques; assuring privacy and confidentiality; allowing for ample, uninterrupted time; and maintaining a nonjudgmental attitude. Addressing the topic of sexuality early in the relationship with a palliative care client legitimizes the issue of intimacy. It portrays the message that this is an appropriate topic for concern within the professional relationship, and it is often met with relief on the part of the client and couple. Often, sexuality concerns are present but unvoiced.

Incorporating several techniques of therapeutic communication enhances the interview. These techniques include asking open-ended questions, using questions that refer to frequency as opposed to occurrence, and "unloading" the question. Following is an example of an open-ended question: "Some people who have an incurable illness are frustrated by their lack of private time with their spouse/sexual partner. Is this a concern for you?" An example of a question that refers to frequency rather than occurrence is "How often do you have intimate relations with your wife/husband/partner?" as opposed to "Do you have intimate relations with your wife/husband/partner?" An example of unloading the question is "Some adolescent boys masturbate on a regular basis, while others seldom or never masturbate. How often do you masturbate?" This technique legitimizes the activity and allows the client to feel safe in responding to the question in a variety of ways.

Gender and age may also play a part in the client's comfort with sexual discussions. An adolescent boy may feel more comfortable discussing sexual concerns with a male health care provider, whereas an elderly woman may prefer to discuss sexual issues with a woman closer to her own age. Assessment of these factors may include statements like the following: "Many young men have questions about sexuality and the effect their illness may have on sexual functioning. This is something we can discuss or, if you'd be more comfortable, I could have one of the male nurses talk to you about this. Which would you prefer?"

If the sexual history reveals a specific sexual problem, a more in-depth assessment is warranted. This would include the onset and course of the problem, the client's or couple's thoughts about what caused the problem, any solutions that have been attempted, and potential solutions and their acceptability to the client/couple. For example, use of a vibrator in the case of male impotence may be entirely acceptable to some couples but abhorrent to others. Determining what is and is not acceptable with regard to potential solutions is part of the logical next step in sexual assessment.

INTERVENTIONS TO AUGMENT SEXUAL HEALTH IN END-OF-LIFE CARE

The specific sexual needs and concerns of the client and couple determine the approach and type of intervention. The intervention can address current needs or focus on potential future needs in the form of anticipatory guidance. Although dated, the P-LI-SS-IT model developed by Annon[7] remains a cornerstone in sexual rehabilitation. The assessment phase, previously outlined, comprises the "P," or permission, phase of this intervention model. Permission simply refers to the openness about discussing sexual concerns. In assessing sexual health, the health care provider has begun intervening in the realm of sexuality. By initiating a discussion about the effects that palliative care may have on an individual's or couple's intimate relations, one legitimizes these concerns.

Limited information regarding actual or potential problems is addressed once the assessment phase of the intervention is complete. This is the "LI" of the acronym. Specific information and suggestions can then be given to assist the client or couple with adapting to changes in intimacy brought on by incurable illness or end-of-life care. Questions can be answered, what is normal can be acknowledged, and myths and misconceptions can be dispelled. False assumptions about intimacy during palliative care can be addressed, and anticipatory guidance regarding what to expect as a result of advancing disease and palliative treatment is included in this discussion.

Specific suggestions ("SS") goes beyond limited information; counseling to rectify specific problems or to attain a mutually stated goal is employed. A stated goal is key to this phase since the resultant plan will aim at attaining that outcome. Specific suggestions usually pertain to the areas of communication, symptom management, and alternate physical expression. Fostering open communication between the couple about sexuality in end-of-life care is essential. Candid discussions regarding their emotional response to this phase of their relationship, their fears and concerns, and their hopes and desires are included in these interactions. Symptom management is essential to optimizing sexual expression. The following section of this chapter addresses specific symptoms, their effect on the expression of intimacy, and strategies to effectively manage them while not compounding sexual problems. Alternate expression of physical intimacy may be necessary if sexual disruption is due to organic changes. If intercourse is difficult, painful, or impossible, the couple may have to expand their sexual repertoire. A thorough discussion of the couple's values, attitudes, and preferences should be done before suggesting alternatives. Using language that is understandable to the client/partner is essential. However, the use of slang or street language may be unacceptable to the health care provider. Therefore, defining terms early in the discussion will alleviate this potential problem.

There are many ways of giving and receiving sexual pleasure; genital intercourse is only one way of expressing physical love. Other suggestions include hugging, massage, fondling, caressing, cuddling, kissing, hand-holding, and masturbation, either mutually or singularly. Sexual gratification may be derived from manual, oral, and digital stimulation. Intrathigh, anal, and intramammary intercourse are also options if the female partner is unable to continue vaginal penetration.

Intensive therapy ("IT") is not usually suggested in end-of-life care. This therapy is generally geared toward couples who have long-standing sexual or marital problems. The feasibility of this type of therapy during palliative care for a terminal illness is questionable.

MANAGEMENT OF ALTERATIONS IN SEXUAL FUNCTIONING DURING END-OF-LIFE CARE

Terminal illness and end-of-life care can interfere with sexual functioning in many ways. Physiological changes; tissue damage; other organic manifestations of the disease; attempts to palliate the symptoms of advancing disease, such as fatigue, pain, nausea and vomiting; and psychological sequelae such as anxiety, depression, and body image changes may impact sexual functioning. Environmental issues that may affect sexual expression were addressed in the previous section. Management of the client's biological and psychological sequelae is addressed below.

Fatigue

Fatigue may be due to an array of factors. In Chapter 7, the etiology and management of fatigue were thoroughly addressed. Fatigue may render a client unable to perform sexually. If fatigue is identified as a factor in the client's ability to initiate or maintain sexual arousal, several strategies may be suggested to diminish these untoward effects. Minimizing exertion during intimate relations may be necessary. Providing time for rest before and after sexual relations is often a sufficient strategy to overcome the detrimental effects of fatigue. Likewise, avoiding the stress of a heavy meal, alcohol consumption, or extremes in temperature may be helpful. Experimenting with positions that require minimal client exertion (male-client, female astride; female-client, male astride) is often helpful. Finally, timing should be taken into consideration. Sexual activity in the morning upon awakening may be preferable over relations at the end of a long day. Planning for intimate time rather than spontaneity can be a beneficial strategy.

Pain

Sexual arousal and performance are often impaired by the presence of pain. Additionally, the use of pain medication (especially opiates) can interfere with sexual arousal.[8] In Chapters 5 and 6, the issues of pain assessment and management are discussed in a comprehensive manner. The goal of pain therapy is to alleviate or minimize discomfort. However, in attaining that goal, sexual responsiveness (i.e., libido or erectile function) may be hindered. Temporarily adjusting pain medications or experimenting with complementary methods of pain management should be explored. For example, relaxation techniques prior to intimacy may be helpful. Romantic music may decrease discomfort through distraction and relaxation while enhancing sexual interest. Sexual activity itself can be viewed as a form of distraction and subsequent relaxation. The couple should be encouraged to explore positions that offer the most comfort. Traditional positions may be abandoned for more comfortable ones, such as sitting in a chair or a side-lying position. Pillows can be used to support painful limbs or to maintain certain positions. A warm bath or shower prior to sexual activity may facilitate pain relief and can be seen as preparatory to intimate relations. Massage can be used as both an arousal technique and a therapeutic strategy for minimizing discomfort. Finally, suggesting the exploration of alternate ways of expressing tenderness and sexual gratification may be necessary if the couple's traditional intimacy repertoire is not feasible due to discomfort.

Nausea and Vomiting

Nausea and vomiting are common during the palliative care trajectory. Chapter 9 delves into the etiology and treatment of these symptoms. Nausea and vomiting negatively impact sexual functioning. There are many medications that suppress nausea; however, they may interfere with sexual functioning due to their sedative effects.[8] If the client complains of sexual difficulties secondary to treatment for nausea and vomiting, an assessment of the prescribed antiemetics may shed light on a pharmocological culprit. Using alternate nonpharmocological methods to control nausea and vomiting or changing to another antiemetic may be warranted. Such strategies include eating small and frequent meals, serving foods at room temperature, avoiding spicy foods, assuring a well-ventilated dining area, and using relaxation and distraction techniques. Providing fresh air through an open window in the bedroom, for example, may decrease noxious olfactory stimuli. As with fatigue, timing may be an important consideration for intimate relations. If the client/couple notes that nausea is more prevalent during a certain time of the day, planning for intimacy at alternate times may circumvent this problem.

Neutropenia and Thrombocytopenia

Neutropenia and thrombocytopenia, per se, do not necessarily interfere with intimacy, but they do pose some potential problems. Sexual intimacy during neutropenic phases may jeopardize the compromised client. Severe neutropenia predisposes a client to infection. Close physical contact may be inadvisable if the sexual partner has a communicable disease, such as an upper respiratory infection or influenza. Specific sexual practices, such as anal intercourse, are prohibited during neutropenic states due to the likelihood of subsequent infection. The absolute neutrophil count, if available, is a good indicator of neutropenic status and associated risk for infection. Client and partner education about the risks associated with neutropenia is essential

Thrombocytopenia and the associated risk of bleeding, bruising, or hemorrhage should be considered when counseling a couple about intimacy issues. Again, anal intercourse is contraindicated due to risk for bleeding. Likewise, vigorous genital intercourse may cause vaginal bleeding. Indeed, even forceful or energetic hugging, massage, or kissing may cause bruising or bleeding. Preventative suggestions might include such strategies as gentle love making with minimal pressure on the thrombocytopenic client or having the client assume the dominant position to control force and pressure.

Dyspnea

Dyspnea is an extremely distressing occurrence in the end-of-life trajectory. In Chapter 13, the management of this symptom is reviewed. Dyspnea, or even the fear of initiating dyspnea, can impair sexual functioning. General strategies can be employed to minimize dyspnea during sexual play. These can include using a waterbed to accentuate physical movements, raising the dyspneic client's head and shoulders to facilitate oxygenation, using supplementary oxygen and/or inhalers prior to and during sexual activity, performing pulmonary hygiene measures before intimacy, encouraging slower movements to conserve energy, and modifying sexual activity to allow for enjoyment and respiratory comfort.

Neuropathies

Neuropathies can be a result of disease progression or complication of prior aggressive treatment. Neuromuscular disturbances are discussed in depth in Chapter 18. Neuropathies can manifest as pain, paresthesia, and/or weakness. Depending on the location and severity of the neuropathy, sexual functioning can be altered or completely suppressed. Management or diminution of the neuropathy may or may not be feasible. If not, creative ways to evade the negative sequelae of this occurrence are necessary. Such strategies might include creative positioning, use of pillows to support affected body parts, or alternate ways of expressing physical love. The distraction of intimacy may temporarily minimize the perception of the neuropathy.

Mobility and Range of Motion

Mobility issues and compromised range of motion may interfere with sexual expression. Similar to issues related to fatigue, a decrease in mobility can inhibit a couple's customary means of expressing physical love. A compromise in range of motion can result in a similar dilemma. For example, a female client may no longer be able to position herself in such a way as to allow penile penetration from above due to hip or back restrictions. Likewise, a male client may have knee or back restrictions that make it impossible for him to be astride his partner. Regardless of the exact nature of the range-of-motion/mobility concern, several suggestions can be offered. Experimenting with alternate positions, employing relaxation techniques before sexual play, massage, warm baths, and exploring acceptable alternative methods of expressing physical intimacy should be encouraged.

Erectile Dysfunction

Erectile dysfunction can be caused by physiological, psychological, and emotional factors. These factors include vascular, endocrine, and neurological causes, chronic diseases, such as renal failure and diabetes; and iatrogenic factors, such as surgery and medications. Surgical severing of the small nerve branches essential for erection is often the untoward effect of radical pelvic surgery, radical prostatectomy, and aortoiliac surgery.[9] Vascular and neurological causes may not be reversible; however, endocrine causes may be minimized. For example, the use of estrogen in advanced prostate cancer may be terminated in palliative care, thus allowing for the return of erectile function. Many medications decrease desire and erectile capacity in men. The most common offenders are antihypertensives, antidepressants, antihistamines, antispasmodics, sedatives or tranquilizers, barbiturates, sex hormone preparations, narcotics, and psychoactive drugs.[8,9] Often, these medications cannot be discontinued to permit the return of erectile function. For those clients, penile implants may be possible. The use of sildenafil (Viagra) has not been researched in the area of terminal care. This medication is classified as a cardiovascular agent. It relaxes smooth muscle, increases blood flow, and facilitates erection.[10] If a vascular component is part of the underlying erectile dysfunction, the use of sildenafil may correct the problem. Certainly, contraindications such as underlying heart disease and other current medications should be taken into consideration. Otherwise, digital or oral stimulation of the female partner may be suggested as well as use of a vibrator, if that is acceptable.

Dyspareunia

Dyspareunia, like erectile dysfunction, can be caused by physiological, psychological, and emotional factors. These factors include vascular, endocrine, and neurological causes as well as iatrogenic factors such as surgery and medications.[9] Again, while vascular and neurological causes may not be reversible, endocrine causes may be minimized. For example, the use of estrogen replacement therapy, vaginal estrogen creams, or water-soluble lubricants may be helpful in diminishing vaginal dryness, which can cause painful intercourse. Gynecological surgery and pelvic irradiation may result in physiological changes which prevent comfortable intercourse. Changes seen postirradiation, such as vaginal shortening, thickening, and narrowing, may result in severe dyspareunia. As with male clients, many medications decrease desire and function in women. These drugs include antihypertensives, antidepressants, antihistamines, antispasmodics, sedatives or tranquilizers, barbiturates, sex hormone preparations, narcotics, and psychoactive drugs.[8,9] Often, these medications cannot be discontinued to permit the return of sexual function. For those clients, digital or oral stimulation of male partner may be suggested, if acceptable. Additionally, intrathigh and intramammary penetration may be suggested to women who find vaginal intercourse too painful.

Body Image Disturbances

Sexuality is closely related to how one views oneself in the physical sense. An incurable illness and concomitant end-of-life care can alter one's physical appearance. Additionally, past treatments for disease often irrevocably alter body appearance and function. Issues such as alopecia, weight loss, cachexia, the presence of a stoma, or amputation of a body part, to name a few, can result in feelings of sexual inadequacy and/or disinterest. End-of-life care can focus on the identification and remediation of issues related to body image changes. Although an altered appearance may be permanent, counseling and behavior modification as well as specific suggestions to minimize or mask these appearances can improve body image to a level compatible with feelings of sexual adequacy and empowerment.

The use of a wig, scarf, or headbands can mask alopecia. Some clients, rather than try to conceal hair loss, choose to emphasize it by shaving the head. Weight loss and cachexia can be masked through clothing and the creative use of padding. The presence of an ostomy can significantly alter body image and negatively affect sexual functioning. Specific interventions geared toward minimizing the effect that the presence of an ostomy has on sexual functioning depend, in part, on the particular type of ostomy. Some ostomies are continent, while others need an appliance attached at all times. If the client has a continent ostomy, timing sexual activity can allow for removal of the appliance and covering the stoma. If the ostomy appliance cannot be safely removed, the patient should be taught to empty the appliance before intimate relations and to use a cover or body stocking to conceal the appliance. Alternate positions may also be entertained, and in the event of a leak, sexual activity can continue in the shower. The United Ostomy Association (http://www.uoa.org) publishes four patient information booklets on sexuality and the ostomate: *Sex, Courtship and the Single Ostomate* by D.P. Binder, *Sex and the Female Ostomate* by G.L. Dickman and C.A. Livingston, *Sex and the Male Ostomate* by E. Gambrell, and *Gay and Lesbian Ostomates and Their Caregivers.* Gay Lesbian Organization.

Anxiety and Depression

Anxiety and depression related to the incurable and terminal aspects of the disease may interfere with sexual desire and response. As two of the most common affective disorders during end-of-life care, they are thoroughly discussed in Chapter 19. Both anxiety and depression have profound effects on sexual functioning.[1] Decreases in sexual desire, libido, and activity are common sequelae of these affective disorders. However, some interventions, especially pharmocological management, can further compromise sexual functioning. A thorough assessment of the client's psychological state and an evaluation of the medications currently prescribed for this condition may reveal the source of the problem. Anxiolytics such as lorazepam and alprazolam are commonly prescribed. Antidepressants, such as tricyclic antidepressants, selective serotonin reuptake inhibitors, and monoamine oxidase inhibitors, are often prescribed. All of these have the potential for interfering with sexual functioning.[8] Unfortunately, one may end up having to choose psychological comfort and compromised intimacy. Alternately, the health care provider may suggest a nonpharmocological approach to the management of these affective disorders, especially if the disorder is mild. Relaxation techniques, imagery, and biofeedback may lower anxiety to a tolerable level. Additionally, the release of sexual tension may resolve anxiety in itself. If desire is maintained and function alone is compromised for male clients, the couple may explore alternate ways of pleasuring each other. For female clients, use of water-soluble lubricants can offset the interference with arousal if interest remains intact. Once again, open communication between both the couple and the health care provider allows for frank discussions and the presentation of possible alternatives to expressing physical affection during palliative care.

SUMMARY

Incurable illness and end-of-life care may result in compromising a couple's intimacy. To prevent or minimize this, health care providers should assume a leading role in the assessment and remediation of potential or identified alterations in sexual functioning. Clearly, not all couples will find intimacy of concern at this point of their life together; however, if intimacy is desired, all attempts should be made to facilitate this important aspect of life. Many find being physically close to the one they love life-affirming and comforting. As clients draw close to the end of life, they remain human and holistic. Their needs, hopes, and concerns remain as intact as all others. If those needs and hopes include maintaining intimacy with a partner, this should be included in the assessment and provision of care. The health care provider's offer of information and support can make a significant difference in a couple's ability to adjust to the changes in intimacy related to end-of-life care.

The realm of sexual functioning and intimacy during end-of-life care remains an area in which further research is warranted. Much of the information presented in this chapter resulted from clinical practice and inferences made from other, tangentially related research. Incorporating intimacy research into end-of-life care research is a natural and much needed marriage.

REFERENCES

1. Varcarolis E. Foundations of Psychiatric Mental Health Nursing, 3rd Ed. Philadelphia: WB Saunders, 1998.

2. Lipson JG, Dibble SL, Minarik PA. Culture and Nursing Care. San Francisco: UCSF Nursing Press, 1996.

3. Cole SW, Kemeny ME, Taylor SE, Visscher BR. Elevated physical health risk among gay men who conceal their homosexual identity. Health Psychol 1996;15:243–251.

4. Matthews AK. Lesbians and cancer support: clinical issues for cancer patients. Health Care Women Int 1998;19:193–203.

5. White JC, Levinson W. Lesbian health care: what a primary care physician needs to know. West J Med 1995;162:463–466.

6. White JC, Dull VT. Health risk factors and health-seeking behavior in lesbians. J Womens Health 1997;6:103–112.

7. Annon JS. The Behavioral Treatment of Sexual Problems. Honolulu: Mercantile Printing, 1974.

8. Cleveland L, Aschenbrenner DS, Venable SJ, Yensen JAP. Nursing Management in Drug Therapy. Philadelphia: Lippincott, Williams & Wilkins, 1999.

9. LeMome P, Burke KM. Medical Surgical Nursing: Critical Thinking in Client Care, 2nd Ed. Menlo Park, CA: Addison-Wesley, 2000.

10. Hodgson BB, Kizior RJ. Saunders Nursing Drug Handbook 2000. Philadelphia: WB Saunders, 2000.

22 Clinical Interventions, Economic Outcomes, and Palliative Care

PATRICK J. COYNE, LAURIE LYCKHOLM, and THOMAS J. SMITH

Whether half full or half empty, it will be a smaller glass.
—Detmer (1997)[1]

The scope of nursing and nursing education has expanded to include multiple domains, many of which overlap with other disciplines, such as wellness and disease prevention and health services administration. Economic outcome is an area in which nursing is essential to the provision of efficient, cost-effective, and appropriate palliative care. In this chapter, we ask several questions regarding the economics of palliative care and provide data from health services research regarding economic outcomes. These data, while limited, may help to set a framework for thinking about how to make palliative care available to everyone in an ethical, economic, and effective manner.

WHY ARE ECONOMIC OUTCOMES IMPORTANT?

Health care spending and health care quality are major problems in the United States. Cancer care costs have risen from $35 billion in 1990[2] to $40 billion in 1994[3] to one estimate of $50 billion by 1996.[4] We are spending a significant amount on high-technology care for the elderly; nearly one-third of all Medicare spending is on patients in their last year of life,[5,6] and those funds cannot be spent on preventive services or chronic disease conditions for the same population.[7] In the largest Virginia insurance plan, the top 1% of the wealthiest population consumes 30% of the resources. The pressure on health care funds will increase due to increased demands for care from an educated elderly population, more elderly long-term survivors, new and expensive technologies, new diseases, and demands for cost cutting. All health care interventions, regardless of intention, active therapy, or palliative care, are delivered at a price. Cost effectiveness of interventions must be continually assessed; less is not necessarily better, but whatever is spent must maximize the resources available.[8] The question of when, where, and why to use high-tech interventions falls into the middle of this debate and must be carefully explored.

The process is not optimal for all patients, and quality of palliative care must improve.[9] The Study to Understand Prognoses and Preferences for Outcomes and Risks of Treatment (SUPPORT) showed that half of all dying patients had unnecessary pain and suffering in their final days of life while in the hospital.[10] Nearly half of patients suffer unnecessary pain, even when cared for by oncologists.[11]

The whole neglected issue of cancer care quality is now under discussion, with active efforts to improve it.[12] The relationship of volume to quality is striking:[13] (*1*) a significant (5% to 10%) overall survival advantage at a breast cancer specialty center versus community hospitals,[14,15] (*2*) better survival for testicular cancer patients treated at specialist centers,[16] (*3*) better survival and fewer complications for ovarian cancer surgery performed by specialist gynecological oncologists rather than general surgeons or gynecologists,[17] and (*4*) better survival for prostate cancer patients at high-volume centers.[18] Until the science of palliative care becomes better known, one can reasonably speculate that palliative care will improve in high-volume or specialized centers.

Clearly, there is a need for additional research to address these questions of quality care. We have identified some important questions about economic outcomes and palliative care, and these are listed in Table 22–1.

THE ETHICS OF ADDING ECONOMIC OUTCOMES

In the modern arena of health care, nonmedical concerns, such as cost control, oversight and audit, utilization review, and decreasing liability risk, have assumed a significant role. Some authorities have argued that such management tools are not inherently unethical.[19] Cost control is certainly not inherently unethical but should be considered secondary to the goal of quality care. The goals of nursing and medicine are grounded in a tradition of promoting health and providing comfort and relief of suffering in a just manner. Cost control through aggressive disease management, or "critical paths," may actually promote these goals by making more and/or better care available if we avoid the current systems which reward/pay for hi-tech interventions while not reimbursing effective low-tech treatments.[20] An example of this is that insurance reimburses a patient-controlled analgesia pump but will not reimburse oral analgesics.

Table 22–1. Types of Needed Health and Service Research Studies

Type of Study	Question Posed
Policy analysis	What outcomes justify treatment? Who should make those decisions?
Type of care: chemotherapy vs. best or other types of supportive care	Does chemotherapy save money compared to best supportive care, when all costs are considered?
Site of service	Is home vs. hospital more effective and less costly?
Structural and process changes in care	Can costs be reduced by changes in how care is delivered, e.g., by inpatient hospice or at home?
Hospice vs. nonhospice	Does hospice improve quality of life and/or reduce costs of care?
Advanced directives and do-not-resuscitate orders	Do advanced directives influence medical treatment decisions and/or change costs?
Nursing ability to impact cost at end of life	Do skilled palliative care nurses have the ability to effectively palliate patients with a savings of resources?

Cost control must be differentiated from profit motivation and entrepreneurship, which have not traditionally been considered the goals of medicine. These activities in the context of health care are unethical in that they may make medical care more expensive and difficult to access, especially for those who are socially disadvantaged. They may also create further conflicts of interest in already precarious fiduciary relationships between clinicians and their patients. A code of ethics that covers all professionals, rather than medicine alone, might be useful.[21]

Tolerance of suboptimal care is an equally important ethical issue and one that is rarely mentioned in either ethical or management studies. Studies such as SUPPORT have revealed that many aspects of end-of-life care are still suboptimal. The national dialogue about physician-assisted suicide might also indicate that end-of-life care has not been optimized, thus resulting in despair and frustration so significant as to urge dying persons to consider suicide to end their suffering. If palliative care can be improved and/or made less costly without sacrificing quality, it must be done in the service of promoting the values of beneficence, compassion, and respect for autonomy. Palliative care has emerged as a national movement, with the advent of several important initiatives [Project on Death in America, Oncology Nursing Society efforts, Education for Physicians on End-of-Life Care by the American Medical Association, established programs such as the Center to Improve Care of the Dying at George Washington University, etc.] and the development of palliative care programs all over the world. The Healthcare Finance Administration's approval of an International Classification of Diseases-9 code for palliative care was hoped by some to indicate its significance in the health care system.[21] The economic outcomes are not known and may be difficult to measure, but regardless, the ethical impetus to correct the deficiency is critical.

Another serious ethical question is the ownership of disease-management models. Should management tools that improve care be protected or available to the general public? If a tool that improved care at markedly lower cost were developed, one could argue that it should be made available for widespread distribution, much like the polio vaccine. Another example would be an algorithm which eased dyspnea rapidly in end-stage disease with minimal economic impact and no requirement for technology.

Some have argued that budgets should not be balanced with penalty to one group, such as the elderly or those on Medicare.[22,23] Many health care goods are rationed justly according to age, such as transplants, coronary bypass, and hemodialysis, based on the theory of equality of opportunity according to ability to benefit from such procedures.[24] However, palliative care is different in that age does not determine whether a person stands to benefit. In this circumstance, the ethic of distributive justice supports the concept that medical and social needs dictate who stands to benefit most from palliative care.

Daniels[25] reported: "it does not seem reasonable to postulate that the medical needs of the elderly terminally ill are any less than those of younger patients, and indeed they may be greater because of multiple additional pathologies associated with aging." Sidgwick's[26] argument that each moment of life is equally valuable no matter when it occurs is most poignant in the instance of palliative care. This would also apply to extending palliative care to neonates expected to live only a short time after birth.

Patients may view benefit and toxicity in ways very different from their health care providers and from those who are well. According to a recent study, dying patients would undergo almost any treatment toxicity for a 1% chance of short-term survival, while their doctors and nurses would not; and these decisions were not changed after patients experienced the toxicity of treatment.[27] A study of palliative radiotherapy for brain tumor patients showed little survival, modest functional benefit, and a substantial decrement in intellectual function; but most patients and families would still want it.[28,29]

WHAT IS THE RIGHT AMOUNT TO SPEND ON HEALTH CARE?

How much to spend on health care cannot be determined without knowing the economic and cultural particulars of a country or even a health system. Blanket statements about a percentage of the gross national product (GNP) may be misleading if a comparison country spends a higher percentage on social net programs but less on direct medical care costs. Comments about health care spending as a percent of the GNP may also reflect opinions about alternative uses, for example, "We should stop spending money on defense and spend it on health care." In the United States, the amount spent on education has declined from 6% to 5% of the GNP, while the amount spent on health care (especially for the elderly) has risen from 6% to about 14%.[30] Clearly, in all countries, the entire system of health care needs to be explored with policies designed to ensure that palliative care is a component of the overall health care system.[31]

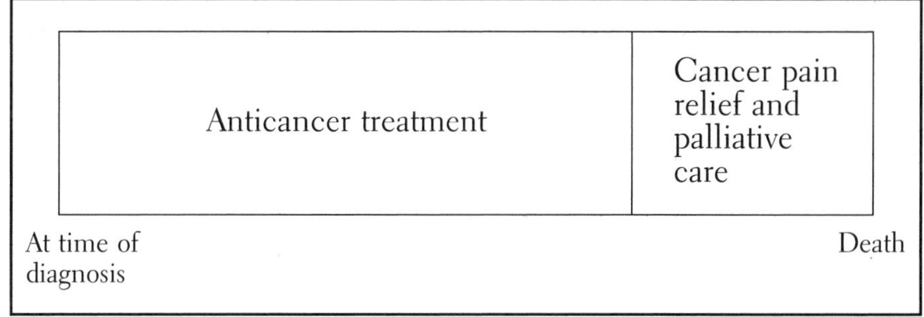

Fig. 22–1. Present allocation worldwide of cancer resources. How worldwide cancer resources are currently allocated. Palliative care must receive more of these resources. (Reproduced by permission of WHO, from: Cancer Pain Relief and Palliative Care. Technical Report Series 304. Geneva: World Health Organization, 1990.[94])

SHOULD THERE BE SPECIAL ECONOMIC OR POLICY CONSIDERATIONS FOR PALLIATIVE CARE?

We believe that, in general, there should be no special considerations for palliative care. Most health care policy analysts and economists would argue that all care should be evaluated equally. For example, a therapy that gains 1 week for 52 patients should be valued as much as a therapy of equivalent cost that gains 52 weeks for 1 patient.[32] Recently, some health economists have argued that time given to those who are most at risk should be valued more (e.g., time added in the last 6 months of life should be given triple value).[33] The analogy was made to food and hunger: a sandwich given to a starving person would be of more intrinsic value than one given to a person who already had many sandwiches. Such discussions, while interesting, are outside the scope of this chapter; but many of the ethical concepts applied to these global discussions have relevance to decisions about palliative care.

The World Health Organization (WHO) has listed priorities for health care. In cancer, palliative care has always been included in the same category as curative therapy. In part, this was done because most palliative care is relatively inexpensive.

As Figures 21–1 through 21–3 illustrate, current allocation of resources greatly favors curative care with less support for palliative care. The WHO advocates a more equal distribution of resources in developed countries and an even greater support of palliative care in developing countries, where most of the population will experience advanced disease rather than cure or long-term survival.

One approach to funding treatments has been based on cost-effectiveness ratios.[32] Laupacis and colleagues[40] in Canada proposed explicit funding criteria: (*1*) treatments that work better and are less expensive should be adopted; (2) treatments with cost-effectiveness ratios of less than $20,000 per additional life year (LY) gained should be accepted, with the recognition that they cost additional resources; (3) treatments with cost-effectiveness ratios of $20,000 to $100,000/LY should be examined on a case-by-case basis with caution; (*4*) and treatments with cost-effectiveness ratios of greater than $100,000/LY should be rejected. These criteria are valid in a system where all resources are shared equally; it is not clear how they apply to other health care systems, where resources may not be shared.[39] Alternatively, patients might be allowed to purchase additional insurance for expensive treatments or pay for them out of pocket. In the United States, there has been no accepted answer, but most authorities have agreed on an implicitly defined benchmark of $35,000 to $50,000/LY saved.[32] For example, an individual with a pathological fracture of a femur is sent to the operating room for pinning. This surgery will aid in relieving pain, improving function, and probably decreas-

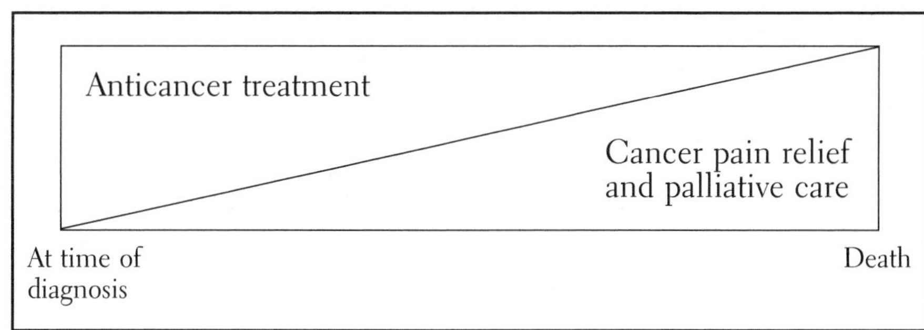

Fig. 22–2. Proposed allocation of cancer resources in developed countries. Curative and palliative care are not mutually exclusive. Resources should be dispensed to allow the greatest benefits for the majority of individuals. (Reproduced by permission of WHO, from: Cancer Pain Relief and Palliative Care. Technical Report Series 304. Geneva: World Health Organization, 1990.[94])

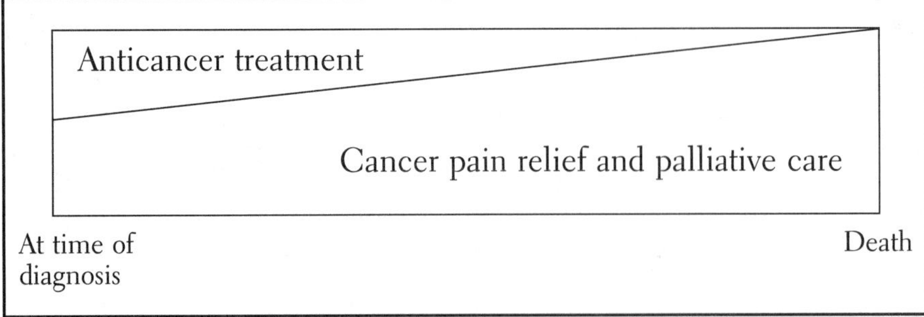

Fig. 22–3. Proposed allocation of cancer resources in developing countries. As developing countries are the least likely to prevent, detect, and cure cancers, the distribution of resources should be further tailored to best meet the needs of their population. (It is a great ethical dilemma: do you cure one to allow 1000 more to suffer?) (Reproduced by permission of WHO, from: Cancer Pain Relief and Palliative Care. Technical Report Series 304. Geneva: World Health Organization, 1990.[94])

ing other potential complications, such as decubitus ulcer and deep venous thrombosis.

WHAT ARE IMPORTANT ECONOMIC OUTCOMES?

Economic outcomes are not different from clinical outcomes, and cost must be considered along with clinical benefit. Only one medical group, the American Society of Clinical Oncology (ASCO), has published recommendations on what benefit is justified to recommend a medical intervention, listed in Table 22–2.[35] Of note, ASCO could not define the lowest amount of benefit that justified an intervention, for example, 2 weeks of quality survival, but recommended that the benefit be weighed against the toxicity and costs. If cost-effectiveness data are not available, then cost consciousness with attention to lowest costs for comparable results would be appropriate; cost alone is not sufficient since more expensive treatments, such as bone marrow transplantation for relapsed leukemia, may give better survival at reasonable cost effectiveness.[32]

The economic data necessary to make decisions about treatment may be collected in much the same way as clinical information, and standard formats for collection and analysis are now available.[36] Some standard definitions are listed in Table 22–3.

It is important to organize data in a way that balances clinical and cost information side by side, as shown in Table 22–4.

Chemotherapy is often thought of as curative, but it is one of several types of palliative care and may be helpful for symptom relief or to prolong survival. Chemotherapy may be a good treatment decision in palliative care as long as the switch to palliative care is made while resources and quality time are still available.[41,42]

It is possible to give chemotherapy and either save money or have a cost effectiveness within accepted limits, as shown in Table 22–5. Patients treated with chemotherapy for non-small-cell lung cancer have a small benefit, estimated at 2 to 4 months in most series,[43,44] and symptom relief in up to 60% of cases.[45] Both the ASCO[46] and the Ontario government[47] recommend consideration of chemotherapy for suitable patients. Jaakimainen and coworkers[48] found that chemotherapy actually saved disease-management costs compared to best supportive care by preventing hospitalizations late in the disease course. The cost-effectiveness ratios ranged from −$8000 (cost saving) to +$20,000 (costs more than supportive care) Canadian for each additional year of life.[48] Chemotherapy with cisplatin and vinorelbine compared to vinorelbine alone or cisplatin and vindesine added substantial clinical benefit[49] at a reasonable cost effectiveness of $15,000 to $17,000/LY.[50] Given the benefit and low cost of the drugs, vinorelbine and cisplatin compared to best supportive care would give results similar to those of Jaakimainen and colleagues.[48] Evans and colleagues[51] used decision analysis to show that chemotherapy in combination with radiation and/or surgery for stage IIIA or IIIB disease in comparison to treatment without chemotherapy would improve survival at a cost of $3348 to $14,958 Canadian per year of life saved. The model showed benefit at a reasonable cost under all situations of reasonable clinical efficacy. The chemotherapy treatments fit existing monetary guidelines for use.[52,53]

A trial of fluorouracil-based chemotherapy for gastrointestinal cancer patients randomized to first-line chemotherapy versus best supportive care, which could include later chemotherapy for symptom control, showed benefit at acceptable cost-effectiveness ratios.[54] For the whole group, chemotherapy enhanced survival by about 5 months at a cost of about $20,000/LY gained, within accepted bounds.[32] For subsets of types of cancer, such as gastric cancer, the treatment was effective at a reasonable cost. For most other subsets, the patient numbers were too small to draw meaningful conclusions about either clinical effect or cost effectiveness.

In a metastatic prostate cancer study,

Table 22–2. Outcomes that Justify a Medical Intervention

Justify	Do not Justify
Improved overall survival	False hope that survival will be improved
Improved disease-free survival	
Improved quality of life	
Less toxicity	
Improved cost effectiveness	Cost alone

Table 22–3. Standard Definitions for Economic Outcome Analysis

Term	Definition	Comment
Resource utilization	Number of units used, e.g., 9 hospital days	Best collected prospectively, using a combination of clinical research forms, hospital bills, and patient diaries for outpatient or off-site events.
Charge	What is billed to the patient	May be fair representation of the cost of service. Can be accurately converted to costs using ratio of charges to cost.[37]
Cost	What it costs society to provide the service	This is different from the charge as many services cost more/less than what may be billed.
Direct medical cost	Cost of standard medical interventions	Usual "cost-drivers" include hospital days, professional fees, diagnostic tests, pharmacy fees, other (blood products, operating room or emergency services, etc.)
Direct nonmedical cost	Costs of medical interventions not usually captured but directly caused	Includes transportation, time lost from work, caregiver costs, etc. Most are not covered by insurance and may be "out-of-pocket" costs.
Perspective	The viewpoint of the analysis	Should be explicitly stated. Most analyses are done from the perspective of society (valuing this intervention vs. other uses of the same money) or a health care system (valuing this intervention against other local health care needs). The perspective of the individual patient or provider may give less attention to the needs of others.[36,39]
Discounting	Adjusts value of intervention for future benefit to present-time amount	Health effects and costs should normally be discounted at 3% per year. Health benefits in the present are worth more than those in the future.

Source: Smith (1993), reference 39.

mitoxantrone added a clinical benefit in terms of pain relief and symptom control in 23 of 80 patients, lasting for 6 months more than prednisone alone, but did not alter survival when compared to prednisone alone.[55] Although initial drug costs were higher, total disease costs were lower in the group that received mitoxantrone as initial treatment,[56] so good chemotherapy palliation could be accomplished at no additional cost to society. Total androgen blockade produced small clinical benefit at an acceptable cost to society compared to single androgen blockade.[57]

There have been no studies on the effectiveness or cost effectiveness of chemotherapy for metastatic breast cancer compared to best supportive care. Hospitalization accounts for the majority of costs, while chemotherapy has been a relatively trivial cost in the United Kingdom.[58] High-dose chemotherapy is commonly used for incurable metastatic disease, and in the one randomized controlled trial, it doubled overall survival from 10.4 to 20.8 months but did not produce a long-term survival plateau.[59] In the only available study of comparative treatment, Hillner and associates[60] compared best standard chemotherapy to high-dose chemotherapy with a stem cell transplant. High dose

Table 22–4. Ways to Balance Clinical Evaluation and Cost Studies

Type of Study	Advantages and Disadvantages
Clinical outcomes only	Ignore costs. Easy to choose among clearly superior therapies such as cisplatin for testicular cancer; harder among all others that give lesser benefits at high costs.
Cost only, e.g., costs of treating febrile neutropenia	Ignores clinical outcomes. Does not help choose among clinical strategies. The cost of colony-stimulating factor (CSF) mobilization of stem cells may be higher than that of bone marrow collection, but it saves money later by reducing hospital stay.[36]
Costs and clinical outcomes together	
• Cost minimization	Assumes that two strategies are equal; lowest cost strategy is preferred.
• Cost effectiveness	Compares two strategies; assigns dollar amount per additional year of life (life year) saved by strategy. Example: at present, CSFs have not improved survival, so cost must be lower for therapy to be cost-effective.
• Cost utility	Compares two strategies; assigns dollar amount per additional year of life (life year) saved by strategy, then estimates the quality of that benefit in cost/quality adjusted life year. No data show significant improvement in quality of life or utilities in patients who have received CSFs, so unlikely to have major impact.
• Cost benefit	Compares two strategies but converts the clinical benefits to money, e.g., a year of life is worth $100,000. This is possible but rarely done due to difficulty in assigning monetary value to benefit; requires assigning a monetary value to human life.

Table 22–5. Chemotherapy vs. Best Palliative Care or Alternative Treatments

Topic	Conclusion
Lung cancer	
Chemotherapy vs. best supportive care in non-small-cell lung cancer[48,50]	Chemotherapy gained 8–13 weeks compared to best supportive care.[48] Chemotherapy generally saved money for the province of Ontario, from a savings of $8000 to an additional cost of $20,000 depending on assumptions. Similar results found for vinorelbine and cisplatin.[50]
Combined modality including chemotherapy vs. radiation or surgery for stage III non-small-cell lung cancer[51–53]	Chemotherapy in combination with radiation or surgery adds clinical benefit; for chemotherapy plus radiation, 1- and 5-year survival rates are increased from 40% to 54% and from 6% to 17%, for instance. The addition of chemotherapy for IIIA patients added cost of $15,866, and addition of chemotherapy to IIIB patients added $8912. The cost/year of life gained was well within accepted bounds at $3348 to $14,958 Canadian.
Alternating chemotherapy for small-cell lung cancer[63]	The alternating chemotherapy arm cost more, but because it was more effective, the marginal cost effectiveness was only $4560/year of life.
Gastrointestinal cancer	
Chemotherapy vs. best supportive care followed by chemotherapy for gastrointestinal cancer patients[54]	Chemotherapy added 5 months median survival if given early rather than late, with symptom palliation for 4 months. The additional cost of about $20,000/life year was within accepted bounds.
Prostate cancer	
Palliative chemotherapy with mitoxantrone plus prednisone vs. prednisone[55,56]	Mitoxantrone did not improve survival but did improve quality of life as measured by several indices, and the mitoxantrone strategy cost less than prednisone supportive care.
Breast cancer	
High-dose chemotherapy for limited metastatic disease vs. standard chemotherapy[60]	High-dose chemotherapy added 6 months at a cost of $58,000, or $116,000/life year; this is palliative care as this treatment has not been shown to be curative.
Other	
Acute myelogenous leukemia[62]	Chemotherapy, compared to supportive care, added additional cost, but the cost effectiveness was $18,000/life year, within acceptable limits.

Source: Smith et al. (1993), reference 32.

chemotherapy added about 6 months at a cost-effectiveness ratio of $116,000/LY gained, outside the bounds of accepted treatments. Of interest, drug costs for most breast cancer patients amount to less than 10% of the total cost.[61]

Acute myelogenous leukemia chemotherapy cost more than supportive care and certain death, and allogeneic transplant was even more effective. The transplant survival benefit of 48% versus 21% at 5 years was sufficient to offset higher costs of treatment and make the cost-effectiveness ratio about $18,000/LY.[62]

The less expensive the setting, the less costly the intervention, as shown in Table 22–6. Home opioid infusions had lower total costs due to lower hospital costs despite higher drug equipment and nursing costs.[64] Outpatient administration of chemotherapy was less expensive than inpatient administration.[65] Home chemotherapy compared to outpatient chemotherapy was accepted well, with only two of 424 patients electing to discontinue home treatment; safe; and no more costly, with an average cost of $50 compared to $116 in hospital and equal total costs.[66]

Disease-management strategies have shown some modest improvements, with better quality of care, less cost, and high patient satisfaction. The available studies are shown in Table 22–7.

Coordinated care may be one of the most successful disease-management strategies. The Medicare Hospice Benefit requires nurse coordination, team management, easy access to low per diem hospital beds for respite or temporary care, and expanded drug coverage.[67,68] Adding a nurse coordinator for terminally ill patients in England did not change any disease outcomes: patients still died, and most still had some unrelieved symptoms; however, patient and family satisfaction was helped slightly.[69] Total costs were reduced from £8814 to £4414 due to decreased hospital days, for a cost savings of 41% in almost all conditions.[70] Home nursing care was associated with more patients dying at home.[71]

One center did a pain-management intervention with enhanced institu-

Table 22–6. Site of Service

Topic	Conclusion
Opioids in home infusion	Opioids at home per diem costs were higher for home patients, but total costs were lower with equivalent palliation.[64]
Inpatient or outpatient	Outpatient administration was less expensive, $184 vs. $223 US.[65]
Home or inpatient/clinic chemotherapy	Home chemotherapy was safe, well accepted, and cost less per treatment.[66]

Table 22–7. Process or Structural Changes in Care

Topic	Conclusion
Reducing uncontrolled pain admissions	A system-wide intervention of focus on pain management, a supportive care consultation team, and a pain resource center. This was associated with a reduction in admissions from 255/5772 (4.4%) to 121/4076 (3.0%), at a project cost savings of $2,719,245.[72]
Presence of nursing care for end of life	Nursing care availability allowed more patients to die at home, consistent with the wishes of most patients.[71]
Clinical practice guidelines for supportive care: antiemetics, treatment of febrile neutropenia, treatment of pain	A division changed practice to standardized oral antiemetics and once-daily ceftriaxone and gentamicin. Cost savings were estimated at $250,000 for each intervention, yearly.[68,77,78]

tional education programs, a highly visible respected consultative team, and a pain-resource center for nurses and families. This was associated with a decrease in admissions and readmissions for pain control and marked cost savings.[72] The study was not randomized and could not account for other significant changes, such as the growth of managed care with restricted admission policies. However, the conclusion must be that this is better pain management and better medical care and probably saves money.[73]

Teaching staff about choices for intensive care unit use can improve economic outcomes. In one setting, an ethicist in the surgical intensive care unit addressed the issues of patient choice about dying and the ethics of futile care. This was associated with a decrease in length of stay from 28 to 16 days, and a decrease in surgical intensive care days from 2028 to 1003, far greater than observed in other parts of the hospital. Cost savings were estimated at $1.8 million.[74] In a similar project, Dowdy and colleagues[75] did proactive ethics consultations for all mechanically ventilated patients beyond 4 days and showed improved length of stay (less use of the intensive care unit, either by discontinuing futile care or transferring the patient to lesser-intensity units) and a decrease in costs.

Clinical practice guidelines for supportive care may decrease costs, but formal data have not been published.[68] Standardization of care can improve the process of care, even if not the outcomes, for most areas studied.[69,76]

While there have been significant anecdotal data and clinical opinion that hospice provides improved quality and decreased cost, the available data do not show that hospice improves care or saves money, as shown in Table 22–8.[68,79,80] A large, randomized, controlled trial of hospice versus standard care showed that hospice did not improve quality of care by any measured benchmark (pain, ability to perform activities of daily liv-

Table 22–8. Hospice vs. Nonhospice Care

Topic	Conclusion
Randomized controlled trial of hospice vs. nonhospice care in Veterans Hospital	Hospice did not improve or worsen quality of care by any measured benchmark (pain, ability to perform activities of daily living). There was no difference in diagnostic procedures. Total costs were $15,000 per patient, with no difference in the arms.[84]
Hospice election vs. standard care, Medicare beneficiaries, 1992	Medicare saved $1.65 for each $1 spent on hospice programs; most of the savings occurred during the last month of life.[81]
Hospice election vs. standard care, Medicare beneficiaries, 1988	Medicare saved $1.26 for each $1 spent on hospice programs; most of the savings occurred during the last month of life.[82]
Total costs from databases	No significant difference in total costs from diagnosis to death, but significant cost savings of 39% for hospice patients who were in hospice over 2 weeks.[85]
Total disease management costs comparing those who elected hospice to those who did not	No difference or slightly higher costs among Medicare beneficiaries who elected hospice. Within the hospice period, average 27 days, costs were slightly lower for those who elected hospice.[68]
Home care	Home care provided by relatives is not much different ($4563 for each 3-month period) from costs in a nursing home or similar setting. The sicker the patient became, the more the cost to the family regardless of diagnosis. Costs were lowest when the patient and caregiver lived in the same household.[86,87]
Matching resource use to the dying patient	Hospice patients more likely to receive more home nursing and spend less time in the hospital than conventional care patients. Conventional care was the least expensive when overall disease management costs were calculated, but hospital-based hospice ($2270) and home care hospice ($2657) were less.

ing). Patients still used many hospital days (48 for controls, and 51 for hospice), but more of the hospice patients were hospitalized on the hospice unit. There was no difference in diagnostic procedures or total costs (about $15,000 per patient).

More recent data suggest that hospice care can be cost-savings.[81] In the 1992 Medicare files, those cancer patients who elected hospice cost less than those who did not elect hospice. For those who enrolled in hospice in the last month of life, typically over half of Medicare hospice patients, Medicare saved $1.65 for each $1 spent. However, those who elected hospice tended to use more resources in the months from diagnosis until about 3 months before death, so the total disease-management savings were close to zero. Similar findings were reported previously.[82]

Hospice may actually not save total disease-management costs but just shift them to costs not captured by our current accounting systems. In our own study of Medicare hospice use in Virginia, total disease-management costs were actually higher for those who eventually elected hospice. Those who elect hospice tend to have resources to absorb more home care costs, more out-of-pocket drug costs, etc. The data are consistent with an affluent group of patients using all of the resources needed for treatment, then using hospice resources in addition. There are no published data on whether the medically underserved use hospice, whether they will accept its philosophy, or how much they will cost the system.[68]

Database studies have shown similar results. In a retrospective study of 12,000 patients at 40 centers, Aiken[83] found that hospice patients were more likely to receive home nursing care and to spend less time in the hospital than conventional care patients. Of the three models of care evaluated, conventional care was the least expensive when overall disease-management costs were calculated, but hospital-based hospice ($2270) and home care hospice ($2657) were less expensive than conventional care ($6100) in the last month of life.

Advanced directives, such as "do-not-resuscitate" (DNR) orders, have been advocated to allow patients to make autonomous choices about their care at the end of life and possibly to reduce costs by preventing futile care. However, as reviewed by Emanuel and Emanuel,[79,88] there has been no cost saving associated with the use of either advanced directives or DNR orders (Table 22–9). These findings have been confirmed in the more recent SUPPORT study.[89]

End-of-life or advanced planning is clearly a part of palliative care and care of the dying. Levinsky[22] has questioned whether end-of-life planning has become an economic strategy as much as a way to respect a patient's wishes: "Confusion between advance planning as a method to find out what the patient wants and advance planning as a mechanism to reduce medical care and thereby contain costs represents a clear danger to the goals of informed consent and autonomy for patients." In a randomized study of 204 patients with life-threatening diseases, it was found that in those who executed an advance directive, there was no significant positive or negative effect on well-being, health status, medical treatments, or medical treatment charges.[90]

NURSING ISSUES

Clearly, many issues related to nursing impact need to be explored. Role utilization and its potential impact will vary within each setting. For example, an entire multidisciplinary palliative care team may be necessary to meet the needs of the population in a large university-based hospital, yet a specially trained nurse may be adequate in a small community hospital. Such impact of services needs to be evaluated in many fields to examine quality of care and cost effectiveness.[92] A cost not truly examined is the out-of-pocket cost that the patient's significant others bear in caring for them, specifically in terms of lost work hours, expended resources, and simple care hours not reimbursed through the health care system. Also to be determined is the increased health care costs of the caregivers due to the stressful, often exhausting requirements.[93]

Nursing needs to continue to advocate for this population while supporting effective quality care, and fair utilization of resources must be frequently assessed. For example, the use of advanced technology, especially expensive diagnostic tests, may be accepted as routine in an acute care hospital, even though it is costly, unnecessary, and not

Table 22–9. Use of Advanced Directives, Do-Not-Resuscitate (DNR) Orders

Study	Conclusion
California durable power of attorney for health care placed on chart[90]	No effect on treatment charges, types of treatment, or health status.
DNR[91]	Average of $57,334 for those without DNR orders, compared to $62,594 for those with DNR orders.
Advanced directives in SUPPORT hospitals[89]	No cost savings with advance directives. For patients prior to the SUPPORT intervention, there was a 23% reduction in cost associated with presence of advance directives, $21,284 with compared to $26,127 without. Intervention patients were more likely to have advance directives documented. Average cost was $24,178 for those without advance directives, $28,017 for those with advanced directives on the intervention arm.

consistent with the goals of palliative care. Consider the following examples.

1. An 82-year-old man with end-stage chronic obstructive pulmonary disease requests removal from a respirator and comfort measures only. He is deemed competent, yet it is questionable if he will be able to survive off the respirator. His wishes are followed, and he is extubated. While adamantly refusing any discussion regarding reintubation, he continues to have arterial blood gases sampled every 2 to 3 hours around the clock. Clearly, use of such sampling is academic as the patient refuses reintubation. Sampling of arterial blood gases is costly and painful and does not contribute to the goals of comfort.
2. A 32-year-old man with widely metastatic colon cancer arrives in your facility with a bowel obstruction related to his disease. He has been in the local hospice program. After evaluation, his prognosis is confirmed as approximately 6 weeks. He has a nasogastric tube placed to relieve persistent nausea, vomiting, and abdominal discomfort. After 4 days of decompression, the surgeon offers to place a gastrostomy tube for drainage and decompression. While the surgery will be costly, placement of the gastrostomy tube meets the goals of both comfort and providing the patient with the ability to return home.
3. A 29-year-old woman with acquired immunodeficiency syndrome is admitted for severe debilitating neuropathic pain, unresponsive to typical adjunctive analgesic agents. The patient is losing her ability to ambulate due to the pain. She is given a trial of epidural opioids with local anesthetics, which offer almost complete pain relief. An intrathecally implanted pump, at a cost of several thousand dollars, is placed. While the initial cost is staggering, the long-term benefits are considerable, including measurable improved functional status, decreased occurrence of depression, decrease in required skilled and nonskilled nursing care hours, decreased opportunistic infection, and improved quality of life for both the patient and her significant others.
4. A 60-year-old woman with multiple myeloma is admitted with an adjusted serum calcium level of 179 mg/dl. The myeloma is now progressing and refractory to therapy. Intravenous fluids, diuretics, biphosphates, and calcitonin are administered, and serum calcium is drawn every 12 hours. The patient's disease is irreversible. The present interventions will perhaps delay an inevitable outcome, but they will cost thousands of dollars while not improving the patient's quality of life and may potentially cause discomfort.

This process of reassessment and recognition should be fostered through education and role modeling and should begin in the very basic nursing courses. It must be integrated throughout the longitudinal nursing curriculum as patients dealing with end-of-life disease processes exist in almost all health care settings. It is imperative that outcomes research accompanies education to ensure the best and most cost-efficient palliative care available.

SUMMARY

Economic outcomes are increasingly important for all types of health care, including palliative care. The few studies show substantial opportunities for improvement by using disease-management strategies. Chemotherapy for some cancers (non-small-cell lung cancer, prostate cancer, and gastrointestinal cancer) is reasonably effective and has acceptable cost-effectiveness ratios; this does not apply to any regimen that has not been formally evaluated. Coordination of palliative care shows no major clinical benefit but major cost savings. Directed, ethically motivated interventions about futile care appear to produce significant cost savings. The use of advance directives or hospice care may be good medical care but has not been shown to produce major economic benefit.

The cost of care is rising due to increasing age of the population, more cancer cases and chronic diseases, increased demand for treatment, and new and expensive technologies. Our limited resources must be rationed wisely so that we can provide both curative and palliative care. The ethical implications of using economic and management outcomes rather than traditional health outcomes include shifting emphasis from helping at all cost to helping at a cost society can afford, as well as how much society is willing to pay, the value of care to the dying versus those with curable illnesses, and tolerance of suboptimal care.

The outcomes of palliative care do not differ from those of other cancer treatment, from the perspective of economics or health service research. For treatment to be justified, there must be some demonstrable improvement in disease-free or overall survival, toxicity, quality of life, or cost effectiveness. Palliative care usually does not change survival, and it does not have a measurable cost-effectiveness ratio since it does not gain years of life. There may be little change in quality-adjusted life years because the improvements in health state are too small to measure with current instruments or are lost in the impact of the disease.

Only a few studies have assessed the economic outcomes of palliative therapy. The major areas of interest include the following: (*1*) palliative chemotherapy versus best supportive care, (*2*) supportive care for cancer symptoms, (*3*) the process and structure of care, (*4*) follow up, and (*5*) hospice care. Palliative first-line chemotherapy for stage III and IV non-small-cell lung cancer, mitoxantrone for prostate cancer, and fluorouracil-based chemotherapy for gastrointestinal cancer have acceptable cost-effectiveness ratios. Supportive care effectiveness and cost for infections, nausea, and pain can be improved. Research outside of cancer is scant. Hospice care saves at best 3% of total care cost but gives care equal to nonhospice care. Coordination of palliative care will save 40% of costs but will not improve the clinical outcomes of dying patients. Nursing clearly has the ability to impact the care and cost for this population and should be in the forefront of these issues.

This work is based on a chapter published in Topics in Palliative Care, Volume 5, edited by R.K. Portenoy and E. Bruera: Economic outcomes and palliative care, by Thomas J. Smith and Laurie Lyckholm. New York: Oxford University Press, 2001, pp. 157–175.

REFERENCES

1. Detmer DE. Half empty or half full, it will be a smaller glass. Inquiry 1997;34:8–10.
2. Brown ML. The national economic bur-

den of cancer. J Natl Cancer Inst 1990;82: 1811–1814.

3. Brown ML, Hodgson TA, Rice DP. Economic impact of cancer in the U.S. In: Schottenfeld D, Fraumeni J, eds. Cacer, Epidemiology, and Prevention. New York: Oxford University Press, 1996:255–266.

4. Rundle RL. Salick pioneers selling cancer care to HMOs. Wall Street J 1996;Aug 12:B1–B2.

5. Lubitz JD, Riley GF. Trends in Medicare payments in the last year of life. N Engl J Med 1993;328:1092–1096.

6. Lubitz J, Beebe J, Baker C. Longevity and Medicare expenditures. N Engl J Med 1995;332: 999–1003.

7. Welch HG, Wennberg DE, Welch WP. The use of Medicare home health care services. N Engl J Med 1996;335:324–329.

8. Brunner D. Cost effectiveness of palliative care. Semin Oncol Nurs 1998;14:164–167.

9. Salt S, Wilson L, Edwards A. The use of specialist palliative care services by patients with human immunodeficiency virus–related illness in the Yorkshire Deanery of the Northern and Yorkshire region. Palliat Med 1998;12:152–160.

10. SUPPORT Principal Investigators. A controlled trial to improve care for seriously ill hospitalized patients. The Study to Understand Prognoses and Preferences for Outcomes and Risks of Treatments (SUPPORT). JAMA 1995;274:1591–1598.

11. Cleeland CS, Gonin R, Hatfield AK, et al. Pain and its treatment in outpatients with metastatic cancer. N Engl J Med 1994;330:592–596.

12. Bevan, G. Taking equity seriously: a dilemma for government from allocating resources to primary care groups. BMJ 1998;316:39–43.

13. Hillner BE, Smith TJ. Hospital volume and patient outcomes in major cancer surgery: a catalyst for quality assessment and concentration of cancer services. JAMA 1998;280:1784.

14. Gillis CR, Hole DJ. Survival outcome of care by specialist surgeons in breast cancer: a study of 3786 patients in the west of Scotland. BMJ 1996;312:145–148.

15. Sainsbury R, Haward R, Rider L, Johnstone C, Round C. Influence of clinician workload and patterns of treatment on survival from breast cancer. Lancet 1995;345:1265–1270.

16. Feuer EJ, Frey CM, Brawley OW, et al. After a treatment breakthrough: a comparison of trial and population-based data for advanced testicular cancer. J Clin Oncol 1994;12:368–377.

17. Nguyen HN, Averette HE, Hoskins W, Penalver M, Sevin B, Steren A. National survey of ovarian carcinoma Part V. The impact of physician's specialty on patient's survival. Cancer 1993; 72:3663–3670.

18. Desch CE, Penberthy L, Newschaffer C, et al. Factors that determine the treatment of local and regional prostate cancer. Med Care 1996; 34:152–162.

19. Berger JT, Rosner F. The ethics of practice guidelines. Arch Intern Med 1996;156:2051–2056.

20. Olson V, Coyne P, Smith V, Hudson C. Critical pathway improves outcomes for patients with sickle-cell disease. Oncol Nurs Forum 1997; 24:1682.

21. Smith R. An ethical code for everybody in health care: a code that covered all rather than single groups might be useful. BMJ 1997;315: 1633–1634.

22. Levinsky NG. The purpose of advance medical planning—autonomy for patients or limitation of care? N Engl J Med 1996;335:741–743.

23. Callahan D. Controlling the costs of health care for the elderly—fair means and foul. N Engl J Med 1996;335:744–746.

24. Randall F. Palliative Care Ethics: A Good Companion. New York: Oxford University Press, 1996.

25. Daniels N. Just Health Care. New York: Cambridge University Press, 1985.

26. Sidgwick H. The Methods of Ethics. London: McMillan, 1907.

27. Slevin ML, Stubbs L, Plant HJ, et al. Attitudes to chemotherapy: comparing views of patients with cancer with those of doctors, nurses, and general public. BMJ 1990;300:1458–1460.

28. Davies E, Clarke C, Hopkins A. Malignant cerebral glioma—I: Survival, disability, and morbidity after radiotherapy. BMJ 1996;313:1507–1512.

29. Davies E, Clarke C, Hopkins A. Malignant cerebral glioma—II: Perspectives of patients and relatives on the value of radiotherapy. BMJ 1996;313:1512–1516.

30. Lamm RD. The ghost of health care future. Inquiry 1994;31:365–367.

31. Coyne P. International efforts in cancer pain relief. Semin Oncol Nurs 1997;13:57–62.

32. Smith TJ, Hillner BE, Desch CE. Efficacy and cost-effectiveness of cancer treatment: rational allocation of resources based on decision analysis. J Natl Cancer Inst 1993;85:1460–1474.

33. Waugh N, Scott D. How should different life expectancies be valued? BMJ 1998;316:1316.

34. Olweny C. Ethics of palliative care medicine: palliative care for the rich nations only! J Palliat Care 1994;10:17–22.

35. American Society of Clinical Oncology Outcomes Working Group (core members). Outcomes of cancer treatment for technology assessment and cancer treatment guidelines. J Clin Oncol 1995;14:671–679.

36. Brown M, Glick H, Harrell F, et al. Integrating economic analysis into cancer clinical trials: The National Cancer Institute–American Society of Clinical Oncology Economics Workbook, 1998:1.

37. Shwartz M, Young DW, Siegrist R. The ratio of costs to charges: how good a basis for estimating costs? Inquiry 1995;32:476–481.

38. Smith TJ, Bodurtha JN. Ethical considerations in oncology: balancing the interests of patients, oncologists, and society. J Clin Oncol 1995; 13:2464–2470.

39. Smith TJ. Which hat do I wear? JAMA 1993;270:1657–1659.

40. Laupacis A, Feeny D, Detsky AS, Tugwell PX. How attractive does a new technology have to be to warrant adoption and utilization? Tentative guidelines for using clinical and economic evaluation. Can Med Assoc J 1992;146:473–481.

41. Smith TJ, Hillner BE, Schmitz N, et al. Economic analysis of a randomized clinical trial to compare filgrastim-mobilized peripheral blood progenitor cell transplantation and autologous bone marrow transplantation in patients with Hodgkin and non-Hodgkin lymphoma. J Clin Oncol 1997;15:5–10.

42. Smith TJ, Desch CE, Hillner BE. Ways to reduce the cost of oncology care without compromising the quality. Cancer Invest 1994;12: 257–265.

43. Blair SN, Kohl HWI, Barlow CE, Paffenbarger RS Jr, Gibbons LW, Macera CA. Changes in physical fitness and all-cause mortality. A prospective study of healthy and unhealthy men. JAMA 1995;273:1093–1098.

44. Souquet PJ, Chauvin F, Boissel JP, et al. Polychemotherapy in advanced non-small cell lung cancer: a meta-analysis. Lancet 1993;342: 19–21.

45. Adelstein DJ. Palliative chemotherapy for non-small cell lung cancer. Semin Onco! 1995; 22:35–39.

46. American Society of Clinical Oncology. Clinical practice guidelines for the treatment of unresectable non-small-cell lung cancer. J Clin Oncol 1997;15:2996–3018.

47. Evans WK, Newman T, Graham I, et al. Lung cancer practice guidelines: lessons learned and issues addressed by the Ontario Lung Cancer Disease Site Group. J Clin Oncol 1997;15:3049–3059.

48. Jaakimainen L, Goodwin PJ, Pater J, Warde P, Murray N, Rapp E. Counting the costs of chemotherapy in a National Cancer Institute of Canada randomized trial in non-small cell lung cancer. J Clin Oncol 1990; 8:1301–1309.

49. Le Chevalier T, Brisgand D, Douillard JY, et al. Randomized study of vinorelbine and cisplatin versus vindesine and cisplatin versus vinorelbine alone in advanced non-small cell lung cancer: results of a European multicenter trial including 612 patients. J Clin Oncol 1994;12:360–367.

50. Smith TJ, Hillner BE, Neighbors DM, McSorley PA, Le Chevalier T. An economic evaluation of a randomized clinical trial comparing vinorelbine, vinorelbine plus cisplatin and vindesine plus cisplatin for non-small cell lung cancer. J Clin Oncol 1995;13:2166–2173.

51. Evans WK, Will BP, Berthelot JM, Earle CC. Cost of combined modality interventions for stage III non-small-cell lung cancer. J Clin Oncol 1997;15:3038–3048.

52. Evans WK, Will BP. The cost of managing lung cancer in Canada. Oncology (Huntingt) 1995;9 (Suppl 11):147–153.

53. Evans WK, Will BP, Berthelot JM, Wolfson MC. The economics of lung cancer management in Canada. Lung Cancer 1996;14:13–17.

54. Glimelius B, Hoffman K, Graf W, et al. Cost-effectiveness of palliative chemotherapy in

advanced gastrointestinal cancer. Ann Oncol 1995;6:267–274.

55. Tannock IF, Osoba D, Stockler MR, et al. Chemotherapy with mitoxantrone plus prednisone or prednisone alone for symptomatic hormone-resistant prostate cancer: a Canadian randomized trial with palliative end points. J Clin Oncol 1996;14:1756–1764.

56. Bloomfield DJ, Krahn MD, Tannock IF, Smith TJ. Economic evaluation of chemotherapy with mitoxantrone plus prednisone for symptomatic hormone resistant prostate cancer (HRPC) based on a Canadian randomized trial (RCT) with palliative endpoints. Proc Am Soc Clin Oncol 1997;17:2272–2279.

57. Hillner BE, McLeod DG, Crawford E, Bennett CL. Estimating the cost effectiveness of total androgen blockade with flutamide in M1 prostate cancer. Urology 1995;45:633–640.

58. Richards MA, Braysher S, Gregory WM, Rubens RD. Advanced breast cancer: use of resources and cost implications. Br J Cancer 1993; 67:856–860.

59. Bezwoda WR, Seymour L, Dansey RD. High-dose chemotherapy with hematopoietic rescue as primary treatment for metastatic breast cancer: a randomized trial. J Clin Oncol 1995;13: 2483–2489.

60. Hillner BE, Smith TJ, Desch CE. Efficacy and cost-effectiveness of autologous bone marrow transplantation in metastatic breast cancer. Estimates using decision-analysis while awaiting clinical trial results. JAMA 1992;267:2055–2061.

61. Holli K, Hakama M. Treatment of the terminal stages of breast cancer. BMJ 1989;298: 13–14.

62. Welch HG, Larson EB. Cost-effectiveness of bone marrow transplantation in acute nonlymphocytic leukemia. N Engl J Med 1989;321: 807–812.

63. Goodwin PJ, Feld R, Evans WK, Pater J. Cost-effectiveness of cancer chemotherapy: an economic evaluation of a randomized trial in small-cell lung cancer. J Clin Oncol 1988;6: 1537–1547.

64. Ferris FD, Wodinsky HB, Kerr IG, Sone M, Hume S, Coons C. A cost-minimization study of cancer patients requiring a narcotic infusion in hospital and at home. J Clin Epidemiol 1991; 44:313–327.

65. Wodinsky HB, DeAngelis C, Rusthoven JJ, et al. Re-evaluating the cost of outpatient cancer chemotherapy. Can Med Assoc J 1987;137: 903–906.

66. Lowenthal RM, Piaszczyk A, Arthur GE, O'Malley S. Home chemotherapy for cancer patients: cost analysis and safety. Med J Aust 1996; 165:184–187.

67. Harris NJ, Dunmore R, Tscheu MJ. The Medicare hospice benefit: fiscal implications for hospice program management. Cancer Manage 1996;May/June:6–11.

68. Smith TJ. End of Life Care: Preserving Quality and Quantity of Life in Managed Care. Alexandria, VA. ASCO: Education Book 33rd Annual Meeting, 1997;303–307.

69. Addington-Hall JM, MacDonald LD, Anderson HR, et al. Randomized controlled trial of effects of coordinating care for terminally ill cancer patients. BMJ 1992;305:1317–1322.

70. Raftery JP, Addington-Hall JM, MacDonald LD, et al. A randomized controlled trial of the cost-effectiveness of a district co-ordinating service for terminally ill cancer patients. Palliat Med 1996;10:151–161.

71. McWhinney IR, Bass MJ, Orr V. Factors associated with location of death (home or hospital) or patients referred to a palliative care team. Can Med Assoc J 1995;152:361–370.

72. Grant M, Ferrell BR, Rivera LM, Lee J. Unscheduled readmissions for uncontrolled symptoms. Nurs Clin North Am 1995;30:673–682.

73. Chandler S, Payne R. Economics of unrelieved cancer pain. Am J Hospice Palliat Care 1998;15:223–225.

74. Holloran SD, Starkey GW, Burke PA, Steele G Jr, Forse RA. An educational intervention in the surgical intensive care unit to improve ethical decisions. Surgery 1995;118:294–298.

75. Dowdy MD, Robertson C, Bander JA. A study of proactive ethics consultation for critically and terminally ill patients with extended lengths of stay. Crit Care Med 1998;26:252–259.

76. Carney PA, Dietrich AJ, Freeman DH Jr, Mott LA. The periodic health examination provided to asymptomatic older women: an assessment using standardized patients. Ann Intern Med 1993;119:129–135.

77. Smith TJ. Reducing the cost of supportive care. I: Antibiotics for febrile neutropenia. Clin Oncol Alert 1996;11:46–47.

78. Smith TJ. Reducing the cost of supportive care. II: Anti-emetics. Clin Oncol Alert 1996; 11:62–64.

79. Emanuel EJ. Cost savings at the end of life. What do the data show? JAMA 1996;275: 1907–1914.

80. Emanuel EJ, Emanuel LL. The economics of dying. The illusion of cost savings at the end of life. N Engl J Med 1994;330:540–544.

81. National Hospice Organization. An Analysis of the Cost Savings of the Medicare Hospice Benefit. Miami: Lewin-VHI, 1997.

82. Kidder D. The effects of hospice coverage on Medicare expenditures. Health Serv Res 1992;27:195–217.

83. Aiken LH. Evaluation and research and public policy: lessons learned from the National Hospice study. J Chronic Dis 1986;39:1–4.

84. Kane RL, Berstein L, Whales J, Leibowitz A, Kaplan S. A randomized control trial of hospice care. Lancet 1984;1:890–894.

85. Brooks CH, Smyth-Staruch K. Hospice home care cost savings to third party insurers. Med Care 1984;22:691–703.

86. Stommel M, Given CW, Given BA. The cost of cancer home care to families. Cancer 1993; 71:1867–1874.

87. Given BA, Given CW, Stommel M. Family and out-of-pocket costs for women with breast cancer. Cancer Pract 1994;2:187–193.

88. Emanuel EJ, Emanuel LL. The economics of dying: the illusion of cost savings at the end of life. N Engl J Med 1994;330:540–544.

89. Teno J, Lynn J, Connors AF Jr, et al. The illusion of end-of-life resource savings with advance directives. SUPPORT Investigators: Study to Understand Prognoses and Preferences for Outcomes and Risks of Treatment. J Am Geriatr Soc 1997;45:513–518.

90. Schneiderman LJ, Kronick R, Kaplan RM, Anderson JP, Langer RD. Effects of offering advance directives on medical treatments and costs. Ann Intern Med 1992;117:599–606.

91. Maksoud A, Jahnigen DW, Skibinski CI. Do not resuscitate orders and the cost of death. Arch Intern Med 1993;153:1249–1253.

92. Kassirer JP. Rationing by any other name. N Engl J Med 1997;336:1668–1669.

93. Levine C. The loneliness of the long-term care giver. N Engl J Med 1999;340:1587–1590.

94. World Health Organization. Cancer Pain Relief and Palliative Care. Technical Report Series 304. Geneva: WHO, 1990.

Part III

Psychosocial Support

23 Establishing Goals: Communication Traps and Treatment Lane Changes

LINDA J. KRISTJANSON

We thought in our own minds that she would be going through more tests and examinations and discussions and so on. . . . But when we sat down with the doctor he just walked in and said, "So you've got the bad news, we've got your surgery scheduled for tomorrow." That was all news and a surprise to us.

—Spouse

According to Stedeford[1] poor communication causes more suffering to cancer patients and their families than any other problems, with the exception of unrelieved pain. If there is confusion about the goals of care, patients, family members, and the health care team are likely to find themselves caught in a tangle of incomplete information, inconsistent care approaches, anxiety, and confusion. Lack of clarity about goals of care can contribute to patients' and families' mistrust in the health care team and may interfere with the quality of care the patient and family receives.[2] Therefore, special attention to communication traps[3] that can occur when trying to establish goals of care is useful. Particular reflection should be paid to moments of "lane changes" when the plan of care shifts from active treatment to palliation. These two issues will be explored in this chapter.

The aim of this chapter is to examine clinical knowledge and relevant research findings about how to establish goals of care in the context of palliative care by:

1. Outlining key elements that underpin communication and applying these to the specific challenge of establishing goals of care,
2. Examining common communication traps that can occur during discussions about goals of care, and
3. Exploring communication approaches when treatment "lane changes" are needed.

The chapter will include reference to relevant research and theoretical literature that examines these issues. As well, patient and family care experiences described in prior qualitative studies will be included to help illustrate the points raised.

FRAMEWORK FOR COMMUNICATION ABOUT GOALS OF CARE

A number of principles underpin communication. According to standard communication theory,[4] any message involving use of words, gestures, or body syntax, has at least three levels—the level of content, the level of emotional expression, and the level of relationships between sender and receiver.

Content Errors

Attention to the content level of a communication exchange involves observance of the accuracy of the information shared and the language used. Lack of attention to the content of the communication exchange can create confusion and errors. The literature consistently documents difficulties that cancer patients and their family members report regarding access to information.[5–7] Patients and family members describe difficulties obtaining specific and straightforward information in a way that they can understand. Use of medical jargon is frequently mentioned as a barrier to adequate communication about the plan of care.[7] Language barriers may also be a problem if patients and family members do not share the same language and cultural background as the health care professional.[8] As well, differences in educational levels between health professionals and patients/families can create problems with exchange of content.[9]

Health professionals may overload family members and patients with large amounts of information or may provide information in small amounts in an effort to not overwhelm patients and families with too much detail.[10] This can create difficulties as patients and families vary in the extent to which they may be able to assimilate and integrate the information shared.[11] The anxiety of the patient and family members may also limit their abilities to integrate information.

Patients and family members may be recipients of messages that appear to contain good amounts of detailed and specific information. However, the distance between hearing the information stated and making meaning of that information may be quite vast, especially if filtered through anxiety, fear, and fatigue. For example, one family member recounted:

The surgeon came and spoke to us after the surgery. He said, "All the lymph nodes, everyone one of them had cancer in it." We were therefore relieved, because we thought that this meant he had removed all of the cancer.

In an effort to comfort the patient or family, health professionals may not communicate as openly and honestly as they might. This can place nurses in a difficult position as they attempt to clarify goals of care without knowing the extent to which information about the prognosis has been honestly communicated to the patient or family.

Content errors may also occur in the reverse direction. Patients and family members may use language and convey messages that are clear to them, but may not be understood by the health care team. Patients and family members also report problems with information sharing when health care providers do not allow them adequate time to describe their symptoms or the patient's or family member's needs. Health professionals who see themselves as the source of information and the transmitters of the treatment plan miss the notion of information exchange as a reciprocal process. For example, one patient stated:

> The doctor never listens to my description of my symptoms—what is bothering me. He just asks questions and gives me no time to say what is bothering me—I think things are worse . . . but it's like he isn't paying attention to that.

Emotional Expression as a Source of Communication Error

The emotional expressions conveyed during a message exchange include tone of voice, body language, facial expressions, and gestures that enhance or detract from the communication. It has been estimated that approximately 80% of communication may occur at the nonverbal level, making this aspect of communication extremely important.[12] Nonverbal communication may convey substantial messages that override verbal statements. A health care professional who appears worried or avoids eye contact may communicate to the patient and family that he/she is discouraged about the plan of care and not optimistic about the patient's abilities to cope with the illness. For example, the husband of a woman with advancing colorectal cancer stated:

> I remember Barbara went back next week to the family doctor and she pointed out the lumps around the neck area . . . and I remember being with her and the doctor looked at her and just sort of shook his head and said, "You're so young." Right away, you know what the situation is.

Health care providers who are abrupt, unusually cheerful, or patronizing in their tone of voice may also communicate messages that are difficult to process.

Relationship Communication Errors

The third level of communication involves the relationship between the sender and receiver. If there is a notable power imbalance, previous history of difficulty communicating, or tension in the relationship, quality of communication will be affected.

An equal and balanced relationship exchange implies that both parties are able to share information, ask questions, and convey emotions and reactions in an open and authentic manner.[13] If this kind of patient–health professional relationship does not exist, it is more likely that one will be allocated the role of imparting information and asking questions, with the other responding in a more passive, reactive manner.

Relationship issues associated with communication are particularly problematic when health professionals are insensitive to the imbalance in power and control patients and families may feel. Family members report a hesitancy to bother busy health professionals with questions about care because they believe that the health care providers are primarily responsible to the patient and that their needs and concerns are tangential.[7]

The importance of communication with the patient and family is partly represented by the time and space created or allotted for this communication exchange. The apparent lack of space for discussion about care plans and goals conveys a message that this interchange is not too important. It is not unusual for patients and families to report communication about treatment and care in the hallways of busy hospitals, over the phone, or in small clinic rooms with little privacy or time for discussion.[8,9] Health professionals may also limit their information sharing with patients and families because of the pace of their busy work schedules, an assumption that the patient or family has understood the information conveyed, and a lack of comfort in knowing how to communicate difficult or bad news.[14–17]

COMMUNICATION TRAPS DURING THE PALLIATIVE CARE ILLNESS TRAJECTORY

It is common in many social interactions for participants who are uncomfortable or nervous to unthinkingly make use of ritualistic communication patterns. Ritualistic communication patterns are familiar to most individuals when they are greeted by someone and are asked, "How are you?" The usual response, regardless of how one is truly feeling, is, "Fine thanks." Individuals may catch themselves and realize that they have answered incorrectly if indeed they are unwell or concerned about something—but the usual pattern is triggered and engages them in the customary reciprocal social banter that may be quite inaccurate and superficial. In most instances this is not a serious predicament. However, when communicating about goals of care in the context of a terminal or advancing progressive illness, perfunctory and prosaic communication patterns may be detrimental and confusing.

Erving Goffman[18] describes ritualistic features of everyday behaviors and in so doing, offers a useful tool for comprehending why health care professionals can become trapped in dysfunctional communication interchanges with patients and families. Use of ritualized interactions leads individuals to unconsciously follow scripts of gestures, body posture, and verbalizations without much considered attention. For example, offering a handshake often prompts an automatic response to grip the person's hand and shake in return. This response ensures that all is well and that the ritual and exchange can continue as expected.[3] A more complicated example is when a person asks a question and the responder provides an answer. The content of the answer is of secondary importance. The act of giving an answer is what counts. Even if the answer-giver thinks the question rude, does not understand the question, or does not know the answer—the pattern of providing an answer in response to a question maintains the expected ritual and the social form continues. Even if the answer-giver responds with an inappropriate answer, the person asking the question usually does not comment, because the critical part of the exchange is that an answer is provided. According to communication experts,[3,18,19] this type of ritualized communication exchange can account for a number of errors in communication. This notion of ritualized communication habits may explain why health professionals who endeavor to discuss sensitive topics or engage in difficult conversations may become trapped in well-known but ineffective ritualistic communication patterns.

In the context of communicating about goals of care, the following communication traps may surface: (*1*) "we all understand each other," (2) "let's be polite," (3) "we should be positive," (*4*) "more of the same," and (5) "can we be clear?" Each of these communication traps is described below.

"We All Understand Each Other"

In the "*we all understand each other*" trap, individuals involved in the care situation assume that the other people involved share a similar understanding of the goals of care and the approach to treatment. This assumed agreement might create conflict within the family or between the health care team and the patient and family. When lack of agreement becomes apparent, anger and mistrust can result.[2] The lack of concordance about the plan of care can also contribute to inconsistent care approaches, confusion about allocation of resources, and inappropriate referrals and care decisions. Nurses can avoid this trap by first being aware of its comfortable seduction, and by simply making explicit the plan of care in a manner that invites clarification and allows for possible discrepancy. For example, the nurse might say, "Sometimes in the process of providing care we may misunderstand each other or mean different things when we talk about treatments and plans. Perhaps you could tell me what you believe the treatment will do and then I can share my view so that we know if we understand each other." It is also often helpful to take responsibility for communications errors that may have occurred to avoid the patient or family feeling inadequate and defensive. For example, if there is a misunderstanding, the nurse might say, "I have probably not been clear enough in describing the plan, let me spend a little more time telling you what I meant." This allows the patient and family to know that the nurse is open to correction and that miscommunications may occur, but are reparable.

"Let's Be Polite"

The "*let's be polite*" trap can occur in situations where patients and families are particularly cognizant of the power imbalance between health care providers and themselves. They may comply with treatment and care approaches with which they are not comfortable, or may use care approaches covertly (e.g., use of alternative therapies) to avoid confrontation or discussion with health care providers about the approach to treatment. This may create particular difficulties if covert care practices and conventional treatments interact. For example, chelation therapy involves intravenous infusion of an amino acid called ethylene diamine tetra-acetic acid (EDTA).[20] Supporters of EDTA argue that chelation therapy removes toxic metals from the body (lead, cadmium, and mercury), which are believed to depress the immune system and promote development and spread of cancer. Supporters believe that the treatment removes undesirable metals from the body, which are believed to cause damage to cell membranes by producing "oxygen free radicals." These free radicals are considered to be contributing factors in diseases such as atherosclerosis, cancer, and diabetes. Advocates argue that once in your blood, EDTA collects the heavy metals in the body, and the agent and metals are then expelled by way of the kidneys.[20] To date, there is no empirical evidence to support the use of this treatment for cancer patients. Adverse effects include immune deficiencies as it removes zinc and other minerals from the body. This therapy may be taken by patients and may cause kidney problems, low blood calcium, insulin shock, hypotension, fever, and cardiac arrhythmia. The treatment should not be used with individuals who have damaged kidneys, liver disease, tuberculosis, brain tumors, or who are pregnant.[20] Thus, if a patient does not disclose use of this alternative therapy serious consequences could occur.

This trap is most evident when patients and family members appear passive and avoid conflict or when health care professionals limit communication and maintain a superficial and cheerful exchange that prevents candid discussions about goals of care. Cultural issues may also trigger this trap. For example, in some cultures it may be especially important to be polite and remain civil despite uncertainty, conflict, and doubt. Cultural barriers between families and the nurse may also create strain, resulting in participants communicating in a cautious, overpolite manner to avoid conflict and not offend. This may create the illusion of harmony, but may in fact be a thin cover for frustration and uncertain aims.

"We Should Be Positive"

The "*we should be positive*" trap occurs when individuals involved in the care hold concerns about "taking away hope" and believe that the most appropriate way to manage an advancing illness is to "fight it" and focus on the positives. This approach is evident when individuals provide incomplete information, overemphasize positive findings and case examples, communicate in dishonest ways about treatment options or anticipated outcomes, maintain an overly lighthearted manner, and avoid detailed discussions about the disease progression. The effect of this type of communication trap may be isolation and loneliness for the patient and/or family members who do not accept the positive spin placed on the treatment plan. There may also be a lack of preparation for impending death, missed opportunities in terms of honest conversations among family members with the patient, and guilt and frustration when communication feels less than honest.

"More of the Same"

The fourth communication trap, "more of the same," occurs when the health care team or patient and family are unwilling to examine or accept a palliative care approach. A particularly difficult juncture for advanced cancer patients and their families may occur when it becomes apparent that the goals of care must shift from those associated with active treatment to goals consistent with palliation. This "lane change" can be particularly difficult to discuss for all involved (patients, family members, and health care providers). The change can be confusing if not all health team members are conscious of the need for it and are in agreement. In many instances health care providers continue to drift down the active treatment lane, hoping that this familiar and charismatic pathway will work a little longer. The effects of this communication trap include an inappropriate use of active treatment at a time when the focus should move to palliation and comfort care and the transmission of "false hope" with the disappointment that may follow.

"Can We Be Clear?"

The fifth communication trap is labeled "can we be clear?" This trap is characterized by a need on the part of the individuals involved (or some of the participants in the exchange) to obtain clarity, precision, and open agreement about the plan of care. Although on the surface this approach to communication may appear to be healthy, overconcern with clarity may create difficulties if the situation is simply not that certain. At times, an eagerness to make a situation understandable, straightforward, and manageable may lead health care providers or others to aim for an unequivocal care goal, when one is not so obvious. This type of communication trap may be evident in situations where there is notable confrontation among health team members and a search for someone to blame for the lack of clarity about the plan of care. Sometimes patients and family members need help to release themselves from this type of trap—the search for precision. In other situations, patients and family members may feel pressured to come to terms with a goal of care that they may not be ready to accept. The effects of this type of communication trap may be a rebound reaction on the part of the patient, family, or health care provider to "try something else"—or to reach out for an alternative approach that is bold and experimental. The patient and family may reject the health care team if they believe that the team is pushing them to "give up" too soon. They may also have later regrets if the exchanges related to care goals were characterized by conflict. In these instances, a tolerance for ambiguity and a slower approach to definition of care goals may be helpful.

Table 23–1 summarizes these traps. As well, the ways in which these traps are evident are shown as "Trap Indicators." Their effects on patients, family members, and the health care team are listed in the column labeled "Trap Consequences."

COMMUNICATION APPROACHES WHEN TREATMENT LANE CHANGES ARE NEEDED

The communication processes needed for a lane change from active treatment

Table 23–1. Communication Traps in the Context of Establishing Goals for Palliative Care

Communication Trap	Evidence of Trap	Trap Consequences
"We all understand each other"	• Lack of explicit discussion of treatment goals	• Confusion • Anger • Inconsistent Treatment • Mistrust
"Let's be polite"	• Avoidance of conflict • Superficial conversations conversations • Short conversations	• Indirect methods of communication used • Conflict • Potential for guilt later
"We should be positive"	• Incomplete information shared • Dishonest communication • Cheerful manner • Avoidance of detailed discussions about illness	• Isolation of patient/family • Lack of preparation for advancing illness • Loneliness • Guilt • Frustration • Missed opportunities
"More of the same"	• Repeated explanations • Focus on same plan of care despite lack of success/resolution	• Inappropriate treatment plans • False hope • Avoidance of in-depth discussion of treatment goals
"Can we be clear?"	• Confrontation • Seeking blame • Questioning approach	• Premature focus on palliative care goals • Rebound reaction of patient/family/health team • Regret

of the disease to palliation of the patient's symptoms are complex and subtle. Use of a simple "goals of care" form will not allow the team to smoothly shift from one lane to the next. A ritualistic script will likely not assist either. However, some lessons from expert palliative care nursing practitioners may provide some useful guidelines about how to facilitate this type of delicate and important transition.[21] Experienced palliative care nurses usually employ a range of strategies to assist patients, family members, and at times, the rest of the health care team to realign goals.[22] These strategies have been labeled "Anticipating the Roadblocks," "Gaining Consensus," "Timing the Transition," and "Shifting Gently."

Anticipating the Roadblocks

Anticipating the roadblocks requires the ability to look ahead to estimate whether the planned care goal is still achievable and whether a change is needed. This strategy is often undertaken by the nurse working in an active treatment setting who may be alert to the quality-of-life concerns of the patient, the patient's symptomatic response to treatment, and the energy level of the patient as he or she copes with the illness. The nurse who anticipates the roadblocks listens carefully to the needs, concerns, and goals of the patient and the family and is able to consult with health team members in a way that takes into account disease factors, treatment approaches, and overall objectives. No one health professional or individual is able to anticipate all of the roadblocks or see far into the distance for each patient's care situation. However, it is often necessary for someone to step outside the usual care pathway to question the merits of continuing down a familiar, but perhaps unhelpful road.

Gaining Consensus

Gaining consensus is a second strategy for assisting movement from one lane of care to another. This strategy requires that patients, family members and health care professionals exchange information, examine implicit care objectives and explore options for care that are consistent with the patient's shifting needs and concerns. Most often this occurs best within the context of a patient conference or family conference, allowing all involved in the care to share their perspectives about the treatment plan. Gaining consensus requires tact, diplomacy, and respect for alternate points of view. A case example helps explain this approach.

Case Study: Mr. W., a Man with Prostate Cancer

Mr. W. was 69-year-old man receiving care on the Palliative Care Unit of a large teaching hospital. He had a primary diagnosis of prostate cancer, with metastasis to bone and lungs. He was described by nursing staff as irritable and closed in his communication. Mr. W. had a history of alcoholism, had been divorced for 15 years and had two adult married daughters. Mr. W. required assistance with personal hygiene, administration of medications, and meal preparation. When the staff made efforts to arrange discharge home with support from home care services augmented by assistance from the two daughters the daughters would repeatedly block the discharge plan. They would identify seemingly small reasons for delaying discharge and were uneasy about learning how to assist with Mr. W.'s personal care. The staff was frustrated and agreed to organize a meeting to discuss the matter. A meeting was held among the daughters, the social worker, and the primary nurse caring for Mr. W. After careful discussion about the practical obstacles associated with discharge, the nurse tactfully inquired about the daughters' relationship with Mr. W. and how that relationship may be affected by the caregiving duties. The daughters then described a history of abuse by Mr. W. when they were young children, which resulted in estrangement and distress for them. They had returned to the relationship with Mr. W. because he was terminally ill, but were not prepared to provide personal care to their father because of their strong feelings about his prior behavior. This disclosure allowed the social worker and nurse to suggest alternate discharge arrangements for the patient to a long-term care facility that would relieve the daughters of the pressure to provide this care. When this was suggested to the patient he agreed and the team shifted its discharge plans, respectfully acknowledging the limits within the family relationships.

Although not all family relationships contain these types of difficulties and may not be resolved as easily, it is important to ensure that some form of consensus and common ground is found so that the best possible plan can be achieved for all involved.

Timing the Transition

Timing the transition requires astute attention to the readiness of patients and families to consider a change from active treatment to palliative care goals. In many instances individuals involved in the care will be at various stages of acceptance regarding the progressive nature of the disease. Therefore, timing the transition will require nondefensive communication skills that allow them to express anger, fear, regret, and perhaps guilt about not pursuing an active treatment plan. Some family members may require more time to assist them to grieve about their loss of hope for recovery. Those who hold on to an active treatment approach may have difficulty imagining how to provide care and support to the patient within a palliative care model. They may feel that acceptance of a palliative care approach means the care has failed and the patient will be abandoned. Continuing support, practical assistance, and specific guidance about how to care for the patient who is receiving palliative care can be extremely helpful.

Shifting Gently

Shifting gently involves use of communication skills that are honest, but gentle and sensitive to the needs of patients and families. This type of shift requires confidence about the palliative care team's ability to provide comfort, to remain present with the patient and family, and to ensure that the patient and family do not feel abandoned or neglected. The knowledge and skills of palliative care teams can be emphasized as a resource that will allow the patient to receive expert comfort care and the family to feel helped. The transition requires well-timed support so that patients and families feel secure in the goal shift. The following example illustrates this approach.

Case Report: Mrs. W., an ICU Patient

Mrs. M. was a 74-year-old woman who had suffered a cerebral vascular accident. She had been admitted to the intensive care unit, was receiving intravenous therapy, was being tube-fed and was receiving chest physiotherapy every two hours. She was unconscious and her breathing was labored. The family was awaiting assessment by the neurologist, who confirmed that the patient had suffered a cerebral hemorrhage to the brain stem region and that recovery was not expected. The palliative care nurse specialist was consulted to assist the ICU staff in preparing the family for a terminal prognosis. The patient's 80-year-old husband had consented to the insertion of a pacemaker and was hopeful that the tube-feeding and chest physiotherapy would revive his wife. The palliative care nurse spent time with the patient and the patient's husband, asking questions about her illness, her care, and her personal background. Through the discussions Mr. M. stated his wife had always said, "If I can't care for myself, don't keep me going." The nurse asked Mr. M. what he understood about the treatments being provided. It was clear that he did not have a good knowledge of the aims of treatments. The nurse carefully explained what each intervention would offer—and through that discussion helped Mr. M. to realize that none of the treatments were curative. Mr. M. agreed to stop the chest physiotherapy, as it appeared to be a futile treatment that was quite disruptive to the patient. When Mr. M. understood that the tube-feeding would not cure his wife, he agreed that she would not wish to die attached to tubes in intensive care. He visited the palliative care unit and was reassured to have the patient moved there so that he and his daughter and grandchildren could spend more time with his wife in a more homelike environment. Mrs. M. died on the Palliative Care Unit one week later. Mr. M. had been by her side throughout the week, was prepared for her death and was grateful for the care transition. The nurse "joined" Mr. M. and timed her information in small doses so that he would be able to shift his understanding of his wife's illness in a way that was tolerable to him.

Much of the literature that describes the process of "breaking bad news" applies to this type of strategy.[14–17] Although palliative care patients have often received the "bad news" of their poor prognosis before being transferred to a palliative care service, it is often the role of the palliative care team to be part of this shift-in-care plan. The palliative care nurse can be particularly helpful in breaking bad news in a way that the patient and family feel supported.

Garg, Buckman, and Maguire[15] have developed and tested a protocol to assist health care providers in breaking bad news. The protocol includes six down-to-earth steps. The first step is labeled, "Getting the setting right" (e.g., eye contact, sitting with the patient, privacy), followed by a step termed, "Finding out what the patient knows already." The authors then recommend that the health care provider "Find out what the patient wants to know" (e.g., by asking the patient if he/she is the type of person who likes to know a good deal about his/her treatment plan). The protocol follows with a step called, "Giving information," which they recommend should be provided using a similar vocabulary to the patient's and in small understandable "chunks" of information. They then emphasize the importance of "Responding to the patient's reactions" by acknowledging his/her responses, using empathy and allowing for expression of negative feelings. The final step is titled "Closing," which requires a summary of the areas discussed, confirmation of whether or not there are unanswered questions, and a clear plan for the next point of contact.[15] These simple steps are useful, can be learned, and are flexible for a range of care situations. Although the steps written from the perspective of communication with patients, the principles apply as well to communication with family members.

GOAL INSTABILITY

The shift may not "hold" in some instances. If patients, family members and health team members are uncertain about the palliative care goals, they may revert to active treatment interventions again. Therefore, the lane change may need to occur more than once and will require careful attention to feelings of loss. The daughter of a woman with advanced breast cancer stated:

> We knew that she was deteriorating and we had agreed that nothing more could be done and then we heard of this doctor who had an experimental treatment that no one knew much about. And so we thought maybe we should give it a chance—you know . . . you can never completely give up hope, even though we knew it was not going to work.

In some instances the patient's status may improve, even briefly, prompting hope for the family and causing them to reconsider the plan of care. Family members may also look longingly for signs of improvement despite their knowledge of a terminal diagnosis. For example, one 50-year-old woman with advanced lung cancer had deteriorated quickly during a six-week period. She had been eating poorly and was quite lethargic and weak. One day she appeared much more alert and was asking her family for a special spicy Caribbean meal that she particularly liked. This request was incongruous with her previous eating abilities, as she had only been tolerating small amounts of bland, blended foods. However, the family responded quickly to her request with confused hope that she might be miraculously cured. The patient enjoyed the meal and conversed in a lively manner with her sons and sister that afternoon, but deteriorated quickly in the following days and died three days later. Family members may feel tossed around by these types of changes and may need help to discuss their observations, make meaning of the patient's illness, and reconcile their hope and acceptance.

COMBINED GOALS

There may be instances where the family or patient is unable to accept a shift to palliative goals of care. This situation may occur when the treatment plan is not very clear or when there is too much resistance to a change in treatment plan to allow a gentle and sensitive shift within the time frame of the patient's illness.

She didn't say much until Robert left. Then she went hysterical for about five minutes. She said, "I don't want to die—what can I do?" She was going sort of mad, like she wanted to tear everything apart.

In these instances, a combination of care goals may be appropriate and is consistent with the definition of palliative care endorsed by the World Health Organization:

Palliative care is the active total care of patients whose disease is not responsive to curative treatment. Control of pain, of other symptoms, and of psychological, social and spiritual problems, is paramount. The goal of palliative care is achievement of the best quality of life for patients and their families. Many aspects of palliative care are also applicable earlier in the course of the illness in conjunction with active treatment.[23]

The WHO definition of palliative care depicts palliative care as a service that can be offered concurrently with active treatment as well as care offered after failure of curative or antidisease treatment. This model is depicted Figure 23–1.

This concurrent model of palliative care and active treatment has yet to be widely embraced by the health care community and reflects the enduring death-denying perspective of society. The association of palliative care approaches with impending death prevents patients from receiving care that can augment active treatment. However, in some instances, patients may benefit from a combination of active treatment interventions together with the expert symptom management and supports of a palliative care model. Detailed discussion about which aspect of care relates to which particular care goal may not be necessary. Rather, a focus on the specific needs of the patient and family with appropriate attention to these needs may be the most useful approach.

CONCLUSION

Establishing care goals requires expert communication skills and attention to communication traps that can occur when health professionals are not alert to ritualistic patterns of interaction. A particular challenge occurs when the patient's goals of care must shift from an active treatment focus to a palliative care approach. Attention to the content, expressive, and relationship issues associated with communication allows nurses to more fully examine communication patterns and exchanges that may be ineffective.

Five common communication traps have been described that may arise when health care professionals endeavor to manage exchanges so that they are socially familiar and "safe." Alertness to signs of communication blocks and a willingness to explore different ways of interacting with patients and families will assist in avoiding these impasses.

Four strategies for facilitating care goal "lane changes" are offered, with acknowledgment that at times there will be periods of goal instability and a need for a combination of seemingly disparate care goals. At these times, those involved in the patient's care need reassurance that comfort care will remain paramount.

There is no simple script for establishing care goals in the context of palliative care. However, attention to the principles of communication and vigilance to communication pitfalls may assist the nurse to stay balanced and open to meaningful dialogues about care goals.

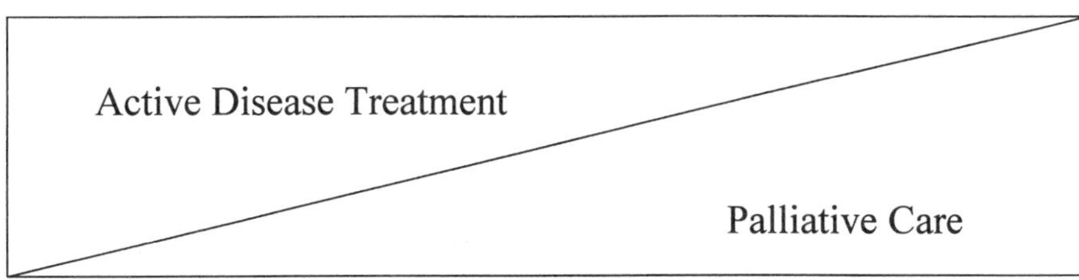

Fig. 23–1. Relationship between active disease treatment and palliative care.

REFERENCES

1. Stedeford A. Couples facing death: Unsatisfactory communication. BMJ 1981;2:1098.
2. Thorne SE, Robinson CA. Reciprocal trust in health care relationships. J Adv Nurs 1988;13:782–789.
3. Kuypers JA, Trute B. The untrapped worker: A precondition for effective family practice. In DS Freeman (Ed). Perspectives on Family Therapy. Vancouver: Butterworth & Co, 1980:57–67.
4. Watzlawick P. Pragmatics of Human Communication. New York: Norton, 1967.
5. Hileman J, Lackey N, Hassanein R. Identifying the needs of home caregivers of patients with cancer. Oncol Nurs Forum 1992;19:771–777.
6. Kristjanson LJ, Ashcroft T. The family's cancer journey: A literature review. Cancer Nurs 1994;17(1):1–17.
7. Northouse PG, Northouse LL. Communication and cancer: Issues confronting patients, health professionals, and family members. J Psychosoc Oncol 1988;5(3):17–45.
8. Northouse L. The impact of cancer on the family: An overview. Int J Psychiatric Med 1984; 14:215–242.
9. Mor V, Masterson-Allen S, Houts P. The changing needs of patients with cancer at home: A longitudinal view. Cancer 1992;69:829–838.
10. Northouse LL, Golden-Peters H. Cancer and the family: Strategies to assist spouses. Semin Oncol Nurs 1993;9(2):74–82.
11. Tayor EJ, Ferrell BR, Grant M, Cheyney L. Managing cancer pain at home: The decisions and ethical conflicts of patients, family caregivers, and homecare nurses. Oncol Nurs Forum 1993; 20,(6), 919–927.
12. Gotcher JM. Interpersonal communication and psychosocial adjustment, J Psychosoc Oncol 1992;10(3):21–39.
13. Artinian BM. Risking involvement with cancer patients. West J Nurs Res 1995;17(3):292–304.

14. Buckman R. I don't know what to say: How to help and support someone who is dying. London: Macmillan, 1998.

15. Garg A, Buckman R, Kason R. Teaching medical students how to break bad news. Can Med Assoc J 1997;156(8):1159–1164.

16. McLauchlan CAJ. Handling distressed relatives and breaking bad news. BMJ 1990;301: 1145–1149.

17. Buckman R, Kason Y. How to break bad news—A practical protocol for healthcare professionals. Toronto: University of Toronto Press, 1992.

18. Goffman E. Interactional Ritual: Essays on Face to Face Behavior. 2nd edition. Harmondsworth: Penguin, 1972.

19. Pepler CJ, Lynch A. Rational messages of control in nurse-patient interactions with terminally ill patients with AIDs and cancer. J Palliat Care 1991;7(1):18–29.

20. Ontario Breast Cancer Information Exchange Project (OBCIEP). A Guide to Unconventional Cancer Therapies. Aurora, Ontario: R & R Bookbar, 1994.

21. Degner LJ, Gow CM, Thompson LA. Critical nursing behaviors in care for the dying. Cancer Nurs 1991;14(5):246–253.

22. Bottorff JL, Gogag M, Engelberg-Lotzkar M. Comforting: Exploring the work of cancer nurses. J Adv Nurs 1995;22(6):1077–1084.

23. World Health Organization. (1990). Cancer pain relief and palliative care. Report of a WHO Expert Committee, Geneva: WHO.

24 The Meaning of Hope in the Dying

MARY ERSEK

This disease—it's kind of an emotional roller-coaster, just sitting here saying that you don't know where you're going to end up. But I can't give up. I've got to have hope, because hope is the key to everything.
—35-year-old man with recurrent cancer

Every time life asks us to give up a desire, to change our direction or redefine our goals; every time we lose a friend, break a relationship, or start a new plan, we are invited to widen our perspectives and to touch, under the superficial waves of our daily lives, the deeper currents of hope.
—Henri Nouwen[1]

Hope has long been recognized as fundamental to the human experience. Many authors have contemplated hope, extolling it as a virtue and an energy that brings life and joy.[1–5] Fromm called hope "a psychic commitment to life and growth"[5] (p. 12). Some authors assert that life without hope is impossible.[6–9]

Despite its positive connotations, hope is intimately bound with suffering.[5,10–11] As the French philosopher Gabriel Marcel observed, "Hope is situated within the framework of the trial"[4] (p. 30). It is this paradox that manifests itself so fully at the end of life.

Indeed, the critical role that hope plays in human life takes on special meaning as death nears.[9] The ability to hope often is challenged, and it can elude patients and families during terminal illness. Hope for a cure is almost certainly destroyed, and even a prolonged reprieve from death is unlikely. Multiple losses are experienced as many patients continue an illness trajectory that is marked by increasing disability and pain.

Even when hope appears to be strong within the dying person or the family, it can be problematic if hopefulness is perceived to be based on unrealistic ideas about the future.[12] Tension grows within relationships as people become subsumed in a struggle between competing versions of reality. Important issues may not be resolved as people continue to deny the reality of impending death.

Despite these somber realities and inevitable suffering, many people do maintain hope as they die, and families recover and find hope even within the experience of loss. How can this be? Part of the reason lies in the nature of hope itself—its resiliency and capacity to coexist with suffering. As witnesses to suffering and hope, palliative care nurses must understand these complexities, and be confident and sensitive in their efforts to address hope and hopelessness in the people for whom they care.

To assist palliative care nurses, this chapter will explore the many dimensions of hope and identify its possible influence on health and quality of life. Nursing assessment and strategies to foster hope will be discussed. In addition, specific issues such as the process of maintaining hope in life-threatening circumstances, "unrealistic hopefulness," and cultural considerations in the expression and maintenance of hope will be explored. The goals of the chapter are to provide the reader with an understanding about this complex but vital phenomenon, offer guidance in the clinical application of this concept to palliative nursing care, and explore some of the controversies regarding hope that challenge clinicians.

DEFINITIONS AND DIMENSIONS OF HOPE

Hope is an important concept for many disciplines, including philosophy, theology, psychology, nursing, and medicine. Many authors have attempted to define hope and describe its attributes.[4–5,13–18] Some are more successful than others in capturing its complexity. A nursing theory of hope, developed by Karin Dufault[19–20] and based on qualitative research involving elderly people with cancer, is particularly notable in its comprehensiveness and expansion of previous psychological models of hope.[17] Dufault described hope as "a multidimensional, dynamic life force characterized by a confident yet uncertain expectation of achieving a future good which, to the hoping person is realistically possible and personally significant"[20] (p. 380). Dufault also theorized that hope has two interrelated spheres: particularized and generalized. Particularized hope is centered and dependent on specific, valued goals, or hope objects. An example is the hope of a terminally ill patient to live long enough to celebrate a particular holiday or event. In contrast, generalized hope is a broader, nonspecific sense of a more positive future that is not directly related to a particular goal or desire. Dufault likened this sphere to an umbrella that creates a diffuse, positive glow on life.

Dufault also postulated several dimensions of hope that were incorporated into later research and theories.[21–23] These dimensions include affective, spiritual, relational, cognitive, behavioral, and contextual aspects of hope. Some of these were identified through research in which people were asked to describe their definitions and sources of hope. Essential components also were confirmed in that the lack or loss of these factors can lead to hopelessness.

The affective dimension of hope encompasses a myriad of emotions. Of course, hope is accompanied by many positive feelings, including joy, confidence, strength, and excitement. The full experience of hope, however, also includes uncertainty, fear, anger, suffering, and sometimes despair.[4,11,24–35] The philosopher Gabriel Marcel, for example, argued that in its fullest sense hope could only follow an experience of suffering or trial.[4] Marcel's thesis is corroborated by the experiences described by people with cancer in which they see their disease as "a wake-up call" that opened their eyes to a greater appreciation for life and an opportunity for self-growth.[21,25–26]

The spiritual dimension is a central component of hope.[5,27–32] Hopefulness is associated with spiritual well-being,[27,33] and qualitative studies have shown that spirituality and spiritual practices provide a context in which to define hope and articulate hope-fostering activities.[20,22–23,34–36] These activities include religious beliefs and rituals, but extend to broader conceptualizations of spirituality that encompass meaning and purpose in life, self-transcendence, and connectedness with a deity or other life-force.[29,37] Although spirituality is nearly always viewed as a hope-fostering influence, serious illness and suffering can challenge one's belief and trust in a benevolent deity, or be viewed as punishment from God; either interpretation of suffering can result in hopelessness.[38]

Relationships with significant others are another important dimension of hope. Interconnectedness with others is cited as a source of hope in virtually every study, and physical and psychological isolation from others is a frequent threat to hope.[19,23,36,39–42] Hope levels are positively associated with social support.[43–44] In addition to family members and friends, patients also have identified nurses as having a significant influence on hope.[19,45–47] Watson[48] acknowledged this role by including the instillation of faith and hope as a primary factor in her nursing theory of caring. Despite being vital sources of hope, others can threaten hope by distancing themselves, showing disrespect, discounting patient's experiences, disclosing negative information, or withholding information.[19,36,41,47]

The cognitive dimension of hope encompasses many intellectual and behavioral strategies, particularly those involving specific goals that require planning and effort to attain. Identification of goals can motivate and energize people, thereby increasing hope.[19,23,31,39] When identifying goals, people assess what they desire and value within a context of what is realistically possible. They appraise the resources necessary to accomplish their goals against the resources that are available to them. They then take action to secure the resources or meet the goal, and decide upon a reasonable time frame in which to accomplish the goal.[19,22–23,31] Active involvement in one's situation and attainment of goals increases the sense of personal control and self-efficacy, which in turn increases hope.[49] When a person repeatedly fails to attain valued goals, hopelessness and passivity can result.[17,50–51]

The goal-focused thoughts and activities that foster hope are similar to the problem-focused coping strategies described by Lazarus and Folkman.[52] This similarity is not surprising, since hope is strongly associated with coping.[21,42,53–56] The exact relationship between the two concepts, however, is unclear.[21,23] Hope has been identified as a foundation for successful coping,[57] a method of coping,[21,42,58] and as an outcome of successful coping.[53] Many strategies that people use to maintain hope have been previously identified as coping methods, and models of maintaining hope overlap substantially with models of coping.[21–22,42,52,59,60] Strategies to maintain hope include problem-focused coping methods (e.g., setting goals, actively managing symptoms, getting one's affairs in order) and emotion-focused strategies (e.g., using distraction techniques, appraising the illness in non-threatening ways).[21–22,23,52]

Contextual dimensions of hope are the life circumstances and abilities that influence hope—for example, physical health, financial stability, and functional and cognitive abilities.[19,20] Common, documented threats to hope include acute, chronic, and terminal illness; cognitive decline; fatigue; and impaired functional status. It is interesting to note that these factors, particularly physical illness and impairment, do not inevitably decrease hope, presumably if people are able to overcome the threat through cognitive, spiritual, relational, or other strategies.[21,23,36,40,61–62]

THE INFLUENCE OF HOPE AND HOPELESSNESS ON ADAPTATION TO ILLNESS

Hope is believed to influence health and adaptation to illness. Although this relationship has been posited in several theories of hope, there also is some research evidence to support this belief. Empirically, diminished hope is associated with poorer quality of life,[53,63] increased severity of suicidal intent[64] and incidence of suicide,[65,66] and decreased adherence to treatment regimens.[67] If hopelessness occurs, anxiety and depression can result.[17,51,63] Lower levels of hope also are associated with lower self-esteem.[43–44]

In addition to its influence on psychological states and behaviors, there is some evidence to suggest that hope affects physical states as well. Some researchers have found an association between hope and immune function,[68] and decreased hope is associated with a worse prognosis in cancer patients.[69–71]

VARIATIONS IN HOPE AMONG DIFFERENT POPULATIONS

The preceding description of the definitions and components of hope is derived from studies involving diverse populations, including children, adolescents, adults, and the elderly. In addition, research has been conducted in inpatient, outpatient, and community settings, with well persons and those with a variety of chronic and life-threatening illnesses. The experiences of families also have been described. Over these diverse populations and settings, many core concepts have been identified that transcend specific groups. However, some subtle but important differences exist. For this reason, hopefulness in selected populations is addressed in the following sections.

Hope in Children and Adolescents

A few investigators have examined hope in pediatric populations. In an early study, Wright and Shontz[72] studied hope in children with chronic disabilities and significant adults in their lives (e.g., parents, teachers, physical therapists). Both the children and the adults were interviewed, allowing for the identification of differences between the two samples. The investigators found that hope for the children in their study was two-dimensional. Hoping involved *(1)* an awareness of the positive and *(2)* a sense of time orientation. For younger children, hope was present-focused, whereas older children had a future-orientation to hope. Younger children also saw adults as being in control of a situation, and were less concerned about assessing how realistic their particular hopes were. In contrast, adults actively assessed the realities of the present, and possibilities for the future.

Artinian[73] explored hope in older children, aged 10–20, who underwent bone marrow transplantation. The findings suggest that ways to reduce stress and instill hope among younger patients and their parents included managing physical discomforts, making children and parents feel cared for, being nonjudgmental when children and parents vented anger, preventing boredom, and assisting with making and altering plans.[23]

A program of research by Hinds and colleagues elucidated the experience of hoping in adolescents.[13–14,47,59,74] Studies were conducted in well adolescents, adolescents undergoing inpatient treatment for substance abuse, and adolescents with cancer. Based on qualitative studies, Hinds defined adolescent hopefulness as "the degree to which an adolescent possesses a comforting or life-sustaining, reality-based belief that a positive future exists for self and others"[14] (p. 85). Interestingly, inclusion of the phrase "and others" arose from the sample of adolescent cancer patients. Hinds found that only in this sample did adolescents express a concern and articulate their hopes for others. Examples of this attribute included such hopes as "my parents will be O.K. if I die," and "there will be a cure soon so patient 'x' will not die"[14] (p. 85). This ability to go beyond oneself and hope for others may be influenced by the adolescents' sense of mortality that accompanies the cancer diagnosis.[14]

Hope and the Elderly

Numerous studies have examined hope in elderly persons.[19,28,39,49,75–77] Religious beliefs and spiritual well-being were strongly associated with elders' hope in the study of Fehring and colleagues;[28] these factors also were prominent themes in qualitative studies.[19,39] The relationships among elders' hope, physical functioning, and health status are unclear; physical functioning and health status were positively correlated with hope in some studies[75,77] but not in others.[39,62]

Herth's qualitative study revealed specific hopes, source of hope, and threats to hope in older persons. She found that older (>80 years) participants usually expressed their hopes in terms of loved ones rather than themselves. When they did refer to themselves, they often focused on "life in the hereafter" (p. 146). Hope-fostering activities included participating in purposeful volunteer activities, reminiscing about past successes, possessing inanimate objects that had personal significance, and connecting with others. Hope-impeding factors consisted of witnessing hopelessness in others, lack of energy, suffering and pain experienced by oneself and others, and impaired cognitive functioning.[39]

Hope from the Family Caregiver's Perspective

Family caregivers are an integral component in palliative care. Patients and families influence each other's hope, and nursing interventions must focus on both groups.[9,78] Often, the physical and psychological demands placed on family caregivers are great, as are threats to hope.[40,79–81] Herth found that threats to caregivers' hope included isolation from support networks and God; concurrent losses, including loss of significant others, health, and income; and inability to control the patient's symptoms. Caregivers with poor health status, high fatigue, multiple losses, and sleep disturbances were significantly less hopeful than caregivers without these problems.[40]

Yates and Stetz found that as awareness of dying increased, caregivers hoped for relief from suffering rather than for a cure.[82] Herth reported that as death became imminent, the need "to do" for the patient was replaced by a wanting simply "to be" with the patient. In addition, little emphasis was placed on the "future" in caregivers' descriptions of hope.[40]

Strategies to maintain hope in family caregivers are similar to those found in patients, with a few differences. Spending time with others in the support network was very important for caregivers. In addition, being able to reprioritize demands helped caregivers to conserve much-needed energy. Caregivers also maintained hope through engaging in relaxing activities such as listening to or playing music, gardening, or watching a sunset.[40]

HOPE IN TERMINALLY ILL PATIENTS: IS HOPE COMPATIBLE WITH DEATH?

Research demonstrates that many people are able to maintain hope during acute and chronic illness. Hope also can thrive during the terminal phase of an illness, despite the realization that no cure is possible. Herth assessed hope levels longitudinally in terminally ill pa-

Table 24–1. Sources of Hope/Hope-Fostering Strategies in Terminally Ill Adults

- Having one or more meaningful, shared relationships in which one feels a sense of "being needed" or "being a part of something"
- Maintaining a feeling of lightheartedness; feeling delight, joy, or playfulness and communicating that feeling; using humor
- Recalling joyous, meaningful events
- Having one's individuality acknowledged, accepted, and honored; having one's worth affirmed by others
- Identifying positive personal attributes such as courage, determination, serenity
- Having spiritual beliefs and engaging in spiritual practices that provide a sense of meaning for their suffering
- Focusing attention and effort on the short-term future
- Thinking about and directing efforts at specific, short-term attainable aims (earlier in terminal illness)
- Thinking about global, positive aims that are focused on others (e.g., support for the bereaved, happiness for their children) (later in terminal illness)
- Desiring serenity, inner peace, eternal rest (last days and weeks of life)

Source: Adapted from Herth.[36]

tients and their caregivers, and found that hope actually *increased* over time;[36,40] it did not diminish as death neared.

Although hope levels may not decrease, the nature of hope often is altered through the dying process. Herth reported that, similar to caregivers, dying patients defined hope more in terms of "being" rather than "doing." Other changes in hope at the end of life include an increased focus on others, and a desire to leave a legacy and to be well remembered.[19] Spirituality also increases in importance during the terminal phases of illness.[19,23] Hope-inspiring strategies for these patients appear in Table 24–1.

MULTICULTURAL VIEWS OF HOPE

Over the past three decades, our understanding of the clinical phenomenon of hope has increased dramatically through theoretical discourse and empirical research. While knowledge regarding the components, processes, and outcomes of hope has grown dramatically, progress in multicultural research on hope has been limited. The samples for many studies that examine hope or hopelessness are ethnically homogenous,[22,54] or the ethnic composition is unknown.[35,83] The studies that do include ethnically diverse samples are small,[19,39,84] thereby precluding making any comparisons or being able to generalize findings.

Existing research, then, may not reflect the experience of hope for people from non-European cultures. Although there is little research to substantiate this hypothesis, several known cultural differences could certainly limit the applicability of these conceptualizations, especially within the palliative care context. Three issues that theoretically could have a major impact on multicultural views of hope are: time orientation, truth-telling, and beliefs in control.

Time orientation is identified as a cultural phenomenon that varies among cultural groups. Some cultural groups, particularly those within the Euro-American culture, tend to be future-oriented. Within these groups, people prefer to look ahead, make short- and long-term plans, and organize their schedules to meet goals.[85] Since hope is defined as being future-oriented, with hopeful people more likely to identify and take action to meet goals, it is possible that members of these future-oriented cultures will appear more hopeful than people who are predominantly present-focused. On the other hand, people who are more focused on the present may be better able to sustain hope at the end of life when the ability to make long-range goals is hindered by the uncertainty surrounding a terminal diagnosis. Additional research is needed to clarify these relationships.

The value for truth-telling in Western health care systems also may affect hope. Current ethical and legal standards demand full disclosure of all relevant healthcare information.[86–87] Informed consent and patient autonomy in medical decision making, two eminent values in American health care, are impossible without this disclosure.[87–88] While few would advocate lying to patients, truth-telling is not universally viewed as helpful or desirable. Some cultures believe that patients should be protected from burdensome information that could threaten hope.[89] Truthful but blunt communication may also be seen as rude and disrespectful in some cultures,[90] and the feeling of being devalued and disrespected has a negative impact on hope.[19,36] In addition to the threats to hope that frank discussion is believed to engender, people who prefer nondisclosure of threatening information may be seen as attempting to cling to unrealistic hopes by refusing to listen to discouraging facts about their condition.

A third cultural concept that may affect hope is control. As described earlier, control is a core attribute in many conceptualizations of hope. Although hope can be relinquished to others, including health care providers or a transcendent power, personal control often is central to the hoping process.[21–23] In Euro-American cultures, applying one's will and energy to alter the course of an illness or to direct the dying process seems natural and desirable.[86–87,91] Advance directives are one culturally sanctioned way in which members of our society exert control over the dying process. This desire and belief in personal control, however, is not a common feature in many other cultures.[87] Especially in cultures where death is viewed as part of the inherent harmony of living and dying, attempting to exert any influence over the dying process may seem unnatural or inappropriate.[92–93] Thus, people from diverse cultures who take a more passive role in their health care, or who do not espouse a desire to control their illness or the dying process, may be viewed as less hopeful than people who manifest a "fighting spirit" and active stance.

More research needs to be conducted to test theories of hope in multicultural groups and ensure the appropriate application of current conceptualizations to diverse cultural groups, or to develop new theories that are relevant for these groups. Until this work is done, palliative care clinicians must be cautious in applying current hope theories, and sensitive to the possible variations in diverse populations.

MODELS OF MAINTAINING HOPE

Several investigators have identified factors that foster hope and strategies that enable people to sustain hope despite life-threatening or chronic illness.[19,22–23,34–36,40,42,59] There is considerable concordance across these studies regarding many of the major themes; however, various models emphasize different styles and strategies that demonstrate the diversity in hope-fostering strategies.

Herth conducted in-depth interviews with 30 terminally ill adults and documented the ways that hope is fostered at the end of life. She described several strategies that are summarized in Table 24–1. These strategies reflect a sense of peace and acceptance of death. The focus is more on "being" than "doing"; time and memories are shared with others in a way that suggests a process of "getting closure."[36]

In contrast, this author's work[21–22] highlights active, cognitive strategies to minimize the psychological distress of life-threatening disease in order to maintain hope. The resulting model emphasizes that maintaining hope requires a dynamic interplay, or dialectic, between two categories of hope-sustaining strategies: "Dealing with It" and "Keeping It in Its Place." "Dealing with It" is defined as the process of confronting the negative possibilities inherent in the illness experience, including death, and allowing the full range of thoughts, behaviors, and emotions resulting from the recognition. "Keeping It in Its Place" is defined as the process of managing the impact of the disease and its treatment by controlling one's response to the disease and therapy. This process occurs after recognizing the serious nature or downside of the illness experience and involves eight groups of hope-sustaining categories (Table 24–2).

The Dialectic of Maintaining Hope model underscores the complex and sometimes contradictory nature of sus-

Table 24–2. Structure of "Keeping It in Its Place": Hope-Maintaining Strategies in People with Life-Threatening Illness

I. Appraising the illness in a nonthreatening manner
1. Seeing the disease/treatment as a challenge or a test
2. Seeing the disease/treatment as a positive influence
   a. Reprioritizing one's life
   b. Becoming altruistic
   c. Looking at the bright side

II. Managing the cognitions related to the illness experience
1. Joking about it
2. Avoiding thinking or talking about the negative
3. Keeping distracted
4. Forgetting about it
5. Not dwelling on it
6. Focusing on loved ones

III. Managing the emotional response to the illness experience
1. Limiting the emotional response
2. Severing the cognitive from the emotional response
3. Shifting from one emotion to another
4. Translating emotional pain into physical pain

IV. Managing the sense of control
1. Maintaining control
   a. Getting information/staying informed
   b. Restraining the disease through exercise, diet, and stress management
   c. Decisional control—making decisions about treatment or other aspects of life to exert control
2. Relinquishing control
   a. To a deity
   b. To the medical and nursing staffs
   c. To medical science

V. Taking a stance toward the illness and treatment
1. Fighting the illness
   a. "Go down fighting"
   b. Imagining the illness as the enemy or an evil being
2. Accepting the illness
   a. "It's God's will"
   b. "It's just part of the process"
   c. Expecting the disease/death

VI. Managing uncertainty
1. Minimizing the uncertainty
   a. "Knowing" the future
   b. "Having to believe"
2. Maximizing the uncertainty
   a. "They (the physicians) could always be wrong"
   b. "I'm not a statistic!"—beating the odds

VII. Managing the focus on the future
1. Living day to day
2. Focusing on long-term goals
   a. Making mutable goals
   b. Establishing interim goals
   c. Using previously met goals as a source of hope
   d. Using unmet goals as a source of hope

VIII. Managing the view of the self in relation to the illness
1. Minimizing the illness and the treatment
   a. "It (the disease) is just a flaw in my system"
   b. "It (the therapy) is just a temporary inconvenience"
2. Maximizing personal strength
   a. Identifying personal attributes of strength
   b. Making downward comparisons with others (e.g., "At least I don't have AIDS")
   c. Focusing on successful others
   d. Identifying a history of personal strength

Source: Adapted from Ersek,[21–22] with permission.

taining hope through serious illness. People use multiple strategies that allow them to confront and to avoid the negative aspects of illness and death.[21–22,59] It also reflects the processes by which people actively negotiate the illness through such means as exerting control and making decisions, seeking information, and "fighting the illness."

This research[21–22] was conducted in a bone marrow transplant setting and its applicability to palliative care has not been investigated. It does provide, however, a model of hope that may elucidate hopefulness in different groups of patients, perhaps those who are in earlier stages of the illness trajectory or for those with coping styles that focus more on active management of the illness and negative emotions.

These different approaches for maintaining hope are important to describe and understand because they assist the palliative care nurse in designing effective strategies to foster hope. They increase clinicians' awareness regarding the various ways that people respond to chronic and terminal illness, and guide clinicians in their interactions with patients and families to sustain hope. They also help palliative care providers understand difficult or troubling responses, such as unrealistic hopefulness.

THE ISSUE OF UNREALISTIC HOPEFULNESS

Reality surveillance is a feature of many conceptualizations of hope.[11,14,16,18–19,46,94] Often, clinicians, researchers, and theorists believe that mentally healthy people should choose and work toward realistic goals. In these frameworks, adhering to unrealistic hopes or denying reality is a sign of maladaptive cognitions that could lead to negative health outcomes. Thus, denial and unrealistic hopes and ideas are discouraged and treated as pathology.[12,95–97]

Clinical examples of unrealistic hopes that cause consternation are numerous and diverse. For instance, one patient with advanced cancer might hope that persistent, severe sciatica is from exercise and overuse rather than spinal metastases. The nurse working with this patient may continually contradict his theory, asserting that his denial of the probable, malignant cause of the pain will delay effective treatment. Another patient might insist that a new cure for her illness is imminent, causing distress for the nurse who knows that it's unlikely that a cure will be found and who believes that the patient's unrealistic hopes will hinder acceptance of and preparation for death.

Despite the concerns of these nurses, however, some investigators argue that these fears may be unfounded. The reason for this perspective is based on findings from studies conducted over the past few decades that have led social psychologists to question the view that denial and unrealistic hopes are always maladaptive. Instead, these researchers argue that human interpretation of information from the environment is *inherently* biased and inaccurate.[98–99]

Shelley Taylor and colleagues developed this idea further in their theory of positive illusions.[99–104] They described positive illusions as general, enduring cognitive patterns involving error and/or bias,[99] that provide a foundation for successful adaptation to many threatening events, including serious illness. Especially important are unrealistically positive evaluations of the self, exaggerated perceptions of control, and unrealistic optimism about the future.[99,100] They support their theory with empirical evidence that denial and positive illusions often are associated with positive outcomes such as better psychological adjustment to illness, less emotional distress, and even decreased mortality.[100,101,103,106–108]

In addition to promoting positive outcomes, unrealistic hopes need to be assessed within the context of uncertainty. No one really does know exactly what the future will bring. So, if a person hopes for something in the future that appears highly unlikely, can it be known for *certain* that it will not occur? Taylor underscored this point:

> By illusions, I do not mean that the beliefs are necessarily opposite to known facts. Rather, their maintenance requires looking at the known facts in a particular light, because a different slant would yield a less positive picture, or the beliefs have yet to yield any factual basis of support.[100] (p. 1161)

Another example is the way in which people exploit uncertainty to maximize hope. For instance, people frequently respond to dire prognostic news with observations that they can always "beat the odds."[21,22] Given the fact that no one can predict the future with absolute certainty, it is impossible to predict which individuals with a 2% chance of remission or recovery will actually be cured. Also, consider the case of a person with life-threatening disease who believes that God can provide a cure. Spontaneous "miracle" cures, however rare, have been documented. We cannot predict with *complete* confidence, then, that there is no possibility of a cure. These observations raise the question: do all people who hope against poor odds need our help to become more "realistic"?

A third argument against aggressive "reality orientation" for all patients and families is the evidence that unrealistic hopes and illusions often are abandoned over time and without intensive intervention from professionals.[19,99,100] In other words, most people acknowledge and accept distressing information, but need to do so on their own schedules.

The preceding discussion may seem to imply that clinicians should not be concerned about unrealistic hopefulness. Of course, that is not the case. Despite their adaptive potential, illusions and denial may result in adverse outcomes.[12,57,99,109] For example, unrealistic hopes may lead to parents to push aggressive therapy, thereby increasing their child's suffering without curing or controlling the disease. Similarly, a person who denies that his illness is terminal may isolate himself from his family to protect his beliefs and avoid contradictory opinions. Unfortunately, in these cases and others, there is insufficient research to inform clinicians fully regarding situations that are potentially maladaptive, and even less guidance about appropriate therapeutic strategies. However, evidence exists that some situations should be viewed with caution and may

Table 24–3. Assessing Unrealistic Hopes

1. Is the focus of the unrealistic hope broad or severe (e.g., complete denial of a disease that has been documented)?
2. Is the persistence of the unrealistic hope severe, i.e., does it persist despite multiple pieces of information from multiple sources (e.g., family, physicians, nurses) that the person is unlikely to realize the hope?
3. Is the person's adherence to the unrealistic hope *complete* (or does the person admit at times that there limitations and acknowledge negative possibilities)? Does the person continually use words such as "knowing" what will happen, rather than acknowledging that what he hopes for might *not* occur?
4. Does the hope cause the person to engage in reckless behaviors?
5. Does the hope cause the person to ignore warning signs (e.g., angina, increased pain) that should be treated promptly?
6. Does the hope cause great distress for family members and other significant others?
7. Has the person become isolated from others, either to avoid their challenges to the unrealistic hope or because others are uncomfortable in responding to the person?
8. Does it appear that adhering to the hope actually is causing distress and anxiety for the person (who may tacitly doubt or disbelieve in the illusion or hope, but is afraid to discuss that possibility with others)?
9. Is death imminent, and the unrealistic hopefulness is hindering efforts to get affairs in order, say good-bye, or receive emotional support?

indicate a need for gentle interventions, such as offering alternative hopes or providing skillful counseling. Table 24–3 lists several questions regarding unrealistic hopes. If the answer to any question is "yes," then further assessment and possible intervention may be necessary.

ASSESSING HOPE

As in all nursing care, thorough assessment of physical and psychosocial factors must precede thoughtful planning and implementation of therapeutic strategies. Thus, consistent and comprehensive evaluations of hope should be included in the palliative nursing assessment. Some conceptual elements of hope, such as those focusing on meaning and purpose in life, are included in a spiritual assessment.[38] Rarely, however, are comprehensive guides to assessing hope included in standardized nursing assessment forms.

Two thorough assessment guides have been developed and published.[110,111] Farran, Wilken, and Popovich's guidelines for the clinical assessment of hope appropriately utilize the acronym HOPE to designate the major areas of evaluation. The areas are: Health, Others, Purpose in Life, and Engaging Process. The engaging process refers to identification of goals, actions taken to achieve goals, a patient's sense of control over the situation, and identification of hope-inspiring factors in the patient's past, present, and future. In Table 24–4, this framework has been adapted and applied to terminally ill patients. It includes examples of questions and probes that can be used to assess hope.

Like pain, hope is a subjective experience and assessment should focus on self-report. However, behavioral cues can also provide information regarding a person's state of hope or hopelessness. Hopelessness is a central feature of depression;[64,112] thus, behaviors such as social withdrawal, flat affect, alcohol and substance abuse, insomnia, and passivity may indicate hopelessness.

As discussed earlier, the patient's terminal illness affects the hope of family caregivers, who in turn influence the hope of the patients.[40,80,82] Thus, assessing the hope of the patients' family caregivers and other significant support people also should occur.

Over the past decades, researchers from several disciplines have developed instruments to measure hope and hopelessness. The theoretical and empirical literature documents the comprehensiveness and face validity of these tools. Advances in psychometric theory and methods have allowed the evaluation of multiple dimensions of validity and reliability. The development and use of well-designed and well-tested tools has contributed greatly to the science of hope. Unfortunately, a thorough discussion of these measures is beyond the scope of this chapter. Table 24–5, however, provides a brief description of several widely used and tested instruments. More complete descriptions and evaluations of these scales can be found elsewhere.[23,113]

NURSING INTERVENTIONS TO MAINTAIN HOPE AT END OF LIFE

Clinicians, theorists, and researchers recognize that nurses play an important role in instilling, maintaining, and restoring hope in people for whom they care.[3,10,15,16,46–48,121,122] Researchers have identified many ways in which nurses assist patients and families to sustain hope during difficult periods,[19,31,47,49,78] including at the end of life.[19,36,40,122]

Table 24–6 provides a summary of nursing approaches to instill hope. A brief perusal of this table reveals an important point about these strategies. For the most part, nursing care to maintain patients' and families' hope fundamentally is about providing excellent physical, psychosocial, and spiritual palliative care. There are few *unique* interventions to maintain hope, and yet there is much nurses *can* do. Because hope is inextricably connected to virtually all facets of the illness experience, including physical pain, coping, anxiety, and spirituality, improvement or deterioration in one area has repercussions in other areas. Attending to these relationships reminds clinicians that virtually every action they take can influence hope, negatively or positively.

Another vital observation about hope-inspiring strategies is that many approaches begin with the patient and family. The experience of hope is a personal one, defined and determined by the hoping person.[19,20] Although others greatly influence that experience, ultimately the meaning and effects of words and actions are determined by the person experiencing hope or hopelessness.

Table 24–4. Guidelines for the Clinical Assessment of Hope in Palliative Care

Interview Question/Probe	Rationale
Health (and Symptom Management)	
1. Tell me about your illness. What is your understanding of the probable course of your illness?	Explore the person's perceptions of seriousness of their illness, and possible trajectories
2. How hopeful are you right now, and how does your illness affect your sense of hope?	Determine the person's general sense of hope and the effect of the terminal illness on hope
3. How well are you able to control the symptoms of your illness? How do these symptoms affect your hope?	Uncontrolled end-of- life symptoms have been found to negatively influence hope (Herth[36,40])
Others	
1. Who provides you with emotional, physical, and spiritual support?	Identify people in the environment that provide support and enhance hope
2. Who are you most likely to confide in when you have a problem or concern?	Identify others in whom the person has trust
3. What kinds of difficulty experiences have you and your family/partner/support network had to deal with in the past? How did you manage those experiences?	Explore experiences of coping with stressful situations
4. What kinds of things do family, support people, health care providers do that make you more hopeful? Less hopeful?	Identify specific behaviors that affect hope Recognize that other people can also *decrease* hope
Purpose in Life	
1. What gives you hope?	Identify relationships, beliefs, and activities that provide a sense of purpose and contribute positively to hope
2. What helps you make sense of your situation right now?	Identify the ways in which the person makes meaning of difficult situations.
3. Do you have spiritual or religious practices or support people that help you? If "yes", what are these practices people?	Identify if and how spirituality acts as a source of hope
4. Has your illness caused you to question your spiritual beliefs? If "yes", how?	Terminal illness can threaten the person's basic beliefs, and test one's faith
5. How can we help you maintain these practices and personal connections with spiritual support people?	Identify ways in which clinicians and others can support spiritual practices that enhance hope
Goals	
1. Right now, what are your major goals?	Identify major goals and priorities Examine whether these goals are congruent with the views of others
2. What do you see are the chances that you will meet these goals?	Explore how realistic the person thinks the goals are; if the goals are not perceived as being attainable, assess the impact on hope
3. What actions can you take to meet these goals?	Identify specific actions the person can take to meet the goals
4. What actions have you already taken to meet these goals?	Identify how active the person has been in attaining the goals
5. What resources do you have for meeting these goals?	Determine other resources to which the person has access for the purpose of attaining goals
Sense of Control	
1. Do you feel that you have much control over your current situation?	Determine if the person feels any ability to control or change the situation. Explore whether the person *wants* to have more control.
2. Are there others that you feel have some control over your current situation? If "yes," who are they and in what ways do they have control?	Determine if the person feels as though trusted others (e.g., health care providers, family, deity) can control or change the situation
Sources of Hope over Time	
1. In the past, what or who has made you hopeful?	Identify sources of hope from the person's past that may continue to provide hope during the terminal phase
2. Right now who and what provides you with hope?	Identify current sources of hope
3. What do you hope for in the future?	Assess generalized and specific hopes for the future

Source: Adapted from Farran, Wilken, and Popovich[110]; Farran, Herth, and Popovich.[23]

Table 24–5. Descriptions of Selected Instruments to Measure Hope and Hopelessness

Instrument Name	Brief Description	Selected References
Beck Hopelessness Scale	• 20-item, true-false format • Based on Stotland's definition of hopelessness: system of negative expectancies concerning oneself and one's future • Developed to assess psychopathological levels of hopelessness; correlates highly with attempted and actual suicides	64,65,66, 112,114
Herth Hope Scale (HHS)	• 30-item, 4-point Likert scale • Designed for well and ill populations • Assesses three overlapping dimensions: *(1)* cognitive-temporal, *(2)* affective-behavioral, *(3)* affiliative-behavioral • Spanish and Thai translations • Shorter 12-item Hope Index is also available	36,40,54,55, 115,116
Hopefulness Scale for Adolescents (Hinds)	• 24-item visual analog scale • Assesses the degree of the adolescent's positive future orientation • Assesses only the relational and rational thoughts processes of hope • Tested in several populations of adolescents: well, substance abusers, adolescents with emotional and mental problems, cancer patients	74,117
Miller Hope Scale	• 40-item scale, 5-point Likert scale • Assesses 10 elements: *(a)* mutuality/ affiliation, *(b)* avoidance of absolutizing, *(c)* sense of the possible, *(d)* psychological well-being & coping, *(e)* achieving goals, *(f)* purpose and meaning in life, *(g)* reality surveillance-optimism, *(h)* mental and physical activation, *(i)* anticipation, *(j)* freedom • Chinese and Swedish versions	28,41,118
Snyder Hope Scale	• 12-item, 4-point Likert scale • Based on Stotland's definition of hope; focus is on goals identification and achievement • Tested in healthy adults, and adults with psychiatric illness • Also has developed tool to measure hope in children[120]	119,120

Ersek found that many of the approaches utilized by bone marrow transplant patients to maintain hope were coping strategies initiated with little influence from others. For example, some people prayed, others distracted themselves with T.V., conversation, or other activities, and many patients used cognitive strategies such as minimizing negative thoughts, identifying personal strengths, and focusing on the positive.[21,22] For many patients and families, then, careful observation and active support of an individual's *established* strategies to maintain hope will be most successful.

A final point is to remind the reader that family caregivers and other support people should be included in these approaches. Ample evidence exists that patients and people within their support system reciprocally influence one another's hope.[23,40,82] In addition, family and significant others are always incorporated into the palliative care plan and considered part of the "unit of care." Maintenance of hope also is a goal following death, in that hope-restoring and -maintaining strategies must be an integral part of bereavement counseling.[94,123]

SPECIFIC INTERVENTIONS

The framework for the following discussion is adapted from Farran, Herth, and Popovich[23,122] who articulated four central attributes of hope: experiential, spiritual/transcendent, relational, and rational thought. These areas encompass the major themes found in the literature, and while they are not mutually exclusive, they provide a useful organizing device. The section also includes a brief discussion of ways in which nurses need to explore and understand their own hopes and values in order to provide palliative care that fosters hope in others.

Experiential Process Interventions

The experiential process of hope involves the acknowledgment and acceptance of suffering, but at the same time using the imagination to move beyond the suffering and to find hope.[23,122] Included in these types of strategies are methods to decrease physical suffering and cognitive strategies aimed at managing the threat of the terminal illness.

Uncontrolled symptoms such as pain, fatigue, dyspnea, and anxiety cause suffering and challenge the hopefulness of patients and caregivers.[19,36,39,40,42] Timely, adept symptom prevention and management, then, is central to maintaining hope. In home care settings, teaching patients and families the knowledge and skills to manage symptoms confidently and competently also is essential.

Other ways to help people find hope in suffering is to provide them a cognitive reprieve from their situation. One powerful strategy to achieve this temporary suspension is through humor. Several studies and lay publications have identified the central place of humor and lightheartedness in promoting hope.[21,22,36,46,47,124] According to patients' views, humor helps put things in perspective, and frees the self, at least momentarily, from the onerous burden of illness and suffering.[36,40] Making light

Table 24–6. Interventions to Foster Hope

Experiential Processes

- Prevent and manage end-of-life symptoms
- Utilize lightheartedness and humor appropriately
- Encourage the patient and family to transcend their current situation
  - Encourage aesthetic experiences
  - Encourage engagement in creative and joyous endeavors
  - Suggest literature, movies, and art that are uplifting and highlights the joy in life
  - Encourage reminiscing
  - Assist patient and family to focus on present and past joys
  - Share positive, hope-inspiring stories
- Support patient and family in positive self-talk

Spiritual/Transcendent Processes

- Facilitate participation in religious rituals and spiritual practices
- Make necessary referrals to clergy and other spiritual support people
- Assist the patient and family in finding meaning in the current situation
  - Assist the patient/family to keep a journal
  - Suggest literature, movies, and art that explore the meaning of suffering

Relational Processes

- Minimize patient and family isolation
- Establish and maintain an open relationship
- Affirm patients' and families' sense of self-worth
- Recognize and reinforce the reciprocal nature of hopefulness between patient and support system
- Provide time for relationships (especially important in institutional settings)
- Foster attachment ideation by assisting the patient to identify significant others and then to reflect on personal characteristics and experiences that endear the significant other to the patient[31]
- Communicate one's own sense of hopefulness

Rational Thought Processes

- Assist patient and family to establish, obtain, and revise goals without imposing one's own agenda
- Assist in identifying available and needed resources to meet goals
- Assist in procuring needed resources; assist with breaking larger goals into smaller steps to increase feelings of success
- Provide accurate information regarding patient's condition and treatment
- Facilitate reality surveillance as appropriate
- Help patient and family identify past successes
- Increase patients' and families' sense of control when possible

of a grim situation brings a sense of control over one's response to the situation, even when one has little influence over it. In one study, a respondent noted, "I may not have much control over the nearness of death, but I do have the power to joke about it"[36] (p. 1225). Of course, the use of humor with patients and families requires sensitivity toward the patient and family, as well as a sense of timing. Otherwise, humor becomes a belittling and hope-destroying mistake. Take cues from the patient and family. Observe how they use humor to dispel stress. Let them take the lead in joking about threatening information and events. In general, focus your humor on yourself or events outside the immediate concerns of the patient and family.

Other ways to move people cognitively beyond their suffering is to assist them in identifying and enjoying that which is joyful in life. Engagement in aesthetic experiences such as watching movies or listening to music that is uplifting can enable people to transcend their suffering. Sharing one's own hope-inspiring stories also can help.

Another strategy is to support people in their own positive self-talk. As noted earlier, many people naturally cope with stress by comparing themselves with people they perceive as less fortunate, or by identifying attributes of personal strength that help them find hope.[21,22,125] For example, an elderly, married woman with advanced breast cancer may comment that, despite the seriousness of her disease, she feels luckier than another woman with the same disease who is younger or without social support. By comparing herself with less fortunate others, she can take solace in recognizing that "things could be worse." Similarly, a person can maintain hope by focusing on particular talents or previous accomplishments that indicate an ability to cope with illness. In one study on hope, a woman asserted that her ability to survive an abusive marriage provided evidence that she could also cope with and manage her illness and treatment.[21] People may also cite their high level of motivation as a reason to feel hopeful about the future. Acknowledgment and validation of these attributes supports hope and affirms self-worth for patients and families.

Spiritual Process Interventions

Several specific strategies can foster hope while incorporating spirituality. These include providing opportunities for the expression of spiritual beliefs, and arranging for involvement in religious rituals and spiritual practices.[19,31,126]

Assisting patients and families to explore and make meaning of their trials and suffering is another useful approach. Encouraging patients and families to keep a journal of thoughts and feelings can help people in this process.[31] Suggesting books, film or art that focuses on religious or existential understandings and transcendence of suffering is another effective way to help people make sense of illness and death.[31]

Palliative care nurses also should assess for signs of spiritual distress and make appropriate referrals to clergy and other professionals with expertise in counseling during spiritual and existential crises.[38,126] Other spiritual and existential strategies are described in chapters 29, 30, and 31 of this text.

Relational Process Interventions

According to Lynch, the true experience of hope requires the recognition and acceptance of the help and support from others that all human beings need.[11] To maximize hope, then, nurses should establish and maintain an open relationship with patients and members of their support network, taking the time to learn what their priorities and needs are, and then addressing those needs in timely, effective ways. Demonstrating respect and interest, and being available to listen and be with people—that is, affirming each person's worth—is essential.[19,42,47,127]

Fostering and sustaining connectedness among the patient, family, and friends can be accomplished by providing time for uninterrupted interactions, which is especially important in institutional settings.[23] Nurses can increase hope by enlisting help from others to help achieve goals. For example, recruiting friends or arranging for a volunteer to transport an ill person to purchase a gift for a grandchild can cultivate hope for everyone involved. It's important to help others realize how vital they are in sustaining a person's hope.[31]

Miller recommended that another method of instilling hope is to foster attachment ideation.[31] Attachment ideation is the preoccupation with significant others such as a child or spouse. To encourage this attachment, a nurse assists a person in identifying and reviewing characteristics that endear and attract the person to the significant other. In this way, the person can focus on the loved one during times of distress or pain, thereby maintaining hope.

Rational Thought Process Interventions

The rational thought process is the dimension of hope that specifically focuses on goals, resources, personal control and self-efficacy, and action.[23,122,128] Interventions related to this dimension include assisting patients and families in devising and attaining goals. Providing accurate and timely information about the patient's condition and treatment helps patients and families decide which goals are achievable. At times, gentle assistance with monitoring and acknowledging negative possibilities will facilitate the choice of realistic goals. Helping to identify and procure the resources necessary to meet goals also is important.

Often, major goals need to be broken into smaller, shorter-term achievements. For example, a patient with painful, metastatic lung cancer might want to attend a family event that is two weeks away. The successful achievement of this goal depends on many factors, for example, adequate pain control, transportation, and ability to transfer to and from a wheelchair. By breaking the larger goal into several smaller ones, the person is able to identify all the necessary steps and resources. Attainment of a subgoal, such as being able to transfer with minimal assistance can empower patients and families and help energize them to reach more difficult and complex goals.

Supporting patients and families to identify those areas of life and death in which they do have real influence can increase self-esteem and self-efficacy, thereby instilling hope.[22,3151,63,128] It also helps to review their previous successes in attaining important goals.

ENSURING THE SELF-KNOWLEDGE NECESSARY TO PROVIDE PALLIATIVE CARE

Providing holistic palliative care requires a broad range of skills. Astute management of physical symptoms and a solid command of technical skills must be matched with an ability to provide psychosocial and spiritual care for patients and families at a time of great vulnerability. To nurture these latter skills, nurses should continually reflect on and evaluate their own hopes, beliefs, and biases[9,38,94,127] and identify how these factors influence their care. Within particular clinical situations, they should evaluate how patients and families' responses and strategies to maintain hope affect them. For example, does it anger or frustrate the nurse that the patient seems to refuse to acknowledge that his disease is incurable? Is this anger communicated nonverbally or verbally to the patient or family? In addition to self-reflection, it is important for palliative care nurses to maintain hopefulness while working with dying patients by engaging in self-care activities.

SUMMARY

Hope is central to the human experience of living and dying, and is integrally entwined with spiritual and psychosocial well-being. Although terminal illness can challenge and even temporarily diminish hope, the dying process does not inevitably bring despair. The human spirit, manifesting its creativity and resiliency, can forge new and deeper hopes at the end of life. Palliative care nurses play important roles in supporting patients and families with this process by providing expert physical, psychosocial, and spiritual care. Sensitive, skillful attention to maintaining hope can enhance quality of life and contribute significantly to a "good death" as defined by the patient and family. Fostering hope is a primary means by which palliative care nurses accompany patients and families on the journey through terminal illness.

REFERENCES

1. Nouwen H, Gaffney W. Aging. New York: Image Books, 1990.

2. Menninger K. Hope. Bull Menninger Clin 1987;51:447–462.

3. Vaillot MC. Hope: The restoration of being. Am J Nurs 1970;70:268–273.

4. Marcel G. Homo Viator: Introduction to a Metaphysic of Hope. New York: Harper and Row, 1962.

5. Fromm E. The Revolution of Hope. New York: Bantam Books, 1968.

6. Dubree M, Vogelpohl R. When hope dies—So might the patient. American J Nurs 1980;80:2046–2049.

7. Engel GL. A life setting conducive to illness: The giving-up–giving-in complex. Ann Intern Med 1968;69:293–300.

8. Limandri BJ, Boyle DW. Instilling hope. Am J Nurs 1978;78:79–80.

9. Scanlon C. Creating a vision of hope: The challenge of palliative care. Oncol Nurs Forum 1989;16:491–496.

10. Laney L. Hope as a healer. Nurs Outlook 1969;17(1):45–46.

11. Lynch WF. Images of Hope: Imagination as Healer of the Hopeless. New York: New American Library, 1965.

12. Ersek M. Examining the process and dilemmas of reality negotiation. Image: J Nurs Scholarship, 1992;24:19–25.

13. Hinds PS. Inducing a definition of 'hope' through the use of grounded theory methodology. J Adv Nurs 1984;9:357–362.

14. Hinds PS. Adolescent hopefulness in illness and health. Adv Nurs Sci 1988;10(3):79–88.

15. Lange SP. Hope. In Carlson CE, Blackwell B, eds. Behavioral Concepts and Nursing Interventions, 2 ed. Philadelphia: JB Lippincott, 1978.

16. McGee RF. Hope: A factor influencing crisis resolution. Adv Nurs Sci 1984;6(4):34–44.

17. Stotland E. The Psychology of Hope. San Francisco: Jossey-Bass, 1969.

18. Pruyser PW. Phenomenology and the dynamics of hoping. J Sci Study Rel 1963;3:86–96.

19. Dufault K. Hope of Elderly Persons with Cancer. Unpublished dissertation. Cleveland: Case Western Reserve University, 1981.

20. Dufault K, Martocchio B. Hope: Its spheres and dimensions. Nurs Clin North Am 1985;20:379–391.

21. Ersek M. The Process of Maintaining Hope in Adults with Leukemia Undergoing Bone Marrow Transplantation. Doctoral dissertation. Seattle: University of Washington, 1991.

22. Ersek M. The process of maintaining hope in adults undergoing bone marrow transplantation for leukemia. Oncol Nurs Forum 1992;19:883–889.

23. Farran CJ, Herth KA, Popovich JM. Hope and Hopelessness: Critical Clinical Constructs. Thousand Oaks, CA: Sage Publications, 1995.

24. Morse JM, Doberneck B. Delineating the concept of hope. Image: J Nurs Scholarship 1995;27:277–285.

25. Morse JM, Penrod J. Linking concepts of enduring, uncertainty, suffering and hope. Image: J Nurs Scholarship 1999;31:145–150.

26. Taylor EJ. Whys and wherefores: Adult patient perspectives on the meaning of cancer. Semin Oncol Nurs 1995;11:32–40.

27. Carson V, Soeken KL, Shanty J, Terry L. Hope and spiritual well-being: Essentials for living with AIDS. Perspect Psychiatric Care 1990;26(2): 28–34.

28. Fehring RJ, Miller JF, Shaw C. Spiritual well-being, religiosity, hope, depression, and other mood states in elderly people coping with cancer. Oncol Nurs Forum 1997;24:663–671.

29. Haase J, Britt T, Coward D, Leidy N, Penn P. Simultaneous concept analysis of spiritual perspective, hope, acceptance and self-transcendence. Image: J Nurs Scholarship 1992;24:141–147.

30. Mickey JR, Soeken K, Belcher A. Spiritual well-being, religiousness, and hope among women with breast cancer. Image: J Nurs Scholarship 1992;24:267–272.

31. Miller JF. Coping with Chronic Illness: Overcoming Powerlessness, 2 ed. Philadelphia: FA Davis, 1992.

32. Raleigh ED. Sources of hope in chronic illness. Oncology Nurs Forum 1992;19:443–448.

33. Carson V, Soeken KL, Grimm PM. Hope and its relationship to spiritual well-being. J Psychol Theol 1988;16:159–167.

34. Hall BA. The struggle of the diagnosed terminally ill person to maintain hope. Nurs Sci Q 1990;3:177–184.

35. Hall BA. Ways of maintaining hope in HIV disease. Res Nurs Health 1994;17:283–293.

36. Herth KA. Fostering hope in terminally-ill people. J Adv Nurs 1990;15:1250–1259.

37. Yates P. Towards a reconceptualization of hope for patients with a diagnosis of cancer. J Adv Nurs 1993;18:701–706.

38. Taylor EJ, Ersek M. Ethical and spiritual dimensions of cancer pain management. In McGuire D, Yarbro CH, Ferrell BR. Cancer Pain Management. 2 ed. Boston, MA: Jones & Bartlett, 1995.

39. Herth KA. Hope in older adults in community and institutional settings. Issues Mental Health Nurs 1993;14:139–156.

40. Herth KA. Hope in the family caregiver of terminally ill people. J Adv Nurs 1993;18: 538–548.

41. Miller JF. Development of an instrument to measure hope. Dissertation Abstracts International, 47, 1B. (University Microforms No. 8705572.), 1986.

42. Miller JF. Hope-inspiring strategies of the critically ill. Appl Nurs Res 1989;2:23–29.

43. Foote A, Piazza D, Holcombe J, Paul P, Daffin P. Hope, self-esteem, and social support in persons with multiple sclerosis. J Neurosci Nurs 1990;22:155–159.

44. Piazza D, Holcombe J, Foote A, Paul P, Love S, Daffin P. Hope, social support and self-esteem of patients with spinal cord injuries. J Neurosci Nurs 1991;23:224–230.

45. Byrne CM, Woodside H, Landeen J, Kirkpatrick H, Bernardo A, Pawlick J. The importance of relationships in fostering hope. J Psychosoc Nurs 1994;32(9):31–34.

46. Hickey SS. Enabling hope. Cancer Nurs 1986;9:133–137.

47. Hinds PS, Martin J, Vogel RJ. Nursing strategies to influence adolescent hopefulness during oncologic illness. J Assoc Pediatr Oncol Nurses 1987;4(1–2):14–22.

48. Watson J. Nursing: The Philosophy and Science of Caring. Boston: Little, Brown and Co., 1979.

49. Mercer S, Kane R. Helplessness and hopelessness among the institutionalized aged: An experiment. Health Social Work 1979;4:91–116.

50. Seligman MEP. Helplessness. San Francisco: Freeman, 1975.

51. Walding MF. Pain, anxiety and powerlessness. J Adv Nurs 1991;16:388–397.

52. Lazarus RS, Folkman S. Stress, Appraisal, and Coping. New York: Springer Publishing, 1984.

53. Brandt BT. The relationship between hopelessness and selected variables in women receiving chemotherapy for breast cancer. Oncol Nurs Forum 1987;14(2):35–39.

54. Herth KA. The relationship between level of hope and level of coping response and other variables in patients with cancer. Oncol Nurs Forum 1989;16:67–72.

55. Herth KA. Relationship of hope, coping styles, concurrent losses, and setting to grief resolution in the elderly widow(er). Res Nurs Health 1990;13:109–117.

56. Korner IN. Hope as a method of coping. J Consulting Clin Psychol 1970;34:134–139.

57. Weisman AD. Coping with Cancer. New York: McGraw-Hill, 1979.

58. Kim T. Hope as a mode of coping in amyotrophic lateral sclerosis. J Neurosci Nurs 1989; 21:342–247.

59. Hinds PS, Martin J. Hopefulness and the self-sustaining process in adolescents with cancer. Nurs Res 1988;37:336–340.

60. Folkman S, Lazarus RS, Dunkel-Schetter C, DeLongis A, Gruen RJ. Dynamics of a stressful encounter: Cognitive appraisal, coping and encounter outcomes. J Personality Soc Psychol 1986;50:992–1003.

61. Rabkin JG, Williams JB, Neugebauer R, et al. Maintenance of hope in HIV-spectrum homosexual men. Am J Psychiatry 1990;147:1322–1326.

62. Rideout E, Montemuro M. Hope, morale and adaptation in patients with chronic heart failure. J Adv Nurs 1986;11:429–438.

63. Prociuk TJ, Breen LJ, Lussier RJ. Hopelessness, internal-external locus of control, and depression. J Clin Psychol 1976;32:299–300.

64. Minkoff K, Bergman E, Beck AT, Beck R. Hopelessness, depression, and attempted suicide. Am J Psychiatry 1973;130:455–459.

65. Beck AT, Brown G, Steer RA. Prediction of eventual suicide in psychiatric inpatients by clinical ratings of hopelessness. J Consulting Clin Psychol 1989;57:309–310.

66. Beck AT, Steer RA, Kovacs M, Garrison B. Hopelessness and eventual suicide: A 10–year prospective study of patients hospitalized with suicidal ideation. Am J Psychiatry 1985;142:559–563.

67. Perley J, Winget C, Placci C. Hope and discomfort as factors influencing treatment continuance. Compr Psychiatry 1971;12:557–563.

68. Udelman DL, Udelman HD. A preliminary report on anti-depressant therapy and its effects on hope and immunity. Soc Sci Med 1985;20:1069–72.

69. Miller T, Spratt JS. Critical review of reported psychological correlates of cancer prognosis and growth. In: Stoll BA, ed. Mind and Cancer Prognosis. Chichester: John Wiley & Sons, 1979.

70. Schmale AH, Iker H. Hopelessness as a predictor of cervical cancer. Soc Sci Med 1971; 5:95–100.

71. Stoll BA. Is hope a factor in survival? In Stoll BA, ed. Mind and Cancer Prognosis. Chichester: John Wiley & Sons, 1979.

72. Wright BA, Shontz FC. Process and tasks in hoping. Rehab Lit 1968;29:329–331.

73. Artinian B. Fostering hope in the bone marrow transplant child. MaternChild Nurs J 1984;13(1):57–71.

74. Hinds PS, Gattuso J. Measuring hopefulness in adolescents. J Pediatr Oncol Nurs 1991; 8:92–94.

75. Farran CJ. A survey of community-based older adults: Stressful life events, mediating variables, hope, and health. (Doctoral dissertation, Rush University, Chicago). Dissertation Abstracts International 46: 113B, 1985.

76. Farran CJ, Salloway JC, Clark DC. Measurement of hope in a community-based older population. West J Nurs Res 1990;12:42–55.

77. Farran CJ, McCann J. Longitudinal analysis of hope in community-based older adults. Arch Psychiatric Nurs 1989;3:272–276.

78. Miller JF. Developing and maintaining hope in families of the critically ill. AACN Clin Issues 1991;2:307–315.

79. Stetz KM. Caregiving demands during advanced cancer. Cancer Nurs 1987;10:160–168.

80. Patel CT. Hope-inspiring strategies of spouses of critically ill adults. J Holistic Nurs 1996; 14:44–65.

81. Vachon MLS. Psychosocial needs of patients and families. J Palliat Care 1998;14:49–56.

82. Yates P, Stetz KM. Families' awareness of and response to dying. Oncol Nurs Forum 1999; 26:113–119.

83. Stoner MH, Keampfer SH. Recalled life expectancy information, phase of illness and hope in cancer patients. Res Nurs Health 1985;8:269–274.

84. Herth K. Hope from the perspective of homeless families. J Adv Nurs 1996;24:743–753.

85. Spector RE. Cultural Diversity in Health and Illness, 4 ed. Stamford, CT: Appleton & Lange, 1996.

86. Delvecchio-Good M, Good BJ, Schaffer C, Lind S. American oncology and the discourse on hope. Culture, Med Psychiatry 1990;14:59–79.

87. Ersek M, Kagawa-Singer M, Barnes D, Blackhall L, Koenig B. Multicultural considerations in the use of advance directives. Oncol Nurs Forum 1998;25:1683–1690.

88. Beauchamp TL, Childress JF. Principles of Bioethics, 4 ed. New York: Oxford University Press, 1994.

89. Muller JH, Desmond B. Ethical dilemmas in a cross-cultural context: A Chinese example. West J Med 1992;157:323–327.

90. Carrese JA, Rhodes LA. Western bioethics on the Navajo reservation: Benefit or harm? JAMA 1995;274:826–829.

91. Siegel BS. Love, Medicine and Miracles. New York: Harper and Row, 1986.

92. Hepburn K, Reed R. Ethical and clinical issues with Native-American elders. End-of-life decision-making. Clin Geriatr Med 1995;11:97–111.

93. Kagawa-Singer M. Cultural diversity in death and dying. Gerontol Geriatr Med 1994;15: 101–112.

94. Adams CL, Proulx JR. The role of the nurse in the maintenance and restoration of hope. In: Schoenberg B, Kutscher AH, Carr AC, eds. Bereavement: Its Psychosocial Aspects, New York: Columbia University Press, 1975.

95. Jahoda M. Current Concepts of Positive Mental Health. New York: Basic Books, 1958.

96. Janis IL, Mann L. Decision-Making. New York: Free Press, 1977.

97. Freud A. The Ego and Mechanisms of Defense. London: Hogarth Press, 1948.

98. Nisbett RE, Ross L. Human Inference: Strategies and Shortcomings of Social Judgment. Englewood Cliffs, NJ: Prentice-Hall, 1980.

99. Taylor SE, Brown J. Illusion and well-being: A social psychological perspective on mental health. Psychol Bull 1988;103:193–210.

100. Taylor SE. Adjustment to threatening events: A theory of cognitive adaptation. Am Psychologist 1983;38:1161–1171.

101. Taylor SE. Positive Illusions: Creative Self-Deception and the Healthy Mind. New York: Basic Books, 1989.

102. Taylor SE, Collins RL, Skokan LA, Aspinwall LG. Maintaining positive illusions in the face of negative information: Getting the facts without letting them get to you. J Soc Clin Psychol 1989;8:114–129.

103. Taylor SE, Armor DA. Positive illusions and coping with adversity. J Personality 1996;64: 873–898.

104. Taylor SE, Brown J. Positive illusions and well-being revisited: Separating fact from fiction. Psychol Bull 1994;116:21–27.

105. Taylor SE, Lichtman RR, Wood JV. Attributions, beliefs about cancer, and adjustment to breast cancer. J Personality Soc Psychol 1984;46: 489–502.

106. Taylor SE, Kemeny ME, Aspinwall LG, Schneider SG, Rodriguez R, Herbert M. Optimism, coping, psychological distress, and high-risk sexual behavior among men at risk for acquired immunodeficiency syndrome (AIDS). J Personality Soc Psychol 1992;63:460–473.

107. Hackett TP, Cassem NH, Wishnie HA. The coronary-care unit: An appraisal of its psychologic hazards. N Engl J Med 1968;279:1365–1370.

108. Stern MJ, Pascale L, McLoone JB. Psychosocial adaptation following acute myocardial infarction. J Chron Dis 1976;29:513–26.

109. Lazarus RS. The costs and benefits of denial. In: Breznitz S, ed. The Denial of Stress. New York: International Universities Press, 1983.

110. Farran CJ, Wilken C, Popovich JM. Clinical assessment of hope. Issues Ment Health Nurs 1992;13:129–138.

111. Penrod J, Morse JM. Strategies for assessing and fostering hope: The hope assessment guide. Oncol Nurs Forum 1997;24:1055–1063.

112. Beck AT, Weissman A, Lester D, Trexler L. The measurement of pessimism: The hopelessness scale. J Consulting Clin Psychol 1974;42: 861–865.

113. Stoner M. Measuring hope. In Stromberg M, Olsen SJ, eds. Instruments for Clinical Nursing Research. 2 ed. Boston: Jones and Bartlett, 1997.

114. Greene SM, O'Mahony PD, Rungasamy P. Levels of measured hopelessness in physically-ill patients. J Psychosomat Res 1982;26: 591–593

115. Herth KA. Development and refinement of an instrument to measure hope. Scholarly Inquiry Nurs Pract 1991;5:39–51.

116. Herth KA. An abbreviated instrument to measure hope: Development and psychometric evaluation. J Adv Nurs 1992;17:1251–1259.

117. Hinds PS, Stoker H. Adolescents' preferences for a scaling format: A validity issue. J Pediatr Nurs 1988;3:408–411.

118. Miller JF, Powers M. Development of an instrument to measure hope. Nurs Res 1988; 37:6–10.

119. Snyder CR, Harris C, Anderson JR, Holleran SA, Irving LM, Sigmon ST, Yoshinobu L, Gibb J, Langelle C, Harney P. The will and the ways: Development and validation of an individual-differences measure of hope. J Personality Soc Psychol 1991;60:570–585.

120. Snyder CR, Hoza B, Pelham WE, Rapoff M, Ware L, Danovsky M, Highberger L, Rubinstein H, Stahl KJ. The development and validation of the Children's Hope Scale. J Pediatr Psychol 1997;22:399–421.

121. Koopmeiners L, Post-White J, Gutknecht S, Ceronsky C, Nickelson K, Drew D, Mackey KW, Kreitzer MJ. How healthcare professionals contribute to hope in patients with cancer. Oncol Nurs Forum 1997;24:1507–1513.

122. Herth K. Engendering hope in the chronically and terminally ill: Nursing interventions. Am J Hospice Palliat Care 1995;12(5):31–39.

123. Cutliffe JR. Hope, counselling and complicated bereavement reactions. J Adv Nurs 1998;28:754–761.

124. Cousins N. Head First: The Biology of Hope and the Healing Power of the Human Spirit, New York: Penguin, 1989.

125. Taylor SE, Lobel M. Social comparison under threat: Downward comparisons and upward contacts. Psychol Rev 1989;96:569–575.

126. Ersek M, Ferrell BR. Providing relief from cancer pain by assisting in the search for meaning. J Palliat Care 1994;10(4):15–22.

127. Cutliffe JR. How do nurses inspire and instill hope in terminally ill HIV patients? J Adv Nurs 1995;22:888–895.

128. Tollett SP, Thomas SP. A theory-based nursing intervention to instill hope in homeless veterans. Adv Nurs Sci 1995;18(2):76–90.

25 Bereavement

INGE B. CORLESS

The individual appears for an instant, joins the community of thought, modifies it and dies; but the species, that dies not, reaps the fruit of his ephemeral existence."[1] *Those who die not and have a close connection with the deceased are bereaved.*

Bereavement takes many forms. It is influenced first and foremost by culture. In Victorian times, bereaved ladies in the northeast United States wore black for a year and used black-edged stationery while men wore a black armband for a matter of days before resuming their regular activities. Bereavement is also influenced by religious practice, the nature of the relationship with the deceased, the age of the deceased, and the manner of death. In this chapter, the impact of social and cultural forces on the form of bereavement will be examined.

Changes have occurred in what is considered appropriate to the expression of grief. The wearing of black by a widow (widow's weeds) for the remainder of her life and the presumption that grief will be "resolved" within a year are no longer societal expectations. There are other expectations, and these expectations color the expressions of bereavement, loss, mourning, and grief. While the greater emphasis will be given to the discussion of bereavement and grief, it behooves us to define these different terms and examine their related elements.

A MATTER OF DEFINITION

Bereavement

With the pronouncement of death, those who have the closest blood or legal connections to the deceased are considered bereaved. Stated simply, "bereavement is defined as the state of having experienced the death of a significant other."[2] Bereavement confers a special status on the individual entailing both obligations and special rights. The obligations concern disposition of the body and any attendant ceremonies as well as disposal of the worldly goods of the deceased unless indicated otherwise in a legal document such as a last will and testament. The rights include dispensation from worldly activities such as work, and, to a lesser degree, family roles, for a variable period of time. Prior to an expanded discussion of bereavement, it is important to distinguish the concept of bereavement from such other related terms as *loss*, *mourning*, and *grief*.

Loss

Loss is a generic term that signifies absence of an object, position, ability, or attribute. More recently it also has been applied to the death of an animal or person. Absence or loss of the same phenomenon has different implications, depending on the strength of the relationship to the owner. For example, loss of a dog with which there was an indifferent relationship, will result in less emotional disruption for the owner than for one that was cherished. The term is often applied to the death of an individual, and it is the bereaved person who is considered to have experienced a loss. Robinson and McKenna[3] note three critical attributes of loss:

1. Loss signifies that someone or something one has had, or ought to have in the future, has been taken away.
2. That which is taken away must have been valued by the person experiencing the loss.
3. The meaning of loss is determined individually, subjectively, and contextually by the person experiencing it.[3]

As is evident from the example given previously of the loss of a dog that wasn't valued, the individual determination of meaning indicates that the second attribute suggested by Robinson and McKenna, namely that what was lost was valued, is not necessarily congruent with the third attribute, which indicates individual evaluation; and is in fact superfluous. A loss occurs and its meaning is determined by the person who sustained the loss. We can reformulate the attributes of loss as follows:

1. Loss signifies the absence of a possession or future possession.
2. Each loss is valued differently and ranges from no or little value to great value.
3. The meaning of the loss is determined primarily by the individual sustaining it.

This suggests that it is wiser not to make assumptions about loss but to query further as to its meaning to the individual.

Mourning

Mourning has been described in various ways. Kagawa-Singer[4] describes mourning as "the social customs and cultural practices that follow a death." This definition highlights the external manifestations of the process of separation from the deceased and the ultimate reintegration of the bereaved into the family and to varying degrees, society. Durkheim,[5] one of the founders of sociology, stated that "mourning is not a natural movement of private feelings wounded by a cruel loss; it is a duty imposed by the group." This duty is participation in the customary rituals appropriate to membership in a given group. Participation in such rituals has meaning for the mourner and group.[6] These rituals and behaviors acknowledge that a loss has occurred for the individual and the group, and that the individual and the group are adjusting their relationships so as to move forward without the presence of the deceased individual.

DeSpelder and Strickland[7] highlight two important aspects of mourning. They state that "Mourning is the process of incorporating the experience of loss into our ongoing lives. . . . Mourning is also the outward acknowledgement of loss." That outward acknowledgment consists of participation in various death and bereavement rituals. As noted, these vary by religious and cultural traditions as well as by personal preferences. Martinson[8] describes the variation in practices in eastern Asia due to the influences of folk practices, Confucianism, Buddhism, and Christianity.

While ancestor worship is important to varying degrees in Asia, Latin cultures believe in "the interdependence between life and death," a belief that reflects "the value that is placed on the continuity of relationships between the living and the dead.[9] This relationship is considered sacred and is expressed openly in some of the ritual practices dedicated to the dead."[9,10] These practices have many functions, including signifying respect for the deceased and providing a mechanism for the expression of feelings by the bereaved.

Grief

Grief has been defined as "a person's emotional response to the event of loss," the "state of mental and physical pain that is experienced when the loss of a significant object, person, or part of the self is realized," and as "the highly personal and subjective set of responses that an individual makes to a real, perceived, or anticipated loss."[11,12,13] There are numerous definitions of grief and these are only illustrative of variations on a theme. The process of grief has been studied and reformulated, phases identified, types proposed (anticipatory, complicated, disenfranchised), and expressions of grief described. Given that nurses work largely with individuals and families but in some cases also with communities, several sections of this chapter will focus on grief as it relates to these different entities. However, even in those sections that putatively deal with associated topics, the subject of grief is related and may be interwoven. With these preliminary definitions as a basis, bereavement, grief, and mourning will be addressed now in greater depth.

THE PROCESS OF BEREAVEMENT

In the process of measuring core bereavement phenomena, Burnett, Middleton, Raphael, and Martinek[14] have identified seventeen items which they consider central to the process of bereavement. These items are categorized under three subscales, namely images and thoughts (e.g., "Do you think about 'x'?"), acute separation (e.g., "Do you find yourself missing 'x'?"), and grief (e.g., "Do reminders of 'x' such as photos, situations, music, places, etc. cause you to cry about 'x'?").[15] While the purpose of this scale is to "assess the intensities of the bereavement reaction in different community samples of bereaved subjects," the bereavement reaction that is being addressed is grief.[16]

The distinction between grief and depression in the bereaved is an important one. As Middleton, Franzp, Raphael, Franzp, Burnett, and Martinek[17] conclude, "The bereaved can experience considerable pain and yet be coping adaptively, and they can fulfill many depressive criteria yet at the same time be experiencing phenomena that are not depressive in nature." Even in individuals with a history of "sadness or irritability" prior to bereavement, although they may have more intense expressions of grief, the rate of recovery is the same as those without such a history.[18] Other authors are not as sanguine and caution that subsyndromal symptomatic depressions are "frequently seen complications of bereavement that may be chronic and often are associated with substantial morbidity."[19] The use of nortriptyline and psychotherapy have been found efficacious in the treatment of bereavement-related major depressive episodes.[20]

Bereavement-related grief is conceptualized by Rubin[21] into two pathways: (*1*) "a dimension concerned with how the bereaved individual functions following loss" and (*2*) "a dimension concerned with the nature of that individual's relational bond to the deceased." He notes further that loss involves disruption of the multiple spheres of the individual's life. Bereavement involves adjustment to these disruptions.

Rubin developed a two-track model of bereavement as a "means of understanding and addressing the bereavement process and its outcome."[22] He states that "Track I focuses on the physiological, somatic, affective, cognitive, social and behavioral factors that are affected by loss—and Track II examines ways of transforming the bereaved's attachment to the deceased and establishing new forms of ongoing relationship to the memories of that person."[23] In essence bereavement involves adjusting to a world without the physical, psychological, and social presence of the deceased.

Bereavement becomes complicated (in the literature and in life) when adjustment is impeded, as in post-traumatic stress disorder.[24] Whether such bereavement occurs as a result of vehicular accident, war, or natural disaster, the suddenness or overwhelming nature of the event dislodges the sense of all being well with the world. Even in such instances where an elective medical procedure such as abortion occurs, the emotional response may not become evident until many years later.

Death before its time, as in children and young and middle-aged adults, affects not only who is bereaved but also the social roles of the survivors, which require readjustment. Hutton and Bradley,[25] in their study of the bereaved siblings of babies who were casualties of sudden infant death, were uncertain as to whether these siblings actually exhibited more behavioral problems or were thought to be doing so by mothers whose perceptions were distorted. The need for greater attention to children who are bereaved was underscored by Mahon,[26] who notes that most of the literature in this area concerns "parental impressions of children's grief and studies of adolescent bereavement." The hesitancy of children to exhibit their own sadness so as not to upset their parents requires that professionals encourage parents to give their children permission to be sad when that is how they feel. By taking care of their parents, children may not receive the attention they require. In a study that sought to identify those factors that helped or hindered adolescent sibling bereavement, a youngster stated: "What helped me the most was my mother who was totally honest with me from the time Sarah got sick through her death. My mother took the time to listen to how I felt as well as understand and hug me."[27]

Formal programs of bereavement for children's support include peer support programs and art therapy programs. Institutions with bereavement programs, whether for children or adults, often send cards at the time of a patient's death, the birthday of the deceased, as well as at 3, 6, 12, and 24 months after the death.[28] Pamphlets with information about grief, a bibliography of appropriate readings, and contact numbers of support groups are also helpful.[29] Lev and McCorkle[30] cite Potocky's[31] finding that short-term programs meeting from two to seven times or as needed were the most effective.

Attention to bereavement support has also been given by institutional trauma programs, in emergency departments, and in critical care departments.[32,33,34] All of these programs maintain contact with the bereaved so as to provide support and make referrals to pastoral care personnel and other professionals as needed. Indeed the combination of "religious psychotherapy" and a cognitive-behavioral approach was observed to be helpful to highly religious bereaved persons.[35] Religious psychotherapy for a group of Malays who adhered to the religion of Islam consisted of discussion and "the reading of verses of the Koran and Hadith, the encouragement of prayers. . . . All patients were given a total of 12–16 psychotherapy sessions."[36] Targeting of the follow-up to the characteristics of the population eschews the notion that one size fits all.

A bereavement support group intervention has been demonstrated to have a significant impact on the grief of both HIV-1 seropositive and seronegative homosexual men.[37] Cognitive processing and finding meaning were found to have immunologic and health benefits independent of the baseline health status of the bereaved HIV-positive homosexual men.[38] This outcome has implications for the approaches nurses use with other bereaved clients.

Cognitive processing and finding meaning can be helpful to a variety of clients. Older persons have been noted, however, to be more reluctant to express their feelings.[39] Nurses can be helpful to these clients by encouraging them to express their feelings and being available when needed.[40]

Aside from such proactive approaches for all bereaved persons, Sheldon[41] notes the following predisposing factors for a poor bereavement outcome: "ambivalent or dependent relationship, multiple prior bereavements, previous mental illness, especially depression and low self-esteem." Billings[42] adds prior physical health problems to these predisposing factors. Around the time of death, Sheldon identifies the following factors: "sudden and unexpected death, untimely death of a young person, preparation for the death, stigmatized deaths—such as AIDS, suicide, culpable deaths, sex of the bereaved person—elderly male widower, caring for the deceased person for over six months, inability to carry out valued religious rituals."[43] Finally, after the death, such factors as "level of perceived social support, lack of opportunities for new interests, stress from other life crises" as well as "dysfunctional behaviors and attitudes appearing early in the bereavement period—consumption of alcohol and drugs, smoking, morbid guilt" and the "professional caregiver's gut feeling that this patient will not do well." are predictive of poor outcomes.[44,45] Knowledge of and alertness to such predisposing factors are useful for the provision of help, both lay and professional, early in the course of the bereavement so as to prevent further debilitating events.

Grief

Rando[46] observes that although Freud was not the first person to examine the effects of bereavement, he nonetheless is taken as an important point of departure. The observation that grief is a normal process and that "a lost love object is never totally relinquished" are congruent with current thinking.[47] The notion that one needs to totally "let go" of the beloved, ascribed to Freud on the basis of some of his work, has influenced professionals to the current day.

The initiation of the modern study of death and dying, especially in America, however, is often attributed to Erich Lindemann, a physician at Massachusetts General Hospital, who responded to the survivors of a fire in Boston's Coconut Grove nightclub. Five hundred persons died as a result of the fire, which took place on Thanksgiving eve, 1942. Lindemann, a psychiatrist, was interested at the time in "the emotional reaction of patients to body disfigurement and plastic surgery."[48] With this background, "Lindemann was struck by the similarity of responses between his patients' reactions to facial disfigurement or loss of a body part and the reactions of the survivors of the fire."[49] Lindemann's study of 101 patients included (*1*) psychoneurotic patients who lost a relative during the course of treatment, (*2*) relatives of patients who died in the hospital, (*3*) bereaved disaster victims (Coconut Grove fire) and their close relatives, and (*4*) relatives of members of the armed forces.[50]

These patients were the basis of his observations of the five indicators that are "pathognomonic for grief."[51] They are: "(1) sensations of somatic distress, such as tightness in the throat, choking and shortness of breath; (2) intense preoccupation with the image of the deceased; (3) strong feelings of guilt; (4) a loss of warmth toward others with a tendency to respond with irritability and anger; and (5) disoriented behavior patterns."[52] Lindemann[53] coined the term *grief work* to describe the process by which individuals attempted to adjust to their loss.

Various theorists have developed a series of stages and phases of grief work.[54,55,56,57] The most well known of these to the general public are those formulated by Elizabeth Kübler-Ross.[58] Proposed for those facing a death, these stages have also been applied to those experiencing a loss. Kübler-Ross identified five stages: denial and isolation, anger, bargaining, depression, and acceptance.[59] The commonality among all theorists of the stages of grief is that there is (*1*) notification and shock; (*2*) experience of the loss emotionally and cognitively; and (*3*) reintegration. Rando,[60] for example, uses the terms *avoidance, confrontation,* and *reestablishment.* Building on the work of Worden,[61] Corr and Doka[62] propose the following tasks:

1. to share acknowledgment of the reality of death
2. to share in the process of working through to the pain of grief
3. to reorganize the family system
4. to restructure the family's relationship with the deceased and to reinvest in other relationships and life pursuits

This latter task has also given rise to some dispute over the degree to which separation from the deceased must occur.

Klass, Silverman, and Nickman[63] make the compelling argument that such bonds continue. They aver "survivors hold the deceased in loving memory for long periods, often forever," and that maintaining an inner representation of the deceased is normal rather than abnormal.[64] The second area of dissension and new consensus is the expectation that grief must be resolved within a year, which is not to say that the expected trajectory of grieving is one in which grief continues at an intense pitch for years. The question of continuing bonds and the length of the grief process will be addressed again at the close of the chapter. In this next section, types of grief will be examined.

TYPES OF GRIEF

The types of grief examined in this section are not exhaustive of all types of grief but rather encompass the major categories.

Anticipatory Grief

Anticipatory grief shares similarities with other forms of grief. It is also different. The onset may be associated with the receipt of bad news such as a terminal diagnosis.[65] Anticipatory grief must be distinguished from the concept of forewarning. An example of forewarning is learning of a terminal diagnosis. Anticipatory grief is an unconscious process, whereas forewarning is a conscious process. With forewarning of a terminal diagnosis the question is "What if we do?" With a death that question has become "What if we had done?" With the former question, there is the potential for hope; with the latter query, there may be guilt. Stephenson[66] describes a roller-coaster effect of hope slashed with experience countered by hope. Even with forewarning, the preparation for loss may not occur, given that this may be perceived to be a betrayal of the terminally ill person. There have also been instances of family members unconsciously preparing for the death of an individual and going through the grieving process only to have that person recover to find no place in the lives of his or her loved ones. This is an example of anticipatory grief.

The question of the utility of forewarning is one of how this time is utilized. If it is utilized to make some preparation for role change, such as becoming familiar with the intricacies of the role the terminally ill person plays in the family—mastering a checking account or other financial aspects of the family—such time may be used to the benefit of all concerned. On the other hand, anticipatory grieving that results in reinvestment of emotional energy prior to the death of the terminally ill person is detrimental to the relationship. Byrne and Raphael[67] found that "widowers who were unable to anticipate their wife's death, even when their wife had suffered a long final illness, had a more severe bereavement reaction." (The term *anticipate* is being used by Byrne and Raphael in the sense of forewarning.)

Duke,[68] in a qualitative study of anticipatory grief, enlarges our understanding not so much of anticipatory grief, but of the status changes of widowhood. She interviewed five spouses in the second year of their bereavement. While the findings may be biased by hindsight, they provide much food for thought. The research identified four areas of change: "role change from spouse to carer during the illness; loss of those roles in bereavement to needing to be cared for; relationship changes from being with spouse to being alone; coping changes from being in suspense to being in turmoil; and change related to experiencing and gathering memories to remembering and constructing memories."[69] It is interesting that these findings reflect the general changes that occur over a terminal illness and not the experience of anticipatory grief. Anticipatory grief as noted previously is unconscious preparation for status change and not a conscious, deliberative process. Anticipatory grief will be contrasted with what is termed *uncomplicated grief.*

Uncomplicated Grief

Uncomplicated grief, or normal grief, is described by Cowles[70] as dynamic, pervasive, highly individualized, and a process. Worthington[71] depicts a linear model of grief which he notes is based on adjustment. In this model, an individual in a normal emotional state experiences a loss causing a reaction and an emotional low. Subsequently the individual begins a recovery to his or her former state. This process of recovery is occasioned by brief periods of relapse, but not to the depths experienced previously. Ultimately the individual moves to adjustment to the loss.[72] While this description simplifies the turmoil that may be experienced, discussion of expressions of grief later in this chapter will capture the physical, psychological, behavioral and social upset that characterizes even uncomplicated grief.

Niemeyer[73] offers a vital new perspective by focusing on meaning reconstruction. He has developed a set of propositions to capture adaptation to loss.

1. Death as an event can validate or invalidate the constructions that form the basis on which we live, or it may stand as a novel experience for which we have no constructions.[74]
2. Grief is a personal process, one that is idiosyncratic, intimate and inextricable from our sense of who we are.[75]
3. Grieving is something we do, not something that is done to us.[76]
4. Grieving is the act of affirming or reconstructing a personal world of meaning that has been challenged by loss.[77]
5. Feelings have functions and should be understood as signals of the state of our meaning-making efforts.[78]
6. We construct and reconstruct our identities as survivors of loss in negotiations with others.[79]

Niemeyer views meaning reconstruction as the central process of grief.[80] The inability to make meaning may lead to complications.

Complicated Grief

In her discussion of complicated mourning, Rando makes observations applicable to complicated grief. She notes that after a suitable length of time the mourner is attempting to "deny, repress, or avoid aspects of the loss, its pain, and its implications and . . . to hold onto and avoid relinquishing, the lost loved one. These attempts or some variants thereof, . . . cause the complications in . . . mourning."[81]

Researchers have identified the diagnostic criteria for complicated grief disorder.[82] These criteria include: "the current experience (more than a year after a loss) of intensive intrusive thoughts, pangs of severe emotion, distressing yearnings, feeling excessively alone and empty, excessively avoiding tasks reminiscent of the deceased, unusual sleep disturbances, and maladaptive levels of loss of interest in personal activities."[83] Other researchers underscore the need for the specification of complicated grief as a unique disorder and have developed an inventory of complicated grief to measure maladaptive symptoms of loss.[84,85,86] The Inventory of Complicated Grief is composed of 19 items with responses ranging from *never* to *rarely*, *sometimes*, *often*, and *always*. Examples of items include: "I think about this person so much that it's hard for me to do the things I usually do; "Ever since s/he died it is hard for me to trust people"; "I feel that it is unfair that I should live when this person died"; "I feel lonely a great deal of the time ever since s/he died."[87] This inventory may be helpful to health care practitioners. Finally, it is the severity of symptomatology and the duration that distinguishes abnormal and complicated responses to bereavement.[88] A caveat: There is some concern among professionals that what is a normal process is being medicalized by health care practitioners. More will be said about this later in the chapter. Bearing this in mind, disenfranchised grief poses different but potentially related problems.

Disenfranchised Grief

Doka[89] defines disenfranchised grief as "the grief that persons experience when they incur a loss that is not or cannot be openly acknowledged, publicly mourned, or socially supported." Doka continues, "The concept of disenfranchised grief recognizes that societies have sets of norms—in effect, grieving rules—that attempt to specify who, when, where, how, how long, and for whom people should grieve."[90] And also, who may publicly grieve and expect to receive support.

Relationships that may not be publicly acknowledged such as those with a mistress or family conceived outside a legally recognized union, or in some cases step-families, colleagues, friends, and so on, are not accorded the deference and support usually accorded the bereaved. Further nonsanctioned relationships, either heterosexual as mentioned above, or homosexual, may result in the exclusion of individuals not legitimated by blood or legal union. Individuals in homosexual relationships of long standing who care for their partners throughout their illness, whether HIV/AIDS or other, may find themselves barred both from the funeral and the home that was shared.[91]

For some time, infection with the human immunodeficiency virus was hidden from the community, thereby depriving both the infected and their caregivers of support. The AIDS quilt has done much to provide a public mourning ritual but has not alleviated the disenfranchised status of homosexual or lesbian partners. The result is what has been termed "modulated mourning."[92] This response to stigmatization constrains the public display of mourning by the griever. In this situation the griever is not recognized. There are other instances when the loss has not been legitimized.

Loss as a result of miscarriage or abortion has not been recognized until more recently. In Japan, a "cemetery" is devoted to letters written by families each year telling the miscarried or aborted about the important events that occurred in the family that year and also expressing their continued grief at the loss.

Grieving in secret is a burden that makes the process more difficult to complete. Disenfranchised grief may also be a harbinger of unresolved grief.

Unresolved Grief

Unresolved grief is a failure to accomplish the necessary grief work. A variety of factors may give rise to unresolved grief, including "guilt, loss of an extension of the self, reawakening of an old loss, multiple loss, inadequate ego development, idiosyncratic resistance to mourning."[93] In addition to these psychological factors such social factors as "social negation of a loss, socially unspeakable loss, social isolation and/or geographic distance from social support, assumption of the role of the strong one, and uncertainty over the loss" (a disappearance or loss at sea, for example) may be implicated in unresolved grief.[94] By helping significant others express their feelings and complete their business prior to the death of a loved one, unresolved grief and the accompanying manifestations can be prevented to some extent.

Eakes, Burke, and Hainsworth[95] question whether closure is a necessary outcome. They explored what they term "chronic sorrow" in bereaved individuals who experienced episodic bouts of sadness related to specific incidents or significant dates. These authors suggest the fruitfulness of maintaining an open-ended model of grief.[96] With this in mind, grief will always be unresolved to some degree and this is not considered pathological but an acknowledgment of a death.

EXPRESSIONS OF GRIEF

In some of the earlier sections of this chapter, various manifestations of grief have been noted. In this section, expressions of grief that are within the range considered normal in this society are described. It is important to note that what is considered appropriate in one group may be considered deviant and even pathological in another.

In Table 25–1, physical, cognitive, emotional, and behavioral symptoms are presented. Table 25–1 is not exhaustive of all of the potential symptoms but rather is illustrative of the expressions and manifestations of grief. What distinguishes so-called normal grief is that it is usually self-limiting. Manifestations of grief at 1 month, 3 months, and 15 months are not the same in intensity. Nor are the outward manifestations that are the expressions of mourning.

Mourning

O'Gorman[97] contrasts death rituals in England with those in Ireland. She recalls the "Protestant hushed respectfulness which had somehow infiltrated and taken over a Catholic community."[98] The body was taken from the home by the funeral director. Children continued with school and stayed with relatives. They were shielded from the death. By way of contrast, she recounts an Irish wake. "The body, laid out by a member of the family, in order to receive a 'special blessing', would be in the parlour of a country house surrounded by flowers from the garden and lighted candles."[99] The children, along with the adult members of the family, view the corpse. "When visitors had paid their last respects they would join the crowd in the kitchen who would then spend all night recounting stories associated with the dead person."[100] O'Gorman notes the plentiful availability of alcohol and states, "By the end of the night to the uninitiated the event would appear to be more like a party than a melancholy event."[101] While O'Gorman initially found this distasteful, she "now believes that rituals like the Irish wake celebrate death as a happy occasion and bestow grace upon those leaving life and upon a community of those who mourn them."[102]

The Irish wake, like the reception held in a church basement, VFW hall, restaurant, or private home, serves not only for the expression of condolences but also as an opportunity to reinforce the connections of the community. Anyone familiar with such events knows that a variety of social and business arrangements are made by mourners both within and outside the immediate family. And while some gatherings are more reserved and others lustier, giving the deceased a good send-off ("good" being defined by the group) is central to each. The good send-off is part of the function of the funeral as piacular rite, that is, as a means of atoning for the sins of the mortal being and as preparation for life in the afterworld.[103] Fulton[104] notes two other functions of funerals, namely integration and separation. The former concerns the living, the latter refers to separation from the loved one as a mortal person. The value of the Irish wake, which in the United States may look more like the Protestant burial O'Gorman describes, is the time spent together sharing stories and feelings. In the Irish wake as practiced in Ireland, one is not alone with one's feelings but in the company of others who are devoting the time to mourning (integration).

This devotion of time to mourning is also found in the Jewish religion, where the bereaved sit "shiva," usually for seven days.[105] In Judaism, the assumption is that the bereaved are to fo-

Table 25–1. Manifestations of Grief

Physical	Cognitive	Emotional	Behavioral
Headaches	Sense of depersonalization	Anger	Impaired work performance
Dizziness	Inability to concentrate	Guilt	Crying
Exhaustion	Sense of disbelief and confusion	Anxiety	Withdrawal
Muscular aches	Idealization of the deceased	Sense of helplessness	Avoiding reminders of the deceased
Sexual impotency	Search for meaning of life and death	Sadness	Seeking or carrying reminders of the deceased
Loss of appetite	Dreams of the deceased	Shock	Overreactivity
Insomnia	Preoccupation with image of deceased	Yearning	Changed relationships
Feelings of tightness or hollowness	Fleeting visual, tactile, olfactory, auditory hallucinatory experiences	Numbness	
Breathlessness		Self-blame	
Tremors		Relief	
Shakes			
Oversensitivity to noise			

Source: Based on K. Doka. Grief, In: R Kastenbaum and B Kastenbaum (Eds.) *Encyclopedia of Death*. Phoenix, Oryx Press, 1989:127.

cus on their loss and the grief of that loss. They are to pay no attention to worldly considerations. This period of time of exemption from customary roles may facilitate the process. Certainly having a minion, where ten men and women (ten men for the Orthodox) say prayers each evening reinforces the reality of the death and the separation. For the Orthodox, the mourning period is for one year.

A very different pattern is practiced by the Hopi in Arizona. The Hopi have a brief ceremony with the purpose of completing the funeral as quickly as possible so as to get back to customary activities.[106] The fear of death and the dead and spirits induces distancing by the Hopi from nonliving phenomena.

Stroebe and Stroebe[107] contrast Shinto and Buddhist mourners in Japan with the Hopi. Both Shinto and Buddhist mourners practice ancestor worship. As a result, the bereaved can keep contact with the deceased, who become ancestors. Speaking to ancestors as well as offering food is accepted practice.[108]

The difference between this Japanese practice and what occurs in the United States is that in the United States, those bereaved who speak with a deceased person do so quietly, hiding the fact from others, believing others will consider it suspect or pathological. It is, however, a common occurrence. Bringing food to the ancestor or, to celebrate the Day of the Dead, to the cemetery, is part of the mourning practice in Hispanic and many other societies.

Practices, however, change with time; although one can often find the imprint of earlier rituals. The practice of saving a lock of hair or the footprint of a deceased newborn may have evolved from the practice in Victorian times of using hair for mourning brooches and lockets. As the salesperson of these items commented, "They liked to be reminded of their dead in those days. Now it's out of sight, out of mind."[109] These practices provide continuing bonds with the deceased and offer a clue to the answer to the question posed for the last section of this chapter: when is it over? Prior to addressing this question, another needs to be raised, and that is of support.

A QUESTION OF SUPPORT

Many of the mourning practices noted previously provide support by the community to the bereaved (see Table 25–2). Formal support is exemplified by the practice of attending a minion for the deceased Jewish person. It expresses support for the living. It is formal in that it is prescribed behavior on the part of observant Jews and incorporates a prayer service. Other examples of formal support include support groups such as the widow-to-widow program and the Compassionate Friends, Inc. for families of deceased children.

The assumption underlying the widow-to-widow program is that grief and mourning are not in and of themselves pathological and that lay persons can be helpful to one another. The widow-to-widow program provides a formal mechanism for sharing one's emotions and experience with individuals who have had a similar experience. The Widowed Persons Service offers support for men and women via self-help support groups and a variety of educational and social activities. The Compassionate Friends, Inc., also a self-help organization, seeks to help parents and siblings after the death of a child. Other support groups may or may not have the input of a professional to run the group.

Support groups may be open-ended, that is, without a set number of sessions, or they may be closed and limited to a particular set of individuals. Support groups with a set number of sessions have a beginning and end and are therefore more likely to be closed to new members until a new set of sessions begins. Open-ended groups have members who stay for varying lengths of time and may or may not have a topic for each session.

Other formal support entails working with a therapist or other health care provider. Arnold[110] suggests the following process for the nurse, namely to assess the "Meaning of loss . . . Nature of the Relationship . . . Expressions and Manifestations of Grief . . . Previous Experience with Grief . . . Support Systems . . . Ability to Maintain Attachments . . . Progression of Grief." Further, Arnold underscores the importance of viewing grief as a healing process (see Table 25–3). She gives the following example of a patient situation and two different approaches to diagnosis.

> A newly widowed woman feels awkward about maintaining social relationships with a group of married couples with whom she had participated with her husband.
>
> **Grief as a pathological diagnosis:** social isolation
>
> **Grief as a healthy diagnosis:** redefinition of social supports.[111]

In addition to conventional talking therapy, such techniques as letter writ-

Table 25–2. Bereavement Practices

Lay	Professional
1. Friendly visiting	1. Clergy visiting
2. Provision of meals	2. Clergy counseling
3. Informal support by previously bereaved	3. Nurse, M.D., psychologist, social worker, psychiatrist counseling
4. Lay support groups	4. Professionally led support groups
5. Participation in cultural and religious rituals	5. Organization of memorial services by hospice and palliative care organizations
6. A friendly listener	6. A thoughtful listener
7. Involvement in a cause-related group	7. Referral to individuals with similar cause-related concerns
8. Exercise	8. Referral to a health club
9. Joining a new group	9. Referral to a bereavement program

Table 25–3. Assessment of Grief

The bereaved often are weary from caring for the deceased. During this period they may not have looked after themselves. An assessment should include:

1. A general health checkup and assessment of somatic symptoms
2. A dental visit
3. An eye checkup as appropriate
4. Nutritional evaluation
5. Sleep assessment
6. Examination of ability to maintain work and family roles
7. Determination of whether there are major changes in presentation of self
8. Assessment of changes resulting from the death and the difficulties with these changes
9. Assessment of social networks

The health care worker needs to bear in mind that there is no magic formula for grieving. The key question is whether the bereaved is able to function effectively. Cues to the need for assistance include:

1. Clinical depression
2. Prolonged deep grief
3. Extreme grief reaction
4. Self-destructive behavior
5. Increased use of alcohol and/or drugs
6. Preoccupation with the deceased to the exclusion of others
7. Previous mental illness
8. Perceived lack of social support

ing, empty chair, guided imagery, and journal writing can be utilized (see Table 25–4).[112] In letter writing, the empty chair technique, and guided imagery, the bereaved is encouraged to express feelings about the past or what life is like without the deceased. These techniques can be helpful as the "wish I had said" becomes said. A journal, on the other hand, is also a vehicle for recording ongoing feelings of the lived experience of bereavement.

Another part of bereavement counseling is the instillation or reemergence of hope. As Cutcliffe[113] concludes, "There are many theories of bereavement counseling, with commonalities between these theories. Whilst the theories indicate implicitly the re-emergence of hope in the bereft individual as a result of the counseling, they do not make specific reference to how this inspiration occurs." Cutcliffe sees the clear need to understand this process.

In her exposition of the concept "hope," Stephenson[114] notes the association made by Frankl with meaning. Stephenson states "Frankl equated hope with having found meaning in life, and lack of hope as have[having] no meaning in life."[115,116] Meaning-making appears key to the emergence of hope, and hope has been associated with coping.[117]

In hospice programs, health care providers encourage dying persons and families to have hope for each day. This compression of one's vision to the here and now may also be useful for the person who is grieving the loss of a loved one. Hope for the future and a personal future is the process that Cutcliffe wishes to elucidate. It may be a process that is predicated on hope for each day, and having found meaning for the past.

A therapist provides a vehicle for the ongoing discussion of the loss that informal caregivers may be unable to provide. A support group of bereaved individuals or periodic contact by an institutional bereavement service may also prove useful. What is helpful depends on the individual and his or her needs and also the informal support that is available.

Informal Support

Informal support that is perceived as supportive and helpful can assist the bereaved to come to terms with life after the death of the beloved. Whether the bereaved is isolated or is part of a family or social group is of tremendous import to the physical, psychological, and social welfare of the individual. Community in a psychosocial sense and a continuing role in the group are key factors in adjustment. In societies where the widow has no role without her husband, she is figuratively if not literally disposed of in one way or another.

It is for this reason that the woman who is the first in her group to experience widowhood has a much more difficult social experience than a woman who is in a social group where several women have become widows. In the former there is no reference group; in the latter there is.

The presence of family and friends takes on added significance after the initial weeks after the funeral. In those initial weeks friendly visiting occurs with provision of a variety of types of foods considered appropriate in the group. After the initial period, friendly visiting is likely to decrease and the bereaved may find themselves alone or the objects of financial predators. The counsel by the health care provider or by family and friends not to make life-altering decisions such as moving, unless absolutely necessary, continues to be valuable advice. On the other hand, the comment that "time makes it easier" is a half truth that is not perceived as helpful by the bereaved.[118,119]

What is helpful is being listened to by an interested person. Quinton[120] dislikes the term *counseling* in that is implies the availability of a person with good counsel to confer. What Quinton considers important is "lots of listening to what the victim wants to off-load."[121] She notes further, "The turning point for me was realizing that I had a right to feel sad, and to grieve and to feel miserable for as long as I felt the need."[122] By owning the grieving process, Quinton provided herself with the most important support for her recovery from a devastating experience—her mother's murder in a massacre by the Irish Republican Army in 1987. The lesson is applicable, however, to any bereaved person re-

Table 25–4. Counseling Interventions

It must be emphasized that grief is not a pathology. It is a normal process that is expressed in individual ways. The following techniques may prove helpful to the individual who is experiencing guilt about things not said or done. This list is not exhaustive, merely illustrative.

A. Letter writing	The bereaved writes a letter to the deceased expressing the thoughts and feelings that may or may not have been expressed
B. Empty chair	The bereaved sits across from an empty chair on which the deceased is imagined to be sitting. The bereaved is encouraged to express his or her feelings
C. Empty chair with picture	A picture of the deceased is placed on the chair to facilitate the expressions of feelings by the bereaved
D. Therapist assumes role of the deceased	In this intervention, the therapist helps the bereaved to explore his or her feelings toward the deceased by participating in a role play
E. Guided imagery	This intervention demands a higher level of skill than, for example, letter writing. Guided imagery can be used to explore situations that require verbalization by the bereaved to achieve completion. Imagery can also be used to recreate situations of dissension with the goal of achieving greater understanding for the bereaved
F. Journal writing	This technique provides an ongoing vehicle for exploring past situations and current feelings. It is a helpful intervention to many
G. Drawing picture	For the artistically and not so artistically inclined, drawing pictures and explaining their content is another vehicle for discussing feelings and concerns
H. Analysis of role changes	Helping the bereaved obtain help with the changes secondary to the death, such as with balancing a checkbook or securing reliable help with various home needs, assists with some of the secondary losses with the death of a loved one
I. Listening	The bereaved has the need to tell his or her story. Respectful listening and concern for the bereaved is a powerful intervention that is much appreciated
J. Venting anger	The professional can suggest the following: • Banging a pillow on the mattress. If combined with screaming it is the best to do with the windows closed and no one in the home • Screaming—at home as above or when parked in a car in an isolated spot with the windows closed • Crying—at home followed by a warm bath and cup of tea or warm milk
K. Normality barometer	Assuring the bereaved that the distress experienced is normal is very helpful to the bereaved

gardless of whether the death was traumatic or anticipated. Quinton's turning point is another clue to answering the question of the last section of this chapter: When is it over?

WHEN IS IT OVER?

To use the colloquial phrase, it's not over until it's over. What does this mean? As long as life and memory persist, the deceased remain part of our consciousness. When is the grieving over? Unfortunately, there is no easy answer and the only reasonable response is "it depends." Lindemann's concept of grief work, mentioned earlier in this chapter, is applicable. Sooner or later that work needs to be accomplished. Delay protracts the time when accommodation is made. And grief work is never over in the sense that there will be moments years hence when an occasion or object revives feelings of loss. The difference is that the pain is not the same acute pain experienced when the loss initially occurred. How one arrives at the point of accommodation is a process termed *letting go.*

Letting Go

The term letting go refers to acknowledgment of the loss of future togetherness—physical, psychological, and social. There is no longer a "we," only an "I" or a "we" without the deceased. Family members speak of the first time a flower or bush blooms, major holidays, birthdays, anniversaries, and special shared times. Corless[123] quotes Jacqueline Kennedy who spoke about "last year" (meaning 1962–1963) as the last time that her husband, John Kennedy, experienced a specific occasion.

> On so many days—his birthday, an anniversary, watching his children running to the sea—I have thought, "but this day last year was his last to see that." He was so full of love and life on all those days. He seems so vulnerable now, when you think that each one was a last time.

Mrs. Kennedy also writes about the process of letting go, although she doesn't call it that.

> Soon the final day will come around again—as inexorably as it did last year. But expected this time. It will find some of us different people than we were a year ago. Learning to accept what was unthinkable when he was alive changes you.[124]

Finally, she addresses an essential truth of bereavement.

> I don't think there is any consolation. What was lost cannot be replaced.[125]

Letting go encompasses recognizing the uniqueness of the individual. It also entails finding meaning in the relationship and experience. It does not mean cutting oneself off from the memories of the deceased.

Continuing Bonds

Klass, Silverman, and Nickman[126] contributed to the reformulation of our thinking on the nature of accommodating to loss. Although theorists postulated that the grief process should be completed in one year and one's emotional energies invested in the living, the experience of the bereaved suggested otherwise. Bereaved persons visit the grave for periodic discussions with the deceased. They gaze at a picture and seek advice on various matters. Such behavior is not pathological.

It is our expectation that teachers in the educational system will have an influence on their students. The students progress and may or may not have continuing contact with those educators. Given that assumption about education, how could we not expect to feel the continuing influence and have memory of those informal teachers in our lives, our deceased family members and friends? Integration of those influences strengthens the individual at any point in his or her life.

A Turkish expression in the presence of death is "May you live."[127] That indeed is the challenge of bereavement.

REFERENCES

1. Byatt AS. Possession—A Romance. (p. 6). New York: Vintage Books. 1990.

2. Warren NA. Bereavement care in the critical care setting. Crit Care Nurs Q 1997;20(2):42.

3. Robinson DS, McKenna HP. Loss: An analysis of a concept of particular interest to nursing. J Adv Nurs 1998;27:782.

4. Kagawa-Singer M. The cultural context of death rituals and mourning practices. ONF 1998; 25(10):1752.

5. Durkheim E. The Elementary Forms of Religious Life. New York: Collier, 1961:443.

6. Stephenson JS. Grief and mourning. In R Fulton, R Bendickson (Eds.), Death and Identity, 3 ed. Philadelphia: Charles Press, 1994:136–176.

7. DeSpelder LA, Strickland AL. The Last Dance 2 ed. Mountain View, CA: Mayfield Publishing Company, 1987:207.

8. Martinson IM. Funeral rituals in Taiwan and Korea. ONF 1998;25(10):1756–1760.

9. Chidester D. Patterns of Transcendence: Religion, Death and Dying. Belmont, CA: Wadsworth, 1990.

10. Munet-Vilaro F. Grieving and death rituals of Latinos. ONF 1998;25(10):1761.

11. DeSpelder and Strickland, loc. cit.

12. Stephenson, loc. cit., p. 136.

13. Doka K. Grief. In R. Kastenbaum and B. Kastenbaum (Eds.). Encyclopedia of Death (p. 127). Phoenix: Oryx Press, 1989.

14. Burnett P, Middleton W, Raphael B, Martinek N. Measuring core bereavement phenomena. Psychol Med 1997;27:49–57.

15. Ibid., p. 56.

16. Ibid., p. 51.

17. Middleton W, Franzp MD, Raphael B, Franzp MD, Burnett P, Martinek N. Psychological distress and bereavement. J Nerv Ment Dis 1997;185:452.

18. Hays JC, Kasl S, Jacobs S. Past personal history of dysphoria, social support, and psychological distress following conjugal bereavement. JAGS 1994;42:712–718.

19. Zisook S, Shuchter SR, Sledge PA, Paulus M, Judd LL. The spectrum of depressive phenomena after spousal bereavement. J Clin Psychiatry 1994;55(4)(suppl):35.

20. Reynolds CF, Miller MD, Pasternak RE, Frank E, Perel JM, Cornes C, Houck PR, Mazumdar S, Dew MA, Kupfer DJ. Treatment of bereavement-related major depressive episodes in later life: A controlled study of acute and continuation treatment with nortriptyline and interpersonal psychotherapy Am J Psychiatry 1999;156: 202–208.

21. Rubin SS, Schecter N. Exploring the social construction of bereavement: Perceptions of adjustment and recovery in bereaved men. Am J Orthopsychiatry 1997;67(2):280.

22. Ibid.

23. Ibid.

24. Stewart AE. Complicated bereavement and posttraumatic stress disorder following fatal car crashes: Recommendations for death notification practice. Death Studies 1997;23(4):289–321.

25. Hutton CJ, Bradley BS. Effects of sudden infant death on bereaved siblings: A comparative study. J Child Psychol Psychiat 1994;55(4): 723–732.

26. Mahon MM. Childhood bereavement after the death of a sibling. Holistic Nurs Pract 1995;9(3):16.

27. Hogan NS, DeSantis L. Things that help and hinder adolescent sibling bereavement. Western J Nurs Res 1994;16(2):137.

28. Coolican MB. Families facing the sudden death of a loved one. Crit Care Nurs Clin North Am 1994;6(3):607–612.

29. Ibid.

30. Lev EL, McCorkle R. Loss, grief and bereavement in family members of cancer patients. Semin Oncol Nurs 1998;4(2):145–151.

31. Potocky M. Effective services for bereaved spouses: A content analysis of the empirical literature. Health Soc Work 1993;18:288–301.

32. Coolican MB, Pearce T. After care bereavement program. Crit Care Nurs Prog North Am 1995;7(3):519–527.

33. Snyder J. Bereavement protocols. J Emerg Nurs 1996;22:39–42.

34. Warren NA. (1997), loc. cit., 42–47.

35. Azhar MZ, Varma SL. Religious psychotherapy as management of bereavement. Acta Psychiatry Scand 1995;91:233–235.

36. Ibid., p. 234.

37. Goodkin K, Blaney NT, Feaster DJ, Baldewicz T, Burkhalter JE, Leeds B. A randomized controlled clinical trial of a bereavement support group intervention in human immunodeficiency virus type 1–seropositive and –seronegative homosexual men. Arch Gen Psychiatry 1999;56: 52–59.

38. Bower JE, Kemeny ME, Taylor SE, Fahy JL. Cognitive processing, discovery of meaning, CD4 decline, and AIDS-related mortality among bereaved HIV-seropositive men. J Consulting Clin Pscyhol 1998;66(6):979–986.

39. Anderson KL, Dimond MF. The experience of bereavement in older adults. J Adv Nurs 1995;22:308–315.

40. Ibid.

41. Sheldon F. ABC of palliative care—bereavement. BMJ 1998;316:456.

42. Billings JA. Useful predictors of poor outcomes in bereavement. In JA Billings, coordinator. Palliative Care Role Model Course, Massachusetts General Hospital, Boston, MA, 1999.

43. Sheldon, loc. cit.

44. Ibid.

45. Billings, loc. cit.

46. Rando TA. Grief and mourning: Accommodating to loss. In H Wass and RA Neimeyer (Eds.). Dying—Facing the Facts. Philadelphia: Taylor and Francis, 1995:211–241.

47. Ibid., p. 213.

48. Fulton R, Bendickson R. Introduction—Grief and the Process of Mourning. In R Fulton and R Bendicksen (Eds.). Death and Identity, 3 ed. Philadelphia: Charles Press Publishers, 1994: 105–109.

49. Ibid., p. 105.

50. Lindemann E. Symptomatology and management of acute grief. Am J Psychiatry (Sesquicentennial Suppl) 1994;151(6):156.

51. Ibid.

52. Ibid.

53. Fulton, loc cit.

54. Gorer G. Death, Grief and Mourning. London: Cresset Press, 1965.

55. Kavanaugh R. Facing Death. Baltimore: Penguin Books, 1974.

56. Raphael B. The Anatomy of Bereavement. New York: Basic Books, 1983.

57. Weizman SG, Kamm P. About Mourning: Support and Guidance for the Bereaved. New York: Human Sciences Press, 1985.

58. Kübler-Ross E. On Death and Dying. New York: Macmillan, 1969

59. Ibid.

60. Rando TA. Grief, Dying and Death—Clinical Interventions for Caregivers. Champaign, IL: Research Press Company, 1984.

61. Worden JW. Grief Counseling and Grief Therapy: A Handbook for the Mental Health Practitioner. 2 ed. New York: Springer, 1991.

62. Corr CA, Doka KJ. Current models of death, dying and bereavement. Crit Care Nurs Clin North Am 1994;6(3):545–552.

63. Klass D, Silverman P, Nickman S. Continuing Bonds. Philadelphia: Taylor and Francis Publishing, 1996.

64. Ibid., p. 349.
65. Stephenson, loc cit., p. 168.
66. Ibid.
67. Byrne GJA, Raphael B. A longitudinal study of bereavement phenomena in recently widowed elderly men. Psychol Med 1994;23:411–421.
68. Duke S. An exploration of anticipatory grief: The lived experience of people during their spouses' terminal illness and in bereavement. J Adv Nurs 1998;28(4):829–839.
69. Ibid., p. 837.
70. Cowles KV. Cultural perspectives of grief: An expanded concept analysis. J Adv Nurs 1996; 23:287–294.
71. Worthington RC. Models of linear and cyclical grief—Different approaches to differenct experiences. Clin Pediatr 1994:297–300.
72. Ibid., pp. 297–298.
73. Neimeyer RA. Meaning reconstruction and the experience of chronic loss. In KJ Doka with J Davidson (Eds.). Living with Grief: When Illness Is Prolonged. Philadelphia: Taylor and Francis, 1997:159–176.
74. Ibid., p. 165.
75. Ibid., p. 167.
76. Ibid., p. 168.
77. Ibid., p. 170.
78. Ibid., p. 172.
79. Ibid., p. 174.
80. Ibid., p. 176.
81. Rando TA. Grief and mourning, loc. cit., p. 239.
82. Horowitz MJ, Siegel B, Holen A, Bonanno GA, Milbrath C, Stinson CH. Diagnostic criteria for complicated grief disorder. Am J Psychiatry 1997;154(7):904–910.
83. Ibid., p. 904.
84. Prigerson HG, Frank E, Kasl SV, Reynolds CF, Anderson B, Zubenko GS, Houck PR, George CJ, Kupfer DJ. Complicated greif and bereavement-related depression as distinct disorders: Preliminary empirical validation in elderly bereaved spouses. Am J Psychiatry 1995;152(1): 22–30.
85. Prigerson HG, Bierhals AJ, Kasl SV, Reynolds CF, Shear MK, Newsom JT, Jacobs S. Complicated grief as a disorder distinct from bereavement-related depression and anxiety: A replication study. Am J Psychiatry 1996;153(11):1484–1486.
86. Prigerson HG, Maciejewski PK, Reynolds CF III, Bierhals AJ, Newsom JT, Fasiczka A, Frank E, Doman J, Miller M. Inventory of complicated grief: A scale to measure maladaptive symptoms of loss. Psychiatry Res 59:65–79.
87. Ibid., p. 79.
88. Krigger KW, McNeely JD, Lippmann SB. Dying, death and grief—Helping patients and their families through the process. Postgrad Med 1997;101(3):263–270.
89. Doka KJ. Disenfranchised grief. In L.A. DeSpelderf and A. L. Strickland (Eds.), The Path Ahead. Mountain View, CA: Mayfield Publishing Company, 1995:271–275.
90. Ibid., p. 272.
91. Corless IB. Modulated mourning: The grief and mourning of those infected and affected by HIV/AIDS. In K.J. Doka and J. Davidson (Eds.). Living with Grief: When Illness Is Prolonged. Philadelphia: Taylor and Francis, 1997: 108–118.
92. Ibid.
93. Rando TA. Grief, Dying and Death, loc. cit., pp. 64–65.
94. Ibid., pp. 66–67.
95. Eakes GG, Burke ML, Hainsworth MA. Chronic sorrow: The experiences of bereaved individuals. Illness Crisis Loss 1999;7(2):172–182.
96. Ibid.
97. O'Gorman SM. Death and dying in contemporary society: An evaluation of current attitudes and the rituals associated with death and dying and their relevance to recent understandings of health and healing. J Adv Nurs 1998;2:1127–1135.
98. Ibid., p. 1133.
99. Ibid.
100. Ibid.
101. Ibid.
102. Ibid.
103. Fulton R. The funeral in contemporary society. In R Fulton and R Bendiksen (Eds.), Death and Identity. 3 ed. Philadelphia: Charles Press Publishers, 1994:288–312.
104. Ibid
105. Stroebe W, Stroebe MS. Is grief universal? Cultural variations in the emotional reaction to loss. In R. Fulton and R. Bendiksen (Eds.), Death & Identity. 3rd ed. Philadelphia: Charles Press, 1994:177–207.
106. Ibid.
107. Ibid.
108. Ibid.
109. Byatt, loc. cit., p. 281.
110. Arnold J. Rethinking—Nursing implications for health promotion. Home Healthcare Nurse 1996;14(10):779–780.
111. Ibid., p. 780.
112. Rancour P. Recognizing and treating dysfunctional grief. ONF 1998;25(8):1310–1311.
113. Cutcliffe JR. Hope, counselling, and complicated bereavement reactions. J Adv Nurs 1998;28(4):760.
114. Stephenson C. The concept of hope revisited for nursing. J Adv Nurs 1991;16:1456–1461.
115. Ibid., p. 1458.
116. Frankl V. Man's Search for Meaning: An Introduction to Logotherapy. New York: Simon and Schuster, 1959.
117. Herth KA. The relationship between level of hope and level of coping and other variables in patients with cancer. ONF 1989;16(1): 62–72.
118. Watson MA. Bereavement in the elderly. AORN J 1994;59(5):1084.
119. Quinton A. Permission to mourn. Nurs Times 1994;90(12):31–32.
120. Ibid., p. 32
121. Ibid.
122. Ibid
123. Corless IB. And when famous people die. In IB Corless, BA Germino, and MA Pittman (Eds.). A Challenge for Living—Dying, Death, and Bereavement. Boston: Jones & Bartlett Publishers, 1995:398.
124. Ibid.
125. Ibid.
126. Klass D, Silverman P, Nickman, S., loc. cit.
127. ——. (1999). Commentary by newscaster on Turkish earthquake, ABC News.

26 Supporting Families in Palliative Care

BETTY DAVIES

I hope someday you'll find a way for families to understand how they should act in order to help a patient. The best help you can get from your family is understanding, for them to listen to you and understand you. . . . To help the family understand the illness, to be a support for the person who is ill: That is the greatest treasure to the person with cancer.

—Daughter

Family-centered care is a basic tenet of palliative care philosophy. Hospice recognizes that terminally ill patients exist within the family system. The patient's illness affects the whole family, and in turn, the family's responses affect the patient.

FAMILY-CENTERED PALLIATIVE CARE

Recognizing the importance of a family focus necessitates clearly defining what we mean by family. Most often, families in palliative care do consist of patients, their spouses, and their children.[1] But in today's world of divorce and remarriage, step relatives must also enter into the family portrait. In other instances, people unrelated by blood or marriage may function as family. Thus, the definition of family must be expanded. The family is a group of individuals inextricably linked in ways that are constantly interactive and mutually reinforcing. For example, Gillis, Highly, and Roberts[2] define a family as a "group of two or more individuals usually living in close geographic proximity; having close emotional bonds; and meeting affectional, socioeconomic, sexual, and socialization needs of the family group or the wider social systems" (p. 72). Moreover, family in its fullest sense embraces all generations—past, present, future; those living, those dead, and those yet to be born.

Palliative care programs are based on the principle that the family is the unit of care. In practice, however, the family is often viewed as a group of individuals who can either prove helpful to or resist efforts to deliver care. Nurses and other health professionals must strive to understand the meaning of the palliative experience to the family. If quality care is to be provided, nurses need to understand how all family members perceive their experience, how the relationships fit together, and that a multitude of factors combine to make families what they are. However, only recently has research gone beyond focusing on the needs of dying patients for comfort and palliation to addressing issues relevant to other family members. And, most of this research has focused on the family's perspective of their needs;[3] experiences and challenges faced;[4,5] adaptation and coping skills required for home care;[6,7] the supportiveness of nursing behaviors;[8,9] and satisfaction with care.[10–13] Most research has focused on families of patients with cancer. Findings make it clear that these family members look to health professionals to provide quality care to the patient. Family members also expect health professionals to meet their own needs for information, emotional support, and assistance with care.[13]

Much of the research that purports to address the impact of cancer on the family is based on the perceptions of individuals—either the patient or adult family members (usually the spouse). As well, many studies were conducted retrospectively, that is, after the patient's death. But even studies conducted during the palliative period frequently exclude the patient—the one who is at the center of the palliative care situation. Examining the palliative experience of the family unit has been rare. Therefore, as a basis for offering optimal support to families in palliative care, this chapter focuses on describing the findings of a research program which prospectively examined the experiences of such families.[14] The research evolved from nurses' concerns about how to provide family-centered palliative care. Nurses in a regional cancer center were constantly having to attend to the needs of not only patients, but patients' families, particularly as they moved back and forth between hospital and home. In searching the literature for guidelines about family-centered care, they found that many articles were about the needs of patients and family members, about levels of family members' satisfaction with care, and about family members' perceptions of nurses, but nothing really described the families' experiences as they coped with the terminal illness of a beloved family member. Research involving families included patients with advanced cancer, their spouses, and at least one of their adult (over 18 years of age) children. Since completing the research, families with AIDS, Alzheimers, and cardiac disease have provided anecdotal validation of the findings for their experience. As well, families of children with progressive, life-threatening illness have provided similar validation. Therefore, it seems that the conceptualization may have relevance for a wide range of families in palliative care.

THE TRANSITION OF FADING AWAY

The common view is that transitions are initiated by changes, by the start of something new. However, as Bridges[15] suggests, most transitions actually begin with endings. This was true for the families in this program of research. Findings generated a theoretic scheme which conceptualized families' experiences as a transition—a transition which families themselves labeled as "fading away." The transition of fading away for families facing terminal illness began with the ending of life as they knew it. They came to realize that the ill family member was no longer living with cancer, but was now dying from cancer.

Despite the fact that family members had been told about the seriousness of the prognosis, often since the time of diagnosis, and they had experienced the usual ups and downs associated with the illness trajectory, the realization that the patient's death was inevitable occurred suddenly: "It struck me hard—it hit me like a bolt. Dad is not going to get better!" The awareness triggered when family members saw, with "new eyes," the patient's weight loss, extreme weakness, lack of mobility, or diminished mental capacity. Realizing that the patient would not recover, family members began the transition of fading away. As one patient commented, "My body has shrunk so much—the other day, I tried on my favourite old blue dress and I could see then how much weight I have lost. I feel like a skeleton with skin! I am getting weaker . . . I just can't eat much now, I don't want to. I can see that I am fading . . . I am definitely fading away."

The transition of fading away is characterized by seven dimensions: redefining, burdening, struggling with paradox, contending with change, searching for meaning, living day by day, and preparing for death. The dimensions do not occur in linear fashion, but are interrelated and inextricably linked to one another. Redefining, however, plays a central role. All family members experience these dimensions, though patients, spouses, and children experience each dimension somewhat differently.

Redefining

Redefining involves a shift from "what used to be" to "what is now." It demands adjustment in how individuals see themselves and each other. Patients maintained their usual patterns for as long as possible, and then began to implement feasible alternatives once they realized that their capacities were seriously changing. Joe, a truck driver altered his identity over time: "I just can't do what I used to. I finally had to accept the fact that the seizures made it unsafe for me to drive." Joe requested to help out at his company's distribution desk. When he could no longer concentrate on keeping the orders straight, Joe offered to assist with supervising the light loading. One day, Joe was acutely aware he didn't have the energy to even sit and watch the others: "I couldn't do it anymore," Joe sighed. "I had reached the end of my work life and the beginning of the end." Joe, as did the other patients, accepted his limitations with much sadness and a sense of great loss. Patients' focus narrowed and they began to pay attention to details of everyday life that they had previously ignored or overlooked. Joe commented, "When I first was at home, I wanted to keep in touch with the guys at the depot; I wanted to know what was going on. Now, I get a lot of good just watching the grandkids out there playing in the yard." Patients were eager to reinforce that they were still the same on the inside, though they acknowledged the drastic changes in their physical appearance. They often became more spiritual in their orientation to life and nature. As Joe said, "I always liked being outside—was never much of an office-type person. But, now, it seems I like it even more. That part of me hasn't changed even though it's hard for some of the fellas (at work) to recognize me now." When patients were able to redefine themselves as Joe did, they made the best of their situation, differentiating what parts of them were still intact. Joe continued, "Yeah, I like just being outside, or watching the kids. And, you know, they still come to their Grandpa when their toy trucks break down—I can pretty much always fix 'em." Patients shared their changing perceptions with family members and others, who then were able to offer understanding and support.

Patients who were unable to redefine themselves in this way attempted to maintain their regular patterns despite the obvious changes in their capacity to do so. They ended up frustrated, angry, and feeling worthless. These reactions distanced them from others, resulting in the patients' feeling alone and, sometimes, abandoned. Ralph, for example, was an educational administrator. Despite his deteriorating health, he insisted that he was managing without difficulty. "Nothing's wrong with me, really . . . We are being accredited this year. There's a lot to do to get ready for that." Ralph insisted on going into the office each day to prepare the necessary reports. His increasing confusion and inability to concentrate made his reports inaccurate and inadequate, but Ralph refused to acknowledge his limitations and delegate the work. Instead, his colleagues had to work overtime to correct Ralph's work after he left the office. According to Ralph's wife, anger and frustration were commonplace among them, but they were reluctant to discuss the issue with Ralph. Instead, they avoided discussions with Ralph and he complained to his wife about his colleagues' lack of interest in the project.

For the most part, spouses took the patient's physical changes in stride. They attributed the changes to the disease, not to the patient personally, and as a result, were able to empathize with the patient. Patients' redefining focused on themselves—the changes in their physical status and intrapersonal aspects; spouses' redefining centered on their relationship with the patient. Spouses did their best to "continue on as normal," primarily for the sake of the patient. In doing so, they considered alternatives and reorganized their priorities.

When patients were able to redefine

themselves, spouses had an easier time. Those patients accepted spouses' offers of support; patients and spouses were able to talk about the changes that were occurring. Spouses felt satisfied in the care that they provided. However, when patients were less able to redefine, then spouses' offers of support were rejected, or unappreciated. For example, Ralph's wife worried about his work pattern and its impact on his colleagues. She encouraged him to cut back, but Ralph only ignored her pleas and implied that she didn't understand how important this accreditation was to the future of his school. Even when Ralph was no longer able to go to the office, he continued to work from home, frequently phoning his colleagues to supervise their progress on the report. His wife lamented, "For an educated man, he doesn't know much. I guess it's too late to teach an old dog new tricks." In such situations, spouses would then avoid talking about or doing anything that reminded the patient of the changes he or she was experiencing but not acknowledging. The relationship between the spouse and patient suffered. Rather than feeling satisfied with their care, spouses were frustrated and angry, though often in silence, and simply "endured" the situation.

Children redefined their ill parent from someone who was strong and competent to someone who was increasingly frail. Children felt vulnerable in ways they had not previously experienced. Most often, children perceived the changes they noted in their ill parent were the result of disease and not intentional: "It's not my father doing this consciously." Younger adult children were particularly sensitive to keeping the situation private, claiming they wanted to protect the dignity of the patient, but seemed to want to protect their own sense of propriety. For example, one young woman in her early twenties, was "devastated" when her father's urinary bag dragged behind him as he left the living room where she and her friends were visiting. It was difficult for some young adults to accept such manifestations of their parent's illness. Adolescents in particular had a difficult time redefining the situation. They preferred to continue on as if nothing was wrong, and to shield themselves against any information that would force them to see the situation realistically.

When the ill parent was able to redefine to a greater degree, then children were better able to appreciate that death is part of life. They recognized their own susceptibility and vowed to take better care of their own health; older children with families of their own committed to spending more quality time with their children. Joe talked, though indirectly, with his son about the situation: "I won't be here forever to fix the kids' toys." Together, Joe and his son reminisced about how Joe had always been available to his son and grandchildren as "Mr. Fix-it." Joe valued his dad's active participation in his life and promised to be the same kind of father to his own sons. When the ill parent was unable to redefine, then children tended to ignore the present. They attempted to recreate the past to construct happy memories they never had. In doing so, they often neglected their own families. Ralph's daughter described her dad as a "workaholic." Feeling as if she had never had enough time with her dad, she began visiting her parents daily, with suggestions of places she could take him. He only became annoyed with her unfamiliar "constant presence . . . it's okay she comes over every day, but enough is enough."

Burdening

The focus of burdening for patients is their concern for the well-being of their family members due to the extra load placed on them by the illness situation. If patients see themselves as purposeless, dependent, and immobile, they have a greater sense of burdening their loved ones. The more patients redefine themselves as they fade away, the more realistic they are in their perceptions of burdening. They acknowledge other family members' effort, appreciate that effort, and encourage family members to rest and take time to care for themselves. Patients who are less able to redefine themselves do not see that they are burdening other family members in any way. They deny or minimize the strain on others. As Ralph said during the last week of his life, "I can't do much, but I am fine really. Not much has changed. It's a burden on my wife, but not much. It might be some extra work . . . she was a nursing aide, so she is used to this kind of work."

Most spouses acknowledge the "extra load" of caring for their dying partner, but indicated that they did not regard the situation as a "burden." They agree that it's "just something you do for the one you love." Spouses of patients who are able to redefine are energized by the patient's acknowledgment of their efforts, and are inspired to continue on. Spouses of patients who are not able to redefine felt unappreciated, exhausted, and confessed to "waiting for the patient to die."

Children, too, experience burdening, but the source stems from the extra responsibilities involved in helping to care for a dying parent superimposed on their work responsibilities, career development, and own families. As a result, adult children of all ages feel a mixture of satisfaction and exhaustion. Their sense of burdening is also influenced by the ill parent's redefining—if the ill parent acknowledges their efforts, they are more likely to feel satisfaction. However, children's sense of burdening is also influenced by the state of health of their well parent. If that parent also is ill or debilitated, the burden on children is compounded. If children are able to prioritize their responsibilities so that they can pay attention to their own needs as well as helping both their parents, they feel less burdened.

Struggling with Paradox

Struggling with paradox stems from the fact that the patient is both living and dying. For patients, the struggle focuses on wanting to believe they will survive and knowing that they will not. On "good days," patients feel optimistic about the outcome; on other days, they succumb to the inevitability of their approaching demise. Often, patients do not want to "give up," but at the same time, they are "tired of fighting." They want to "continue on" for the sake of their families, but want "it to end soon" so their families can "get on with their lives." Patients cope by hoping for miracles, fighting for the sake of their families, and focusing on the good days. As Joe said, "I like to think about the times when things are pretty good. I enjoy those days. But, on the bad days, when I'm tired, or when the pain gets the best of me, then I just wonder if it wouldn't be best to just quit. But you never know—maybe I'll be the one in a million who makes it at the last minute. Hmmm, big chance of that."

Spouses struggle with a paradox of their own: they want to care for and spend time with the patient, and also want a "normal" life. They cope by juggling their time as best they can, and usually put their own life on hold. Spouses who managed to find ways of tending to their own needs usually were less exhausted and reported fewer health problems than spouses who neglected their own needs. For years, Joe and his wife had been square dancers. They hadn't been dancing together for many months when his wife resumed going to "dance night as a sub" or to prepare the evening's refreshments. "Sometimes, I feel guilty for going and leaving Joe at home, but I know I need a break. When I did miss dance night, I could see I was getting really bitchy—I need to get out for a breather so I don't suffocate Joe."

Children struggle with hanging on and letting go to a greater extent than their parents. They want to spend time with their ill parent and also "get on with their own life." Feeling the pressure of dual loyalties (to their parents and their own young families), the demands of both compound the struggle that children face.

Contending with Change

Those facing terminal illness in a family member experience changes in every realm of daily life—relationships, roles, socialization, work patterns. The focus of the changes differ among family members.

Patients face changes in their relationships with everyone they know. They realize that the greatest change of their life is under way and that life as they know it will soon be gone. They tend to break down tasks into manageable pieces, and increasingly focus inwards. The greatest change that spouses face is in their relationship with the patient. They cope by attempting to keep everything as normal as possible. Changes that children must contend with are more all-encompassing. They cannot withdraw as their ill parent does, nor can they prioritize their lives to the degree that their well parent can. They easily become exhausted. As Joe's son explained, "It's a real challenge coming by this often—I try to come twice a week and then bring the kids on the weekends. But I just got a promotion at work this year so that's extra work too. Seems like I don't see my wife much—but she's a real trooper. Her dad died last year so she knows what it's like."

Searching for Meaning

Searching for meaning has to do with seeking answers to help in understanding the situation. Patients tend to journey inward, reflect on spiritual aspects, deepen their most important connections, and become closer to nature: "The spiritual thing has always been at the back of my mind, but it's developing more . . . When you're sick like that, your attitude changes toward life. You come not to be afraid of death."

Spouses concentrate on their relationship with the patient. Some search for meaning through personal growth while others search for meaning by simply tolerating the situation. Some focus on spiritual growth while others adhere rigidly to their religion with little, if any, sense of inner growth or insight. Joe's wife commented, "Joe and I are closer than ever now. We don't like this business, but we have learned to love each other even more than when we were younger—sickness is a hard lesson that way." In contrast, Ralph's wife said with resignation, "He's so stubborn—always has been. I sometimes wonder why I stayed. But, here I am."

Children tend to reflect on and reevaluate all aspects of their lives: "It puts in perspective how important some of our goals are . . . having financial independence and being able to retire at a decent age . . . those things are important, but not at the expense of sacrificing today."

Living Day to Day

Not all families reached the point of living day to day. If patients were able to find some meaning in their experience, then they were better able to adopt an attitude of living each day. Their attitude was characterized by "making the most of it." As one patient described, "There's not much point in going over things in the past; not much point in projecting yourself too far into the future either. It's the current time that counts." Patients who were unable to find much meaning in their experience, or who didn't search for meaning, focused more on "getting through it." As Ralph said with determination, "Sure, I am getting weaker. I know I am sick . . . but I will get through this!"

Spouses who searched for meaning focused on "making the best of it" while making every effort to enjoy the time they had left with their partner. Other spouses simply endured the situation without paying much attention to philosophizing about the experience. Children often had difficulty concentrating on living day to day since they were unable to defer their obligations and so were constantly worrying about what else needed to be done. However, some children were still able to convey an attitude of "Live for today, today. Worry about tomorrow, tomorrow."

Preparing for Death

Preparing for death involved concrete actions that would have benefit in the future, after the patient died. Patients had their family's needs uppermost in their minds and worked hard to teach or guide family members with regard to various tasks and activities that the patient would no longer be around to do. Patients were committed to leaving legacies for their loved ones, not only as a means of being remembered, but also as a way of comforting loved ones in their grief. Joe spent time "jotting down a few Mr. Fix-it pointers" for his wife and son. Ralph's energy was consumed by focusing on the work he still had to do, so he was unable to consider what he might do for his wife and daughter.

Spouses concentrated on meeting the patient's wishes. Whatever the patient wanted, spouses would try to do. They attended to practical details and anticipated their future in practical ways. Children offered considerable help to their parents with legal and financial matters. They also prepared their own children for what was to come. A central aspect was reassuring the dying parent that they would take care of the surviving parent. Children also prepared for the death by envisioning their future without their parent: "I think about it sometimes . . . about how my children will never have a grandfather. It makes me so sad. That's why the photos we have been taking are so important to me . . . they will show our children who their grandfather was."

GUIDELINES FOR NURSING INTERVENTIONS

Much of the nursing literature which provides guidelines for nursing care addresses the importance of four major interventions:

1. *Maintain hope in patients and their family members.* As families pass through the illness trajectory, the nature of their hope changes from hope for cure, to hope for remission, to hope for comfort, to hope for a good death. Offering hope during fading away can be as simple as assuring families that everything will be done to ensure the patient's comfort. Talking about the past also can help some families by reaffirming the good times spent together and the ongoing connections that will continue among family members. Referring to the future beyond the immediate suffering and emotional pain can also sustain hope. For example, when adult children reassure the ill parent that they will care for the other parent, the patient is hopeful that the surviving spouse will be all right.

2. *Involve families in all aspects of care.* Include them in decision making and encourage active participation in the physical care of the patient. This is their life—they have the right to control it as they will. Involvement is especially important for children when a family member is very ill. The more children are involved in the care during the terminal phase, and in the activities that follow the death, the better able they are to cope with bereavement.[16]

3. *Offer information.* Tell families about what is happening and what they can expect to happen. Doing so also provides them with a sense of control. Initiate the discussion of relevant issues that family members themselves may hesitate to mention. For example, the nurse might say, "Many family members feel like they are being pulled in two or more directions, when a loved one is very ill. They want to spend as much time as possible with the patient, but also feel the pull of their own daily lives, careers, or families. How does this fit with your experience?"

4. *Communicate openly.* Open communication with nurses and other health professionals is frequently the most important need of families. They need to be informed; they need opportunities to ask questions and to have their questions answered in terms that they can comprehend. Open communication among team members is basic to open communication with families. Unfortunately, this is an aspect that is often taken for granted; communication among colleagues must be conscientiously supported.

It is not an easy task for the family to give up their comfortable and established views of themselves as death approaches. The nurse's challenge is to help family members anticipate what lies ahead without violating their need to relinquish old orientations and hopes at a pace they can handle. These four broad interventions assist the nurse in providing good palliative care; the following guidelines offer further direction. They are derived from the direct accounts of the patients, spouses, and children about the strategies they used to cope with the dimensions of fading away.

Redefining

Supporting patients and other family members with redefining requires that nurses appreciate how difficult it is for family members to relinquish familiar perceptions of themselves and adopt unfamiliar, unwelcome, and unasked for changes into their self-perceptions. Disengagement from former perceptions and the adoption of new orientations occur over time. The nurse is challenged to help family members anticipate and prepare for what lies ahead, while not pushing them at a pace that threatens their sense of integrity. All family members will redefine at their own pace; the nurse must tailor interventions according to the individual needs of each. At the same time, the nurse supports the family as a unit by reassuring family members that their varying coping responses and strategies are to be expected.

The nurse should provide opportunities for patients to talk about the losses incurred by the illness, the enforced changes, the adaptations they made, and their feelings associated with these. Reinforce their normal patterns of living as long as possible and as appropriate. When they can no longer function as they once did, focus on what patients still can do and reinforce those aspects of self that remain intact. Acknowledge that roles and responsibilities may be expressed in new and different ways and suggest new activities, appropriate to the patient's interest and current capabilities.

The nurse's focus with spouses and children centers on explaining how the disease or treatment contributes to changes in the patient physically, psychologically, and socially. Provide opportunities for spouses to talk about how changes in the patient affect their marital relationship. Help children appreciate their parent from another perspective, such as in recalling favorite memories or identifying the legacies left. Discuss how they can face their own vulnerability by channelling concerns into positive steps for self-care. Reinforce the spouses' and children's usual patterns of living for as long as possible and as appropriate; when former patterns are no longer feasible, consider adjustments or alternatives. Provide opportunities for spouses to discuss how they may reorganize priorities in order to be with and care for the patient to the degree they desire. Consider resources that enable the spouse to do this, such as with the assistance of volunteers, home support services, or additional nursing services. Teach care-giving techniques if the spouse shows interest. With the children, discuss the degree to which they want to be open or private about the patient's illness with those outside of the family. Acknowledge that family members will vary in their ability to assimilate changes in the patient and in their family life.

Burdening

Nurses can help patients find ways to relieve their sense of burden. Provide patients with opportunities to talk about their fears and concerns, and to consider with whom they want to share their worries. In this way, patients may avoid their concern for putting excessive demands on family members. Explain the importance of a break for family members and suggest that patients accept assistance from a volunteer or home support services at those times to relieve family members from worry. Explain that when patients affirm family members for their efforts, this contributes to family members' feeling appreciated and reduces their sense of burden.

Nurses can assist spouses with burdening by supporting the spouse's reassurances to the patient that he or she is not a burden. Acknowledge spouses' efforts when they put their own needs on hold to care for the patient; help them to appreciate the importance of taking care of themselves as a legitimate way of sustaining the energy they need for the patient. Talk with spouses about how they might take time out and consider the various resources they might use. Acknowledge the negative feelings spouses may have about how long they can continue; do not negate their positive desire to help.

For children, acknowledge the reorganization and the considerable adjustment in their daily routines. Explain that ambivalent feelings are common—the positive feelings associated with helping and the negative feelings associated with less time spent on careers and their own families. Acknowledge that regular communication with their parents by phoning or visiting more often are all part of the "work" of caring and should not be underestimated; encourage children to take time out for themselves.

Struggling with Paradox

Facing the usual business of living and directly dealing with dying is a considerable challenge for all members of the family. The nurse's challenge is to appreciate that it is not possible to alleviate completely the family's psychosocial and spiritual pain. To do so, nurses must face their own comfort level in working with families facing paradoxical situations and the associated ambivalent feelings. Like family members, nurses, too, may want to avoid the distress of struggling with paradox. They may feel unprepared to handle conversations where no simple solution exists and where strong feelings abound.

Nurses can support patients and other family members by providing opportunities for all family members to ventilate their frustrations; do not minimize their pain and anguish. On the good days, rejoice with them. Listen to their expressions of ambivalence, and be prepared for the ups and downs and changes of opinion that are sure to occur. Reassure them that their ambivalence is a common response. Encourage "time out" as a way to replenish depleted energy.

Contending with Change

Nurses must realize that not all families communicate openly or work easily together in solving problems. Therefore, nurses can support patients and family members to contend with change by creating an environment in which families explore and manage their own concerns and feelings according to their particular coping style. Providing information so families can explore various alternatives helps families to determine what adjustments they can make. Make information available not only verbally, but in writing as well. Or, tape-record information discussions so that families can revisit what they have been told.

Searching for Meaning

Nurses help families search for meaning by enabling them to tell their personal story and make sense of it. It is essential that nurses appreciate the value of storytelling—when families talk about their current situation and recollections of the past, it is not just idle chatter. It is a vital part of making sense of the situation and coping with it. Nurses must appreciate that much of searching for meaning involves examining spiritual dimensions, belief systems, values, and relationships within and outside of the family. Nurses can be supportive by suggesting approaches for personal reflection, such as journal writing or writing letters.

Living Day to Day

In living day to day, families make subtle shifts in their orientation to living with a dying member. They move from thinking there is no future, to making the most of the time they have left. This is a good time for the nurse to review the resources available to the family to ensure that they are utilizing all possible sources of assistance so that their time together is optimally spent.

Preparing for Death

In helping families prepare for death, nurses must be comfortable talking about the inevitability of death, describing the dying process, and helping families make plans for wills and funerals. It is important not to push or force such issues; it is equally important not to avoid them because of the nurse's personal discomfort with dying and death. Encourage such discussions among family members while acknowledging how difficult they can be. Affirm them for their courage to face these difficult issues. Encourage patients to attend to practical details, such as finalizing a will and distributing possessions. Encourage them to do "last things," such as participating in a special holiday celebration. Provide information to spouses and children about the dying process. If the plan is for death at home, provide information about what procedures will need to be followed and the resources that are available. Provide opportunities for family members to express their concerns and ask questions. Encourage them to reminisce with the patient as a way of saying "good-bye" and acknowledge the bittersweet quality of such remembrances. Provide information to the adult children about how they can help their own children with the impending death.

The foregoing guidelines are intended to assist nurses in their care of individual family members. The guidelines are summarized in Table 26–1. In addition, family centered care means that nurses must also focus on the family as a unit. Nurses must appreciate that the family as a whole has a life of its own that is distinct but always connected to the individuals who are part of it. Both levels of care are important.[17] The families in the fading-away study also provided insights about how family functioning plays a role in how families cope with terminal illness in a family member.

FAMILY FUNCTIONING AND FADING AWAY

Families experienced the transition of fading away with greater or lesser difficulty, depending on their level of functioning according to eight dimensions: integrating the past, dealing with feelings, solving problems, utilizing resources, considering others, portraying family identity, fulfilling roles, and tolerating differences. These dimensions occur along a continuum of functionality; family interactions tend to vary along this continuum rather than being positive or negative, good or bad.

Some families acknowledge the pain of past experience with illness, loss, and other adversity and integrate previous learning into how they manage their current situation. These families express a range of feelings, from happiness and satisfaction, through uncertainty and dread, to sadness and sorrow. Family members acknowledge their vulnerabilities and their ambivalent feelings. All topics are open for discussion. There are no clear-cut rights and wrongs, and no absolute answers to the family's problems. They apply a flexible approach to problem solving and openly exchange all information. They engage in mutual decision making, considering each member's point of view and feelings. Each family member is permitted to voice both positive and negative opinions in the process of making decisions. They agree on the characteristics of their family and allow individual variation within the family. They allocate household and patient care responsibilities in a flexible way. These families are often amenable to outside intervention and are comfortable in seeking and utilizing external resources. Such families are often appealing to palliative care nurses and other personnel since they openly discuss their situation, share their concerns, and accept help willingly.

Other families are more challenging for palliative care professionals. These are families who hang on to negative past experiences and continue to dwell on the painful feelings associated with the event. They appear to avoid the feelings of turmoil and ambivalence, shielding themselves from the pain, often indicating that they do not express their feelings. These families approach problems by focusing more on why the problem occurred and who was at fault rather than generating potential solutions. They often are unable to communicate their needs or expectations to each other or to health care professionals and are angry when their wishes are not fulfilled. They express discrepant views only in individual interviews, not when all members are present, and tend not to tolerate differences. Varying approaches by health care workers are not generally well tolerated either. They do not adapt easily to new roles nor do they welcome outside assistance. Such families show little concern for others. They use few resources since family members are often unable or reluctant to seek help from others. These families often present a challenge for nursing care. Nurses must realize expecting such families to "pull together" to cope with the stresses of palliative care are unrealistic. It is essential not to judge these families, but rather to appreciate the family is coping the best it can under very difficult circumstances. These families need support and affirmation of their existing coping strategies, not judgmental criticisms.

Nurses are encouraged to complete assessments of level of family system functioning early in their encounters with families.[17,18] This is the best time to begin to develop an understanding of the family as a whole as a basis for the services to be offered. Assessment of family functioning provides a basis for effective nursing interactions to ensure a family-focused approach in palliative care nursing. The eight dimensions of family functioning provide a guideline for assessment. Table 26–2 summarizes these dimensions and gives examples of the range of behaviors evident in each dimension. The table summarizes those behaviors that, on one end of the continuum are more helpful, and on the other end are less helpful to families facing the transition of fading away. Understanding the concept of family functioning will enhance the nurse's ability to assess the unique characteristics of each family. An assessment of family functioning enables the nurse to interact appropriately with the family and to help them solve problems more effectively (see Table 26–3). For example, in families where communication is open and shared among all members, the nurse can be confident that communication with one family member will be accurately passed on to other members. In families where communication is not

Table 26–1. Dimensions of Fading Away: Nursing Interventions for Family Members

Redefining

Appreciate that relinquishing old and comfortable views of themselves occurs over time, and does not necessarily occur simultaneously with physical changes in the patient

Tailor interventions according to the various abilities of family members to assimilate the changes

Reassure family members that a range of responses and coping strategies is to be expected within and among family members

Provide opportunities for patients to talk about the illness, the enforced changes in their lives, and the ways in which they have adapted; for spouses to talk about how changes in the patient affect their marital relationship; and for children to talk about their own feelings of vulnerability and the degree to which they want to be open or private about the situation

Reinforce normal patterns of living for as long as possible and as appropriate. When patterns are no longer viable, consider adjustments or alternatives

Focus on the patient's attributes that remain intact, and acknowledge that roles and responsibilities may be expressed differently. Consider adjustments or alternatives when former patterns are no longer feasible

Help spouses consider how they might reorganize priorities and consider resources to help them do this

Help children appreciate their parent from another perspective, such as in recalling favorite stories or identifying legacies left

Burdening

Provide opportunities for patients to talk about fears and anxieties about dying and death, and to consider with whom to share their concerns

Help patients stay involved for as long as possible as a way of sustaining self-esteem and a sense of control

Assist family members to take on tasks appropriate to their comfort level and skill and share tasks among themselves

Support family members' reassurances to patient that he or she is not a burden. Explain that when patients reaffirm family members for their efforts, this contributes to their feeling appreciated and lessens the potential for feeling burdened

Explain the importance of breaks for family members. Encourage others to take over for patients on a regular basis so family members can take a break

Acknowledge the reorganization of priorities and the considerable adjustment in family routines and extra demands placed on family members. Acknowledge the "work" of caring for all family members

Realize that family members will vary in their ability to assimilate the changes and that a range of reactions and coping strategies is normal

Struggling with Paradox

Appreciate that you, as a nurse, cannot completely alleviate the psycho-social-spiritual pain inherent in the family's struggle

Assess your own comfort level in working with people facing paradoxical situations and ambivalent feelings

Provide opportunities for family members to mourn the loss of their hopes and plans. Do not minimize these losses; help them modify their previous hopes and plans and consider new ones

Listen to their expressions of ambivalence, and be prepared for the ups and downs of opinions

Ensure effective symptom management as this allows patients and family members to focus outside the illness

Explain the importance of respite as a strategy for renewing energy for dealing with the situation

Contending with Change

Create an environment in which family members can explore and manage their own concerns and feelings. Encourage dialogue about family members' beliefs, feelings, hopes, fears, and dilemmas so they can determine their own course of action

Recognize that families communicate in well-entrenched patterns and their ability to communicate openly and honestly differs

Normalize the experience of family members and explain that such feelings do not negate the positive feelings of concern and affection

Provide information so families can explore the available resources, their options, and the pros and cons of the various options. Provide information in writing as well as verbally

Explain the wide-ranging nature of the changes that occur within the patient's immediate and extended family

Searching for Meaning

Appreciate that the search for meaning involves examination of the self, of relationships with other family members, and of spiritual aspects.

Realize that talking about the current situation and their recollections of past illness and losses is part of making sense of the situation

Encourage life reviews and reminiscing. Listen to the life stories that family members tell

Suggest approaches for self-examination such as journal writing, and approaches for facilitating interactions between family members such as writing letters

Living Day to Day

Listen carefully for the subtle shifts in orientation to living with a dying relative and gauge family members' readiness for a new orientation

Ensure effective control of symptoms so that the patient can make the most of the time available. Assess the need for aids

Without minimizing their losses and concerns, affirm their ability to appreciate and make the most of the time left

Review resources that would free family members to spend more time with the patient

Preparing for Death

Assess your own comfort level in talking about the inevitability of death, describing the dying process, and helping families make plans for wills and funerals

Provide information about the dying process

Discuss patients' preferences about the circumstances of their death. Encourage patients to discuss these issues with their family. Acknowledge how difficult such discussions can be

Encourage patients to do important "last things", such as completing a project as a legacy for their family

Provide opportunities for spouses and children to express their concerns about their future without the patient. Provide them with opportunities to reminisce about their life together. Acknowledge such remembrances will have a bittersweet quality

Source: Davies et al.[14]

Table 26–2. Dimensions of Family Functioning: Examples of the Range of Behaviors

More Helpful	Less Helpful
Integrating the Past	
Describe the painful experiences as they relate to present experience	Describe past experiences repeatedly
Describe positive and negative feelings concerning the past	Dwell on painful feeling associated with past experiences
Incorporate learning from the past into subsequent experiences	Do not integrate learning from the past to the current situation
Reminisce about pleasurable experiences in the past	Focus on trying to "fix" the past to create happy memories which are absent from their family life
Dealing with Feelings	
Express a range of feelings including vulnerability, fear, and uncertainty	Express predominately negative feelings, such as anger, hurt, bitterness, and fear
Acknowledge paradoxical feelings	Acknowledge little uncertainty or few paradoxical feelings
Solving Problems	
Identify problems as they occur	Focus more on fault finding than on finding solutions
Reach consensus about a problem and possible courses of action	Dwell on the emotions associated with the problem
Consider multiple options	Unable to clearly communicate needs and expectations
Open to suggestions	Feel powerless about influencing the care they are receiving
Approach problems as a team rather than as individuals	Approach problems from individual perspective rather than as a family
	Display exaggerated response to unexpected events
	Withhold or inaccurately share information with other family members
Utilizing Resources	
Utilize a wide range of resources	Utilize few resources
Open to accepting support	Reluctant to seek help or accept offers of help
Open to suggestions regarding resources	Receive help mostly from formal sources rather than from informal support networks
Take the initiative in procuring additional resources	
Express satisfaction with results obtained	Express dissatisfaction with help received
Describe the involvement of many friends, acquaintances, and support persons	Describe fewer friends and acquaintances who offer help
Considering Others	
Acknowledge multidimensional effects of situation on other family members	Focus concern on own emotional needs
Express concern for well-being of other family members	Fail to acknowledge or minimize extra tasks taken on by others
Focus concern on patient's well-being	
Appreciate individualized attention from health care professionals, but do not express strong need for such attention	Display inordinate need for individualized attention
Direct concerns about how other family members are managing rather than with themselves	
Identify characteristic coping styles of family unit and of individual members	Describe own characteristics coping styles rather than the characteristic way the family as a unit coped
Demonstrate warmth and caring toward other family members	Allow one member to dominate group interaction
Consider present situation as potential opportunity for family's growth and development	Lack comfort with expressing true feelings in the family group
Value contributions of all family members	Feign group consensus where none exists
Describe a history of closeness among family members	Describe few family interactions prior to illness

(continued)

Table 26–2. Dimensions of Family Functioning: Examples of the Range of Behaviors (*Continued*)

More Helpful	Less Helpful
Fulfilling Roles	
Demonstrate flexibility in adapting to role changes	Demonstrate rigidity in adapting to role changes and responsibilities
Share extra responsibilities willingly	Demonstrate less sharing of responsibilities created by extra demands of patient care
Adjust priorities to incorporate extra demands of patient care and express satisfaction with this decision	Express resentment over perceived lack of support in caregiving Refer to caregiving as a duty or obligation Criticize or mistrust caregiving provided by others
Tolerating Differences	
Allow differing opinions and beliefs within the family	Display intolerance for differing opinions or approaches of caregiving
Tolerate different views from people outside the family	Demonstrate critical views of friends who fail to respond as expected
Willing to examine own belief and value systems	Adhere rigidly to belief and value systems

Source: Originally published in Davies, B., Reimer, J., and Maartens, N. (1994). Family functioning and its implications for palliative care. *Journal of Palliative Care,* 10(1):35–36. Reprinted with permission.

Table 26–3. Family Functioning: Guidelines for Interventions in Palliative Care

Assessing Family Functioning

Use dimensions of family functioning to assess families. For example: Do members focus their concern on the patient's well-being and recognize the effect of the situation on other family members or do family members focus their concerns on their own individual needs and minimize how others might be affected? Putting your assessment of all the dimensions together will help you determine to what degree you are dealing with a more cohesive family unit or a more loosely coupled group of individuals, and hence what approaches are most appropriate.

Be prepared to collect information over time and from different family members. Some family members may not be willing to reveal their true feelings until they have developed trust. Others may be reluctant to share differing viewpoints in the presence of one another. In some families. Certain individuals take on the role of spokesperson for the family. Assessing where everyone in the family shares the viewpoints of the spokesperson, or whether different family members have divergent opinions but are reluctant to share them, is a critical part of the assessment.

Listen to the family's story and use clinical judgment to determine where intervention is required. Part of understanding a family is listening to their story. In some families, the stories tend to be repeated and the feelings associated with them resurface. Talking about the past is a way of being for some families. It is important that the nurse determine whether family members are repeatedly telling their story because they want to be better understood or because they want help to change the way their family deals with the situation. Most often the stories are retold simply because family members want the nurse to understand them and their situation better, not because they are looking for help to change the way their family functions.

Solving Problems

Use your assessment of family functioning to guide your approaches. For example, in families where there is little consensus about the problems, rigidity in beliefs, and inflexibility in roles and relationships, the common rule of thumb of offering families various options so they may choose those that suit them best tends to be less successful. For these families, carefully consider which resource provides the best possible fit for that particular family. Offer resources slowly, perhaps one at a time. Focus considerable attention on the degree of disruption associated with the introduction of the resource and prepare the family for the change that ensues. Otherwise, the family may reject the resource as unsuitable and perceive the experience as yet another example of failure of the health care system to meet their needs.

Be aware of the limitations of family conferences and be prepared to follow up. Family conferences work well for more cohesive family units. However, where more disparity exists among the members, they may not follow through with the decisions made, even though consensus was apparently achieved. Though not voicing their disagreement, some family members may not be committed to the solution put forward and may disregard the agreed-upon plan. The nurse needs to follow up to ensure that any trouble spots are addressed.

Be prepared to repeat information. In less-cohesive families, do not assume that information will be accurately and openly shared with other family members. You may have to repeat information several times to different family members and repeat answers to the same questions from various family members.

Evaluate the appropriateness of support groups. Support groups can be a valuable resource. They help by providing people with the opportunity to hear and perspective of others in similar situations. However, some family members need more individualized attention than a support group provides. They do not benefit from hearing how others have experienced the situation and dealt with the problems. They need one-to-one interaction focused on themselves with someone with whom they have developed trust.

Adjust care to the level of family functioning. Some families are more overwhelmed by the palliative care experience than others. Understanding family functioning can help nurses appreciate that expectations for some families to "pull together" to cope with the stress of palliative care may be unrealistic. Nurses need to adjust their care according to the family's way of functioning and be prepared for the fact that working with some families may be more demanding and the outcomes achieved are less optimal.

Source: Davies et al.[14]

as open, the nurse must take extra time to share the information with all members. Or, in families who dwell on their negative past experiences with the health care system, nurses must realize that the establishing trust will likely require extra effort and time. Families who are open to outside intervention are more likely to benefit from resource referrals; other families may need more encouragement and time to open their doors to external assistance.

The nurse must remember that each family is unique and comes with its own life story and circumstances; listening to their story is central to understanding the family. There may be threads of commonality, but there will not be duplicate experiences. Assist family members to recognize the essential role they are playing in the experience and acknowledge their contributions. Most importantly, nurses must realize that each family is doing the best it can. Nurses must sensitively, creatively, and patiently support families as they encounter one of the greatest challenges families must face—the transition of fading away.

REFERENCES

1. Ferrell BR. The family. In Oxford Textbook of Palliative Medicine (D. Doyle, G. Hanks, and N. MacDonald, eds.). Oxford: Oxford University Press, 1998:909–917.

2. Gilliss CL, Highly BL, Roberts BM. Toward a Science of Family Nursing. Menlo Park, CA: Addison-Wesley Publishing Co, 1989.

3. Tringali CA. The needs of family members of cancer patients. Oncol Nurs Forum 1986;13: 65–70.

4. Thorne S. The family cancer experience. Cancer Nurs 1985;8:285–291.

5. Woods NF, Lewis FM, Ellison ES. Living with cancer: Family experiences. Cancer Nurs 1989;12:28–33.

6. Hull M. Coping strategies of family caregivers in hospice homecare. Oncol Nurs Forum 1992;19:1179–1187.

7. Stajduhar K, Davies B. Palliative care at home: Reflections on HIV/AIDS family caregiving experiences. J Palliat Care 1998;14:14–22.

8. Dyck S, Wright K. Family perceptions: The role of the nurse throughout an adult's cancer experience. Oncol Nurs Forum 1985;12:53–56.

9. Raudonis B, Kirschling M. Family caregivers' perspectives on hospice nursing care. J Palliat Care 1996;12:14–19.

10. Hays RD, Arnold S. Patient and family satisfaction with care for the terminally ill. Hospice J 1986;2:129–150.

11. Kristjanson LJ. Indicators of quality of care from a family perspective. J Palliat Care 1986; 5:8–17.

12. Kristjanson LJ. Quality of terminal care: Salient indicators identified by families. J Palliat Care 1989;5:21–30.

13. Kristjanson LJ, Leis A, Koop P, Carriere KC, Mueller B. Family members' care expectations, care perceptions, and satisfaction with advanced cancer care: Results of a multi-site pilot study. J Palliat Care 1997;13:5–13.

14. Davies B, Chekryn Reimer J, Brown P, Martens N. Fading Away: The Experience of Transition in Families with Terminal Illness. Amityville, NY: Baywood Publishing Co, 1995.

15. Bridges W. Transitions: Making Sense of Life's Changes. Reading, MA: Addison-Wesley, 1980.

16. Davies B. Environmental factors affecting sibling bereavement. In B Davies, Shadows in the Sun: Experiences of Sibling Bereavement in Childhood. Philadelphia: Brunner/Mazel. 1999: 123–148.

17. Jassak P. Families: An essential element in the care of the patient with cancer. Oncol Nurs Forum 1992;19:871–986.

18. Gulla J. Family assessment and its relation to hospice care. Am J Hospice Palliat Care 1992; July/August:30–34.

27 Complementary Therapies

HOB OSTERLUND and PATRICIA BEIRNE

A significant and growing trend in American health care is the integration of many complementary and alternative medicine (CAM) approaches. The *Journal of the American Medical Association* reported in 1998 that use of alternative therapies in the United States increased from 33.8% in 1990 to 42.1% in 1997.[1] In October of 1998, Congress established the National Center for Complementary and Alternative Medicine (NCCAM), promoted from its former status as the Office of Alternative Medicine. With a $50 million annual budget, NCCAM will support research and disseminate information on CAM to both professionals and the public. Multiple CAM studies were reported at the 1998 Twelfth World AIDS Conference in Geneva, and nurses all over the country have begun to integrate such complementary practices into the care of their patients.

The term *CAM* actually refers to a broad and complex combination of interventions, and is also interchangeably called holistic, unorthodox, unconventional, natural, traditional, or nontraditional, depending upon your cultural perspective.[2] These interventions can be distinguished from contemporary biomedicine by examining some of the underlying assumptions that support them. Biomedicine uses Newtonian and Cartesian theories as its foundation, and believes that the mechanics of everyday experience can be explained by physically measurable data. Another key assumption is called "objectivism" and refers to the belief that the *observer* is separate from the *observed*.

According to biomedicine, the way something is "known" is by its predictability within scientific law, and its ability to be reduced to simple phenomena. Generally, if biomedicine cannot scientifically explain the impact of CAM therapies, it assumes that the research used to measure these therapies is erroneous, unscientific or "soft."

The perspective of CAM practice is quite different from that of biomedicine. Complementary practitioners emphasize wellness rather than the treatment of disease, and focus on engaging inner resources of each individual as an active participant in his or her own health.[1] In addition, "health" is not *provided* to the individual as a result of the medical practitioner's intervention, but results from a balance of the individual's internal resources and the interplay between the external physical and social environment. The same factors are equally important for the practitioner's own health and ability to have a positive impact on the health of another.

The CAM emphasis is also upon the whole person, rather than systems of the body. This whole person is generally viewed as unique, with his or her own set of internal resources. In addition, more significance is given to *healing* rather than *curing*. The original meaning of "healing" is "to make whole." Since an individual can be cured without being healed and healed without being cured, and since cure in palliative care is no longer the focus, it has become apparent that many CAM interventions have the possibility for exploration within the context of palliative care (Table 27–1).

Neither biomedicine nor CAM interventions have all the answers, nor are they as mutually exclusive as they might sound. Ultimately the balance of the brain, the heart, the organs of the body, and the immune system, and perhaps an understanding of matter and energy, is what both disciplines seek.

The options shown in Table 27–2 are not intended to be exhaustive of the CAM interventions that have been shown to be helpful in palliative care, but rather serve as examples of strategies that might be chosen. They are also not intended to be used exclusive of biomedicine, but to be both complementary to biomedicine as well as specifically tailored to the individual being treated. Five of these strategies are discussed in some depth in the pages that follow:

GUIDED IMAGERY

Guided imagery and hypnosis have been used for many years as techniques to relieve symptoms and encourage many levels of healing. Institutions and agencies such as Marin General Hospital in California,[2] the Queen's Medical Center in Honolulu, and San Diego Hospice have utilized guided imagery for many purposes and with positive results.

For our purposes, the term *guided imagery* (GI) will be used, and is defined as *access to the imagination through a guide.*[2] This "guide" is often a nurse, social worker, chaplain, or clinical psychologist who has been trained in the use of GI. In imagery, the mind affects the body and the body affects the mind. This relationship was proposed more than a century ago by William James, considered the father of American psychology.[3] Much research has been done over the most recent decades to explore this reversal of the Cartesian belief in mind–body separation.

Messages such as feelings, attitudes, or beliefs that are suggested to the mind have to be translated by the right hemisphere of the brain before they can be understood by the involuntary or autonomic nervous system.[5] Once trans-

Table 27–1. Uses of Complementary Therapies

Enable self-care
Control symptoms
Reduce treatment side effects
Enhance well-being
Improve quality of life
Reduce fear and anxiety
Reduce pain

lated, a bridge between conscious processing of information and physiologic change has, at least in theory, been created. Because GI uses mind modulation to tap the unlimited capabilities of the human body–mind–spirit entity, imagery can be used for a number of purposes in palliative care.

The primary purposes of GI include (*1*) inducing physiologic changes, (*2*) raising psychological insight, and (*3*) increasing emotional awareness. In the management of physiologic symptoms, for example, imagery has been successfully used to reduce pain, nausea, and vomiting associated with chemotherapy, reduce allergic responses and blood pressure, relieve gastrointestinal symptoms, and modify cardiac arrhythmias.[6]

Each of these symptoms evokes its own stress response. In addition to stress, anxiety and fatigue can further decrease pain tolerance, making the pain itself even more intense. Imagery can interrupt this cycle that begins with a primary pain and continues to perpetrate secondary pains resulting from stress and fatigue. Relaxation from imagery, for example, directly reduces muscle tension and related muscle spasms. It promotes rest and sleep, which further increases pain tolerance.

Table 27–2. Examples of Complementary Therapies Used to Enhance Quality of Life

Guided imagery/hypnosis
Healing touch/therapeutic touch
Reflexology
Acupuncture
Massage
Acupressure
Music therapy
Art therapy
Aromatherapy/essential oils
Meditation/prayer
Biofeedback
Humor therapy
Reiki
Polarity therapy

Imagery can also serve as distraction. In several studies evaluating procedure-related cancer pain, imagery was useful in altering the patient's perception of pain.[7–9] To reduce pain, imagery can use a *transformational* focus, which involves transformation of either the painful sensation itself or the context of the pain. *Dissociative* imagery uses the imagination to disconnect or dissociate from the pain experience itself. Even short break periods from pain can help to interrupt the difficult cycle of pain that confines many cancer patients.

Guided imagery can also be specific to the treatment modality, the disease or the age group. GI was found to be effective for enhancing the comfort of women undergoing radiation therapy for early-stage breast cancer.[9] In this research, the imagery was designed specifically for the disease and the treatment as well as for the symptoms associated with the interventions used. Dozens of studies reveal the impact of hypnosis and GI on children with cancer.[10]

Overall, imagery techniques have been shown to be clinically effective and economically feasible. Often these services are provided by volunteer practitioners and are of no cost to the patient. They can reduce physical symptoms and increase emotional and spiritual well-being. The well-informed palliative care practitioner might consider these techniques for any appropriate, consenting patient.

HEALING TOUCH

Healing Touch (HT) is one of many techniques that uses the hands for the purpose of providing comfort. In general, these interventions are based on the theoretical presence of *universal energy*. The basic premise is that our world of physical matter is surrounded by and penetrated with a fluid world of radiating energy, constantly moving and changing. This energy is seen as the basic constituent and source of all life. It permeates all space, animate, and inanimate objects and connects all objects to each other. The "human energy field" (HEF) is a manifestation of universal energy that is intimately involved with human life. The HEF is defined as the field around the human body and can be influenced by attention and intention. Many cultures have rich and complex traditions around this concept, which include *prana* in India, *qi* in China, and *mana* in Hawaii. The energy can be sensed and influenced, and this kind of work is gaining growing acceptance within many medical settings.

Healing through touch is as old as civilization itself. Egyptian, Chinese, Indian, Greek, Polynesian, Native American, and Roman cultures have recorded its use, and there are many references to healing through touch in the Bible. Traditional healers and shamans used touch widely until the rise of the Puritan culture.[11]

Interventions other than HT which are actively being used for health care include therapeutic touch, polarity, Reiki, Jorei, Chinese energetic medicine, and others. Regardless of the practitioner's training, common beliefs include (*1*) there is only one energy and (*2*) the energy has a beneficent power which is available to everyone.

Healing touch and therapeutic touch techniques may be performed by physical touch and/or through the use of hand movements and placement inches or feet from the recipient's body. Treatment times vary from a few minutes to an hour or more, according to the setting, the presenting problem, and the practitioner's skill.

The two most prominent of these interventions involving touch within nursing are HT and therapeutic touch (TT). Healing touch is endorsed by the American Holistic Nursing Association and consists of several levels of training leading to the option of national certification. Therapeutic touch, which provided the essentials out of which HT grew, is endorsed by the Nurse Healers-Professional Associates and refers to the

Kreiger-Kunz method. This method is referred to as a modern interpretation of several ancient healing techniques, historically called "laying on of hands."[12] To be effective, the practice of either intervention requires an ordered approach that includes the following steps:

- Centering oneself
- Assessing the healee
- Unruffling the energy field
- Direction and modulation of the energy
- Reassessment and closure

Although HT blossomed from TT's roots, it has quickly become a larger hybrid, combining both traditional and modern healing techniques. It relies on the practitioner's ability to interpret the energy of the recipient and to choose appropriate techniques based on those findings. Its growth in popularity has been rapid, with more than 40,000 practitioners trained internationally in the 1990s. Many of these practitioners are nurses, previously skeptical about how simple hand movements might have an impact on the well-being of their patients. Nurses, however, are relentlessly interested in what makes their patients feel better. Despite the controversy that these techniques might sometimes incite, nurses by the thousands have learned to incorporate HT and TT into their busy work schedules simply because so many patients have told them what a difference it makes in their comfort.

Practitioners are not limited to nurses. At The Queen's Medical Center (QMC) in Honolulu, where thousands of inpatients have received HT since the program began in 1991, volunteer HT practitioners have included airline pilots, active-duty policemen, retired Broadway performers, models, accountants, real estate agents, medical students, and television producers. Along with HT training, each of these individuals brings a certain devotion to the relief of human suffering, and each is willing to offer time to contribute to that outcome.

At the same time, all HT/TT practitioners are trained to detach from outcomes, so as to not bring personal needs or expectations to the bedside. This approach leaves the patient free to respond to treatment without concern for the practitioner's own feelings or beliefs, and often find positive and sometimes unexpected responses. At San Diego Hospice, where Reiki and HT/TT are used, patients often experience a reduction in anxiety and pain after a treatment. In addition, there is an inexplicable "letting go" and simultaneous emotional comfort that cannot be explained by physical relaxation alone.

At QMC 200 inpatients were interviewed after receiving HT. The average decrease in pain was 2.8 (0–10 scale) and average increase in relaxation was 1.8 on a 1–4 scale. In most situations, these reflected 20- to 30-minute sessions done in a hospital room by a practitioner the patient has never met. Comments such as "I could finally tolerate my chemotherapy" or "I didn't need as much pain medicine" were common. Visitors observed the response of their loved ones: "My little boy could finally get some sleep," said one mother. A son commented his mother "could finally die in peace." "Her cancer didn't go away, but she wasn't afraid anymore," said a husband.

Some practitioners find a spirituality in HT/TT that resonates with their own path. Sister Rita Jean DuBrey,[13] a Catholic nun who ministers at the Wellness Institute of St. Mary's Hospital in Amsterdam, New York, says that in her HT work she humbly serves as a "conduit for God's healing energy" and assists patients in self-healing. Joan Stemple, admissions nurse from Carondelet Hospice Services in Tucson, tells of a terminally ill man who suffered from unrelieved agitation despite their best pharmaceutical interventions. Healing touch was given by a Catholic sister hospice volunteer while the patient continued to struggle to get out of bed and to have severe muscular tremors. During the one-hour treatment his agitation gradually diminished until he fell asleep and his symptoms ceased. Thirty minutes later, he died peacefully, surrounded by his loved ones.

There are countless stories such as these. In addition, many research projects are investigating the impact of HT/TT. Among other positive impacts, therapeutic touch has been shown to decrease chemotherapy-induced symptoms, decrease agitation and anxiety, alleviate pain, and enhance wound healing.[14] It seems particularly beneficial in the terminally ill, alleviating symptoms such as dyspnea, coughing, hiccoughs, diarrhea, cramping abdominal pain, constipation, fever, pain, and anxiety associated with AIDS.[15]

Dozens of similar studies are investigating the impact of HT,[16] including two studies at QMC looking at pain reduction in patients immediately after mastectomies and at the impact of HT on pain and function on employees with work-related back injuries. Other studies have investigated the positive impact of HT on depression, pain, and mobility after joint replacements, chronic pain, recovery after hysterectomies, and wound infection. Many of these studies are as yet unpublished, and the process of HT's integration is just now emerging in the literature.[17]

Since no adverse effects have been noted, HT/TT can be used on almost any consenting adult. Exceptions may include actively psychotic or paranoid patients. Any practitioner trained in HT/TT will take the time to be sure the patient wishes to proceed with a treatment, and that he or she may stop at any time for any reason.

Finally, central to the work of HT/TT practitioners is *intention*. Practitioners focus on their intention for the optimal benefit by the recipient, and separate themselves from specific expectations about how that benefit might look. Patients feel that compassion, and are often soothed by its presence. For people experiencing distress, as many people in palliative care settings are, relief of any kind is welcome. Since comfort and compassion are the main goals of palliative care, further work of this nature is encouraged.

In the basic procedures of HT/TT, the practitioner must become centered with full attention and intention on assisting the patient. By assessing the patient's "energy field" for feelings of congestion, imbalances, or obstructions, the specific techniques are ascertained. These techniques are varied and many, such as "unruffling" the field, directing and modulating the energy, and "clearing" excess blockage. All of this requires a strong knowledge base of HT/TT and a physically, mentally, emotionally, and spiritually aware practitioner. The experience with each patient is unique and the energy exchange between the patient and the practitioner enhances the well-being of both. As we learn more about the impact of energy healing, perhaps one day we will understand exactly *how* it works. In the meantime, however, *that* it works is enough to encourage us to continue to explore its greatest benefits.

AROMATHERAPY

Aromatherapy is to the use of essential oils which are extracted from plants and whose fragrance is used for therapeutic purposes. It is conjectured that an essential oil is to a plant what blood is to a human being: it is not the whole plant, but is a whole organic entity unto itself, without which the organism cannot live.[18]

Essential oils can be extracted from roots, stalks, flowers, leaves, and bark of certain plants. They are then distilled and are applied topically to the soles of the feet, wrist, temples, or other parts of the body depending on the symptom and the type of oil used. Oils can also be used as a compress or for massage. They can be used in conjunction with other modalities such as reflexology, healing touch, or other energy therapies, or with acupuncture. They can be mixed with ointment and inserted into an orifice of the body, or inhaled via a cold air diffuser, vaporizer, or humidifier. When mixed with baths or used on washcloths they can be very effective. Even a few drops of essential oil in water distillers have been used for specific purposes. At the same time, it's important to keep in mind that there is a wide range of essential oil grades, and the purity and quality of the essential oil can make a big difference on its therapeutic impact. The use of pure, nonsynthetic oils is crucial. In purchasing these oils it is most important to look for a distributor of essential oils or someone trained in their use.

Unfortunately the Food and Drug Administration does not currently require precise labeling of the ingredients in essential oils. As a result, only specific laboratories can determine exact ingredients. Testing of an oil can be done by a "gaschromatogram" that can give a profile of an oil in exact percentage of the individual constituents of that oil, and provide a certificate of analysis.

Aromatherapy began as a specific branch of science in France in 1928. Prior to that, oils were used in the ancient civilizations of Egypt, China, Greece, Rome, and the Arab countries. There are many biblical references to their use. Moses was commanded by God to make a holy anointing oil (Exodus 30:22–25) of myrrh, cinnamon, calamus, cassia, and olive oil; in particular, Westerners are familiar with frankincense and myrrh as gifts to the infant Jesus (Matthew 2:11). Sixteenth-century European pharmacopeias listed at least 80 essential oils for the treatment of various conditions, and Native American shamans bathe their patients in scents for the purpose of personal transformation.[18]

The French chemist Maurice-René Gattefosse[19] was initially responsible for the reintroduction of aromatherapy into modern science. Having suffered from a burn after a chemical explosion in his laboratory, he applied lavender essential oil to the burn. The burn healed so quickly and completely that he began to investigate the nature and properties of many of the essential oils and was the first person to officially catalog and classify the oils. Jean Valnet,[20] a World War II army doctor, recognized the antibacterial and antiviral properties of essential oils on wounds and in France, Madame Maury described aromatherapy as an allopathic medicine available to physicians as well as a beauty treatment.[18]

Essential oils, like many other CAM therapies, experienced a rise in popularity in the 1990s. Fifty books were published on aromatherapy from 1988 to 1995 in the United Kingdom alone, and essential oils are used there in a variety of settings for a number of purposes. These include relaxation, the relief of pain and anxiety, treatment for insomnia, restlessness, wound healing, and shortness of breath.

In a palliative care aromatherapy study,[21] 51 patients were given massages with Roman chamomile and compared to a group of patients who were massaged without the oil. Those in the aromatherapy group experienced significant decreases in physical symptoms and anxiety, while reported increases in quality of life. In another randomized controlled study, 100 cardiac surgery patients reported significant anxiety reduction after receiving foot massages with oil of neroli citrus compared with patients whose foot massages were done with vegetable oil. In general, however, more research would be helpful in determining the impact of these oils.

In theory, it is the human response to fragrances that makes aromatherapy both appealing and compelling. The neurons of the olfactory system are found in the limbic area of the midbrain. The limbic system extends to the hypothalamus into a portion of the forebrain which is responsible for visceral functions and emotional expression. As a result, aromatherapy's impact on an individual's emotional and psychological state can be both quick and profound.[18]

San Diego Hospice (SDH) which serves as the palliative medicine and hospice care teaching facility for the School of Medicine at the University of California at San Diego, has been experimenting with a variety of essential oils as part of their exploration of CAM. Patricia Mittendorff, M.A., P.A.-C, the staff member responsible for coordinating the use of aromatherapy, reports successful use of oils for balancing mood and emotion, for relaxation, and for the relief of obsessive thinking, fear of death, nausea, and shortness of breath. Many of these uses are supported in the literature. Table 27–3 lists some essential oils associated with various uses.

Table 27–3. Essential Oils and Their Uses

To Reduce Fear

Roman chamomile (*Chamaemelum nobile*)
Cypress (*Cupressus sempervirens*)
Frankincense (*Boswellia carterii*)
Geranium (*Pelargonium* x *Asperum*)
Lavender (*Lavandula officinalis*)
Marjoram (*Origanum majorana*)
Melissa (*Melissa officinalis*)
Orange (*Citrus aurantium*)
Patchouli (*Pogostemon cablin*)
Rose (*Rosa damascena*)
Sandalwood (*Santalum album*)
Spruce (*Picea mariana*)
Ylang-ylang (*Cananga odorata*)

To Reduce Pain

Birch (*Betula allegheniensis*) for muscle, bone pain
Basil (*Ocimum basilicum*) for nerve pain, migraines, muscle spasms
Cypress (*Cupressus sempervirens*) for bone pain
Eucalyptus (*Eucalyptus citriodora*) for muscle pain
Ginger (*Zingiber officinale*) for muscle pain
Lavender (*Lavandula officinalis* or *augustifolia*) for nerve pain, headache, pain associated with anxiety/agitation
Marjoram (*Origanum majorana*) for muscular pain
Peppermint (*Mentha piperita*) bone pain, headaches
Tangerine (*Citrus nobilis*) for discomfort related to stagnant fluids, edema

To Reduce Nausea

Basil (*Ocimum basilicum*)
Caramon (*Elettaria cardamomum*)
Fennel (*Foeniculum vulgare*)
Ginger (*Zingiber officinale*)
Lavender (*Lavandula officinalis* or *augustifolia*)
Melissa (*Melissa officinalis*)
Peppermint (*Mentha piperita*)
Rose (*Rosa damascena*)
Sandalwood (*Santalum album*)
Tarragon (*Artemisia album*)

To Reduce Shortness of Breath

Cypress (*Cupressus sempervirens*)
Eucalyptus (*Eucalyptus globulus* and other species)
Frankincense (*Boswellia carterii*)
Lavender (*Lavandula augustifolia* or *officinalis*)
Marjoram (*Origanum marjorana*)
Melissa (*Melissa officinalis*)
Ravensara (*Ravensara aromatica*)

To Relieve Fatigue

Basil (*Ocimum basilicum*) for mental fatigue
Clove (*Eugenia caryophyllus*)
Frankincense (*Boswellia carterii*)
Jasmine (*Jasminum officinale*)
Lavender (*Lavandula officinalis*)
Melissa (*Melissa officinalis*)
Nutmeg (*Myristica fragrans*)
Mountain savory (*Satureja montana*)
Peppermint (*Mentha piperita*)

Essential oils listed in Tables 27–3 can be applied by placing about three drops in a basin of bathwater; used as a mist with a spray bottle or diffused into the air; dropped on a cotton pad and placed on the chest for inhaling; or massaged into the feet. Chaplains can use the oils to anoint and palliative care staff can use them for the purpose of symptom reduction. Family members can also participate in this manner, relieving some of their own feelings of helplessness in the process. Special "synergy" blends can be created or purchased to relieve multiple concerns. *It is always important to keep in mind the quality, purity, and consistency of the oils*; with this focus and patient comfort in mind, it is likely that oils will routinely join our tool chest of low-cost and quick-acting interventions. However it is used, aromatherapy has a promising future in the field of palliative care.

MUSIC THERAPY

It's difficult to overestimate the power, mystery, and impact of music. Music has been a part of human expression and language since ancient times, and has been documented as a treatment modality for more than 4000 years.[27] Egyptians observed that incantation improved female fertility. In the Bible, David used the harp to treat King Saul's depression, and both Plato and Aristotle prescribed music for the treatment of medical conditions. Music has been used to treat hyperactive children, behavior difficulties, and mental illness. Florence Nightingale noted the healing nature of music in the care of patients.[27]

As a distinct health profession, music therapy began in the 1940s. Since then, music therapists have been responsible for describing and using the therapeutic power of music within health institutions. They have discovered means to offer controlled use of music to influence physiologic, psychologic, and emotional integration and balance, and thereby have a therapeutic impact on illness.[28]

Modern use of music in palliative care is also now its own discipline. Since music has already been shown to reduce pain, stress, and anxiety, to alter mood, to promote relaxation, to facilitate grief, and to help the transition from life to death,[29] its place in palliative care is obvious. In addition *music thanatology* has emerged as an important modality by which music is used to serve the dying in homes, hospitals, and hospices.

The best-known American music thanatologist is singer and harpist Teresa Schroeder-Sheker,[30] who founded and directs the Chalice of Repose Project in Missoula, Montana. Its goals are to "lovingly serve the physical and spiritual needs of the dying with the delivery of prescriptive music, live, at the bedside of the dying patient." Housed at St. Patrick Hospital in Missoula, music thanatology has become a standard element of care for patient services. Endorsed by the medical staff as a full medical modality, the program has 27 harps and singing harpists-in-training.

Schroeder-Sheker describes six educational assumptions that are fundamental to music thanatologists. These include the beliefs that

- death is a spiritual process which represents an opportunity for growth;
- that "musical midwifery" is not merely a technical musical skill but also a contemplative practice with clinical applications that requires inner work on the part of the caregiver;
- death is not the enemy, but an important chapter in a person's biography;
- the way a person dies is as important as the way that person has lived, and that beauty, reverence, and intimacy can be a natural part of the experience;
- music thanatology is much more *service* than it is a career;
- music thanatologists support education of individuals and communities about the importance of restoring dignity to the dying and grieving process.

"The sole focus of the music is to help the person move toward completion and to unbind from anything that prevents, impedes or clouds a tranquil passage," says Schroeder-Sheker.[31] As a result, each bedside application of this music is highly individualized. The Chalice workers respond to referrals from nurses, physicians, chaplains, and other professionals. They often arrive in teams of two and begin the process of *sound anointing* with their harps. This continues for over an hour, and the workers are often profoundly moved by the peaceful atmosphere that accompanies and follows their work.

Music thanatology and music therapy are not identical, but are allies in the treatment of discomfort and illness. Music therapy focuses on the alleviation of symptoms and the promotion of relaxation and communication, while music thanatology is rooted in palliative care and is one-pointed in its focus on treating the complex needs of the dying. In music thanatology, the patient is seen as a chalice that simply receives, and is not required to respond to a relationship or connection with the therapist. In the former, the connection between the therapist and the patient might be vital. Music for the living is intended to engage people; music for the dying is meant to free them.[32]

Such distinctions may be subtle. At San Diego Hospice, where there is a formal affiliation with the International Harp Therapy Association, harpists come in to play for any patient that the charge nurse believes can benefit. Patients may be chosen because of anxiety, fear of death, family difficulties, personality conflicts, shortness of breath, and many other potential indications. As with HT/TT, we look at the human energy field. Many healers use music to effect change in this field. We find some music soothes the energy field while some charges it. For instance, drum music may be very grounding, while love songs may help us to connect with others at a heart level. The harp seems to resonate with our essence and can take us into a spiritual experience. Many times, loved ones and staff involved in a music presentation feel comforted as well. A trained musician can use any instrument to take us through all levels of human experience.

San Diego Hospice also has an extensive library of music. Patricia Mittendorff, M.A., P.A.-C, says that they sometimes focus on music for a specific purpose, and even have a "music mattress" which vibrates to the music and resonates throughout the patient's body. The system has been effective in reducing pain and anxiety, and doesn't even require melodic content as much as the vibration itself. The staff might also choose to play music from the culture or era from which the patient comes, thereby making the therapy as individual as possible. At Hospice Hawai'i, Arthur Harvey, Ph.D., is the coordinator of Therapeutic Music Services. He sits at the bedside of patients, singing songs from their own era. One recent patient requested "cowboy music," and died peacefully while listening to "Red River Valley." At the Hospice Hawai'i inpatient facility, harpists come to play ambient music for the whole staff. Staff, patients, and families all feel the impact of such resonant, peaceful sounds.

Dr. Harvey says most researchers find that two generic types of music seem to be most beneficial, Baroque-Classical and New Age music. However, many other types and styles of music have proven to be therapeutic and rehabilitative, depending on the person's perceptual style and music background.[33] The components of music that affect us mostly are (*1*) the tempo (slow to fast), (*2*) the volume (soft to loud), (*3*) the degree of dissonance (calm consonance to cacophony), and (*4*) the quality of sound (range, timbre, and presence). While studies show live performance is better than recorded music, practical constraints may necessitate the use of taped music.[34]

Music has also been shown to be an effective adjunct to pharmacologic antiemetic therapy.[35] In this study, patients were randomly assigned to receiving music along with the usual antiemetic protocol for high-dose chemotherapy in a bone marrow transplant unit. Patients listened on headphones to 45-minute CDs of self-selected music at 6, 9, and 12 hours after the start of each chemotherapy infusion. Patients in the experimental group had significantly less nausea and vomiting than patients in the control group. Patients who listened to music in the immediate postoperative period have also been found to feel more relaxed, have less anxiety, and be more distracted than patients undergoing the same procedures who did not listen to music.[36] In this study, nurse researchers evaluated the effect of music played through headphones on patients during the last 30 minutes of their surgical procedures and during the first hour in the postanesthesia care unit.

Palliative care workers are encouraged to investigate further use of music in their own settings. Music therapy has the opportunity to be both clinically effective and cost-effective, requiring few resources and opening the door for reduced symptoms and increased patient comfort and satisfaction. Music at the time of death may add a positive component that we are not able to quantify, but that we feel richly. And perhaps, as Deforia Lane[37] teaches us, music may truly be a "gift without measure."

HUMOR THERAPY

As with music, it's difficult to underestimate the power of humor. Laughter releases tension, creates harmony, is a social harmonizer, overcomes obstacles, thrives in an atmosphere of intimacy, and gives us the strength and courage to face impossible odds. What pharmaceutical company could boast of a product that produces all accomplishments? Yet even as recently as 25 years ago, humor and nursing were considered contradictory. Perhaps professional distance was the greater goal. Fortunately, this norm has naturally evolved into a much greater appreciation for humor's therapeutic power for everyone concerned. Patients, families, and nurses alike benefit from its impact.

Ever since Norman Cousins[38] testified about the positive impact of humor on his painful illness in *Anatomy of an Illness* in 1979, belief in the analgesic power of humor has become common. In one survey, Fritz[39] asked participants with chronic cancer pain to rate the effectiveness of all their nondrug techniques. They rated laughter as the most effective. Other studies have demonstrated that humor may not only increase tolerance to pain, but also may assist pain tolerance in lasting beyond the humorous event itself.[40]

We know there is much more to the power of humor than distraction. To begin with, humor creates an entire series of physiological changes, including the increase of oxygen exchange, heart rate, and muscular activity; it also stimulates the sympathetic nervous system and the production of catecholamines. This stimulated state is closely followed by a period of greater relaxation and lower blood pressure, a state resembling the body after physical exercise.[41] Other studies have demonstrated the impact of laughter on salivary immunoglobulin A (S-IgA), an immune system protein that is vital to the body's defense against respiratory illness.[42] One study by Martin and Dobbin[43] used self-report humor scales and showed a greater negative relationship between stress and S-IgA with subjects who had low humor scores than those with higher humor scores. The researchers concluded that those subjects with a strong sense of humor experienced less mood disturbance and impairment in immune function after stressful events than their more serious counterparts. Similar results were found by Lambert and Lambert[44] when studying S-IgA levels and fifth-grade students.

Berk and colleagues[45] at Loma Linda University School of Medicine have researched the impact of laughter on the neuroendocrine system, stress hormones, and immune parameters. A complex series of responses to laughter suggests that it may be an antagonist to the human stress response. It lowers cortisol levels, increases activated T-lymphocytes, and increases the activity of killer cells. In essence, laughter counteracts the immunosuppressive effects of stress by stimulating the immune system.

Even if none of this were known, humor would still be a powerful tool. In fact, its ability to bring light into a dark moment is nearly miraculous. It enhances the well-being of everyone in its vicinity. It levels hierarchies and provides a oneness to events that might otherwise have been perceived as separate, even opposite experiences. The nurse who laughs with her patients creates an intimacy and telegraphs an understanding of "there but for fortune." The wise nurse understands that the only real difference between the patient and her is the clothing. Otherwise, she could just as easily be the hospice patient; and perhaps one day she will be. Empathic laughter with the patient, then, is also being empathic with one's own self.

These moments of laughter are largely spontaneous, and take a certain sensitivity to the patient's receptivity to humor. True humor is always unifying and never derogatory, never creating more separation or less worthiness. As a result, the safest humor either comes from one who is teasing her own self, or simply witnesses the absurdities of life. It also allows room for humor to be interjected by the patient or family whenever they feel such an urge. At the deathbed of her mother, a daughter weeps openly while the nurse stands lovingly by her side. At one point the daughter looks up and smiles through her tears: "My mother preferred denial. I used to prefer obsession. Now she's dead and only now I understand her . . . I want denial too!" Together they laugh softly, and the intimacy carries them both, offering courage and strength.

For the nurse who feels less able to participate in spontaneous humor, there are other methods to offer humor to the interested patient: videos such as the "Chuckle Channel" previously available at the Queen's Medical Center in Honolulu; comedy audiotapes specific to the patient's taste; professional clowns; San Diego Hospice pet therapy with the black Labrador dressed up as a cowgirl; children who come to act out a skit or sing a song—all these can bring lifesaving humor to the patient. Comedy videos such as *"Ivy Push, RN"* can be offered to staff and patients alike. Inquiries about this video may be addressed to hosterlund@queens.org.

SUMMARY

Complementary and alternative medicine (CAM) represents one of the most exciting evolutions in health care for the twenty-first century. Often inexpensive and noninvasive, various CAM therapies show tremendous promise for symptom relief, emotional support, and spiritual enhancement. No less important than the therapies listed above, we suggest further investigation into the promising work in acupuncture, prayer, massage, art therapy, long-distance healing, homeopathy, herbal medicine, and Ayurvedic medicine. A wealth of articles can be found in *Alternative Therapies in Health and Medicine*, a peer-reviewed journal devoted to high-quality exploration of these methods.

REFERENCES

1. Eisenberg D, Davis RB, Ettner SL, et al. (1998). Trends in alternative medicine use in the United States, 1990–1997. *JAMA* 280(18):1569–1575.

2. Nienstedt BC (1998). The definitional dilemma of alternative medicine. In *Alternative Therapies* (R.J. Gordon, B.C. Nienstedt, and W.M. Gesler, eds.), pp. 13–24. Springer Publishing Co., New York.

3. Micozzi MS (1996). Characteristics of complementary and alternative medicine. In *Fundamentals of Complementary and Alternative Medicine* (M.S. Micozzi, ed.), pp. 3–8. Churchill Livingstone, New York.

4. Moore N (1997). Humanizing medicine: The humanities program at Marin General Hospital. Alt Ther Health Med 3:4.

5. Dossey B (1995). Imagery: Awakening the inner healer. In *Holistic Nursing: A Handbook for Practice* (B. Dossey, L. Keegan, C. Guzzetta, and L. Kolkmeier, eds.), pp. 609–666. Aspen Publishers, Baltimore.

6. Post-White J (1998). Imagery. In *Complementary/Alternative Therapies in Nursing* (M. Snyder and R. Lundquist, eds.), pp. 103–122. Springer Publishing Co., New York.

7. Kellerman J, Zeltzer L, Ellenberg L, Dash L (1983). Adolescents with cancer: hypnosis for the reduction of acute pain and anxiety associated with medical procedures. J Adolesc Health Care 4:85–90.

8. Hilgard E, LeBaron S. (1987). Relief of anxiety and pain in children and adolescents with cancer: Quantitative measures and clinical observations. Int J Clin Exp Hypn 30:417–442.

9. Kolcaba K, Fox C. (1999). The effects of guided imagery on comfort of women with early stage breast cancer undergoing radiation therapy. Oncol Nurs Forum 26(1):67–72.

10. Steggles S, Damore-Petingolas S, Maxwell J, et al. (1997). Hypnosis for children and adolescents with cancer: An annotated bibliography, 1985–1995. J Pediatr Oncol Nurs 14(1):27–32.

11. Sayre-Adams J. (1995). Therapeutic touch. In *The Nurses Handbook of Complementary Therapies* (D. Rankin-Box, ed.), pp. 158–161. Churchill Livingstone, London.

12. Slater VE. (1996). Healing touch. In *Fundamentals of Complementary and Alternative Medicine* (M.S. Micozzi, ed.), pp. 121–135. Churchill Livingstone, New York.

13. DuBrey RJ. (1999). Healing touch: A ministry of love and compassion. Supportive Voice, 4(2):9–10.

14. Egan EC. (1998). Therapeutic touch. In *Complementary/Alternative Therapies in Nursing* (M. Snyder and R. Lindquist, eds.), pp. 49–62. Springer Publishing Co., New York.

15. Newshan MA. (1989). Therapeutic touch for symptom control in persons with AIDS. Holistic Nurs Pract 3(4):45–51.

16. Pitorak EF. (1999). The challenge of pain management in the elderly patient in hospice care. J Hospice Palliat Nurs 1(1).

17. Osterlund H. (1999). Healing touch at the Queen's Medical Center in Honolulu, Hawaii. In *Fundamentals of Contemporary Nursing Practice* (C.A. Lindeman and M. McAthie, eds.), pp. 951–953. W.B. Saunders Company, Philadelphia.

18. Stevensen C. (1996). Aromatherapy. In *Fundamentals of Complementary and Alternative Medicine* (M. Micozzi, ed.), pp. 137–147. Churchill Livingstone, New York.

19. Gattefosse R-M. (1993). *Gattefosse's Aromatherapy* (R. Tisserand, ed.). C.W. Daniel Company, Essex, England.

20. Valnet J. (1980). *The Practice of Aromatherapy: A Classic Compendium of Plant Medicines and Their Healing Properties* (R.Tisserand, ed.). Healing Arts Press, Rochester, Vermont.

21. Wilkinson S. (1995). Aromatherapy, therapeutic use of essential oils. Int J Palliative Nurs 1(1):21–30.

22. Stevensen CJ. (1994). The psychophysiological effects of aromatherapy massage following cardiac surgery. Comple Ther Med 2:27–35.

23. Friedmann T. (1998). *Freedom through Health.* Harvest Publishing, Northglenn, CO.

24. Price S. (1993). *Shirley Price's Aromatherapy Workbook: Understanding Essential Oils from Plant to Bottle.* HarperCollins Publishers, San Francisco.

25. Tisserand R. (1977). *The Art of Aromatherapy: The Healing and Beautifying Properties of the Essential Oils of Flowers and Herbs.* Healing Arts Press, Rochester, Vermont.

26. Young D. (1996). *Aromatherapy: The Essential Beginning.* Essential Press Publishing, Salt Lake City.

27. Chlan L. (1998). Music Therapy. In *Complementary/Alternative Therapies in Nursing* (M. Snyder and R. Lindquist, eds.), pp. 243–252. Springer Publishing, New York.

28. Beck SL. (1991). The therapeutic use of music for cancer-related pain. Oncol Nurs Forum 18:1327–1337.

29. Rykov M, Salmon D. (1998). Bibliography for music therapy in palliative care, 1963–1997. Am J Hospice Palliat Care 15(3):174–180.

30. Schroeder-Sheker T. (1998). Anointing the dying with sound: Music thanatology and the care of the dying. Caduceus 40:23–27.

31. Schroeder-Sheker T. (1993). Music for the dying: A personal account of the new field of music thanatology: History, theories and clinical narratives. Adv J Mind-Body Health 9(1).

32. Schroeder-Sheker T. (1994). Music for the dying. J of Holistic Nurs 12(1).

33. Harvey A, Rapp L. (1988). Music soothes the troubled soul. AD Nurse, March/April (19): 19–22.

34. Harvey A. (1999). Music: Rx for pain. HMEA Bull September, pp. 16–20.

35. Ezzone S, Baker C, Rosselot R, Terepka E. (1998). Music as an adjunct to antiemetic therapy. Oncol Nurs Forum 25:1551–1556.

36. Heiser RM, Chiles K, Fudge M, Gray SE. (1997). The use of music during the immediate postoperative recovery period. AORN J 65(4): 777–778, 781–785.

37. Lane D. (1992). Music therapy: A gift beyond measure. Oncol Nurs Forum 19:863–867.

38. Cousins N. (1979). Anatomy of an Illness as Perceived by the Patient. W.W. Norton, New York.

39. Fritz D. (1988). Noninvasive pain control methods used by cancer outpatients. Oncol Nurs Forum 15(suppl):108.

40. Hudak D, Dale JA, Hudak MA, DeGood DE. (1991). Effects of humorous stimuli and sense of humor on discomfort. Psychol Rep 69:779–786.

41. Fry W. (1971). Mirth and oxygen saturation of peripheral blood. Psychother Psychosomat (19):76–84.

42. Dillon K, Minchoff B, Baker K. (1985). Positive emotional states and enhancement of the immune system. Int J Psych Med 15(1):13–17.

43. Martin R, Dobbin J. (1988). Sense of humor, hassles, and immunoglobulin evidence for a stress-moderating effect of humor. Int J Psych Med 18(2):93–105.

44. Lambert R, Lambert N. (1995). The effects of humor on secretory immunological A levels in school-aged children. Pediatr Nurs 21(1): 16–19.

45. Berk L, Tan S, Fry W. (1989). Neuroendocrine and stress hormone changes during mirthful laughter. Am J Med Sci 298(6):390–396.

28 Planning for the Actual Death

PATRICIA BERRY and JULIE GRIFFIE

Twenty-four hours before he died, his right arm pointed and waved upward. My father cried out for his long-ago dead mother, "Mae! Mae! Mae!" His speech had become slurred and was most often incomprehensible. When he spoke more, I strained to hear. "Dad, I'm sorry I couldn't understand what you just said. Would you please tell me again?" Clearly, strongly, and with utmost certainty he replied, "My mother would have understood me!" He did not repeat himself and I smiled.

Now, an overwhelming calm enveloped me as I looked at my father finally lying so much at peace. Daddy was gone; he had taken his last living breath only moments before. A tortuous and tumultuous five-week ordeal with brain cancer had ended for him and our family. All was quiet, even my tears.

—A daughter

Issues and needs at the time of death are exceedingly important and, at the same time, exceedingly personal. While the physiology of dying may be the same for most expected deaths, the psychological, spiritual, cultural, and family issues are as unique and varied as the patients and families themselves. As death nears, the goals of care must be discussed and, as appropriate, redefined. While some treatments may be discontinued, symptoms may intensify, subside, or even appear anew. Physiological changes as death approaches must also be defined, explained, and interpreted to the patient, whenever possible, as well as to the patient's family, close others, and caregivers. The nurse occupies a key position in assisting patients' family members at the time of death by supporting or suggesting death rituals, caring for the body after death, and facilitating early grief work. Most of the focus on death and dying in the past has been on dying in general, making the need for a chapter focused specifically on the actual death even more important.

Terminally ill persons are cared for in a variety of settings, including home with hospice care or traditional home care, hospice residential facilities, traditional home care, nursing homes, hospitals, intensive care units, and group homes. Deaths in intensive care settings may present special challenges—for example, restrictive visiting hours, and lack of space and less privacy for families—shortcomings that may be addressed by thoughtful and creative nursing care. Likewise, death in a nursing home setting may also offer unique challenges. Regardless of the setting, dying persons *can* be managed in such a way as to minimize distressing symptoms and maximize quality of life. Families can be supported in a way that optimizes use of valuable time and lessens distress during the bereavement period. Like it or not, we as health professionals only have one chance to "get it right" when caring for dying persons and their family, as death nears. In other words, there is no dress rehearsal for the time surrounding death; extensive planning ensures the least stressful and best possible outcome for all involved.

The patient's family is especially important as death nears. Family members may become full- or part-time caregivers, daughters and sons may find themselves in a position to "parent" their parents, and family issues, long forgotten or ignored, may surface. While we often think of "family" in traditional terms, a family may take on several forms and configurations. For purposes of this chapter the definition of family recognizes many patients have nontraditional families and may be cared for by a large extended entity, for example, a church community, a group of supportive friends, or the staff of a health care facility. Family is defined broadly to include not only persons bound by biology or legalities but also those whom the patient defines or who define themselves as a "close other" with another person, or those who function for the patient in "familistic" ways. These functions can include nurturance, intimacy, and economic, social, and psychological support in times of need, support in illness (including dealing with those outside the family), and companionship.[1,2]

The research regarding uncontrolled symptoms at end of life is misleading. It is most often performed in palliative care units or other settings dedicated to end-of-life care where goals of care are focused on assuring maximal symptom management. Most studies demonstrate that, unfortunately, the majority of people do not have a death where symptoms are well managed.[3] Up to 52% of persons have refractory symptoms at the very end of life that, at times, require terminal sedation.[4,5,6,7] Dyspnea may worsen as death approaches, while the notion of a final crescendo of pain is supported in some studies and not in others. Many patients experience a higher frequency of noisy and moist breathing, urinary incontinence and retention, restlessness, agitation, delirium, and nausea and vomiting.[5,6] Less frequently, symptoms such as sweating, myoclonus, and confusion have also been reported.[6] Ventafridda and colleagues[6] report that while most patients (91.5%) die peacefully, 8.5% experience symptoms requiring additional intervention in the final 24 hours, such as hemorrhage or hemoptysis (2%), respiratory distress (2%), restlessness (1.5%), pain (1%), myocardial infarction (1%), and regurgitation (1%). The wide variation in frequency of symptoms and reported "good deaths" may result from differing populations and sites of care (e.g., home, a specialized palliative care unit, or an inpatient hospice), differing measurement protocols or instruments, and the participants' cultural variations in reporting symptoms and approaching death. In most studies, symptoms requiring maximum diligence in assessment, prevention, and aggressive treatment during the final day or two before death are pain, dyspnea, restlessness, and agitation. The nurse plays a key role in educating family members and other caregivers in assessment, treatment, and continual evaluation of these symptoms.

Regardless of individual patient and family needs, attitudes, and "unfinished business," the nurse's professional approach and demeanor at the time near death is crucial and worthy of close attention. Patients experience total and profound dependency at this stage of their illness. Families are often called upon to assume total caregiving duties, often disrupting their own responsibilities for home, children, and career. While there may be similarities, all patients and families experience this time through the lens of their own perspective and thus, form their own unique meaning.

Some authors suggest theories and guidelines as the basis for establishing and maintaining meaningful, helpful, and therapeutic relationships with patients/clients and their families. One example is Carl Rogers's theory of helping relationships, in which he proposes the characteristics of a helping relationship are empathy, unconditional positive regard, and genuineness.[8] These characteristics, defined below as part of the nurse's approach to patients and families, are essential in facilitating care at the end of life. We have also added "attention to detail" because we feel, as do others, that this additional characteristic is essential for quality palliative care.[9,10] We urge you to consider the following characteristics in the context of your own practice, as a basis for facilitating and providing supportive relationships:

- *Empathy:* the ability to put oneself in the other person's place, trying to understand the patient/client from his or her own frame of reference; it also requires the deliberate setting aside of one's own frame of reference and bias.
- *Unconditional positive regard:* a warm feeling toward others, with a nonjudgmental acceptance of all they reveal themselves to be; the ability to convey a sense of respect and esteem at a time and place in which it is particularly important to do so.
- *Genuineness:* the ability to convey trustworthiness and openness that is real rather than a professional facade; also the ability to admit that one has limitations, makes mistakes, and does not have all the answers.
- *Attention to detail:* the learned and practiced ability to think critically about a situation and not make assumptions. The nurse, for example, discusses challenging patient and family concerns with colleagues and other members of the interdisciplinary team. The nurse considers every "what if" before making a decision and, in particular, any judgment. Finally, the nurse is constantly aware of how one's actions, attitudes, and words may be interpreted—and even misinterpreted—by others.[9]

The events and interactions—positive as well as negative—at the bedside of a dying person set the tone for the patient's care and form lasting memories for family members. The time of death and the care received by both the person who has died and family members present are predominant aspects of the survivor's memory of this momentous event.[11] Approaching patients and families with a genuine openness characterized by empathy and positive regard will ease the way in making this difficult time meaningful, individualized, and deeply profound.

In the pages ahead, we will discuss some key issues surrounding the death itself, including advanced planning, the changing focus of care as death nears, common signs and symptoms of death and their management, and care of the patient and family at time of death. We will conclude with two case examples illustrating the chapter's content.

ADVANCED PLANNING: EVOLVING CHOICES AND GOALS OF CARE

Health care choices related to wellness are generally viewed as clear-cut or easy. We have an infection, we seek treatment, and the problem resolves. Throughout most of the life span, medical treatment choices are obvious. As wellness moves along the health care continuum to illness, choices become less clear and consequences of choices have a significantly greater impact.

Many end-of-life illnesses present with well-known and well-documented natural courses. Providing the patient and family with information on the natural course of the disease at appropriate intervals is a critical function of health care providers, such as nurses. Providing an opening for discussion such as, "Would you like to talk about the future?" "Do you have any concerns that I can help you address?" or "It seems you are not as active as you were before," may open a much-needed discussion of fears and concerns about impending death. Family members may request information that patients do not wish to know at certain points in time. With the patient's permission, discussions with the family may occur in the patient's absence. Family members may also need coaching to initiate end-of-life discussions with the patient. End-of-life goal setting is greatly enhanced when the patient is aware of the support of family.

End-of-life care issues should always be discussed with patients and family members. The competent patient is always the acknowledged decision maker. The involvement of family assures maximal consensus for patient support as decisions are actually implemented. Decisions for patients who lack decision-making capacity should be made by a consensus approach, using family conference methodology. If documents such as a durable power of attorney for health care or a living will are available, they can be utilized as a guide for examining wishes that influence decision making and goal setting. The decision maker, usually the person named as health care power of attorney (HCPOA) or the patient's primary family members, should be clearly identified. This approach may also be used with patients who are able to make their own decisions.

To facilitate decision making, a family conference of the decision makers (decisional patient, family members, and the HCPOA), patient's physician, nurse, chaplain, and social worker is initiated. A history of how the patient's health care status evolved from diagnosis to the present is reviewed. The family is presented with the natural course of the disease. Choices on how care may proceed in the future are reviewed. Guidance or support for the choices is provided based on existing data and clinical experience with the particular disease in relation to the current status of the patient. If no consensus for the needed decisions occurs, decision making is postponed. Third-party support by a trusted individual or consultant may then be enlisted. Personal fundamental values of the patient, family, and physician should be recognized and protected throughout this process.[12]

Decisions by patients and families cross the spectrum of care. They range from continuing treatment for the actual disease, such as undergoing chemotherapy or renal dialysis or utilization of medications, to initiating cardiopulmonary resuscitation (CPR). The health care provider may work with the patient and family, making care decisions for specific treatments and timing their discontinuance within a clear and logical framework. A goal-setting discussion may determine a patient's personal framework for care such as:

- treatment and enrollment in any clinical studies for which I am eligible
- treatment as long as statistically there is a greater than 50% chance of response
- full treatment as long as I am ambulatory and able to come to the clinic or office
- treatment only of "fixable" conditions like infections, blood glucose levels
- treatment only for controlling symptomatic aspects of disease

Once a goal framework has been established with the patient, the appropriateness of interventions such as CPR, renal dialysis, or intravenous (IV) antibiotics is clear. For instance, if the patient states a desire for renal dialysis as long as transportation to the clinic is possible without the use of an ambulance, the end point of dialysis treatment is quite clear. At this point the futility of CPR would also be apparent. Allowing a patient to determine when the treatment is a burden unjustified by his or her value system and communicating this to family and caregivers is perhaps the most pivotal point in management of the patient's care.

Changing the Focus of Care as Death Nears

Vital Signs. As nurses, we derive a good deal of security in performing the ritual of measurement of vital signs, one of the hallmarks of nursing care. When death is approaching, we need to question the rationale for measuring vital signs. Are interventions going to change by discovering the patient has experienced a drop in blood pressure? If the plan of care no longer involves intervening in changes in blood pressure and pulse rates, the measurements should cease. The time spent taking vital signs, then, can be channeled to assessment of patient comfort and provision of family support. Changes in respiratory rate are visually noted, and do not require routine monitoring of rates, unless symptom management issues develop that could be more accurately assessed by vital signs. The measurement of body temperature using a non-invasive route should continue on a regular basis until death, allowing for the detection and management of fever, a frequent symptom that may cause distress and require management.

Fever often suggests infection. As death approaches, goal setting should include a discussion of the nontreatment of infection. Indications for treatment of infection are based upon the degree of distress and patient discomfort.[13] Pharmacological management of fever should be available with antipyretics, including acetaminophen, and nonsteroidal anti-inflammatory drugs for all patients. Ice packs, alcohol baths, and cooling blankets should be used cautiously as they often cause more distress than the fever itself.[14]

Fever may also suggest dehydration. As with the management of fever, interventions are guided by the degree of distress and patient discomfort. The appropriateness of beginning artificial hydration for the treatment of fever is based upon individual patient assessment.

Cardiopulmonary Resuscitation. Patients and family members may need to discuss the issue of the futility of CPR when death is expected from a terminal illness. Developed in the 1960s as a method of restarting the heart in the event of sudden, unexpected clinical death, CPR was originally intended for circumstances when death was unexpected or accidental. It is not indicated in certain situations, such as cases of terminal irreversible illness where death is not unexpected; resuscitation in these circumstances may represent an active violation of a person's right to die with dignity.[15,16] Over the years, predictors of the success of CPR have become apparent, along with the predictors of the burden of CPR. In general, a poor outcome of CPR is predicted in patients with advanced terminal illnesses, patients with dementia, and patients with poor functional status who depend upon others for meeting their basic care needs. Poor outcomes or physical problems resultant from CPR include broken ribs, punctured lung, brain damage if anoxia has occurred for too long, and permanent unconsciousness or persistent vegetative state.[17] Most importantly though, the use of CPR negates the possibility of a peaceful death. This is considered the gravest of poor outcomes.

Artificial Fluids. The issue of artificial hydration is emotional for many patients and families because of the role that giving and consuming fluids plays in our culture. When patients are not able to take fluids, concern surfaces among caregivers. A decision must be reached regarding the appropriate use of fluids within the context of the patient's framework of goals. Beginning artificial hydration is a relatively easy task, but the decision to stop is generally much more problematic given the emotional implications. Ethical, moral, and most religious viewpoints state there is no difference between withholding and withdrawing a treatment such as artificial hydration. However, the emotional response attached to withdrawing a treatment adds a world of difference to the decision to suspend. It is therefore much less burdensome to not begin treatment, if this decision is acceptable in light of specific patient circumstances.[18]

Most patients and families are aware that without fluids, death will occur quickly. Current literature suggests that fluids should not be routinely administered to dying patients, nor automatically withheld from them. Instead the decision should be based upon careful, individual assessment. Zerwekh[19] suggests consideration of the following when the choice to initiate and continue hydration is evaluated:

- Is the patient's well-being enhanced by the overall effect of hydration?
- Which current symptoms are being relieved by artificial hydration?
- Are other end-of-life symptoms being aggravated by the fluids?
- Does hydration improve the patient's level of consciousness? If so, is this within the patient's goals and wishes for end-of-life care?
- Does it appear to prolong the patient's survival? If so, is this within the patient's goals and wishes for end-of-life care?
- What is the effect of the infusion technology on the patient's well-being, mobility, ability to interact and be with family?
- What is the burden of the infusion technology on the family in terms of caregiver stress, finance? Is it justified by benefit to the patient?

An important study by Fainsinger and Bruera[20] suggests that while some dying patients may benefit from dehydration, others may manifest symptoms such as confusion or opioid toxicity that may be corrected or prevented by parental hydration. Regardless, the uniqueness of the individual situation, the goals of care, and the comfort of the patient must always be considered when this issue is addressed.

Terminal dehydration refers to the process in which the dying patient's condition naturally results in a decrease in fluid intake. A gradual withdrawal from activities of daily living may occur as symptoms such as dysphagia, nausea, and fatigue become more obvious. Families may commonly ask if the patient will be thirsty as fluid intake decreases. In a study at St. Christopher's Hospice in Sydenham, England, although patients reported thirst, there was no correlation between thirst and hydration, resulting in the assumption that artificial hydration to relieve symptoms may be futile.[21] Artificial hydration has the potential to result in fluid accumulation, resulting in distressful symptoms such as edema, ascites, nausea and vomiting, and pulmonary congestion. Does artificial hydration prolong life? Smith cites two studies that reported longer survival times with no artificial hydration.[22] Health care providers need to assist patients and family members to refocus on the natural course of the disease, and the notion that the patient's death will be caused by the disease, not dehydration, a natural occurrence in advanced illness and dying. Nurses may then assist families in dealing with symptoms caused by dehydration.

Dry mouth, a consistently reported distressing symptom of dehydration, can be relieved with sips of beverages, ice chips or hard candies.[23] Another simple comfort measure for dry mouth is spraying normal saline into the mouth with a spray bottle or atomizer. (Normal saline is made by mixing one teaspoon of table salt in a quart of water.) Meticulous mouth care must be administered to keep the patient's mouth clean. Family members can be instructed to anticipate this need. The nurse can assist the family by assuring the necessary provisions are on hand to assist the patient.

Medications. Medications unrelated to the terminal diagnosis are generally continued as long as their administration is not burdensome. When swallowing pills becomes too difficult, the medication may be offered in a liquid or other form if available, considering patient and family comfort. Continuing medications, however, may be seen by some patients and families as a way of normalizing daily activities and therefore should be supported. Considerable tact, kindness, and knowledge of the patient and family are needed in assisting them to make decisions about discontinuing medications. Medications that do not contribute to daily comfort should be evaluated on an individual basis for possible discontinuance. Medications such as antihypertensives, replacement hormones, vitamin supplements, iron preparations, hypoglycemics, long-term antibiotics, anti-arrythmics, laxatives, and diuretics, unless they are essential to patient comfort, can and should be discontinued unless doing so would cause symptoms or discomfort.[24] Customarily, the only drugs necessary in the final days of life are analgesics, anticonvulsants, antiemetics, antipyretics, anticholenergic medications, and sedatives.[24]

Implantable Cardioverter Defibrillator. Implantable cardioverter defibrillators (ICDs) are used to prevent cardiac arrest due to ventricular tachycardia or ventricular fibrillation. Patients with ICDs who are dying of another terminal condition may choose to have the defibrillator deactivated, or turned off, so there is no interference from the device at the time of death. Patients with ICDs who enter a hospice or palliative care program with the diagnoses such as advanced terminal cancer or end-stage renal disease and have decided to stop dialysis are candidates for such consideration. Patients with ICDs have been instructed to carry a wallet identification card at all times that provides the model and serial number of the implanted device.[25] The identification card will also have the name of the physician to contact for assistance. Deactivating the ICD is a simple, noninvasive procedure. Standard practice calls for the patient to sign a consent. The device is tested after it is turned off to assure it is no longer operational, and the test result is placed in the patient record. Patients who are at peace with their impending death find this procedure important to provide assurance that death indeed with be quiet and easy, when it does occur.

Corticosteroids in Patients with Intracranial Malignancy. In most cases, the patient with an intracranial malignancy will be maintained on a corticosteroid such as dexamethasone to control headaches and seizures caused by intracranial swelling. When the patient is nearing death and no longer able to swallow, the corticosteroids may be discontinued with minimal or no tapering.[24] Discontinuation of the corticosteroid may lead to increased cerebral edema, and thus, headache and progressive neurological dysfunction.[26] Addition or adjustment of analgesics and anticonvulsant medications may be needed for the patient's continued comfort.

A patient who is still able to swallow medications may also request to stop treatment with corticosteroids because of continued deterioration and poor quality of life. Should this occur, the drug can be tapered, at the same time an oral anticonvulsant medication is increased. Careful assessment and control of headache and discomfort should be done twice a day, preferably by the same person. Resumption of the drug at any point is always an option that should be offered to patient and family members if the need becomes apparent.[7]

Renal Dialysis. Renal dialysis is a life-sustaining treatment, and as death approaches, it is important to recognize and agree upon its limitations. Discontinuing dialysis should be considered in the following cases:

- patients with acute, concurrent illness, who, if they survive, will be burdened with a great deal of disability as defined by the patient and family,
- progressive and untreatable disease or disability, and/or
- dementia or severe neurological deficit.[27]

There is general agreement dialysis should not be used to prolong the dying process.[28] The time between discontinuing dialysis and death varies widely, between hours and days (for patients with acute illnesses, described above) to days, weeks, and even longer, if some residual renal function remains.[27,29] Opening a discussion of the burden of treatment, however, is a delicate task. There may be competing opinions among the patient, family, and even staff about the tolerability or intolerability of continuing treatment. The nurse who sees the patient and family on a regular basis may be the most logical person to recognize the discrete changes in status. Gently validating these observations may open a much-needed discussion regarding the goals of care.

The discussions and decisions surrounding discontinuing or modifying treatment are never easy. Phrases like "there is nothing more that can be done" or "we have tried everything" have no place in end-of-life discussions with patients and families. Always assure the patient and family members—and be prepared to follow through—that you will stand by them and do all you can to provide help and comfort.[9] This is essential to ensure that palliative care is not interpreted as abandonment.

COMMON SIGNS AND SYMPTOMS OF IMMINENT DEATH AND THEIR MANAGEMENT

There usually are predictable sets of processes that occur during the final stages of a terminal illness due to gradual hypoxia, respiratory acidosis, metabolic consequences of renal failure, and the signs and symptoms of hypoxic brain function.[7,30,31] These processes account for the signs and symptoms of imminent death and can assist the nurse in helping the family plan for the actual death.

The following signs and symptoms provide cues that death is only days away:[7,24]

- Profound weakness (patient is usually bedbound; requires assistance with all or most of cares)
- Gaunt and pale physical appearance (most common in persons with cancer when corticosteroids have not been used as treatment)
- Drowsiness and/or a reduction in awareness, insight, and perception (often extended periods of drowsiness; extreme difficulty in concentrating; severely limited attention span; unable to cooperate with caregivers; often disoriented to time and place)
- Increasing lack of interest in food and fluid with diminished intake
- Increasing difficulty in swallowing oral medications

During the final days, the signs and symptoms above become more pronounced, and as oxygen concentrations drop, new symptoms also appear. We in no way advocate measuring oxygen concentration in the dying person, as this will add discomfort and not alter the course of care. Knowing, however, the signs and symptoms associated with decreasing oxygen concentrations can assist the nurse in guiding the family as death nears.[32] As oxygen saturation drops below 80%, signs and symptoms related to hypoxia appear. As the dying process proceeds, special issues related to normalizing the dying process for the family, symptom control, and patient/family support present themselves. Table 28–1 summarizes the physiological process of dying and suggests interventions for both patients and families.

As the imminently dying person takes in less fluid, third spaced fluids clinically noted as peripheral edema, acites, or pleural effusions, may be reabsorbed. Breathing may become easier, and there may be less discomfort from tissue distention. Accordingly, as the person experiences dehydration, swelling is often reduced around tumor masses. Patients may experience transient im-

Table 28–1. Symptoms in the Normal Progression of Dying and Suggested Interventions

Symptoms	Suggested Interventions
Early Stage	
Sensation/perception • Impairment in the ability to grasp ideas and reason; periods of alertness along with periods of disorientation and restlessness are also noted	• Interpret the signs and symptoms to the patient (when appropriate) and family as part of the normal dying process, for example, assure them the patient's "seeing" and even talking to persons who have died is normal and often expected • Urge family members to look for metaphors for death in speech and conversation (for example, talk of a long journey, needing maps or tickets, or in preparing for a trip in other ways)[33] and using these metaphors as a departure point for conversation with the patient • Urge family to take advantage of the patient's periods of lucidity to talk with patient and ensure nothing is left unsaid • Encourage family members to touch and speak slowly and gently to the patient without being patronizing • Maximize safety; for example, use bedrails and schedule people to sit with the patient
• Some loss of visual acuity • Increased sensitivity to bright lights while other senses, except hearing, are dulled	• Keep sensory stimulation to a minimum, including light, sounds, and visual stimulation; reading to a patient who has enjoyed reading in the past may provide comfort • Urge the family to be mindful of what they say "over" the patient, as hearing remains present; also continue to urge family to say what they wish not to be left unsaid
Cardiorespiratory: • Increased pulse and respiratory rate • Agonal respirations or sounds of gasping for air without apparent discomfort • Apnea, periodic, or Cheyne-Stokes respirations • Inability to cough or clear secretions efficiently, resulting in gurgling or congested breathing (sometimes referred to as the "death rattle")	• Normalize the observed changes by interpreting the signs and symptoms as part of the normal dying process and assuring the patient's comfort • Assess and treat respiratory distress as appropriate • Assess use and need for parenteral fluids, tube feedings, or hydration. (It is generally appropriate to either discontinue these at this point in time or greatly decrease them) • Reposition the patient in a side-lying position with the head of the bed elevated • Suctioning is rarely needed, but when appropriate, suction should be gentle and only at the level of the mouth, throat, and nasal pharynx • Administer anticholinergic drugs (transdermal scopolamine, hyoscyamine) as appropriate, recognizing and discussing with the family that they will not decrease already existing secretions.
Renal/Urinary • Decreasing urinary output, sometimes urinary incontinence or retention	• Insertion of catheter and/or use of absorbent padding • Careful assessment for urinary retention as restlessness can be a related symptom
Musculoskeletal • Gradual loss of the ability to move, beginning with the legs, then progressing	• Repositioning every few hours as appropriate • Anticipate needs such as sips of fluids, oral care, changing of bed pads and linens, etc.

(*continued*)

Table 28–1. Symptoms in the Normal Progression of Dying and Suggested Interventions (*Continued*)

Symptoms	Suggested Interventions
Late Stage	
Sensation/perception	
• Unconsciousness • Eyes remain half open, blink reflex is absent; sense of hearing remains intact and may slowly decrease	• Interpret the patient's unconsciousness to the family as part of the normal dying process • Provide for total care, including incontinence of urine and stool • Encourage family members to speak slowly and gently to the patient with the assurance hearing remains intact
Cardiorespiratory	
• Heart rate may double, strength of contractions decrease, rhythm becomes irregular • Patient feels cool to the touch, and becomes diaphoretic. • Cyanosis is noted in the tip of the nose, nail beds, and knees; extremities may become mottled (progressive mottling indicates death within a few days); absence of a palpable radial pulse may indicate death within hours.	• Interpret these changes to family members as part of the normal dying process • Frequent linen changes and sponge baths may enhance comfort
Renal/Urinary	
• A precipitous drop in urinary output	• Interpret to the family the drop in urinary output as a normal sign that death is near • Careful assessment for urinary retention; restlessness can be a related symptom

provements in comfort, including increased mental status, and decreased pain. The family needs a careful and compassionate explanation regarding these temporary improvements and encouragement to make the most of this short but potentially meaningful time.

There are multiple patient and family education tools available to assist families to interpret the signs and symptoms of approaching death (Fig. 28–1). However, as with all aspects of palliative care, consideration of the individual perspective and associated relationship of the patient/family member, the underlying disease course trajectory, anticipated symptoms, and the setting of care is essential for optimal care at all stages of illness, but especially during the final days and hours.

CARE AT TIME OF DEATH, DEATH RITUALS AND FACILITATING EARLY GRIEVING

At the time of death, the nurse has a unique opportunity to provide information helpful in making decisions about organ and body donation and autopsy. In addition, the nurse can also support the family's choice of death rituals, gently care for the body, assist in funeral planning, and facilitate the early process of grieving.

Family members' needs around the time of death change just as the goals of care change. During this important time, plans are reviewed and perhaps refined. Special issues affecting the time of death, such as cultural influences, decisions regarding organ or body donation, or need for autopsy, are also reviewed. Under U.S. federal law, if death occurs in a hospital setting, staff must approach the family decision maker regarding the possibility of organ donation.[34] While approaching family at this time may seem onerous, the opportunity to assist another is often comforting. Some hospital-based palliative care programs include information about organ donation in their admission or bereavement information. We urge you to review your own organization's policies and procedures.

Regardless, it is important to clarify specifically with family members what their desires and needs are at the time of death. Do they wish to be present? Do they know of others who wish to now say a final goodbye? Have they said everything they wish to say to the person who is dying? Do they have any regrets? Are they concerned about anything? Do they wish something could be different? Every person in a family has different and unique needs that unless explored, can go unmet. Family members recall the time before the death and immediately afterward with great acuity and detail. As we mentioned above, there is no chance for a dress rehearsal—we only have the one chance to "get it right"—and make the experience an individual and memorable one.

While an expected death can be anticipated with some degree of certainty, the exact time of death is often not predictable. Death often occurs when there are no health care professionals present. Often, dying people seem to determine the time of their death—for example, waiting for someone to arrive, a date or event to pass, or even family members to leave—even if the leave-taking is brief. Because of this, it is crucial to ask family members who wish to be present at the time of death if they have thought about the possibility they will not be there. This opens an essential discussion regarding the time of death; while it can be predicted to some degree, we never know when death will actually occur. Gently reminding family members of that possibility can assist them in preparing for any eventuality.

Determining Death Has Occurred

Death often occurs when health professionals are not present at the bedside or in the home. Regardless of the site of death, a plan must be in place for who will be contacted, how the death pronouncement will be handled, and how the body will be removed. This is especially crucial for deaths outside a health care institution. Death pronouncement procedures vary from state to state, and sometimes, from county to county within states. In some states, nurses can pronounce death, and in others, they cannot. In inpatient settings, the organization's policy and procedures are followed. In hospice home care, generally the nurse makes a home visit, assesses lack of vital signs, contacts the physician who verbally agrees to sign the death certificate, and then contacts the funeral home or mortuary.[35] Local customs, the ability of a healthcare agency to assure the safety of a nurse during the home visit, and provision for "do-not-resuscitate" orders outside a hospital setting, among other factors, account for wide variability in the practices and procedures surrounding pronouncing death in the home. Although the practice varies widely, the police or coroner may be called if the circumstances of the death were unusual, were associated with trauma (regardless of the cause of the death), or occurred within 24 hours of a hospital admission.[36] The practice of actual death pronouncement varies widely and is not often taught in medical school or residencies.[36] The customary procedure[36,37] is to, first, identify the patient, then note the following:

- general appearance of the body
- lack of reaction to verbal or tactile stimuli
- lack of pupillary light reflex (pupils will be fixed and dilated)
- absent breathing and lung sounds
- absent carotid and apical pulse (in some situations, listening for an apical pulse for a full minute is advisable)[37]

Likewise, documentation of the death is equally important and should be thorough and clear. The following guidelines are suggested:[36,37]

- patient's name and time of call
- who was present at the time of death and at the time of the pronouncement
- detailed findings of the physical examination
- date and time of death pronouncement (either by the nurse or the time physician either assessed the patient or was notified)
- who else was notified and when—for example, additional family members, attending physician, or other staff members
- if the coroner was notified, rationale and outcome, if known
- special plans for disposition and outcome (for example, organ or body donation, autopsy, special care related to cultural or religious traditions)

Care of the Body after Death

Regardless of the site of death, care of the body is an important nursing function. In gently caring for the body, the nurse can continue to communicate care and concern for the patient and family members and model behaviors that may be helpful as the family members continue their important grief work. Caring for the body after death also calls for an understanding of the physiological changes that occur. By understanding these changes, the nurse can interpret and dispel any myths and explain these changes to the family members and therefore, assist the family in making their own personal decisions about the time immediately following death and funeral plans. A time-honored and classic article regarding postmortem care, the only one published in the nursing literature since 1978, emphasizes that while postmortem care may be a ritualized nursing procedure, the scientific rationale for the procedure rests upon the basics of the physiological changes after death.[38] These changes occur at a regular rate depending on the temperature of the body at the time of death, the size of the body, the extent of infection, if any, and the temperature of the air. These three important physiological changes, rigor mortis, algor mortis, and postmortem decomposition are discussed in turn along with the relevant nursing implications in Table 28–2.

Care of and respect for the body after death by nursing staff should clearly communicate to the family that the person who died was indeed important and valued. Often, caring for the body after death provides the needed link between family members and the reality of the death, recognizing everyone present at the time of death and soon after will have a different experience and a different sense of loss. Many institutions, however, no longer require nursing staff to care for the person after death or perform "postmortem" care.[40] Further, the only published resources related to postmortem care are a series of three articles describing the procedure of "last offices" published in a British journal in 1998.[41,42,43] In a recent review of nursing textbooks, only 26% covered this important aspect of nursing care.[44] Family members will long remember the actions of the nurse after the death. A kind, gentle approach and meticulous attention to detail are imperative.

Encourage rituals the family members and others present find comforting. Rituals are practices within a social context that facilitate and provide ways to understand and cope with the contradictory and complex nature of human existence. They provide a way to express and contain strong emotions, ease feelings of anxiety and impotence, and provide structure in times of chaos and disorder.[45] Rituals can take many forms—a brief service at the time of death, a special preparation of the body as in the Orthodox Jewish tradition, an Irish wake, where, after paying respect to the person who has died, family and friends gather, sometimes all night, to share stories, food, and drink.[46] Of utmost importance, however, is to ensure that family members see this ritual as comforting and meaningful. It is the family's needs and desires that direct this activity—not the nurse's. There are, again, no rules that govern the appropriateness of rituals; rituals are comforting and serve to begin the process of healing and acceptance.

To facilitate the grieving process it is often helpful to create a pleasant, peaceful, and comfortable environment for family members who wish to spend time with the body, according to their desires and cultural or religious traditions. Consider engaging family members in after-death care and ritual by inviting them to either comb the hair or wash the hands and face, or more, if they are comfortable. Parents can be encouraged to hold and cuddle their baby or child. Including siblings or other involved children in rituals, traditions, and other end-of-life care activities according to their developmental level is also essential. During this time, invite talk about their family member and encourage them to reminisce—valuable rituals that can help persons begin to work through their grief.[47] Encourage family to touch, hold, and kiss the person's body, as they feel comfortable. Parents may wish to clip and save a lock of their child's hair as a keepsake. Offer to dress the person's body in something other than a hospital gown or other nightclothes. Wrap babies snugly in a blanket. Many families may choose to dress the body in a favorite article of clothing before removal by the funeral home. Note that when turning a body, at times, air escapes from the lungs, producing a "sighing" sound. Informing family members of this possibility is wise. Again, modeling gentle and careful handling of the body can communicate the care and concern on the part of the nurse, and facilitate grieving and the creation of positive and long-lasting memories.

Postmortem care also includes, unless an autopsy or the coroner is involved, removing any tubes, drains, and other devices. In home care settings, these can be placed in a plastic bag and given to the funeral home for disposal as medical waste or simply double-bagged and placed in the family's regular trash. Placing a waterproof pad, diaper, or adult incontinence brief on the patient often prevents soiling and odor as the patient's body is moved and the rectal and urinary bladder sphincters relax. Packing the rectum and vagina is considered unnecessary, as it increases the rate of bacterial proliferation that naturally occurs when these areas are not allowed to drain.[39]

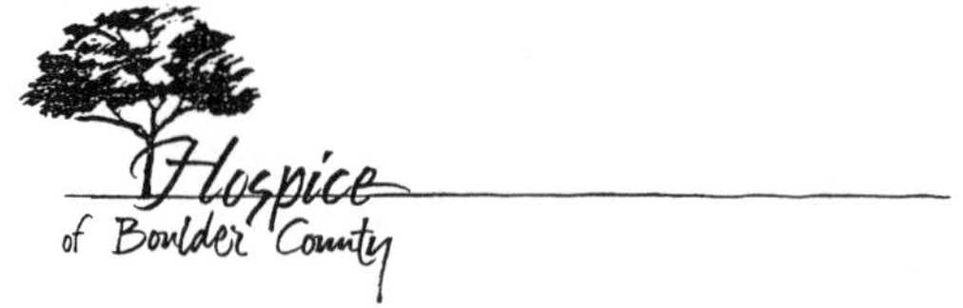

SIGNS AND SYMPTOMS OF APPROACHING DEATH

This list of symptoms and what to do about them may appear frightening, but knowing what to expect may reduce some of your anxiety about the approaching death.

Each person approaches death in their own way, bringing to this last experience their own uniqueness. Our list of "Symptoms and What To Do" is a map to the goal of a peaceful death. Like all maps, there are many different routes to the same destination.

You may see all of these symptoms or none. Death will come in its own time, and its own way to each of us. It is important to remember that **dying is a natural process.**

1.	Withdrawal - Physical and emotional, and increased sleep.	Natural process of withdrawing from everything outside of one's self, looking inward, reviewing one's self and one's life. Your loved one may turn inward, withdraw physically and emotionally. This occurs in an attempt to cope with the many changes that are occurring.
2.	Reduced food and fluid intake.	Decreased need because body will naturally begin to conserve energy which is expended on these tasks. Dehydration is a natural comfort measure requiring body to handle less fluids in all the systems. At no time should food/fluids be forced.
3.	Confusion/Agitation can vary from mild to the end stage agitation which may include trying to get out of bed, picking at covers, seeing things that are not apparent to us.	Talk calmly and assuredly. Keep lights on, use times when patient is alert for meaningful conversation. Music can be very calming. Medication often used to control this symptom.

(*continued*)

Fig. 28–1. Hospice of Boulder County, Colorado, handout for families responsible for end-of-life care.

Occasionally families, especially in the home care setting, may wish to keep the person's body at home to perhaps wait for another family member to come from a distance and ensure that everyone has adequate time with the deceased. If the family wishes the body embalmed, this is best done within 12 hours. If embalming is not desired, the body can remain in the home for approximately 24 hours before further decomposition and odor occurs. Suggest to the family they make the immediate area cooler to slow down the natural decomposition by either turning down the furnace or turning up the air conditioning.[39] Be sure, however, to inform the funeral director that the family has chosen to keep the body at home a little longer. Finally, funeral directors are a reliable source of information regarding post-death changes, local customs, and cultural issues.

4.	Change in breathing patterns.	This is common. You may see irregular breathing: very rapid, very slow, and/or 10 to 30 seconds of no breathing at all (called apnea). These symptoms are very common and indicative of a decrease in circulation. It does not mean that your loved one is uncomfortable or struggling.
5.	Oral secretions collect in back of throat causing noisy respiration.	Swallowing reflex may be absent. Patient may be breathing through the secretions - this may be more uncomfortable for us as observers than patient experiencing it - Elevate head of bed or turning patient on side.
6.	Incontinence of urine and stool.	Reduced intake results in reduced output with darker color. Bedpads and diapers can be used to protect bed linens. Cleanse patient and change linens frequently to maintain comfort and protect skin.
7.	Changes in skin temperature and color.	Decreased circulation can cause coolness and discoloration of skin. Use light covers, turn side to side frequently to maintain comfort and prevent skin breakdown (bedsores). Heating pads and electric blankets NOT recommended.

Hearing is the last sense to be lost, so the patient can hear all that is being said - This is a good time to say good-bye, reassure them that you will be all right even though you will miss them greatly. (You may tell them it's OK to "let go".) This permission is often helpful for a peaceful death.

How would you know death has occurred?
1. No breathing
2. No heartbeat or pulse

If you believe that death has occurred, call Hospice at 651-3922 (Longmont) or 449-7740 (Boulder). **Do not call 911 or the physician.** We will come to your home to help you. (You may want to use the time until we arrive to say your last good-byes.)

Fig. 28–1. *(Continued)*

The care of patients and families near to death and afterward is an important nursing function—arguably one of the most important. As you review the following case studies, consider how the nurse interceded in a positive manner, mindful of the changing tempo of care, and the changing patient and family needs, desires, and perspectives.

Case Study: Mrs. B, an Elderly Woman with Generalized Seizure

Mrs. B was admitted to the acute care setting for obstipation. She was a 95-year-old woman with advanced dementia who had been cared for by her 75-year-old daughter in her home. Her Karnofsky performance score was 35, indicating greatly limited function. On the day of admission, her daughter was also admitted for treatment of a chronic illness. Mrs. B's obstipation was corrected and discharge was planned for her to return to her family. Her functional status had not changed in the course of the hospitalization. The morning before the scheduled discharge, she experienced a generalized seizure and required high doses of a benzodiazepine to stop the seizure, allowing her finally to sleep. Twelve hours after the seizure, she had not awakened. A computerized tomography (CT) scan showed no cause for the seizure. Twelve hours post generalized seizure, the family gathered for information and to discuss the following issues:

- Will she awaken?
- Will she die?
- What will the plan of care be in the hours ahead?

Framework of care: "watchful waiting."

The family was informed that all efforts would be made to control seizures and keep Mrs. B comfortable. Artificial hydration would be maintained. The plan was that the family would meet again with the physician in 72 hours if there was no change in her status. In the interim, they agreed to a no-code status for the patient.

Seventy-two hours later, there was no change in Mrs. B's status. She remained unresponsive, with no further seizure activity. The family gathered again to discuss changes in the plan of care, particularly treatment of infections and artificial feedings. The family clearly stated that they desired to "support life," and wanted feeding begun through a nasogastric tube and IV antibiotics prescribed if fever/infection were present.

Framework of care: A trial of interventions for life support (nutritional support), with the plan to meet again in three to four days to revisit the issues if Mrs. B remained unresponsive.

Seven days post initial seizure, Mrs. B's neurological status remained unchanged. Mrs. B developed pneumonia and treatment with IV antibiotics began, but fevers continued to occur. The family was told that the prognosis was poor, and that hope for the patient to return to her previous functional status decreased with each day. The family again stressed that they wanted "everything done"—relating that they felt this was an important part of their religious value system. Information was provided to all family members on prognosis based upon the known natural course of current medical problems. All members were clearly confronted with information that Mrs. B was not expected to recover, and that death was anticipated. The family was invited to consider other care options such as home hospice. They choose to continue in the acute care setting.

Framework of care: Clearly there were mixed feelings among family members as to the aggressiveness of care desired. The family was urged to talk among themselves and speak with their minister. Leaders emerged among the family group who spoke privately to family members who desired aggressive care. Plans were made to meet with the family in 72 hours. At that time, a discussion of the ap-

Table 28–2. Normal Postmortem Physiological Changes and Their Implications for Nursing

Change	Underlying Mechanisms	Nursing Implications
• Rigor mortis	Approximately two to four hours after death, adenosine phosphate (ATP) ceases to be synthesized due to the depletion of glycogen stores. ATP is necessary for muscle fiber relaxation, so the lack of ATP results in an exaggerated contraction of the muscle fibers that eventually immobilizes the joints. Rigor begins in the involuntary muscles (heart, GI tract, bladder, arteries) and progresses to the muscles of the head and neck, trunk and lower limbs. After approximately 96 hours, however, muscle chemical activity totally ceases, and rigor passes. Persons with large muscle mass (for example, body builders) are prone to more pronounced rigor mortis. Conversely, frail elderly persons, or persons who have been bed bound for long periods of time, are less subject to rigor mortis[39]	In many cultures, the body is viewed within 24–48 hours after death. Therefore, post-death positioning becomes of utmost importance. In many cases, it is important to be sure the eyelids and jaw are closed and dentures are place in the mouth. (Rolling a towel and placing it under the jaw often helps to keep it closed.) The position of the hands is also important. Position all limbs in proper body alignment. If rigor mortis does occur, it can often be "massaged out" by the funeral director.[39] Finally, by understanding this physiology, the nurse can also reassure the family about the myth that due to rigor mortis, muscles can suddenly contract and the body can appear to move
• Algor mortis	After the circulaton ceases and the hypothalamus stops functioning, internal body temperature drops by approximately 1° C or 1.8° F per hour until it reaches room temperature. As the body cools, skin loses its natural elasticity. If a high fever was present at death, the changes in body temperature are more pronounced and the person may appear to "sweat" after death. Body cooling may also take several more hours[39]	The nurse can prepare family members for the coolness of the skin to touch or the increased moisture by explaining the changes that happen after death. The nurse may also suggest kissing the person on their hair instead of their skin. The skin, due to loss of elasticity, becomes fragile and easily torn. If dressings are to be applied, it is best to apply them with either a circular bandage or paper tape. Handle the body gently as well, being sure to not place traction on the skin
• Postmortem decomposition or "liver mortis"	Discoloration and softening of the body are due largely to the breakdown of red blood cells and the resultant release of hemoglobin that stains the vessel walls and surrounding tissue. This staining appears a mottling, bruising, or both in the dependent parts of the body as well as parts of the body where the skin has been punctured (for example, intravenous or chest tube sites).[39] Often this discoloration becomes extensive in a very short time. The remainder of the body has a gray hue. In cardiac-related deaths, the face often appears purple in color regardless of the positioning at or after death[39]	As the body is handled, for example, while bathing and dressing, the nurse informs the family member about this normal change that occurs after death

propriateness of continuing IV antibiotics and artificial feeding was presented.

Ten days post initial seizure, Mrs. B's neurological status remained unchanged. The pneumonia had not responded to treatment but her fever was controlled with scheduled antipyretics. The family was advised that death was expected and that in order to make Mrs. B as comfortable as possible, it was suggested that artificial feeding be discontinued. Because feedings were not causing uncomfortable symptoms, the family chose to continue until symptoms of distress were noted. They were advised, however, that IV antibiotics had been ineffective and would be discontinued, and that all efforts would focus on control of seizures and fever and other issues of patient and family comfort.

Framework of care: Symptom management only, with support for family grieving. Planning for funeral is begun with a focus on "celebration of life."

Critical Points

- Coming to grips with death is a process. If the goals of care related to the death process have not previously been discussed with family members and close others, time will be needed for this to take place.
- Frameworks of care must be clear at all points in the treatment process.
- Family values or perceptions of the meaning of care interventions vary and may not encompass a vision of end-of-life care. Families may not have considered what this vision is. If so, they will need assistance from chaplain, ministers, and supportive loved ones who can talk them through discovering this meaning.

- Prognostic information must be presented clearly and realistically. This information is needed to guide family members in their decision making.
- Futility and burdens of treatment must openly be addressed within the framework of care.

Case Study: Joe, a Patient with Malignant Melanoma

Joe was a 35-year-old English professor with a two-year history of malignant melanoma metastatic to the liver. After unsuccessful treatment, including participation in clinical trials, Joe, with the blessing of his wife, Ann, and their sons, Andy, age 16, and Josh, age 12, decided to focus on symptom management and assuring the quality of his remaining life. However, when his oncologist suggested hospice, he resisted, claiming that "hospice" was synonymous with death, and while he knew he was dying, he did not feel the need to talk about it outside of his immediate family, did not want to "give up," and wanted to finish a book he was writing as well as leave some sort of a written legacy for his sons. The oncologist consulted the palliative care team at the hospital where Joe had received care and Joe and Ann agreed to meet with the palliative care clinical nurse specialist that day.

Framework of care: Gentle and respectful explanation of the options open to them—and their meaning for care, first understanding and then incorporating Joe and his family's goals and needs.

After meeting with the clinical nurse specialist, Joe and Ann agreed they would think about a referral to the local hospice program. The following week they enrolled and became acquainted with the hospice staff that would be overseeing their care. Joe also decided to update his durable power of attorney for health care and formalize his wish to not be resuscitated by wearing a bracelet communicating his wishes to the area emergency medical services. Joe's pain was well controlled with oral medications. He worked on his book diligently and nearly finished it. Although rapidly losing strength, he also expressed a wish to visit his parents, grandparents, siblings, and an important professional mentor who was quite ill and near death himself—all of whom lived in a distant state.

Framework of care: Though felt to be inadvisable, the hospice staff chose to facilitate and honor Joe's wishes despite his progressive illness. They advocated for him and his family with the airline and arranged for a local hospice program to be "on call" in the event of any need.

Joe and his family had an incredible time. Joe and Ann even took a two-day camping trip to the mountains where they had honeymooned 17 years earlier. The wildflowers were in bloom—both Ann and Joe's favorite time in the mountains. Joe was able to spend time with all his family and even mend some old issues and hurts with his oldest sister. Soon after their return, Joe became increasingly weak and found walking difficult and most other activities exhausting.

Framework of care: The hospice staff revisited Joe's goals in the context of his declining strength, understanding that there may indeed be things Joe wanted to accomplish before he died. They held a family meeting with Joe, Ann, Andy, and Josh to address these concerns, answer questions, and discuss how his illness may progress.

The hospice provided volunteers who assisted Joe in the completion of his book. With the advice of the hospice social worker and help from volunteers, Joe made books for each of his sons as reminders of him for them to treasure. He remained steadfast in his desire to not talk with anyone outside his family about his dying—and the hospice staff honored his feelings. The hospice team contacted Andy and Josh's school and met with their teachers and fellow students. As his illness worsened, his parents and siblings took turns coming and staying with Joe, Ann, and the boys. This gave Ann needed respite from caregiving and Joe time alone with his parents—which rarely happened—as well as time alone with each of his siblings. The nurse was able to inform the family when his death neared, so all his family members were present, as Joe had wished, when he died. Ann and their children were so prepared for Joe's death that they didn't call the nurse until each had the time alone with him they wanted. During the visit at the time of Joe's death, Ann, Andy, and Josh helped the nurse prepare Joe's body for transportation to the mortuary, even choosing to dress Joe in his favorite flannel shirt. Andy and Josh picked wildflowers in a nearby field and placed them in Joe's hands. The nurse and Joe's wife, children, parents, and siblings reflected back how they had worked together and had empowered each other so they could make this difficult experience Joe's very own.

Framework of care: The goals of care changed again to assisting Joe with accomplishing his final wishes and insuring that his continued care needs were addressed. At the same time, Joe's family began to prepare for his death by participating in early grief work.

Critical Points

- Coming to grips with death is a process and cannot be rushed. It is different for everyone.
- Joe's *and* family's needs were listened to, honored, and not questioned or challenged. He and his family remained in charge and in control.
- Time-of-death rituals—i.e., bathing and dressing the body—can often be comforting and memorable for family members.
- The care of a patient and family at end of life includes *all* family members—not just immediate family. By supporting Joe's entire family, memorable and comforting memories were ensured.

Assisting and walking alongside dying patients and their families especially close to and after death, is an honor and privilege. Nowhere else in the practice of nursing are we invited to be companions on such a remarkable journey as that of a dying patient and family. Likewise, nowhere else in the practice of nursing are our words, actions, and guidance more remembered and cherished. Caring for dying patients and families is indeed the essence of nursing. Take this responsibility seriously, understanding while it may be stressful and difficult at times, it comes with personal and professional satisfaction beyond measure. Listen to your patients and their families. They are the guides to this remarkable and momentous journey. Listen to them with a positive regard, empathy, and genuineness, and approach their care with an acute attention to every detail. They—in fact all of us—are counting on you.

REFERENCES

1. Settles BH. A perspective on tomorrow's families. In: Sussman MB, Steinmetz SK, eds. Handbook of Marriage and the Family. New York: Plenum, 1987:157–180.

2. Matocha LK. Case study interviews: Caring for a person with AIDS. In: Gilgun JF, Daly

K, Handel G, eds. Qualitative Methods in Family Research. Newbury Park, CA: Sage, 1992:66–84.

3. SUPPORT Study Principle Investigators. A controlled trial to improve care for seriously ill hospitalized patients: A study to understand prognoses and preferences for outcomes and risks of treatments (SUPPORT). JAMA 1995; 274:1591–1598.

4. Fainsinger R, Miller MJ, Brurera E, Hanson J, Maceachern T. Symptom control during the last week of life on a palliative care unit. J Palliat Care 1991; 7(1):5–11.

5. Lichter I, Hunt E. The last 48 hours of life. J Palliat Care 1990; 6(4):7–15.

6. Ventifridda V, Ripamonti C, De Conno F, Tamburini M, Cassileth BR. Symptom prevalence and control during cancer patients' last days of life. J Palliat Care 6(3):7–11.

7. Twycross R, Lichter I. The terminal phase. In: Doyle D, Hanks GWC, MacDonald N, eds. Oxford Textbook of Palliative Medicine. 2nd ed. Oxford: Oxford University Press, 1998:977–992.

8. Rogers C. On Becoming a Person: A Therapist's View of Psychology. Boston: Houghton Mifflin, 1961.

9. Twycross R. Symptom Management in Advanced Cancer. 2nd ed. Oxan, UK: Radcliffe Medical Press, 1997.

10. Du Boulay S. Cicely Saunders: Founder of the Modern Hospice Movement. London: Hodder and Stoughton, 1984.

11. Berns R, Colvin ER. The final story: Events at the bedside of dying patients as told by survivors. ANNA 1998; 25:583–587.

12. Karlawish HT, Quill T, Meier D (for the ACP-ASIM End of Life Care Consensus Panel). A consensus-based approach to providing palliative care to patients who lack decision making capacity. Ann Inter Med 1999; 130:835–840.

13. Cleary J. Fever and sweats: Including the immunocompromised hosts. In: Berger A, Portenoy R, Weissman D. Principles and Practice of Supportive Oncology. New York: Lippincott-Raven, 1998:119–31.

14. Brody H, Campbell ML, Faber-Langendoen K, Ogle KS. Withdrawing intensive life-sustaining treatment: Recommendations for compassionate clinical management. N Engl J Med 1997; 336:652–657.

15. National Conference for Cardiopulmonary Resuscitation (CPR) and Emergency Cardiac Care (ECC). Standards of CPR and ECC. JAMA 1974; 227:864–866.

16. Tomlinson T, Brody H. Sounding board: Ethics and communication in do-not-resuscitate orders. N Engl J Med 1988; 318:43–46.

17. McIntyre KM. Failure of predictors of CPR outcomes to predict CPR outcomes (editorial). Arch Intern Med 1993; 153:1293–1296.

18. Dunn H, Hard Choices for Loving People. 3rd ed. Herndon, VA: A & A Publishers, 1994.

19. Zerwekh J. Do dying patients really need IV fluids? Am J Nurs 1997; 97(3):26–31.

20. Fainsinger RL, Bruera E. When to treat dehydration in a terminally ill patient? Supportive Care in Cancer, 1997; 5(3):205–211.

21. Ellershaw JE, Sutcliffe JM, Saunders CM. Dehydration and the dying patient. J Pain Sympt Manage 1995; 10:192–197.

22. Smith SA. Patient induced dehydration: Can it ever be therapeutic? Oncol Nurs Forum 1995; 22:1487–1491.

23. McCann RM, Hall WJ, Groth-Juncker A. Comfort care for terminally ill patients: The appropriate use of nutrition and hydration. JAMA 1994; 272:1263–1266.

24. Working Party on Clinical Guidelines in Palliative Care. Changing Gear—Guidelines for Managing the Last Days of Life. London: National Council for Hospice and Specialist Palliative Care Services, 1997.

25. Medtronic Inc. Restoring the Rhythms of Life: Your Implantable Defibrillator. St. Paul: Medtronic, Inc., 1994

26. Weissman D. Glucocorticoid treatment for brain metastases and epidural spinal cord compression: A review. J Clin Oncol 1988;6:543–551.

27. DeVelasco R, Dinwiddie LC. Management of the patient with ESRD after withdrawal from dialysis. ANNA J 1998; 25:611–614.

28. Moss A. Ethics in ESRD patient care: To use dialysis appropriately: The emerging consensus on patient election guidelines. Adv Renal Replace Ther 1998; 2:175–183.

29. Campbell ML. Forgoing Life-Sustaining Therapy. Aliso Viejo, CA: AACN Critical Care Publications, 1998.

30. Kelly C, Yetman L. At the end of life. Canad Nurse 1987; 83(4):33–34.

31. Smith JL. The process of dying and managing the death event. In: Schoenwetter RS, Hawke W, Knight CF. Hospice and Palliative Medicine Core Curriculum and Review Syllabus. Dubuque, IA: Kendall/Hunt, 1999.

32. Kelly C, Yetman L. At the end of life. Canad Nurse 1987; 83(4):33–34.

33. Callahan M, Kelley P. Final Gifts: Understanding the Special Awareness, Needs, and Communications of the Dying. New York: Bantam Books, 1993.

34. Conditions of participation for hospitals. Conditions of participation: Organ, tissue and eye procurement. Federal Register 1998; section 482. 45.

35. Berry PH, Zeri K, Eagan K. The Hospice Nurses Study Guide: A Preparation for the CRNH Candidate. Pittsburgh: Hospice Nurses Association, 1997.

36. Marchand LR, Siewert L. Death pronouncement: Survival tips for residents. Am Fam Physician 1998; 58:284–285.

37. Heidenreich C, Assistant Professor of Medicine, Medical College of Wisconsin, Milwaukee, WI, personal communication.

38. Pennington EA. Postmortem care: more than ritual. Am J Nurs 1978; 75(5):846–847.

39. Hron J. Funeral Director, Gunderson Funeral Home, Madison, WI, personal communication.

40. Speck P. Care after death. Nursing Times 1992; 88:20.

41. Nearny L. Practical procedures for nurses: Last offices—1. Nursing Times 1998; 94(26): insert.

42. Nearny L. Practical procedures for nurses: Last offices—2. Nursing Times 1998; 94(27): insert.

43. Nearny L. Practical procedures for nurses: Last offices—2. Nursing Times 1998; 94(28): insert.

44. Ferrell B, Virani R, Grant M. Analysis of end of life content in nursing textbooks. Oncol Nurs Forum 1999; 26(5):869–876.

45. Romanoff BD, Terenzio M. Rituals and the grieving process. Death Stud 1998; 22:697–711.

46. O'Gorman SM. Death and dying in contemporaty society: an evaluation of current attitudes and the rituals associated with death and dying and their relevance to recent understanding of health and healing. J Adv Nurs 1998; 27: 1127–1135.

47. Passagno RA. Postmortem care: Healing's first step. Nursing 97 1997; 24(4):32a–32b.

Part IV

Spiritual Care

Spiritual distress or "soul pain" is a common experience in those who are dying. The dimensions are complex, varied, and individual, and if left un-addressed may stifle the opportunity for growth at the end of life, lead to poorly controlled symptoms, and result in an "unquiet" death. The following four chapters focus on the spiritual dimensions of palliative care nursing. The first three address spiritual assessment, spiritual interventions, and meaning in illness. The final chapter consists of a personal reflection on the role of the chaplain in end-of-life care.

29 Spiritual Assessment

ELIZABETH JOHNSTON TAYLOR

Unless there was one of those miracles that people talk about of, of religious belief, there was no hope for a long life together. You know my only hope was that the life that Mark had left would be comfortable and pain free . . . And, if that miracle comes, I'll be any religion anybody wants me to be.

—Spouse

To solve any problem, one must first assess what the problem is. Consequently, the nursing process dictates that the nurse begin care with an assessment of the patient's health needs. Although palliative nurses are accustomed to assessing patients' pain experiences, hydration status, and so forth, they less frequently participate in assessing patients' and family members' spirituality.

Because spirituality is an inherent and integrating—and often extremely valued—dimension for those who receive palliative nursing care, it is essential that palliative care nurses know to some degree how to conduct a spiritual assessment. This chapter will review models for spiritual assessment, present general guidelines on how to conduct a spiritual assessment, and discuss what the nurse ought to do with data from a spiritual assessment. These topics will be prefaced by arguments supporting the need for spiritual assessments, descriptions of what spirituality "looks like" among the terminally ill, and risk factors for those who are likely to experience spiritual distress. But first, a description of spirituality is in order.

WHAT IS SPIRITUALITY?

Nurses who are researching spirituality typically emphasize aspects of spirituality when they attempt to define it, including transcendence, interconnectedness, and meaning.[1] For example, Reed[2] proposed that spirituality involves meaning-making through intrapersonal, interpersonal, and transpersonal connection. Fehring, Miller, and Shaw[3] summarized the definitions found in nursing literature when they defined the concept:

> Spirituality . . . generally connotes harmonious relationships or connections with self, neighbor, nature, God, or a higher being that draws one beyond oneself. . . . Spirituality provides a sense of meaning and purpose, enables transcendence, and empowers individuals to be whole and to live fully. (p. 663)

Usually spirituality is differentiated from religion—the organized, codified, and often institutionalized beliefs and practices that express one's spirituality. Likewise, care is often taken to allow for an open interpretation of what a person considers to be divine, or a transcendent Other. Although health care literature frequently uses phrases such as "higher power" in addition to "God," demographers of religion find that over 90% of Americans report belief in "God."[4]

WHY IS IT IMPORTANT FOR A PALLIATIVE CARE NURSE TO CONDUCT A SPIRITUAL ASSESSMENT?

There is mounting empirical evidence to suggest that persons with terminal illnesses consider aspects of spirituality to be one of the most important contributors to quality of life.[5,6] For example, in a quantitative study of 911 cancer patients (albeit, not necessarily terminally ill), Wan[7] observed "spiritual beliefs" to be the greatest determinant of health-related quality of life. The potential for spiritual distress is also thought to increase among many facing death.[8–11] Yet there is also evidence that those who face death become more spiritually aware and well.[12–15] Reed[14–15] found increased spiritual perspective among terminally ill cancer patients compared with non-terminally ill hospitalized patients. Religious beliefs and practices (e.g., prayer, beliefs that explain suffering or death) are also known to be valued and frequently used as helpful coping strategies among those who suffer from physical illness.[10,16–18] Family caregivers of seriously ill patients also find comfort and strength from their spirituality that assists them to cope.[19–22]

The above themes from research imply that attention to the spirituality of terminally ill patients and their caregivers is of utmost importance. That is, if patients' spiritual resources assist them to cope, and if imminent death precipitates heightened spiritual awareness and concerns, and if patients view their spiritual health as most important to their quality of life, then spiritual assessment that initiates a process promoting spiritual health is vital to effective palliative care.

But why should palliative care nurses be conducting spiritual assessments? Yeadon[23] proposed that all members of a hospice team are spiritual caregivers. In surveying hospice team members, Millison and Dudley[24] found nurses are often the ones responsible for completing spiritual assessments. Other nurse authors imply that nurses are pivotal in the process of spiritual assessment.[25–28] Indeed, considering nurses' frontline position, coordination role, and intimacy with the concerns of patients; the holistic perspective on care; and even their lack of religious cloaking, nurses are ideal professionals for completing a spiritual assessment.

However, nurses must recognize that they are not specialists in spiritual assessment and caregiving; they are generalists. Most oncology and hospice nurses perceive they do not receive adequate training in spiritual assessment and care.[29–31] In fact it is this lack of training that nurses often cite as a barrier to their completing spiritual assessments.[23,32–34] When a nurse's assessment indicates need for further sensitive assessment and specialized care, a referral to a specialist (e.g., chaplain, clergy, patient's spiritual director) is in order.

HOW DOES SPIRITUALITY MANIFEST?

To understand how to assess spirituality, the palliative care nurse must know what to look for. What subjective and objective observations would indicate spiritual disease or health? To approach an answer, it is helpful to consider the various aspects of spirituality. Conceptualizations of spirituality often include the following as aspects of spirituality: the need for purpose and meaning, forgiveness, love and relatedness, hope, creativity, religious faith and its expression.[35–37] Dudley and colleagues[38] found hospice spiritual assessment forms often include more specific spiritual problems such as fear of death or abandonment, spiritual emptiness, unresolved grief, unresolved past experiences, confusion or doubts about beliefs, and the need for reconciliation, comfort, or peace.

These aspects of spirituality can manifest among terminally ill persons in a myriad of ways. For example, one indication of a spiritual need is the asking of questions about "why?" (e.g., "Why do I have to suffer?"). Another illustration of spiritual need may be found when a patient states remorse about life ("I wish I had spent more time helping others when I could"). Spiritual need may also be found among patients who express difficulty accepting self or others ("I'm not good enough" or "I don't deserve to be treated so lovingly"). Often the need to reciprocate love in a relationship precipitates patients' feeling that they are a burden to their family. Other manifestations of spiritual need can include a depressed affect or behaviors, and statements of doubt related to religious or spiritual beliefs ("I wonder if there really is a Heaven, or if I'll be saved"). Questions about the efficacy of spiritual practices can also arise ("I wonder why God didn't answer my prayers for a cure?"). But spiritual needs can also be of a positive nature. For example, patients can have a need to express their joy about sensing closeness to others, or have a need to pursue activities that allow expression of creative impulses (e.g., artwork, music making, writing). Although the following models for conducting a spiritual assessment will provide more understanding of how spirituality manifests, the reader is referred to Carpenito[39] and Highfield[35] for further concrete indicators of spiritual distress or need.

SPIRITUAL ASSESSMENT MODELS

Health care professionals from multiple disciplines offer models for spiritual assessment. Selected models from chaplaincy and pastoral counseling (which has been strongly influenced by psychiatry), medicine, and nursing will be presented here.

Chaplaincy/Pastoral Counseling

Over the past several decades as the field of chaplaincy and pastoral counseling have advanced, there have been several models for spiritual assessment published. However, most discussions of spiritual assessment in this field reflect the ideas of the Christian psychologist Pruyser.[40]

Pruyser proposed seven dimensions or traits to spirituality.[40–42] Each dimension can be considered a continuum with negative and unhealthy versus positive and healthy ends. These dimensions are presented in Table 29–1 with statements that terminally ill patients or their loved ones might make to illustrate each end of the continuum. Where a patient is on these continuums can change over time. Malony[42] asserted that one more dimension needs to be added to Pruyser's seven, a trait Malony labels "openness in faith." That is, a positive, healthy sense of openness in faith allows an individual to not be rigid or resistant to new ideas in their spiritual beliefs. Although Pruyser and Malony acknowledge this model as being molded by Christian perspectives, much of the model still offers non-Christians insight into what spiritual dimensions can encompass.

More recently, Fitchett[43] developed the "7 by 7" model for spiritual assessment. In addition to reviewing seven dimensions of a person (medical, psychological, psychosocial, family system, ethnic and cultural, societal issues, and spiritual dimensions), Fitchett advances seven spiritual dimensions to include in an assessment: beliefs and meaning (i.e., mission, purpose, religious and nonreligious meaning in life), vocation and consequences (what persons believe they should do, what is their calling), experience (of the divine or demonic) and emotion (the tone emerging from one's spiritual experience), courage and growth (the ability to encounter doubt and inner change), ritual and practice (activities that make life meaningful), community (involvement in any formal or informal community that shares spiritual beliefs and practices), and authority and guidance (exploring where or with whom one places trusts, seeks guidance). An example of how this model was applied to a patient is shown in the following case study.

Case Study: Fitchett's Model Applied: The Story of Lynne

Lynne is a 43-year-old Roman Catholic woman of Italian descent living with recurrent breast cancer metastasized to the spine. Excepts from an interview conducted by this author provide a partial picture of Lynne's spirituality:

"When I was feeling well, I was doing

Table 29–1. Pruyser's Spiritual Dimensions

Spiritual Dimension	Patient Statements: Negative, Less Healthy	Patient Statements: Positive, More Healthy
Awareness of the Holy or God (sense of awe, reverence for that which is divine)	"When I hear the birds sing, they mock me; I see nothing sacred in nature—or anything else."	"I feel very close to God now and am dependent on God's help to face my death."
Acceptance of God's grace and steadfast love (experience of God as benevolent and unconditional in loving)	"I don't need or deserve any help or kindness; I'll handle things alone."	"Thank you for caring for me so tenderly; you mirror God for me."
Being repentant and responsible (openness to change, acceptance of responsibility for own feelings and behaviors)	"It's not my fault I feel bitter."	"How can I deal with my situation better?"
Faith (open, committed, and positive attitude toward life)	"There are some things in life I'd be afraid to do."	"I've enjoyed every minute of life! I try anything new."
Sense of providence (experience of God's leadership and direction)	"Where has God been for me? He left me when I got sick."	"I trust that God's will will be done in my life and dying."
Involvement in spiritual/religious community, and experience of communion	"Why should I have to ask for help from my church? They don't bother to even call me!"	"I still feel connected to my church because I know that they are praying for me."
Flexibility and commitment to living an ethical life	"There is no reason for me to still live. Let's pull the plug here."	"How I am choosing to die reflects my respect for the sacredness of my life; I have much to offer even while I'm in the process of dying."

Source: Interpretations of Pruyser by Malony[24] and Kloss.[22]

things and I was able to maintain my good spirits. Now I am going to the Wellness Center every Monday. And I dragged myself there this Monday even though I had a pounding headache, I was determined . . . to go, and I get a lot from going. So I went. I felt like doodoo, but I went [laughs]! Yeah, my emotional state is really tied into my physical state. Yeah, I've been thinking about that myself, 'I've got to do something about that.' It might be something I want to talk to the group about.

"I am in a body that is unsafe. Safety had to come from someplace besides controlling every single thing, and my body. [NURSE: So where does this safety come from?] I'm not sure yet. Really. That's why I go to the Wellness Center. I'm really not sure. I think it deals with spirituality. And I'm not a real religious person, but it has something to do with me that's not physical. . . .

"I haven't done art work in years. And I thought well maybe that's something I can do. So far, I can still use my hands; I mean you don't have to lift, push, or pull, or bend. So my friend bought me a big hunk of clay and I'm thinking of doing some sculpture. And at least it'll be something. I feel like I'm not productive. I don't know why I feel I have to be productive every minute?! I mean that's part of my old neurosis. . . .

"I was always involved in work (prior to teaching) that involved other people's tragedies. Like I was a patient consultant at the Hart Hospital for five years. So I had to deal with people who had cancer, had heart problems, parents of children with congenital defects. I worked for the city with inner city youth, who had lots of problems—as you can well imagine! And so, I thought I was a really good problem-solver, but I really never had to solve problems for myself, because I was never challenged. But I dunno, what's to solve here? [sarcastic voice] It's all that inner stuff, that spiritual stuff, gets back to that. So I don't know.

"All the things I want to be involved in [cries] with my son. Taking him to school. Being able to give him advice. He'll have a dad, grandmother, [pause] but he won't have me. And then, part of me says that's really arrogant. . . .

"Trying to search for meaning and why you have cancer is a lot like chasing your tail [voice about to crack]. I alternate between thinking it's a crapshoot—a celestial crapshoot, perhaps, but a crapshoot none-theless. That it could be the lady across the street as well as me. And then other times I think there has to be a reason for this [voice even more unsteady now]. I wish I could figure out what it is. I know I am more able to let people do things for me. And maybe that's what I need to learn in life [cries]. . . ."

- *Belief and Meaning:* Lynne explicitly describes her distress caused by questions of meaning, the meaning of her illness, her life, and her eventual death. Is she a victim of a "celestial crapshoot" or a purposeful, ordered universe? Although not explicit in these excerpts, Lynne's beliefs reflected those of a critical Roman Catholic.
- *Authority and Guidance:* Lynne saw herself prior to illness as being able to answer satisfactorily the questions of life; now authority in self is challenged. She wonders where to turn for comfort, security, direction, and answers. She did mention that since her diagnosis, she has begun to pray to her grandmother whom she saw as a saint. She does find guidance from her support group, relaxation tapes, and books on coping with cancer.
- *Experience and Emotion:* Lynne's spiritual issues manifest in anger and anxiety. Amidst Lynne's distress, there is an appreciation for the self-insight she has gained from her cancer experience. She also recognizes a direct relationship between how she feels physically and her "spirits."
- *Fellowship:* Lynne's pre-cancer involvement in her community (which gave her a great sense of purpose), is cur-

tailed due to her cancer. However, she does thrive on her relationships with her husband and son, and the friends who have remained loyal.

- *Ritual and Practice:* Presently, most religious practices fail to bring comfort to Lynne. However, her art work will allow her to pray, to express herself in a meaningful way. Her art work is also a way for her to leave a legacy, another way to create a sense of meaning for her life.
- *Courage and Growth:* Lynne's courage is exhibited by her ability to enter spiritual doubt, to face the "dark night of the soul." Although she is not satisfied with the answers (or lack thereof) to her many spiritual questions, she is allowing for spiritual maturation by entering into struggle. It is struggle and doubt that precedes breakthrough, turnarounds, learning, growth.
- *Vocation:* What duties and obligations make Lynne's life purposeful? Lynne finds meaning in being a mother, wife, friend, and creating beauty and joy for others through her art work.*

*Reprinted from Taylor, E. J. (1998). Caring for the spirit. In: Burke C., ed. *Psychosocial Oncology Nursing*. Pittsburgh: Oncology Nursing Society Press.

Using an approach less complex than Fitchett's, van der Poel[44] offers five general questions for organizing the assessment of an incurably ill patient: What is the place of God in the patient's life? What is the patient's attitude toward self? How is the patient's relationship with family and friends? What is the patient's understanding of and interest in prayer? What is the patient's attitude toward his or her religion? Van der Poel does specify substatements for each of these questions, but offers them in a tool that quantifies (using five-point response options) patient responses.

Hospice chaplain Muncy[10] assesses three dimensions of patients' spirituality. First, patient's self-understanding and attitudes about others are explored, since, in Muncy's view, how a patient views self and others frequently portrays their view of God. Second, religious and spiritual history, including sense of purpose, are assessed. Last, patients are asked about their spiritual goals; this allows the clinician to discuss with the patient a plan for spiritual care.

Medicine

Family physician T. A. Maugens[45] offers the mnemonic SPIRIT for remembering six components to cover during a spiritual assessment, or "history" (to use Maugens's physician terminology). "**S**piritual belief system" refers to religious affiliation and theology. "**P**ersonal spirituality" refers to the spiritual views shaped by life experiences that are unique to the individual and not necessarily related to one's religion. "**I**ntegration and involvement with a spiritual community" reminds the clinician to assess for a patient's membership and role in a religious organization or other group that provides spiritual support. "**R**itualized practices and restrictions" are the behaviors and lifestyle activities that influence one's health. "**I**mplications for medical care" reminds the nurse to assess how spiritual beliefs and practices influence the patient's desire and participation in health care. "**T**erminal events planning" reminds the clinician to assess end-of-life concerns. Maugens provides examples of questions that probe the above dimensions; some of these are found in Table 29–2.

Nursing

The nurse authors who have written about spiritual assessment are influenced by the writings of chaplains and pastoral counselors. However, they often go beyond a discussion of what dimensions to include in an assessment, to concrete suggestions about how to incorporate spiritual assessment into nursing care. However, it is instructive to continue with a review of what some nurse authors have suggested as spiritual dimensions for which to assess.

In what is now a classic article, Stoll[28] suggests four areas for spiritual assessment: the patient's concept or God or deity, sources of hope and strength, religious practices, and the relationship between spiritual beliefs and health. Carpenito's[39] questions for collecting data to make a nursing diagnoses of "spiritual distress" or "potential for enhanced spiritual well-being" reflect Stoll's approach. In addition to questions that simply ascertain a patient's religious af-

Table 29–2. Selected Questions from Maugens's "SPIRITual History"

S (spiritual belief system)
  What is your formal religious affiliation?
P (personal spirituality)
  Describe the beliefs and practices of your religion or spiritual system that you personally accept.
  What is the importance of your spirituality/religion in daily life?
I (integration with a spiritual community)
  Do you belong to any spiritual or religious group or community? What importance does this group have to you?
  Does or could this group provide help in dealing with health issues?
R (ritualized practices and restrictions)
  Are there specific elements of medical care that you forbid on the basis of religious/spiritual grounds?
I (implications for medical care)
  What aspects of your religion/spirituality would you like me to keep in mind as I care for you?
  Are there any barriers to our relationship based on religious or spiritual issues?
T (terminal events planning)
  As we plan for your care near the end of life, how does your faith impact on your decisions?

Source: Maugens (1996), reference 45.

filiation, supportive clergy and helpful religious books, and source of strength and meaning, questions which explore the link between spirituality and health are given (e.g., "What effect do you expect your illness (hospitalization) to have on your spiritual practices or beliefs?" "How can I help you maintain your spiritual strength during this illness?").

Dossey's[46] spiritual-assessment tool uses language that is less traditional (i.e., less overtly religious). This tool includes questions designed to assess meaning and purpose ("a person's ability to seek meaning and fulfillment in life, manifest hope, and accept ambiguity and uncertainty") and inner strength ("a person's ability to manifest joy and recognize strengths, choices, goals, and faith"). The tool also contains questions that assess interconnections, or what Dossey describes as "a person's positive self-concept, self-esteem, and sense of self; sense of belonging in the world with others; capacity to pursue personal interests; and ability to demonstrate love of self and self-forgiveness." Selected questions from Dossey's tool are found in Table 29–3, many in an adapted form.

Highfield[47] presents a model for spiritual assessment that focuses not on the dimensions of spirituality, but on assessment and care that reflect four increasingly complex tiers. The level of assessment the nurse conducts is to be based on the unique concerns of the patient and the level of ability of the nurse. The first tier of the PLAN model involves gaining permission, letting the patient know that it is appropriate to discuss their spiritual concerns with a nurse. Next, the nurse can provide limited information in response to the concerns raised. The third and fourth tiers involve activating resources (based on a more in-depth spiritual assessment) to assist the patient toward spiritual well-being and making nonnursing referrals when the nurse needs assistance to address the patient's spiritual concerns.

Table 29–3. Selected Questions Adapted from Dossey's Spiritual-Assessment Tool

Meaning and Purpose:

What gives your life meaning?
How does your illness interfere with your life goals?
How eager are you to get well—or to die?
What is the most important or powerful thing in your life?

Inner Strengths

What brings you joy and/or peace in your life?
What makes you feel alive and full of spirit?
What traits do you like about yourself? And how have these traits helped you to cope with your current situation?
Although physical healing may not be possible, what would help you to heal emotionally or spiritually?
How does your faith play a role in your health? In your preparation for death?

Interconnections

With Self
How do you feel about yourself right now?
What do you do to love yourself, or forgive yourself?
What do you do to heal your spirit?

With Others
Who are the people to whom you are closest? How can they help you now? How can you help them now?
How able are you to ask for help? To receive that help graciously?
How able are you to forgive others?

With Transcendent Other, Divinity
How important is it to you to worship a higher power or God? What forms of worship are most helpful to you now?
Does prayer, meditation, relaxation, or guided imagery, or anything like these, help you? How do they help you? E.g., How are your prayers answered?

With the Environment, Nature
How connected to the earth do you feel?
Do you have spiritual insights when you enjoy nature's beauty?
How does your environment stress you, or contribute to your illness?

Source: Questions selected and adapted from Dossey (1998), reference 46.

SUMMARY

The above summaries of various models for spiritual assessment identify spiritual dimensions which may be included in a spiritual assessment. Many of the dimensions identified in one model are observed (often using different language) in other models. The method necessary for completing the assessment generally requires the professional to make observations while asking questions, and listening for the patient's response. The vast majority of questions recommended for use in following such a model are open-ended. Several of the questions—indeed, the dimensions of spirituality—identified in this literature use "God language" or assume a patient will have belief in some transcendent divinity. The medical and nursing models explicitly suggest assessment questions should address the linkage between spirituality and health, while the pastoral counseling models do not. All the models are developed by professionals who are influenced predominantly by Western, Judeo-Christian ways of thinking.

GENERAL OBSERVATIONS AND SUGGESTIONS FOR CONDUCTING A SPIRITUAL ASSESSMENT

Qualitative and Quantitative Approaches

Whereas researchers assess individuals' spirituality quantitatively with "paper and pencil" questionnaires, health care professionals generally assess spirituality using qualitative methods (e.g., participant observations, semistructured interviews). However, it is possible to use questionnaires during the clinical spiritual-assessment process (e.g., Salisbury, Ciulla, & McSherry,[48], van der Poel[44]). This approach to conducting a spiritual assessment allows for identification, and possibly measurement, of what one believes and how one behaves (versus the semistructured interview approach, which assesses the function and experience of spirituality).

A quantitative tool that impresses this author is that used by Chaplain Robert Engstrom at Florida Hospital in Orlando, Florida (see Fig. 29–1 for a modified version). This type of tool should not "stand alone" in the process of spiritual assessment; rather it can be the springboard for a more thorough assessment and deeper encounters with a patient. A quantitative tool should never replace human contact; instead, it should facilitate it. Although this tool may not be perfect for each clinical setting, it certainly provides insight for the development of other tools that would fit a palliative care setting.

When to Assess

Dudley and colleagues[38] found that 100 of 117 hospices surveyed acknowledged that they did spiritual assessments routinely. In practice, if spiritual assessment is a routine, it generally occurs during the initial intake assessment. However, some experts agree that spiritual assessment should be an ongoing process.[45,49] The nurse does not complete a spiritual assessment simply by asking some questions about religion or spirituality during an intake interview. Instead, spiritual assessment should be ongoing throughout the nurse–patient relationship.

Stoll,[28] recognizing the significance of timing when asking patients questions about spirituality, suggested that spiritual assessment be separated from a sexual assessment because both topics are so sensitive and intimate. However, both spiritual and sexual assessment should occur during the general assessment. Several authors remind their readers that spiritual assessments can only be effectively completed if the health care professional has first established trust and rapport with the patient.[27,28,49]

Burkhardt and Nagai-Jacobson[25] and Highfield[26] imply a two-tiered approach to assessment that suggests the nurse conduct a basic spiritual assessment for all patients, and pursue an in-depth or focused assessment upon observing indicators of spiritual distress. For example, if a nurse observes a terminally ill patient's spouse crying and stating, "Why does God have to take my sweetheart?" then the nurse would want to understand further what factors are contributing to or may relieve this spiritual pain. To focus the assessment on the pertinent topic, the nurse would then ask questions that explore the spouse's "why" questions, beliefs about misfortune, perceptions of God, and spiritual coping strategies.

Prefacing the Spiritual Assessment

Because spirituality and religiosity are sensitive and personal topics (as are most other topics nurses assess), it is polite for a nurse to preface a spiritual assessment with an acknowledgement of the sensitivity of the questions and an explanation for why such an assessment is necessary.[28,45] For example, Maugens[45] suggested this preface:

> Many people have strong spiritual or religious beliefs that shape their lives, including their health and experiences with illness. If you are comfortable talking about this topic, would you please share any of your beliefs and practices that you might want me to know as your physician. (p.12)

Such a preface undoubtedly will help both the patient and the clinician to feel at ease during the assessment.

Assessing Nonverbal Indicators of Spirituality

Although this discussion of spiritual assessment has thus far focused on how to frame a verbal question and allow a patient to verbalize a response, the nurse must remember that most communication occurs nonverbally. Hence, the nurse must assess the nonverbal communication and the environment of the patient. A chaplain mentor instructed the author to observe the ABCs of spiritual assessment (personal communication, John Pumphries, October 1986). The observer must assess the **a**ffect, **b**ehaviors, and **c**ommunication of the patient and think, "Are these elements congruent?" An incongruency between affect and words indicates an area requiring care and further assessment. To illustrate, a patient who responds to "How are you?" with "Fine"—but with an angry tone of voice and demeanor and avoidance of eye contact, is sending incongruent messages. Such a patient is likely angry.

Assessment of the patient's environment can also provide clues about spiritual state.[49] Are there religious objects on the bedside table? Are there religious paintings or crucifixes on the walls? Get-well cards or books with spiritual themes? Are there indicators that the patient has many friends and family providing love and a sense of community? Are the curtains closed and the bedspread pulled over the face? Does the patient appear agitated or angry? Many of the factors a palliative care nurse usually assesses will provide data for a spiritual assessment as well as the psychosocial assessment.

Language: Religious or Spiritual Words?

One barrier to spiritual assessment is the nurses' fear of offending a nonreligious patient by using religious language. However, when one remembers the nonreligious nature of spirituality, this barrier disappears. Patients' spirituality can be discussed without "God language" or reference to religion.

To know what language will not be offensive during a spiritual assessment, the nurse must remember two guidelines. First, the nurse can begin the assessment with questions which are general and unrelated to religious assumptions. For example, "What is giving you the strength to cope with your illness now?" or "What spiritual beliefs and practices are important to you as you cope with your illness?" Second, the nurse must listen for the language of the patient, and use the patient's language when formulating more-specific

SPIRITUAL ASSESSMENT FORM

Dear Client,
Below you will find questions and suggested choices to help you identify what are your spiritual needs right now. Your answers will also help us as staff in providing you vital support as you move forward in your spiritual journey.

You do not have to respond to every question. Just fill out what is important to you. You may write comments about any answer on the back side of this sheet.

When you are finished, or if you need help with this form, please call ________________.

YOUR NAME: ________________________________

CONTACT INFORMATION FOR THE SPIRITUAL COMMUNITY WITH WHICH YOU RELATE MOST:

____

____

1. I have recently experienced God (or whatever name you give to a higher power) . . .
   __ as punishing, hurtful
   __ as not involved in my life
   __ as loving, accepting, helpful
   __ as ________________

2. How I view God (or my higher power) relating to my problems and illness:
   __ No help at all
   __ Not much help
   __ Will heal me completely
   __ Will heal me gradually
   __ Will help me find peace and growth, in spite of what won't change.

3. What is the relationship between what you believe and how you behave?
   __ I don't live up to what I believe.
   __ I live up to my beliefs part of the time.
   __ My life closely reflects what I believe.

4. Who has helped you most to get closer to God (or your spiritual core)? How?

   Has someone hurt you in a way related to your spiritual or religious life? In what way?

5. What beliefs have helped you? In what way?

   Are there religious beliefs that hurt you? Explain.

6. What spiritual or religious activities have helped you? How?

   Are there any spiritual or religious activities that cause you problems? Explain.

7. Has your spirituality changed because of your illness? How? Why?

8. What do you need most from God/higher power? Your spiritual community?

9. What is the most important goal in your spiritual life?

MY SPIRITUAL CARE PLAN NEEDS TO INCLUDE THE FOLLOWING:
__ Help understanding my spiritual needs.
__ Hope-building discussions or activities.
__ Finding meaning and purpose for my life.
__ Identifying and developing my special spiritual talents.
__ Finding inner peace, strength, or my spiritual center.
__ Learning to meditate.
__ Learning to pray effectively.
__ Learning to understand Scripture, holy writings.
__ Finding a supportive spiritual community.
__ Help in dealing with frightening feelings or thoughts.
__ To accept forgiveness.
__ To forgive myself.
__ To forgive people who have hurt me.
__ Spiritual help in healing weak or broken relationships.
__ Other needs
(please comment below and on the back side of this sheet as needed).

Fig. 29–1. Engstrom's Spiritual Assessment Form (modified and used with permission).

follow-up questions. If a patient responds to a question with "My faith and prayers help me," then the nurse knows "faith" and "prayer" are words that will not offend this patient. If a patient states that the "Great Spirit guides," then the sensitive nurse will not respond with, "Tell me how Jesus is your guide."

Asking Questions

Because asking a patient questions is an integral part of most spiritual assessments, it is good to remember some of the basics of formulating good questions. Asking close-ended questions that allow for short factual or yes/no responses is helpful when a nurse truly has no time or ability for further assessment. Otherwise, to appreciate the uniqueness and complexity of an individual's spirituality, the nurse must focus on asking open-ended questions. The best open-ended questions begin with how, what, when, who, or phrases like "Tell me about . . ." Generally, questions beginning with *why* are not helpful; they are often mixed with a sense of threat or challenge (e.g., "Why do you believe that?").

Listening to the Answers

Although it is easy to focus and worry about what to say during an assessment, the palliative care nurse must remember the importance of listening to the patient's responses. Although a discussion of active listening is beyond the scope of this chapter, a few comments are in order. Remember that silence is appropriate when listening to a patient's spiritual and sacred story. Listen for more than words; listen for symbols, listen for where the patient places energy, listen for emotion in addition to cognitions. The nurse will do well to listen to his or her own inner response. This response will mirror the feelings of the patient.

Overcoming the Time Barrier

Health care professionals may believe that they do not have enough time to conduct a spiritual assessment. Indeed, Maugens[45] observed that completing his SPIRITual history with patients took about 10–15 minutes. Although this is much less time than Maugen and his colleagues expected it to take, it is still a considerable amount of time in today's health care context. One response to this time barrier is to remember that spiritual assessment is a process which develops as the nurse gains the trust of a patient. The nurse can accomplish the assessment during "clinical chatterings."[45] Furthermore, data for a spiritual assessment can be simultaneously collected with other assessments or during interventions (e.g., while bathing or completing "hs" [or bedtime] care). And finally, it can be argued that nurses do not have time to not conduct a spiritual assessment, considering the fundamental and powerful nature of spirituality.

Overcoming Personal Barriers

Nurses can encounter personal barriers to conducting a spiritual assessment. These barriers can include feelings of embarrassment or insecurity about the topic, or can result from projection of unresolved and painful personal spiritual doubts or struggles. Every nurse has a personal philosophy or worldview that influences his or her spiritual beliefs. These beliefs can color or blind the nurse's assessment techniques and interpretation. Hence, an accurate and sensitive spiritual assessment requires that the nurse be spiritually self-aware. Nurses can increase their comfort with the topic and their awareness of their spiritual self if they ask themselves variations on the questions they anticipate asking patients. For example, "What gives my life meaning and purpose?" "How do my spiritual beliefs influence the way I relate to my own death?" "How do I love myself and forgive myself?"

Assessing Impaired Patients

Although verbal conversation is integral to a typical spiritual assessment, some terminally ill patients may not be able to speak, hear, or understand a verbal assessment. Patients who are unable to communicate verbally may feel unheard. In such situations, the nurse again must remember alternative sources of information. The nurse can consult with the family members and observe the patient's environment and nonverbal communications. Alternative methods for "conversing" of course can be used also. For patients who can write, paper-and-pencil questionnaires can be very helpful. Always be patient and be unafraid of the tears which can follow. Questions which demonstrate concern for their innermost well-being may release their floodgates for tears.

Assessing Children

While assessing children, it is vital to consider their stage of cognitive and faith development.[50] Questions must be framed in age-appropriate language. (A four-year-old will likely not understand what "spiritual beliefs" means!) Again, building trust and rapport over time with children is essential to completing a helpful spiritual assessment. Children are especially capable of ascertaining an adult's degree of authenticity. Children also are less likely to be offended by a question about religion. If a nurse creates a comfortable and nonjudgmental atmosphere in which a child can discuss spiritual topics, then the child will talk. The nurse may also need to be more creative in formulating questions if the child's vocabulary is limited. For example, instead of asking the child about "helpful religious rituals," the nurse may need to ask questions about what they do to get ready to sleep or what they do on weekends. When asking, "Does your mommy pray with you before you go to sleep?" or "What do you do on Sunday or Sabbath mornings?" the nurse can learn whether prayer or religious service attendance are a part of this child's life. Never underestimate the profoundness of a child's spiritual experience, especially a dying child's.

THE NEXT STEP: WHAT TO DO WITH A SPIRITUAL ASSESSMENT

Making a Diagnosis

The North American Nursing Diagnosis Association (NANDA) includes "spiritual distress" and "potential for enhanced spiritual well-being" as validated diagnoses.[39,51] However, other language can be used to label a spiritual problem. For example, the NANDA diagnoses of "anxiety," "impaired adjustment," "infective family coping," "dysfunctional grieving," "fear," "hopelessness," "loneliness," "social isolation," "ineffective coping," and "defensive coping" can also refer to what may be essentially spiritual problems. O'Brien[52] offered a more complete taxonomy for spiritual problems which were identified during research on spirituality during life-threatening illness. O'Brien's labels for spiritual problems include: spiritual pain, spiritual alienation, spiritual anxiety, spiritual guilt, spiritual anger, spiritual loss, and spiritual despair.

O'Brien's[52] list of potential spiritual problems begins to show the variety of diagnoses one patient could be given. Indeed, the NANDA primary diagnoses offer only a vague description; it is essential that the secondary or "related to" element of the NANDA diagnosis be determined.[39] Without specific identification of a spiritual problem, appropriate and effective interventions are less likely to be implemented.

Documentation

Although assessments of physiologic phenomenon are readily documented in patient charts, assessments and diagnosis of spiritual problems are less frequently documented. However, for many reasons, spiritual assessments and care should be documented. These reasons include: to facilitate the continuity of patient care among palliative care team members, and to document for the monitoring purposes of accrediting bodies, researchers, quality management teams, and so forth.

Formats for documenting spiritual assessments and diagnoses can vary. Some institutions encourage staff to use SOAP (**s**ubjective, **o**bjective, **a**ssessment, **p**lan) or similar formatting in progress notes shared by the multidisciplinary team. Others have developed quick and easy checklists for documenting spiritual and religious issues. Perhaps, an assessment format which allows for both rapid documentation and optional narrative data is best. However, merely documenting one's religious affiliation and whether one desires a referral to a spiritual care specialist certainly does not adequately indicate a patient's spiritual status and need.

A summary of assessment forms created by professionals at hospices is reported by Dudley, Smith, and Millison.[38] These researchers synthesized the spiritual assessment forms from 53 hospices, finding questions about religious affiliation and rituals, religious problems or barriers, and questions about spiritual (nonreligious) topics—that is, questions void of overtly religious language. While Dudley and colleagues summarize the content of these forms, they do not review the format for documentation on these forms.

CONCLUSION

Spirituality is an elemental and pervading dimension for persons, especially those for whom death is imminent. Spiritual assessment is essential to effective and sensitive spiritual care. Indeed, spiritual assessment is the beginning of spiritual care. While the nurse questions a patient about spirituality, the nurse is simultaneously assisting the patient to reflect on the innermost and most important aspects of being human. The nurse is also indicating to the patient that grappling with spiritual issues is normal and valuable. The nurse also provides spiritual care during an assessment by being present and witnessing what is sacred for the patient.

REFERENCES

1. Emblen JD. (1992). Religion and spirituality defined according to current use in nursing literature. J Prof Nurs 8:41–47.

2. Reed PG. (1992). An emerging paradigm for the investigation of spirituality in nursing. Res Nurs Health 15:349–357.

3. Fehring RJ, Miller JF, and Shaw C. (1997). Spiritual well-being, religiosity, hope, depression, and other mood states in elderly people coping with cancer. Oncol Nurs Forum 24:663–671.

4. Gallup G, Jr. (1999). Religion in America. Morehouse Publishing, Harrisburg, PA.

5. Buchholz WM. (1996). Assessment of quality of life. N Engl J Med 335:520–521.

6. Swenson CH, Fuller S, and Clements R. (1993). Stages of religious faith and reactions to terminal cancer. J Psychol Theol 21:238–245.

7. Wan GJ. (1997). The influence of social and clinical factors on health-related quality of life reports in ethnically diverse cancer patients. Ph.D. dissertation, St. Louis University. DAI 59-01B, p. 149.

8. Francis MR. (1986). Concerns of terminally ill adult Hindu cancer patients. Cancer Nurs 9:164–171.

9. McCracken AL, and Gerdsen L. (1991). Sharing the legacy: Hospice care principles for terminally ill elders. J Gerontol Nurs 17:4–8.

10. Muncy JF. (1996). Muncy comprehensive spiritual assessment. Am J Hospice Palliat Care 13:44–45.

11. Taylor EJ. (1997). The spiritual and ethical "end of life" decisions of cancer survivors. In: Groenwald S.L., Frogge M.H., Goodman M., Yarbro C.H., eds. Cancer Nursing: Principles and Practice. Jones and Bartlett, Boston.

12. Hall BA. (1997). Spirituality in terminal illness: An alternative view of theory. J Holistic Nurs 15:82–96.

13. Fryback PB. (1993). Health for people with a terminal diagnosis. Nurs Sci Q 6:147–159.

14. Reed PG. (1986). Religiousness among terminally ill and healthy adults. Res Nurs Health 9:35–41.

15. Reed PG. (1987). Spirituality and well-being in terminally ill hospitalized adults. Res Nurs Health 10:335–344.

16. Fleming C, Scanlon C, and D'Agostino NS. (1987). A study of the comfort needs of patients with advanced cancer. Cancer Nurs 10:237–243.

17. Raleigh EDH. (1992). Sources of hope in chronic illness. Oncol Nurs Forum 19:443–448.

18. Reed PG. (1991). Preferences for spiritually related nursing interventions among terminally ill and nonterminally ill hospitalized adults and well adults. Applied Nurs Res 4: 122–128.

19. Stiles MK. (1990). The shining stranger: Nurse-family spiritual relationship. Cancer Nurs 13:235–245.

20. Forbes EJ. (1994). Spirituality, aging, and the community-dwelling caregiver and care recipient. Geriat Nurs 15:297–302.

21. Rabins PV, Fitting MD, Eastham J, and Zabora J. (1990). Emotional adaptation over time in care-givers for chronically ill elderly people. Age and Ageing 19:185–190.

22. Picot SJ, Debanne SM, Namazi KH, and Wykle ML. (1997). Religiosity and perceived rewards of black and white caregivers. Gerontologist 37:89–101.

23. Yeadon BE. (1986). Spiritual assessment for a community-based hospice. Caring 5(10):72–75.

24. Millison M, and Dudley JR. (1992). Providing spiritual support: A job for all hospice professionals. Hospice J 8(4):49–65.

25. Burkhardt MA, and Nagai-Jacobson MG. (1985). Dealing with spiritual concerns of clients in the community. J Community Health Nurs 2: 191–198.

26. Highfield MF. (1993). PLAN: A spiritual care model for every nurse. Quality of Life 2(3): 80–84.

27. McSherry W. (1996). Raising the spirits. Nurs Times 92(3):48–49.

28. Stoll RI. (1979). Guidelines for spiritual assessment. Am J Nurs 79:1574–1577.

29. Peterson L. (1996). A survey of hospice nurses: Attitudes and beliefs regarding spiritual care. Masters thesis, Georgia Southwestern College.

30. Taylor EJ, and Amenta MO. (1994). Midwifery to the soul while the body dies: Spiritual care among hospice nurses. Am J Hospice Palliat Care 11(6):28–35.

31. Taylor EJ, Amenta MO, and Highfield MF. (1995). Spiritual care practices of oncology nurses. Oncol Nurs Forum 22:31–39.

32. Narayanasamy A. (1993). Nurses' aware-

ness and educational preparation in meeting their patients' spiritual needs. Nurse Educ Today 13: 196–201.

33. Ross LA. (1996). Teaching spiritual care to nurses. Nurse Educ Today 16:38–43.

34. Boutell KA, and Bozett FW. (1987). Nurses' assessment of patients' spirituality: Continuing education implications. J Cont Educ Nurs 21:172–176.

35. Highfield MF, and Cason C. (1983). Spiritual needs of patients: Are they recognized? Cancer Nurs 6:187–192.

36. Donley R. (1991). Nursing's mission: Spiritual dimensions of health care. J Contemporary Health Law and Policy 1:207–217.

37. Haase J, Britt T, Coward D, Leidy N, and Penn P. (1992). Simultaneous concept analysis of spiritual perspective, hope, acceptance and self-transcendence. Image 24:141–147.

38. Dudley JR, Smith C, and Millison MB. (1995). Unfinished business: Assessing the spiritual needs of hospice clients. Am J Hospice and Palliat Care 12(2):30–37.

39. Carpenito LJ. (2000). Nursing diagnosis: Applications to clinical practice. 7th ed. Lippincott, Philadelphia.

40. Pruyser PW. (1976). The minister as Diagnostician. Westminster Press, Philadelphia.

41. Kloss WE. (1988). Spirituality: The will to wellness. Harding J Relig Psychiatry 7:3–8.

42. Malony HN. (1993). Making a religious diagnosis: The use of religious assessment in pastoral care and counseling. Pastoral Psychol 41:237–246.

43. Fitchett G. (1993). Assessing Spiritual Needs: A Guide for Caregivers. Augsburg, Minneapolis.

44. van der Poel CJ. (1998). Sharing the Journey: Spiritual Assessment and Pastoral Response to Persons with Incurable Illnesses. Liturgical Press, Collegeville, MN.

45. Maugens TA. (1996). The SPIRITual history. Arch Fam Med 5:11–16.

46. Dossey BM. (1998). Holistic modalities and healing moments. Am J Nurs 98:44–47.

47. Highfield MF. (1997). Spiritual assessment across the cancer trajectory: Methods and reflections. Semin Oncol Nurs 13:237–241.

48. Salisbury SR, Ciulla MR, and McSherry E. (1989). Clinical management reporting and objective diagnostic instruments for spiritual assessment in spinal cord injury patients. J Health Care Chaplaincy 2:35–64.

49. Peterson EA. (1987). How to meet your clients' spiritual needs. J Psychosoc Nurs 25:34–39.

50. Hart D, and Schneider D. (1997). Spiritual care for children with cancer. Semin Oncol Nurs 13:263–270.

51. Lindeman CA, and McAthie M. (1999). Fundamentals of Contemporary Nursing Practice. Saunders, Philadelphia.

52. O'Brien ME. (1999). Spirituality in Nursing: Standing on Holy Ground. Jones and Bartlett, Boston.

30 Spiritual Care Interventions

CHARLES KEMP

When death is near, many people turn instinctively to faith, to God. Spiritually and philosophically, death—the enemy, the end—becomes "an invitation to new life."

—J. P. Carse[1]

But an invitation is not a map, nor a companion for the journey. The invitation may be only the explication of the need for a new life, without the understanding that a new life is possible, or how it can be found. Spiritual care helps in exploring that possibility, and achieving it.

—Charles Kemp[2]

This chapter addresses the challenges of providing effective spiritual care to patients with terminal illness. The chapter is structured around the basic spiritual needs; and is based on the certainty that there often is no one in a better position to provide spiritual care than the informed and committed nurse.

DEFINITIONS

There are many definitions of spirituality, religion, faith, and spiritual needs. For the purposes of this chapter, these terms are defined as follows:[2,3]

- Religion: An organized effort, usually involving ritual and devotion, to manifest spirituality.
- Faith: The acceptance, without objective proof, of something, e.g., God.
- Spirituality: The incorporation of a transcendent dimension in life; usually, but not always, involving faith and religion.
- Spiritual needs: Human needs for transcendence that are addressed by most religions. The basic spiritual needs are meaning, hope, relatedness, forgiveness (or acceptance), and transcendence.

Popular psychology or postmodern standards of political correctness often focus on spirituality without religion, faith, or God. However, in the real world of death and dying and suffering, it is religion, faith, and God to which the huge majority of people turn.

PREPARATION

Providing spiritual care at the end of life can (and perhaps should) be a daunting task. Even the most academically and clinically prepared chaplain or counselor sometimes feels her or his own inadequacy to intervene effectively with a person facing the end of life. Many nurses receive little or no education or training in spiritual care. This lack of preparation coupled with the enormity of death and the nurse's personal doubts and uncertainties may result in a reluctance to attempt to provide spiritual care—even when the need is apparent.

Preparation to provide spiritual care includes clarification of goals, knowledge of spiritual needs, personal exploration, and willingness to apply knowledge of some basic interventions.

Clarification of Goals

The primary goal of spiritual care is to increase the opportunity for reconciliation with God (or a higher power) and self. This goal is based on the ideas that (*1*) life does indeed come from God and (2) for many people, the process of living includes some degree of felt separation from God and faith. In the Western world, approximately 95% of people claim to believe in God,[4,5] so this goal would logically be as basic to persons with terminal illness as would relieving pain, dyspnea, and other symptoms. More-specific goals might be related to the spiritual needs, such as decreasing a sense of meaninglessness or hopelessness; or increasing a sense of relatedness, forgiveness, or acceptance. In terms of nursing diagnoses, the goal would likely be relieving spiritual distress, but the previously stated goals are more specific and function as etiologies (e.g., "spiritual distress related to hopelessness"). Note that the goal in spiritual care is not to provide one's own answers to ultimate questions or for the patient to achieve a particular belief. Most of the interventions and goals given here can apply to persons of any faith, or even persons of no faith.

Knowledge of Spiritual Needs

Each of the spiritual needs is discussed below. Hope is also discussed more extensively in another chapter.

- *Meaning* includes the reason for an event or events; the purpose of life; and the belief in a primary force in life.[3] Meaning may be sought in a review of life achievements; in a review of relationships; in a moral or spiritual search, especially of life as it was lived; and in an effort to discern the meaning of dying, of human existence, of suffering, and of the remaining days of life.[6]
- *Hope* is for the "expectation of a good that is yet to be."[7] There often is hope to not die; and failing that, hope to live and die in a way perceived to be good. In the cru-

cible of the physical and other exigencies of terminal illness, spiritual hope may be distilled into achieving the purpose of life: reconciliation with God, with self, and with others.

- *Relatedness* for Christians, Jews, and Muslims is to God; and for Hindus and Buddhists, relatedness may also be to (*1*) God or a god or (2) a system of spiritual faith or belief. Here, God is defined as supreme or ultimate reality, infinite, eternal, universal, all-knowing, and Being Itself. Relatedness for persons of any faith may also include relatedness to a religion or faith community.
- *Forgiveness* by God is often seen in the West as a concept of Christianity, Judaism, or Islam. However, the Buddhist and Hindu concepts of karma and transmigration of souls also directly address forgiveness or at least another chance to rectify mistakes. *Acceptance* is related to forgiveness, and meets the underlying need to deal with mistakes or misfortune in life.[2]
- *Transcendence* is that which takes one beyond self and suffering—or attachment to self and suffering—beyond death. Transcendence can occur as a result of other spiritual needs being met *or* as grace or manifestation of the divine; and thus may be seen as the outcome of spiritual needs or as the ultimate spiritual need.

Understanding or working toward understanding these needs provides a framework for understanding and intervening in spiritual distress. Not every person fits neatly into spiritual distress related to one or more of these (unmet) needs, but at a minimum, these needs give nurses and others a place to start looking in a mindful manner at the spiritual dimension in terminal illness.

Personal Exploration

Working in palliative care is emotionally and spiritually challenging. Regardless of profession or role, those who work in palliative care operate at least some of the time at the very edge of human existence and are often confronted by deep human suffering in all spheres of being (physical, psychological, social, and spiritual). To work gracefully and effectively in these circumstances, it is essential to explore one's own losses, grief, and fears. Such an exploration brings the practitioner face-to-face with existential challenges such as the inevitability and finality of death, the isolation and separateness that are part of every life, and, if the truth be known, the inability to truly "deal with it." Sooner or later, personal exploration may then evolve into a spiritual search. Here again, though, the searcher may be found wanting. One may then look to the *refuge* intrinsic in every major faith. For here is the truth: Few of us in palliative care would presume to think "I can do the whole of the physical care"—in terms of the care for a particular patient, much less in terms of developing and putting into practice the theory and principles of palliative care! Few of us (clergy included) should then presume to think "I can do the whole of the spiritual care"—either in terms of the care for a particular patient, much less in terms of confronting and understanding the enormity of human existence, including death.

Personal spiritual exploration may lead to exploration of spiritual and religious resources such as church, synagogue, mosque, or temple. Of course there are those who are spiritually well-grounded and able to provide quality spiritual care, but who do not participate in religious activities. However, a greater number do find that participation in spiritually based activities, specifically in religious activities where "universal values" are served by tradition,[8] increases the capacity to provide spiritual care.[2] In their seminal study of the spiritual practices of oncology nurses, Taylor, Amenta, and Highfield[9] found that 65% of oncology nurses surveyed attended religious services "frequently," ranging from one to three times per month (21%) to weekly or more often (44%). Both nurses and their patients benefit from the strongest possible spiritual foundation.[2,5]

Willingness to Apply Knowledge of Some Basic Spiritual Care Interventions

While interventions related to basic spiritual needs are presented below, it is vital to keep in mind that the critical and most fundamental intervention is to remain present (to "watch" through the night) in the face of suffering, fear, despair, and all the physical/emotional/social/spiritual trials of dying.[10] Being present on a consistent basis through the process of dying is *primary spiritual care*, and addresses the most fundamental spiritual need: The need for transcendence. Granted, neither the patient nor the nurse may necessarily feel transcendent. Still, there is an undeniable element of transcendence in the willingness to go beyond self and suffering and there is an undeniable need for this presence. The Bible presents the need for this presence in stark and universal terms: "My soul is very sorrowful, even to death; remain here, and watch with me" (Matthew 26:38).[11] And so the nurse and others working in palliative and hospice care have this opportunity to provide primary spiritual care that does not require understanding, answers, acceptance, or conquering; all that is required is to "watch with me." There are, of course, other interventions.

INTERVENTIONS: SPIRITUAL NEEDS, PROBLEMS, AND PRACTICES

Each of the spiritual needs is examined below, including a discussion of the need, manifestations of the unmet need, and interventions to help in meeting the need. In actual practice, there often is overlap among problems resulting from the unmet needs. This may include needs that are never assessed and needs that are met or neglected to varying degrees. As with other frameworks for practice, patients and families do not always fit neatly into certain categories. In general, unmet spiritual needs may be expressed by direct statements of hopelessness, meaninglessness, guilt, and so on. Indirect expressions of unmet spiritual needs may include anxiety, sadness/depression, fear, irritation, loneliness, and anger. (See Chapter 29, "Spiritual Assessment," for discussion of these signs.)

MEANING

For many people, serious questions about meaning of life typically arise in the late teen years and into the early twenties. After that, for most people, these questions are set aside or put into the background as the day-to-day struggles of life ensue: work, relationships, raising children, and other life demands tend to take precedence over philosophical pursuits. Often, decisions are made and paths taken without regard to any component of meaning or other such concerns. In life, one does what one must do. Later, as the end of life approaches, questions of meaning may again arise.

Few people go through the process of terminal illness without experiencing some form of life review. It is important to note that those whose physical symptoms are unmanaged without remission are often unable to address meaning and other spiritual issues as they are more likely to focus only on physical needs and suffering. That life review, whether conscious or unconscious, brings forth the question of, "What did my life mean and how well did I live it?" If the answer is, "My life was full of meaning and I lived it well," then meaning is more likely to be found in the last days and those days are more likely to be lived well. If, on the other hand, the answer is, "My life had little meaning and I did not live it well," then meaning is less likely to be found in the last days and those days are less likely to be lived well. The old adage of palliative care is again illustrated: Without skilled intervention, most people die in a manner very similar to that of the rest of their lives.

However, there are those whose lives are characterized by spiritual emptiness and pain who then find meaning in life even as life draws to an end. For these, terminal illness may serve as a motivation to reach beyond self and suffering. To participate in such a process of spiritual growth is a privilege. Much of this chapter is focused on promoting this growth.

A sense of meaninglessness in life as a whole may be first addressed by the nurse through assisting the patient through a mindful life review. Previously it was noted that unless physical problems are overwhelming, almost everyone who is dying goes through some sort of life review. The problem with such life reviews is that many times they are undertaken in a time of despair and/or they tend to focus on the negative. More importantly, these reviews are unproductive. This writer is probably not alone in a tendency to awaken in the night obsessing about a problem or personal deficit (in the midst of a life of plenty) and spend an hour or more going over and over and over that problem or deficit with little or no progress or insight achieved. The result is a sleepless night with nothing to show for the distress.

"Mindful life review" means that the nurse or other staff suggests to the patient a deliberate and thoughtful verbal or written review of the patient's life, including relationships, achievements, failures, high points, low points, and so on. It is essential to understand that such a review is not a one-time activity, nor something that occurs early in the relationship, but rather is one valued aspect of an ongoing nurse–patient relationship. For example, in a home care setting the nurse might ask the patient to think about one important relationship that was or is positive and one that was or is less positive and to talk about those during the next home visit. At that next home visit, the nurse listens to what the patient says about the relationships, helps the patient explore them in greater depth, and helps identify ways in which the relationships might be redefined or viewed in a more realistic manner. Specific to spiritual matters and meaning, the nurse might ask the patient to think about something that has been full of meaning in the patient's life and conversely, to think of something important that seemed meaningless or possessed of negative meaning. The interventions are contained (*1*) in the patient's explication of the issue or issues and (2) in the nurse's help to the patient in breaking out of repetitious thinking about the issue(s).

The search for meaning in life as it has been lived is facilitated by asking the patient the very serious question, "If you had your life to live over again, what would you like to be different and what would you like to be the same?" In certain close and therapeutic relationships, this question can serve as a framework for the therapeutic aspect of the relationship. In a home care setting, for example, the question can be rephrased to address the various dimensions of a person's life (e.g., "In terms of your spiritual life, what would you . . ." or "In terms of relationships . . ."

This "If you had your life to live over" question is often painful for the patient. Who among us does not have painful memories and regrets? But the pain is not caused by the question. Most likely the pain was already there, perhaps suppressed or perhaps just hidden from others. This question serves not only to look at the past and the meaning of a person's life, but also to present circumstances, the future, and what meaning might emerge.

The meaning of dying, suffering, and death are difficult, if not impossible to understand in terms of psychological explanation. These meanings can be addressed by questions such as, "What does it mean to you that this (dying or suffering) is happening?" This is a very serious question, and often gets serious answers. The suffering of the dying is not in any way an academic issue. The question of, "Why me; why am I suffering; why am I dying?" is not one for the nurse or others to answer. Rather, it is a question to which the response is to stay with the patient in her or his time of questioning and doubt. Many times, providing an answer only stifles the patient's exploration of the suffering and its meaning.

Every religion acknowledges and deals with the problem of suffering and death and every religion is rich in examples of compassionate reaction to human suffering and death.

On Him let man meditate
Always, for then at the last hour
Of going hence from his body he will be strong
In the strength of this yoga, faithfully followed:
The mind is firm, and the heart
So full, it hardly knows its love."

—The Way to Eternal Brahman[12]

Buddha's compassion is equal toward all people; but it is expressed with special care toward those, who, because of their ignorance, have heavier burdens of evil and suffering to bear.

Buddha's Relief and Salvation for Us[13]

"I lift up my eyes to the hills.
From whence does my help come?
My help comes from the Lord, who made heaven and earth.
He will not let your foot be moved, he who keeps you will not slumber.
Behold, he who keeps Israel will neither slumber nor sleep.
The Lord is your keeper; the Lord is your shade on your right hand.
The sun shall not smite you by day, nor the moon by night.
The Lord will keep you from all evil; he will keep your life,
The Lord will keep your going out and your coming in from this time forth and for evermore.

—Psalm 121[11]

Let not your hearts be troubled; believe in God, believe also in me. In my Father's house are many rooms; if it were not so, would I have told you that I go to prepare a place for you? And when I go and prepare a place for you, I will come again and take you to myself, that where I am you may be also. And you know the way where I am going.

—John 14:1–4[11]

We heard his prayer and relieved his affliction. We restored to him his family and as many more with them: a blessing from Ourself and an admonition to worshipers.

—The Prophets[14]

For many patients, help in finding and discussing passages from the sacred books of their own faiths may provide the best kind of answer to the question of the meaning of suffering and death. Of course worship, ritual, prayer, and meditation are or should be part of the spiritual care milieu. Encouraging these is important, both for the patient's and family's life, and for promoting their presence in the life of the institution or organization in which one practices.

Most people confront the questions of meaning in life, suffering, and death from the point of view of their *own* existence. The human condition and its tendency to isolation leads to the idea that the feelings of meaningless, emptiness, and brokeness are unique to the one who is experiencing them. Of course these feelings are not unique! Exploration of how and why a person feels this way, coupled with a gentle reminder that the person is not alone in these feelings may be helpful. Here again the questions and responses lead to the realms of spirituality and religion: For Christian and Jewish patients, certain Psalms (e.g., 6, 32, 38, 39, 41, 51, 61, 69, 88, 91, 102, 103, 130, and 143) are appropriate to read and discuss with respect to the meaning of suffering.

Contemplating and exploring the questions of meaning in life, suffering, and death noted above is likely to lead to other questions: about forgiveness, acceptance, punishment, and even transcendence. Once again the questions and responses lead to the realms of spirituality and religion. These questions may lead also to questions and exploration of the meaning of the remaining days of life and to the question of what might be done to make the most of that time, both in the present and in the future. As noted earlier, the primary goal of spiritual care is to increase the opportunity for reconciliation with God (or a higher power) and self; and indeed, the very purpose of life is reconciliation: with God, with self, and with others. It is not overly directive to suggest that a person looking at a very limited future on earth might consider whether one or all three of these reconciliations are worth serious contemplation for at least part of future direction.

Finding meaning in the process of dying is largely dependent upon the degree to which the patient finds some meaning in his or her life when reviewing it. Looking at the question of what one would like to have done different in life is critical to a fulsome review of life—the good and the bad. Bringing the whole of one's life into consciousness and applying sacred literature, worship, and prayer to the process of dying may lead directly to increased meaning in the present and future (Table 30–1). "What our patients need is unconditional faith in unconditional meaning."[8]

Table 30–1. Notes on the Search for Meaning: The Patient, Family, and Nurse

- Mindfully review life: the good and the bad.
- Integrate the sacred into the process of dying: prayer, reading, worship, ritual.
- Set realistic goals for the remaining days: improving a relationship, reading portions of a sacred book, praying regularly.
- The nurse and others consistently dispense loving and competent care, regardless of the extent to which the patient does or does not find meaning in the process.

HOPE

Although Chapter 24 is devoted to hope, hope in a solely spiritual sense is also discussed here. Themes or "universal components of hope" include finding meaning through faith or spirituality, having affirming relationships, relying on inner resources, living everyday life, and anticipating survival.[15] Not all these may be achieved in the context of terminal illness—at least in a physical sense—but all are applicable to many people going through a terminal illness. Despite the realities and challenges of terminal illness, there may be much to hope for: to live another day; for relief from suffering; for a greater understanding of life; for a good death with dignity; for a healed relationship; to see a loved one; to not die at all; or simply to be able to go through the ordeal of dying.

Hope in terminal illness can be addressed directly by asking, "What do you hope for . . . in this illness (or situation)? . . . from others? . . . at this point in your life? . . . in or for yourself? . . . in your faith (or religion or spiritual life)?" These questions are very powerful at a time like this and can facilitate expression of deep feelings and issues. What a question to ask and issue to raise—hope in terminal illness! The answers to the questions are often a mix of hope and resignation. The critical point is to bring up directly the concept of hope for exploration and discussion.

Hope in this context includes hope for reconciliation with God and self. This does not, in any way, diminish the importance of hope in relation to other matters, especially hope to heal relationships with other people. Hearkening back to the earlier discussion of meaning and reconciliation, one quickly sees that making progress toward reconciliation will have a direct impact on the presence or absence of hope, whether spiritual or otherwise—or more commonly, on the waxing and waning of hope.

Case Study: Mrs. P, a Patient with Cervical Cancer

Mrs P. had a terribly difficult life. She grew up poor and in her middle years survived war, torture, forced labor, and became a refugee several times over. When I met her she was an alcoholic and abusive to her children. She lived in a run-down one-bedroom apartment with her husband (also an alcoholic), a son who was a gangster, another son with Down syndrome, and a 12-year-old daughter who was the primary caregiver. Mrs. P. spent most of her days and nights lying on a small couch in the apartment living room.

She had cervical cancer with many complications. Symptom and disease management were complicated by both alcoholism, poverty, and Mrs. P.'s limited English proficiency. Overall and considering the circumstances, her symptoms were relatively well managed.

It was clear to all concerned that Mrs. P. was spiritually bereft and without hope. Using both Buddhist and Christian translators, we tried counseling to address hope and other spiritual issues in several different ways. Although she was nominally Buddhist, she refused offers of transportation to the temple. On several occasions she accepted gifts of objects sacred to Buddhists, but after a few days would put them away. Several Christian missionaries visited on a regular basis and, although she did not resist these visits, neither did she respond to them. Everything we tried seemed to fail. She did, however, show appreciation for our efforts to care for her and her family.

The only thing that seemed to affect her was when one day a nursing student knelt unbidden beside Mrs. P.'s couch and prayed. Although Mrs. P. understood little of the prayer, tears began to run down her cheeks as the young woman prayed. Afterward, Mrs. P. whispered, "Thank you."

As far as I know, this patient's spiritual needs were never met, and I never saw any evidence of hope or reconciliation. So what is the point of this case study? Where are the effective interventions and the insights? Unfortunately they are not to be found—except that those of us who tried to be effective and insightful never gave up. Though none of the caregivers, the patient, or the family ever experienced much in the way of transcendence, in retrospect, there were two years of transcending the desire to quit.

The week before she died I went out of town for a conference. I returned late Sunday. On Monday I left for work early so I could see Mrs. P. first. I walked into her apartment and at that moment, she died.

There are two great hopes offered to the dying and to all others by faith and religion:

1. The hope to live more fully and deeply—after all these years of superficiality. All the major faiths provide clear guidelines for living in connection to faith and God or whatever one calls ultimate reality. All the major faiths say without equivocation that living in this manner brings the greatest possible fulfillment.[2]
2. The hope for a life beyond this one. All the major world religions have definitive and hopeful beliefs in outcome, i.e., in what happens or can happen after death. In fact, it is only religious belief that offers any possibilities about the future after death—other than the recyclable nature of our basic molecule, carbon.

Increasing or reaching these two great hopes begins with exploration of hope and hopelessness, and thence to sources of knowledge and insight into hope and truth. After looking at what hope and hopelessness exists, one may then in partnership with the patient begin looking at the patient's faith tradition for hope that may be found there (Table 30–2).

Die, and you win heaven. Conquer and you enjoy the earth. Stand up now, son of Kunti, and resolve to fight. Realize that pleasure and pain, gain and loss, victory and defeat, are all one and the same: then go into battle. Do this and you cannot commit any sin.

—The Yoga of Knowledge[12]

Table 30–2. Notes on Hope: The Patient, Family, and Nurse

- Understand common hopes in the process of dying.
- Understand that two great hopes are offered by faith and religion: (*1*) to live fully and deeply and (*2*) for life after death.
- Ask direct questions about and explicate the presence or absence of hope.
- Integrate the sacred into the process of dying: prayer, reading, worship, ritual.
- The nurse and others faithfully "watch through the night," whether the patient or others have or do not have hope.

RELATEDNESS

Relatedness in the spiritual sense is to faith, religion, and especially to God (or with whatever represents God) or to all three. Existentially, of course, many people feel very much alone in life and in the universe. The same holds true in terms of faith and/or religion. Just as the quest for meaning in life may have been put into the background, so may a quest for spiritual growth or for a deep connection with faith been put away. In some people there is a deep feeling of having been failed by their faith and the faith community. The result of any or all of these is a sense of isolation from faith and from God or anything greater than this—this life, this inadequacy, this suffering, this transience. It is possible, and even not unusual to spend an entire lifetime trying to avoid dealing with existential and spiritual isolation. Those who constantly seek sensation (drugs, sex, adventure, etc.) may be trying to deal with isolation and separateness more than anything else.

Terminal illness tends to bring everything into sharper focus, and loneliness or meaninglessness that once seemed a bearable part of life may come to the forefront after years of suppression. The need for reconciliation or reconnection then becomes a driving force in the remaining days of life.

For most people of most faiths, the reconnection is to God. Whether referred to as Yahweh, God, Lord, or Allah, the God of Judaism, Christianity, and Islam is clearly explicated. Contrary to some conceptions of Hinduism, Hindus also believe in "One God, who can be understood and worshipped in many different forms."[16] In the Buddhist canon, relatedness is to the faith and philosophy. However, in practice, many Buddhists believe in a divine "force" or "being," as expressed by the Buddha or existing as mystery and never explicated, but never denied in the teachings of the Buddha. From a psychological perspective, Carl Jung[17] wrote with deep insight that the presence or acknowledgment of God among virtually all peoples of all religions through all times is evidence of God as a universal archetype or "living psychic force" and that the imprint of God in this manner "presupposes an imprinter."

Given the incomplete and unenlightened nature of most of us, the primary way then to relatedness to or reconciliation with God is through religion and religious practice, including prayer, ritual, and worship. A noted physician and ethicist suggests that prayer may be gently introduced into a patient care encounter by asking, "Would it be okay if we have a prayer. Even if it won't help you, it will help me."[18] Readers will readily see that such a request also is likely to have a salutary effect on the relationship between the patient and provider.

Ritual and worship are sometimes constrained, not so much by patient circumstances, but more by a lack of imagination on the part of regular sources of spiritual care. Thus a church may not think to bring communion to the patient's home, nor a temple to offer an opportunity to give alms to monks. The nurse or other provider can then act as an advocate for the patient by giving direct suggestions to the source of spiritual care. The nurse may also in some cases provide/participate in ritual. Of course the presence of chaplains on palliative care and hospice services is of great benefit to many patients in need of spiritual support, including ritual and worship.

Another form of relatedness is to a belief system and/or religion, which, paradoxically, may not necessarily mean a strong sense of relatedness to God. In some cases, God seems too much to comprehend or relate to: If God is indeed "ultimate reality" then how are we to comprehend? In other cases, there may simply be an inability to take the leap to belief. Nevertheless, relatedness to a religion or a faith community may be a step toward relatedness to God, or if not relatedness to God, then toward spiritual comfort to the patient and family.

Ideally, the patient's source of help in finding or increasing a sense of relatedness is the patient's own faith and clergy. For a variety of reasons such help is not always available, which tends to further increase a sense of separation. The nurse or others can explore with the patient her or his faith history, especially times when faith and relatedness were strong and when they were weak; and what influenced those changes (Table 30–3). As in other aspects of palliative care, it often is the nurse's willingness to bring up and explore difficult issues that is the most therapeutic measure taken. One cannot confer relatedness to God. But what can be conferred is the possibility that there is, indeed, something beyond this suffering and isolation. Here again, the ancient and priestly act of watching through the night of fear, suffering, and isolation may be the only spiritual care possible—not to mention, the best spiritual care available. Prayer, with the patient, for the patient, or for the nurse or other caregivers is an important part of spiritual care in this and other issues. For Christians and Jews, the Psalms are especially appropriate and helpful readings.

Table 30–3. Notes on Relatedness: The Patient, Family, and Nurse

- Understand the common problem of existential and/or spiritual isolation.
- Relatedness may be to God or to religion or faith community.
- Explore the patient's faith history to help rekindle a sense of relatedness—or uncover reasons for a lack of relatedness.
- When relatedness does not seem possible, the primary spiritual care is to watch with the patient through the night.
- Prayer with or for the patient, and for the caregivers is important.

> "Oh God, thou hast rejected us, broken our defenses; thou hast been angry; oh, restore us . . ."
>
> —Psalm 60[11]

FORGIVENESS OR ACCEPTANCE

Every religion has rules and sanctions related to how one lives in the world and how one practices the religion and its precepts. Every religion also acknowledges that humans fail to fully follow its rules and has provisions for such failures. In Hinduism and Buddhism there are cycles of birth and rebirth based on actions in life (we are born to be healed). Although sin and attendant suffering are issues in these faiths, the focus of practicing the faiths is more on acceptance of self and suffering than on forgiveness. In Judaism, Christianity, and Islam there is the concept of forgiveness of sins.

> To those who avoid the grossest sins and indecencies and commit only small offenses, your Lord will show abundant mercy. He knew you well when He created you of earth and when you were hidden in your mother's wombs. Do not pretend to purity; He knows best those who guard themselves against evil.
>
> —The Star[14]

Psychologically, there may also be a need for forgiveness or acceptance of self. While routinely considered psychological issues, the need for self-forgiveness or self-acceptance may be tied to spiritual issues. In most cases, a sense of forgiveness or acceptance from either source (self or God) promotes the same from the other source.

Earlier, it was suggested that persons who are dying (and others as well) benefit from a mindful life review that includes both the "good" and the "bad" of the person's life. Such a review inevitably leads to consideration of mistakes and/or unfortunate aspects of life. In many cases, there is at least some crumbling of defenses that functioned to hide certain painful aspects of life. Guilt is often the result; and it does not seem to matter whether the issue is something

Table 30–4. Notes on Forgiveness or Acceptance: The Patient, Family, and Nurse

- Understand the universality of sin, regret, and guilt.
- Not all guilt is related to the patient's own doing.
- A life review almost always includes elements of the need for forgiveness or acceptance.
- Forgiveness and/or acceptance cannot be conferred by another; but the practice of mercy is a manifestation of forgiveness and acceptance.
- Integrate the sacred into the process of dying: prayer, reading, worship, ritual.

one did, such as a pattern of dishonesty, or if the issue is something that was experienced, such as growing up in an alcoholic family.

In the discussion of meaning it was strongly suggested that the nurse employ the question, "If you had your life to live over again, what would you like to be different?" Clearly this question has direct application to the issue of forgiveness or acceptance. In the sort of deep and open relationship for which we strive in hospice and palliative care, this question often brings a strong response that may include a deep sense of regret or guilt. The question is really less of an assessment question than a starting point in a search for understanding and ultimately, forgiveness or acceptance (Table 30–4).

Case Study: Mrs. K, a Patient with Lung Cancer

Mrs. K was dying from small cell carcinoma of the lung with metastases to brain and bone. Treatment of the primary tumor and metastases included several courses of chemotherapy and radiation, both initiated and discontinued at appropriate times. Her primary symptoms were pain, fatigue, and nausea, all of which were well managed. She lived in a cottage behind the house where her son, daughter-in-law, and grandson lived. She enjoyed warm, supportive relationships with her family and others. She had no financial worries.

However, there was an element of low-level unhappiness and vague suffering through much of her illness. In a series of difficult interactions in which she and her son struggled to share their deepest feelings about her life and their relationship she was finally able to say truthfully how she saw herself: "I'm naked and ugly and skinny. I'm lying in the bottom of a pit and it's dirty and there are cigarette butts all around me." Her son responded, "That's not you—it's what you feel like, but it's not you." She replied by begging for forgiveness for the mistakes she had made. Her son told her not to beg, that he forgave her and hoped that she forgave him; but more importantly, God forgave her.

She felt a great sense of peace afterward and began making detailed plans for her funeral. Her choices of scripture and hymns were a lovely expression of her past and her future. She spent many hours talking about what these passages and hymns meant to her.

The role of the nurse or chaplain or other caregivers is not to try to confer forgiveness or acceptance or convince a patient that her or his faith offers forgiveness. It is possible, however, to manifest forgiveness and acceptance through providing consistent loving care, and thereby hold out to the patient the possibility that forgiveness and acceptance are possible. This practice of mercy is a high ethical demand in nursing and related fields and may be seen in terms of beneficence, fidelity, and justice.[2] Similarly to the care in other spiritual issues, the nurse may help connect the patient to the sacred and the practice of faith: prayer (in this case for forgiveness or acceptance), reading (especially passages that acknowledge the reality of sin and forgiveness), and worship and ritual (especially ritual related to purification).

TRANSCENDENCE

"Transcendence is a quality of faith or spirituality that allows one to move beyond, to 'transcend' what is given or presented in experience—in this case, the suffering and despair so often inherent in dying."[2]

Beyond, beyond
Beyond that beyond
Beyond the Beyond.

—Buddhist mantra

Transcendence is certainly more than resignation and is also more than what many think of as acceptance in the process of dying. At its highest level, there is an element of beauty or numinousness in transcendence. At its most basic level, transcendence is the means by which one finds meaning "retroactively . . . even in a wasted life."[8] Even more than the need for forgiveness or acceptance, transcendence resists being conferred by others or problem-solving approaches. "Man is never helped in his suffering by what he thinks of for himself; only suprahuman, revealed truth lifts him out of his distress."[17]

Transcendence can occur in at least one of two ways:

1. The other spiritual needs are met and transcendence then is an outcome.
2. Transcendence occurs through grace, or as Jung would state it, through "suprahuman, revealed truth," and thus may exist independently of other spiritual needs; or of work, actions, or human interventions. In this latter case, we see that through transcendence, all other spiritual needs are met.

Transcendence is a profound issue that cannot be approached from a problem-solving perspective and there are no specific interventions that lead to transcendence. One "watches" with the patient and practices mercy and is grateful when transcendence occurs.

It is well worth considering that there may be elements of transcendence in the practice of hospice and palliative care. Those who practice in this field operate at the very edge of human existence. Sometimes we see that the practice also has elements of our own denial and fear of death; but sometimes, in the deep heart of the night, we transcend our own denials and fears and become—if only for a moment—a manifestation of the transcendent beauty seen when there is reconciliation with God, with self, and with others (Table 30–5).

GENERAL NOTES ON PROVIDING SPIRITUAL CARE

The following are general suggestions for providing spiritual care. Not all are

Table 30–5. Notes on Transcendence: The Patient, Family, and Nurse

- Integration of the sacred into the process of dying may lead to transcendence.
- Transcendence is beyond human intervention.
- Take note of the times when transcendence occurs in the practice of hospice and palliative care.

applicable in every case and some may never be applicable to a particular patient or in a particular person's practice. They are offered here as ideas or suggestions that readers may add to in the effort to provide quality spiritual care.

- Remember that there often is nobody better placed or better qualified than the nurse to provide spiritual care.
- Integration of the sacred into the process of dying should probably always be attempted, even if only in the nurse's life and the institution's milieu.
- There are situations in which the patient cannot physically tolerate going to a place of worship for a complete service, but can stay for a limited time. When this is the case, (*1*) the patient may need help to choose which part of the service to attend and (*2*) the place of worship may need help in accommodating the patient's participation in the service. In some cases, the patient may need additional medication or portable equipment to make it through even part of the service.
- When, because of physical or other limitations, it becomes difficult for the patient to visit a place of worship, home or hospital visits from clergy should be considered. It is sometimes necessary for the nurse or other staff to make repeated appeals to the patient's clergy for such visits.
- Other religious activities that can take place at home or hospital include prayer, ritual, reading, and other spiritually oriented activities, including music. Music can be very helpful to the patient and others, and might by provided by a few choir members coming to the home or by tapes or CDs of religious music.
- The presence of a religious book in the patient's home or room provides the opportunity for the nurse to pick up the book and discuss it with the patient. It is helpful for the nurse to actually take the book in hand when initiating discussion. It also is helpful to ask the patient to read aloud passages that are most important to her or him. If the patient is unable to read, the nurse or other caregiver can do the reading. (If the book is the Koran, the nurse should wash his or her hands before taking it in hand.)
- There is an understandable tendency for people to want to do things for the person who is dying. It is important to encourage the person who is dying to also do things for others. Creating or affirming memories and leaving a legacy is suggested by Lynn.[19] This might include the patient giving a copy of the holy book of her or his faith to a loved one (e.g., a grandchild), planning the funeral service, making a point of reconciling with others, spending time to consider a mindful good-bye, and other means of making connection with others.
- Everyone dies, and while it is of no help to trivialize an individual's experience by pointing this out in a heedless manner, it may be helpful to carefully introduce the universality of the experience—especially the fact that many others have struggled with pain, fear, guilt, and other core issues in dying and death. All the major religions address the universality of death and suffering.
- Recall that hospice and palliative care emerged, in part, as humane responses to the increasingly technological nature of dying and death in the modern world. The serious question arises, how can the spiritual and sacred become more a part of the process, both in terms of a particular patient and in terms of institutions.

And finally, the practice of mercy—of watching through the night—is central to hospice and palliative care and to the practice of every faith.

REFERENCES

1. Carse JP. (1980). Death and Existence. John Wiley and Sons, New York.
2. Kemp CE. (1999). Terminal Illness: A Guide to Nursing Care. Lippincott-Williams and Wilkins, Philadelphia.
3. Baylor University School of Nursing (1991). Report of Self-Study. Baylor University School of Nursing, Dallas.
4. Burton LA. (1998). The spiritual dimension of palliative care. Semin Oncol Nurs 14: 121–128.
5. Gallup International Institute (1997). Spiritual Beliefs and the Dying Process. Gallup International Institute, Princeton, NJ.
6. Speck PW. (1993). Spiritual issues in palliative care. In Oxford Textbook of Palliative Medicine (D. Doyle, G.W.C. Hanks, and N. MacDonald, eds.), pp. 517–525. Oxford University Press, Oxford.
7. Nuland S. (1994). How We Die. Alfred A. Knopf, New York.
8. Frankl V. (1969). The Will to Meaning. New American Library, New York.
9. Taylor EJ, Amenta M, Highfield M. (1995). Spritual care practices of oncology nurses. Oncol Nurs Forum 22:31–39.
10. Saunders CM. (1978). Appropriate treatment, appropriate death. In The Management of Terminal Disease (C.M. Saunders, ed.), pp. 1–18. Edward Arnold, London.
11. The Bible. Revised standard edition.
12. Bhagavad-Gita. (1991). Translated by Swami Prabhavananda and C. Isherwood. Mentor Religious Classics, New York.
13. The Teaching of Buddha. (1981). Bukkyo Dendo Kyokai, Tokyo.
14. The Koran. Translated by N.J. Dawood (1990). Penguin Books, New York.
15. Post-White J, Ceronsky C, Kreitzer MJ, Nickelson K, Drew D, Mackey KW, Koopmeiners L, and Gutknecht S. (1996). Hope, spirituality, sense of coherence, and quality of life in patients with cancer. Oncol Nurs Forum 23:1571–1579.
16. Green J. (1989). Death with dignity: Hinduism. Nursing Times 85(6):50–51.
17. Jung CG. (1953). Psychology and alchemy. In C.G. Jung: Psychological Reflection (J. Jacobi and R.F.C. Hull, eds.), pp. 338–339. Princeton University Press, Princeton, NJ.
18. Foster D. (1999). Personal communications.
19. Lynn J, Harrold J, and the Center to Improve Care of the Dying. (1999). Handbook for Mortals. Oxford University Press, New York.

31 Meaning in Illness

TAMI BORNEMAN and KATHERINE BROWN-SALTZMAN

I still question, sometimes . . . but then I also do believe that she's still here for a reason. God has not taken her home yet for a reason.
—Husband of a cancer patient

In the driest whitest stretch
Of pain's infinite desert
I lost my sanity
And found this rose.
—Galal al-Din Rumi; Persia, 1207–1273

Is it possible to adequately articulate and give definition to meaning in illness? Or is meaning in illness better described and understood through using symbolism and metaphors such as the above poem? To try and define that which is enigmatic and bordering on the ineffable seems almost sacrilegious. The unique individual journey of finding meaning in illness experienced by each patient and their family caregiver facing the end of life would seem to be diminished by the very process that seeks to understand through the use of language.

Is it that we seek to find meaning in illness or is it that we seek to find meaning in the life that is now left and in those relationships and things we value? Do we seek to find meaning in illness itself as an isolated event or that which is beyond the illness such as how to live out this newly imposed way of life? Terminal illness forces us to look at and possibly reappraise the meaning *in* our life and the meaning *of* our life.[1] If we allow space in our lives for the process of meaning in illness to unfold, we then move from the superficial to the profound.

Terminal illness also forces us at some point to look directly at death, yet we resist getting in touch with the feelings that arise. Everything in us seeks life. Everything in us hopes for life. Everything in us denies death. There is something very cold, very unmoving, and very disturbing about it all. Does the end of one's human existence on earth need to be the sole metaphor for death?

Even though end-of-life issues have progressed nearer to the forefront of healthcare, the dying patient is still the recipient of an impersonal, detached, and cure-focused system, thereby exacerbating an already catastrophic situation. As necessary as it is for nurses to use the nursing process, it is not enough. The patient's illness odyssey beckons us to go beyond assessment, diagnosis, intervention, and evaluation to a place of vulnerability, not in an unprofessional manner but rather in a way that allows for a shared connectedness unique to each patient–nurse relationship. We need to be willing to use feelings appropriately as part of the therapeutic process. Separating ourselves from touching and feeling in order to protect ourselves, only serves to make us more vulnerable because we have then placed our emotions in isolation. Nurses can be a catalyst for helping the patient and family find meaning in the illness, and, in the process, help themselves define or redefine their own meaning in life, illness, and death.

MEANING DEFINED

Johnston-Taylor[2] presents several definitions for *meaning* (Table 31–1). In the dictionary[3] one finds *meaning* simply defined as "Something that is conveyed or signified" or as "An interpreted goal, intent, or end." But it is the etymology of the word *mean* that helps nursing come to understand our potential for supporting patients in the process of finding meaning in their lives, even as they face death. *Mean* comes from the Old English *maenan*, "to tell of." One does not find meaning in a vacuum; it has everything to do with relationships, spirituality, and connectedness. While the process of finding meaning depends greatly on an inward journey, it also relies on the telling of that journey. The telling may use language, but it may also be conveyed by the eyes, through the hands, or just in the way the body is held. Frankl[4] reminds us that the "will to meaning" is a basic drive for all of humanity and is unique to each individual. A life-threatening illness begs the question of meaning with a new urgency and necessity.

Cassell[5] tells us that "all events are assigned meaning," which entails judging their significance and value. Meaning cannot be separated from the person's past; it requires the thought of future, and ultimately influences perception of that future (p. 67). Finding meaning is not a stagnant process, it changes as each day unfolds and the occurrences are interpreted. As one patient reflected upon her diagnosis, "Cancer changes your perception of your world

Table 31–1. Definitions of Meaning

Meaning	"refers to sense, or coherence. . . . A search for meaning implies a search for coherence. 'Purpose' refers to intention, aim, function. . . . However, 'purpose' of life and 'meaning' of life are used interchangeably."[38]
	"a structure which relates purposes to expectations so as to organise actions. . . . Meaning . . . makes sense of actions by providing reasons for it."[39]
[Search for] meaning	"is an effort to understand the event: why it happened and what impact it has had . . . [and] attempts to answer the question(s), What is the significance of the event? . . . What caused the event to happen? . . . [and] What does my life mean now?"[40]
	"is an attempt to restore the sense that one's life is orderly and purposeful."[41]
Personal search for meaning	"the process by which a person seeks to interpret a life circumstance. The search involves questioning the personal significance of a life circumstance, in order to give the experience purpose and to place it in the context of a person's total life pattern. The basis of the process is the interaction between meaning in and of life and involves the reworking and redefining of past meaning while looking for meaning in a current life curcumstance."[1]

and life."[6] Coming face to face with one's mortality not only defines what is important, but also the poignancy of the loss of much of what has been meaningful.

One's spirituality is often the key to transcending those losses, finding ways of maintaining those connections. Whether it is the belief that one's love, work, or creativity will remain after the physical separation or the belief that one's spirit goes on to an afterlife or through reincarnation. Meaning in life concerns the individual's realm of life on earth. It has to do with one's humanness, the temporal, and the composites of what one has done in life to give meaning. Meaning of life has more to do with the existential. It is looking beyond one's earthly physical existence to an eternal, secure, and indelible God or spiritual plane. The existential realm of life provides a sense of security whereby one can integrate experiences.[7]

Spirituality has been defined as a search for meaning.[8] One of the Hebrew words for meaning is *biynah* (bee-naw), which is understanding, knowledge, meaning, wisdom. It comes from the root word *biyn* (bene), to separate mentally or to distinguish.[9] How is it that one can come to knowledge and understanding? Patients receiving palliative care often describe a sense of isolation and loneliness. They frequently have endless hours available while at the same time experiencing a shortening of their life. It is here that nursing has a pivotal role as the listener, for when the ruminations of the dying are given voice, there is an opportunity for meaning. Important life themes are shared and the unanswerable questions are at least asked. As the stranger develops intimacy and trust, meaning takes hold.

Suffering creates one of the greatest challenges to uncovering meaning. For the dying patient, suffering comes in many packages: physical pain, unrelenting symptoms (nausea, pruritis, dyspnea, etc.), spiritual distress, dependency, multiple losses, and anticipatory grieving. Even the benefits of medical treatments given to provide hope or palliation can sometimes be outweighed by side effects (e.g. sedation and constipation from pain medication), inducing yet further suffering. The dictionary[3] defines *suffering* in this way: "To feel pain or distress; sustain loss, injury, harm, or punishment." But once again it is the root word that moves us to a more primitive understanding, the Latin *sufferre*, which comprises *sub*, "below," and *ferre* "to carry." The weight and isolation of that suffering now becomes more real at the visceral level. Cassell[5] reminds us that pain itself does not foreordain suffering; it is in fact the meaning that is attributed to that pain that determines the suffering. In his clinical definition, "Suffering is a state of severe distress induced by the loss of the intactness of person, or by a threat that the person believes will result in the loss of his or her intactness" (p. 63), suffering is an individual and private experience and will be greatly influenced by the personality and character of the person, so for example the patient who has needed control during times of wellness will find the out-of-control experience of illness as suffering.[5] In writing about cancer pain and its meaning, Ersek and Ferrell[10] provide a summary of hypotheses and theses from the literature (Table 31–2).

Although it is not always recognized it is the duty of all who care for patients to alleviate suffering and not just treat the physical dimensions of the illness. This is no small task, for first professionals must be free from denial and the need to self-protect in order to *see* the suffering of another. Then they must be able to attend to it, without trying to fix it or simplify it. The suffering needs to be witnessed; in the midst of it, presence and compassion become the balm and hope for its relief.

THE PROCESS OF FINDING MEANING IN ILLNESS

From years of working with terminally ill patients and their families, the authors have found that the process of finding meaning in illness invokes many themes. The title given to each theme is an attempt to represent observed transitions that many terminally ill patients seem to experience. Not all patients experience the transitions in order, and not all transitions are experienced. However, we have observed that these transitions are experienced by the majority of patients. Issues faced by family caregivers and health care professionals are

Table 31–2. Summary of Hypotheses and Theses from the Literature on Meaning

Hypothesis/Thesis	Source
The search for meaning is a basic human need.	Frankl 1959[4]
Meaning is necessary for human fulfillment.	Steeves and Kahn 1987[42]
Finding meaning fosters positive coping and increased hopefulness.	Ersek 1991;[43] Steeves and Kahn 1987;[42] Taylor 1983[40]
One type of meaning-making activity in response to threatening events is to develop causal attributions.	Gotay 1983;[44] Haberman 1987;[45] Steeves and Kahn 1987;[42] Taylor 1983;[40] Chrisman and Haberman 1977[46]
Meaning making can involve the search for a higher order.	Ersek 1991;[43] Ferrell et al 1993;[47] Steeves and Kahn 1987[42]
Making meaning often involves the use of social comparisons.	Ferrell et al. 1993;[47] Taylor 1983;[40] Ersek 1991;[43] Haberman 1987[48]
Meaning can be derived through construing benefits from a negative experience.	Ersek 1991;[43] Haberman 1987;[45] Taylor 1983[40]
Meaning sometimes focuses on illness as challenge, enemy, punishment.	Barkwell 1991;[48] Ersek 1991;[43] Lipowski 1970[49]
Pain and suffering often prompt a search for meaning.	Frankl 1959;[4] Steeves and Kahn 1987;[42] Taylor 1983[40]
Uncontrolled pain or overwhelming suffering hinder the experience of meaning.	Steeves and Kahn 1987[42]
One goal of care is to promote patients' and caregivers' search for and experiences of meaning.	Ersek 1991;[43] Ferrell et al. 1993;[47] Steeves and Kahn 1987;[42] Haberman 1988[50]

discussed in later sections. The themes shared in this section are the imposed transition, loss and confusion, dark night of the soul, randomness and absence of God, brokenness, and reappraisal. In experiencing some or all of these transitions, one can perhaps find meaning in this difficult time of life.

The Imposed Transition

Being told that you have a terminal illness can be like hearing the sound of prison doors slam shut. Life will never be the same. The sentencing has been handed down and there is no reversing the verdict. Terminal illness is a loss and there is nothing we can do to change the prognosis even though we may be able to temporarily delay the final outcome. The very essence of our being is shaken and our souls are stricken with a panic unlike any other we have ever felt. For the first time, we are faced with an "existential awareness of nonbeing."[11] For a brief moment, the silence is deafening, as if suspended between two worlds, the known and the unknown. As one "regains consciousness" so to speak, the pain and pandemonium of thoughts and emotions begin to storm the floodgates of our faith, our coping abilities, and our internal fortitude while simultaneously the word "terminal" reverberates in our heads. There is no easy or quick transition into the acceptance of a terminal diagnosis.

Facing the end of life provokes questions. Not only is the question "why me?" asked, but questions regarding the meaning *in* one's life as well as the meaning *of* one's life.[1] Whether we embrace with greater fervor the people and things that collectively give us meaning in life or we view it all as now lost, the loss and pain are real. Nothing can be done to prevent the inevitable. There is a sense of separation or disconnectedness in that while *I* am the same person, *I* have also become permanently different from you. Unless you become like me, diagnosed with a terminal illness, we are in this sense, separated. In a rhetorical sense, the meanings we gain in life from relationships and the material world serve to affirm us as participants in these meanings.[11] When these meanings are threatened by a terminal diagnosis, we fear the loss of who we are as functioning productive human beings. The affirmations we received from our meanings *in* life are now at a standstill.

A 38-year-old man with cancer, facing the end of life, shared that many of the people he thought were his friends stopped coming by to see him. These people included those from his work in the fishing industry, and childhood friends. This man was struggling already with who he was because he no longer could work or enjoy fishing. He was also well known in the fishing industry. So for him, not being able to "do" affected his meaning in life as a contributer to society. In addition, feeling abandoned by friends and colleagues affected his sense of "being." He was no longer giving or receiving from them, both of which affect one's meaning in life.

In addition to questioning meaning *in* life, those facing the end of life also question the meaning *of* life. A life-threatening illness makes it difficult to maintain an illusion of immortality.[12] What happens when we die? Is there really a God? Is it too late for reconciliation? For those believing in life after death, the questions may focus on uncertainty of eternal life, fear of what eternal life will be like or the possibility of this being a test of faith. No matter what the belief system, the existential questions are asked. We reach out for a connection with God or something beyond one's self in order to obtain some sense of security and stability. Then, in this ability to transcend the situation, ironically, we somehow feel a sense of groundedness. Frankl[4] states, "It denotes the fact that being human always points, and is directed, to something or someone, other than oneself—be it a meaning to fulfill or another human being to encounter." There is an incredibly strong spiritual need to find meaning in this new senseless and chaotic world.

Loss and Confusion

One cancer patient stated, "Our lives are like big run-on sentences and when cancer occurs, it's like a period was placed at the end of the sentence. In reality, we all have a period at the end of the sentence, but we don't really pay attention to it."[13] With a terminal diagnosis, life is changed forever, for however long that life may be. Each day life seems to change as one is forced to experience a new aspect of the loss. There is a sense of immortality that pervades our lust for life, and when we are made to look at our mortality, it is staggering. With all of the many losses, coupled with the fear of dying, one can be left feeling confused from the infinite possibilities of the unknown. The panorama of suffering seems to be limitless.

The pain of loss is as great as the pleasure we derived from life.[14] The pain is pure and somewhat holy. The confusion comes not only from one's world having been turned upside down, but also from those who love us and care about us. It is not intentional, nevertheless its impact is greatly felt. In trying to bring encouragement or trying to help one find meaning, the loss and pain are sometimes minimized by comparing losses, attempting to save God's reputation by denying the one hurting the freedom to be angry at God, or, by immediately focusing on the time left to live. The hurting soul needs to feel the depth of the loss by whatever means it can. The pain from loss is relentless, like waves from a dark storm at sea crashing repeatedly against rocks on the shoreline.

A 65-year-old woman with terminal lung cancer experienced further physical decline each day. She was surrounded by a family who lovingly doted on her. She was one who loved life and loved people. Many losses were experienced due to her condition. What added to these losses was the fact that her family wanted her to focus on life and not her disease or death. They knew she was going to die but felt that her quality of life would be better if these issues were not discussed. The patient had many thoughts and feelings to sort through and wanted to talk, but no one was listening. Her loss was not just physical, it also was an imposed emotional loss caused by a loving family trying to do the right thing. The communications with her family were different, constantly reminding her that nothing was the same, and in turn reminded her of her losses and impending death.

"Dark Night of the Soul"

The descent of darkness pervades every crack and crevice of one's being. One now exists in the place of Nowhere, surrounded by a nothingness which is void of texture and contour. One's signature is seemingly wiped away, taking with it the identification of a living soul.[14] Job states, "And now my soul is poured out within me; days of affliction have seized me. At night it pierces my bones within me, and my gnawing pains take no rest. . . . My days are swifter than a weaver's shuttle, and come to an end without hope."[15] "One enters the abyss of emptiness—with the perverse twist that one is not empty of the tortured *feeling* of emptiness."[16] This is pain's infinite desert.

Darkness looms as one thinks about the past, full of people and things that provided meaning in life, and will soon have to be given up. Darkness looms as one thinks about the future because death precludes holding on to all which is loved and valued. Darkness consumes one's mind and heart like fire consumes wood. It makes its way to the center with great fury where it proceeds to take possession, leaving nothing but a smoldering heap of ashes and no hope of recovering any essence of life.[17]

A woman in her mid-forties with metastatic bone cancer was at the end of her emotional rope. She had suffered several losses within a relatively short period of time and now her cancer was actively progressing. This woman shared that the bottom line is that she didn't want to die but she felt her body giving up. She didn't want to die, but without a sense of purpose and meaning in her present life, she had nothing to hope for. She definitely did not want to be alone when she died and presently felt forsaken and desolate.

Though one might try, there are no answers theological or otherwise to the "why's" that engulf one's existence. Death moves from an "existential phenomenon to a personal reality."[18] All our presuppositions about life fall away and we are left emotionally naked. There is neither the physical, the emotional, nor the spiritual strength to help our own fragility. The world becomes too big for us and our inner worlds are overwhelming.[14] The enigma of facing death strips order from one's life, creating fragmentation and leaving one with the awareness that life is no longer tenable.

Randomness and the Absence of God

The pronouncement of a terminal diagnosis provokes inner turmoil and ruminating thoughts from dawn to dusk. Even in one's chaotic life, there was order. But order does not always prevail. A young athlete being recruited for a professional sport is suddenly killed in a tragic car accident. A mother of three small children is diagnosed with a chronic debilitating disease that will end in death. An earthquake levels a brand-new home that a husband and wife had spent years saving for. A playful young toddler drowns in a pool. There seems to be no reason. It would be different if negligence were involved. For example, if the young athlete was speeding, or driving drunk, although still quite devastating, a "logical" reason could be assigned to the loss. But randomness leaves us with no "logical" explanation.[16]

The word *random* comes from the Middle English word *randoun*, which is derived from the Old French word *randon*, meaning violence and speed. The word connotes an impetuous and haphazard movement, lacking careful choice, aim, or purpose.[3] The feeling of vulnerability is overwhelming. In an effort to find shelter from this randomness, meaning and comfort is sought from

God or from something beyond one's self, but how do we know that God or something beyond ourselves is not the cause of our loss? Our trust is shaken. Can we reconcile God's sovereignty with our loss?[16] Can we stay connected to and continue to pull or gain strength and security from something beyond ourselves that may be the originator of our pain? There is a sense of abandonment by that which has been our stronghold in life. Yet to cut ourselves off from that stronghold out of anger would leave us in a state of total disconnection. A sense of connection is a vital emotion necessary for existence, no matter how short that existence may be. But facing death forbids us to keep our existential questions and desires at a distance. Rather, it seems to propel us into a deeper search for meaning as the questions continue to echo in our minds.

Brokenness

Does one come to a place of acceptance within brokenness? Is acceptance even attainable? Sometimes. Sometimes not. Coming to a place of acceptance is a very individual experience for each person. Kearney,[19] in a wonderful analogy of acceptance, states, "Acceptance is not something an individual can choose at will. It is not like some light switch that can at will be flicked on or off. Deep emotional acceptance is like the settling of a cloud of silt in a troubled pool. With time the silt rests on the bottom and the water is clear" (p. 98). Brokenness does however, open the door to relinquish the illusion of immortality. Brokenness allows the soul to cry and to shed tears of anguish. It elicits the existential question "why" once again, only this time not to gain answers, but to find meaning.

A woman in her mid-sixties, dying of lung cancer, shared how she came to a place of acceptance. When she was first diagnosed, the cancer was already pretty advanced. Her health rapidly declined and she was more or less confined to bed or sitting. Out of her frustration, anger at God, sadness, and tears, came the desire to paint again. It was her way of coping, but it became more than that. It brought her to a place of peace in her heart. She had gotten away from painting due to business and was now learning to be blessed by quietness. She was very good at replicating Thomas Kinkade paintings, and her final picture which was to be a gift, included many beautiful flowers. She was always surrounded by flowers.

If we go back to the poem at the beginning of this chapter, it wasn't until "sanity" was lost that the rose was found. A gradual perception takes place whereby we realize that the way out is by no longer struggling.[19] When we come to the end of ourselves and the need to fight the inevitable that is death, we give space for meaning to unfold. It isn't that we give up the desire, but we relinquish the *need* to emotionally turn the situation around and to have all our questions answered. Sittser,[16] a minister who experienced a sudden loss of several immediate family members, states, "My experience taught me that loss reduces people to a state of almost total brokenness and vulnerability. I did not simply feel raw pain; I *was* raw pain" (p. 164). Pain and loss are still profound but in the midst of these heavy emotions, there begins to be a glimmer of light. Like the flame of a candle, the light may wax and wane. It is enough to begin to silhouette those people and things that still can provide meaning.

Reappraisal

It is here where one begins to realize that something positive can come from even a terminal diagnosis and the losses it imposes. The good that is gained does not mitigate the pain of loss, but rather fosters hope. Hope that is not contingent on healing but on reconciliation, on creating memories with loved ones, on making the most of every day, on loving and being loved.[20] It's a hope that transcends science and explanations, and changes with the situation. It is not based on a particular outcome but rather focuses on the future, however long that may be. Despair undermines hope, but hope robs death of despair.[21]

A male patient in his late thirties, facing the end of life after battling leukemia and having gone through a bone marrow transplant, shared that he knew he was going to die. It took him a long time to be able to admit it to himself. The patient recalled recently visiting a young man who had basically given up and did not want his last bag of chemotherapy. He talked a while with this young man and encouraged him to "go for it." He told him that there's nothing like watching the last drop of chemo go down the tube and into his body, and the sense of it finally being all over. The patient shared with the young man that when he received his own last bag of chemo, he stayed up until three in the morning to watch the last drop go down the tube. While the chemotherapy did not help him to the extent that he wanted, he wanted to encourage the young man to hope and not give up. Life was not yet over. He had tears in his eyes when he finished the story.

Facing end of life with a terminal diagnosis will never be a happy event. It will always be tragic because it causes the pain and loss to everyone involved. But at a time unique to each person facing death, a choice can be made as to whether one wants to become bitter and devalue the remaining time, or value as much as possible the time that is left.

An important choice to be made during this time is whether to forgive or to be unforgiving, toward oneself, others, God, or one's stronghold of security in life. Being unforgiving breeds bitterness and superficiality. As we face the end of life we need both an existential connection and a connection with others. Being unforgiving separates us from those connections, and it is only through forgiveness that the breech is healed. Forgiveness does not condone another's actions nor does it mean that this terminal diagnosis is fair. Rather, forgiveness is letting go of expectations that one somehow will be vindicated for the pain and loss. Whether by overt anger or by emotional withdrawal, in seeking to avoid being vulnerable to further pain and loss, we only succeed in making ourselves more vulnerable. Now we have chosen a deeper separation that goes beyond facing the death of the physical body—that of the soul.[16] Positive vulnerability through forgiveness provides a means of healing, and when possible, reconciliation with others. It always provides healing and reconciliation with one's God or one's stronghold of security. Forgiveness allows both physical and emotional energy to be used for creating and enjoying the time left for living.

There are many emotions and issues with which those facing death must contend. It is not an easy journey and the process is wearing; nevertheless the rose can be found.

IMPACT OF THE TERMINAL ILLNESS ON THE PATIENT–CAREGIVER RELATIONSHIP

Each of us comes to every new situation with our life's experiences and the meanings we have gained from them. It is no different when being confronted with illness and the end of life. However, in this special episode of life, there are often no personal "reruns" from which to glean insight. Patient and family come together as novices, each helping the other through this unknown passage. As there exist different roles and relationships, the impending loss will create different meanings for each person involved.

Facing the loss of someone you love is very difficult. The process of finding meaning by the family caregiver can either be facilitated or hindered by the meaning held by the one facing death.[22] One example experienced by one of the authors of this chapter involved a wife's short discussion with her terminally ill husband on the subject of heaven. She asked him if he thought he was going to heaven and if he was, would she be able to be with him even though she was from a different religion. He assured her that they would someday be together in heaven, and an immediate sense of peace came over his wife. He was not looking forward to dying, but for him, his death was not the end. He would see her again. His own meaning of death helped create a whole new meaning for his wife. He imparted to her a sense of eternal connection that allayed her fears of eternal separation from the most important person in her life. She could now face his death, with sorrow, but without fear.

In another example a woman helped her family create meaning for themselves from the picture she had painted of herself sitting on the beach as a little girl next to a little boy. She explained that the little boy had his arm around her as they stared out at the sea. Each time the waves covered the surface of the beach and then retreated, the sea would carry with it bits and pieces of her fears and disease. The birds circling overhead would then swoop down to pick up and carry off any pieces not taken by the sea. The little boy's arm around her signified all the loving support she had received from others. When the time would come for her to die, she would be ready because she had been able to let go of life as she knew it. She had let the waves slowly carry that way of life out to sea and yet had learned to hold on to the meaning that that life had represented. In doing so, she enabled her family to hold on to the meaning of their relationship with her and to realize that they would never be separated from that meaning.[23]

A final poignant story offers a different perspective: A 53-year-old woman with stage IV ovarian cancer was very angry at everyone and everything and could not seem to find any positive meaning. She was angry that her life would be cut short and she would not live to see her grandchildren grow. She and her husband had made plans to travel and now she was too ill to make even one of the trips. She made life difficult for those who loved her. She made loving her and caring for her difficult. No one could seem to do anything right. She was bothered by company yet wanted someone with her all the time, and she did not like the intrusion of health care professionals in her home. She felt that her physician and family had given up on her and she resented it. She died a very angry and unhappy woman. This was very difficult for her family. The family was left feeling rather fragmented. What exactly *did* all of this mean? They had spent so much time trying to please the patient, which was almost impossible, that they never had time to synthesize the events and their feelings regarding the whole terminal illness trajectory. Not only did the family have their own pain from loss, they were left with final memories that created negative meanings. For example, various family members had begun to withdraw emotionally from the patient out of hurt and frustration, yet felt guilty for "abandoning" her. After her death, those family members still felt guilty because they had really wanted to be with her.

These actual patient stories were given to exemplify how the patient's meaning in illness affects the meaning held or created by family members. Differing or divergent meanings can be detrimental in a relationship or they can be used to strengthen it, thereby increasing the quality of time left together. That is not to imply that the patient is *responsible* for the meaning created by family members, but how one affects the other. Germino, Fife, and Funk[22] suggest that the goal is not merely converging meanings within the patient–family dyad but rather encouraging a sharing of individual meanings so that all can learn, and relationships can be deepened and strengthened.

There are many issues that family caregivers face in caring for a loved one nearing the end of life. They are discussed at length in the literature. There is one issue, however, that warrants more attention—the loss of dreams. The loss of dreams for a future with the person is in addition to the loss of the person. It is the loss of the way one used to imagine life, and how it would have been with that person. It is the loss of an emotional image of oneself and the abandonment of chosen plans for the future and what might have been.[24]

When asked about what dreams would be lost, a retired male caregiver shared, "Well, we had hoped that we would have a good twenty years or so of just being golf course bums, going around the country visiting golf courses having a good time. That's lost. She's had a real full life. It's just that it's not nearly as long . . . as we had thought.

And so that's what we've lost, I guess longevity."[25] This caregiver had also shared that given his family's health history, he had always thought that he would die first. He had never imagined himself as a single man. His wife's impending death propelled him into creating a different meaning in life as a single man. He would continue to carry with him the meaning in life they had held together, but in addition, now he would have to create his own meaning. His wife had been a wonderful support in helping him to see that in looking at the future and finding meaning in a different way, he was not abandoning all that they had together.

The loss of dreams is an internal process, spiritual for some, seldom recognized by others as needing processing.[24,26,27] Nurses have a wonderful opportunity at this point to verbally recognize the family caregivers' loss of dreams and to encourage them in their search to find meaning in the loss. The ability to transcend and connect to God or something greater than one's self, helps the healing process.

TRANSCENDENCE: STRENGTH FOR THE JOURNEY THAT LIES AHEAD

Transcendence is defined as lying beyond the ordinary range of perception; being above and independent of the material universe. The Latin root is *trans-*, "from or beyond," plus *scandere*, "to climb."[3] The images are many, the man in a pit climbing his way out one handhold at a time, the story of Job as he endured one defeat after another and yet found meaning, the climber who reaches the mountaintop, becoming closer to the heavens while still having the connection to the earth, or the dying patient who in peace is already seeing into another reality. The ability to transcend truly is a gift of the human spirit and often comes after a long struggle and out of suffering. It is often unclear which comes first—does meaning open the door for transcendence or, quite the opposite, does the act of transcendence bring the meaning? More than likely it is an intimate dance between the two. One fueling the other. In the Buddhist tradition, suffering and being are a totality, and integrating suffering in this light becomes an act of transcendence.[28]

Transcendence of suffering can also be accomplished by viewing it as reparation for sins while still living, preparing the way for eternity, as in the Islamic tradition. In other traditions transcendence is often relationship based, the connection to others and sometimes to a higher power.[4] For example, the Christian seeing Christ on the cross connects one to the relationship and endurance of God and the reality that suffering is a part of life. For others it is finding meaning in relating to others, even the act of caring for others. And for some that relationship may be with the earth, a sense of stewardship and leaving the environment a better place. It is rare that patients reach a state of transcendence and remain there through their dying. Instead it is for most a process in which there are moments when they reach a sense of expansion that supports them in facing death. The existential crisis does not rule, because one can frame the relationship beyond death, for example, "I will remain in their hearts and memories forever, I will live on through my children, or my spirit will live beyond my limited physical state."

NURSING INTERVENTIONS

If one returns to the root word of *meaning, maenan*, "to tell of," this concept can be the guide that directs the nurse toward interventions. Given the nature of this work, interventions may not be the true representation of what is needed. For intervention implies action that the nurse has an answer and she can direct the course of care by intervening. It is defined as "To come, appear, or lie between two things. To come in or between so as to hinder or alter an action."[3] But finding meaning is process oriented; while finely honed psychosocial skills and knowledge can be immensely helpful, there is no bag of tricks. One example would be of a chaplain who walks in the room and relies only on offering prayer to the patient, preventing any real discourse or relationship building. The patient's personhood has been diminished and potentially more harm than good has been done.

So let us revisit "to tell of." What is required of the professional who enters into the healing dimension of a patient's suffering and search for meaning? It would seem that respect may be the starting point, respect for that individual's way of experiencing suffering and attempts of making sense of the illness. Secondly, allowing for an environment and time for the telling. Even as this is written, the sighs of frustration are heard, "We have no time!" If nursing fails at this, if nurses turn their backs on their intrinsic promise to alleviate suffering, then nursing can no longer exist. Instead the nurse becomes simply the technician and the scheduler, the nurse becomes a part of the problem. She has violated the Code for Nurses, which states, "Nursing care is directed toward the prevention and relief of the suffering commonly associated with the dying process . . . and emphasizes human contact."[29]

In the midst of suffering if patients receive the message, nonverbal or directly, that there is no time, energy, or compassion, they will in their vulnerability withdraw or become more needy. Their alienation becomes complete. On the other hand, if privacy and a moment of honor and focused attention is provided, this allows for the tears to spill or the anguish to be spoken. Then the alienation is broken and the opportunity for healing one dimension is begun. The terminally ill are a vulnerable population. They die and do not complete patient satisfaction surveys; their grievances, and their stories die with them. But the violation does not, for each nurse now holds that violation, as does society as a whole. The wound begets wounds, the nurse sinks further into the protected and unavailable approach, alienated herself. The work holds no rewards, only endless days and demands. She has nothing left to give. The patient and family are ultimately abandoned. In the work of Kahn and Steeves[30] one finds a model for the nurse's role in psychosocial processes and suffering. It represents the dynamic relationship of caring, acted out in caregiving as well as in the patient's coping, which transform each other.

In order for the nurse to provide this level of caregiving, she must understand the obstructions that may interfere. It is essential that the nurse undergo her own journey, visiting the intense emotions around the dying process and the act of witnessing suffering. In the words of Younger, "Being fully present is the ability to convey that personal fears and ego needs have been laid aside in deference to those of the other."[31] Presence may in fact be our greatest gift to these patients and their families. Still, imagine charting or accounting for presence on an acuity system! Presence "transcends role obligations and acknowledges the vulnerable humanness of us all . . . to be present means to unconceal, to be aware of tone of voice, eye contact, affect, and body language, to be in tune with the patient's messages."[31] Presence provides confirmation, nurturing, and compassion and is an essential transcendent act.

Touch becomes one of the tools of presence. Used with sensitivity, it can be as simple as the holding of the hand, or as powerful as the holding of the whole person. Sometimes, because of agitation or pain, direct touch becomes intrusive; even then touch can be invoked, by the touching of a pillow, the sheet, or the offering of a cold cloth. Healing touch takes on another level of intention through the directing energy or prayer.

If a key aspect of meaning is to tell, then one might be led to believe that the spoken word would be imperative. Yet over and over, it is silence that conveys the meaning of suffering, "a primitive form of existence that is without an effective voice and imprisoned in silence." Compassionate listeners in respect and presence become mute themselves.[31] They use the most intuitive of skills to carry the message. This may also be why other approaches that utilize symbols, metaphors, and the arts are the most potent in helping the patient to communicate and make sense of meaning. The arts, whether writing, music, or visual arts, often help the patient not only gain new insight, but convey that meaning to others. There are many levels on which this is accomplished. Whether it is done passively, through reading poetry, listening to music, or viewing paintings, or actively through creation, thoughts can be inspired, feelings moved, and the sense of connectedness and being understood can evolve. What once was ubiquitous can now be seen outside of one's soul, as feelings become tangible. It can be relational, as the act of creation can link one to the creator, or it can downplay the role of dependency, as the ill one now cares for others with a legacy of creational gifts.[32]

Meditation is another act of transcendence that can be extremely powerful for the dying.[33,34] Even those who have never experienced a meditational state can find that this new world in many ways links them to living and dying. The relaxation response that allows the anxious patient to escape into a meditative state, experiencing an element of control while relinquishing control. Many patients describe it as a floating state, a time of great peace and calm. Some, who have never had such an experience, can find the first time frightening, as the existential crisis, quelled so well by boundaries, is no longer confined. Most, given a trusting and safe teacher, will find that meditation will serve them well. The meditation can be in the form of prayer, guided imagery, breathing techniques, or mantras.

Prayer is well documented in the literature[35,36] as having meaning for patients and families; not only does it connect one to God, but it also again becomes a relational connection to others. Knowing that one is prayed for not only by those close at hand, but by strangers, communities, and those at a great distance can be deeply nurturing. Often forgotten is the role the patient can be empowered in, that of praying for others. One of the authors experienced her patient's prayers for her as the tables were turned, and the patient became the healer. The patient suddenly left behind the sense of worthlessness and glowed with joy.

Leaving a legacy may be one of the most concrete ways for patients to find meaning in this last stage of their lives.[37] It most often requires the mastering of the existential challenges, in which the person knows that death is at hand and chooses to direct their course and what they leave behind. For some patients, that will mean going out as warriors, fighting till the end; for others it will mean end-of-life planning that focuses on quality of life. Some patients will design their funerals, using rituals and readings that reveal their values and messages for others. Others will create videos, write letters, or distribute their wealth in meaningful ways. Parents who are leaving young children sometimes have the greatest difficulty with this aspect. On one hand the feelings of horror at "abandoning" their children are so strong that they have great difficulty facing their death. Still there is often a part of them that has this need to leave a legacy. The tug of war between these two willful emotions tends to leave only short windows of opportunity to prepare. The extreme can be the young father who began to push his toddler away, using excuses for the distancing. It was only after a trusting relationship had been established with one of the authors that she could help him to see how this protective maneuver was in fact harming the child. The father needed not only to see what he was doing, but to see how his love would help the child and how others would be there for the child and wife in their pain and grief. With relief, the father reconnected to his young son, creating living memories and a lifetime protection of love.

Another courageous parent anticipating the missed birthdays, bought cards and wrote a note in each one, so that the child would be touched not only by the individual messages, but the knowledge that the parent found a way to be there for him with each new year. A mother wrote a note for her young daughter, so that if she should ever marry, she would have a gift to be opened on her wedding day. The note described the mother's love, wisdom about marriage, and her daughter's specialness, already known through a mother's eyes. An elderly person may write or tape an autobiography or even record the family tree lest it be lost with the passing of a generation. The nurse can often be the one who inspires these acts, but always it must be done with great care so as not to instill a sense of "should" or "must," which would add yet another burden.

THE HEALTH CARE PROFESSIONAL

While the health care professional can be educated about death and grieving, like the patient and family, it is in living out the experience that understanding is reached. It is a developmental process and the nurse is at great risk, given the demands of the work, for turning away from her feelings. There is often little mentoring that accompanies the first deaths, let alone formal debriefing or counseling. How can it be that we leave such important learning to chance? And what about accumulative losses and the years of witnessing suffering? Health care needs healing rituals for all of its healthcare professionals to support and guide them in this work. Individual institutions can develop programs that address these needs.

At one institution "Teas for the Soul," sponsored by the Pastoral Care Department, provide respite in the workplace on a regular basis as well as after difficult deaths or traumas. A cart with cookies and tea and soft music is provided as physical nurturance, as well as nurturing the emotions of the staff and legitimizing the need to come together in support. Another support is a retreat, the "Circle of Caring." This retreat supports health care professionals from a variety of institutions in a weekend of self care, integrating spirituality, the arts, and community building. The element of suffering is a focal point for a small group process that unburdens cumulative effects of the work and teaches skills and rituals for coping with the ongoing demands.

Clearly, there is much that can be done in this area to support nurses individually and to support organizations. There are many opportunities for assisting nurses in their own search for meaning and enhancing the care of patients and families. When the nurse takes the time to find meaning in this work, she is finding a healthy restorative practice that will protect her personally and professionally. Like the patient, she will need to choose this journey and find pathways that foster and challenge her.

As long as we can love each other,
and remember the feeling of love we had,
we can die without ever really going away.
All the love you created is still there.
All the memories are still there.
You live on—in the hearts of everyone you have
touched and nurtured while you were here.
—Morrie Schwartz

REFERENCES

1. O'Connor A., Wicker C., Germino B. (1990). Understanding the cancer patient's search for meaning. Cancer Nurs 13(3), 167–175.
2. Johnston-Taylor E. (1995). Whys and wherefores: Adult patient perspectives of the meaning of cancer. Semin Oncol Nurs 11(1), 32–40.
3. The American Heritage Dictionary (3rd ed.). (1996). Boston: Houghton Mifflin Co.
4. Frankl V.E. (1959). Man's Search for Meaning: An Introduction to Logotherapy. Boston: Beacon.
5. Cassell E.J. (1989). The relationship between pain and suffering. Adv Pain Res Ther 11: 61–70.
6. Eick-Swigart J. (1995). What cancer means to me. Seminars in Oncology Nursing 11(1): 41–42.
7. Koestenbaum P. (1976). Is There an Answer to Death? Englewood Cliffs, NJ: Prentice-Hall.
8. Jones CPE. (1979). In C. Jones, G. Wainwright, E. Yarnold (eds.). The Study of Spirituality. Oxford: Oxford University Press.
9. Strong's Exhaustive Concordance. (1995). Nashville: Thomas Nelson Publishers.
10. Ersek M., Ferrell BR. (1994). Providing relief from cancer pain by assisting in the search for meaning. J Palliat Care 10(4), 15–22.
11. Tillich P. (1952). The Courage to Be. New Haven, CT: Yale University Press.
12. Benson H. (1997). Timeless Healing. New York: Simon and Schuster.
13. Putnam C. (1999). Personal communication.
14. O'Donohue J. (1999). Eternal Echoes. New York: HarperCollins Publishers.
15. New American Standard Bible. (1977). Anaheim, CA: J.B. McCabe Company.
16. Sittser G. (1995). A Grace Disguised. Grand Rapids, MI: Zondervan Publishing House.
17. St. John of the Cross. (1542). Dark Night of the Soul. Kila, Montana: Kessinger Publishing Company.
18. Kritek P. (1997). Reflections on Healing. New York: NLN Press.
19. Kearney M. (1996). Mortally Wounded. New York: Simon and Schuster.
20. Martins L. (1992). The silence of God: The absence of healing. In Spiritual, Ethical and Pastoral Aspects of Death and Bereavement (GR Cox and RJ Fundis, eds.), pp. 25–31. Amityville, NY: Baywood Publishing Company.
21. Pellegrino E., Thomasma D. (1996). The Christian Virtues in Medical Practice. Washington, DC: Georgetown University Press.
22. Germino B., Fife B., Funk S. (1995). Cancer and the partner relationship: What is its meaning? Semin Oncol Nurs 11(1):43–50.
23. Smith E. (1995). Addressing the psychospiritual distress of death as reality: A transpersonal approach. Social Work 40(3):402–413.
24. Bowman T. (1997). Facing loss of dreams: A special kind of grief. Int J Palliat Nurs 3(2):76–80.
25. Personal interview, (1997).
26. Rando TA. (1993). Treatment of Complicated Mourning. Champaign, IL: Research Press.
27. Garbarino J. (1996). The spiritual challenge of violent trauma. Am J Orthopsychiatry 66(1):162–163.
28. Kallenberg K. (1992). Is there meaning in suffering? An external question in a new context. Proceedings: Cancer Nursing Changing Frontiers. (Vienna), pp. 21–24.
29. American Nurses Association. (1996). American Nurses Association Code for Nurses with Interpretive Statements. American Nurses Publishing, Washington, DC.
30. Kahn DL, Steeves RH. (1995). The significance of suffering in cancer care. Semin Oncol Nurs 11(1):53–72.
31. Younger JB. (1995). The alienation of the sufferer. Adv Nurs Sci 17(4):53–72.
32. Bailey S. (1997). The arts in spiritual care. Semin Oncol Nurs 13(4):242–247.
33. Brown-Saltzman K. (1994). Tending the spirit. Oncol Nurs Forum 21(6):1001–1006.
34. Brown-Saltzman K. (1997). Replenishing the spirit by meditative prayer and guided imagery. Semin Oncol Nurs 13(4):255–259.
35. Coward D. (1997). Constructing meaning from the experience. Semin Oncol Nurs 13(4): 248–251.

36. Johnston-Taylor E. (1998). Caring for the spirit. In Burke C. (ed.) Psychosocial Dimensions of Oncology Nursing Care. Pittsburgh: Oncology Nursing Press.

37. Davies B. (1993). Sibling bereavement: research-based guidelines for nurses. Semin Oncol Nurs 9(2):107–113.

38. Yalom ID. (1980). Existential Psychotherapy. New York: Basic Books.

39. Marris P. (1986). Loss and Change (2nd ed.). London: Routledge and Kegan Paul.

40. Taylor SE (1983). Adjustment to threatening events: A theory of cognitive adaptation. Am Psychology 38:1161–1173.

41. Thompson SC, Janigian AS (1988). Life schemes: A framework for understanding the search for meaning. J Soc Clin Psychol 7:260–280.

42. Steeves RH, Kahn DL (1987). Experience of meaning in suffering. Image: J Nurs Scholarship 19(3):114–116.

43. Ersek M (1991). The process of maintaining hope in adults with leukemia undergoing bone marrow transplantation. Unpublished doctoral dissertation, University of Washington, Seattle, Washington.

44. Gotay CC (1985). Why me? Attributions and adjustment by cancer patients and their mates at two stages in the disease process. Soc Sci Med 20(8):825–831.

45. Haberman MR (1987). Living with leukemia: The personal meaning attributed to illness and treatment by adults undergoing bone marrow transplantation. Unpublished doctoral dissertation, University of Washington, Seattle, Washington.

46. Chrisman H (1977). The health seeking process: An approach to the natural history of illness. Culture, Med Psychiatry 1(4):351–377.

47. Ferrell BR, Taylor EJ, Sattler GR, Fowler M, Cheyney BL (1993). Searching for the meaning of pain: Cancer patients', caregivers', and nurses' perspectives. Cancer Pract 1(3):185–194.

48. Barkwell DP (1991). Ascribing meaning: A critical factor in coping and pain attenuation in patients with cancer-related pain. J Palliat Care 7(3):5–10.

49. Lipowski Z (1970). Physical illness, the individual and their coping processes. International Journal of Psychiatr Med 1(9):101.

50. Haberman MR (1988). Psychosocial aspects of bone marrow transplantation. Semin Oncol Nurs 4(1):55–59.

32 The Role of the Nurse Chaplain: A Personal Reflection

CAROL WENZL

"I would like you to become a hospital chaplain. Your understanding of and involvement with holistic care, your experience with pain management for fifteen years, the incredible experience you have had with Mercy Hospice, your care of patients over many years . . . this is what makes you a perfect candidate for hospital chaplain."

With that statement from the director of Pastoral Services at Mercy Health Center, Oklahoma City, my career took a giant leap into unknown territory. I responded by saying, "I have no credentials, no real experience, no clear understanding of the chaplain role, and I am retired." In answer to my protestations, the director said, "You have cared for the very sick and the dying for 20 years. You understand holistic care and are accustomed to sitting with patients and families that are troubled. You are comfortable discussing grave issues, and you have a faith-filled life. You are just the person I need."

I knew that to become a chaplain I would have to go through some type of formal training such as clinical pastoral education (CPE) and/or a masters of divinity program. However, when I asked about chaplaincy training programs, the director suggested that I delay formal training and experience chaplaincy firsthand and then decide if I wanted to continue the role and pursue further training. I reluctantly agreed and began my on-site orientation as a chaplain.

My background is in education. In many ways, my entire nursing career was training grounds for my new role as chaplain. I graduated in 1976 and began my nursing career at Mercy Health Center as a "float" nurse, working on different floors. One day the nursing supervisor assigned me to an area on the third floor, and asked me to tell her what I thought of the day once my shift ended. I discovered that the area I was assigned to was the Oncology Unit, which at the time housed nineteen beds. That day two patients died—one was a nurse that everyone knew and loved. The other patient, whom I took care of, was a woman in her forties with three teenage children and a husband at her bedside.

It was a complex day that totally challenged me but I loved the experience. When I visited with my supervisor after the shift I said, "That was the most difficult nursing day I have ever experienced. Two patients died, three teenagers and a husband needed help from me when their mother and wife died. A nurse died—one that everyone knew, except me. But today, I also encountered the best nursing care I have ever experienced. The nurses cared for each other, and the patients and families cared for one another and helped each other." After that day, I was consistently assigned to the Oncology Unit and later I became part of the regular staff.

Later, I was asked to join the Oncology Outpatient Department, where nurses administered chemotherapy to outpatients and inpatients, and conducted clinical trails. We counseled patients and families regarding their diagnosis and long-term care. Later, I became head nurse of the department. It was exciting and challenging to serve these special patients and to work with an outstanding group of dedicated nurses. In the early 1980s we became aware that new techniques of pain relief were possible. We arranged a week at Memorial Sloan-Kettering Cancer Center in New York City, so that we could learn more about the newest advances in pain-management approaches. With their help we initiated the "pain team" at Mercy Health Center. In July of 1981 we trained the outpatient cancer nurses to be active members of the Mercy pain team.

My interest in palliative care took a leap forward as my work extended beyond the pain service to hospice care. After years of planning, Mercy opened the first hospital-owned home-based hospice in the Oklahoma City area, and asked me to manage it. One of my fondest memories is of Robert, a patient diagnosed with lung cancer. He was a tough, burly, in-control kind of man, who was told he had only one to two months to live. He asked me, "Is there a place or an organization that can help me die because this will be very hard for my wife." There was no hospice available at the time. He asked to be kept informed of his status so that when death was imminent he might be admitted to the hospital, in order that his wife, Mary, wouldn't have bad memories of his death at home. He was admitted for his last 36 hours of life. I received a phone call from Mary, his wife, saying, "Bob had just died—I wanted to call you so you wouldn't come bounding into his room and find him gone." I thanked her and was profoundly affected by her graciousness in caring for *my* needs in her deepest grief. This couple helped motivate me in the planning of hospice.

Initiating Mercy Hospice was a labor of love—working with so many patients and their families, a wonderful staff, huge challenges every day, Medicare evaluations, savoring the true multidisciplinary team. So many stories and so much love. After six years of hospice I decided to retire. At this point I had my conversation with the director of Pastoral Care at Mercy Health Center. Two weeks after my retirement, I began my orientation to a whole new world of care.

I deeply believe that God has a mission and a purpose for each of us. He gives us special, unique gifts, and we must continually seek his mission for us and how we can better serve others through this mission. Looking back now after $3^1/_2$ years of experience as a hospital chaplain—three of those years as a hospice chaplain—I can identify different roles and responsibilities that I believe are important.

ROLES AND RESPONSIBILITIES

My first consideration must always be the patient and family. The patient is the reason I am present. Very shortly after my orientation, I was asked if I felt comfortable working in the oncology area. Yes, of course I was, but would the nurses accept me as a chaplain rather than a nurse? I asked for the nurses' input—would it and could it work? How could I help? What would they like me to do? We discussed my change in roles and I knew I needed to prove myself to them and to myself. I would be working one on one with patients, families, and staff, to offer spiritual support as a representative of the community of faith. I would not be involved with a congregation like a minister; rather, my focus would be those in the hospital.

One of the strongest influences on my transition to the role of chaplain has been the work of the late Henri Nouwen.[1–3] Nouwen, a Catholic priest, and prolific writer, describes the basic principles of Christian leadership to include personal concern, a deep-rooted faith in the value and meaning of life, and an ongoing hope.[3]

For me, such principles open the door to seek the gifts that God has shared with us, and become involved in his mission. We must recognize our greatness and share it. I believe that God has gifted me to be a caring, concerned person who can offer my presence to those who need it. With regard to Nouwen's first principle, personal concern, I become involved in an intimate way with those I minister to. I try to share myself, to be real, and to be open to the other person. It is amazing how the sharing of oneself can open the door for conversation and sharing.

My approach with patients and their families is to introduce myself and then ask how they are feeling and what the doctor has told them. I seek to see if something is troubling the patient or family by asking, "Is there some way I can be of help?" If appropriate, and often it is, I tell them that I have worked with persons diagnosed with cancer for 23 years. I tell them that I started my work on the oncology unit, and they asked me to become a chaplain after I retired because of my great love for these special people. I share of myself and of my experiences. I try to be real. This type of sharing is often very effective.

Openness with each person—to listen, to get them to feel comfortable, to trust you—helps them to share their pain. I have witnessed great healing of the spirit even as the body deteriorates. I have come to know spiritual pain just as I knew physical pain, and I have learned to respond to the combined experience of this pain. This attention to the person and involvement as a caregiver is described by Berggren-Thomas and Griggs:[4] "It is important to realize that spiritual care is an essential part of holistic care. Nurses must meet clients on their individualized spiritual path and enhance that journey in any way possible. Whether it be through attentive listening, prayer for or with them or mere conversation, nurses allow their spirits to touch those of the clients and assist them along their path of spiritual growth. What is needed is not so much a new model of spiritual care, but a new mind-set of what it means to care for the spirit."

As a nurse chaplain, I feel increasingly comfortable in this role. I see it as my mission to help patients find their faith and values in their lives. I allow the patients to discuss these values openly, if they choose, and I encourage their hope, depending upon their faith belief. Some days it may be the patient's needs and often it is the family that needs my support. I try to just be there—to be present to them—to let them know I have time and I wish to share and be with them, if they wish. Having time to sit with patients is a luxury that I enjoy as a chaplain that was impossible in my nursing positions.

Nurse chaplain skills are integral to the skills of any palliative care nurse. They are not unique to the nurse chaplain. All of us have different gifts and talents, even within the area of palliative nursing. However, skills are rare in the sense that people don't take the time to use them. Part of who I am as a chaplain stems from my formal training as a nurse and from my experiences over 23 years of nursing. I have found that patients are not really concerned about my training for the chaplaincy role. They just want me to pull up a chair, hold their hand, and ask how they are doing. They want my presence. There are times, though, when it is important for them to know I am also a nurse. When they talk about the effects of chemotherapy, their low white counts, and other clinical concerns, they are relieved to know I've had many years of experience working with other patients who had similar issues. In some ways, being a nurse gives credibility to my role as a chaplain and vice-versa. They need to feel as if they can gain something from the conversation. While my intent and focus is spiritual, sometimes the most spiritual thing I can do for them is to answer their clinical questions. Without faith, though, all my training is rather empty. Every time I enter a patient's room, I pray. It's a faith that recognizes that I am not the one in charge. I am simply open.

I remember Mrs. Lyons, her daughter, May, and her husband, Ben. Mrs. Lyons was an inpatient with stomach cancer who was near death, weak, but talked with me quietly about her life and faith. She was ready to die, but her husband had lung cancer and was receiving chemotherapy. He was fatigued and depressed about his cancer and his wife's illness. May, a social worker, was anxious to solve issues, and by her own admission did not have a very good relationship with her mom. No one was talking with the other.

May began to attack the staff, complaining about specific nurses; stating that she needed the same nurses for her mother each shift. She complained to one nurse about another, basically displacing her anger, her fear, and her concern for her mom and dad on the oncology staff. The staff asked me to talk with the family and offer assistance to both parties. May talked for over 90 minutes with me while I just listened. She said, "you don't understand, my mom is dying and we haven't talked about it. My dad has lung cancer and I'm afraid I am going to lose both parents, and I don't know what to do." Again, I just listened and offered my presence and suggested she just be a daughter and not a social worker, and to tell her mom she loves her, and wants to be with her, no matter what happens. Three days later, I learned that Mrs. Lyons had died that same day, peacefully, with her husband, and daughter present. I received a call from May that day and she said she wanted to see me at the hospital. She said, "You really helped me. I sat with mom and just tried to be a loving daughter. Dad and I both did—and mom talked of her peace and her faith. She died with a smile on her face shortly after. Thank you. We appreciate you and all of the hospice staff."

Pain comes in many different forms. As a member of the pain team for fifteen years, I recognize that it is not likely that patients will discuss spiritual needs when they are hurting or experiencing other distressing symptoms. As Dr. Derek Doyle states, "First we must recognize that seldom if ever does a dying patient raise spiritual issues when his physical, emotional and social problems remain unsolved. Our first responsibility is to relieve pain and other suffering, to deal with every emotional problem . . . then, and only then, can we look at spiritual matters . . . spiritual and many psychosocial problems only surface when the shackles of pain, vomiting, dyspnea and terror have been relieved and released."[5] Sometimes spiritual distress is expressed as pain. This pain will not be relieved until spiritual distress is relieved.

Nurses and nurse chaplains need to provide an openness—a touch—a sense of care that allows a patient and a patient's family to seek help if they wish to have it. We all must provide this help within the patient's agenda—not our own. Nurse thanatologist Joy Ufema suggests that nurses use a "cushion of caring": "By that I mean a relationship of trust and an honest exchange of feelings. It is imperative that you understand each patient's perception of his/her situation. That means listening from your heart, your spirit, not your religion . . . let him/her know that it's okay to pray or practice his/her own comforting spiritual rituals in your unit. When a sick and dying fellow human being honors you by sharing what's deep in his/her marrow, you will know the difference between religion and spirituality."[6]

After support of the patient and the family, I believe that staff support is essential. Sometimes the staff has just lost a special long-term patient. They need just to talk and to be listened to. I must be present to them, to let them know I care. A typical patient was David—a patient diagnosed with colon cancer. He was receiving chemotherapy—fighting infection, weakness, lack of appetite and the frustration of having to come in for chemotherapy for four days in a row. He would "ride" his IV pole down the hall and joke with everyone and try to make their days brighter. David developed metastases to his lungs and his liver. Only 32 years old, David was a joyful, hopeful person, and he had a tough time dealing with the concept of his death, as did the staff. It was a difficult loss for me, too. We all shared our loss together—and we all grew as a result of the sharing. We all learned, developed, and matured, because we all shared David, his life and his death.

As previously stated, I believe that my role as chaplain has benefited from my background as a nurse with an oncology background and palliative care experience, and because I worked with patients on the inpatient unit and hospice patients at home. As a chaplain, I have the best of all the "options" because I have more time to spend with the patients, families, and staff. When it is very busy on the oncology unit, I ask the staff how I can be of help—who can I spend time with that can free up the nurses. Sometimes I can help with discharge planning, when the nurses cannot get free from their other patients. Because I know the patients, I can often answer questions the social worker has about their discharge. If appropriate, I retrieve pillows, blankets, ice, water, coffee, chairs—whatever it takes to help the nurses and make the patients and families more comfortable. Sometimes it is necessary for me to cross back over the line and do nursing functions to truly be of service. At times I also check with our ethicist for additional help.

Widerquist[7] describes the common ground of nurses and chaplains in stating, "Pastoral care workers and nurses share a holistic view of a person which sees individuals as psychosocial, biological—spiritual entities. . . . An evaluation of pastoral qualities in nursing provides an interesting approach—both pastoral care workers and nurses may use approaches which (a) provide concern and comfort, (b) assist the patient and family to find meaning in the illness, (c) provide hope, (d) facilitate expression of feelings, (e) respond to spiritual distress, and (f) promote actions aimed at seeking forgiveness. Both the nurse and the pastoral care worker are responding to the call to care and are present to the suffering patient or client."[7]

Widerquist also describes nursing as a ministry, but not of a particular faith tradition. Widerquist emphasizes that by providing intimate bodily care as the original basis of nursing, the nurse adds psychosocial and spiritual knowledge for a holistic approach.[7]

If I can be of help to the staff in whatever way, I feel I have accomplished my mission for that day. When I hear them say, "Thanks for being with Mary and her husband—she was much more peaceful, and accepting after your visit. He died last night—it was good, thanks." Or when they say, "The Doctor just told

Jerry that the treatment is not working any more—and there is no other treatment available. He is upset and withdrawn. Please see him." I am sure I am doing what I am supposed to be doing.

After working for one year as a hospital chaplain, I was asked to assist the hospice minister with the spiritual care of the patients, in their home or in a nursing home. That opened up another avenue for me to serve the needs of others—what a challenge! Because hospice is my first love, I cherished the opportunity to be with the patients and their caregivers. As mentioned previously, Nouwen's principles of Christian leadership include personal concern, faith in the meaning of life, and hope.[1]

Nouwen describes the Christian leader as an artist who can bind together many people by his courage in giving expression to an individual's most personal concern. Nouwen contends that concerns can only be heard by one who has a deep-rooted faith in the value and meaning of life and by recognizing that life is not a static given, but a "mystery which reveals itself in the ongoing encounter between man and his world."[1] He describes hope as "an act of discipleship in which we follow the hard road of Christ, who entered death with nothing but bare hope."[1]

The chaplain is often called a 'wounded minister,' as described by Nouwen in his book *The Wounded Healer.*[1] He states that the Christian way of life does not take away our loneliness; it protects and cherishes it as a precious gift. Nouwen says that the awareness of loneliness is a gift we must protect and guard because our loneliness reveals to us an inner emptiness that can be destructive when misunderstood, but filled with promise for those who can tolerate it. When the chaplain lives with false expectations he prevents himself from claiming his own loneliness as a source of human understanding and is unable to offer real service to those who do not understand their own suffering."[1]

Nouwen considers two factors important in a helping relationship—hospitality and concentration, and hospitality and community. He cautions, "Anyone who wants to pay attention without intention, has to be at home in his own house—that is, he has to discover the center of his life in his own heart." Concentration, which leads to meditation and contemplation, is the necessary precondition for true hospitality. He believes that when our souls are restless and we are driven by thousands of different stimuli, we cannot possibly create the space where someone else can enter without feeling himself an unlawful intruder.[1]

With regard to hospitality and community, Nouwen states, "No minister can save anyone. He can only offer himself as a guide to fearful people, yet paradoxically, it is precisely in this guidance that the first signs of hope become visible. This is so because a shared pain is no longer paralyzing but mobilizing."[1] I believe that we must recognize our brokenness and our forgiveness—and to share that great gift with those we encounter. I recognize that we are to offer our presence, our openness, our care and our time, to let the patient and family set the agenda. I try to let them see that they can leave their "spirit," their "gifts" to those they leave behind when they die. Their "fruits" will live on in those that they have loved and cared for. This may be a great source of strength for them in their dying.

It is God's love that gives us the power to help others. An example of the wounded helping others is the Alcoholics Anonymous (AA) organization, as Girzone[8] describes. "Members of the twelve step program develop an attachment to God that is touching in its humility and wonderfully childlike in its simplicity. It is big and grand enough to embrace people of all religions and races and every variety of pain and sin. It has the all embracing goodness of God."

I have found that our best approach to helping patients is to ignore the religious concerns and seek to help spiritually. Sometimes it is not the patient, but the caregiver who needs help. Many times, we help the patient by assisting the caregiver. Sometimes we need to facilitate their conversation. I remember a patient, Martha, in her last few weeks of life. She confided in me that she needed to talk to her daughter, but the daughter didn't want to discuss her death. She was concerned with putting her house in her daughter's name. I asked if I could talk with the daughter, and perhaps help them both. Martha agreed. I visited with Mary, the daughter, and told her the situation. She said that she didn't want to talk with her mom about her death, because she felt uncomfortable with the subject. Gradually, after I spoke with both of them at length, I brought them together and said they needed to talk about Martha's death, the house, and all the other important things they needed to share. As they began to talk, I left the room. They had a wonderful conversation, and later a lawyer came and all the financial issues were settled. This effort to facilitate discussion about the house created an openness for both of them to talk and share their love for one another. This process of facilitating conversations, of being present and sharing my presence, of honestly caring, is something I have gradually learned and grasped as I have matured as a person, as a nurse, and as a spiritual being.

Nouwen's *Out of Solitude* describes the term *care* in its roots in the Gothic *Kara,* which means "lament." The basic meaning of *care* is to grieve, to experience sorrow, to cry out with. One of my favorite excerpts from Nouwen's work is the following: "When we honestly ask ourselves which persons in our lives mean the most to us, we often find that it is those who, instead of giving much advice, solutions, or cures, have chosen rather to share our pain and touch our wounds with a gentle and tender hand. A friend who can be silent with us in a moment of despair, or confusion, who can stay with us in an hour of grief and bereavement, who can tolerate not-knowing, not-curing, not-healing and face with us the reality of our powerlessness, that is the friend who cares."[2] This is a reminder of the importance of listening and being with patients.

This presence, this caring, this friendship, this staying . . . this is what my ministry is all about. We must help the patient's and family members' suffering by sharing it, and being human—only then will their spiritual needs be met. Many authors have affirmed the importance of presence as a component of ministry by any professional.[9–13] These sources remind me of the need to enter the suffering with the patient. I find that this requires totally giving of oneself, for the time involved, and it takes time. Humility helps and prayer is essential.

Phyllis was a 70-year-old, elegant, graceful, gracious lady with metastatic lung cancer. I repeatedly called to arrange to visit her, and after a few tries, she agreed to let me come for a few moments. I discovered she had a tracheostomy that she kept covered with a loose scarf. It was obvious to me that this distressed her a great deal. She immediately apologized for the "smell" of her "hole," and for the mucus that she needed to constantly remove. I asked if I could sit with her for a while. I told her I had been a cancer nurse and had cared for many people with tracheostomies and I felt very comfortable with her. I told her I had retired and that I had become a chaplain. I also confided that while I was quite new in the role and uncertain, I had time!

Gradually Phyllis began to open up more and more. She told me of a very happy marriage to Allen, three daughters that shared a mutual love, an active social life, and "having everything." That was changed when her husband of 25 years divorced her. She lost her home and her lifestyle and she needed to begin work to make a life for herself and her daughters. She talked for hours.

Often I would suggest getting a "minister" to be with her and to talk about her funeral plans. She said, "I am a Christian, but I have no 'home church' and did not want to get involved in one now. I continued to offer Phyllis my presence, my humanness, my mistakes, my own relationship with God, my care. In time, I met Phyllis's three daughters, as well as other family and friends. Toward the end, Phyllis was confined to bed rest, so I would just sit by the bed, hold her hand, and tell her of God's great love for her and of his total forgiveness, if she chose to accept it. She wrote to me, "I am at peace with God, I am ready to go to Him. I want you to speak at my funeral." With those words, I felt that my ministry had been what Phyllis needed. Just before she died, her former husband came, made peace with her, and received her last hug. She died peacefully.

At the funeral, I read I Corinthians 13 about love and caring. I spoke about Phyllis's love of butterflies—she had them all over her house and yard. I suggested that her life had been like a butterfly—that has moved from the larva that lives in a cocoon (life on earth), entrapped with our humanness, our limits, but also with our gifts, that we are to share with others—From that level, to a butterfly, that emerges and is free (life in heaven). Phyllis is free from this life and has flown to God.

DIFFERENT AREAS OF INVOLVEMENT

As a hospital chaplain, when I work on weekends or evenings, I am responsible for the whole hospital. On my very first night as a new chaplain, after I had seen all my assigned patients, I went home. Two hours later my pager went off and I was advised of a full code being admitted to the emergency room. A 72-year-old man was being admitted, with dyspnea. I checked in with the ER nurses to see how the patient was doing, to let them know I was there and to ask them what they wanted me to do. They asked me to stay with the wife and they would be checking in.

I found her, introduced myself, and asked her to tell me what had happened. She said, "He has lung cancer . . . has had one course of chemotherapy . . . was at home and suddenly could not catch his breath. I called the ambulance and here we are." I prayed a quick prayer for guidance, as I always do, and then told her that I had been a cancer nurse at the hospital and I had dealt with many lung cancer patients. She began to relax and talk to me. She told me her husband's entire story of having cancer. I just listened and held her hand and we prayed together.

Every 20 minutes or so I would go back to the ER to check on him. This made her feel better and let her know how much all of us cared. I stressed that the doctors and the nurses were working aggressively to help him. About two hours later, a doctor came out and very gently told her they had not been able to save him, and he was very sorry. I sat with her—took her back to see him when the nurses said it was okay—then I made phone calls for her. I stayed with her and offered my presence. She told me that I had helped her, just by being able to answer some of her questions and knowing that I had been a nurse. I was grateful to be a nurse chaplain. I believe my experience with this special lady was the beginning of my understanding of how valuable my nursing role is to my evolving chaplain role.

Sometimes I work in the preoperative area, early in the morning, before I go to the oncology unit. I talk to patients and their families prior to their surgeries. Many times I encounter cancer patients in whom have been found metastases, and they discuss their plans to stop treatment. I try to help them with this important transition and with palliative care decisions.

I have found that to be of service to others, I must face suffering. An excellent resource is the work of a nurse who states, "I have ached, cried and lamented when I have suffered for others, but only my own experiences of suffering have I experienced first hand . . . this journey into spirituality manifests itself in the offering of true compassion and love between and among family members and nurse. Likewise, these efforts to alleviate suffering cross the border into healing; a healing that is not reserved only for family members but also for nurses."[14]

I care for patients and their families as newly diagnosed cancer patients, patients with recurrent cancer that are palliative, crisis patients, terminal patients, hospice patients, and some bereavement families. Regardless of which patient or family I am dealing with, the same approach must be taken. I listen, am present, show I care, and am concerned; I use only their agenda, seeking their minister or rabbi if they wish, and I always tell them of God's love for them. These actions, I believe, offer relief from suffering.

I try to be a "spiritual companion" for them, offering the "four Rs for the Spirit":

1. Remembering—to take time to reflect on your life and its events
2. Reassessing—take time to see your life as a whole
3. Reconciling—try to be at peace with yourself
4. Reuniting—try to be at peace with those you love[15]

ADVANTAGES OF THE NURSE CHAPLAIN

While moving into the chaplain role has been challenging, I also have found many strengths in this role of nurse chaplain. I am open to all faiths. I am not a minister in a certain faith. I try to meet their needs or to find someone who they can identify with. I help the patient and family to identify any rituals that they would like to take part in, and try to make that possible for them.

I understand, at least in part, their physical condition, because I am a nurse, and many times that opens the door, gradually, to more in-depth spiritual conversation, if they wish. The nurses tend to trust my involvement because I have worked with most of them in the past. They can give me a little information, and I can begin to work with the patient, and they don't have to worry that I will do or say something inappropriate. The doctors know me and have worked with me for years. Many times we talk together about a patient and family, to try to help them through a set of circumstances, or I am there when their patient dies, to help their families.

Working as a nurse chaplain requires great care. I must not use my R.N. title to get too involved with the physical care of the patient. If, for example, I encounter a patient that is in pain, I tell the patient's nurse immediately. I do not get involved in actual pain management, and the nurses appreciate this.

As I mature and grow and reflect on God's words I come to a peace about my role with each person I encounter. I try to be God's instrument. I remember a new hospice patient, Mike, and his wife, Helen, who called and were anxious to see the hospice chaplain. Mike had been diagnosed with gastric cancer. Both of them had been married before, but they had celebrated 41 years of marriage and they were very close. Gradually, over a four-month period, visiting each week, our relationship grew. Mike was a very quiet man who let Helen do most of the talking. I remember him sitting on a twin bed in the family room, very alert, "weaving" his oxygen tubing into complex knots! I asked if he was used to working with his hands. He told me of his work on car engines—that he was really good at what he did. Then his lung problems started and he had to retire, so he started working on lawnmowers, and other small engines, out of the house, always helping other people. As Mike was placed on oxygen, he had to give up the small engine work, and remain in the house, so he began to make and repair clocks! When I first visited him he had over 200 clocks throughout their small home.

After I had been visiting them for three months, Helen said to me, "Mike wants to be baptized, and so do I." I sat with Mike and asked him about this. He said, "As a child, my family always went to church, many different ones, but we always went. And as a young adult, we went as well. Finally, I decided church was not where I felt comfortable, because everyone seemed to be using the church to gain new jobs, or gain politically, etc., so I left, and I worship God within me. I am Christian, but not a church-going Christian, and I have never been baptized."

The same was true with Helen. I asked her if I could get a 'real' minister to baptize them, but they refused. I decided to set up a simple ceremony, read from the Gospel of John, chapter 15, which describes the vine and the branches, and how we must cling to God and let him bear his fruit through us, and then I baptized both of them.

Our visits continued and their faith appeared to grow. I brought them a Bible with the newer translation, which they enjoyed. They both seemed to be at peace with God. Mike died at home, and Helen asked me to do a memorial service at the cemetery. Mike had a son, who had died. He had recorded some songs, so we began the service with his song. I then thanked God for all the blessings he had shared with all of us, for the blessing of Mike, and all that he had shared with others, asking God to be with Helen and their family. Then I read a short obituary telling of his birth, his marriage, his children, grandchildren, his war experience, his coming to Oklahoma, his work on car engines, then small engines, and finally his work on clocks, when most of his energy had diminished. I went on to say that he had always kept busy, had always served and had always given to others. He had always encouraged others in his own quiet way. Mike hoped to be an organ donor, but this was not possible due to medical problems. Mike was a donor to each of us, donating his love, his caring, his sharing, his service. He was a donor for God.

Mike's granddaughter had written him a letter and had given it to him two months before he died. In the letter she told him how much she loved him, how good he had always been to her and so many others. I read this at the close of the service. All of the family seemed very pleased with the service, and Helen said, "It was just what Mike would have wanted." I felt that I had ministered effectively to Mike and Helen and their entire family.

I experienced a true miracle. I went to see Val, who lives on the outskirts of southwest Oklahoma City, about 25 miles from the Mercy Hospice office. As I drove closer to their home, I saw damage from the tornado that struck the area on May 3, 1999. There were trees down, homes destroyed, cardboard signs nailed up identifying the name of the place where each house used to be, so that people could tell where they were in the midst of all the destruction.

As I entered their house, Lou, Val's wife, greeted me, along with their granddaughter. She appeared to be very stressed. She showed me their backyard. "We lost between 75 and 100 large trees—gone," she said, and she was crying. All around the outside of their house, you could see destruction, but inside their house, with many glass plates hanging up, glass figurines adorning shelves, and so on, not one item was out of place or broken. I said, "Lou, this was a miracle". "Yes," she said, "when the storm got closer, one of our son-in-laws came over to take us away. But Val said he would not go, so I climbed into bed with him, and covered both us up with quilts, and prayed and we rode out the storm together."

We talked a lot about God's grace and goodness and miracles. I listened to her and learned about love, grace, caring, giving, and trusting. These are some of the reasons I most love my job as a nurse chaplain.

SPIRITUALITY AND SUFFERING

One of the things I try to do is to encourage the oncology staff, the hospice staff, the other wonderful chaplains I work with, and everyone I encounter to develop their spirituality—individually—for themselves. I try to help them look at opportunities to get away, to reflect, to ponder life, to seek their direction and their own mission. Each person is given gifts from God, and He wants us to use our gifts to help others. We must ponder, be quiet, pray, read God's word, and seek his will for us.

I annually attend a four-day retreat, and some of the staff members from the hospital join me. I try to encourage others to do something like this. I daily ask for God's help in all that I do, especially in my role as a nurse chaplain. I ask to be God's instrument, as St. Francis did:

Lord, make me an instrument of thy peace,
where there is hatred,
let me sow love;
where there is injury, pardon;
where there is doubt, faith;
where there is despair, hope;
where there is darkness, light;
and where there is sadness, joy.
O Divine Master,
Grant that I may not so much seek to be consoled,
As to console;
To be understood,
As to understand;
To be loved,
As to love.
For it is in giving, that we receive,
It is in pardoning, that we are pardoned,
And it is in dying, that we are born to eternal life.[16]

I try to share, through my actions, how to give of my presence to another. Even in a short time, I try to let them know that I care, and that I am here for them. I encourage patients and their families to tell their "story"—to each other, to their nurses, nursing assistants, anyone who will listen and that they want to tell the story to. This allows the patient to reflect on his or her life and to share their spirit with those who will live after them. I often talk to the staff about spiritual pain and suffering as well as spirituality. What is spiritual pain? "The state in which the individual experiences a disturbance in the belief or value system that provides strength, hope and meaning to his life."[12] We address spiritual pain and suffering best when we have tended to our own spirit.[9,17–21]

Suffering

We must nurture our own spirit before we can help our patients and their families with their spiritual needs. Many nurses say that the key to their entering the spiritual dimension of nursing practice has been taking their own spiritual journey—to learn to better know themselves and the spirit that is the essence of self. We need to ask ourselves:

- What do I believe?
- What do I value?
- What is the meaning and purpose of my life?
- For what do I hope?
- Who loves me?
- Whom do I love?
- How is my love returned?

We must learn and we must love. When we love, we receive all that is good and we are spiritually nourished. Cardinal Bernadin writes, "I have also grown spiritually by extensive reading."[21]

Henri Nouwen and his many books have influenced me greatly. Another person whom I have learned much from is Mother Teresa of Calcutta. She writes, "There are different kinds of poverty. In India some people live and die in hunger. But in the West, you have another kind of poverty . . . spiritual poverty. This is far worse. People do not believe in God, do not pray. People do not care for each other. You have the poverty of people who are dissatisfied with what they have, who do not know how to suffer, who give in to despair. This poverty of heart is often more difficult to relieve and to defeat."[22]

I have also learned about spiritual care through other nurses. One palliative care nurse leader, Katherine Brown-Saltzman,[9] describes her own spiritual growth as well as the importance of setting limits. She shares, "Many years ago, I had a heavy heart from all of the care taking. At that time I heard a familiar story from the Bible about the loaves and the fishes. I came to understand that I needed only to do what I could during the course of a day, no more. In doing that, by taking what was done in a day and asking God to bless it, to multiply and extend it, I came to know that it was enough. I have learned with this blessing that I am enough."

This explains why it is so important to care for the dying. To care for the dying is to help the dying, make that hard move from action to passion, from success to fruitfulness, from wondering how much they can still accomplish, to making their very lives a gift for others. Caring for the dying means helping the dying discover that, in their increasing weakness, God's strength becomes visible. But as a community of care, we can remind each other that we will be fruits far beyond the few years we have to live. As a community of care, we trust that those who live long after we have lived will still receive the fruits of the seeds we have sown in our weakness and find new strength from them. As a community of care, we can send the Spirit . . . to each other. Thus, we become the fruit bearing people of God who embrace past, present and future and thus are a light in the darkness.[1]

"Pastoral persons need to be spiritual persons who are comfortable with God and comfortable talking about Him, and sincerely striving to live by His principles. However, it is necessary for us to be comfortable with ourselves, to feel good about who we are. There is an old adage, 'you can't give what you don't have'. In the area of spirituality, this means that we pastoral persons can't assist others in relating to God unless we ourselves have a relationship with Him. It means that only a person who has experienced the Lord's love can speak convincingly about that love."[13]

SUGGESTIONS FOR SPIRITUAL CARE

My own learning as a nurse chaplain has been vast but continues to grow. The greatest lessons I have learned can be summarized as follows:

1. competence
2. care and concern
3. offering of presence (giving of self)
4. be open to *their* faith discussion (i.e. assess cultural needs)
5. encourage hope (remember . . . God is in charge!)
6. listen actively
7. allow trust and honesty
8. prayer if requested by family or patient, and if appropriate
9. personal touch
10. openness
11. seek forgiveness (closure of past issues)
12. LOVE

I am privileged to be an oncology nurse and now a chaplain. My own mission statement is that I am human; I have gifts and I have failings. But what I can do, I must do, and it is enough and it is good.

I would like to pay special tribute to May Cordry, the Head Librarian at the Mercy Health Center Library, who spent many hours doing a literature search for this chapter. I would also like to thank Sr. Francella, Director, Pastoral Care, all Chaplains, and the patients, their families, and all the staff who contributed to this chapter, as well as my daughter, Sandi McDermott, RN, who assisted me with the production of this manuscript.

REFERENCES

1. Nouwen H.J.M. (1972). The Wounded Healer, pp. 52–65. Doubleday & Co., Garden City, NY.
2. Nouwen H.J.M. (1974). Out of Solitude, p. 34. Ave Maria Press, Notre Dame, IN.
3. Nouwen H.J.M. (1996). Our Greatest Gift, p. 99. HarperCollins, San Francisco.
4. Berggren-Thomas P., and Griggs M. (1995). Spirituality in aging: Spiritual need or spiritual journey? J Gerontol Nurs March: 9.
5. Doyle D. (1992). Have we looked beyond the physical and psychosocial? J Pain Sympt Manage 7(5):304.
6. Ufema J. (1997). Insights on death and dying. Nursing 97 March: 66.
7. Widerquist J., and Davidhizar R. (1994). The ministry of nursing. J Adv Nurs 19:647–652.
8. Girzone J. (1994). In Never Alone, p. 71. Doubleday Dell Publishing Group, New York, NY.
9. Brown-Saltzman K. (1994). Tending the spirit. Oncol Nurs Forum 21(6):1004.
10. Burns S. (1998). Spiritual care at the end of life. Health Progr May/June: 49.
11. Donley R. (1994). Spiritual dimensions of health care, nursing's mission. Nurs Health Care April: 179.
12. Murray C. (1995). Addressing your patient's spiritual needs. Am J Nurs November: 160.
13. Nicklas G.R. (1981). The Making of a Pastoral Person. Alba House, New York, p. 158.
14. Wright L. (1997). Suffering and spirituality: The soul of clinical work with families. J Family Nurs 3(1):3–14.
15. Lynn J., and Harrold J. (1999). Handbook for Mortals: Guidance for People Facing Serious Illness. Oxford University Press, New York, pp. 28–30.
16. Prayer of St. Francis of Assisi, The Catholic Prayer Book, Ed. T. Castle. Servant Publications, Ann Arbor, Michigan, 1986, p. 150.
17. Carson V. (1997). Spiritual care: The needs of the caregiver. Semin Oncol Nurs 13(4): 271–274.
18. Laukhuf G., and Werner, H. (1998). Spirituality: The missing link. J Neurosci Nurs 30(1): 60–67.
19. Ferrell B.R. (1996). Suffering. Oncology Nursing Society, Jones and Bartlett Publishers, Sudbury, MA.
20. Zerwekh J. (1997). The practice of presencing. Semin Oncol 13(4):260–262.
21. Bernadin J. (1997). In The Gift of Peace, pp. 126–128. Loyola Press, Chicago.
22. Teresa M. (1998). In Everything Starts with Prayer, p. 8. White Cloud Press, Ashland, OR.

Part V

Special Patient Populations

33 Elderly Patients

SUSAN DERBY and SEAN O'MAHONY

Being elderly and sick is very frightening . . . your children have moved far away and many of your friends have died. Making decisions without support is frightening and lonely.

—An elderly woman, dying of cancer

Aging is a normal process of life. Aging is not a disease and infirmity and frailty do not always have to accompany being old. It is expected that most of us will live well into our seventies or eighties, and the aging of the population is projected to continue well into the next century. Projected growth for the elderly population is staggering. During the next 20 years the fastest-growing segment of the population will be in the group aged 85 years and older. Over the past decades this increase in life expectancy has been mainly due to improvements in sanitation and infectious disease control through vaccinations and antibiotics. Now the older population is growing older because of trends in treatment of chronic diseases—cardiovascular and neurologic disease, as well as cancer. This "swelling" of the older segments of the population reinforces the need for nurses, physicians, and all health care professionals to understand the special palliative care needs of the elderly.

COMORBIDITY AND DISABILITY

The elderly have many comorbid medical conditions contributing an added symptom burden to this palliative care population. The presence of existing comorbidities and disabilities renders them more susceptible to the complications of new illnesses and their treatments. The presence of chronic medical conditions is associated with disability, and increased health care utilization including institutionalization and hospitalization in the elderly (Table 33–1). Forty percent of community-dwelling adults older than 65 report impairment in their daily activities secondary to chronic medical conditions.[1] Sixteen percent of adults older than 65 report impairment in walking; increasing to over 32% in those older than 85. Comorbidity is highly prevalent in people over 65 years. In the United States, 49% of noninstitutionalized people over 60 have two or more chronic conditions. Much higher percentages of adults older than 65 are residing within a nursing home or are hospitalized.[1–11]

SITES OF RESIDENCE AND PLACE OF DEATH

Sixty-six percent of older noninstitutionalized persons live in a family setting; this decreases with increasing age. Three out of every five women older than 85 live outside of a family arrangement. Rates of institionalization are estimated to be 4% to 5% in the United States; this increases to 23% in the over-85 population. The wide range of care settings for the elderly is reflected in the sites of death of the elderly.[8,12–15]

Over the past hundred years, the site of death has shifted from the home to institutions. Data from the National Institute on Aging–funded "Survey of the Last Days of Life" (SLDOL) indicate that 45% of the elderly who died spent the night prior to death in a hospital and 24% in a nursing home. Forty-five percent died in hospital, 25% died in a nursing home and 30% died at home. There was a significant drop in the proportion of patients in the older age group for both men and women who died in hospital and increase in proportions dying at home or nursing homes. Almost one-third of older women died in nursing homes. Interestingly, the National Mortality Follow Back Survey reported that only 8.7% of decedents were receiving home hospice and less than 0.5% were receiving inpatient hospice care.[8–9]

In several studies, cancer and dementia are predictive of death at home rather than in institutions. Death in hospice appears to correlate with the local availability of hospice beds as well as cancer as a diagnosis. The availability of home visits by physicians correlates with a higher rate of death at home in patients with a preference for death at home. In patients expressing an initial wish to die at home, caregiver burnout and unrelieved symptoms are predictive of death in hospitals and hospice.[12–15] The available data suggest that with limited increase in the allocation of nursing support, dying patients' wishes to die at home can be met. Elderly women are more than twice as likely to be living alone than are elderly men. Over half of women 75 and older live alone.[12–15] Those living alone rely more heavily on the presence of social supports and assistance for the provision of health care.[12–15]

PALLIATIVE CARE IN NURSING HOMES

End-of-life care in long-term-care settings is described in greater detail in Chapter 38. It is estimated that for per-

Table 33–1. Age-Specific Prevalence of Chronic Medical Conditions in Noninstitutionalized U.S. Adults (per 1000)

	18–44 Years	45–64 Years	65–74 Years	Older Than 75
Arthritis	52.1	268.5	459.3	494.7
Hypertension	64.1	258.9	426.8	394.6
Heart disease	40.1	129.0	276.8	349.1
Hearing impairment	49.8	159.0	261.9	346.9
Deformity/orthopedic impairment	125.3	160.6	167.9	175.5
Chronic sinusitis	164.4	184.8	151.2	160.0
Visual impairment	32.8	43.7	76.4	128.8
Diabetes	9.1	51.9	108.9	95.5
Cerebrovascular disease	1.9	17.9	54.0	72.6
Emphysema	1.6	15.2	50.0	38.9

Source: Seeman T, Guralnik J, Kaplan G, Knudsen L, Cohen R. (1989). The health consequences of multiple morbidity in the elderly. The Alameda County Study. *J Aging Health.* 1: 50–66. (27)

sons who turned 65 years old in 1990, 43% will enter a nursing home before they die.[16] Because the fastest-growing segment of the population is those over 85 years, it is likely that these individuals will require long-term care in these settings. Pain management and end-of-life care in nursing homes represent management of the frailest individuals, often with minimal physician involvement. As many as 45%–80% of nursing home residents have pain that contributes significantly to impaired quality of life.[17] Most mild pain in nursing homes is related to degenerative arthritis, low back disorders, diabetic and postherpetic neuropathy. Cancer pain accounts for the majority of severe pain.[18]

Barriers to palliative care in the nursing home include institutional, patient, and staff-related barriers (Table 33–2). One of the most difficult concerns expressed by staff who care for nursing home residents is the difficulty in assessing pain in the cognitively impaired elderly resident.

Table 33–2. Barriers to Palliative Care in Nursing Homes

Institution-Related

Low priority given to palliative care management by administration
Limited physician involvement in care, weekly or monthly assessments
Limited pharmacy involvement, no onsite pharmacy
Limited R.N. involvement in care; inadequate nurse–patient staff ratios
Primary care being administered by nonprofessional nursing staff
Limited radiological and diagnostic services, which impair determination of a pain diagnosis

Patient-Related

Physiologic changes of aging which impact on distribution, metabolism, and elimination of medications
Multiple chronic diseases
Polypharmacy
Impaired cognitive status and dementia of the Alzheimer's type
Underreporting of pain due to fear of addiction, lack of knowledge, fear of being transferred
Sensory losses which impede assessment
Increased incidence of depression that may mask reporting and assessment of pain

Staff-Related

Lack of knowledge of symptom management at the end of life
Lack of knowledge in the assessment and management of chronic cancer pain
Lack of knowledge in use of opioid drugs, titration, and side effect management
Fear of using opioids in elderly residents
Misconceptions about use of opioids in elderly patients (e.g., fear of addiction, "elderly feel less pain")
Lack of knowledge in using nonpharmacological techniques
Lack of experience with other routes of administration including patient-controlled analgesia, transdermal, rectal, subcutaneous and intravenous routes

Source: Adapted from: Stein W., Barriers to Effective Pain Management in the Nursing Home. In: Pain in the Nursing Home. Clinics in Geriatric Medicine Pain Management. (Eds) Ferrell B. WB Saunders, Philadelphia, 1996; 12(3);604.

ECONOMIC CONSIDERATIONS IN CARING FOR THE ELDERLY

The higher rates of disability and comorbidity in the elderly result in considerable costs to the health care system with the associated requirement for the provision of long-term residential care as well as home care.

Health Care Financing Administration data indicate that 6%–8% of Medicare enrollees die annually and account for 27%–30% of annual Medicare expenses.[19] However, spending on aggressive interventions is not a major component of the hospital costs incurred in hospital costs in the dying in elderly. Only 3% of Medicare beneficiaries who die sustain high costs associated with aggressive interventions such as surgery, chemotherapy, or dialysis.

While hospital costs in the last days of life are lower for the oldest old, the percentage of Medicare and Medicaid expenditure for nursing home care rises from 24% for the young old (65 to 74 years) to 62% for the oldest old (over 85 years).[24–26] Much of this requirement for residential care occurs in the last days of life. The average cost of nursing home care for the elderly in the last three months of life is reported to be $1700.[24]

DETERMINATION OF PROGNOSIS AND THE PROVISION OF PALLIATIVE CARE

The provision of palliative care to elderly patients is limited by the uncertain prognoses of many chronic illnesses in this population (congestive heart failure, chronic obstructive pulmonary disease, cerebrovascular disease, dementia). Because of difficulty in accurate prognostication and many other factors, most patients who have fatal illnesses do not use the Medicare hospice benefit until shortly before death.[26] Even the most complex prognostic scoring systems, such as the APACHE (Acute Physiology Age Chronic Health Evaluation), provide little information for the likelihood of individual patients dying.

The uncertain prognoses of chronic nonmalignant medical conditions can affect clinical decision making. It may also lead to overutilization of health care resources in acute care settings even when death is imminent. An analysis of Medicare claim data for 6451 elderly hospice patients demonstrated that median survival after enrollment was only 36 days with 15.6% dying within 7 days.[20–23]

FAMILY/CAREGIVER ISSUES

Who Are the Caregivers for the Elderly?

The term *caregiver* refers to anyone who provides assistance to someone else who needs it. *Informal caregiver* is a term used to refer to unpaid individuals such as family members and friends who provide care. These persons can be primary or secondary caregivers, full or part time, and can live with the person being cared for, or live separately. Formal caregivers are volunteers or paid care providers associated with a service system. Estimates vary on the numbers of caregivers in the United States.

According to the most recent National Long Term Care Study (NLTCS), over 7 million people are informal caregivers, defined here as spouses, adult children, other relatives, and friends who provide unpaid help to older people with at least one limitation in their activities of daily living. An estimated 15% of American adults are providing care for seriously ill or disabled adults.[27] Of these, an estimated 12.8 million Americans need assistance to carry out activities such as eating, dressing, and bathing. About 57% are aged 65 or older (7.3 million). Spouses accounted for about 62% of primary caregivers. Approximately 72% of caregivers are female.[28] The majority of caregivers provide unpaid assistance for one to four years; 20% provide care for five years or longer.[28]

According to the 1996 National Hospice Care Survey (NHCS), 55% of patients enrolled in hospice programs were women, and 45% were men. The majority (78%) were 65 years or older, and a significantly larger portion of women than men were 85 years of age or older. At the time of the survey, 78% were living in a private or semiprivate residence, and 11% were residents of an inpatient facility. Men were more likely to have a spouse as their primary caregiver while women were more likely to be cared for by a child or child-in-law. The most common diagnosis for most of the hospice care patients included neoplasm, heart disease, and chronic obstructive pulmonary disease.

Involving Family in Caregiving for the Elderly: What Is the Burden?

The burden of caregiving has been well documented in the literature and includes a greater number of depressive symptoms, anxiety, diminished physical health, financial problems, and disruption in work. The amount of concrete needs the patient has strongly relates to family and caregiver psychological distress and burden of care.[29] Elderly patients who are dying require varying levels of assistance with personal care, meal preparation, shopping, transportation, paying bills, and submitting forms related to health care. The level of physical care may be tremendous and include bathing, turning and positioning, wound care, colostomy care, suctioning, medication administration, and managing incontinence. If the patient is confused or agitated, the strain is even greater as 24-hour care may be necessary. In the palliative care setting, where the treatment goals are supportive and often include management of symptoms including pain, respiratory distress, and delirium, the patient is often confined to home, with a greater burden being placed on the live-in spouse or child.

In one study comparing the impact of caregiving in curative and palliative care settings, two study groups were evaluated—267 patients receiving active, curative treatment, and 134 patients receiving palliative care through a local hospice. Patients in the palliative care group were more physically debilitated, and had poorer performance status. The mean age for the curative group was 59.7 and for the palliative care group the mean was 57.9. Caregiver quality-of-life measures demonstrated that family caregivers of patients receiving palliative care had lower quality-of-life scores and worse overall physical health than family caregivers of patients receiving curative care.[30] Families with low socioeconomic status and those with less education were more distressed by the patient's illness.

In another study of 231 caregivers of patients with cancer pain who were at home, the goals were to evaluate family caregivers' quality of life, financial burden, and experience of managing cancer pain in the home.[31] Family caregivers scored worse in areas of difficulty coping, anxiety, depression, happiness, and feeling in control. In areas of physical well-being, the greatest problems were sleep changes and fatigue. Other quality-of-life disruptions included interference with employment, support from others, isolation, and financial burden. The estimated average time spent caregiving was over 12 hours per day, the estimated time for pain management was more than 3 hours per day. Family caregivers reported worse outcomes than patients in their perception of the pain intensity, pain distress to themselves, feeling able to control the pain, and family concern about pain in the future. Caregivers reported fear of future pain, fear of tolerance, and concern about addiction and harmful effects of analgesics. The authors concluded that educational programs in pain management are needed and that further educational efforts should also address the emotional aspects of managing cancer pain in the home.

Interventions directed toward improvement in the quality of life of direct caregivers include educational programs, improvement in homecare supports, psychoeducational programs and improved access to healthcare professionals providing symptom management and end-of-life care.

Family grief therapy during the palliative phase of illness has also been shown to improve the psychosocial quality of life of caregivers. Kissane and colleagues[32] utilized a screening tool to identify dysfunctional family members and relieve distress through a model of family grief therapy sessions. Smeenk and colleagues[33] demonstrated improved quality of life of direct caregivers after implementation of a transmural home care intervention program for terminal cancer patients. Macdonald[34] demonstrated that massage as a respite intervention for caregivers was successful in reducing physical and emotional stress, physical pain, and sleep difficulties. This nonpharmacologic and noninvasive intervention is highly valued and accepted by caregivers due to its simplicity and beneficial effects.

PHARMACOLOGIC CONSIDERATIONS

Pharmacological intervention is the mainstay of treatment for management of symptoms in palliative care of the elderly patient. Knowledge of the parameters of geriatric pharmacology can prevent serious morbidity and mortality when multiple drugs are used to treat single or multiple symptoms, or when, in the practice of chronic pain management, trials of sequential opioids (opioid rotation, or opioid switch) are used.

Pharmacokinetics

The four components of pharmacokinetics are absorption, distribution, metabolism and excretion. In the absence of malabsorption problems and obstruction, oral medications are well tolerated in the elderly population. With aging there is some decrease in gastric secretion, absorptive surface area, and splanchnic blood flow. Most studies show no difference in oral bioavailability—the extent to which a drug reaches its site of action. There is little literature on the absorption of long-acting drugs in the elderly, including controlled or sustained-release opioids, and transdermal opioids commonly used in the treatment of chronic cancer pain in the elderly patient. Controlled-release dosage forms are generally more appropriate with drugs that have short half-lives (less than four hours) and include many of the shorter-acting opioids including morphine and hydromorphone. Generally, it is safer to use opioids that have shorter half-lives in the elderly cancer patient.

Distribution refers to the distribution of drug to the interstitial and cellular fluids after it is absorbed or injected into the bloodstream. There are several significant physiologic factors that may influence drug distribution in the elderly palliative care patient. An initial phase of distribution reflects cardiac output and regional blood flow. The heart, kidneys, liver, and brain receive most of the drug after absorption. Delivery to fat, muscle, most viscera, and skin is slower; it may take several hours before steady-state concentrations are reached. Although cardiac output does not change with age, chronic conditions including congestive heart failure may contribute to a decrease in cardiac output and regional blood flow.

This second phase of drug distribution to the tissues is highly dependent upon body mass. Body weight generally decreases with age, but more importantly, body composition changes with age. Total body water and lean body mass decrease, while body fat increases in proportion to total body weight. The volume of distribution changes are mostly for highly lipophilic and hydrophilic drugs, and the elderly are most susceptible to drug toxicity from drugs that should be dosed on ideal body weight or lean body weight. Theoretically, highly lipid-bound drugs, for example, long-acting benzodiazepines and transdermal fentanyl, both commonly prescribed to elderly patients, may have an increased volume of distribution and a prolonged effect if drug clearance is constant.[35] Water-soluble drugs (e.g., digoxin) may have a decreased volume of distribution and increased serum levels and toxicity if initial doses are not conservative. To avoid possible side effects in a frail elderly patient, it may be safe to start with one-half the dose usually prescribed for a younger patient.

Another host factor that influences drug distribution is plasma protein concentrations.[36,37] Most drugs, including analgesics, are extensively bound to plasma proteins. The proportion of albumin among total plasma proteins decreases with frailty, catabolic states and immobility, commonly seen in many elderly patients with chronic conditions. A decrease in serum albumin can increase the percentage of free (unbound) drug available for pharmacologic effect and elimination. In this setting, standard doses of medications lead to higher levels of free (unbound) drug and possible toxicity.

The liver is the major site of drug metabolism. Hepatic metabolism of drugs is dependent on drug-metabolizing enzymes in the liver. The hepatic microenzymes are responsible for this biotransformation. With advanced age there is a decrease in liver weight by 20%–50% and liver volume decreases by approximately 25%.[38] In addition, a nondrug marker for hepatic functional mass, galactose clearance, is decreased by 25% in advanced age. Associated with these changes in liver size and weight is a decrease in hepatic blood flow, normalized by liver volume, this corresponds to a decrease in liver perfusion of 10%–15%. Drugs absorbed from the intestine may be subject to metabolism and the first-pass effect in the liver, accounting for decreased amounts of drug in the circulation after oral administration. The end result is decreased systemic bioavailability and plasma concentrations.[38]

The process of biotransformation in the liver is largely dependent upon the P-450 cytochrome. During biotransformation the parent drug is converted to a more polar metabolite by oxidation, reduction, or hydrolysis. The resulting metabolite may be more active than the parent drug. The cytochrome P-450 has been shown to decline in efficiency with age. These altered mechanisms of drug metabolism should be considered when treating the elderly palliative care patient with opioids, long-acting benzodiazepines, and neuroleptics.

The effect of age on renal function is quite variable. Some studies show a linear decrease in renal function, amounting to decreased glomerular function; other studies indicate no change in creatinine clearance with advancing age.[38] Renal mass decreases 25%–30% in advanced age, and renal blood flow decreases 1% per year after age 50.[38] There are also decreases in tubular function, and reduced ability to concentrate and dilute the urine. In general, the clearance of drugs that are secreted or filtered by the kidney is decreased in a predictable manner.

For example, delayed renal excretion of meperidine's metabolite normeperidine, may result in delirium, central nervous system stimulation, myoclonus, and seizures. Meperidine is not recommended for chronic administration in any patient but is of special concern for elderly patients with borderline renal function. Other drugs that rely on renal excretion include nonsteroidal anti-inflammatory agents, digoxin, aminoglycoside antibiotics, and contrast media.

Table 33–3. Risk Factors for Medication Problems in the Elderly Palliative Care Patient

1. Multiple health care prescribers (e.g. multiple physicians, nurse practitioners)
2. Multiple medications
3. Automatic refills
4. Age-related physiologic pharmacokinetic changes
5. Age-related pharmacodynamic changes
6. Sensory losses: visual, hearing
7. Cognitive defects: delirium, dementia
8. Depression
9. Anxiety
10. Knowledge deficits related to indication, action, dosing schedule, and side effects of prescribed medication
11. Complex dosing schedule or route of administration
12. Comorbid medical conditions: frailty, cerebrovascular disease, cardiac disease, musculoskeletal disorders, advanced cancer
13. Self-medication with over-the-counter medications, herbal remedies
14. Lack of social support or lives alone
15. Alcoholism
16. Financial concerns
17. Illiteracy
18. Misconceptions about specific medications (e.g. addiction)
19. Language barrier

Source: Adapted from: Walker MK, Marquis DF, NICHE Faculty. Ensuring medication safety for older adults. In: Geriatric Nursing Protocols for Best Practice. Eds: Abraham I, Bottrell M, Fulmer T, Mezey MD. Springer Publishing Co., Inc. New York, NY. 1996;(10)131–144.

Medication Use in the Elderly: Problems with Polypharmacy

Older individuals use three times more medications than younger people. They account for approximately 25% of physician visits and approximately 35% of drug expenditures. Elderly patients are more likely to be prescribed inappropriate medications than younger patients.[39] Advancing age alone does not explain the risk of adverse drug reactions and polypharmacy is a consistent predictor. As noted earlier, in the palliative care setting, elderly patients often have more than one comorbid medical condition necessitating treatment with many medications, which places them at greater risk of adverse drug reactions. In addition, new medications not only place the elderly at risk of adverse drug reactions; they also increase the risk of significant drug interactions. For example, the addition of an antacid to an elderly patient already on corticosteroids for bone pain may significantly decrease the oral corticosteroid effect due to decreased absorption.

Understanding pharmacodynamics in relationship to age-related physiological changes can assist the clinician in evaluating the effectiveness and side-effect profile in the elderly palliative care patient (Table 33–3). When multiple drugs are used to treat symptoms, the side-effect profile may increase, potentially limiting the use of one or more drugs. For example, when using an opioid and a benzodiazepine in treating chronic pain and anxiety in the elderly patient, excessive sedation may occur, limiting the amount of opioid that can be administered. Table 33–4 outlines the components of a comprehensive

Table 33–4. Medication Assessment in the Elderly Palliative Care Patient

1. Identify prior problems with medications.
2. Identify other health care providers who prescribe medications.
3. Obtain a detailed history of present medication use at all patient contacts. Include over-the-counter and herbal remedies and dosage, frequency, expected effect, and side effects. When assessing efficacy of pain management, ask about p.r.n. "rescue" doses.
4. Identify "high-risk "medications and assess for side effects or drug-drug interactions.
5. Evaluate the need for drug therapy by performing a comprehensive physical examination, symptom assessment and obtain appropriate laboratory data.
6. Assess functional, cognitive, sensory, affective and nutritional status.
7. Review patient's and family member's level of understanding about indications, dosing, side effects.
8. Identify any concerns about medications (cost, fears, misconceptions).
9. Identify presence of caregiver or support person and include in all assessments.
10. Implement strategies to increase support if lacking (e.g. skilled or nonskilled home care nursing support, community groups, other family members, community-based day programs).

Source: Adapted from: Walker MK, Marquis DF, NICHE Faculty. Ensuring medication safety for older adults. In: Geriatric Nursing Protocols for Best Practice. Eds: Abraham I, Bottrell M, Fulmer T, Mezey MD. Springer Publishing Co., Inc. New York, NY. 1996;(10)131–144.

medication assessment in the elderly palliative care patient.

SYMPTOM MANAGEMENT DURING THE LAST WEEKS OF LIFE: SPECIAL CONCERNS

Numerous studies have evaluated symptoms during the last weeks of life and indicate that patients experience a high degree of symptom distress and suffering. In one study by Seale and Cartright[40] there were age-related difference in the incidence of mental confusion, loss of bladder and bowel control as well as seeing and hearing difficulties. There was no age-related difference in patients reporting pain (72%), trouble breathing (49%), loss of appetite (47%), drowsiness (44%), and other symptoms including sleeplessness, constipation, depression, vomiting, and dry mouth.

Studies have documented the most prevalent and difficult-to-manage symptoms in dying patients including pain, dyspnea, and confusional states.[41,42,43] In one evaluation of the symptom burden of seriously ill hospitalized patients in five tertiary care facilities, pain, dyspnea, anxiety, and depression caused the greatest symptom burden.[44] In this study, patients for whom hospital interviews were not available had more dependencies in daily living and more comorbidities, were older, sicker, and poorer, and more often had respiratory failure and multiorgan system failure.

The complex symptomatology experienced by elderly patients, especially those with cancer and multiple comorbidities demands that an aggressive approach to symptom assessment and intervention be utilized. Devising a palliative plan of care for the elderly patient who is highly symptomatic or who is actively dying requires ongoing communication with the patient and family; assessment of patient and family understanding of goals of care and religious, cultural and spiritual beliefs; access to community agencies; psychological assessment; and patient and family preferences regarding advance directives. Dimensions of a palliative care plan for the elderly are outlined in Table 33–5. The management of three prevalent and distressing symptoms experienced by the elderly at the end of life—dyspnea, pain, and delirium—is discussed below. Each of these symptoms is discussed in greater detail in other chapters.

Table 33–5. Dimensions of a Palliative Plan of Care for the Elderly Patient

1. Assess extent of disease documented by imaging studies and laboratory data.
2. Assess symptoms including prevalence, severity, and impact on function.
3. Identify coping strategies and psychological symptoms including presence of anxiety, depression, and suicidiality.
4. Evaluate religious and spiritual beliefs.
5. Assess overall quality of life and well-being. Does the patient feel secure that all that can be done for them is being done? Is the patient satisfied with the present level of symptom control?
6. Determine family burden. Is attention being paid to the caregiver so that burnout does not occur? If the spouse or caregiver is elderly, are they able to meet the physical demands of caring for the patient?
7. Determine level of care needed in the home if the patient is dying.
8. Asses financial burden on patient and caregiver. Is an inordinate amount of money being spent on patient and will there be adequate provisions for the elderly caregiver when the patient dies?
9. Identify presence of advance care planning requests. Have the patient's wishes and preferences for resuscitation, artificial feeding, and hydration been discussed? Has the patient identified a surrogate decision maker who knows their wishes? Is there documentation regarding advance directives?

Source: Adapted from Improving Care at the End of Life. In: Approaching Death. (Eds) Field MJ, Cassel CK. 1997;50–86.

DYSPNEA

Dyspnea may be one of the most frightening and difficult symptoms an elderly patient can experience. A subjective feeling of breathlessness or the sensation of labored or difficult breathing, dyspnea contributes to severe disability and impaired quality of life. Dyspnea and fear of dyspnea produces profound suffering for dying patients and their families. This section will outline the special needs for elderly patients, with a focus on physiological factors which increase the risk of dyspnea.

Physiological Correlates in the Elderly That Increase Risk of Dyspnea

The effects of aging produce a clinical picture in which respiratory problems can develop. With aging the elastic recoil of the lungs during expiration is decreased due to less collagen and elastin. Alveoli are less elastic, and develop fibrous tissue. The stooped posture and loss of skeletal muscle strength often found in the elderly contribute to the reduction in the vital capacity and an increase in the residual volume of the lung. Table 33–6 outlines the pulmonary risk factors for the development of dyspnea in the elderly palliative care patient.

Respiratory muscle weakness may play a major role in some types of dyspnea. Palange and colleagues[45] found that malnutrition significantly affected exercise tolerance in patients with chronic obstructive pulmonary disease (COPD) by producing diaphragmatic fatigue. In patients with cachexia, the maximal inspiratory pressure, an indicator of diaphragmatic strength is severely impaired. Cachexia and asthenia occur in 80%–90% of patients with advanced cancer, and are also very prevalent in elderly patients with multiple comorbid psychiatric and medical conditions. These mechanisms may affect the development of dyspnea and fatigue in the elderly who have advanced nonmalignant and malignant disease. Ripamonti and Bruera[46] have suggested that in some patients dyspnea may be a clinical presentation of overwhelming cachexia and asthenia.

The multiple etiologies of dyspnea in the dying elderly patient include both malignant (e.g. tumor infiltration, superior vena cava syndrome, pleural ef-

Table 33–6. Risk Factors for Dyspnea in the Elderly Palliative Care Patient

Risk Factor	Comment
Structural	
Increased chest wall stiffness	Increase in the work of breathing
Decrease in skeletal muscle, barrell chest, increase in anteroposterior diameter	Decrease in maximum volume expiration
Decrease in elasticity of alveoli	Decrease in vital capacity
Other	
Anemia	
Cachexia	
Dehydration	Drier mucous membranes, increase in mucous plugs
Ascites	
Atypical presentation of fever	Reduced febrile response, decreased WBC response
Heart failure	
Immobility	Increased risk of aspiration, DVT, PE
Obesity	
Recent abdominal, pelvic, or chest surgery	Increased risk of DVT, PE
Lung disease (chronic obstructive pulmonary disease, lung cancer)	

Sources: Adapted from Eliopoulos, C. Respiratory Problems. Gerontological Nursing, Fourth Edition. Lipincott, New York. 1996;277–290. Additional Source: Palange P., Forte S., Felli A., et al. (1995). Nutritional State and Exercise Tolerance in Patients with COPD. *Chest* 107:1206–1212.

fusion), treatment-related (Adriamycin-induced cardiomyopathy, radiation-induced pneumonitis, pulmonary fibrosis), and nonmalignant causes (e.g. metabolic, structural).

Two causes of dyspnea, deep vein thrombosis (DVT) and pulmonary embolism (PE), are prevalent in the elderly and are often unrecognized and undiagnosed. They may present as pleuritic chest pain with or without dyspnea and hemoptysis. The risk factors in the elderly include increased venous stasis in the legs, impaired fibrinolysis, coagulopathies, recent surgery, immobility, and congestive heart failure. Treatment is dependent on accurate diagnosis, and an estimate of risks versus benefits should be considered in deciding on a course of action. Ventilation-perfusion scans are the most reliable indicator of whether a PE has occurred, and the identification of a DVT as the source of the PE can be accomplished through noninvasive Doppler studies of the legs. Whether it is prudent or compassionate to perform these studies in the elderly patient who is dying should be considered. In the elderly patient who is not actively dying, diagnostic tests can be safely performed. Treatment with anticoagulants in addition to supportive symptom management will reduce the symptom burden and suffering.

Treatment of Dyspnea

When possible, relief of dyspnea is aimed at treatment of the underlying disease process, whether malignant or nonmalignant in origin. Symptomatic interventions are used when the process is not reversible. Both pharmacologic and nonpharmacologic interventions should be employed. One patient may present with multiple etiologies, therefore multiple interventions are indicated.

Therapeutic interventions are based on the etiology and include pharmacologic (e.g., bronchodilators, steroids, diuretics, vasodilators, opioids, sedatives, antibiotics), procedural (e.g., thoracentesis, chest tube placement), nonpharmacological (e.g., relaxation, breathing exercises, music), radiation therapy, and oxygen. At the end of life the pharmacological use of benzodiazepines, opioids, and corticosteroids remain the primary treatment. The use of morphine to control dyspnea at the end of life is advocated by many palliative care professionals.[46–49] Often there is reluctance among staff to use opioids and sedatives in the elderly due to unfamiliarity with these medications, lack of experience in treating dyspnea in dying patients, low priority given to this symptom, and fear that these drugs may hasten death in the elderly. Table 33–7 outlines management guidelines based on presenting symptoms.

Case Study: Management of Dyspnea in an 80-Year-Old Woman with Metastatic Lung Cancer

An 80-year-old woman with metastatic lung cancer to bone, mediastinum, and lung has persistent dyspnea related to lymphangitic spread of disease. She has received radiation therapy to the mediastinum, and she completed a course of chemotherapy two months ago. She is still at home receiving morphine sulfate 30 mg. p.o. every 4 hours which has been very effective for bone pain. She tried long acting morphine but did not like the way it made her feel. She is also receiving prednisone 30 mg. p.o. two times daily for bronchospasm and albuterol inhaler which she occasionally uses. Physical examination reveals breath sounds decreased bilaterally, occasional rhonchi, but no rales or crackles present. She has no distended neck veins, gallop or peripheral edema. Her respiratory rate is 24 per minute at rest, and she complains of feeling breathless and anxious. She is also very fatigued and cannot sleep at night. She refuses to go to the hospital and says she wants to die in her own bed at home. She also is refusing further aggressive intervention and has signed a home DNR order.

Suggestions for Assessment and Intervention

What further symptom management can be offered to this patient?

1. Determine the etiology of the dyspnea in this patient. In the terminally ill patient, dyspnea is often due to multiple causes. A thorough history and physical examination should be performed and will assist in determining specific interventions. In this patient the probable cause of the dyspnea is lymphangitic spread of the malignancy.

Table 33–7. BREATHES Program for Management of Dyspnea in the Elderly Palliative Care Patient

B—*bronchospasm.* Consider nebulized albuterol and or steroids.
R—*rales/crackles.* If present, reduce fluid intake. If patient is receiving IV hydration, reduce fluid intake or discontinue. Consider gentle diuresis with lasix 20–40 mg p.o. daily ± spironalactone (aldactone) 100 mg p.o. daily.
E—*effusion.* Determine on physical examination or chest x-ray. Consider thoracentesis or chest tube, if appropriate.
A—*airway obstruction.* If patient is at risk or has had aspiration from food, puree solid food, avoid thin liquids, and keep the patient upright during and after meals for at least one hour.
T—*tachypnea and breathlessness.* Opioids reduce respiratory rate and feelings of breathlessness as well as anxiety. Assess daily. If patient is opioid naïve, begin with morphine sulfate 5–10 mg p.o. q 4 hours and titrate opioids 25%–50% daily—every other day as needed. Consider nebulized morphine, and anxiolytic such as ativan 0.5–2 mg p.o. b.i.d.–t.i.d. Use of a fan may reduce feelings of breathlessness.
H—*hemoglobin low.* Consider a blood transfusion if anemia is contributing to dyspnea.
E—*educate* and support the patient and family during this highly stressful period.
S—*secretions.* If secretions are copious consider a trial of a scopalamine patch q 72 hours, atropine 0.3–0.5 mg s.c. q 4 hours p.r.n., glycopyrrulate (Robinul) 0.1–0.4 mg IM.SQ q 4–12 hours p.r.n.

Sources: Adapted from Storey P, Knight CF. Unipac Four: Management of selected nonpain symptoms in the terminally ill. A self-study program. Gainesville, Fla.: American Academy of Hospice and Palliative Medicine. 1996, Dyspnea p. 25–32. *Additional sources:* Ripamonti, C. Management of dyspnea in advanced cancer patients. Support Care Cancer 1999; 7(4):233–243. Tobin, M. Dyspnea: Pathophysiolgic basis, clinical presentation, and management. Arch Intern Med Vol 150, Aug. 1990; 1604–1613. Kuebler, K.K. Dyspnea. Hospice and Palliative Care Clinical Practice Protocol, Fall 1996.

2. Excessive fatigue is present in this patient and a complete blood count will determine if anemia is contributing to fatigue and dyspnea. Consider a trial of a low-dose stimulant such as Ritalin 2.5–5 mg. p.o. daily in the morning. This may decrease fatigue and give her more energy during the day.
3. Infection can be ruled out with a complete blood count. If pneumonia is suspected, try to arrange for a chest x-ray if the patient agrees or empirically initiate a trial of oral antibiotics. Although this patient has no signs of congestive heart failure on physical examination, it should be ruled out.
4. If available, use pulse oximetry to determine benefits of oxygen therapy or try nasal O_2 at 3 L/minute.
5. The patient is presently receiving morphine sulfate for pain. Increase her opioids by 25%–50% to a dose of 40–45 mg p.o. q4 hours to assist with tachypnea and anxiety.
6. Consider a trial with an anxiolytic such as ativan 0.5 mg p.o. q8–12 hours.
7. Consider increasing the prednisone to treat the bronchospasm.
8. Encourage use of an Albuterol inhaler t.i.d.–q.i.d. for bronchospasm.
9. If oral morphine cannot be titrated to effect, consider a trial of nebulized morphine 2.5–5.0 mg q4 hours p.r.n., if available.
10. Consider the benefit versus burden of additional interventions that are employed. The patient has stated that no further interventions are to be used. Review the goals of care with the patient and family members.
11. Assess functional status and reduce the need for physical exertion. Provide for assistance with daily activities, positioning techniques, and frequent rest periods.
12. Address anxiety, provide support and reassurance. Determine level of support from family and friends, and spiritual and religious beliefs. Reassure patient that symptoms can be controlled.
13. Incorporate nonpharmacological interventions (e.g., progressive relaxation, guided imagery, and music therapy).

PAIN

The physiological changes accompanying advanced age have been discussed in this chapter, however it is important to emphasize that the elderly are more sensitive to both the therapeutic and toxic effects of analgesics. The principles of drug selection, route of administration and management of side effects are the same in the elderly population as for younger adults.

Opioid Selection

In elderly patients with moderate to severe pain who have limited prior treatment with opioids, it is best to begin with a short-half-life agonist (morphine, hydromorphone, oxycodone). Shorter-half-life opioids are easier to titrate than longer-half-life opioids such as levorphanol or methadone, and in the elderly may have fewer side effects. Morphine can be administered as a controlled release tablet every 8 to 12 hours; however, plasma clearance decreases with age.[50] Consequently, the metabolite of morphine, morphine-6 glucuronide, may accumulate with repeated dosing, especially in the setting of impaired renal or hepatic function.[51] This may mean that morphine is not the most suitable opioid in the elderly. If after several days of treatment with morphine, the elderly patient develops side effects including sedation, confusion or respiratory depression, it may mean that there is an accumulation of these metabolites and the opioid should be changed.

Opioids with longer half-lives such as methadone can be safely used in the elderly provided they are carefully monitored. Controlled-release morphine and oxycodone are now available and may be very convenient for some elderly patients who have difficulty taking pills throughout the day.

As in younger individuals, the use of meperidine for the management of chronic cancer pain is not recommended. The active metabolite of meperidine is normeperidine, which is a proconvulsant. The half-life of normeperidine is 12 to 16 hours. With repeated dosing, accumulation of normeperidine can result in central nervous system excitability with possible tremors, myoclonuses, and seizures. Table 33–8 outlines guidelines for opioid use in the elderly patient.

The fentanyl patch can be used safely in the elderly palliative care patient but patients should be monitored carefully. If after initiation with the fentanyl patch side effects develop, it is im-

Table 33–8. Opioid Use in the Elderly Patient at the End of Life

Opioid	Comments
Morphine	Observe for side effects with repeated dosing. Continuous or sustained release may not be tolerated even after a trial with immediate release
Hydromorphone (Dilaudid)	Short half-life opioid; may be safer than morphine
Propoxyphene (Darvon, Darvocet)	Avoid use, metabolite causes CNS and cardiac toxicity
Codeine	May cause excessive constipation, nausea and vomiting
Methadone	Use cautiously, long half-life may produce excessive side effects; requires careful monitoring especially during first 72 hours after initiation. If it is indicated, it may be safer to use a short-acting opioid as a rescue dose
Pentazocine (Talwin)	Opioid agonist/antagonist should not be used; may cause CNS side effects (delirium, agitation)
Transdermal fentanyl patch	Long half-life (12–24 hours) is used cautiously in the frail elderly or in elderly with multiple comorbid conditions; cannot titrate easily. If side effects develop will last for at least 12–24 hours after patch is removed
Meperidine	Avoid use in elderly due to CNS toxicity
Oxycodone	Useful for moderate to severe pain control

Source: Adapted from: McCaffery M, Pasero, C. Pain: Clinical Manual, pp. 179–180. Mosby, 1999. St. Louis, Missouri.

portant to remember that they may persist for long periods (hours or even days) after the patch is removed. The frail elderly, who have experienced multiple side effects from opioids may not do well with this route of administration.

Parenteral routes of administration should be considered in elderly patients who require rapid onset of analgesia, or require high doses of opioids that cannot be administered orally. They may be administered in a variety of ways including the intravenous and subcutaneous route using a PCA (patient-controlled analgesia) device. A careful evaluation of the skin in the elderly patient should be done prior to initiation of the subcutaneous route of administration. If the patient has excessive edema, a very low platelet count, or skin changes related to chronic steroid use, absorption may be impaired or subcutaneous tissue may not sustain repeated dosing even with a permanent indwelling butterfly catheter. Infusion devices with the capability of patient-administered rescue dosing can be safely used in the elderly cancer patient. It is important to remember that severe cognitive impairment should not deter the use of the intravenous route of administration, especially in the elderly patient at the end of life. Choice of analgesics and routes of administration must be based on individual assessment of each patient.

Dose Titration

After initiation with an opioid a stepwise escalation of the opioid dose should be done until adequate analgesia or intolerable side effects develop. The increased sensitivity of the elderly to opioid side effects suggests that careful titration and escalation should be performed.[52] It is generally safe to begin with a dose 25%–50% less than the dose for a younger adult, especially if the elderly patient is frail or has a history of side effects from prior opioid use. Generally, it is safe to titrate opioids 25%–50% every 24–48 hours, although a less aggressive approach may be necessary in elderly patients.

Case Study: An 80-Year-Old Man with Bladder Cancer

An 80-year-old man with bladder cancer and extensive intraabdominal and pelvic disease is receiving hydromorphone 6 mg p.o. every 4 hours and is reporting inadequate pain relief with a pain intensity of 7/10. He also is having intermittent nausea and vomiting. He has been on this dose for about 6 weeks and is reporting having some confusion for the past week, which his wife has corroborated. He is also having periods of severe incidental pain related to movement. He has no p.r.n. rescue doses ordered. For the past 2 weeks he has been in bed most of the time. He also reports constipation with no bowel movement for 5 days.

Case Analysis

What evaluation of this patient should be done and what changes in his opioid regimen should be made?

1. The etiology of the confusion should be determined. A careful review of all medications should be done and all centrally acting medications discontinued. In this patient his only additional medication is digoxin.
2. A digoxin level and appropriate laboratory data should be obtained to determine if he is digoxin toxic and if there is any metabolic etiology for his confusion. His digoxin level is normal, and his electrolytes, and renal and liver function studies are normal.
3. A change in opioid is indicated, as this may be contributing to his confusion.
4. An evaluation for the etiology of the nausea and vomiting should be done. A history of onset, duration, temporal characteristics, and exacerbating/relieving factors should be obtained. A thorough physical examination is performed with special attention to the abdominal and rectal examination. In this patient physical examination reveals that bowel sounds are present and rectal exam reveals retained feces in the rectal vault.
5. An abdominal x-ray is done and shows extensive retained feces but no bowel obstruction. Abdominal CAT scan done one month ago revealed extensive intrapelvic and intraabdominal disease.
6. It has been determined that the etiology of the nausea and vomiting is related to severe constipation and may be worsened

by intermittent extrinsic compression of the bowel by tumor infiltration.
7. The severe constipation may also be contributing to the development of confusion.
8. The decision is made to switch the patient to another opioid. In selecting another opioid, factors to consider include half-life, duration of action, and route of administration. The decision is made to start the patient on a continuous infusion of morphine until the nausea and vomiting resolve and then convert the patient to oral morphine. The equianalgesic dose table should be used as a guide. Because of the existence of incomplete cross-tolerance between drugs, advanced age, and cognitive changes, the alternative opioid should be reduced by 50%–75%.
9. Disimpaction was attempted but could not be tolerated. A bowel regimen of an oil retention enema followed by a Fleets enema was tolerated and the patient had a large bowel movement. The patient was also started on an oral regimen of Senekot 2 tabs p.o. b.i.d. and Colace 300 mg p.o. daily.

Management of Side Effects Related to Opioids

The elderly who have multiple medical conditions, who are frail and bedbound are at greatest risk for potential side effects of opioids due to age-related alterations in pharmacokinetics, specifically distribution and elimination. Avoiding side effects by "starting low and going slow" is common advice given to many clinicians in treating elderly patients, but this may run the risk of undertreatment of pain. Careful monitoring and frequent assessment can prevent a minor side effect from becoming life-threatening in the elderly.

Suggestions in the management of mild nausea and vomiting, sedation, or confusion is to decrease the 24-hour total dose by 25% if the patient has adequate analgesia and is taking only a minimal number of p.r.n. rescue doses in a 24-hour period. This strategy avoids a complete change in opioid, although anecdotally, this approach may be useful for a limited time only; if the pain escalates, this will necessitate a titration of the opioid and the side effects will return.

Treating the side effect can be very effective but the risk of polypharmacy remains. If, for example, the elderly patient is experiencing sedation from the opioid, it may be wiser to decrease the 24-hour total dose rather than add a psychostimulant, which can produce irritability, tremors, anxiety, and insomnia. If decreasing the dose cannot be done, a small dose of a psychostimulant such as Ritalin 2.5 mg p.o. twice a day, can be very effective in controlling daytime sedation. Changing the opioid can be another strategy to minimize or treat side effects. This can be very effective in the management of opioid-induced nausea and vomiting, especially if the patient has only been exposed to one or two opioids and there are other opioids to switch to. Again, this strategy eliminates the use of an additional medication with its own potential side effects.

The addition of an adjuvant such as a nonsteroidal anti-inflammatory agent (NSAID) has been shown to be very effective in reducing the opioid requirement, thus allowing a reduction in the 24-hour opioid dose. Table 33–9 outlines commonly used adjuvant drugs in the elderly palliative care patient.

The elderly are particularly susceptible to opioid-induced constipation,

Table 33–9. Common Adjuvant Drugs for Use in the Elderly

Drug	Approximate Adult Daily Dose Range	Common Side Effects
Antidepressants		
Amitriptyline	25–150 mg p.o.	Sedation, constipation, urinary retention, dry mouth, hypotension, blurred vision. If conduction disorders do not use in elderly. Angle closure glaucoma, prostatism, glaucoma May need to start at 10 mg po qhs.
Doxepin	25–150 mg p.o.	Same as for Amitriptyline
Imipramine	20–100 mg p.o.	Same as for Amitriptyline
Trazodone	75–225 mg p.o.	Same as for Amitriptyline
Anticonvulsants		
Carbamazepine	200–1200 mg p.o.	Nausea, dizziness, somnolence, hepatic and hematopoietic dysfunction (leukopenia and thrombocytopenia). Rarely, CHF, hyponatremia
Phenytoin	300–500 mg p.o.	Nausea, dizziness, somnolence, ataxia, dermatitis, gingival hyperplasia, seizures, hepatoxicity
Clonazepam	1–3 mg p.o.	Drowsiness, ataxia, confusion, depression, dizziness
Gabapentin	600–3600 mg p.o.	Short-term memory loss, sedation, ataxia, confusion
Local Anesthetics		
Lidocaine	5 mg/kg IV	Light-headedness, nervousness, confusion, dizziness, bradycardia
Mexiletine	300–600 mg p.o.	Nausea, dizziness, tremor, coordination difficulties. Use if CHF rhythm disorders

Source: Adapted from McCaffery M, Pasero C, Commonly Used Adjuvant Analgesics. In: Pain: Clinical Manual. Mosby, St. Louis, Missouri, 1999, 342–344.

and laxative and stool softener should be prescribed whenever an opioid is prescribed.[53] Constipation can be life-threatening in the debilitated elderly patient, especially if it is unrecognized and untreated. The initial presentation of opioid-induced constipation may be confusing. Abdominal signs and symptoms including pain, distension, and nausea may be absent and the patient may present with confusion, depressed mood, and loss of appetite. Assessment of the elderly patient should include all medications including over-the-counter drugs—iron preparations, antacids, and drugs with anticholinergic properties.

Nonsteroidal Anti-inflammatory Agents

NSAIDs are useful as initial therapy for mild to moderate pain and can be used as an additive with opioids and nonopiods. In particular, NSAIDs are useful in the treatment of nociceptive pain related to bone or joint disease. When used concurrently with opioids, lower doses of opioids may be an additional benefit.

Elderly patients with a history of ulcer disease are most vulnerable to the side effects of these drugs, which can cause renal insufficiency and nephrotoxicity. Cognitive dysfunction has been reported with the use of salicylates, indomethacin, naproxen, and ibuprofen. Also, NSAIDs are problematic in elderly patients with congestive heart failure, peripheral edema, or ascites. In the palliative setting, consideration of the risks versus the benefits to the elderly patient should be done. If, for example, the use of NSAIDs provides effective analgesia, and the life expectancy of the patient is limited (days to weeks), it is probably prudent to initiate this therapy.

Invasive Approaches

Anesthetic and neurosurgical approaches are indicated when conservative measures utilizing opioids and adjuvant analgesics have failed to provide adequate analgesia, or when the patient is experiencing intolerable side effects. The use of these approaches is not contraindicated in the elderly. The clearest indication for these approaches is intolerable central nervous system toxicity. These procedures include regional analgesia (spinal, intraventricular, and intrapleural opioids), sympathetic blockade and neurolytic procedures (celiac plexus block, lumbar sympathetic block, cervicothoracic [stellate] ganglion block), or pathway ablation procedure (chemical or surgical rhizotomy, or cordotomy). At the end of life these approaches may be useful in some elderly patients who have intractable pain that cannot be managed with systemic treatment.

Nonpharmacological Approaches: Complementary Therapies

Physical and psychological interventions can be used as an adjunct with drugs and surgical approaches to manage pain in the elderly. These approaches carry few side effects and, when possible, should be tried along with other approaches. In selecting an approach in the dying patient, factors that should be considered include physical and psychological burden to the patient, efficacy and practicality. If the patient has weeks to live, these strategies may allow for a reduction in systemic opioids and diminish adverse effects.

Cognitive-behavioral interventions include relaxation, guided imagery, distraction, and music therapy. The major advantages of these techniques are that they are easy to learn, safe, and readily accepted by patients. Cognitive and behavioral interventions are helpful to reduce emotional distress, improve coping, and offer the patient and family a sense of control.

The Cognitively Impaired Elderly: Problems in Assessment and Fear of Treating Pain and Other Symptoms

Cognitively impaired nursing home residents present a special barrier to pain assessment and management.[54–59] Residents of nursing homes exhibit very high rates of cognitive impairment.[60] Most studies of nursing home residents reveal that cognitively impaired nursing home residents are prescribed and administered significantly less analgesic medication, both in number and in dosage of pain drugs than their more cognitively intact peers.[60,61]

Assessment of pain in cognitively impaired elderly at the end of life remains a special challenge. Mild to moderate cognitive impairments seem to be associated with a decrease in propensity to report pain.[60] In severely cognitively impaired individuals assessment is often difficult as these individuals often cannot verbalize their reports of pain. Ferrell and colleagues[62] found in their evaluation of 217 elderly patients with significant cognitive impairment, 83% could complete at least one pain scale, with the McGill Present Pain Intensity Scale having the highest completion rate, and 32% were able to complete all of the scales presented.

The best way to assess pain is to ask the individual. As previously stated there is often a general bias among many older individuals to report or express their pain. The ability of caregivers, either family or staff, to assess pain in this population is thereby crucial. In one study of caregiver perceptions of nonverbal patients with cerebral palsy, more than 80% used aspects of crying and moaning to alert them to a pain event.[63] In another study evaluating a measurement tool for discomfort in noncommunicative patients with advanced Alzheimer's disease, indicators of pain included noisy breathing, negative vocalizations, facial expression (content, sad, or frightened), frown, body language (relaxed, tense, or fidgeting).[55]

There is some evidence that cognitively impaired elderly individuals' facial expressions of pain depend on the cause of the underlying cognitive disorder, including hemispheric dysfunction and type of dementia, however facial expressions and body language can be very useful indicators of pain.

DELIRIUM AT THE END OF LIFE

In all settings, delirium is a common symptom in the elderly medically ill and cancer patient. The presence of delirium contributes significantly to increased morbidity and mortality. Estimates of the prevalence of delirium range from 25% to 40% in patients with cancer at some point during their disease and in the terminal phases of disease the incidence increases to 85%.[64–66] In elderly hospitalized patients, delirium prevalence ranges from 10% to 40% and up to 80% at the end of life. One of the major problems in the treatment of delirium in the elderly patient is lack of assessment by hospital staff, especially if the patient is quiet and noncommunicative.

Predisposing and Etiologic Factors

The etiology of delirium in the medically compromised and dying elderly patient is often multifactorial and may be nonspecific. In an elderly patient delirium is often a presenting feature of an acute physical illness or exacerbation of a chronic one, or of intoxication with even therapeutic doses of commonly used drugs.[67] A number of factors appear to make the elderly more susceptible to the development of delirium (Table 33–10).

Delirium can be due to the direct effects of the disease on the central nervous system, metabolic reasons including organ failure, electrolyte imbalance, infection, hematological disorders, nutritional deficiencies, paraneoplastic disorders, hypoxemia, chemotherapeutic agents, immunotherapy, vascular disorders, hypothermia, hyperthermia, uncontrolled pain, sensory deprivation, sleep deprivation, medications, alcohol or drug withdrawal, diarrhea, constipation, or urinary retention. A variety of drugs can produce delirium in the medically ill or elderly patient (Table 33–11). In the palliative care setting, multiple medications are generally required to control symptoms at the end of life. To reduce the risk of polypharmacologically induced delirium, it is prudent to add one medication at a time, evaluating its response, before adding another medication.

Delirium in the elderly patient is often undertreated for several reasons including lack of assessment tools, inadequate knowledge of early signs of confusion and inadequate time spent with the patient to determine cognitive function—all factors which lead to underdiagnosis. Behavioral manifestations include a variety of symptoms that may be interpreted as depression, psychosis, or dementia.

A multifactorial model of delirium in the elderly, with baseline predisposing factors and the addition of various insults has been established by Inouye.[68] The factors that he has identified to be contributory to baseline vulnerability in the elderly include visual impairment, cognitive impairment, severe illness, and an elevated blood urea nitrogen/creatinine ratio of 18 or greater. Other factors which have been identified in the elderly include advanced age, depression, electrolyte imbalance, poor functional status, immobility, foley catheter, malnutrition, dehydration, alcohol, and medications including neuroleptics, opioids, and anticholinergic drugs. Lastly, delirium in an elderly patient is often a precursor to death, and should be viewed as a grave prognostic sign.

Many elderly persons abuse alcohol. Alcoholism is often missed in elderly hospitalized patients. In one study, organic mental syndromes were diagnosed in over 40% of elderly alcoholics admitted for alcohol abuse and alcohol withdrawal delirium was found in about 10% of these.[69] Illness, malnutrition, concurrent use of a hepatotoxic drug, or one that is metabolized by the liver may result in increased sensitivity of the elderly to alcohol. Alcohol, combined with other medication, especially centrally

Table 33–10. Factors Predisposing the Elderly to Delirium

Factor	Comments
Age-related changes in the brain	Atrophy of gray and white matter Senile plaques in hippocampus, amygdala, middle cerebral cortical layers Cell loss in frontal lobes, amygdala, putamen, thalamus, locus ceruleus
Brain damage	Alzheimer's disease, cerebrovascular disease
Reduced regulation and resistance to stress	
Sensory changes	Visual, hearing loss
Infection	Prolonged immobility, foley catheters,
Intravenous lines	
	Pulmonary and urinary tract infections
Impaired pharmacokinetics	Reduced ability to metabolize and eliminate drugs
Malnutrition	Vitamin deficiency as a result of prolonged illness Folate deficiency may directly cause delirium
Multiple comorbid diseases	Cancer and cardiovascular, pulmonary, renal, and hepatic disease Endocrine disorders including hyperthyroidism and hypothryoidism Fluid and electrolyte abnormalities
Reduced thirst	Hypovolemia
Reduction of protein-binding of drugs	Enhanced effects of opioids, diuretics
Polypharmacy	Use of sedatives, hypnotics, major tranquilizers

Sources: Adapted from Lipowski Z. (1990). Delirium in geriatric patients In *Delirium: Acute Confusional States.* pp. 413–441.Oxford University Press. New York. Additional source: Inouye S., Charpentier P.A., et al. (1996). Precipitating factors for delirium in hospitalized elderly persons: predictive model and interrelationship with baseline vulnerability. *JAMA* 275: 852–857.

Table 33–11. Drugs Commonly Causing Delirium in the Elderly

Classification	Example
Antidepressants	Amitriptyline, doxepin
Antihistamines	Chlorpheniramine, diphenhydramine, hydroxyzine, promethazine
Diabetic agents	Chlorpropamide
Cardiac	Digoxin, dipyridamole
Antihypertensives	Propranolol, clonidine
Sedatives	Barbiturates, chlordiazepoxide, diazepam, flurazepam, meprobamate
Opioids	Meperidine, pentazocine, propoxyphene
Nonsteroidal anti-inflammatory agents	Indomethacin, phenylbutazone
Anticholinergics	Atropine, scopolamine
Antiemetics	Trimethobenzamide, phenothiazine
Antispasmodics	Dilomine, hyoscyamine, propantheline, belladonna alkaloids
Antineoplastics	Methotrexate, mitomycin, procarbazine, Ara-C, Carmustine, Fluorouracil, Interferon, Interleuken-2, L-Asparaginase, Prednisone
Corticosteroids	Prednisone, dexamethasone
H2 receptor antagonists	Cimetidine
Lithium	
Acetaminophen	
Salicylates	Aspirin
Anticonvulsant agents	Carbamazepine, diphenylhydantoin, phenobarbital, sodium valproate
Antiparkinsonian agents	Amantadine, levodopa
Alcohol	

Source: Adapted from Lipowski Z. (1990). Delirium in geriatric patients. In: *Delirium: Acute Confusional States.* pp. 229–276, 413–441. Oxford University Press. New York.

acting medications, can produce delirium in the elderly.

The diagnosis of delirium in an elderly patient carries with it serious risks. An agitated delirious patient may climb out of bed; pull out foley catheters, intravenous lines, and sutures; and injure staff in an attempt to protect themselves from perceived threat. Mental status questionnaires are relatively easy to administer and an examination should be performed on all patients with mental status changes. The Mini-Mental State Exam, a 10-item test is easy to administer to an elderly patient.[70]

Delirium and Dementia

Delirium may often be superimposed upon dementia in the elderly patient. In clinical practice it is important to distinguish whether the delirious patient has an underlying dementia. When an elderly demented patient becomes delirious, it should be assumed that an organic precipitating factor—metabolic, drug-induced, acute illness is the cause and the patient should be evaluated for the etiology and treated. The distinction is not always apparent. Both delirium and dementia feature global impairment in cognition. Obtaining a careful history from family members or caregivers to obtain the onset of symptoms is probably the most important factor in making the distinction. In general, acute onset of cognitive and attentional deficits and abnormalities, whose severity fluctuates during the day and tends to increase at night, is typical of a delirium. Delirium in general is a transient disorder that seldom lasts for more than a month, while dementia is a clinical state that lasts for months or years.[67] Dementia implies impairment in short or long-term memory associated with impaired thinking and judgment, with other disturbances of higher cortical function, or with personality change.[71] The presence and severity of cognitive deficits and attentional disturbances should be further established by a comprehensive mental status examination.

Treatment of Delirium

Treatment of delirium includes an identification of the underlying cause, correction of the precipitating factors and symptom management of the delirium. In the very ill or dying patient, however, the etiology may be multifactorial, and the cause is often irreversible.

If delirium is occurring in the dying elderly patient and the goal of care has been identified as the promotion of comfort and relief of suffering, diagnostic evaluations (imaging and laboratory studies) would not prove beneficial.

Interventions that may be helpful include restoration of fluid and electrolyte balance, environmental changes, and supportive techniques such as elimination of unnecessary stimuli, provision of a safe environment, and measures which reduce anxiety. In many cases the etiology of delirium may be pharmacologic, especially in the elderly patient. All nonessential and central nervous system depressant drugs should be stopped.

Pharmacologic treatment includes the use of sedatives and neuroleptics. Breitbart and Jacobsen[72] have demonstrated that the use of lorazepam alone in controlling symptoms of delirium was ineffective and contributed to worsening cognition. These authors advocate the use of a neuroleptic such as haloperidol along with a benzodiazepine in the control of an agitated delirium. Other neuroleptics, risperidone and Olanzapine, have also been used to treat delirium in the elderly, and may have fewer side effects. The oral route is preferred, although in cases of severe agitation and delirium the parenteral route should be used.

SUMMARY

Caring for the elderly patient at the end of life will continue to be a challenge to clinicians. The twenty-first century will bring new opportunities as well as problems in providing care to the elderly at the end of life. Older adults will constitute a larger proportion of the population than today, and the total number of dying elderly will be greater. Most deaths occur in institutions, mainly hospitals, fewer in nursing homes. The number of people dying at home is increasing, placing a greater burden on friends and family and places them at great risk for psychological distress and physical decline.

Elderly patients who are dying should be able to receive skillful and expert palliative care. This means that caregivers must become knowledgeable about the aging process—the physiological changes that normally occur with aging and the impact of progressive disease on an already frail system. Management of symptoms at the end of life in the elderly patient is different because of their altered response to medications, their fear of taking medication, and the need to involve and educate informal and formal caregivers who are often elderly themselves.

Pain, respiratory distress, and delirium are the three most common symptoms in the elderly patient who is dying. Relief of these symptoms is a basic priority for care of the dying elderly patient. Management of these symptoms requires knowledge of appropriate pharmacological and nonpharmacological interventions. Continued assessment of the patient will allow for drug changes, dose adjustments, and relief of distressing symptoms. Providing distress from these symptoms will facilitate a comfortable death, one that is remembered, with peace and comfort, by family and friends.

REFERENCES

1. Rabin D., Stockton P. (1987). Long-Term Care of the Elderly: A Factbook. New York, Oxford University Press.

2. National Center for Health Statistics (1989). Advance report of final mortality statistics, 1987. Monthly Vital Statistics Reports, 38(5 Supp).

3. National Center for Health Statistics (1989). Advance report of final mortality statistics, 1987. Monthly Vital Statistics Reports 38 (5 supp.).

4. Foley D., Brock D. (1998). Demography and epidemiology of dying in the US with emphasis on deaths of older persons. Hosp J 13(1-2): 49–60.

5. National Center for Health Statistics (1995). Monthly Vital Statistics Report 43(13).

6. Grulich A., Swerdlow A., Dos Santos Silva I., Beral V. (1995). Is the apparent rise in cancer mortality in the elderly real? Analysis of changes in certification and coding of cause of death in England and Wales, 1970–1990. Int J Cancer 63(2):164–168.

7. National Center for Health Statistics (1986). Moss A, Parson V. Current estimates from the National Health Interview Survey, United States 1985. In: Vital Health Statistics, ser. 10, no. 160, pp. 13, 82–83, 106, 118. DHHS Pub. No. (PHS) 860-1588. Washington, DC: Public Health Service.

8. Foley D.J., Miles T.P., Brock D.B., Phillips C. (1995). Recounts of elderly deaths: endorsements for the Patient Self-Determination Act. Gerontologist 35(1):119–121.

9. Seeman I. National Mortality Followback Survey: 1986 summary. United States. Vital Health Statistics, ser. 20, no. 19. DHHS Pub. No. (PHS) 92-1656. Hyattsville, MD: National Center for Health Statistics.

10. Foley D., Brock D. (1998). Demography and epidemiology of dying in the US with emphasis on deaths of older persons. Hosp J 13(1-2): 49–60.

11. Wallace R, Woolson R, eds. (1992). The Epidemiological Study of the Elderly. New York: Oxford University Press.

12. Fried T., Pollack D., Drickamer M., Tinetti M. (1999). Who dies at home? Determinants of site of death for community-based long-term care patients. J Am Geriatr Soc 47: 25–29.

13. Groth-Janucker A., McCusker J. (1983). Where do elderly patients prefer to die? Place of death and patient characteristics of 100 elderly patients under the care of a home healthcare team. J Am Geriatr Soc 31:457–461.

14. McWhinney I.R., Bass M., Orr V. (1995). Factors associated with location of death (home or hospital) of patients referred to a palliative care team. CMAJ 152(3): 361–367.

15. Townsend J., Frank A., Fermont D., Dyer S., Karran O., Walgrove A., Piper M. (1990). Terminal cancer and patients' preference for place of death: A prospective study. BMJ 301(6749): 415–417.

16. Kemper P., Murtaugh C.M. (1991). Lifetime use of nursing home care. N Engl J Med 324: 595–600.

17. Stein W.M., Ferrell B.A. (1996). Pain in the nursing home. Clin Geriatr Med 12(3): 601–613.

18. Ferrell B.A., Ferrell B.R., Osterweil D. (1990). Pain in the nursing home. J Am Geriatr Soc 38: 409–414.

19. Gornick M., McMillan A., Lubitz J. (1993). A longitudinal perspective on patterns of Medicare payments. Health Aff (Millwood) 12(2): 140–150.

20. Knaus W., Wagner D.P., Draper E.A., Zimmerman J.E., Bergner M., Bastos P.G., Sirio C.A., Murphy D.J., Lotring T., Damiano A. (1991). The APACHE prognostic system: Risk prediction of hospital mortality for critically ill hospitalized adults. Chest 100(6): 1619–1636.

21. Christakis N.A., Escarce J.J. (1996). Survival of Medicare patients after enrollment in hospice programs. N Engl J Med 18;335(3):172–178.

22. Rosenthal M.A., Gebski V.J., Keffors R.F., Stuart Harris R.C. (1993). Prediction of life-expectancy in hospice patients: Identification of novel prognostic factors. Palliat Med 3(7): 199–204.

23. Bruera E., Miller M., Kuehn N., MacEachern T., Hanson J. (1992). Estimate of survival of patients admitted to a palliative care unit: A prospective study. J Pain Symptom Manage 7: 82–86.

24. Perls T.T., Wood E.R. (1996). Acute costs and the oldest old. Arch Intern Med 156: 759.

25. Riley G., Potosky A., Lubitz J., Kessler L. (1995). Medicare payments from diagnosis to death for elderly cancer patients. Med Care 33(8): 828–841.

26. Riley G., Lubitz J., Prihoda R., Rabey E. (1987). The use and costs of Medicare services by cause of death. Inquiry 24(3): 233–244.

27. Otten, A. (1991). About 15% of U.S. adults care for ill relatives. Wall Street Journal, April 22, B1.

28. Stone R., Cafferata G.I., Sangl J. (1987). Caregivers of the frail elderly: A national profile. Gerontologist 27(5): 616–626.

29. Schott-Baer D., Fisher L, Gregory C. (1995). Dependent care, caregiver burden, hardiness, and self-care agency of caregivers. Cancer Nurs 18(4): 299–305.

30. Weitzner M.A., McMillan S., Jacobson P. (1999). Family caregiver quality of life: Differences between curative and palliative cancer treatment settings. J Pain Sympt Manage 17(6): 418–428.

31. Ferrell B.R., Grant M., Borneman T., Juarez G., Ter Veer A. (1995). Family caregiving in cancer pain management. J Palliat Med 2: 185–195.

32. Kissane D.W., Block S., McKenzie M., McDowell A.C., Nitzan R. (1998). Family grief therapy: A preliminary account of a new model to promote healthy family functioning during palliative care and bereavement. Psychooncology 7(1): 14–25.

33. Smeenk F.W., de Witte L.P., Van Haastregt J.C., Schipper R.M., Biezeman H.P., Crebolder H.F. (1998). Transmural care of terminal cancer patients. Nurs Res 47(3): 129–136.

34. Macdonald G. (1998). Massage as a respite intervention for primary caregivers. Am J Hosp Palliat Care 15(1): 43–47.

35. Greenblatt D.J., Harmatz J.S., Shader R.I. (1991). Clinical pharmacokinetics of anxiolytics and hypnotics in the elderly: therapeutic considerations. Clin Pharmacokinet 21: 165–177, 262–273.

36. Vestal R.F., Montamat S.C., Nielson C.P. (1992). Drugs in special patient groups: The elderly. In: Clinical Pharmacology: Basic Principles in Therapeutics (K.L. Melmon, H.F. Morrelli, B.B. Hoffman, D.W. Nierenberg, eds.). 3rd edition, pp. 851–874. New York: McGraw-Hill.

37. Avorn J., Gurwitz H.H. (1997). Principles of pharmacology. In: Geriatric Medicine (C.K. Cassel, H.J. Cohen, E.B. Larson, D.E. Meier, N.M. Resnick, L.Z. Rubenstein, L.B. Sorenson, eds.). 3rd edition, pp. 55–70. New York: Springer.

38. Vestal R.E. (1997). Aging and pharmacology. Cancer 89(7): 1302–1310.

39. Aparasu R.R., Sitzman S.J. (1999) Inappropriate prescribing for elderly outpatient. Am J Health Syst Pharm 56(5): 433–439.

40. Seale C., Cartwright A. (1994) The Year Before Death. Brookfield VT: Ashgate Publishing Company.

41. Fainsinger R., Miller M.J., Bruera E. (1991). Symptom control during the last week of life on a palliative care unit. J Palliat Care 7(1): 5–11.

42. Ventafridda V., Ripamonti C., DeConno F., Tamburini M., Cassileth B.R. (1990). Symptom prevalence and control during cancer patients' last days of life. J Palliat Care 6(3): 7–11.

43. Coyle N., Adelhardt J., Foley K., Portenoy R. (1990). Character of terminal illness in the advanced cancer patient: Pain and other symptoms during the last four weeks of life. J Pain Sympt Manage (5)2: 83–93.

44. Desbiens N.A., Mueller-Rizner N., Connors A.F., et al. (1999). The symptom burden of seriously ill hospitalized patients. J Pain Sympt Manage 17(4): 248–255.

45. Palange P., Forte S., Felli A., et al. (1995). Nutritional state and exercise tolerance in patients with COPD. Chest 107: 1206–1212.

46. Ripamonti C, Bruera E (1997). Dyspnea: Pathophysiology and assessment. J Pain Sympt Manage 13(4): 220–232.

47. Cowcher K., Hanks G.W. (1990). Long-term management of respiratory symptoms in advanced cancer. J Pain Sympt Manage 5(5): 320–330.

48. Farncombe M., Chater S. (1993). Case studies outlining use of nebulized morphine for patients with end-stage chronic lung and cardiac disease. J Pain Sympt Manage 8(4): 221–225.

49. Fishbein D., Kearon C., Killian K.J. (1989). An approach to dyspnea in cancer patients. J Pain Sympt Manage 4(2): 76–81.

50. Allard P., Lamontagne C., Bernard P., Tremblay C. (1999). How effective are supplementary doses of opioids for dyspnea in terminally ill cancer patients? A randomized continuous sequential clinical trial. J Pain Sympt Manage 17(4): 256–265.

51. Kaiko R.F.,Wallenstein S.L., Rogers A.G., et al. (1982). Narcotics in the elderly. Med Clin N Am 66(5): 1079–1089.

52. Sjogren P. (1993). Myoclonic spasms during treatment with high doses of intravenous morphine in renal failure. Pain 55(1): 93–97.

53. Popp B., Portenoy R.K. (1996). Management of chronic pain in the elderly: pharmacology of opioids and other analgesic drugs. In: B.R. Ferrell and B.A. Ferrell (eds.). Pain in the Elderly. Pp. 21–34. Seattle: IASP Press.

54. Derby S., Portenoy R. (1997). Assessment and management of opioid-induced constipation. In: Topics in Palliative Care (R.K. Portenoy and E. Bruera, eds.). Vol. 1, pp. 95–112. New York: Oxford University Press.

55. Farrell M.J., Katz B., Helme R.D. (1996). The impact of dementia on the pain experience. Pain 67: 7–15.

56. Hurley A.C., Volicer B.J., Hanrahan P.A., et al. (1992). Assessment of discomfort in advanced alzheimer patients. Res Nurs Health 15:369–377.

57. Porter F.L., Malhotra K.M., Wolf C.M., et al. (1996). Dementia and response to pain in the elderly. Pain 68(2-3): 413–421.

58. Sengstaken E.A., King S.A. (1993). The problem of pain and its detection among geriatric nursing home residents. J Am Geriatr Soc 41: 541–544.

59. Stein W.M., Ferrell B.A. (1996). Pain in the nursing home. Clin Geriatr Med 12(3): 601–613.

60. Kaasalainen S., Middleton J., Knezacek S., et al. (1998). Pain and cognitive status in the institutionalized elderly: Perceptions and interventions. J Gerontol Nurs 24(8): 24–31.

61. Parmelee A. (1996). Pain in cognitively impaired older persons. Clin Geriatr Med 12(3): 473–487.

62. Ferrell B.A., Ferrell B.R., Rivera L. (1995). Pain in cognitively impaired nursing home patients. J Pain Sympt Manage 10(8):591–598.

63. Ferrell B.R., Grant M., Chan J, Ahn C, Ferrell B.A. (1995). The impact of cancer pain education on family caregivers of elderly patients. Oncol Nurs Forum 22: 1211–1218.

64. McGrath P.J., Rosmus C., Campbell M.A., et al. (1998). Behaviours caregivers use to determine pain in non-verbal, cognitively-impaired individuals. Dev Med Child Neurol 40: 340–343.

65. Breitbart W., Bruera E., Chochinov H., Lynch M. (1995) Neuropsychiatric syndromes and psychological symptoms in patients with advanced cancer. J Pain Sympt Manage 10: 121–141.

66. Foreman M.D. (1993). Acute confusion in the elderly. Annu Rev Nurs Res 11: 3–30.

67. Lipowski Z. (1990). Delirium in geriatric patients. In: Delirium: Acute Confusional States. Pp. 413–441. New York: Oxford University Press.

68. Inouye S., Charpentier P.A., et al. (1996). Precipitating factors for delirium in hospitalized elderly persons: Predictive model and interrelationship with baseline vulnerability. JAMA 275: 852–857.

69. Finlayson R.E., Hurt R.D., Davis L.J., et al. (1988). Alcoholism in elderly persons: A study of the psychiatric and psychosocial features of 216 inpatients. Mayo Clin Proc 63(8): 761–768.

70. Folstein M.F., Folstein S.E., McHugh P.E. (1975). "Mini-Mental Status": A practical method for yielding the cognitive state of patients for clinicians. J Psych Res 12: 189–198.

71. Costa P.T., William T.F., Somerfield M., et al. (1996). Recognition and Initial Assessment of Alzheimer's Disease and Related Dementias. Clinical Practice Guideline No. 19. Pub. No. 97-0702. Rockville, MD: U.S. Department of Health and Human Services, Public Health Service, Agency for Health Care Policy and Research.

72. Breitbart W., Jacobsen P.B. (1996). Psychiatric symptom management in terminal care. Clin Geriatr Med 12(2): 329–347.

34 End-of-Life Decision Making in Pediatric Oncology

PAMELA S. HINDS, LINDA OAKES, and WAYNE FURMAN

We could have continued with the standard drugs which I'm not too crazy about because she has side effects and the side effects are unpleasant for her. And she can't be cured, so why do it? Why be miserable for what time you have to live? We were given the option of experimental drugs, which are just that. I would have considered them but she wanted to come home. So it's kind of like, we've devoted the last eight months to cure and now she's doing what she wants to do.

—Mother of a 15-year-old with incurable leukemia who decided to end all treatment efforts and instead take her daughter home to die

Ending a life . . . ending a child's life . . . deciding to end a child's life . . . involving a child in deciding to end his life. As startling as those phrases may be, we in pediatric oncology participate in those considerations with parents, patients, and other members of the health care team as a part of providing the highest-quality care for the child or adolescent with incurable cancer. Participating in end-of-life decisions is life-altering for the child or adolescent and for the family, but it can also be life-altering for the health care provider. Clinical anecdotes suggest that the way in which patients, family members, and health care providers complete end-of-life decision making can color all of their preceding treatment-related interactions, and may influence how well parents emotionally survive the dying and death of their child. The manner in which end-of-life decision-making processes are completed may also contribute to the survival of health care providers as compassionate and fully competent professionals.

Despite the significant immediate and longer-term impact of participating in end-of-life decision making for a child or adolescent with incurable cancer, there are no guidelines for making or for facilitating such decisions. Preparation for participating in end-of-life decision making is rarely a formal part of a health care provider's education and is rarely addressed in preceptoring or mentoring relationships. There is clearly a great need for information that can be used to develop such guidelines. The purposes of this chapter are (*1*) to offer a review of the current literature (both clinical and research-based) on end-of-life decision making in pediatrics, with a special emphasis on pediatric oncology and (*2*) to propose guidelines for the use of health care professionals in assisting children, adolescents, their parents, and other health care professionals in making such decisions. Table 34–1 defines key terms used in this chapter.

BACKGROUND

Advances in pediatric oncology have significantly increased the survival rates of patients during the past decade. The disease once thought to be universally fatal for children and adolescents is now viewed as a life-threatening, chronic illness that is potentially curable for many.[1–3] With these advances come more treatment options and more treatment-related decisions for patients, their parents, and their health care providers.[4] Although certain decisions, such as whether to have a permanent venous access device implanted, and which type to use, are made early in treatment, parents and health care providers report that the most challenging decision making in pediatric oncology occurs when efforts to cure the cancer have failed.[5] A few parents report that end-of-life decision making was not complicated for them because they had already decided what they would do *if* their child's cancer did not respond to treatment. However, the majority of parents and health care providers involved in the decision process describe this time as extraordinarily difficult. They attribute the difficulty to multiple and complex factors that must be considered, including the differing preferences of those involved in the actual decision making or affected by it, and to intense emotions at a time when the parents' energy is depleted.

NEONATAL AND OTHER PEDIATRIC SPECIALTIES

End-of-life decision making in pediatric oncology has been influenced by clini-

Table 34–1. Key Terms Used in This Chapter

Term	Definition
Decision	The final choice between two or more treatment-related options
Phase I study	The initial stage of human testing of a drug, in which the the maximum tolerated dose is established; in oncology, the subjects are usually patients who have refractory disease
Do not resuscitate	An order written in the medical record directing that no cardiopulmonary resuscitation is to be performed in the case of an acute event such as cardiac, respiratory, or neurological decompensation
Withdrawal of life-support	Stopping a life-sustaining medical treatment such as mechanical ventilator therapy, pharmacological support of blood pressure, or dialysis, after it has been initiated
Life-sustaining medical treatment	Interventions that may not control the patient's disease but may prolong the patient's life; these may include not only ventilator support, dialysis, and vasoactive infusions, but also antibiotics, insulin, chemotherapy, and nutrition and hydration provided by tubes and intravenous lines
Supportive care	Comfort measures that exclude curative efforts but could include symptom management such as pain relief and hydration or symptom prevention such as limited blood product support

cal and research reports from neonatal and other pediatric specialties and organizations. The growing commitment by professional associations to include pediatric patients and parents in end-of-life decisions marks a notable shift in care philosophy. Expectations that patients and their parents should be involved in these decisions have been formalized in policy statements of organizations such as the American Academy of Pediatrics,[6] the American Nurses Association,[7] the American Association of Critical Care Nurses,[8] and the United Hospital Fund in its report on end-of-life care in New York.[9] In these published statements, the recommended patient and parental involvement is described as participative and mutual with health care providers. Legislative rulings and legal decisions in some states and Canadian provinces support the participation of adolescents or mature minors in medical decision making and in creating advance directives.[10–14]

The actual extent to which patients and parents participate in end-of-life decision making varies and can be influenced by the personal and professional preferences of the health care provider.[15,16] For example, the way the health care provider frames or words information about treatment options may influence the way a patient and family perceive the available alternatives.[17,18] Some advocate that the physician should assume the final responsibility for the decision,[19–21] whereas others believe that the parents should be the primary decision maker.[22–24] Yet another view, which is not espoused by many authors, is that the adolescent patient should be the primary decision maker, with his or her parents serving as a consultant.[25] Even fewer sources advocate that children should be the primary decision makers, but several advocate that children as young as 6[26] or 7[10] should be involved in the decision making.

The available reports on end-of-life decision making that involves parents and health care providers are predominantly from neonatal settings. End-of-life decisions in these settings often reflect the presenting condition of the infant. The decisions primarily considered include (*1*) limiting care, (2) withdrawing life-support, or (3) withholding life-support for infants who are extremely premature or have severe congenital abnormalities.[27–32] Most reports describe the decision making as having been initiated when the intensivist determined that the infant had no chance for survival or no chance for quality of life. In most cases parents agreed with the recommendations of the intensivist or the infant's attending physician. These descriptive reports are based on review of medical records. No information was obtained from parents about the factors they considered when making an end-of-life decision on behalf of their infant.

Two notable exceptions exist. In the first, Able-Boon and colleagues[33] interviewed parents and health care providers of seriously ill infants regarding medical decision making and the provision of health care information. The parents emphasized their need and desire to be honestly informed of their child's health status. They expressed special appreciation of health care professionals who drew pictures to convey technical information rather than relying only on words. Parents also expressed a strong need for information that is coordinated by the health care team so that it is not confusing or contradictory.

The second study that recorded the values of parents in end-of-life decisions is the grounded-theory study in which Rushton[34] interviewed 31 parents of 20 hospitalized neonates with life-threatening congenital disorders about their decisions for or against implementing or continuing life-sustaining measures for their infants. Rushton concluded that the parents made these decisions based on their understanding of what it means to be a "good parent" for a neonate with a life-threatening congenital disorder. According to these parents, the characteristics of good parents for such neonates include putting the needs of the neonate first, not giving up, not taking the "easy" way out despite the self-sacrifice involved, and courage to pursue a "good" outcome for the child.

Reviews of the medical records of patients who have died in pediatric intensive care units (PICUs) show that withdrawal of life-support was chosen in 8% to 32% of cases,[35–37] and that limitation of supportive care (described as not escalating care efforts but providing hydration and pain comfort measures) was chosen in 26% to 46% of cases.[35,37] The wide range of these percentages may reflect cultural, ethnic, or religious differences: the lowest rate of withdrawal of life-support reported was from a PICU in Malaysia and the highest rates were from PICUs in Europe, the United States, and the United Kingdom. Even within a single PICU setting, decision making can reflect cultural differences. For example, the report from the Malaysian setting noted that Muslim parents declined end-of-life options at significantly higher rates than did non-Muslim parents.[35]

PARTICIPATION OF CHILDREN AND ADOLESCENTS

Children and adolescents have not routinely been involved in making end-of-life decisions on their own behalf, largely because of doubt on the part of parents and health care providers that the child or adolescent has sufficient understanding of the clinical situation.[38–41] This doubt is based in part on adults' belief that children and adolescents are unable to appraise their well-being and are unaware of their life goals and values.[22] Buchanan and Brock[38] described children who are 9 or more years of age as competent to make certain decisions, but they did not study children's competence in end-of-life decision making. The same authors also indicated that children of that age may be competent to make some decisions but not others and that competence thus depends on the specific decision. According to Ariff and Groh,[42] a child's competence to make medical decisions is an ongoing developmental process that parallels other cognitive, moral, and emotional processes and is influenced by environment and by physical and mental illness. The capacity to make an end-of-life decision cannot be determined, then, on the basis of the child's or adolescent's competence in a different situation or decision. Instead, competence must be determined for each specific decision at a defined time point and under specific circumstances.[10] Recent cognitive studies on adolescent decision making indicate that although adolescents are able to make decisions, they may be unaware of all possible options or may be unable to identify all possible consequences of those options.[43] Therefore, adolescents may need assistance in identifying, considering, and selecting end-of-life options.

Experiencing a life-threatening illness like cancer and seeing others suffer and die from it may help a child to understand death and his or her own end-of-life circumstances.[14,44,45] Although they acknowledged that the competence to participate in decision making differs with age and cognitive abilities, Burns and Truog[45] recommended that children and adolescents be involved early in the process of medical decision making, including end-of-life decisions. In fact, Burns and Truog warned that if a child or adolescent is not involved early in the decision-making process, his or her ability to express an opinion may be lost before it can be exercised.

Our combined clinical and research experiences have convinced us that as a general rule, seriously ill patients aged 10 years and older are able to understand that they are participating in decisions about their cancer-related treatment and their lives, and are able to understand the options and the likely outcomes. Of course, some younger patients may also understand these issues and be competent to participate in end-of-life decisions, whereas some older patients may be less competent. Because of these very possible differences in understanding, each child needs to be individually assessed for his or her competence to participate. An assumption that a child is or is not competent to participate made without the assessment is not in the child's best interest.

Others have provided compelling support for the involvement of younger children in end-of-life decision making. Nitschke and colleagues[26] reported that patients as young as 6 years of age participated in end-of-life discussions in their pediatric oncology treatment setting. They described care conferences held with 43 families over a six-year period in which children and adolescents with end-stage cancer, and their families, participated in discussions of therapeutic options, disease progression, lack of effective therapies, improbability of cure, and imminent death. The patients (who were 6 to 20 years of age) and their parents were offered the choice of Phase II investigational drugs or supportive care. According to this report, it was the patients who most frequently made the final decision. Fourteen chose further chemotherapy, 28 chose supportive care only, and 1 made no decision. Nitschke and colleagues also noted that patients younger than age 9 understood that they were going to die soon of their disease. The authors concluded that children with cancer do have an advanced understanding of death and recommended that children as young as 5 years of age have the capacity to make decisions about whether to continue therapy. This team did not investigate the specific factors considered by the patients, parents, and health care providers and did not describe ways in which providers may have attempted to facilitate patient and parent decision making.

A health care team member who has established a relationship of trust with the child or adolescent and who has observed the child or adolescent in various challenging clinical situations is likely to be the best judge of competence in end-of-life decision making. However, before initiating this assessment, the health care team should discuss the purpose and process of the assessment, first as a group and then with the patient's parent or parents, and identify any areas of actual or potential disagreement between the team and the parents. Disagreements should be openly discussed, and participants should be allowed sufficient time to weigh the issues—another reason for initiating the end-of-life discussions in a timely manner. After the team and the parents agree on the intent and timing of the competence assessment, the team member, parent(s), and child or adolescent choose the location for the discussion. Most children younger than eleven years of age prefer to have their parents present for this discussion.

Determining the child or adolescent's competence requires establishing whether he or she understands the seriousness of the medical condition and understands that a decision point is at hand. If asked to explain the seriousness of the situation, the child or adolescent will use words or describe events that have personal symbolic or literal meaning. The health care team can then use these same words to communicate with the patient about decision making. Throughout the assessment, the child or adolescent will need reassurance from the health care team member that the serious situation is not the fault of the child or adolescent.[47] The child or adolescent must also be able to indicate an understanding of the choices, including the potential consequences of each. In addition, the child or adolescent must show an understanding of how each choice made now could change future options. As McCabe and colleagues[13] emphasized, the health care team member conducting the assessment must ensure that the child or adolescent does not feel coerced to make a certain choice. The team member should also ensure that the child or adolescent has access to the information needed to make a competent decision.[48] It is especially important that the team member assess to what extent the child or adolescent wants to be included in the decision making. That preference should be honored regardless of the personal preferences of team members.

Our experience is that children (some as young as 7 years of age) have definite preferences regarding whether to participate in a Phase I clinical trial. Preferences most commonly reflect a desire to be home, to play with a sibling or a friend, or to not feel sickly. Preferences regarding do-not-resuscitate status, although quite firmly expressed by some adolescents, tend to require more patient contemplation time. By the time this kind of end-of-life decision making needs to be considered, the members of the health care team are very familiar with the child and the family and already have established a style of interacting. However, it is generally useful to preface the assessment of patient preference with a statement that conveys the important nature of what is about to be said, such as, "May I ask you to be quite serious with me for a few moments? I want to tell you something important about your [insert here the term used by the child when referring to the illness]. And I want you to tell me something, too." If the child conveys an inability to be serious at that moment, the team member needs to clarify whether that means the child only wants the "serious and important" topics to be discussed with the child's family, or if it means the child wants to try to be serious at a later time.

COMPETENCE OF SURROGATES

Concern about patients' competence to participate in end-of-life decisions, although valid, may sometimes be exaggerated. As Levetown and Carter[48] wrote, it is relatively easy to usurp the autonomy of children and adolescents in end-of-life decision making. This threat lends special importance to the use of guidelines for making end-of-life decisions. Guidelines could serve as formal reminders to health care professionals to consider the preferences of children and adolescents to the extent that is possible or advisable. Of equal or greater concern is the competence of parents and health care providers to make such decisions on behalf of the child or adolescent. Making these decisions competently requires an understanding of their own values, the patient's values and goals, the treatment options, the likely outcome of each option, and the nature of the life-threatening illness. This imposes a short-term and a longer-term burden of unknown proportions on the parents and the health care providers.

There are few empirically based or theoretically based guidelines for involving children, adolescents, or their parents in end-of-life decisions. Instead, it is generally assumed that children younger than age 10 are not competent to participate in such decision making *and* that their parents are both competent and attentive to the best interests of their child.[13,22,46] This assumption is crucial, because it tends to ensure that end-of-life decisions are made for seriously ill children and adolescents by their parents and health care professionals. The role of parents as surrogates in this circumstance is supported by legal rulings and common health care practices; it is rarely challenged, and health care providers or others replace parental authority only in exceptional circumstances.[46] In order to feel competent, to be competent, and to be satisfied with their performance as surrogate decision makers, parents and health care providers need opportunities to exchange information about the child's preferences, the family's preferences, the child's chances of survival, and the progression of the disease. They also need to reflect on previous efforts to achieve cure and to question previous decisions.

PARTICIPATION OF PATIENTS AND PARENTS

Previous studies indicate that the more informed parents become about their seriously ill child's condition, the more they are able to participate in making decisions and advocating for their child.[49,50] Parents report that information is most helpful when it is provided gradually and repeatedly.[51] Stevens[52] recommends that parents be allowed to make tape recordings or bring friends or family members to the treatment-related discussions to help them later recall the details of the discussion. Other investigators suggest that parents differ in how much detailed information they desire[53] and in how much they want to participate in the actual decision making[54] during periods of crisis in their child's illness. However, parental preferences about participation in end-of-life decision making have not been well-studied.

In an international feasibility study, parents from pediatric oncology settings in Australia, Hong Kong, and the United States were interviewed about their decision making on behalf of their ill child. There were clear differences among the countries in parental preference for involvement in decision making. Mothers in Hong Kong were reluctant to participate in end-of-life decisions because of either their gender ("Women cannot make these decisions") or their lack of expert knowledge ("I am only the mother. The doctor is the expert and he should decide").[55] It remains unknown whether these parental preferences change between diagnosis and end of life. Regardless of their preference, all parents need reassurance from the health care team that their child's condition is not their fault.[52]

The factors that parents consider at decision points in the treatment of their seriously ill child have only recently been studied. Using a phenomenological approach, Kirschbaum[56] interviewed 20 parents of children who had died in the previous 6 to 12 months. The parents had all made life-support decisions on behalf of their ill child. A variety of diagnoses were represented, including trauma, cancer, septic shock, liver failure, and congestive heart disease. Nine factors were identified as having influenced the parental decisions: (*1*) wanting life as the principal good for their child, (*2*) avoiding suffering and pain, (*3*) considering current and future quality of life, (*4*) respecting the individuality of the child, (*5*) defining and redefining the family, (*6*) having spiritual beliefs and explanations, (*7*) believing in natural or biological explanations, (*8*) considering the child's unique personality, and (*9*) having a favorable view of technology in health care.

In a retrospective study that conducted telephone interviews with 39 parents of 37 pediatric oncology patients who had died in the previous 6 to 24 months, Hinds and colleagues[5] were able to identify the factors most frequently considered by parents in end-of-life decision making. The end-of-life decisions that were reported most frequently by these parents were choosing between a Phase I drug study and no further treatment (n = 14), maintaining or withdrawing life support (n = 11), and giving more chemotherapy or ending treatment (n = 8). The factor most considered in the parents' decision making was "information received from health care professionals." This information included facts, explanations, and opinions about their child's disease status, likelihood of survival, and complexities of continued care. Other factors parents frequently reported were "feeling supported by and trusting of the staff," which reflected the parents' sense that the health care team listened and responded to their or their child's concerns and respected the parents' decisions, and "making decisions together with my child." This factor reflected the parents' comfort in having known and respected their child's wishes.

The parents also completed a 15-item questionnaire about the importance of each factor considered in their decision making. The parents rated eight items as "very important" at least 50% of the time. The highest rated factors included "recommendations received from health care professionals," "things my child had said about continuing or not continuing treatment," "information received from healthcare professionals," "my child's breathing problems," and "sensing that my child was no longer himself (herself)." These findings clearly indicate that information and recommendations received from health care professionals are very important to parents who are making end-of-life decisions on behalf of their child, as is feeling certain of their child's desires about treatment.

The same research team has prospectively studied end-of-life decision making by conducting interviews of parents, physicians, and, when possible, the children or adolescents with incurable disease who had participated in making an end-of-life decision within the past week. The same factors noted in the retrospective study—related to trust, support, information, and advice—were also identified in the prospective study.

Case Study: A Decision Agreement Between Parents and the Health Care Team

A 12-month-old infant girl has been treated for an aggressive form of leukemia. It is clear that the disease is not responding to the chemotherapy. She was transferred to the pediatric intensive care unit when she began to experience respiratory distress. Initially, oxygen was administered by simple mask but her breathing difficulties persisted and became more evident within a few hours. The possibility of endotracheal intubation was first discussed among the health care team members and then with the parents. During the meeting with the parents, the current symptoms of the little girl were discussed, the current disease status and its unresponsiveness to treatment were reviewed, and options of intubating or not intubating were considered. The parents then discussed the options privately with each other and in less than 30 minutes reached the decision that ventilatory support not be a part of their daughter's medical care. The parents' stated that knowing that their daughter was not going to be cured of the leukemia and understanding that the ventilator would help reduce their daughter's respiratory distress but not the leukemia were both factors that assisted them in making the decision. They credited their discussions with the doctors as key: "From the discussion we had with the doctors, we felt if it came to that point the only reason for using a ventilator would be just to keep her breathing." An additional factor identified by the parents as influencing their decision making was support from the health care team. "Chaplain X and Dr. Y were real patient with us and understood the situation that we were in and did not seem to put pressure one way or another, or seem to think that we were making the wrong decision one way or another . . . they told us the decision was actually ours. They let us know that, but they were supportive and also gave us their opinions."

In addition, parents cited these factors: wishing for the child's survival, reassuring themselves of the correctness of their decisions, questioning certain statements or behaviors of health care professionals, and making decisions that would allow them to maintain communication with their dying child for as long as possible (Table 34–2).

Case Study: Disagreement

An adolescent with incurable cancer had been hospitalized for three weeks, the past 8 days in the intensive care unit. His physical deterioration and suffering had created anguish in his father and in the health care

Table 34–2. Guidelines for the Health Care Team to Use in Assisting Parents with End-of-Life Decision Making

1. At the time of diagnosis and throughout treatment, actively seek opportunities to provide information to the parent about treatment and the patient's response to treatment.
2. At the time of diagnosis and throughout treatment, involve the parent in treatment-related discussions and decision making. Be available to discuss and rediscuss decisions and related concerns.
3. Encourage parents to talk with parents of other pediatric oncology patients.
4. Verbally and nonverbally reassure the parents that they are "good" parents who are committed to the well-being of their child.
5. Give assurances that everything that can be done to help the patient is being done and being done well.
6. As the child's disease progresses, provide clear verbal (and written, if desired by the parent) explanations of the child's status.
7. Inform parents of treatment options as they become available in the treating institution or elsewhere.
8. Include more than one health care team member in end-of-life discussions with the parents.
9. When discussing end-of-life options with parents,
   a. strongly emphasize the team's commitment to the patient's comfort and to providing expert care at all times,
   b. offer professional recommendations,
   c. describe how their child is likely to respond to each option (the child's physical appearance, ability to communicate, etc.), and
   d. give information about other support resources (ethics committees, social services, other health care professionals, etc.).
10. When discussing end-of-life options with parents, anticipate
    a. parents' vacillation between certainty and uncertainty about the decision,
    b. parents' need for clarification and additional information to resolve their uncertainties,
    c. parents' need for practical information about ways to explain the end-of-life decision to other family members, and
    d. being asked to give personal advice.
11. Allow parents private time to consider the options.
12. Maintain sensitivity to any specific ethnic, cultural, or religious preferences during the terminal stage.
13. Convey respect for the parents' right to change decisions, when clinically feasible.
14. Demonstrate commitment to maintaining the child's comfort and dignity, and to affirming the parents' role.
15. Do not question the parents' decision after it has been made.

team. The attending physician discussed with the father the likelihood of the adolescent having a cardiac arrest, described the actions the team would take for a full resuscitation as well as the varying levels of resuscitation approved by the treatment setting, which included a do-not-resuscitate option, and asked the father to express his preferences regarding resuscitation. The father initially chose the do-not-resuscitate status for his son and completed all of the official paperwork to implement that decision. During the next 12 hours, the father actively solicited from nursing and medical staff their definitions of do-not-resuscitate. He then contacted the attending physician to rescind his decision, choosing instead to have a full resuscitation order in place. He explained his decision change as, "When I saw that the nurses and doctors did not all define resuscitation in the same way, I decided that I would not leave that in their hands. I am my son's father and I will be his father to the end." This new decision was enacted and over the next four days, the young patient showed clear signs of dying. His father stayed with him in the intensive care unit and witnessed the changes in his son's physical appearance. He began commenting on those changes and on his son's obvious suffering. Within two hours of his son's death, the father told the nurse that he did not want his son to be resuscitated. This information was immediately conveyed to the health care team and a brief discussion with the physician, father, and nurse was convened to affirm this decision.

Ten patients participated in individual interviews about the end-of-life decision they had made. The factors most frequently considered in their decisions included "information from my doctor or my parents," "wanting to be done with treatment," and "worrying about my family." These factors convey the interconnectedness between children or adolescents with incurable disease and their families and health care providers. All are affected by the decision-making process and the outcomes of the decision. This interconnectedness among the seriously ill child or adolescent, the family, and the health care providers contributes to more agreements on end-of-life decisions than disagreements. Although rare, disagreements between the patient and parent, or between parents and health care providers, do occur and are especially difficult for all involved. Disagreeing with a health care professional who is deemed essential for their child's well-being and with whom a care alliance is desired is at best troubling for parents, but at worst, disruptive to relationships and problem solving. When circumstances exist that allow a delay in the contested decision making, a consultation with an ethicist or ethics board can facilitate consensus making. Involving the family, the patient who is deemed competent to participate in end-of-life decision making, and the health care team in the same meeting with the ethicist or ethics board is particularly helpful, as all perspectives can be considered. When a family and a health care team do not have agreement, special measures must be initiated by the team leaders to support team members in their efforts to continue to deliver excellent care to the patient and family. Measures can include brief meetings with an esteemed institutional leader who openly acknowledges the sizable difficulty that the team is facing, having information-sharing or cathartic sessions with the ethicist, and developing strategies for handling similar future difficulties. Likewise, similar support measures need to be implemented for the family. In addition, regular opportunities to interact with the health care team (such as care conferences) need to be established so that trust between the family and team can be fostered.

Case Study: Involving an Ethicist to Assist a Team in Anticipation of, During, or after an End-of-Life Decision

A 7-year-old boy had a second recurrence of acute lymphoblastic leukemia. His leukemia was first diagnosed when he was 19 months old. The first recurrence occurred less than a year after completing the three-year treatment protocol, and the second recurrence occurred 8 months after completing the treatment for relapsed leukemia. As his mother pointed out to the treating team, her son had had very few months in his life of feeling healthy. She conveyed reluctance to continue any curative efforts, preferring instead to have her son discharged from the inpatient unit so that she could take him home. The attending physician, an internationally recognized expert in the treatment of leukemia, strongly disagreed with the mother's stated preference and offered her information on the likelihood of cure (admittedly low) and emphasized his desire to continue curative efforts. When the mother firmly declined the option of further treatment, the physician told the mother that he considered the discharge to be "against medical orders" and noted that in the medical record. A nurse on the team later approached the physician and proposed a meeting with the team and an ethicist to discuss the decision. The physician agreed and the full team met a week later with an ethicist. The physician honestly acknowledged his sadness about the child's incurable disease, his liking of the child, and his concern that because the mother disagreed with his recommendation of further treatment, the health care team might think less of him as a physician. The team and the ethicist reacted with surprise at the last admission and conveyed instead their strong respect for him and his efforts to be a good doctor and for the mother's efforts to be a good parent. The physician offered to write a letter to the mother expressing the team's support of her and her child and that the child would always have complete access to all of the care setting's resources. The mother telephoned the physician after receiving the letter to express her relief. Three weeks later, the mother brought her son to the hospital to die.

FACTORS CONSIDERED BY HEALTH CARE PROVIDERS

The factors considered by health care professionals in end-of-life decision making on behalf of children and adolescents reveal important similarities and differences between nurses and physicians. Current reports indicate that nurses are more likely to reflect on the moral balance of the decision, i.e., the goodness or lack thereof of extending a child's life if doing so also extends or increases the child's suffering,[57] whereas physicians first consider whether the child's life can be saved.[5] This difference can create tension within the health care team and merits discussion by the team members. Nurses and physicians also identified a factor they both consider frequently in end-of-life decision making for pediatric oncology patients: "respecting the patient's and family's preferences." This factor reflected the health care professionals' efforts to inform the patient and family of all options and then to respect the choice they made. In a survey completed by 21 health care professionals in pediatric oncology (16 physicians, 3 nurses, and 2 chaplains) regarding end-of-life decisions for patients with incurable cancer, the factors rated as most important included "discussions with the family of the patient," "thinking the patient would never get any better," "the belief that nothing else could help the patient," and "things the patient had said about continuing or not continuing treatment." Most of the participating health care professionals also indicated that they did not make end-of-life decisions alone but sought the input of other team members.[5]

STRATEGIES FOR FACILITATING CHILD, ADOLESCENT, AND PARENT INVOLVEMENT

End-of-life decision making is a process that very likely begins at the time of diagnosis, when the patient and the parents are exposed to the seriousness of the illness, the possible risks of treatment, and the uncertainty of short-term and long-term treatment outcomes. When faced with the actual decision-making, a few parents and patients express a preference seemingly without hesitation or anguish. They are likely to have gained an earlier understanding of the situation; often, patients and parents who observe others undergoing end-of-life experiences begin to reflect on their own life values. More often, however, patients and parents require time to think after becoming aware of the impending decision point and treatment options.[20] In both the briefer and longer contemplation periods, the decision-making capability evolved as treatment continued and understanding of the patient's situation increased. As noted in the American Academy of Pediatrics guidelines on forgoing life-sustaining treatment,[58] end-of-life decision making is not a single event or one well-defined point in time.

It is essential that health care providers realize that the end-of-life decision-making process begins early in treatment and evolves with each interaction between the provider, the patient, and the parent, and with each observation of or encounter with other seriously ill patients and their parents (see Fig. 34–1). Each interaction provides an opportunity for the health care provider to build the patient's and family's trust in him or her as a source of information and support and as a care expert who can be relied on to do what is best for the patient.[5] Each interaction is also an opportunity for the provider to facilitate parents' efforts to function fully as parents—a role that becomes increasingly uncertain as parents deal with unfamiliar decisions. Feeling competent in their parenthood is especially crucial to parents who face end-of-life decisions on behalf of their child. Believing that they have acted as "good parents" in such a situation is likely to be very important to their emotional recovery from the dying and death of their child.

Decision making by patients and parents is influenced not only by their interactions with the health care team but also by the impressions they form through observations of and encounters with other patients and families in the care setting. As patients and parents learn about the treatment experiences and the positive or negative outcomes of other patients, they contemplate what it would be like to experience those situations themselves. A second type of personal experience that prompts this kind

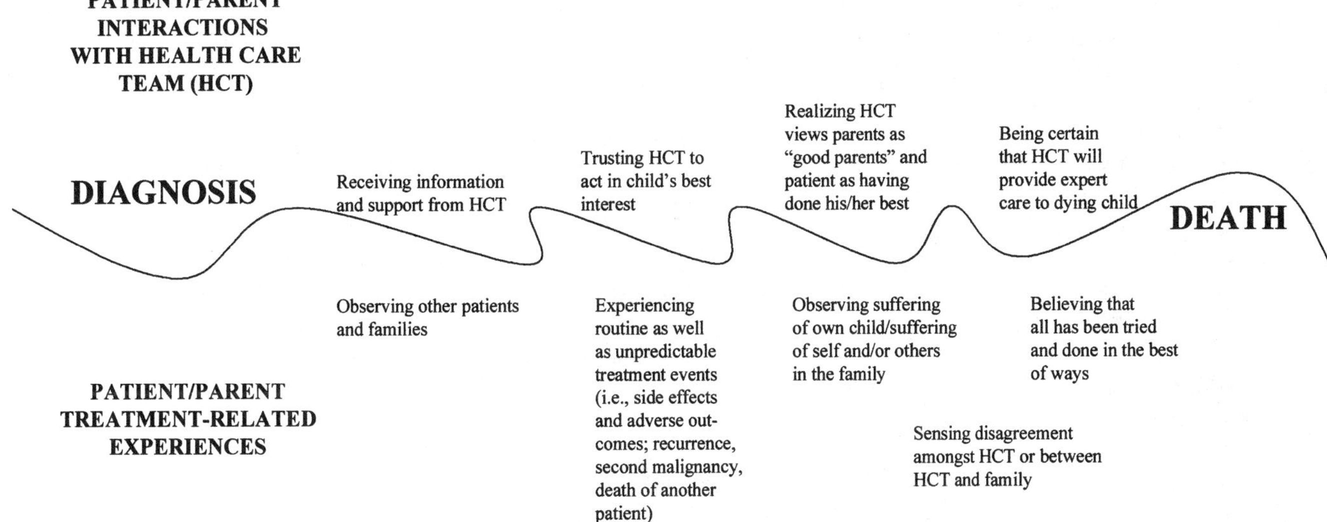

Fig. 34–1. The interactions and experiences of pediatric oncology patients, their parents, and the members of their health care team (HCT) from the point of diagnosis forward that influence end-of-life decision making.

of reflection is an unexpected negative response to treatment, such as an adverse reaction or even disease progression, after positive responses. When patients and parents feel well-informed by health care team members about disease response to treatment and are routinely involved in treatment discussions and other decisions, they are being prepared for end-of-life decision making, should it become necessary.

A third experience that prepares the patient and parents for end-of-life decision making is the patient's experience of suffering and the parent's experience of witnessing that suffering and being unable to adequately relieve it. In our research with parents of children and adolescents who are experiencing a first or second recurrence of cancer, parents and guardians are more likely to contemplate ending curative efforts when they see their child in pain, unable to enjoy favorite activities, places, and people, or unable to find comfort.[53] Parents may react to the same experiences in different—even opposite—ways. The mother of a child treated for acute lymphocytic leukemia wrote in her guide for parents, friends, and health care providers that an end-of-life decision is an "intensely personal decision."[59] Some parents seek to exhaust all possible treatments, whereas others hope only for sufficient time to prepare themselves and their child for the dying and death. A study by Hollen and Brickle[60] suggested that the socioeconomic status of parents of well adolescents helps to predict the quality of the parents' decision making about their teenaged children. However, no similar data are available that identify relationships between characteristics of parents whose child is seriously ill and their end-of-life decisions on behalf of their child.

THE NURSE'S ROLE

The American Nurses Association's Position Statement on Nursing and the Pa-

Table 34–3. Guidelines for the Health Care Team to Use in Assisting Each Other with End-of-Life Decision Making

1. Know the guidelines offered by specific disciplines regarding roles in end-of-life decision making (i.e. the American Nurses Association's official statements on what the nurse is expected to do to help parents and patients make decisions), as it is possible that the guidelines differ from expectations held by others outside the discipline.
2. Before initiating end-of-life discussions with patients* and parents, all members of the health care team should discuss and agree on
   a. the need for such a discussion,
   b. which options are appropriate and available,
   c. whether outside consultants, such as an ethics committee or external oncology expert, are needed to identify which options are in the best interest of the patient,
   d. which other team members will participate in the discussion with the parents and patient,
   e. the time of the discussion and specific staff members who will participate,
   f. which staff member will document the discussions in the medical record, and
   g. availability of the appropriate staff time and resources to address any questions parents and patients may have. Communicate to the team members who were not present at the patient and parent discussion what specific language was used to provide support to the parents and patient in making this decision.
3. Be available to team members and to the patient and parents to discuss and rediscuss decisions and related concerns.
4. Explore with the team all appropriate options to ensure that all that can be done is being done and being done well.
5. Inform other team members if feedback from or assessment of the patient, parents, or both indicates that any decision needs clarification or reconsideration.

* When considering whether the patient should be present during such discussions, evaluate the developmental stage of the patient and the severity of illness and symptoms at the time of the discussion.

tient Self-Determination Act[7] asserts that nurses have a professional responsibility to facilitate informed decision making by patients about end-of-life options. The statement does not specify patient age, but other wording, such as that describing the nurse's responsibility for knowing state laws about advance directives, suggests that the statement is oriented toward adult patients. The document also asserts that the nurse is responsible for ensuring that advance directives are current and reflect the patient's choices. The ANA makes equally explicit assertions about the nurse's role in its position statement "Nursing Care and Do-Not-Resuscitate Decisions."[7] That position statement urges nurses to assume principal responsibility for ensuring that competent patients' preferences regarding resuscitation are honored, even if those preferences conflict with those of other health care professionals and family members. Nurses are further urged to facilitate explicit discussions of the resuscitation order with the patient, family members, and health care team, and to document the decisions clearly.

Several general studies about how nurses, physicians, and other health care team members perceive end-of-life decision making have revealed differences in role responsibilities and interpretations of care priorities.[30,61–65] These differences contribute to tension among team members. It is important that team members be aware of official statements issued by each discipline's professional association about role expectations. For example, the Guidelines on Forgoing Life-Sustaining Medical Treatment issued by the American Academy of Pediatrics[6] indicates that physicians are expected to provide adequate information to patients, parents, and "other appropriate decision makers" about therapeutic options and their risks, discomforts, adverse effects, projected financial costs, potential benefits, and likelihood of success. In addition, physicians are expected to offer advice about which option to choose and to elicit questions from the patients and parents. Nurses should openly discuss expectations and team functions with other team members (Table 34–3) to prevent misunderstanding or disappointment about their perceived roles.

GUIDELINES FOR END-OF-LIFE DECISION MAKING IN PEDIATRICS

End-of-life decision making for children and adolescents who have been seriously and chronically ill necessitates consistent and careful attention to their most meaningful relationships.[66] The relationships of obvious importance are the relationship of child or adolescent with self and with family. Less obvious but also meaningful relationships are those between the patient and the health care professionals, and between the family and health care professionals (those who provide care for the child or adolescent or for the family). Because of the importance of these relationships in end-of-life decision making, separate (although overlapping) guidelines are provided addressing how members of the

Table 34–4. Guidelines for the Health Care Team to Use in Assisting Pediatric Patients with End-of-Life Decision Making

1. Seek input of parents as to the timing and extent of information that should be offered to the patient about diagnosis, treatment options, and the likely response to treatment.
2. At the time of diagnosis and throughout treatment, actively seek opportunities to provide information to the children or adolescents that is appropriate to their developmental stage.
   - For a child, assure parental presence during such discussions.
   - For an adolescent, assure a discussion that includes the parents but offer to discuss with the patient alone as well.
3. Be available to discuss and rediscuss decisions and related concerns in a manner appropriate to the developmental stage of patients.
4. With parental agreement, encourage patients to interact with other pediatric oncology patients.
5. Convey verbally and nonverbally the recognition that patients are trying their best and that the health care team is committed to the patients' well-being.
6. Give assurances that everything that can be done to help the patient is being done and being done well.
7. As a patient's disease progresses, provide clear verbal (and written, if desired by the patient) explanations of the patients' status.
8. With parental agreement, inform patients of treatment options as they become available in the treating institution or elsewhere.
9. Assess patient suffering and the need to change interventions to relieve such suffering.
10. When end-of-life options should be discussed with patients, consult parents about the appropriate depth and timing of such discussions.
11. After receiving input from the parents and exploring the patient's readiness for information, discuss the end-of-life options with:
    a. a strong emphasis on the team's commitment to the patient'comfort and to providing expert care at all times,
    b. professional recommendations,
    c. descriptions about how the the patient is likely to respond to each option (physical appearance, ability to communicate, etc.), and
    d. information about other support resources such as chaplains and ethicists.
12. Include more than one health care team member in end-of-life discussions with the patients.
13. Allow the patients private time to consider the options with their parents.
14. Reassess the appropriateness of the chosen end-of-life options on an ongoing basis, remaining aware that patients will
    a. vacillate between certainty and uncertainty about the decision, and
    b. need clarification and additional information to resolve uncertainties.
15. Convey respect for the patients' right to change decisions, when such changes are clinically feasible.
16. Maintain sensitivity to any specific ethnic, cultural, or religious preferences during the terminal stage.
17. Demonstrate continued commitment to providing symptom management, support of quality of life, and assurance of the parents' well-being.

health care team can assist parents, patients (Table 34–4), and each other in making end-of-life decisions. The overlap in the guidelines reflects the parallel, and at times interacting, decision-making processes experienced by children, adolescents, and their parents. Health care professionals will be most effective in implementing these guidelines if they first reflect on their feelings and concerns about the dying and death of children and adolescents and about participating in end-of-life decision making. Research findings to date consistently indicate that when the child or adolescent participates as fully as possible in end-of-life decision making, parents and health care providers are more certain and more comfortable about the decision that is made.[4,5,55] Their belief that the decision reflects the child's or adolescent's preferences helps parents and health care providers to make the decision and to recover emotionally from this painful experience.

The authors express sincere appreciation to Linda Watts Parker for her careful formatting of this chapter, to Erin E. Downs, S.N., for her helpful questioning, and to Sharon Naron for her thoughtful editing.

REFERENCES

1. United States Department of Education, National Center for Educational Statistics (1993). Youth Indications 1993: Trends in the Well-Being of American Youth. Washington, D.C.: Government Printing Office.

2. Karian V.E., Jankowski S.M., and Beal J.A. (1998). Exploring the lived-experience of childhood cancer survivors. J Pediatr Oncol Nurs 15(3): 153–162.

3. Kazak A.E. (1993). Psychological research in pediatric oncology (editorial). J Pediatr Psychol 18(3):313–318.

4. Hinds P., Oakes L., Quaragnenti A., Furman W., Sandlund J., Bowman L., Olson M., and Heideman R. (1998). Challenges and issues in conducting descriptive decision-making studies in pediatric oncology: A tale of two studies. J Pediatr Oncol Nurs 15(3):10–17.

5. Hinds P., Oakes L., Furman W., Foppiano P., Olson M.S., Quargnenti A., Gattuso J., Powell B., Srivastava D.K., Jayawardene D., Sandlund J.T., and Strong C. (1997). Decision making by parents and health care professionals for pediatric patients with cancer. Oncol Nurs Forum 24: 1523–1528.

6. American Academy of Pediatrics, Committee on Bioethics (1994). Guidelines on foregoing life-sustaining medical treatment. Pediatrics 93(3):532–536.

7. American Nurses Association, Task Force on the Nurse's Role in End-of-Life Decisions. (1991). Compendium of Position Statements on the Nurse's Role in End-Of-Life Decisions. Washington, D.C.: American Nurses Association, pp. 1–14.

8. Lindquist R, Banasik J, Barnsteiner J, et al. (1993). Determining AACN's research priorities for the 90's. Am J Crit Care 2:110–117.

9. Zuckerman C. and Mackinnon A. (1998). The challenge of caring for patients near the end of life: Findings from the Hospital Palliative Care Initiative. (March). United Hospital Fund of New York. New York.

10. Awong L. (1988). Ethical dilemmas: When an adolescent wants to forgo therapy. Am J Nurs 98(7):67–68.

11. Kluge E.H. (1995). Informed consent by children: The new reality. CMAJ 152(9):1495–1497.

12. Mayo T.W. (1997). Withholding and withdrawing life-sustaining care: Legal issues. In Essentials of Pediatric Intensive Care. D. Levin and F. Morriss eds. New York: Churchill Livingstone, vol. 1, pp. 1091–1103.

13. McCabe M.A., Rushton C.H., Glover J., Murray M.G., and Leikin S. (1996). Implications of the Patient Self-Determination Act: Guidelines for involving adolescents in medical decision making. J Adolesc Health 19(5):319–324.

14. Weir R.F. and Peters C. (1997). Affirming the decisions adolescents make about life and death. Hastings Center Rep 27(6):29–34.

15. Edwardson S.R. (1983). The choice between hospital and home care for terminally ill children. Nurs Res 32(1):29–34.

16. Kollef M.H. (1996). Private attending physician status and the withdrawal of life-sustaining interventions in a medical intensive care unit population. Crit Care Med 24(6): 968–975.

17. Miller D.K., Coe R.M., and Hyers T.M. (1992). Achieving consensus on withdrawing or withholding care for critically ill patients. Journal of Gen Intern Med 7:475–480.

18. Overbay J.D. (1996). Parental participants in treatment decisions for pediatric oncology ICU patients. Dimensions Crit Care Nurs 15(1): 16–24.

19. Campbell A. and McHaffie H. (1995). Prolonging life and allowing death: Infants. J Med Ethics 21:339–344.

20. Nelson L. and Nelson R. (1992). Ethics and provision of futile, harmful, or burdensome treatment to children. Crit Care Med 20:427–433.

21. Raffin T.A. (1995). Withdrawing life support: How is the decision made? JAMA 273(9): 738–739.

22. Rushton C. and Glover J (1990). Involving parents in decisions to forego life-sustaining treatment for critically ill infants and children. AACN clinical issues. Crit Care Nurs 1(1):206–214.

23. Rushton C. and Lynch M (1992). Dealing with advance directives for critically ill adolescents. Crit Care Nurs 12:31–37.

24. Zaner R.M. and Bliton M.J. (1991). Decisions in the NICU: The moral authority of parents. Child Health Center 20(1):19–25.

25. Ross L.F. (1997). Health care decision making by children: Is it in their best interest? Hastings Center Rep 27(6):41–45.

26. Nitschke R., Humphrey G., Sexauer C., Catron B., Wunder S., and Jay S. (1982). Therapeutic choices made by patients with end-stage cancer. J Pediatr 10(3):471–476.

27. Cook L.A. and Watchko J.F. (1996). Decision making for the critically ill neonate near the end of life. J Perinatol 16(2):133–136.

28. De Leeuw R., Beaufort A.J., de Kleine M.J., van Harrewijn K., and Kollee L.A. (1996). Foregoing intensive care treatment in newborn infants with extremely poor prognoses. J Pediatr 129(5):661–666.

29. Ragatz S.C. and Ellison P.H. (1983). Decisions to withdraw life support in the neonatal intensive care unit. Clin Pediatr 22(11):729–736.

30. Van der Heide A., van der Maas P.J., van der Wal G., de Graaff C.L., Kester J.G., Kollee L.A., de Leeuw R., and Holl R.A. (1997). Medical end-of-life decisions made for neonates and infants in the Netherlands. Lancet 350(9073):251–255.

31. Wall S.N. and Partridge J.C. (1997). Death in the intensive care nursery: physician practice of withdrawing and withholding life support. Pediatrics 99(1):64–70.

32. Whitelaw A. (1986). Death as an option in neonatal intensive care. Lancet 2(8502):328–331.

33. Able-Boone H., Dokecki P.R., and Smith M.S. (1989). Parent and health care provider communication and decision making in the intensive care nursery. Child Health Care 18(3):133–141.

34. Rushton C. (1994). Moral Decision Making by Parents of Infants Who Have Life-Threatening Congenital Disorders. Ph.D. dissertation, School of Nursing, Catholic University of America, Washington, D.C.

35. Goh A.Y., Lum L.C., Chan P.W., Bakar F., and Chong B.O. (1999). Withdrawal and limitation of life support in pediatric intensive care. Arch Disabled Child 80(5):424–428.

36. Lantos J.D., Berger A.C., and Zucker A.R. (1991). Do-not-resuscitate orders in a children's hospital. Crit Care Med 21:52–55.

37. Vernon D.D., Dean J.M., Timmons O.D., Banner W., and Allen-Webb E.M. Modes of death in the pediatric intensive care unit: Withdrawal and limitation of supportive care. Crit Care Med 21(11):1798–1802

38. Buchanan A. and Brock D. (1989). Deciding for Others: The Ethics of Surrogate Decision-Making. Cambridge: Cambridge University Press, 1989.

39. Foley M. (1989). Children with cancer: Ethical dilemmas. Seminars in Oncol Nurs 5(2): 109–113.

40. Weithorn L. and Campbell S. (1982). The competency of children and adolescents to make informed treatment decisions. Child Dev 53:1589.

41. President's Commission for the Study of Ethical Problems in Medicine and Biomedical and Behavioral Research. (1983). Deciding to Forego Life-Sustaining Treatment: A Report on the Ethical, Medical and Legal Issues in Treatment Decisions. Washington, D.C.: U.S. Government Printing Office.

42. Ariff J.L., Groh D.H. (1996). In the best interests of the child: Ethical issues. In Critical Care Nursing of Infants and Children. M. Curley, J. Smith, and P. Moloney-Harmon eds. Philadelphia: Saunders, pp. 126–141.

43. Beyth-Marom R. and Fischhoff B. (1997). Adolescents' decisions about risks: A cognitive perspective. In Health Risks and Developmental Transitions During Adolescence. J. Schulenberg, J. Maggs, and K. Hurrelmann eds. Cambridge: Cambridge University Press, pp. 110–135.

44. Hinds P. and Martin J. (1988). Hopefulness and the self-sustaining process in adolescents with cancer. Nurs Res 37(6):336–340.

45. Hinds P. (1990). Quality of life in children and adolescents experiencing cancer. Semin Oncol Nurs 6(4):285–291.

46. Burns J. and Truog R. (1997). Ethical controversies in pediatric critical care. New Horizons 5(1):72–84.

47. Goldman A. (1998). Life threatening illnesses and symptom control in children. In Oxford Textbook of Palliative Medicine. Second edition, D. Doyle, G. Hanks, and N. MacDonald eds. New York: Oxford University Press, pp. 1033–1043.

48. Levetown M. and Carter M (1998). Child-centered care in terminal illness: An ethical framework. In Oxford Textbook of Palliative Medicine. Second edition, D. Doyle, G. Hanks, and N. MacDonald eds. Oxford: Oxford University Press, pp. 1107–1117.

49. James L.S. and Johnson B. (1996). The needs of pediatric oncology patients during the palliative care phase. J Pediatr Oncol Nursing 14(2):85–95.

50. Martinson I.M. and Cohen M.H. (1988). Themes from a longitudinal study of family reactions to childhood cancer. J Psychosoc Oncol 6(3/4):81–98.

51. Chesler M.A. and Barbarin O.A. (1984). Difficulties of providing help in a crisis: Relationships between parents and children with cancer and their friends. J Soc Issues 40:113–134.

52. Stevens M.M. (1998). Care of the dying child and adolescent: Family adjustment and support. In Oxford Textbook of Palliative Medicine. Second edition, D. Doyle, G. Hanks, and N. MacDonald, eds. Oxford: Oxford University Press, pp. 1057–1075.

53. Hinds P.S., Birenbaum L., Clarke-Steffen L., Quargnenti A., Kreissman S., Kazak A., Meyer W., Pratt C., Mulhern R., and Wilimas J. (1996). Coming to terms: Parents response to a first cancer recurrence. Nurs Res 45(3):148–153.

54. Pyke-Grimm K.A., Degner L., Small A., and Mueller B. (1999). Preferences for participation in treatment decision making and information needs of parents of children with cancer: A pilot study. J Pediatr Oncol Nurs 16(1):13–24.

55. Hinds P.S., Drew D., Martinson I.M., Oakes L., Quargnenti A., Furman W., Bowman L., Gilger E., and Gattuso J. (2000). An international feasibility study on parental decision making in pediatric oncology. Abstract, J Pediatr Oncol Nurs. 17(2):910.

56. Kirschbaum M.S. (1996). Life support decisions for children: What do parents value? Adv Nurs Sci 19(1):51–71.

57. Davies B., Deveau E., deVeber B., Howell D., Martinson I., Papadatou D., Pask E., and Stevens M. (1998). Experiences of mothers in five countries whose child died of cancer. Cancer Nurs 21(5):301–311.

58. American Academy of Pediatrics, Committee on Bioethics (1995). Informed consent, parental permission, and assent in pediatric practice. Pediatrics 95:314–317.

59. Keene N. (1997). Childhood Leukemia: A Guide for Families, Friends and Caregivers. Sebastopol: O'Reilly & Associates.

60. Hollen P.J. and Brickle B.B. (1998). Quality parental decision making and distress. J Pediatr Nurs, 13(3):140–150.

61. Phillips R.S., Rempusheski V.F., Puopolo A.L., Naccarato M., and Mallatratt L. (1990). Decision making in SUPPORT: The role of the nurse. J Clin Epidemiol 43(Supplement):55S–58S.

64. Randolph A.G., Zollo M.B., Wigton R.S., and Yeh T.S. (1997). Factors explaining variability among caregivers in the intent to restrict life-support interventions in a pediatric intensive care unit. Crit Care Med 25(3):435–439.

63. Randolph A.G., Zollo M.B., Egger M.J., Guyatt G.H., Nelson R.M., and Stidham G.L. (1999). Variability in physician opinion on limiting pediatric life support. Pediatrics 103(4):s43.

64. Solomon M.Z., O'Donnell L., Jennings M.A., Guilfoy V., Wolf S.M., Nolan K., Jackson R., Koch-Weser D., and Donnelley S. (1993). Decisions near the end-of-life: Professional views on life-sustaining treatments. Am Public Health 83(1):14–23.

65. Walter S.D., Cook D.J., Guyatt G.H., Spanier A., Jaeschke R., Todd T.R., and Streiner D.L. (1998). Confidence in life-support decisions in the intensive care unit: A survey of healthcare workers. Crit Care Med 26(1):44–49.

66. Hume M. (1998). Improving care at the end of life. Quality Letter for Healthcare Leaders 10(10):2–10.

35 The Poor and Underserved

ANNE HUGHES

I can beat this.

—Joe, a 57-year-old man recently diagnosed with stage IV squamous cell cancer of the base of the tongue, who is proud that he has stable housing and is clean and sober for 6 years after 34 years of alcohol abuse

Poverty is inextricably linked to increased morbidity, premature mortality, and limited access to both preventive health care and ongoing medical care. Persons who are poor constitute a *vulnerable population,* a term used in community health to describe social groups at greater risk for adverse health outcomes.[1] According to Flaskerud and Winslow, the root causes of this vulnerability are typically low economic status and social status and poor access to resources.[1]

Persons with limited life expectancy because of a life-threatening illness or injury also constitute a vulnerable population. In recent years the SUPPORT study underscored the vulnerability of the hospitalized seriously ill, not only as it related to anticipated mortality but more compellingly as it related to the manner of dying these persons and their families experienced. The Study to Understand Prognoses, Preferences for Outcomes and Risks of Treatments (SUPPORT) was a multisite intervention study, funded by the Robert Wood Johnson Foundation, designed to improve care of seriously ill persons in the hospital.[2]

To be poor *and* to have a progressive, life-threatening illness presents more challenges than either one of these conditions alone. As Taipale[3] elegantly notes, "Poverty means the opportunities and choices most basic to human development are denied" (pg. 54). When you do not have a home or you live in a rodent-infested room without a toilet or kitchen facilities, what type of death do you hope for? When death is a way of life and survival a moment to moment goal, what is the meaning of illness and death?

The purpose of this chapter is to examine characteristics of the poor and underserved population that place them at particular risk when the need for palliative care is identified. In particular this chapter will look at a subset of the poor who are homeless or marginally housed and how this affects both access to and quality of end-of-life care. The literature and research in end of life issues for the poor and underserved is extremely sparse, which is symbolic of the neglect of this population. Case studies will be used to illustrate concepts discussed.

EPIDEMIOLOGY OF POVERTY IN UNITED STATES

According to the U.S. Census Bureau, there are 35.6 million Americans whose incomes fall below the poverty level.[4] This figure equals just over 13% of the entire population (see Table 35–1 for list of states whose poverty level exceeds the national average). Of all poor, 46% are white, 26.5% are black, and 27% Hispanic. Children make up 40% of the poor but only 26% of the population. Almost 74% of the poor are families. Over 75% of the poor live within metropolitan areas and 42.5% of the poor live within central cities.

Most of the poor have access to some type of housing or shelter, even if the basic accommodations (cooking and refrigeration, heat, water, private toilet and bathing facilities) are inadequate. However, for a small subset housing is marginal or unavailable.

DEFINITION AND PREVALENCE OF HOMELESSNESS

Homelessness is defined as a condition under which persons lack fixed, regular and adequate night-time residence or reside in temporary housing such as shelters and welfare hotels (Stewart B. McKinney Homeless Assistance Act of 1987 as reported in Fellin).[5] Calculating the number of Americans homeless or marginally housed is extremely difficult. Most cross-sectional studies fail to capture persons transiently homeless, the hidden homeless staying with family members, those living in cars or encampments, and others living in single-room occupancy hotels (SROs), sometimes known as welfare hotels. Additionally many of the poor and in particular the homeless avoid contact with social and health services.

According to the National Law Center on Homelessness and Poverty, approximately 700,000 Americans each night are homeless, and 3% of the population in major metropolitan cities are estimated to be homeless.[6] Persons who are homeless are not members of a homogenous group. Some are street people and chronically homeless while others are homeless because of a financial crisis that put them out of more stable housing. Street people may be more reluctant to accept services and may have much higher rates of concurrent substance abuse and mental illness (the so-called dual diagnosed).[5]

Table 35–1. States Whose Poverty Rates Exceed National Average

State	People in Poverty (%)
Alabama	14.8
Arizona	18.8
Arkansas	18.4
California	16.8
District of Columbia	23.0
Florida	14.3
Georgia	14.7
Kentucky	16.4
Louisiana	18.4
Mississippi	18.6
Montana	16.3
New Mexico	23.4
New York	16.6
Oklahoma	15.2
South Dakota	14.1
Tennessee	15.1
Texas	16.7
West Virginia	17.5

Source: U.S. Census Bureau, Current Population Studies, March 1998.[4]

HEALTH PROBLEMS ASSOCIATED WITH POVERTY

A number of health problems are associated with poverty. Many of these problems are related to environmental factors such as exposure to weather conditions, poor ventilated spaces, unsafe hotels and street conditions, and high-crime neighborhoods where the poor tend to live. Health problems (see Table 35–2) of the poor include: malnutrition (contributing to dental problems, tuberculosis, wasting); lack of access to shelter and bathing facilities (skin infections, cellulitis, podiatric problems, hypothermia); problems related to drug and alcohol use (overdose, seizures, delirium, sexually transmitted infections such as HIV, Hepatitis B, Hepatitis C, trauma); chronic mental illness (paranoid ideation; antisocial behaviors, psychosis, and suicide); and violence-related injuries (assaults, homicides, trauma, rape). One-third of the homeless may have a psychiatric illness.[5] Many of the homeless and the other poor abuse drugs and alcohol. In some instances drugs and alcohol are used to self medicate distressing psychiatric symptoms (e.g., anxiety, depression). Persons who are poor on average have a shorter life expectancy than national population surveys; some have suggested that homeless poor in the United States have life expectancy rates comparable to developing countries.[7]

Table 35–2. Health Problems Associated with Homelessness

Causes	Manifestations
Malnutrition	Dental problems, tuberculosis, wasting
Lack of shelter and access to bathing facilities	Skin infections, lice, cellulitis, podiatric problems, hypothermia, tuberculosis
Drug and alcohol use	Overdose, seizures, delirium, sexually transmitted infections such as HIV, hepatitis B, hepatitis C, trauma, falls, cirrhosis, heroin nephropathy, esophageal varices
Chronic mental illness	Paranoid ideation, antisocial behaviors, psychosis, suicide
Violence-related injuries	Assaults, homicides, rape

CLINICAL PRESENTATIONS OF ADVANCING DISEASE IN THE POOR

Persons who are poor frequently present with advanced disease. In addition to the late-stage disease presentation, many of these persons have significant comorbidities (concurrent illnesses) that affect both the course of each illness and the therapy available. The case below illustrates this point:

Case Study: Debbie

Debbie is a 38-year-old white woman living in a single-room occupancy hotel admitted with fever, SOB, hemoptysis, and fatigue. While being ruled out for tuberculosis she tests positive for HIV antibody. Debbie reluctantly shares with the HIV test counselor that she often exchanged sex for crack cocaine. Her CD 4 lymphocyte count at the time of presentation is 75 cells/μg (indicating severe immune suppression and qualifying as an AIDS indicator condition). Her chest radiograph is reviewed by the radiologist, who suspects a malignancy; her biopsy is positive and staging work-up reveals stage III non-small-cell lung cancer. She has no primary health care provider. Debbie's social situation is complicated. She recently stopped using crack cocaine when her respiratory symptoms worsened. She has three children staying with her mother; she has no primary relationship. Debbie is ashamed by her AIDS diagnosis and relieved to also have a lung cancer diagnosis. She insists that her AIDS diagnosis not be disclosed to her family, who are told only that Debbie has advanced lung cancer. Debbie is counseled about the additive bone-marrow-suppressive effects of chemotherapy and antiretroviral therapy. She chooses not to have treatment for her HIV infection.

In many instances comorbidities, especially those related to drug use, complicate the differential diagnosis.[8] As Debbie's case study points out there were several competing diagnoses that might explain her presenting illness: tuberculosis, community-acquired pneumonia, lung cancer and crack cocaine use (associated with pulmonary fibrosis).

Comorbidities also affect the health care providers' ability to realistically estimate prognosis and the nature of symptoms or problems that might occur down the road. Charting the dying trajectory for the chronic progressive illness may be conceivable, but superimposing the acute illnesses and injuries that the very poor live with and manage creates jagged peaks and valleys in a downward course. How quickly the life-threatening illness will progress becomes a prognostication puzzle; some persons living on the street truly seem to have had nine lives.

Persistent alcohol or drug dependence may or may not affect the ability of the person to comply with a treatment plan. The case study which follows describes such a scenario.

Case Study: Jeremiah

Jeremiah is a 57-year-old African American man who has injected heroin for over 40 years. As a result of his heroin use he developed end-stage renal disease and required hemodialysis. Jeremiah keeps about 35% of his outpatient dialysis appointments.

When he has not been treated for several weeks he is brought into the emergency room with altered mental status, uremic and unable to care for himself. Prior to this admission, he was found in the street by the paramedics and has laboratory evidence of rhabdomyolysis (muscle destruction and serious metabolic derangement due to prolonged immobility). Jeremiah receives acute dialysis, is stabilized and returns to the community.

Jeremiah's heroin use affected his ability to adhere to the burdens of his hemodialysis schedule. Furthermore his drug use compounded his delirium when he presented acutely uremic; and compromised his medical decision-making capacity. In the absence of a surrogate decision maker directing the medical team otherwise about Jeremiah's wishes, emergent treatment was intiated.

The management of symptoms associated with progressive illness is complicated. End organ diseases may alter pharmacokinetics of medications used to palliate symptoms. Clinically significant drug–drug and drug–nutrient interactions may occur. Determining whether the person is experiencing an adverse drug reaction is not easy when the person has comorbidities, has rapidly progressive disease, is malnourished, or may be continuing to use alcohol or other substances. In the case described above, Jeremiah's confusion may be due to an elevated creatinine level, the heroin he shot up 48 hours ago that remains in his system, or his not having had sufficient food or fluids for 36 hours prior to admission. At what point in Jeremiah's illness should an ethics consultation assist with the decisions related to whether he is terminal, and whether further therapy, even hemodialysis, is futile or clearly not acceptable to him? In some instances from a resource allocation perspective, his nonadherence to hemodialysis may serve as justification for his discharge from this life-supporting therapy.

Despite the prevalence of substance abuse in this population lack of attention to self-care activities cannot be assumed in all drug users. Some persons who use drugs and are homeless or marginally housed manage complex HIV antiretroviral regimens that require scrupulous attention to when to eat, which other medications may or may not be taken at the same time and the several times a day dosing is necessary.[9] Race, class, and housing status cannot be used as surrogate predictors of who abuses drugs and alcohol nor who will adhere or not adhere to treatment demands.

Other psychosocial issues complicate symptom management in persons who are poor and living with a life-threatening illness. Persons known to be chemically dependent are often denied treatment for pain because of providers' concerns of aberrant or drug-hoarding behaviors. Local pharmacies that stock opioid and sedative-hypnotic agents may not be available in the high-crime areas where the poor usually live. Access to medications may be limited to hospital pharmacies that may or may not be geographically near the person. If an antiemetic prescribed to relieve the chronic nausea experienced by a person with pancreatic cancer is not covered on the Medicaid formulary, or the person is not eligible for any drug assistance program, the range of medications used to manage the nausea will be severely limited. Additionally, use of high-tech methods to control symptoms are probably not an option for the person who lives in a tent encampment. Many poor persons require placement in a hospital or long-term care to manage moderate to severe symptoms that cannot be managed sufficiently on the street or in the shelter.

PSYCHOSOCIAL FACTORS INFLUENCING PALLIATIVE CARE AVAILABLE TO THE POOR AND HOMELESS

Health care professionals committed to support their patients' right to a "good death" may be challenged working with the poor and the homeless. The good death is described as: (*1*) free from avoidable distress and suffering, (*2*) in accord with the patient and family's wishes, and (*3*) consistent with clinical, cultural, and ethical standards.[10] Bad deaths, in contrast, include those accompanied by neglect, violence, or unwanted and senseless medical interventions.[10] Most persons who are poor or homeless are at great risk for a bad death.

Basic survival needs (food, shelter, clothing, protection) are the primary concern of the poor; often of greater and more pressing importance than the existential crisis of facing one's own mortality. Seeing others die prematurely, often under violent or disturbing circumstances may be an all too common experience for this population. Table 35–3 lists challenges to providing a good death in this population. The lack of resources, both economic and human, limit the palliative options available to the person who is poor. In the movie *The Wizard of Oz*, Dorothy's refrain,

Table 35–3. Psychosocial Challenges in Providing Palliative Care to the Poor

- Homeless or unstable housing with inadequate basic facilities (phone, private bathroom, refrigerator and cooking facilities) or rodent infested.
- Fragile or nonexistent support system (no family primary caregiver, estranged from family, history of family violence/abuse).
- Many persons have encountered rejection, or shame when accessing health care services and therefore avoid contact. May be slow to trust even well-meaning caregivers. Compounded because of the history of racism in care and research.
- Most health care or specialized palliative care services are geographically remote; some service providers may curtail services to the poorest communities because of concerns about staff safety.
- Behavioral difficulties (e.g., drug hoarding, selling prescriptions, hostility, psychiatric illness, substance abuse) may affect their relationships with health care providers
- Decision-making capacity and patient's goals are difficult to assess when intoxicated, brain-injured, and lacking an advance directive.
- Generally this population is excluded from clinical trials; therefore little evidence is available on which to base therapeutic interventions.

"There's no place like home, there's no place like home," speaks of an almost far-away magical experience that many who are poor and dying cannot even imagine.

Relationships with health care professionals may be strained when patients feel stigmatized for their appearance or lack of hygiene. Sometimes the presence of body odor may be offensive to some health care professionals and lead to rejection.

Historical events or traditional roles can also affect such relationships. For example, the African American experience with the medical care system includes the Tuskegee experiment and other instances of abuse, and many people continue to mistrust the predominantly white health care establishment. Discussions about limiting therapy or do-not-resuscitate decisions may be regarded as a dominant culture withholding possibly life-sustaining therapy. Some individuals and communities fear being treated "like a guinea pig" and refuse to participate in clinical trials when offered.

An issue that may strain the drug user's willingness to trust health care providers is the criminalization of his or her lifestyle. Health care providers sometimes may be regarded as moralistic authority figures, not to be trusted.[11] Some of the behavioral problems exhibited by this population may frustrate, anger, and at times intimidate health care professionals. How the professional maintains a sense of caring and calm when threatened or subject to hostility is a complex issue.

Indeed finding those with chronic mental or substance-abuse-related illness for follow-up care may require expert detective ability and contacts in the community. For some persons on the street who have sustained brain injury, whether because of chronic alcohol or drug use or related to trauma, minor illnesses may lead to delirium and impaired decision-making capacity. When no longer intoxicated or medically stabilized the competent person may decide to return to the street rather than consider the loss of freedom associated with institutional placement or the need to stop using drugs.

WHERE AND FROM WHAT CAUSES DO MOST HOMELESS PEOPLE DIE?

Limited data is available regarding the socioeconomic factors, places of death, and immediate causes of death of the homeless. In 1992, 57% of all U.S. deaths occurred in hospitals, 17% in nursing homes, 20% in residences, and 6% elsewhere.[10] Given these statistics for the general population, it is came be assumed that most poor people, like those who are not poor, die in institutions. For those who are homeless dying on the street or in jail is another fact of life.[17]

Data from the Centers for Disease Control and Prevention and the San Francisco Department of Public Health provides additional information.[12–15] In San Francisco,157 homeless persons died in 1997 (see Table 35–4).[15] The average age of this cohort was 42.3 years, males predominated (85%), and the ethnic composition of those who died included more whites and African Americans than live in the city. Data reported to the CDC corroborates the role of chronic alcohol abuse and acute alcohol intoxication as a cause of death in the homeless in Georgia.[12] In addition hypothermia-related deaths have been reported in Chicago and in Georgia.[12,14] Accidental deaths due to fires, falls, pedestrian–motor vehicle accidents and drowning and violent deaths related to homicide and suicide were also reported in the homeless.[12]

Table 35–4. Known Causes of Death in 1997 in Homeless Persons in San Francisco

Causes	Numbers of Persons
Acute Drug Poisoning (Heroin, Cocaine, Poly Drug, Alcohol)	62
Accidents	13
Alcohol Related	10
Heart Disease	7
Suicide	7
Severe Infection	4
Other	10
Total	**141**

Source: Aragon.[15]

STRATEGIES FOR WORKING WITH THE POOR AND HOMELESS WHO HAPPEN TO BE DYING

Kemp[16] believes working with the very poor may be challenging because of generations of internalized hopelessness and poor self-awareness, differing perceptions of time (everything seeming to take much longer), and difficulties navigating the many bureaucracies necessary to obtain services. He suggests that modifying expectations to these realities and recognizing small successes may be a strategy to address these background factors.

On the other hand, for many persons who live on the street survival skills are keenly developed. Knowing when a food bank opens, where to get clothing, when shelter bed waiting lines begin to form, or how to get benefit checks without an address requires remarkable ingenuity and discipline. Needless to say, as with persons who are not poor, wide variations in abilities, resources, and relationships with health care professionals exist.

Given the lack of studies about best practices working with the very poor diagnosed with a life-threatening illness, clinical experience, often of a trial-and-error nature usually guides practice. Additionally the harm reduction model of working with active drug users may assist the clinician to develop therapeutic relationships with difficult-to-engage clients or the poor. Harm reduction seeks to reduce or eliminate the risk of HIV infection by changing high-risk behaviors. It accepts the client how and where he is. It does not mandate abstinence but instead explores the negative and positive consequences of the high risk behavior on the person's life.[11]

Developing therapeutic relationships with the poor and homeless requires (*1*) expecting the person's trust to be earned over time (sometimes a long time) and not automatically taken for granted; (2) respecting the person's hu-

Table 35–5. Helpful Suggestions When Engaging a Difficult-to-Engage Client

- Address anyone over 40 years of age by the title of Mr. or Ms. Ask permission to be on a first-name basis.
- Do not hestitate to shake hands.
- Be prepared to meet people more intelligent and perceptive, and more wounded than you expect.
- Be tolerant. How would you react if you were in that situation?
- Don't make promises you can't keep.
- Don't take it personally.
- Taking time out helps prevent burnout.
- Get to know the community.
- If you feel you have to save the human race, do it one person at a time.
- Direct material assistance (e.g., clean socks, food, hygiene kits) opens people up.
- Usually the most difficult clients are those most in need. Throw the word *noncompliant* out of your vocabulary.
- Make eye contact. If the person does not like eye contact or becomes agitated, avoid using it.
- Keep in mind that people who live intense lives may not particularly like unasked-for physical contact.
- Don't be afraid to ask stupid questions; answers are better than assumptions.
- Adjust your expectations and accept small victories with satisfaction.

Source: Patchell (1997), reference 19.

manity, no matter how they look, what they say and the feelings in us they may evoke; (3) appreciating the person's story as influencing the response to the illness, and finally (4) recognizing and addressing maladaptive behaviors.[17,18] Table 35–5 includes a list of helpful suggestions to reach a difficult-to-engage client. The case studies below illustrate some of these points.

Case Study: Jose

Jose is a 40-year-old man who has presented to the Emergency Department 50 times in the past year for alcohol- and drug-related problems. He has occasionally obtained care at a community clinic serving a poor neighborhood. He lives on the street and has had frequent battles with other street residents, the police, and even other patients when hospitalized. He threatened to strike a nurse on a prior admission when the nurse threatened to withhold pain medication because " it was not time yet" and did not offer any alternative. Jose was counseled at the time of this incident that physical attacks would not be tolerated, and the nurse worked with the medical team to come up with a better pain management regimen. After three unsuccessful referral attempts over a two-year period, Jose agreed to a case management program to link him to stable housing, community resources for food and clothing, and medical and alcohol treatment. He tells the case manager that his life had become too much for him to bear. He described to the case manager a life of living on the streets since he was 12 years old, having to prostitute himself to get money for food and shelter, countless attacks, having no family or friends and no job, no future. Despite increasing medical problems (diagnosis of AIDS, hepatitis, and cirrhosis), Jose has a hotel room, is receiving welfare benefits, and has begun antiretroviral therapy. He has had one relapse but called his case manager and has remained sober for eight months, his longest period of sobriety in 22 years.

Jose's story illustrates that a "reachable moment" was achieved after years of chemical dependency, referrals for treatment, and episodic use of medical care services. Additionally his story reminds us of the years of child sexual abuse that may be part of a difficult-to-engage patient's history. Many abused persons use drugs and alcohol to self-medicate psychic or emotional trauma.

Alcohol and drug intoxication and serious mental illness usually affects the health care professional's ability to meaningfully interact with a client facing a life-threatening illness. As one clinical expert commented, "How can you reason with someone who is intoxicated that they are dying and (ask them what their wishes are)?" Advance care planning may not be realistic expectation as the case study below demonstrates.

Case Study: Michael

Michael is a 26-year-old Native American man who lives in an SRO. He has drunk alcohol, sometimes one or two quarts of whiskey daily, since he was 14 years old. He has had frequent hospitalizations related to his alcohol use—hypothermia, injuries due to assaults, or falling down on sidewalks. He has no primary care provider but is known to the outreach workers who work with the homeless, to the police who have picked him up for disorderly conduct, and to the emergency room staff who feel they "patch him up to go right back drinking." He has not seen nor spoken to his family in years. Michael is brought into the hospital and diagnosed with severe diabetic ketoacidosis and rhabdomyolysis. He is transferred to the ICU, ventilated, and acutely dialyzed. Subsequently he develops sepsis. The treating team have been unable to locate a family member or surrogate decision makers. Despite volumes of medical records there is no mention of what Michael would want done if he was critically ill. Ultimately, given the overwhelming sepsis unresponsive to treatment and multiorgan failure, further medical care is determined to be futile. Life-support therapy is withdrawn and he dies in the ICU alone.

Michael's story underscores the terminal nature of alcoholism. Regretfully access to and acceptance of alcohol treatment is limited. In some instances poor patients lack any family or friends, and the medical care team becomes the patient's support system. Many persons who are poor and have had episodic contact with the health care system during acute illnesses or life-threatening trauma wind up receiving life-saving therapies such as mechanical ventilation, vasopressors, dialysis, and other therapies. All too often the client does not have an advance directive or a surrogate decision maker to articulate his or her wishes. Furthermore the technological imperative of hospitals and physicians in training may see saving a life at any cost of greater value in the absence of a competent patient or family directing otherwise.[10]

In addition to the interpersonal interventions to engage the client in a therapeutic interaction, nurses are often required to become knowledgeable about the availability of and the services provided by community agencies. Knowing which agencies or services are involved with a client and communicating with them assures consistency of approach and continuity of care. In many instances advocacy may be required to access services such as pain management, substance abuse treatment, mental health services, and social services for housing and money management.

CONCLUSION

Providing palliative care to the poor, especially the homeless, is extremely challenging. Comorbid illnesses, illnesses associated with poverty, and clarifying the etiology of presenting symptoms may seem almost impossible at times. Psychosocial risk factors and strained relationships with health care providers sometimes result in the client receiving futile or unwanted medical interventions at an advanced stage of illness. Clarifying with a patient what constitutes a good death for him can be humbling when the patient tells you he wants simply to have shelter and to feel safe and to be forgiven for mistakes he has made. As palliative care improves by innovations in both research and the education of health care providers, the unique needs of vulnerable populations such as the poor and the homeless must be examined and addressed.

REFERENCES

1. Flaskerud J.H., Winslow B.J. (1998). Conceptualizing vulnerable populations health-related research. Nursing Research 47:69–78.

2. SUPPORT Principal Investigators (1995). A controlled trial to improve care for seriously ill hospitalized patients: The Study to Understand Prognoses and Preferences for Outcomes and Risks of Treatment (SUPPORT). JAMA 274:1591–1598.

3. Taipale V. (1999) Ethics and allocation of health resources: The influence of poverty on health. Acta Oncologica 38:51–55.

4. U.S. Census Bureau, Department of Commerce, Web site: www.census.gov

5. Fellin P. (1996). The culture of homelessness. In The Cross-Cultural Practice of Clinical Case Management in Mental Health (P. Manoleas, ed.), pp. 41–77. Haworth Press, New York.

6. National Coalition for the Homeless Web site: http://nch.ari.net.

7. Kushel M. (1999). Personal communication, August 3.

8. O'Connor P.G., Selwyn P.A., Schottenfeld R.S. (1994). Medical care for injection drug users with human immunodeficiency virus infection. New England Journal of Medicine 331:450–459.

9. Bangsberg D., Tulsky J.P., Hecht F.M., Moss A.R. (1997). Protease inhibitors in the homeless. Journal of the American Medical Association 278:63–65.

10. Institute of Medicine (1997). Approaching Death: Improving Care at the End of Life, pp. 24. National Academy Press, Washington D.C.

11. Fisk S. (1996). Substance Users. In ANAC's Core Curriculum for HIV/AIDS Nursing (K. Casey, F. Cohen, A. Hughes, eds.), pp. 305–306. Nursecom, Philadelphia.

12. Centers for Disease Control (1987). Deaths among the homeless—Atlanta, Georgia. Morbidity and Mortality Weekly Report 36: 297–299.

13. Centers for Disease Control (1991). Deaths among the homeless persons—San Francisco, 1985–90. Morbidity and Mortality Weekly Report 40: 877–80.

14. Centers for Disease Control (1991). Hypothermia-Related Deaths—Cook County, Illinois, November 1992–March 1993. Morbidity and Mortality Weekly Report 42:917–919.

15. Aragon T. (1998). Report on Homeless Death Review, 1998. San Francisco Department of Public Health. Report to the San Francisco Health Commission, December 10, 1998.

16. Kemp C. (1999). Terminal Illness: A Guide to Nursing Care. 2nd edition. Philadelphia: Lippincott, Williams and Wilkins.

17. Patchell T. (1996). Nowhere to run: Portraits of life on the street. Turning Wheel Fall: 14–21.

18. Patchell T. (1999). Personal communication, August 2.

19. Patchell T. (1997). Suggestions for more effective outreach. San Francisco Department of Public Health. Homeless Death Prevention Project, 1997.

36 Patients with Acquired Immune Deficiency Syndrome

DEBORAH WITT SHERMAN

My life will never be what it was. I'm living with AIDS and I have to deal with it and struggle. My philosophy is taking one day at a time. Some days the quality of my life is so low that I wonder what is the point because I am so tired of suffering. When I'm physically suffering, I pray for relief. Yet on days when I'm feeling good, I pray for strength.

—a patient

Acquired immune deficiency syndrome (AIDS) has stimulated the need for evaluation of clinical practice at the interface of curative and palliative care and raises some interesting and interconnected issues in the care of individuals with life-threatening, progressive illnesses.[1] Within the last few years, both the public and health professionals have been troubled by the reality of overtreatment and undertreatment of pain and symptoms in individuals with life-threatening illness, and particularly at the end of life.[2] Such concern extends to the care of patients with human immunodeficiency virus (HIV) and the resultant illness of AIDS, as no cure has yet been found. The focus of care must therefore be on improving quality of life by providing palliative care for the management of pain and other physical symptoms, while addressing the emotional, social, and spiritual needs of patients and their families throughout the illness trajectory. Even though current therapies have increased the life expectancy of people with HIV/AIDS, the chance of their experiencing symptoms related not only to the disease but from the effects of therapies also increases. Furthermore, palliative measures can be beneficial in ensuring tolerance of and compliance with difficult pharmacologic regimens.[3]

Although in the past little attention has been given to palliative care as a component of AIDS care, it is now realized that the palliation of pain, symptoms, and suffering must occur throughout the course of a life-threatening disease not just in the final stages, near the end of life. This chapter will provide an overview and update of the comprehensive care related to HIV/AIDS, and will address the palliative care needs of individuals and families living with and dying from this illness. With this information, nurses and other health care professionals will gain the knowledge to provide effective and compassionate care, recognizing the need for both curative and aggressive care, as well as supportive and palliative therapies to maximize the quality of life of patients and their family caregivers.

OVERVIEW AND UPDATE: INCIDENCE, HISTORICAL BACKGROUND, EPIDEMIOLOGY, AND PATHOGENESIS

Incidence of HIV/AIDS

HIV/AIDS is a worldwide epidemic affecting more than 24 million people globally, and with over 688,299 reported cases in the United States since the beginning of the epidemic.[4] At the end of 1997, approximately 270,000 persons in the United States had a diagnosis of AIDS, which was a 12% increase from 1996 as a result of improved survival for patients receiving treatment and a decrease in the number of deaths.[4] The human immunodeficiency virus (HIV) is the leading cause of death of all Americans between the ages of 25 and 44 years, with the highest incidence and prevalence now among African Americans, women, and heterosexuals.[4] To date, nearly 9 million have died from the infection. Statistical models indicate that 40,000 Americans are infected each year and approximately the same number die from the disease annually.[5] It was further estimated that by the year 2000, nearly 70 million adults will be infected worldwide.[6] Given that there are no approved vaccines against HIV/AIDS or cures for the disease, AIDS remains a life-threatening and progressive illness that marks the final stage of a chronic viral illness identified by the occurrence of particular opportunistic infections, cancers, and neurological manifestations.[7]

Historical Background of HIV/AIDS

In the early 1980s, cases were reported of previously healthy homosexual men who were diagnosed with *Pneumocytis carinii* pneumonia and an extremely rare tumor known as Kaposi sarcoma (KS). As the number of cases doubled every six months, and with the further occurrence of unusual fungal, viral, and parasitic infections, it was realized that the immune systems of these individuals were being compromised. Over time, the Centers for Disease Control (CDC) learned that a complex of diseases that produced immunocompetence was being experienced outside of the homosexual community, among heterosexual partners, intravenous substance users, persons with hemophilia, individuals receiving infected blood products, and children born to women with the disease. These epidemological changes alerted health professionals to the existence of an infectious agent that was transmitted via infected body fluids, particularly through sexual transmission and blood products.[8]

Origins of HIV can be traced through serum studies to 1959 when crossover mechanisms between humans and primates through animal bites or scratches in Africa led to HIV transmission. In 1981 the virus was identified and named lymphadenopathy-associated virus (LAV). By 1984 the termed had been changed to human T-lymphocytic virus type III (HTLV-III), and renamed in 1986 the human immunodeficiency virus type 1 (HIV-1). HIV-1 accounts for nearly all the cases reported in the United States, while a second strain, HIV-2, accounts for nearly all the cases reported in West Africa. There have only been 17 cases of HIV-2 reported in the United States with the majority being immigrants from Africa.

Globally, AIDS is characterized as volatile, unstable, and dynamic epidemic that has spread to new countries around the world; has become increasingly complex due to the viruses' ability to mutate; and crosses all socioeconomic, cultural, political, and geographic borders.[5] To date, scientific progress has been made in combating the infection: (*1*) the virus has been identified; (2) a blood screening program has been implemented; (3) vaccines are being tested; (*4*) biologic and behavioral cofactors have been identified related to infection and disease progression; (5) prophylactic treatments are available to prevent opportunistic infections; (6) newly developed HIV RNA quantitative assays, which measure viral load, have become available to guide the treatment of the disease; and (7) the latest advances in treatment involve the use of combination antiretroviral therapies, including protease inhibitors, early in the disease to limit viral replication and decrease viral loads to undetectable levels.[5] However, epidemiologic evidence heightens concern regarding changes in the population affected, and the morbidity and mortality still associated with the disease.

HIV Epidemiology

From an epidemiological perspective, the percentage of the total number of AIDS cases in the ten metropolitan statistical areas in the United States has declined since 1991, yet there is a spread to smaller cities and rural areas in the United States and Southeast.[5] A decline is reported in the proportion of newly reported AIDS cases in the United States from a annual total of 66% in 1985 to 42% in 1995. There has been a decline in the occurrence of AIDS among whites from 60% in 1985 to 40% in 1998.[9] Although there has been a 34% decrease in the infection rate in the number of young, white homosexual men, there is a 19% and 24% increase, respectively, in the infection rate for homosexual African American and Latino men.[10] Indeed, there has been a substantial increase in the HIV infection rate among all African Americans, from 25% in 1985 to 33% in 1997, and in Latinos, from 15% to 19% over the same 12-year period. Currently, the rate of infection among female adults and adolescents has also risen from 7% in 1985 to 19% in 1997, with the majority of infections occurring in heterosexual women.[9] Epidemiologic studies have also confirmed that HIV-1 is transmitted through semen, cervical and vaginal secretions, breast milk, contaminated drug equipment, transfusions and blood products, tissue transplants, perinatal exposure, and occupational exposure in health care settings.[4]

HIV Pathogenesis and Classification

Like all viruses, the HIV virus survives by reproducing itself in a host cell, upsurping the genetic machinery of that cell and eventually destroying the cell.[11] The HIV is a retrovirus whose life cycle consists of (*1*) attachment of the virus to the cell, which is affected by cofactors that influence the virus's ability to enter the host cell; (2) uncoating of the virus; (3) reverse transcription by an enzyme called reverse transcriptase which converts two strands of viral RNA to DNA; (*4*) integration of newly synthesized proviral DNA into the cell nucleus, assisted by the viral enzyme, integrase, and which becomes the template for new viral components; (5) transcription of proviral DNA into messenger RNA; (6) movement of messenger RNA outside the cell nucleus where it is translated into viral proteins and enzymes; and (7) assembly and release of mature virus particles out of the host cell.[12]

The host cell therefore produces viral proteins instead of the cell's normal regulatory proteins, and results in the eventual destruction of the host cell. Given that the virus has an affinity for CD4 molecules, any cells that have the CD4 molecule on their surface, such as T lymphocytes and macrophages, become major viral targets. Recently, research has identified chemokines and chemokine receptors as playing important roles in HIV pathogenesis by inhibiting HIV infection. Given that CD4 cells are the master coordinator of the immune response, chronic destruction of these cells severely compromises individuals' immune status, leaving them susceptible to opportunistic infections. Macrophages are also directly targeted by the virus and may serve as reservoirs for the virus for months after initial infection, as well as contributing to HIV-related dementias and other neurological syndromes.[12]

HIV and AIDS are not synonymous terms but refer to the natural history or progression of the infection, ranging from asymptomatic infection to life-threatening illness characterized by opportunistic infections and cancers. This continuum of illness is associated with a decrease in CD4 cell count and a rise in HIV RNA viral load.[13] In monitoring disease progression, it should be noted, however, that although low CD4 cell counts are generally correlated with high viral loads, some patients with low CD4 counts have low viral loads and vice versa. The most reliable current measurement of HIV activity is therefore the viral load, and the more consistent surrogate marker is the percentage of lymphocytes that are CD4 cells rather than the absolute CD4 cell count.[14]

In 1993 the CDC reclassified HIV disease according to the CD4 T lymphocyte count and clinical conditions associated with HIV infection. The classification of HIV disease is as follows:[5,11]

Primary or acute infection occurs when the virus enters the body and replicates in large numbers in the blood. This leads to an initial decrease in the number of T cells. Viral load climbs during the first two weeks of the infection. Within 5 to 30 days of infection the individual experiences flulike symptoms characteristic of a viremia such as fever, sore throat, skin rash, lymphadenopathy, and myalgia. The production of HIV antibodies results in seroconversion that generally occurs within 6 to 12 weeks of the initial infection. The amount of virus present after the initial viremia and the immune response is called the viral set point.

Clinical latency refers to the chronic, clinically asymptomatic state in which there is a decreased viral load and resolution of symptoms of the primary infection. It was previously thought that in this period, the virus laid dormant in the host cells for a period of 5 to 7 years. However, recent advances in the understanding the pathogenesis of the virus reveal that there is continuous viral replication in the lymph nodes. As more than 10 billion copies of the virus can be made every day during this period, early medical intervention with combination antiretroviral therapy is recommended.[15]

Early symptomatic stage occurs after years of infection and is apparent by conditions indicative of primarily defects in cell-mediated immunity. Early symptomatic infection occurs when CD4 counts fall below 500 cells/mm^3 and the HIV viral load copy count increases above 10,000/ml up to 100,000/ml, which indicates a moderate risk of HIV progression and a median time to death of 6.8 years.

Late symptomatic stage begins when the CD4 count drops below 200 cells/mm^3 and the viral load increases above 100,000/ml. This CD4 level is recognized by the CDC as the case definition for AIDS. Severe opportunistic infections or cancers characterize this stage and result in multiple, severe symptoms. In addition to such illness as Kaposi sarcoma, *Pneumocystis carinii* pneumonia, HIV encephalopathy, and HIV wasting, diseases such as pulmonary tuberculosis, recurrent bacterial infections, and invasive cervical cancer have been added to the list of AIDS-indicative illnesses.[4]

Advanced HIV disease stage occurs when the CD4 cell count drops below 50 cells/mm^3 and the immune system is so impaired that death is likely within one year. Unfortunately, persons with advanced HIV disease diagnosed with AIDS increasingly represent persons whose diagnosis was too late for them to benefit from treatment, persons who either did not seek or had no access to care, or persons for whom treatment failed.[4] In the late stages of the disease, most individuals have health problems such as pneumonia, oral candidiasis, depression, dementia, skin problems, anxiety, incontinence, fatigue, isolation, bed dependency, wasting syndrome, and significant pain.[16]

Research regarding AIDS patients experiencing advanced disease confirm the multitude of patient symptoms and factors that contribute to mortality. In a study of 83 hospitalized AIDS patients, factors contributing to higher mortality include the type of opportunistic infections, serum albumin level, total lymphocyte count, weight, CD4 count, and neurological manifestations.[17] Of 363 patients with AIDS referred to community palliative care services, the most severe problems throughout care were patient and family anxiety and symptom control.[18] In the last month of life, a retrospective study of 50 men who died from AIDS indicated that the most distressing symptoms included pain, dyspnea, diarrhea, confusion, dementia, difficulty swallowing and eating, and loss of vision. Dehydration, malnutrition, and peripheral neuropathy were also important problems.[19]

PALLIATIVE CARE AS A NATURAL EVOLUTION IN HIV/AIDS CARE

From the earliest stages of HIV disease, symptom control becomes an important goal of medical and nursing care to maintain patients' quality of life. Palliative care for patients with HIV/AIDS should therefore be viewed not as an approach to care in only the advanced stage of the illness, but as an aspect of care that begins in the early stage of illness and continues as the disease progresses.[20]

With the occurrence of opportunistic infections, specific cancers, and neurological manifestations, AIDS involves multiple symptoms from not only the disease processes, but from the side effects of medications and other therapies. Patients with AIDS present with complex care issues, as they experience bouts of severe illness and debilitation, alternating with periods of symptom stabilization.[21] In one model of care, AIDS palliation begins when active treatment ends. Although this model limits service overlap and is economical, it creates not only the ethical issue of when to shift from a curative to a palliative focus, but promotes discontinuity of care and possible discrimination. In contrast, a second model of AIDS care recognizes that AIDS treatment is primarily palliative, directed toward minimizing symptoms and maximizing the quality of life, and necessitates the use of antiretroviral drugs, treatment of infections and neoplasms, and provision of high levels of support to promote the patient's quality of life over many years of the illness.[22]

Although thousands of individuals have suffered and died from AIDS each year, the palliative care needs of HIV/AIDS patients has been largely neglected by organizations involved in medical care.[23] This has occurred because the division between curative-aggressive care and supportive-palliative care is less well defined and more variable than in other life-threatening illnesses such as cancer.[16] With HIV/AIDS, the severity, complexity, and unpredictability of the illness trajectory have blurred the distinction between curative and palliative care.[24] Other challenges associated with HIV/AIDS are the societal stigmatization of the disease and, therefore, the greater emotional, social, and spiritual needs of those experiencing the illness, as well as their family and professional caregivers who experience their own grief and bereavement processes.

Resources aimed at prevention, health promotion and maintenance, and end-of-life care must be available through health care policies and legislation.[25] Not only the treatment of chronic debilitating conditions, but also the treatment of superimposed acute opportunistic infections and related symptoms is necessary to maintain quality of life. For example, intravenous therapy and blood transfusions, as well as health prevention measures such as ongoing intravenous therapies to prevent blindness from CMV retinitis, must be available to patients with AIDS to maintain their quality of life.

Palliative care is therefore a natural evolution in AIDS care. Core issues of comfort and function, fundamental to palliative care, must be addressed throughout the course of the illness, and may be concurrent with restorative or curative therapies for persons with AIDS.[21] The management decisions for patients with advanced AIDS will revolve around the ratio between benefits and burdens of the various diagnostic and treatment modalities, and the patient's expectations and goals, as well as anticipated problems.[26] In the face of advanced HIV disease, health care providers and patients must determine the balance between aggressive and supportive efforts, particularly when increasing debility, wasting, and deteriorating cognitive function is evident.[27] At this point the complex needs of patients and families with HIV/AIDS require the coordinated care of an interdisciplinary palliative care team, involving physicians, advanced practice nurses, staff nurses, social workers, dieticians, physiotherapists, and clergy.[3,28]

Given that in palliative care the unit of care is the patient and family, the palliative care team offers not only support for patients to live as fully as possible until death, but offers support to the family to help them to cope during the patient's illness and in their own bereavement.[29] Palliative care core precepts of respect for patient goals, preferences, and choices; comprehensive caring; and acknowledgment of caregivers' concerns[30] supports the holistic and comprehensive approach to care needed by individuals and families with HIV/AIDS.

Although the hospice and palliative care movement developed as a community response to those who were dying, primarily of cancer, the advent of the AIDS epidemic made it necessary for hospices to begin admitting patients with AIDS. This meant applying the old model of cancer care to patients with a new infectious, progressive, and terminal disease.[31] Unlike the course of cancer, which is relatively predictable once the disease progresses beyond cure, AIDS patients experience a series of life-threatening opportunistic infections. It is not until wasting becomes apparent that the course of AIDS achieves the predictability of cancer.[31] Furthermore, while the underlying goal of AIDS care remains one of palliation, short-term aggressive therapies are still needed to treat opportunistic infections.[32] Also, unlike cancer palliation, AIDS palliation deals with a fatal infectious disease of primarily younger people, which requires ongoing infection control and the management of symptoms.[33]

Barriers to Palliative Care

The neglect of the palliative care needs of patients with HIV disease also relates to certain barriers to care such as reimbursement issues. Specifically, public and private third-party payers have reimbursed end-of-life care only when physicians have verified a life expectancy of less than six months to live.[23] Given the unpredictability of the illness trajectory, many patients with AIDS have been denied access to hospice care. Currently, these policies are under review and the six-month limitation is being extended so that patients with AIDS will be eligible for comprehensive care with control of pain and other symptoms along with psychological and spiritual support offered by hospice/palliative care.

As a second barrier to hospice/palliative care, patients with AIDS have been denied access because of the need to continue antiretroviral therapies and other medications to prevent opportunistic infections. Given that the estimated cost of treatment for AIDS patients in hospices could amount to twice the cost of treating patients with cancer, particularly when the costs of medications are included, cost remains a financial issue for hospices.[29] Financing of such therapies for patients with AIDS is now being discussed and addressed by hospice/palliative care organizations.

The third barrier to palliative care is the patients themselves, many of whom are young, cling to the hope of a cure for AIDS, and are unwilling to accept hospice care. However, the current emphasis on beginning palliative care at the time of diagnosis of a life-threatening illness may shift the perception of palliative care as only end-of-life care, and promote palliative care as an aggressive approach to care throughout the course of the illness to insure their quality of life. Indeed, media and internet coverage of government and private initiatives to improve the care of the seriously and terminally ill in the United States is informing patients, families, and nurses of the philosophy and precepts of palliative care, the access to palliative care for life-defining illnesses, and the rights of patients to receive excellent end of life care, as well as the obligations of health professionals to provide such care across health care settings.

Criteria for Palliative Care

Grothe[31] suggests that four criteria be considered regarding the admission of AIDS patients to hospice: Functional ability, statistical prognosis, CD4 count and viral load, and history of opportunistic infections. These criteria give a better understanding of the patient's prognosis and needs. The complex needs of patients with advanced AIDS also indicate the need for an interdisciplinary approach to care offered by hospice/palliative care. Bloom and Flannery[34] encourage the continual review of hospice policies in accordance with the changes in the disease and encourage change in the community to provide an effective continuum of care. Indeed, developing different models of care such as enhanced home care, hospice care, day care, or partnerships with community hospitals or agencies and conducting cost-benefit analysis will be important in meeting the health care needs of patients with AIDS and their families in the future.[16]

Important advances are currently being made in the field of palliative medicine and nursing, involving an active set of behaviors that continue throughout the caregiving process to manage the pain and suffering of individuals with HIV/AIDS. Health professionals have the responsibility to be knowledgeable about the various treatment options and resources available for pain and symptom management. They must know about pharmacologic agents' actions, side effects, and interactions, as well as alternative routes of medication administration. And they must be able to inform patients of their options for care—documenting their preferences, wishes, and choices; performing a complete history and physical assessment; and collaborating with other members of the interdisciplinary team to develop and implement a comprehensive plan of care.[28]

HEALTH PROMOTION AND MAINTENANCE IN PROMOTING THE QUALITY OF LIFE OF PERSONS WITH HIV/AIDS

As palliative care becomes an increasingly important component of AIDS care from diagnosis to death,[25] and given the definition of palliative care as the comprehensive management of the physical, psychological, social, spiritual, and existential needs of patients with incurable progressive illness,[30] palliative care must involve ongoing prevention, health promotion, and health maintenance to promote the patient's quality of life throughout the illness trajectory. With HIV/AIDS, health promotion and maintenance involves promoting behaviors that will prevent or decrease the occurrence of opportunistic infections and AIDS-indicator diseases, promoting prophylactic and therapeutic treatment of AIDS-indicator conditions, and preventing behaviors that promote disease expression.[5]

With no current prospect for cure, the health management of patients with HIV/AIDS is directed toward prolonging survival and maintaining quality of life.[35] Nurses generally refer to quality of life as the impact of sickness and health care on an ill person's daily activities and sense of well-being.[36] Furthermore, quality of life varies with disease progression from HIV to AIDS. To understand quality of life means to understand the patient's perceptions of his or her ability to control the physical, emotional, social, cognitive, and spiritual aspects of the illness.[37] Quality of life is therefore associated with health maintenance for individuals with HIV/AIDS, particularly as it relates to functioning in activities of daily living, social functioning, and physical and emotional symptoms.[38]

Health promotion and maintenance for patients with HIV/AIDS must therefore acknowledge patients' perceived health care needs. Based on a study of 386 HIV-infected persons, it was determined that the health care challenges perceived by patients with HIV/AIDS across hospital, outpatient, home, and long-term-care settings included decreased endurance, physical mobility, and sensory perception, as well as financial issues—specifically lack of income and resources to cover living and health care expenses.[39] Often, meeting these and other health care challenges, particularly managing pain and other symptoms, becomes a major goal of primary care as the illness progresses. Enhancing immunocompetence is critical at all stages of illness, as well as treating the symptoms brought on by the disease or related to prophylatic or treatment therapies. Palliation of physical, emotional, and spiritual symptoms, particularly as experienced in the late symptomatic and advanced stages of HIV disease, is considered the final stage of a health and disease prevention approach and will be discussed later on in this chapter.[5]

Through all stages of HIV disease, health can be promoted and maintained through diet, micronutrients, exercise, reduction of stress and negative emotions, symptom surveillance, and the use of prophylactic therapies to prevent opportunistic infections or AIDS-related complications.

Diet

A health-promoting diet is essential for the optimal functioning of the immune system. Deficiencies in calorie and protein intake impair cell-mediated immunity, phagocytic function and antibody response. Adequate nutrition is a challenge for individuals with HIV/AIDS due to diseases of the mouth and oropharynx, such as oral candidiasis, anular cheilitis, gingivitis, herpes simplex, and hairy leukoplakia.[40] Incidence of diseases of the gastrointestional tract such as cytomegalovirus, mycobacterium avium complex, cryptosporidiosis, and Kaposi sarcoma increases for individuals with CD4 counts of 50 or less and may adversely affect their nutritional status.[41] The Task Force on Nutrition in AIDS (1989) recommended that the goals of sound nutritional management should include: (*1*) provision of adequate nutrients; (*2*) preservation of lean body mass; and (*3*) minimization of symptoms associated with malabsorption. A diet with a variety of foods from the five basic food groups, including 55% of calories from carbohydrates, 15% to 20% of calories from proteins, and 30% of calories from fats, is important in supporting immune function.[42] Each day it is recommended to have two or three servings from the protein and dairy group, seven to twelve servings from the starch and grain group, two servings of fruits and vegetables rich in vitamin C, as well as three servings of other fruits and vegetables.[5]

Micronutrients

Research has indicated that HIV-infected individuals have lower levels of magnesium, total carotenes, total choline, and vitamins A and B6, yet higher levels of niacin than noninfected individuals.[43] A linkage has been reported between vitamin A (beta carotene) deficiency and elevated disease progression and mortality.[44] Correcting both vitamin A and B6 deficiencies has been hypothesized to restore cell-mediated immunity, and vitamin supplement trials are under way. Current research supports the increase in dietary intake of n-3 polyunsaturated fatty acids, arginine, and RNA to increase body weight and stave off wasting owing to malabsorption. Increase in concentrations of amino acids such as arginine has also been found to preserve lean muscle mass.[43]

Exercise

A consistent outcome of the effects of exercise on immune function is the increase in natural killer cell activity, though variable results are reported on the effects of exercise on neutrophil, macrophage, and T and B cell function and proliferation.[45] In a review of exercise studies, LaPerriere, Klimas, and Fletcher[46] reported a trend in CD4 cell count elevation in all but one study, with the greatest effect from aerobic exercise and weight training. The CDC[47] recommend a physical exercise program of 30 to 45 minutes, four or more times a week as a health-promoting activity to increase lung capacity, endurance, energy, flexibility, and improve circulation.

Massage has also be linked to natural killer cell activity and overall immune regulation as reported in a research study of 29 HIV-infected men who received daily massages for one month.[48] Patient reports of less anxiety and greater relaxation related to exercise and massage are regarded by both patients and practitioners as important as laboratory markers.[43]

Stress and Emotions

Stress and negative emotions have also been associated with immunosuppression and vulnerability to disease. Stress of living with HIV/AIDS is related to the uncertainty regarding illness progression and prognosis, stigmatization and discrimination, and financial concerns as disabilities increase with advancing disease. Persons with AIDS frequently site the avoidance of stress as a way of maintaining a sense of well-being.[49] The use of exercise and massage and other relaxation techniques such as imagery, meditation, and yoga are reported as valuable stress management techniques.[50]

Health promotion also involves health beliefs and coping strategies that support well-being despite protracted illness. A study of 53 patients diagnosed with AIDS demonstrated that long-term survivors used numerous strategies to support their health, such as having the will to live, positive attitudes, feeling in charge, a strong sense of self, expressing their needs, and sense of humor. Other health promotion strategies frequently used by these patients included remaining active, seeking medical information, talking to others, socializing and pursuing pleasurable activities, good medical care, and counseling.[51] Health promotion may also involve financial planning and identification of financial resources available through the community and the public assistance offered through Medicaid.

It must also be recognized that additional physical and emotional stress is associated with the use of recreational drugs such as alcohol, chemical stimulants, tobacco, and marijuana, as such agents have an immunosuppressant effect and may interfere with health-promoting behaviors.[52] The use of such substances may also have a negative effect on interpersonal relationships and are associated with a relapse to unsafe sexual practices.[53] Interventions toward health promotion include encouraging patients to participate in self-health groups and harm reduction programs to deal with substance abuse problems.

Symptom Surveillance

Throughout the course of their illness, individuals with HIV disease require primary care services to identify early signs of opportunistic infections and minimize related symptoms and complications. This includes a complete health history, physical examination, and laboratory data including determination of immunologic and viral status.

Health History. In the care of patients with HIV/AIDS, the health history should include the following.[14]

- *History of present illness,* including a review of those factors that lead to HIV testing
- *Past medical history,* particularly those conditions that may be exacerbated by HIV disease or its treatments such as diabetes mellitus, hypertriglyceridemia, or chronic or active hepatitis B infection
- *Childhood illnesses and vaccinations* in preventing common infections such as polio, DPT, measles
- *Medication history,* including the patient's knowledge of the types of medications, side effects, adverse reactions, drug interactions, and administration recommendations
- *Sexual history,* regarding sexual behaviors and preferences and history of sexually transmitted diseases which can exacerbate HIV disease progression
- *Lifestyle habits,* such as the past and present use of recreational drugs, such as alcohol, which may accelerate progression of disease; cigarette smoking, which may suppress appetite or be associated with opportunistic infections such as oral candidiasis, hairy leukoplakia, and bacterial pneumonia
- *Dietary habits,* including risks related to food-borne illnesses such as hepatitis A
- *Travel history,* to countries in Asia, Africa, and South America where the risk of opportunistic infections increase
- *Complete systems review,* to provide indications of clinical manifestations of new opportunistic infections or cancers, as well as AIDS-related complications both from the disease and its treatments

Physical Examination. A physical exam should begin with a general assessment of vital signs and height and weight, as well as overall appearance and mood. A complete head-to-toe assessment is important and may reveal various findings common to individuals with HIV/AIDS such as:[14]

- *Oral cavity assessment* may indicate candida, oral hairy leukoplakia, or Kaposi sarcoma.
- *Fundoscopic assessment* may reveal visual changes associated with cytomegalovirus retinitis; glaucoma screening annually is also recommended.
- *Lymph node assessment* may reveal adenopathy detected at any stage of disease, yet indicative of disease progression.
- *Dermatologic assessment* may indicate various cutaneous manifestations that occur throughout the course of the illness such

as HIV exanthem, Kaposi sarcoma, or infectious complications such as dermtomycoses.

- *Neuromuscular assessment* may indicate various central, peripheral, or autonomic nervous systems disorders and signs and symptoms of conditions such as meningitis, encephalitis, dementia, or peripheral neuropathies.
- *Cardiovascular assessment* may reveal cardiomyopathy related to the use of antiretroviral therapy.
- *Gastrointestional assessment* may indicate organomegaly, specifically splenomegaly or hepatomegaly, particularly in patients with a history of substance abuse, as well as signs related to parasitic intestional infections; annual stool of guiac and rectal examination, as well as sigmoidoscopy every five years is also a part of health maintenance.
- *Reproductive system assessment* may reveal occult sexually transmitted diseases or malignancies, as well vaginal candidiasis, cervical dysplasia, pelvic inflammatory disease, or rectal lesions in women with HIV/AIDS, as well as uretheral discharge and rectal lesions or malignancies in HIV-infected men. Health maintenance in individuals with HIV/AIDS also includes annual mammograms in women, as well as testicular exams in men and prostate-specific antigen (PSA) annually.

Laboratory Data

- Immunologic and virologic determinations. CD4 counts, both the absolute numbers and the CD4 percentages, should be evaluated to assist the health practitioner in therapeutic decision making about treatments of opportunistic infections and antiretroviral therapy. Quantitative RNA determination or viral load (VL) is also an important marker for disease progression and to measure the effectiveness of antiretroviral therapy.[14] Furthermore it is recommended for patients with an initially high CD4 cell count and VL below the limits of quantification and on no therapy, to take both measurements every 4 to 6 months. During therapy initiation, CD4 cell counts and VL should be measured every 4 weeks until a good response and then every 3 months. After a change in therapy, CD4 cell counts and VL should be measured every 4 to 8 weeks.[14]
- Other laboratory determinations. The decision regarding laboratory testing is based on the stage of HIV disease, the medical processes warranting initial assessment or follow-up, and consideration of the patient-benefit-to-burden ratio. Complete blood counts are often measured with each VL determination or with a change of antiretroviral therapy, particularly with patients on drugs known to cause anemia. Chemistry profiles are done to assess liver function, lipid status, and glycemia every 3 to 6 months or with a change in therapy and are determined by the patient's antiretroviral therapy, baseline determinations, and coinfections. Abnormalities in these profiles may occur as a result of antiretroviral therapy. Increasing hepatic dysfunction is evident by elevations in the serum transaminases (AST, ALT, ALP, LDH).

Urine analysis should be done annually unless the person is on antiretroviral therapy, which may require more frequent follow-up to check for toxicity. Annual Papanicolaou (PAP) smears are also indicated, with recommendations for PAP smears every 3 to 6 months in HIV-infected women who are symptomatic. Syphilis studies should be done annually; however, patients with low positive titers should have follow-up testing at 3, 6, 9, 12, and 24 months. Gonorrhea and chlamydia test are encouraged every 6 to 12 months if the patient is sexually active. In addition, cytomegalovirus (CMV) serology for patients with CD4 cell counts under 100 cells/mm^3 should be measured every 6 months.[14] Individuals with CD4 cell counts below 100 cells/mm^3 and who had negative toxoplasmosis antibiodies at baseline should also be tested and started on TMP-SMZ (Bactrim) for prophylaxis.

Annual tuberculin skin testing (TST) is also important for HIV-infected individuals. A TST is considered positive in patients with induration of greater than or equal to 5 mm. With a positive TST, a yearly chest radiograph is warranted.

Prophylaxis

The primary strategy to prevent the development of opportunistic infections is to avoid exposure to microorganisms in the environment. Secondly, the immune system can be supported and maintained through the administration of prophylactic and/or suppressive therapies, which decrease the frequency or severity of opportunistic infections.[54] Primary prophylaxis is the administration of a pharmacologic agent to prevent initial infection, while secondary prophylaxis is the administration of a pharmacologic agent to prevent future occurrences of infection.[55] Table 36–1 describes the common opportunistic infections and recommended prophylactic and alternative regimens. In the late symptomatic and advanced stages of HIV disease, when CD4 counts are low and viral load may be high, prophylaxis remains important to protect against opportunistic infections. Therefore, throughout the illness trajectory, and even in hospice settings, patients may be taking prophylactic medications, requiring sophisticated planning and monitoring.[31]

At the sixth Conference on Retroviruses and Opportunistic Infections, reports indicated that patients with good CD4 cell responses to antiretroviral therapy (ART) were able to discontinue cytomegalovirus maintenance successfully. However, relapses did occur in several patients who failed ART therapy. Similarly, patients who responded to potent ART demonstrated restored immune responses to mycobacterium avium complex. Further studies are needed to determine the safety of discontinuation of prophylaxis in the case of low viral loads and high CD4 cell counts.[56] In addition, HIV-infected individuals are at risk for severe diseases that are vaccine preventable, such as hepatitis A and B, tetanus, influenza, pneumoccocal and measles, rubella and mumps. Table 36–2 presents vaccine-preventable illness and interventions. Von Gunten and colleagues [57] suggest the continuation of prophylaxis in hospice and palliative care settings for patients with AIDS as long as patients are able to take oral medications. This is because there is a high risk of reactivation and dissemination of diseases that can result in high number of symptoms. Suppressive therapy for herpes infections is also continued to prevent painful

Table 36–1. Opportunistic Infections and Treatments: Prophylaxis to Prevent First Episode of Opportunistic Disease in Adults and Adolescents Infected with Human Immunodeficiency Virus

Pathogen	Preventive Regimens		
	Indication	First Choice	Alternatives
Strongly Recommended as Standard of Care			
*Pneumocystis carinii**	CD4+ count <200/μL or oropharyngeal candidiasis	Trimethoprim-sulfamethoxazole (TMP-SMZ), 1 DS p.o. q.d. (AI) TMP-SMZ, 1 SS p.o. q.d. (AI)	Dapsone, 50 mg p.o. b.i.d. *or* 100 mg p.o. q.d. (BI); dapsone, 50 mg p.o. q.d. *plus* pyrimethamine, 50 mg p.o. q.w. *plus* leucovorin, 25 mg p.o. q.w. (BI); dapsone, 200 mg p.o. *plus* pyrimethamine, 75 mg p.o. *plus* leucovorin, 25 mg p.o. q.w. (BI); aerosolized pentamidine, 300 mg q.m. via Respirgard II nebulizer (BI); atovaquone, 1500 mg p.o. q.d. (BI); TMP-SMZ, 1 DS p.o. t.i.w. (BI)
Mycobacterium tuberculosis Isoniazid-sensitive†	TST reaction ≥5mm *or* prior positive TST result without treatment *or* contact with case of active tuberculosis	Isoniazid, 300 mg p.o. *plus* pyridoxine, 50 mg p.o. q.d. × 9 mo (AII) or isoniazid, 900 mg p.o. *plus* pyridoxine, 100 mg p.o. b.i.w. × 9 mo (BI); rifampin, 600 mg *plus* pyrazinamide, 20 mg/kg p.o. q.d. × 2 mo (AI)	Rifabutin 300 mg p.o. q.d. *plus* pyrazinamide, 20 mg/kg p.o. q.d. × 2 mo (BIIt); rifampin 600 mg p.o. q.d. × 4 mo (BIII)
Isoniazid-resistant	Same; high probability of exposure to isoniazid-resistant tuberculosis	Rifampin 600 mg *plus* pyrazinamide, 20 mg/kg p.o. q.d. × 2 mo (AI)	Rifabutin, 300 mg *plus* pyrazinamide 20 mg/kg p.o. q.d. × 2 mo (BIII); rifampin, 600 mg p.o. q.d. × 4 mo (BIII); Rifabutin, 30 mg p.o. q.d. × 4 mo (CIII)
Multidrug-(isoniazid and rifampin) resistant	Same; high probability of exposure to multidrug-resistant tuberculosis	Choice of drugs requires consultation with public health authorities	None
Toxoplasma gondii§	IgG antibody to *Toxoplasma* and CD4+ count <100/μL	TMP-SMZ, 1 DS po q.d. (AII)	TMP-SMZ, 1 SS po q.d. (BIII): dapsone, 50 mg po q.d. *plus* pyrimethamine, 50 mg p.o. q.s. *plus* leukovorin, 25 mg po q.w. (BI); atovaquone, 1500 mg p.o. q.d. with or without pyrimethamine, 25 mg po q.d. *plus* leukovorin, 10 mg p.o. q.d. (CIII)
Mycobacterium avium complex¶	CD4+ count <50/μL	Azithromycin, 1,200 mg p.o. q.w., (AI) or clarithromycin, 500 mg p.o. b.i.d. (AI)	Rifabutin, 300 mg p.o. q.d. (BI); azithromycin, 1,200 mg p.o. q.w. *plus* rifabutin, 300 mg p.o. q.d. (CI)
Varicella zoster virus (VZV)	Significant exposure to chickenpox or shingles for patients who have no history of either condition or, if available, negative antibody to VZV	Varicella zoster immune globulin (VZIG), 5 vials (1.25 mL each) im, administered ≤96 h after exposure, ideally within 48 h (AIII)	
Generally Recommended			
*Streptococcus pneumoniae***	All patients	Pneumococcal vaccine, 0.5 mL im (CD4+ ≥200/μL [BII]; CD4+ <200/μL [CIII])-might reimmunize if initial immunization was given when CD4+ <200/μL and if CD4+ increases to >200/μL on HAART(CIII)	None

(continued)

Table 36–1. Opportunistic Infections and Treatments: Prophylaxis to Prevent First Episode of Opportunistic Disease in Adults and Adolescents Infected with Human Immunodeficiency Virus (*Continued*)

	Preventive Regimens		
Pathogen	Indication	First Choice	Alternatives
Hepatitis B virus[††]	All susceptible (anti-HBc-negative) patients	Hepatitis B vaccine: 3 doses (BII)	None
Influenza virus[††]	All patients (annually, before influenza season)	Whole or split virus, 0.5 mL im/yr (BIII)	Rimantadine, 100 mg p.o. b.i.d. (CIII), or amantadine, 100 mg p.o. b.i.d. (CIII)
Hepatitis A virus[††]	All susceptible (anti-HAV–negative) patients with chronic hepatitis C	Hepatitis A vaccine: two doses (BIII)	None
Not Routinely Indicated			
Bacteria	Neutropenia	Granulocyte-colony–stimulating factor (G-CSF), 5–10 μg/kg sc q.d. × 2–4 w or granulocyte-macrophage colony-stimulating factor (GM-CSF), 250 μg/m^2 iv over 2 h q.d. × 2–4 w (CII)	None
Cryptococcus neoformans[§§]	CD4+ count <50/μL	Fluconazole, 100–200 mg p.o. q.d. (CI)	Itraconazole, 200 mg p.o. q.d. (CIII)
Histoplasma capsulatum[§§]	CD4+ count <100/μL, endemic geographic area	Itraconazole capsule, 200 mg p.o. q.d. (CI)	None
Cytomegalovirus (CMV)[¶¶]	CD4+ count <50/μL and CMV antibody positivity	Oral ganciclovir, 1 g p.o. t.i.d. (CI)	None

Notes: Information included in these guidelines might not represent Food and Drug Administration (FDA) approval or approved labeling for the particular products or indications in question. Specifically, the terms "safe" and "effective" might not be synonymous with the FDA-defined legal standards for product approval. The Respirgard II nebulizer is manufactured by Marquest, Englewood, Colorado. Letters and Roman numerals in parentheses after regimens indicate the strength of the recommendation and the quality of evidence supporting it.

Abbreviations: Anti-HBc = antibody to hepatitis B core antigen; b.i.w. = twice a week; DS = double-strength tablet; HAART = highly active antiretroviral therapy; HAV = hepatitis A virus; HIV = human immunodeficiency virus; im = intramuscular; iv = intravenous; po = by mouth; q.d. = daily; q.m. = monthly; q.w. = weekly; SS = single-strength tablet; t.i.w. = three times a week; TMP-SMZ = trimethoprim-sulfamethoxazole; sc = subcutaneous; and TST = tuberculin skin test.

*Prophylaxis should also be considered for persons with a CD4+ percentage of <14%, for persons with a history of an AIDS-defining illness, and possibly for those with CD4+ counts >200 but <250 cells/μL. TMP-SMZ also reduces the frequency of toxoplasmosis and some bacterial infections. Patients receiving dapsone should be tested for glucose-6 phosphate dehydrogenase deficiency. A dosage of 50 mg q.d. is probably less effective than that of 100 mg q.d. The efficacy of parental pentamidine (e.g., 4 mg/kg/month) is uncertain. Fansidar (sulfadoxine-pyrimethamine) is rarely used because of severe hypersensitivity reactions. Patients who are being administered therapy for toxoplasmosis with sulfadiazine-pyrimethamine are protected against *Pneumocystis carinii* pneumonia and do not need additional prophylaxis against PCP.

†Directly observed therapy is recommended for isoniazid, 900 mg b.i.w.; isoniazid regimens should include pyridoxine to prevent peripheral neuropathy. Rifampin should not be administered concurrently with protease inhibitors or nonnucleoside reverse transcriptase inhibitors. Rifabutin should not be given with hard-gel saquinavir or delavirdine; caution is also advised when the drug is coadministered with soft-gel saquinavir. Rifabutin may be administered at a reduced dose (150 mg q.d.) with indinavir, nelfinavir, or amprenavir; at a reduced dose of 150 mg q.o.d. (or 150 mg three times weekly) with ritonavir; or at an increased dose (450 mg q.d.) with efavirenz; information is lacking regarding coadministration of rifabutin with nevirapine. Exposure to multidrug-resistant tuberculosis might require prophylaxis with two drugs; consult public health authorities. Possible regimens include pyrazinamide plus either ethambutol or a fluoroquinolone.

§Protection against toxoplasmosis is provided by TMP-SMZ, dapsone plus pyrimethamine, and possibly by atovaquone. Atovaquone may be used with or without pyrimethamine. Pyrimethamine alone probably provides little, if any, protection.

¶See footnote † regarding use of rifabutin with protease inhibitors or nonnucleoside reverse transcriptase inhibitors.

**Vaccination should be offered to persons who have a CD4+ T-lymphocyte count <200 cells/μL, although the efficacy might be diminished. Revaccination 5 years after the first dose or sooner if the initial immunization was given when the CD4+ count was <200 cells/μL and the CD4+ count has increased to >200 cells/μL on HAART is considered optional. Some authorities are concerned that immunizations might stimulate the replication of HIV. However, one study showed no adverse effect of pneumococcal vaccination on patient survival (McNaghten AD, Hanson DL, Jones JL, Dworkin MS, Ward JW, and the Adult/Adolescent Spectrum of Disease Group. Effects of antiretroviral therapy and opportunistic illness primary chemoprophylaxis on survival after AIDS diagnosis. AIDS 1999;13:1687–1695).

††These immunizations or chemoprophylactic regimens do not target pathogens traditionally classified as opportunistic but should be considedred for use in HIV-infected patients as indicated. Data are inadequate concerning clinical benefit of these vaccines in this population, although it is logical to assume that those patients who develop antibody responses will derive some protection. Some authorities are concerned that immunizations might stimulate HIV replication, although for influenza vaccination, a large observational study of HIV-infected persons in clinical care showed noadverse effect of this vaccine, including multiple doses, on patient survival (J. Ward, CDC, personal communication). Hepatitis B vaccine has been recommended for all children and adolescents and for all adults with risk factors for hepatitis B virus (HBV). Rimantadine and amantadine are appropriate during outbreaks of influenza A. Because of the theoretical concern that increases in HIV plasma RNA following vaccination during pregnancy might increase the risk of perinatal transmission of HIV, providers may wish to defer vaccination until after antiretroviral therapy is initiated. For additional information regarding vaccination against hepatitits A and B and vaccination and antiviral therapy against influenza see CDC. Prevention of hepatitis A through active or passive immunization: recommendations of the Advisory Committee on Immunization Practices (ACIP). *MMWR* 1996;45(No. RR-15); CDC. Hepatitis B virus: a comprehensive strategy for eliminating transmission in the United States through universal childhood vaccination: recommendations of the Advisory Committee on Immunization Practices (ACIP). *MMWR* 1991;40(No. RR-13); and CDC. Prevention and control of influenza: recommendations of the Advisory Committee on Immunization Practices (ACIP). *MMWR* 1999;48(No. RR-4).

§§In a few unusual occupational or other circumstances, prophylaxis should be considered; consult a specialist.

¶¶Acyclovir is not protective against CMV. Valacyclovir is not recommended because of an unexplained trend toward increased mortality observed in persons with AIDS who were being adminsitered this drug for prevention of CMV disease.

Source: From Centers for Disease Control and Prevention.[109]

Table 36–2. Vaccine-Preventable Illness

Condition	Evidence Requiring Intervention	Intervention
Hepatitis A *consider in nonimmune sexually active patients*	Hepatitis A antibody-negative	Hepatitis A vaccine. Doses given at 0 and 6 months
Hepatitis B	Hepatitis B antibody-negative	Hepatitis B vaccine. Doses given at 0, 1, and 6 months
Tetanus	No serologic test available	Consider booster if not vaccinated within 10 years
Hib	No serologic test available available	Routine vaccination has not been demonstrated to be beneficial; however, vaccine is inexpensive
Influenza	No serologic test available	Vaccine should be offered annually in the fall
Pneumococcal	No serologic test available	Vaccine is given at baseline and every 6–8 years
MMR	Measles, rubella, and mumps titer-negative or nonimmune	Vaccination not routinely given but may be required in those never immunized, particularly students, teachers, health care workers, and other care providers

Source: Adapted from Centers for Disease Control and Prevention (1993). Recommendations of the Advisory Committee on Immunization Practices (ACIP): Use of vaccines and immune globulins in persons with altered immunocompetence. *Morbidity and Mortality Weekly Report* 42(RR-5):5.

lesions. Von Gunten and colleagues[57] also recommend the following plan regarding prophylaxis and suppressive therapy in hospice/palliative care:

1. If the patient is clinically stable and wants to continue prophylaxis, continue drug therapy.
2. If side effects occur, and the patient continues to be otherwise stable, consider alternative regimens.
3. If patient is intolerant of prophylaxis and/or the regimens are burdensome, discontinue medications.

Indications for Antiretroviral Therapy Across the Illness Trajectory. Without a cure for HIV disease, all treatments are essentially palliative in nature to slow disease progression and limit the occurrence of opportunistic infections, which adversely affect quality of life. The CD4 cell count and viral load are used in conjunction to determine the initiation of antiretroviral therapy. With the introduction of highly active antiretroviral therapy (HAART), the basic principle is to begin therapy as early as possible to limit damage to the immune system. Therapy is therefore recommended by the International AIDS Society for all patients who manifest an acute primary infection or are symptomatic regardless of their CD4 cell count; for individuals who are asymptomatic but whose CD4 cell counts are below 350 cells/mm^3, irrespective of HIVRNA level, and for individuals who have an HIVRNA level above 30,000 copies/ml of plasma, irrespective of CD4 cell count.[5] Therapy is also indicated for patients with low detectable HIVRNA level (<5,000 to 10,000 copies) but who have a low CD4 cell count (<500 cells/mm^3) and for those who CD4 cell counts are above 500 cells/mm^3 but who have an HIVRNA level in the 5000 to 30,000 copies range.[58]

Recommended Antiretroviral Therapy. Monotherapy is no longer the accepted standard of care for HIV/AIDS.[58] Currently, triple drug therapy is a first-line option in lowering viral load and limiting the destruction of the immune system.[56] Clinical trials indicate that the most effective course of treatment is by combining three or more drugs from the following three categories:

- nucleoside-analog reverse transcriptase inhibitors (NRTIs)
- nonnucleoside reverse transcriptase inhibitors (NNRTIs)
- protease inhibitors

The nucleoside-analog reverse transcriptase inhibitors (NRTIs) were the first class of antiretroviral agents approved for the treatment of HIV disease and included the drug known as AZT, otherwise known as zidovudine. NRTIs limit HIV replication early in the HIV life cycle by inhibiting the enzyme, reverse transcriptase, necessary for transcription of viral RNA into DNA. For many years zidovudine was used as monotherapy. It is now recognized that since viral replication continues from the point of initial infection, the virus must be challenged early in the course of illness. NRTIs include zidovudine (AZT, ZVD, Retrovir), didanosine (ddi, Videx), zalcitabine (ddc, Hivid), stavudine (d4t, Zerit), lamivudine (3TC, Epivir), and a new agent, abacavir (Ziagen).[56] The NRTI abacavir, in combination with ZDV and 3TC, appears to suppress viral load to a similar degree when compared to a protease inhibitor (PI) plus two NRTIs after 48 weeks of follow-up. However, abacavir is associated with potentially life-threatening hypersensitivity syndrome.[58] To date, insufficient clinical data is available to guide the optimal use of Abacavir as a potent NRTI in combination with PIs and/or NNRTIs.[58]

To limit the number of medications taken, thereby promoting medication adherence, a combination antiretroviral drug called combivir, which combines two NRTIs, lamivudine 150 mg and zidovudine 300 mg, is available as a single tablet. Combivir is often taken with a protease inhibitor.

The second category of antiretrovirals developed were the nonnucleoside reverse transcriptase inhibitors (NNRTIs). Like the NRTIs, they function by inhibition of the enzyme reverse transcriptase. Because of the potential risk of resistance, these drugs are not recommended for monotherapy, but can be used as triple drug therapy along with an NRTI and protease inhibitor. The NNR-

TIs are nevirapine (Viramune), delavirdine (Rescriptor), and efavirenz (Sustiva). However, not all PIs can be given with NNRTIs; for example, saquinavir should not be given with efavirenz.

The third category of antiretrovirals are the protease inhibitors (PI), which are highly potent with limited toxicity. Protease inhibitors function by inhibiting the action of protease by binding to the cleavage site of replicating HIV and halting the production of new infectious virons. The protease inhibitors include saquinavir (Fortovase), nelfinavir (Viracept), ritonavir (Norvir), indinavir (Crixivan), and a new investigational drug, amprenavir, which has a unique resistance profile and high tolerability. A summary of the current antiretroviral medications is presented in Table 36–3.

To achieve maximal viral suppression, treatment with one potent PI and two NRTIs has proven effective in initial therapy. The NNRTI efavirez used in combination with two NRTIs has also been shown to produce maximal viral suppression.[58] Another first-line option is two PIs, such as saquinavir and ritonavir, plus one or two NRTIs. Other alternatives are available and many be used in selected settings. However, they are considered by many to be less likely to produce maximal viral suppression.[58] These alternative options include:

- triple NRTIs combination
- one NNRTI (Nevirapine) plus two NRTIs
- a combination of one PI, one NNRTI, and one NRTI[58]

Change from one potent induction regimen to another potent regimen may be necessary if the patient's triglyceride and cholesterol levels become elevated, as lipodystrophy can be induced by protease inhibitors. If the initial response to a drug regimen is good but not optimal, or if there is a need to promote the durability of response in a successful regimen, intensification of treatment can occur by adding a drug to the regimen.[59] Although the addition of hydroxyurea to certain antiretroviral regimens may enhance the activity of these agents, the role of hydroxyurea in HIV treatment remains uncertain given the relative lack of information from controlled trials, and the number of toxicities.[58]

A log change in plasma HIV-1 RNA level is the most clinically sensitive marker of antiretroviral failure. If a suboptimal response is apparent by viral load, intensification of drug regimen as described above is a consideration, while an early viral rebound may motivate a change of at least two if not all components of a failing regimen.[59] The change of agents should be to new agents that are not likely to show cross-resistance with drugs given previously.[58]

Concern Regarding Drug Interactions. Considerations are also to be given to possible drug interactions such as pharmacokinetic interactions, which occur when administration of one agent changes the plasma concentration of another agent, and pharmacodynamic interactions which occur when a drug interacts with the biologically active sites and changes the pharmacologic effect of the drug without altering the plasma concentration. For example in palliative care, drug interactions have been reported for patients who are receiving methadone for pain management and who begin therapy with an NNRTI, nevirapine. These individuals have reported symptoms of opioid withdraw within 4 to 8 days of beginning nevirapine due to its effect on the cytochrome P-40 metabloic enzyme CYP3A4 and its induction of methadone metabolism.[60] See Table 36–3 on antiretroviral medications for dosages, common side effects, special instructions, and drug interactions.

Use and Continuation of Antiretrovirals in the Hospice/Palliative Care Setting and in Patients with Organ Failure. At present the aims of antiretroviral therapy are to prevent progression to AIDS, prevent the direct effects and symptoms of HIV disease, such as anemone, dementia, neuropathy, and diarrhea, and prevent the complications of AIDS. According to Von Gunten and colleagues,[57] the continuation of antiretroviral therapy in hospice or palliative settings is often contingent on the feelings of patients regarding the therapy. Patients can be asked, "How do you feel when you take your antiretroviral medications?" As medications may still symbolize hope, patients who enter hospice may have a greater acceptance of their mortality and wish to stop antiretrovirals because of the side effects. Other patients may wish to continue antiretroviral therapy because of its symptom relief and the prevention of future symptoms related to opportunistic infections. Von Gunten and colleagues[57] suggest the following plan:

1. If the drug causes burdensome symptoms, discontinue.
2. If the patient no longer wants the drug, discontinue.
3. If the patient is asymptomatic and wants the drug, continue with close clinical assessment.
4. Discontinue the measurement of viral loads and CD4 counts and help the patient focus on relief of symptoms.

The use of antiretrovirals must also be seriously considered for patients who have organ dysfunction or failure, given changes in hepatic and renal function and the effects on drug elimination. For example, patients with renal impairment may be at greater risk for zidovudine-induced hematologic toxicity due to lowered production of erythropoietin. In addition, because of the markedly decreased clearance of ZVD and increased drug half-life, it is recommended that the daily dosage of ZVD be reduced by approximately 50% in patients with severe renal dysfunction (CrCL < 25mL/min), for those receiving hemodialysis, and for those with hepatic dysfunction.[61] In addition, due to reduced drug clearance, patients should be monitored for ZVD-related adverse effects.

Although specific dosage recommendations are available for some of the early developed antiretrovirals for patients with organ dysfunction or failure, there are no specific studies that provide guidelines for the dosing of many of the new antiretroviral agents. As many of the antiretroviral agents are metabolized by the liver and excreted by the kidney, knowledge of pharmacokinetic properties of antiretroviral drugs is recommended to monitor drug therapy for efficacy and safety.[61] The suggested dosing recommendations for antiretroviral

Table 36–3. Antiretroviral Medications

Name	Dosage	Common Side Effects	Special Instructions	Drug Interactions
Nucleoside Reverse Transcriptase Inhibitors				
Zidovudine (ZVD, AZT, Retrovir)	200 mg t.i.d. or 300 mg b.i.d. (higher doses may be necessary for neurologic disease)	Neutropenia, anemia, nausea, myalgia, malaise, headache, insomnia	Take with meals to decrease nausea, and myalgias	Increased risk of neutropenia with ganciclovir and trimethoprimsulfamethoxole. Methadone increases blood levels. Stavudine may decrease effectiveness. Phenytoin alters metabolsim (may increase or decrease levels)
Didanosine (ddI, Videx)	>60 kg: 2 100 mg tablets or 250 mg powder; <60 kg: 125 mg in 2 tablets or 167 mg powder every 12 hours	Peripheral neuropathy, abdominal pain, dry mouth, altered taste, diarrhea, pancreatitis, rash	Always take both tablets or all the powder to ensure correct dosage. Take with about 4 oz. of water. Should be taken on an empty stomach (one half hour before meals or 1–2 hours after a meal). Avoid alcohol. Dapsone, ketoconazole, intraconazole should be taken 2 hours after didanosine. Report any numbness, burning, or tingling. Tetracycline and fluoroquinole should be administered 2 hours before or after ddI. Indinavir should be administered at least 1 hour before or after ddI on an empty stomach. Ritonavir should be administered at least 2 hours before or after ddI	Buffer affects dapsone, ketoconazole, protease inhibitors, and quinolones. Ganciclovir increase blood blood levels. Concomitant administration of pentamidine increases the risk of pancreatitis
Zalcitabine (ddC, Hivid)	0.75 mg t.i.d.	Peripheral neuropathy, pancreatitis, rash, fever, apthous ulcer, anemia, elevated liver enzymes	Avoid alcohol. Report any numbness, burning or tingling. Should be taken on an empty stomach	Similar toxicity to didanosine and stavudine
Stavudine (D4T, Zerit)	>60 kg: 40 mg b.i.d.; <60 kg: 30 mg b.i.d.	Peripheral neuropathy, elevated liver enzymes, nausea, diarrhea, myalgia	Avoid alcohol. Report any numbness, burning, or tingling	Similar toxicity to zalcitabine and didanosine
Lamivudine (3TC, Epivir)	150 mg b.i.d.	Mild rash, headache, diarrhea, hair loss, neutropenia	Can be taken with food	Trimethohprim-sulfa increases blood levels
Abacavir (Ziagen)	300 mg b.i.d.	Fatal hypersensitivity reactions. Common side effects: nausea, vomiting, diarrhea, anorexia, insomnia, fever, headache, skin rash	Taken with or without food	Alcohol decreases the elimination of abacavir causing an increase in overall exposure
Lamivudine/ zidovudine (Combivir)	1 tab b.i.d. (150 mg of lamivudine and 300 mg of zidovudine per tablet)	Headache, malaise, fatigue, nausea, diarrhea, cough	Can be taken with food to decrease nausea	Coadministration of ganciclovir, interferon-alpha or other bone-marrow-suppressive or cytotoxic agents may increase the hematoxicity of ZVD

(continued)

Table 36–3. Antiretroviral Medications (*Continued*)

Name	Dosage	Common Side Effects	Special Instructions	Drug Interactions
Nonnucleoside Reverse Transcriptase Inhibitors				
Nelvirapine (Viramune)	200 mg, every day for 2 weeks, then 200 mg every 12 hours	Rash, puritus, fever, thrombocytopenia, elevated liver enzymes	Discontinue if severe rash develops. Monitor liver function tests. Should not be used concurrently with hormonal contraception.	Decreases protease inhibitor levels (induces cytochrome P450 enzymes)
Delavirdine (Respirtor)	400 mg t.i.d.	Rash, fever, elevated liver enzymes	Take on an empty stomach. Monitor liver function test. Should be taken 1 hour before or after ddI or antacids	Increases protease inhibitors, clarithromycin, dapsone, rifabutin, ergot alkaloids, dihydropyrides, quinidine, and warfin levels (inhibits cytochrome P450 enzymes)
Efavirenz (Sustiva)	600 mg p.o. with protease inhibitor or NRTI	Psychiatric and nervous system symptoms such as dizziness, abnormal dreams, impaired concentration, delusions, insomnia, abnormal behavior, and rash	Taken with or without food. If taken with food, a high-fat meal should be avoided. If taken at bedtime, there is improved tolerabilty of nervous system side effects	Drugs that induce CYP3A4 activity such as phenobarbital, rifampin, and rifabutin, would be expected to increase the clearance of efavirenz therefore resulting in lower plasma concentrations. Warfin plasma concentrations and effects are potentially increased or decreased with efavirenz. The dose of indinavir should be increased from 800 mg to 1000 mg if coadministered with efavirenz. Saquinavir and clarithromycin plasma concentrations are decreased by efavirenz
Protease Inhibitors				
Indinavir (Crixivan)	800 mg t.i.d.	Nephrolithiasis, hyperbilrubinemia, fatigue, headache, nausea, abdominal pain	Lactose-intolerant patients should take with lactaid tablets. Should be taken on an empty stomach or with light, low to nonfat meal. Increase water intake each day (at least 48 oz of fluid in adults). Never take double doses unless instructed	Inhibits cytochrome P450. Ketoconazole increases blood levels; rifabutin and rifampin decrease blood levels; astemizole, terferadine, cisapride, and triazolam increases the risk of dysrhythmias
Nelfinavir (Viracept)	750 mg t.i.d.	Mild diarrhea, elevated liver enzymes	Never take double doses unless instructed. Should be taken with a meal or light snack. Should be adminsitered 2 hours before of 1 hour after ddI	Inhibits cytochrome P450. Rifabutin and rifampin decrease blood levels; astemizole, and cisapride increase risk of dysrhythmias
Ritonvir (Norvir)	600 mg b.i.d.	Nausea, vomiting, diarrhea, taste alterations, paresthesias (hands, feet, and lips), elevated triglycerides	Therapy should be started at a low dose and increased over 5 days to decrease nausea. Never take double doses unless instructed. Monitor liver function test. Evaluate patient's medications profile before administering	Inhibits cytochrome P450. Numerous drug interactions

(*continued*)

Table 36–3. Antiretroviral Medications (*Continued*)

Name	Dosage	Common Side Effects	Special Instructions	Drug Interactions
Saquinavir (Invirase [hard gel capsule] and Fortvase [soft gel capsule]).	600 mg t.i.d.	Headache, nausea, diarrhea	Should be taken within 2 hours of a full meal. Never take a double dose unless instructed. Lactose intolerant patients should take with lactaid tablets	Inhibits cytochrome P450. Rifabutin and rifampin decrease blood levels; ketoconazole, itraconazole, and ritonavir increase blood levels; terfenadine and astemiazole increase risk of dysrhythmias

Source: Adapted from Porche.[55]

agents in patients with organ dysfunction is presented in Table 36–4.

Adherence to Therapy. A major obstacle to the success of antiretroviral therapy in suppressing viral replication is that partial suppression facilitates the emergence of resistant viral strains.[62] Adherence, which is "the extent to which a person's behavior coincides with medical and health advice,"[63] is therefore essential to health maintenance for patients with HIV/AIDS. Nonadherence to antiretroviral therapy may lead not only to resistance to a whole class of drug, especially protease inhibitors, but may affect systemic drug concentration, intracellular drug concentration, drug potency, viral resistance, and viral inhibition.[64]

Medication adherence is defined as the ratio of medication doses taken to those prescribed with a cutoff of 80% to categorize the patient as adherent.[64] However, there is concern that with HAART therapy viral replication suppression may not be ensured even with 80% adherence. Assessment of adherence is most often done by self-report, with studies showing that it is a valid indicator of adherence.[65] Asking patients to bring their medications to a health visit, to describe their pill-taking regi-

Table 36–4. Dosing Recommendations for Antiretroviral Agents in Patients with Organ Dysfunction

	Renal Dysfunction Creatinine Clearance (mL/min)					
	≥50	26–49	10–25	<10	Hemodialysis	Hepatic Dysfunction
Zidovudine	200 mg q8h	200 mg q8h	100 mg q8h	100 mg q8h	100 mg q8h	100 mg q8h
Didanosine						
≥60 kg†	200 mg q12h	200 mg q24h	100 mg q24h	100 mg q24h	100 mg q24h*	Consider empiric dosage reduction in moderate to severe disease‡
<60 kg†	125 mg q12h	125 mg q24h	50 mg q24h	50 mg q24h	50 mg q24h*	
Zalcitabine	0.75 mg q8h	0.75 mg q12h	0.75 mg q12h	0.75 mg q24h	0.75 mg q24h*	0.75 mg q8h
Stavudine						
≥60 kg†	40 mg q12h	40 mg q24h	20 mg q24h	20 mg q24h	20 mg q24h*	40 mg q12h‡
<60 kg†	30 mg q12h	30 mg q24h	15 mg q24h	15 mg q24h	15 mg q24h*	30 mg q12h‡
Lamivudine	150 mg q12h	150 mg q24h	150 mg × 1, then 100 mg q24h	150 mg × 1, then 25–50 mg q24h	150 mg × 1, then 25–50 mg q24h*	150 mg q12h‡
Nevirapine	200 mg q12h	200 mg q12h	200 mg q12h	200 mg q12h	NR*	Consider empiric dosage reduction‡
Delavirdine	400 mg q8h	400 mg q8h	400 mg q8h	400 mg q8h	NR*	Consider empiric dosage reduction‡
Efavirenz	600 mg q24h	600 mg q24h	600 mg q24h	600 mg q24h	NR*	Consider empiric dosage reduction‡
Saquinavir§	600 mg q8h	600 mg q8h	600 mg q8h	600 mg q8h	NR*	Consider empiric dosage reduction‡
Ritonavir	600 mg q12h	600 mg q12h	600 mg q12h	600 mg q12h	NR*	Consider empiric dosage reduction‡
Indinavir	800 mg q8h	800 mg q8h	800 mg q8h	800 mg q8h	NR*	Mild to moderate: 600 mg q8h Severe: consider further dosage reduction‡
Nelfinavir	750 mg q8h	750 mg q8h	750 mg q8h	750 mg q8h	NR*	Consider empiric dosage reduction‡

*Administer daily dose after completion of hemodialysis.
†Dosage based on body weight.
‡No specific recommendations available. Patients should be carefully monitored for adverse effects.
§Data shown for hard gelatin capsule formulation. Dosage or soft gelatin capsule is 1200 mg q8h.
NR = No recommendations.
Source: Hilts and Fish.[61]

Table 36–5. Interventions to Improve Antiretroviral Medication Adherence

Type of Intervention	Specific Examples
Interventions addressing the patient	
Key patient education topics	Dynamics of HIV infection Purpose of antiretroviral therapy All names of medications Reasons for dose and administration requirements Potential side effects Techniques for managing side effects
Cues and reminders for patient	Detailed daily schedule Doses planned to coincide with daily habits (favorite TV program, morning news) Medication boxes and timers (available from some pharmaceutical companies) Prepoured medications Unit of use packaging
Patient involvement in therapeutic plan	Contributes to choice of antiretroviral combination Self-control of medications for side effects Anticipatory planning for weekends, vacations
Rewards and reinforcements	Positive feedback: falling HIV RNA level, rising CD4 cell count, fewer clinic appointments
Social support for adherence	Involvement of significant others Support groups Peer counseling and buddy plans Treatment of concomitant conditions such as substance abuse, depression Case management and financial assistance Home visits and telephone follow-up
Interventions addressing the clinician	
Continuing education regarding	Importance of adherence Factors associated with adherence Techniques to increase adherence Teaching skills Communication skills Effective management of side effects
Cues and reminders for the clinician	User-friendly medication review forms Tables and checklists in the clinical chart Patient teaching tools
Social support	Involvement of colleagues Team approach Administrative approval for additional time spent with patient on adherence concerns
Interventions addressing the regimen	Once or twice-a-day dosing regimens Use of fewer pills per day Use of smaller pills or capsules Improved taste Simpler storage requirements Fewer side effects Increased effectiveness Decreased cost

Source: Williams.[64] A. B. (1999). Adherence to highly active antiretroviral therapy. In *HIV/AIDS update* (D. W. Sherman, ed.), pp. 113–127. Nursing Clinics of North America; W. B. Saunders Co., Philadelphia, PA.

mens, review of the number of doses taken in 24 hours, and asking about troubles taking the medications and the effects of medications are important aspects of assessment.[64] Factors not predictive of adherence include age, sex, race, education, occupation, and socioeconomic status,[66] while factors predictive of adherence include[67]

1. patient characteristics such as physical and emotional health, material resources, cultural beliefs, self-efficacy, social support, personal skills, and HIV knowledge
2. clinician factors including interpersonal style availability, as well as assessment, communication and clinical skills
3. medication regimen factors such as the frequency, number and size of pills, taste of pills, storage, side effects, effectiveness, and cost
4. illness factors including symptoms duration, severity, and stigma.

Adherence to medication regimens can be improved through educational, behavioral, and social interventions, specific to the patient, clinician, and medication regimen.[64] (See Table 36–5.) An established partnership and an open, trusting, and supportive relationship between patients and clinicians remain key factors in promoting not only adherence to medication regimens, but support of all health promotion and management initiatives to delay disease progression, and AIDS-related complications.

AIDS-RELATED OPPORTUNISTIC INFECTIONS AND MALIGNANCIES

Opportunistic infections are the greatest cause of morbidity and mortality in individuals with HIV disease. Given the compromised immune system of HIV-infected individuals, there is a wide spectrum of pathogens that can produce primary, life-threatening infections, particularly when the CD4 cell counts fall below 200 cells/mm^3. Given the weakened immune systems of HIV-infected persons, even previously acquired infections can be reactivated. Most of these opportunistic infections are incurable and can at best be palliated to control the acute stage of infection and prevent recurrence through long-term suppressive therapy. In addition, patients with HIV/AIDS often experience concurrent or consecutive opportunistic infections, which are severe and cause a great number of symptoms. In Table 36–6, the various categories of opportunistic infections and malignancies are reviewed with regard to epidemiology/pathogenesis, presentation and assessment, diagnosis and interventions.[5,11]

Table 36–6. Opportunistic Infections and Malignancies Associated with HIV/AIDS

Types of Infections and Malignancies	Epidemiology/ Pathogenesis	Presentation and Assessment	Diagnosis	Interventions
Fungal Infections				
Candida albicans	Ubiquitious organism. Occurs with immunosuppression/ alteration in mucus membranes or skin. Early manifestation of HIV. Predictor of disease progression. Human-to-human transmission possible. Oropharyngeal candidiasis common	Oral *Candida* presents as pseudomembranous white patches, easily removed, leaving erythematous or bleeding mucosa. Vaginal candidiasis presents with pruritus and curdlike vaginal discharge. Esophageal candidiasis presents with dysphagia. Candida leukoplakia cannot be removed	Often presumptive by tissue inspection. Wet mount and/or potassium hydroxide (KOH) smear showing budding hyphae. Esophageal diagnosis by endoscopy with biopsy. Diagnosis by culture is unreliable	Mucotaneous infection treated locally with Clotrimazole troches, Nystatin suspension, Fluconazole, Miconazole, or Amphoterician B
Coccidioides immitis (Coccidioidomycosis)	Endemic to southwestern US. Acquired by inhalation of spores. Occurs with CD4 <250 mm^3	May be asymptomatic or with progressive signs of fever, malaise, weight loss, cough, fatigue	Chest radiographs may show diffuse interstitial or nodular infiltrates. Definitive diagnosis by culture or direct visualization of the organism in sputum, urine, or CSF	Systemic Amphotericin B, followed by lifelong suppressive therapy with oral Fluconazole
Cryptococcus neoformans (Cryptococcosis)	Ubiquitious organism. Aerosolized and inhaled. Most common life-threatening infection in AIDS. *Cryptococcus* meningitis has high mortality rate	Meningitis is most common clinical manifestation, presenting with headache, fever, stiff neck, photophobia, lethargy, and confusion. Symptoms develop over 2–4 week period. Cranial nerve palsies occur. Decreased vision. Can lead to blindness. Cryptococcal pneumonia may present with cough, dypsnea. Infection may disseminate to bone marrow, kidney, liver, spleen, lymph nodes, heart, oral cavity, and prostate	Serum cryptoccal antigen is 99% indicative. Examination of CSF. Infection of extrameningeal sites diagnosed with India ink and culture of tissues, and specimens. MRI or CT scan can show cryptococcoma. Chest radiographs show diffuse or focal infiltrates with or without mediastinal adenopathy	Acute therapy with Amphotericin B with or without Fluconazole and life-long suppression with Fluconazole
Histoplasma capsulatum	Endemic to midwest and south central US. Spores are inhaled. Occurs with CD4 counts <100/mm^3	Cough with fever. Often disseminated disease rather than pneumonitis Signs and symptoms include fever, weight loss, night sweats, nausea, diarrhea, abdominal pain	Chest radiograph show diffuse bilateral interstitial infiltrates. One-third have normal chest-xray. 5–10% have cutaneous lesions	Amphotericin B for serious illness or itraconazole or Fluconazole for mild disease. Life-long therapy of Itraconazole or Fluconazole

(*continued*)

Table 36–6. Opportunistic Infections and Malignancies Associated with HIV/AIDS (*Continued*)

Types of Infections and Malignancies	Epidemiology/ Pathogenesis	Presentation and Assessment	Diagnosis	Interventions
Mycobacterial Infections				
Mycobacterium tuberculosis (TB)	Increase in infections attributable to the high incidence of HIV-infection. HIV-infection may lead to reactivation of latent TB infection. Outbreaks of multidrug-resistant TB. Caused by inhalation of infectious particles that are aerosolized. Can have latent infection with no symptoms of active TB. Extrapulmonary TB may occur in 70% of HIV infected HIV infected TB decrease CD4 count and increases viral load	Fever, weight loss, night sweats, fatigue are initial complaints. With pulmonary TB, dyspnea, hemoptysis and chest pain may occur. Extrapulmonary sites such as lymph nodes, bones, bone marrow, joints, liver, spleen, skin, cerebrospinal fluid may show TB	Positive PPD is defined as >5 mm of induration at 48 to 72 hours using Mantoux intradermal method. Check for anergy with use of mumps and Candida. Chest radiographs show apical or cavitary infiltrates, and may show intrathoracic adneopathy. Diagnosis confirmed by sputum for acid-fast bacilli (AFB) stain. Blood cultures for AFB should be obtained.	Four-drug regimen with Isoniazid, Rfampin, Pyrazinamide, and either Streptomycin or Ethambutol. Prophylaxis with Isoniazid or Rifampin for individuals without current active TB
Mycobacterium avium intracellulare (MAC)	MAC composed of M. avium and M. intracellulare- two related species. Exist in water, soil, and foodstuffs. Person to person transmission is not likely. Most common cause of systemic bacterial infection in AIDS. Disseminated disease frequently cause of mortality in advanced HIV disease	Respiratory symptoms uncommon with MAC. MAC bacteremia is the most common syndrome. Fever, fatigue, weight loss, anorexia, nausea and vomiting, night sweats, diarrhea, abdominal pain, hepatosplenomegaly, and lymphadenopathy are common symptoms	Positive cultures from normally sterile sites, such as blood, bone marrow, or lymph nodes. Confirmed by biopsy with AFB stain. Lab studies usually demonstrate anemia and elevated alkaline phosphatase	Macrolide (Clarithromycin or Azithromycin) and Rifabutin, and Ethambutol for acute treatment. Prophylaxis with Rifabutin or Clarithromycin, or Azithromycin
Viral Infections				
Cytomegalovirus (CMV)	Ubiquitious, human herpesvirus. Most common cause of serious opportunistic disease in AIDS. May have contracted primary infection in childhood or young adulthood. Occurs in more than 40% of patients with CD 4 count $<50/mm^3$	CMV retinitis most common form and untreated can quickly lead to blindness. May be asymptomatic or with painless loss of visual acuity and symptoms of floaters or visual field defects, or conjunctivitis. Gastrointestinal tract second most common site with symptoms of dysphagia, abdominal pain, odynophagia, fever, bloody diarrhea and colitis	CMV retinitis on opthalmoscopic exam shows creamy yellow-white exudate with retinal hemorrhage. GI CMV demonstrated by endoscopy showing ulceration and tissue biopsy	High doses of Ganciclovir or Foscarnet, followed by life-long daily intravenous infesions with maintenance doses of one of these two medications

(*continued*)

Table 36–6. Opportunistic Infections and Malignancies Associated with HIV/AIDS (*Continued*)

Types of Infections and Malignancies	Epidemiology/ Pathogenesis	Presentation and Assessment	Diagnosis	Interventions
Herpes simplex virus (HSV)	HSV-1 transmitted primarily by contact with mucus membranes and salivary secretions HSV2- spread by sexual transmission. Risk with CD4 count $<100/mm^3$	Cutaneous ulcerative, vesicular painful lesions on any part of the body, particularly face, genitals, or perianal. May cause esophagitis with dysphagia and odynophagia	Visual infection with confirmation by viral swab culture. If vesicle present, it should be unroofed with 18 gauge needle and swabbed over the base of the ulcer	Acyclovir is used in primary therapy. Intravenous Acyclovir for severe HIV infections or HSV encephalitis. Topical Acyclovir ointment to relieve subjective symptoms. Maintenance therapy to prevent reactivation with acyclovir.
Varicella zoster (Herpes zoster) (VZV) [shingles]	Herpes virus may be initial presentation of HIV infection. Recurrent or disseminated seen with advanced HIV disease. Primary VZV is chicken pox	Radicular pain, a localized burning, followed by localized maculopular rash along a dermatone progressing to a fluid-filled continuous vesicles. May have postherpatic neuralgia for months after lesions have healed. Visceral dissemination to lung, liver, or CNS is life threatening	Clinical appearance. Cutaneous scrapings stained with fluorescein-conjugated monoclonal antibodies to confirm presence of VZV antigens	Acyclovir or Famciclovir, or Ganciclovir or Foscarnet for acute treatment
Human papilloma virus (HPV)	Most prevalent STD. Occurs with increased frequency with immunocompromised patients	Genital and perianal warts in men and women. May also have internal warts	Cytological dysplasia evident on smears	Trichloroacetic acid 50% or Podophyllin 25% or Podofilox or 5-Fluorouracil cream for acute treatment. Electrosurgery or surgical excision
Protozoal Infections				
Cryptosporidium parvum	Transmitted through fecally contaminated water or food. May have person to person spread in HIV-infected individuals. Oocyts can remain active outside the body for 2–6 months. Major cause of diarrhea when CD4 count $<200/mm^3$	Profuse, watery diarrhea, severe crampy abdominal pain, nausea, flatuance, weight loss, electrolyte imbalance, dehydration. May lead to malabsorption and wasting syndrome	Confirmed by modified acid fast or fluorescent antibody stain of stool specimen or small bowel biopsy	Restore immune system with HAART. No currently approved specific agent. Paromomycin or nitrazoxanide may be beneficial
Toxoplasma gondii	Occurs worldwide in humans and domestic animals, particularly cats. Oocytes transmitted in infected meats, eggs, vegetables or other food products. Major cause of neurological morbidity and mortality especially with individuals with CD4 <100 mm^3	Toxoplasmosis encephalitis most common with headache, fever, altered mental status, focal neurological deficits and seizures	Laboratory studies non-specific. CT scan with contrast or brain MRI shows multiple diffuse mass lesions with edema. Examination of CSF is usually not helpful	Pyrimethamine and Folinic acid as first line treatment for acute infection. Second line treatment with Clindamycin or Atovaquone or Clarithromycin or Azithromycin. Life-long prophylaxis with Trimethoprim-sulfamethoxozole for those with CD4 $<$ $100/mm^3$

(*continued*)

Table 36–6. Opportunistic Infections and Malignancies Associated with HIV/AIDS (*Continued*)

Types of Infections and Malignancies	Epidemiology/ Pathogenesis	Presentation and Assessment	Diagnosis	Interventions
Isospora belli	Distributed throughout the animal kingdom and endemic to parts of Africa, Chile, and Southeast Asia. Transmission through direct contact with infected animals, persons, or contaminated water. Shed in the stool of humans or host animals. Latino and foreign born persons at greater risk	Profuse, watery diarrhea, with stool output averaging 8–10 bowel movements a day, steatorrhea, headache, fever, malaise, abdominal pain, vomiting, dehydration, and weight loss	Identification of oocytes in the stool. Suggest minimum of 4 stool specimens taken for patients with AIDS A rapid auto-fluorescence technique may help in making a more rapid and reliable diagnosis	Trimethoprim-sulfamethoxazole or Pyrimethamine for acute treatment. Maintenance treatment with either agent
Microsporidia	Includes multiple species that are pathogenic to humans. Worldwide distribution. Occurs with CD4 count $<100/mm^3$. Fecal-oral transmission by ingestion of spores. Can live outside body for for up to 4 months	Profuse, watery diarrhea with crampy abdominal pain, malabsorption, weight loss, and wasting	Poor staining qualities. Detection requires endoscopy with small bowel biopsy	HAART has led to the resolution of this infection. Albendazole and Octreotide have been proven to be beneficial
Bacterial Infections				
Streptococcus pneumoniae and *Hemophilus influenzae* (Community acquired)	Most common causes of bacterial pneumonia in HIV infected individual. Occurs five times more frequently in individuals with CD4 $<200/mm^3$. Reach the lungs through inhalation, aspiration of secretions from mouth or oropharynx, or spread by blood to the lungs from another site	Abrupt onset with fever, cough with purulent sputum, and systemic toxic effects	Chest radiograph shows dense segmental or lobar consolidation. Chest radiograph may show nodular patterns, or diffuse interstitial infiltrates	Clarithromycin or azithromycin used to treat or prevent infection. Low dose trimethoprim-sulfamethoxazole as secondary prophylaxis for sinopulmonary infections. Vaccination against H. Influenzae in persons with HIV infection
Pseudmonas aeruginosa	Important pathogen in late HIV disease. Isolated from soil, water, plants, and animals. Most frequently acquired nosocomial pulmonary or cutaneous infection. Associated with a high rate of relapse in those who survive initial infection	Fever, cough, dyspnea, chest pain, sinusitis. May have recurrent cellutitis	Blood and sputum cultures. Focal chest x-rays similar to other bacterial pneumonias	Optimize immunologic status since PCP or MAC prophylaxis is not effective in prevention of *Pseudmonas.* Treatment requires two or more anti-pseudomonal agents

(*continued*)

Table 36–6. Opportunistic Infections and Malignancies Associated with HIV/AIDS (*Continued*)

Types of Infections and Malignancies	Epidemiology/ Pathogenesis	Presentation and Assessment	Diagnosis	Interventions
Salmonella species	Gram-negative bacteria pathogenic in both animals and humans. *Salmonella* typhi cause typhoid fever. Non-typhoid *Salmonella* species causes infection in patients with AIDS. Transmitted person to person by oral-fecal route, and infection in animals such as chickens. *Salmonella* gastroenteritis results from exposure to infected pets or animal derived food stuff such as poultry or eggs. HIV-infected patients are at risk for *Salmonella* bacteremia with or without gastrointestional disease	Bacteremia without signs of localizing infection and nonspecific signs of septicemia. Gastrointestinal presentation includes diarrhea or abdominal pain	Bacterial culture of blood. *Salmonella* enteritis is diagnosed by positive stool cultures. Other localized diagnosed by culture of CSF or aspirated fluid	Ampicillin or Fluoroquinolone or Ciprofloxacin or Cefotaxime or Ceftriaxone or Trimethoprim-sulfamethoxazole for acute treatment. Trimethoprim-sulfamethoxazole or Amoxicillin for maintenance treatment
Pneumocystis Infections				
Pneumocystis carinii (PCP)	One of most common OIs in HIV infection. Most common cause of pulmonary disease. Without prophylaxis, occurs with CD4 less than 200/mm^3	Fever, dyspnea, a non-productive cough. 2% of patients develop spontaneous pneumothorax	Sputum induction, bronchoalveolar lavage. Arterial blood gases show hypoxia. LDH elevated	Trimethoprim-sulfamethoxazole or Dapsone as first line drugs. Penatmidine or Clindamycin as second line drugs. Trimethoprim-sulfamethoxazole used for prophylaxis
Malignancies				
Non-Hodgkin's Lymphoma (NHL)	Rate of NHL is 73 times higher in HIV infected individual than the general population. Greater chance of NHL with CD4 count <50/mm^3 and in older white males. Caused by uncontrolled proliferation of lymphatic tissue, usually arising in the lymph nodes, spleen, liver, and bone marrow. Brain is the most common site of involvement. In patients with HIV disease, 80–90% of the NHL is extranodal, making lymph node based tumors uncommon	Nonspecific symptoms of unexplained fever, weight loss, and night sweats. Elevated serum lactate dehydrogenase level. Localizing symptoms depending on the site of the tumor. Neurological deficits if NHL of the brain. NHL of GI tract presents with abdominal pain, weight loss, or gastrointestinal bleeding. Small bowel lymphoma may lead to obstructive jaundice and small-bowel intussusception	Biopsy of specimens or cytological examination of tissue fluid. CT scan of brain or abdomen	CNS lymphoma treated with radiation with poor survival of only 3 months. Disease outside CNS treated with chemotherapy. Assess and treat for neutropenia secondary to chemotherapy. Antiretroviral agents may enhance clinical response to chemotherapy

(*continued*)

Table 36–6. Opportunistic Infections and Malignancies Associated with HIV/AIDS (*Continued*)

Types of Infections and Malignancies	Epidemiology/ Pathogenesis	Presentation and Assessment	Diagnosis	Interventions
Kaposi sarcoma (KS)	Rare, unusual neoplasm which usually affected older men of Jewish and Mediterranean ancestory (Classic KS). Classic KS different from KS of HIV infection. KS most frequently seen in HIV-infected men who have sex with men and is the most common HIV-associated malignancy. It is associated with specific sexual practices and geographic locations	Seen in any tissue but most often found in GI tract, mucus membranes, lymph nodes, and skin. Identified as patch, plaque and/or nodular lesions of any size, color or configuration on the trunk, arms, head or neck. Lesions in GI tract may be associated with bleeding pain, weight loss and diarrhea	GI lesions visualized by barium studies and are best evaluated endoscopically. Histological examination of tissue biopsy to confirm the diagnosis	Treatment based on immunological status and symptoms. KS lesions are highly sensitive to radiation therapy. Isolated KS lesions can be treated with cryotherapy or laser surgery. Interferon alpha with antiretroviral agents may be beneficial, as well as single agent or combination chemotherapy
Cervical invasive cancer	HIV-infected women have a 7 to 10 greater chance of developing precancerous or cancerous cervical lesions and a higher rate of recurrence following cervical intraepithelial neoplasia (CIN) excisions. Progression of CIN referred to as cervical dysplasia, to carcinoma of the cervix is a slow process in immunocompromised women. Appears to have higher incidence of AIDS defining cervical cancer in women who are injecting substance users, black, and live in the south	Early stages are asymptomatic and usually identified by PAP smear. Vaginal bleeding, usually post-coital, most common symptom. Metrorrhagia and malodorous, blood-tinged vaginal discharge may be present. Advanced disease may experience pelvic, back or leg pain, as well as hematuria, rectal bleeding or bladder and bowel involvement	PAP smear to determine the presence of abnormal cells, visible lesions, or both. Recommended that HIV infected women have a PAP smear twice in the first year after diagnosis. If both are negative then a yearly PAP smear is recommended. If PAP smear is abnormal than a colposcopy is recommended	Treatment of CIN and cervical cancer is carbon dioxide laser therapy, conization, cryosurgery or electrocautery. Treatment of invasive cancer depends on the stage of the disease and may include, surgery, radiation or chemotherapy

PAIN AND SYMPTOM MANAGEMENT IN HIV DISEASE

Patients with HIV/AIDS require symptom management not only for chronic debilitating opportunistic infections and malignancies, but from the side effects of treatments and other therapies. There are five broad principles fundamental to successful symptom management: (*1*) taking the symptoms seriously, (*2*) assessment, (*3*) diagnosis, (*4*) treatment, and (*5*) ongoing evaluation.[68]

- Taking the symptoms seriously implies that symptoms are often not observable and measurable. Therefore, self-report of the patient should be taken seriously by the practitioner and acknowledged as a real experience of the patient. An important rule in symptom management is to anticipate the symptom and attempt to prevent it.[23]
- Assessment and diagnosis of signs and symptoms of disease and treatment side effects requires a thorough history and physical examination. Questions as to when the symptom began and its location, duration, severity, and quality, as well as factors that exacerbate or alleviate the symptom, are important to ask. Patients can also be asked to rate the severity of a symptom by using a numerical scale from 0 to 10, with 0 being "no symptom" to 10 "extremely severe." Such scales can also be used to rate how much a symptom interferes with activities of daily life with 0 meaning "no interference" and 10 meaning "extreme interference."
- Many patients seek medical care for a specific symptom, which requires a focused history, physical exam, and diagnostic testing. Throughout the continuum of HIV disease, CD4 counts and percentages, viral loads, and blood counts and chemistries may provide useful information in the management of the disease and its symptoms. Assessment of current medications and complementary therapies, including vitamin therapy, past medical ill-

ness which may be exacerbated by HIV disease, and the administration of chemotherapy and radiation therapy should also be ascertained to determine the effects of treatment, side effects, adverse effects, and drug interactions. However, when treatment is no longer effective in the case of extremely advanced disease, practitioners must reevaluate the benefits verses burden of diagnostic testing and treatments, particularly the need for daily blood draws, or more invasive and uncomfortable procedures. When the decision of the practitioners, patient, and family is that all testing and aggressive treatments are futile, their discontinuation is warranted.

- Treatment of opportunistic infections and malignancies often requires support of the patient's immune system, antiretroviral therapy to decrease the viral load and improve CD4 cell counts, and medications and therapies to cure the patient of opportunistic infections or merely palliate the associated symptoms. Indeed, the treatment of symptoms to improve quality of life plays an important role in the management of HIV disease throughout the course of the illness.[20] In the case of many infections, acute treatment is followed by the regular dosing or maintenance therapy to prevent symptom recurrence. To maximize the quality of life, each patient's treatment regimen and plan of care should be individualized, with documentation of the treatment response and ongoing evaluation.
- Ongoing evaluation is key to symptom management and to the determination of the effectiveness of traditional, experimental, and complementary therapies. Changes in therapies are often necessary as concurrent or sequential illness or conditions occur.[68]

Pain Management. Pain management must become more integrated in the comprehensive care offered to patients with AIDS, as nearly two-thirds of patients with HIV/AIDS report increasing pain as the disease progresses.[69] General estimates of the prevalence of pain in HIV-infected individuals range between 25% and 80%, which is associated with psychological and functional morbidity.[70] Shofferman and Brody[71] reported that over half of the patients cared for in hospice with advanced AIDS experienced pain. In a study by Breitbart and colleagues[72] only 8% of patients who reported severe pain (score of 8 to 10 on a pain intensity scale) in an AIDS patient cohort received a strong opioid, as recommended by the World Health Organization (WHO) pain management guidelines. Cleeland and colleagues[73] also reported significant undermedication of pain in AIDS patients (85%), far exceeding the published reports of undertreated pain in cancer populations.

The inadequate assessment and treatment of pain often occurs because of societal, practitioner, and patient barriers and limitations. For example, with regard to pain management, society fears addiction to opioids and has not distinguished between the legitimate and illegal use of drugs. Practitioners may have inadequate knowledge and misconceptions about pain management, while patients often fear pain as suggesting advanced disease and are reluctant to report pain with the desire to be perceived as "good" patients.[29]

Pain syndromes in patients with AIDS are diverse in nature and etiology. For patients with AIDS, pain can occur in more than one site, such as pain in the legs (peripheral neuropathy reported in 40% of AIDS patients), which is often associated with antiretroviral therapy such as AZT, as well as pain in the abdomen, oral cavity, esophagus, skin, perirectal area, chest, joints, muscles, and headache.[24] Pain is also related to HIV/AIDS therapies such as antiretroviral therapies, antibacterials, chemotherapy such as vincristine, radiation, surgery, and procedures.[70] Following a complete assessment, including a history and physical examination, an individualized pain management plan should be developed to treat the underlying cause of the pain, often arising from underlying infections associated with HIV disease.[74]

The principles of pain management in the palliative care of patients with AIDS are the same as for patients with cancer, and include regularity of dosing, individualization of dosing, and using combinations of medications.[24] The three-step guidelines for pain management, as outlined by WHO, should be utilized for patients with HIV disease.[75] This approach advocates for the selection of analgesics based on the severity of pain. For mild to moderate pain, anti-inflammatory drugs such as NSAIDS or acetaminophen are recommended. However, the use of NSAIDS in patients with AIDS requires awareness of toxicity and adverse reactions, as they are highly protein-bound and the free fraction available is increased in AIDS patients who are cachetic or wasted.[70] For moderate to severe pain that is persistent, opioids of increasing potency are recommended, beginning with opioids such as codeine, hydrocodone, or oxycodone (each available with or without aspirin or acetaminophen), and advancing to more potent opioids such as morphine, hydromorphone (Dilaudid), methadone (Dolophine), or fentanyl (Duragesic) either intravenously or transdermally. In conjunction with NSAIDS and opioids, adjuvant therapies are also recommended such as:[70]

- tricyclic antidepressants, heterocyclic and noncyclic antidepressants and serotonin reuptake inhibitors for neuropathic pain
- psychostimulants to improve opioid analgesia and decrease sedation
- phenothiazine to relieve anxiety or agitation
- butyrophenones to relieve anxiety and delirium
- antihistamines to improve opioid analgesia and relieve anxiety, insomnia and nausea
- corticosteroids to decrease pain associated with an inflammatory component or with bone pain
- benzodiazepines for neuropathic pain, anxiety, and insomnia

Caution is however noted with use of protease inhibitors as they may interact with some analgesics. For example, Ritonavir has been associated with potentially lethal interactions with meperidine, propoxyphene, and piroxican. PIs must also be used with caution inpatients receiving codeine, tricyclic antidepressants, Sulindac, and indomethacin to avoid toxicity. Furthermore, for patients with HIV disease who have high fevers, the increase in body temperature to may lead to increased absorption of transdermally administered fentanyl.[76]

To insure appropriate dosing when changing the route of administration of opioids or changing from one opioid to another, the use of an equianalgesic conversion chart is suggested. As with all patients, oral medications should be used if possible with round-the-clock dosing at regular intervals, and the use of rescue doses for breakthrough pain. Often, controlled-released morphine or oxycodone are effective drugs for patients with chronic pain from HIV/AIDS. In the case of neuropathic pain, often experienced with HIV/AIDS, tricyclic antidepressants such as amitriptyline, or anticonvulsants such as neurontin can be very effective.[24] However, the use of neuroleptics must be weighed against an increased sensitivity of AIDS patients to the extrapyramidal side effects of these drugs.[70] If the cause of pain is increasing tumor size, radiation therapy can also be very effective in pain management by reducing tumor size, as well as the perception of pain. Tables 36–7 and 36–8 present the nonopiate analgesics for pain management in patients with AIDS and opioid analgesics for the management of mild to moderate pain and from moderate to severe pain in patients with AIDS, respectively.

Tolerance, Dependence, and Addiction. Physiologic tolerance refers to the shortened or diminished effect of a drug due to exposure to the drug, and thereby the need for increasing doses to maintain effect. In the case of opioids, tolerance to analgesic properties of the drug appears to be uncommon in the clinical setting, while tolerance to adverse effects such as respiratory depression, somnolence, and nausea is common and favorable. Most patients can remain on stable doses of opioids for prolonged periods of time. If an increase in opioid dosage is needed, it is usually because of disease progression. Another expected physiological response to opioids is physical dependence, which occurs after three to four weeks of opioid administration, as evidenced by withdrawal symptoms after abrupt discontinuation. If a drug is to be discontinued, halving the daily dose every one to two days until the dose is equivalent to 15 mg of morphine will reduce withdrawal symptoms.[29] Tolerance to opioids does not imply addiction, as addiction is a compulsive craving for a drug for effects other than pain relief and is extremely uncommon in patients who are terminally ill. Furthermore, studies have demonstrated that although tolerance and physical dependence commonly occur, addiction (psychological dependence) is rare and almost never occurs in individuals who do not have histories of substance abuse.[70]

Health care providers in palliative care are often concerned with the administration of opioids to patients with a history of substance abuse, who are in methadone maintenance programs or currently abusing drugs. As a result, these patients often receive ineffective pain management. Consistent use of a standard pain scale and regular monitoring of drug consumption by one nurse and one physician can be helpful in ongoing assessment and pain management as it limits potential abuse. Oral administration of medications also lowers abuse potential. Given that substance-abusing patients have greater tolerance to morphine derivatives and benzodiazepines because of previous exposure to these drugs, increased dosage may be necessary for effective pain management or the interval between doses should be shortened. Furthermore, the dosages of medications should be carefully monitored to avoid overdosing, given the possibility of hepatic failure in substance-abusing patients. Simultaneous use of agonists and antagonists are avoided in all populations because they provoke withdrawal symptoms.

Alleviating Opioid Side Effects. Although opioids are extremely effective in pain management for patients with HIV disease, their common side effects must be anticipated and minimized. Given that in medically fragile populations such side effects may also result from other comorbid conditions rather than from opioid analgesia itself, a complete assessment is war-

Table 36–7. Nonopioid Analgesics for Pain Management in Patients with AIDS

Analgesic Nonopiate	Starting Dose (mg/d)	Plasma Duration (hours)	Half-Life (hours)	Comments
Aspirin	650	4–6	3–12	The standard for comparison among nonopoids. GI toxicity. May not be as well tolerated as some newer analgesics
Ibuprofen	400–600	4–8	3–4	Can inhibit platelet function
Acetaminophen	650	4–6	2–4	Overdosage produces hepatic toxicity. Not antiinflammatory. Lack of GI and platelet toxicity
Choline magnesium trisalicylate	700–1500	12	8–12	Believed to have less GI toxicity than other NSAIDS. No effect on platelet aggregation
Naproxen	250–500	8–12	13	Lower incidence of side effects than other agents
Indomethacin	25–75	8–12	4–5	Available in sustained release in the U.S.
COX 2 inhibitor: Celecoxib	100–200 mg o.d. or b.i.d.	3–5	11	Not used for patients under 18 years of age. Maximum daily dose of 400 mg
Vioxx	12.5–25 mg ood.	2–9	17	Fewer GI effects than other NSAIDS

Portenoy, R. K. (1997). *Contemporary Diagnosis and Management of Pain in Oncologic and AIDS Patients.* Pennsylvania: Handbooks in Health Care Co.

Table 36–8. Opioid Analgesics for Mild to Moderate to Severe Pain in Patients with AIDS

	Recommended Dose (mg)	Peak Effect (hours)	Duration (hours)	Plasma Half-Life (hours)	Comments
For Mild to Moderate Pain					
Codeine (with or without acetaminophen) Tylenol #2 acetaminophen 300 mg + codeine 15 mg Tylenol #3 Acetaminophen 300 mg + codeine 30 mg; Tylenol #4 Acetaminophen 300 mg + codeine 60 mg	30–60 p.o.	1–2	3–4	2–3	Metabolized to morphine, often used to suppress cough. When acetaminophen is added, there is a ceiling dose of 4 gm per day
Hydrocodone (with acetaminophen combinations in Lorcet, Lortab, Vicodin, others)	30 p.o.	1–2	3–6	2–4	When acetaminophen is added, there is a ceiling dose of 4 gm per day
Oxycodone (Roxicodone—a single entity oxycodone) or Oxycodone (with acetaminophen) Percoset (Oxycodone 5 mg + acetaminophen 325 mg) Roxicet (Oxycodone 5 mg + acetaminophen 500 mg)	20–30 p.o.	1–2	3–6	2–3	Toxicity is the same as morphine. used with acetaminophen for moderate pain. Available as a single agent for severe pain. Equianalgesic to morphine when not combined with acetaminophen
Oxycodone (sustained release) (Oxycodone SR)	20–40 p.o.	1	8–12	2–3	No comment
Oxycodone (controlled release) (OxyContin)	20–30 p.o.	3–4	8–12	2–3	No comment
For Moderate to Severe Pain					
Morphine (immediate release)	20–60 p.o. 10 IM, IV, SC	1–2 0.5–1	3–6 3–4	2–3 2–3	Standard of comparison for the opioid analgesics. Constipation, nausea, sedation common side effects. Respiratory depression rare
Morphine (controlled release) (MS Contin)	20–60 p.o.	3–4	8–12	2–3	
Morphine (sustained release) (Kadian, Oramorph SR)	20–60 p.o.	4–6	24	2–3	Kadian is only q day dosing
Hydromorphone (Dilaudid)	7.5 p.o. 1.5 IM, IV	1–2 0.5–1	3–6 3–4	2–3 2–3	Short half-life for elderly patients. Toxicity is the same as morphine
Methadone (Dolophine)	20 p.o. 10 IM	1–2 0.5–1.5	4–>8 4–>8	12>150 12>150	Requires close monitoring for toxicity due to long half-life and careful titration
Levorphanol (Levo-Dromoran)	4 p.o. 2 IM	1–2 0.5–1	3–6 3–6	12–15 12–15	Long half-life requiring careful titration in the first week
Fentanyl	—	—	—	7–12	Can be administered as a continuous IV or SC infusion, 100 μg/h is roughly equianalgesic to morphine 4 mg/h

(*continued*)

Table 36–8. Opioid Analgesics for Mild to Moderate to Severe Pain in Patients with AIDS (*Continued*)

	Recommended Dose (mg)	Peak Effect (hours)	Duration (hours)	Plasma Half-Life (hours)	Comments
Fentanyl transdermal (Duragesic)	—	—	48–72	16–24	100 μg/h transdermal system is approximately equianalgesic to morphine 4 mg/h. Not suitable for rapid titration. If patient has pain after 48 hours increase the dose or change the patch every 48 hours
Fentanyl transmucosal (Actiq)	200 m.c.g. (1–2 units) q3h p.r.n. but no more than 4 units/day. The unit is to be sucked and not chewed. Redosing within a single pain episode can occur 15 minutes after the previous unit has been completed or 30 minutes after the start of the previous unit	0.5	—	7	Unit is administered as a "lozenge" on a stick that is to be sucked. Used for breakthrough pain as a rescue dose for cancer patients. Not to be used with opioid-naïve patients due to life-threatening hypoventilation. Recent research findings suggest that the onset of effect is faster than oral morphine and the same as IV morphine

Portenoy, R. K. (1997). *Contemporary Diagnosis and Management of Pain in Oncologic and AIDS Patients.* Pennsylvania: Handbooks in Health Care Co.

ranted. Medications and treatments to alleviate opioid side effects include:

- *Nausea and vomiting,* treated with prochlorperazine (Compazine), metoclopramide (Reglan), haloperidol (Haldol), hydroxyzine (Vistaril), lorazepam (Ativan), granistron (Kytril), and odansetron (Zofran). A change in the opioid may also be necessary.
- *Constipation,* treated by an increase in fiber in the diet, stimulating cathartic drugs such as bisacodyl, senna, or hyperosmotic agents like sorbitol or lactulose.
- *Sedation,* treated by reducing the opioid in each dose or decreasing the frequency, as well as the ingestion of caffeine, and administration of dextroamphetamine, or methylphenidate. Again, a change in the opioid may be warranted.
- *Confusion,* treated by lowering the opioid dose, changing to a different opioid or Haldol.
- *Myoclonus,* treated with clonazepan (Klonopin), diazepan (Valium), and baclofen (Lioresal), or a change in the opioid.
- *Respiratory depression,* prevented by starting at a low dose in opioid-naïve patients, and being aware of relative potencies when changing opioids, as well as differences by routes of administration. Naloxone (Narcan) may be administered to reverse respiratory depression but should be used with caution in patients who are opioid tolerant because of the risk of inducing a withdrawal state. Dilute one ampule of naloxone (0.4 mg) in 10 ml of normal saline and titrate to the patient's respirations.[70]

Management of Other Symptoms Experienced with HIV Disease. For patients with HIV/AIDS, suffering occurs from the many symptoms experienced at the various stages of the illness. Fantoni and colleagues[77] reported, based on a sample of 1128 HIV-infected patients, that the most commonly experienced symptoms were fatigue (65%), anorexia (34%), cough (32%), and fever (29%). In a study to assess the predominant symptoms in 72 patients with AIDS, the most common symptoms were pain (97%), weakness (78%), and weight loss (53%).[78] Based on a sample of 207 patients with AIDS, Holzemer, Henry, and Reilly[79] also found that 50% of the participants experienced shortness of breath, dry mouth, insomnia, weight loss, and headaches. The records of 50 men who died of AIDS between 1988 and 1992 indicated the distressing symptoms of dyspnea, diarrhea, confusion, dementia, difficulty eating, and swallowing. Therefore, care in the last month of life was often directed at the palliation of symptoms.[19] Indeed, the last stage of HIV infection is often marked by increasing pain, gastrointestinal discomfort, and depression.[5] Patients may be suffering from inflammatory or infiltrative processes and somatic and visceral pain. Neuropathic pain is commonly a result of the disease process or the side effect of medications.[80] Avis, Smith, and Mayer[81] also reported, based on a sample of 92 HIV-positive men, that quality of life was more related to symptoms, measured by the Whalen's HIV Symptom Index, than CD4 counts or hemoglobin. With the myriad of symptoms experienced by patients with HIV disease across the illness trajectory, health care practitioners need to understand the causes, presentations, and interventions of common symptoms, as presented in Table 36–9, to enhance the quality of life of patients.

Table 36–9. Selected Symptoms Associated with HIV/AIDS

Symptom	Cause	Presentation	Interventions
Fatigue (asthenia)	• HIV infection • Opportunistic infections • AIDS medications • Prolonged immobility • Anemia • Sleep disorders • Hypothyroidism • Medications	• Weakness • Lack of energy	• Treat reversible causes • Pacing activities • Rest periods/naps • Adequate nutrition • Relaxation exercises • Meditation • Warm rather than hot showers or baths • Cool room temperatures • Administer dextroamphetamine 10mg/day p.o.
Anorexia (loss of appetite) and cachexia (wasting)	• Metabolic alterations caused by cytokines and interleukin-1 • Opportunistic infections • Nutrient malabsorption from intestines • Chronic diarrhea • Depression • Taste disorders	• Diminished food intake • Profound weight loss	• Treat reversible causes • Consult with dietitian about choice of food • Make food appealing by color and texture • Avoid noxious smells at mealtime • Avoid fatty, fried, and strong-smelling foods • Offer small frequent meals and nutritious snacks • Encourage patients to eat whatever is appealing • Provide high-energy, high-protein liquid supplements • Use appetite stimulants such as megesterol acetate 800 mg/day p.o. or Dronabinol 2.5 mg p.o. q.d. or b.i.d. • Testosterone administered by 5 mg transdermal patch to increase weight gain and muscle mass
Fever (elevated body temperature)	• Bacterial toxins • Viruses • Yeast • Antigen–antibody reactions • Drugs • Tumor products • Exogenous pyrogens	• Body temperature greater than 99.5 F (oral), 100.5 F (rectal), or 98.5 F (axillary) • Chills, rigor • Sweating, night sweats • Delerium • Dizziness • Dehydration	• Treat reversible causes • Maintain fluid intake • Loose clothing and sheets with frequent changing • Avoid plastic bed coverings • Exceptionally high temperature may require ice packs or cooling blankets. • Around-the-clock antipyretics such as acetaminophen or ASA 325-650 mg p.o. q 6–8 hrs
Dyspnea (shortness of breath) and cough	• Bronkospasm • Embolism • Effusions • Pulmonary edema • Pneumothorax • Kaposi sarcoma • Obstruction • Opportunistic infections • Anxiety • Allergy • Mechanical or chemical irritants • Anemia	• Productive or nonproductive cough • Crackles • Stridor • Hemoptysis • Inability to clear secretions • Wheezing • Tachypnea • Gagging • Intercostal retractions • Areas of pulmonary dullness • Anxiety	• Treat reversible causes • Elevate bed to Fowlers or high Fowlers position • Provide abdominal splints • Administer humidified oxygen therapy to treat dyspnea • Use fans or open windows to keep air moving for dyspnea • Remove irritants or allergens such as smoke • Teach pursed lips breathing for patients with obstructive disease • Frequent mouth care to decrease discomfort from dry mouth. • Treat bronchospasm

(continued)

Table 36–9. Selected Symptoms Associated with HIV/AIDS

Symptom	Cause	Presentation	Interventions
			• Suppress cough with dextromethorphan hydrobromide 15–45 mg p.o. q4h p.r.n. or opioids such as codeine 15–60 mg p.o. q4h even if taking other opioids for pain or hydrocodone 5–10 mg p.o. q4–6h p.r.n. or morphine 5–20 mg p.o. q4h p.r.n. (may be increased) to relieve dyspnea, relieve cough, and associated anxiety • For hyperactive gag reflex use nebulized lidocaine 5 ml of 2% solution (100 mg) q3–4 hrs p.r.n.
Diarrhea	• Idiopathic HIV enteropathy • Diet • Bowel infections (bacteria, parasites, protozoa) • Chronic bowel inflammation • Medications • Obstruction with overflow incontinence • Stress • Malabsorption	• Flatulence • Multiple bowel movements/day • Cramps/colic • Hemorrhoids	• Treat reversible causes • Maintain adequate hydration • Replace electrolytes by giving Gatorade or Pedialyte. • Give rice, bananas, or apple juice to reduce diarrhea • Increase protein and calories • Avoid dairy products, alcohol, caffeine, extremely hot or cold foods, spicy or fatty foods • Maintain dignity while toileting • Provide ready access to bathroom or commode • Maintain good perianal care • Administer medications such as Lomotil 2.5–5.0 mg q4–6 hrs; Kaopectalin 60–120 ml q4–6 hrs (max 20 mg/day); Immodium 2–4 mg q6 hr (max 16 mg/day) or paregoric (tincture of opium) 5–10 ml q4–6 hrs
Insomnia (inability to fall asleep or stay asleep)	• Anxiety • Depression • Pain • Medications • Delirium • Sleep disorders such as sleep apnea • Excess alcohol intake • Caffeine	• Early morning awakening • Night-time restlessness • Fear • Nightmares	• Treat reversible causes • Establish a bedtime routine • Reduce daytime napping • Avoid caffeinated beverages and alcohol • Take a warm bath 2 hours before bedtime • Use relaxation techniques • Provide an environment conducive to sleep (dark, quiet, comfortable temperature) • Administer anxiolytics such as benzodiazapines (use for less than 2 weeks because of dependency), antidepressants (helpful over long term) or other sedatives such as Benadryl
Headache	• Infections such as encephalitis, herpes zoster, meningitis, toxoplasmosis • Sinusitis	• Pain in one or more areas of the head or over sinuses	• Treat reversible causes • Suggest chiropractic manipulation • Provide massage therapy • Use relaxation therapy • Apply TENS • Use stepwise analgesia • Administer corticosteroids to reduce swellings around space-occupying lesions

Ropka M. E., and Williams A. B. (1998). HIV Nursing and Symptom Management. Sudbury, Mass: Jones and Bartlett Publishers.
Unzarski, P.J., and Flaskerud, J. H. (1999). HIV/AIDS A Guide to Primary Care Management, Philadelphia, PA: W. B. Saunders Company.

Nonpharmacologic Interventions for Pain and Symptom Management. Nonpharmacologic interventions for pain and symptom management can also be effective in the care of patients with HIV disease. Bed rest, simple exercise, heat or cold packs to affected sites, massage, transcutaneous electrical stimulation (TENS), and acupuncture can be effective physical therapies with this patient population. Psychological interventions to reduce pain perception and interpretation include hypnosis, relaxation, imagery, biofeedback, distraction, and patient education. In cases of refractory pain, nerve blocks and cordotomy are available neurosurgical procedures for pain management. Increasingly, epidural analgesia is an additional option that provides continuous pain relief.[70]

The ten most commonly used complementary therapies and activities reported by 1106 participants in the Alternative Medical Care Outcomes in AIDS study were aerobic exercise (64%), prayer (56%), massage (54%), needle acupuncture (48%), meditation (46%), support groups (42%), visualization and imagery (34%), breathing exercises (33%), spiritual activities (33%), and other exercise (33%).[82] Clearly, patients with HIV disease seek complementary therapies to treat symptoms, slow the progression of the disease, and enhance their general well-being. Nurses' knowledge, evaluation, and recommendations regarding complementary therapies are important aspects of holistic care.

PSYCHOSOCIAL ISSUES FOR PATIENTS WITH HIV/AIDS AND THEIR FAMILIES

Uncertainty is a chronic and pervasive source of psychological distress for persons living with HIV disease, particularly as it relates to ambiguous symptom patterns, exacerbation and remissions of symptoms, selection of optimal treatment regimens, the complexity of treatments, and the fear of stigma and ostracism. Such uncertainty is linked with negative perceptions of quality of life and poor psychological adjustment.[83] However, many practitioners focus on patient's physical functioning and performance status as the main indicators of quality of life, rather than on the symptoms of psychological distress such as anxiety and depression.[84] In a study of the problems and needs of HIV/AIDS patients during the last weeks of life, Butters, Higginson, and George[85] determined, based on the Support Team Assessment Schedule (STAS), that symptom control, patient and family anxiety, spiritual needs, and communication between patient and family were their greatest needs. Furthermore, Friedland, Renwick, and McColl[86] identified the determinants of quality of life in a sample of 120 individuals with HIV/AIDS. Income, emotional support, and problem-oriented and perception-oriented coping were positively related to quality of life, while tangible support and emotion-focused coping were negatively related.

Ragsdale and Morrow[36] emphasized the importance of focusing on the psychosocial aspects of life in patients with HIV/AIDS as patients reported a repetitive cycle of emotional changes with slight physical changes. Disfigurement, the symptoms associated with the disease and its treatment, and the contagious nature of the disease add to the psychological distress associated with HIV/AIDS.

Nurses must also be cognizant of such issues as the experience of multiple losses, complicated grieving, substance abuse, stigmatization, and homophobia, which contribute to patients' sense of alienation, isolation, hopelessness, loneliness, and depression. Such emotional distress often extends to the patient's family caregivers as they attempt to provide support and lessen the patient's suffering, yet are often suffering from HIV disease themselves. Reciprocal suffering is experienced by family caregivers with the need to also improve their quality of life through palliative care, as well as the patients.[87]

Psychosocial Assessment of Patients with HIV Disease

Psychosocial assessment of patients with HIV disease is important throughout the illness trajectory, particularly as the disease progresses and there is increased vulnerability to psychological distress. Psychosocial assessment includes the following:

- *past social, behavioral and psychiatric history*, which includes the history of interpersonal relationships, education, job stability, career plans, substance use, preexisting mental illness and individual identity
- *crisis points* related to the course of the disease as anxiety, fear, and depression intensify and a risk of suicide exists
- *life cycle phase* of individuals and families which influences goals, financial resources, skills, social roles, and the ability to confront personal mortality
- *influence of culture and ethnicity*, including knowledge and beliefs associated with health, illness, dying, and death, as well as attitudes and values toward sexual behaviors, substance use, health promotion and maintenance, and health care decision making
- *past and present patterns of coping*, including problem-focused and/or emotion-focused coping
- *social support*, including sources of support, types of supports perceived as needed by the patient/family, and perceived benefits and burdens of support
- *financial resources*, including health care benefits, disability allowances, and the eligibility for Medicaid/Medicare

Depression and Anxiety in Patients with HIV Disease

Given that AIDS is a life-threatening, chronic, debilitating illness, patients are at risk for such psychological disorders as depression and anxiety. Among persons living with HIV/AIDS, the prevalence of depression has been estimated at 10% to 25%,[88] and is characterized by depressed mood, low energy, sleep disturbance, anhedonia, inability to concentrate, loss of libido, weight changes, and possible menstrual irregularities.[89] It is also important to assess whether depressed patients are using alcohol, drugs, and opioids.

Patients with HIV disease who are diagnosed with depression should be treated with antidepressants which target their particular symptoms. For example, tricyclic antidepressants are indicated for anxious depression, insomnia, low daytime energy, and neuropathic pain; selective serotonin reuptake inhibitors (SSRIs) are indicated for lethargy, hopelessness, and hypersomnia; and stimulants are indicated for fatigue, hypersomnia, poor appetite, and to improve cognitive function.[90] It is noted that monoamine oxidase (MAO) inhibitors may interact with multiple medications used to treat HIV disease, and therefore should be avoided.

Anxiety may also be associated with the stresses of HIV, or may result from the medications used to treat HIV disease such as anticonvulsants, sulfonamides, NSAIDS, and corticosteroids.[91] Generalized anxiety disorder is manifested as worry, trouble falling asleep, impaired concentration, psychomotor agitation, hypersensitivity, hyperarousal, and fatigue.[92]

The treatment for patients with anxiety is based on the nature and severity of the symptoms and the coexistence of other mood disorders or substance abuse. Short-acting antidepressants, such as lorazepam (Ativan), and alprazolam (Xanax) are beneficial for intermittent symptoms, while buspirone (Buspar), and clonazapam (Klonopin) are beneficial for chronic anxiety.[90]

For many patients experiencing psychological distress associated with HIV disease, participation in therapeutic interventions such as skills building, support groups, individual counseling, and group interventions using meditation techniques can provide a sense of psychological growth and meaningful ways of living with the disease.[92–94] Such interventions are particularly helpful for patients with HIV/AIDS who may not have disclosed their sexual orientation or substance-abusing history to their families. Often, significant stress is associated with sharing such information and particularly when such disclosures occur during the stage of advanced disease. However, the need for therapeutic communication and support from all health professionals caring for the patient and their family exists throughout the illness continuum. Furthermore, fear of disclosure of the AIDS diagnosis and stigmatization in their communities often raises concern in the family about the diagnosis stated on death certificates. Practitioners may therefore write a nonspecific diagnosis on the main death certificate and sign section B on the reverse side to signify to the registrar general that further information will be provided at a later date.

Given the transmission of the disease to sexual partners and through childbirth, often many members of a single family are infected and die. In the homosexual community and substance-abusing community, multiple deaths have also resulted in complicated mourning. The anxiety, depression, sadness, and loneliness associated with these multiple deaths and unending experiences of loss must be recognized and support offered. Community resources and referrals to HIV/AIDS support groups and bereavement groups are important in emotional adjustment to these profound losses.

SPIRITUAL ISSUES IN AIDS

The spiritual care of the patient and the ability of the community to support patients with HIV/AIDS may be unique opportunities for both personal and societal growth and transcendence. Mellors, Riley, and Erlen[96] examined the relationship of self-transcendence and quality of life in a sample of 46 individuals with HIV/AIDS. The results demonstrated that overall self-transcendence for this sample was relatively high. Quality of life was higher than reported in previous research, yet those with disease progression, evident by the diagnosis of AIDS, had lower quality of life than those who were asymptomatic or symptomatic with CD4 counts greater than 200 cells/mm^3. There was no significant difference in self-transcendence between groups, but those with AIDS were more inclined to accept death and refrained from dwelling on the past or unmet dreams. There was a moderate positive correlation ($r = 0.46$, $p < 0.01$) between self-transcendence and quality of life.

As health professionals, assessment of patient's spiritual needs is an important aspect of holistic care. Learning about patients' spiritual values and needs and religious perspectives is important in understanding their perspectives regarding their illness and their perception and meaning of life and its purpose, suffering, and eventual death. According to Elkins and colleagues,[97] spirituality is a way of being or experiencing that comes about through an awareness of a transcendent dimension and identifiable life values with regard to self, others, nature, and God. An understanding of the patient's relationship with self, others, nature, and God can inform interventions that promote spiritual well-being and the possibility of a "good death" from the patient's perspective.

Patients living with and dying from HIV disease have the spiritual needs of meaning, value, hope, purpose, love, acceptance, reconciliation, ritual, and affirmation of a relationship with a higher being.[90] Assisting patients to find meaning and value in their lives, despite adversity, often involves a recognition of past successes and their internal strengths. Respectful behavior toward patients demonstrates love and acceptance of the patient as a person. Encouraging open communication of patient and family is important to reconciliation and the completion of unfinished business.

Case Study: John

John Bowman was a 45-year-old gay male admitted to the inpatient palliative care unit for recurrence of a high grade non-Hodgkins lymphoma (NHL) of the gastrointestional tract. His original diagnosis with NHL was made four months earlier at which time he presented with a 35 lb weight loss over a three month period, night sweats, and rectal bleeding. As a differential diagnosis, he was also tested for HIV disease. Findings indicated a CD4 count of 35 cells/mm^3 and a viral load of 140,000 ml indicative of the advanced stage of HIV disease. Physical examination revealed two enlarged inguinal lymph nodes, with the diagnosis of non-Hodgkins lymphoma of the GI tract determined by biopsy and an abdominal CAT scan.

John was treated with chemotherapy for the non-Hodgkins lymphoma and was also begun on antiretroviral agents to improve his immune status, as well as to enhance his clinical response to chemotherapy. He was begun on a highly active antiretroviral

(HAART) regimen of one potent protease inhibitor and two nucleoside reverse transcriptase inhibitors, specifically Ritonavir (PI), and Zidovudine and Didanosine (ddI)(both NRTIs). However, he developed persistent neuropathic pain, characterized as burning, tingling sensations in his lower extremities, from the antiretroviral therapy.

John moved eight months ago from San Francisco to New York to "get away from all the ghosts." John expressed a sense of displacement due to relocation and found it difficult living in a five-story walk-up. His partner was also diagnosed with AIDS and received disability benefits, as did John. John cried when he spoke of his rejection by his family when he disclosed his AIDS diagnosis, and rejection by his church when he admitted his sexual orientation. He stated, "My life has no meaning. I actually wish it were all over so I wouldn't have to deal with it every day." During the day, he most often laid in bed with night blinders covering his eyes. A tricyclic antidepressant was suggested to offer some relief from his neuropathic pain, and hopefully to improve his emotional state. However, the medication was refused by John, who remarked, "That will only get at the tip of the iceberg."

Given John's severe immunocompromised state, further chemotherapy was not recommended, and a palliative care approach was decided upon by the patient. Neurontin, an anticonvulsant effective in the management of neuropathic pain, was begun with the dosage increased to 300 mg t.i.d., which gave him substantial relief. Roxanol 10 mg p.o. q3h was ordered for breakthrough pain. Antiretroviral therapies were continued to prevent opportunistic infections, which would further compromise his quality of life, but ddI was changed to 3TC, which is not associated with the development of peripheral neuropathy. Counseling by an advanced practice palliative care nurse was begun and John began to discuss his various losses related to his diagnosis of advanced cancer and AIDS, including his sense of grief, displacement, isolation, and rejection. The nurse, noticing a carousel of slides on his bedstand, asked John about them. Sitting straight up in bed and taking off his blinders, he showed her his artwork, which expressed the meaning of living with HIV/AIDS. Having developed a therapeutic relationship and with new insights into his thoughts and fears, she was able to provide emotional, as well as spiritual support. Although John was a Roman Catholic, he found comfort in the visits from an Episcopal priest, who was a member of the palliative care team. Father Matthews visited John regularly and discussed with him many spiritual issues that were sources of distress. The administration of an antidepressant was again suggested and now accepted by John. After two weeks, John was looking forward to returning home with support from a community hospice team. The social worker was also exploring other housing options, which he requested, so that he could maintain a sense of independence and functional status, not possible in a five-story walk-up. Although no cure could be offered for his progressive, life-threatening diseases, John found a new sense of meaning and appreciation for each day. In his last weeks of life, he sent a copy of his lastest artwork to the members of the palliative care team. It was titled *Breaking Through the Ice.* He thanked the team for their compassionate and comprehensive care that enabled him to live as fully as possible until death.

As with many life-threatening illnesses, patients with AIDS may express anger with God. Some may view their illness as a punishment, or are angry that God is not answering their prayers. Expression of feelings can be a source of spiritual healing. Clergy can also serve as valuable members of the palliative care team in offering spiritual support and alleviating spiritual distress. The use of mediation, music, imagery, poetry, and drawing may offer outlets for spiritual expression and promote a sense of harmony and peace.

Hope often shifts from hope that a cure will soon be found to hope for a peaceful death with dignity, with the alleviation of pain and suffering, by determining one's own choices, by being in the company of family and significant others, and with the knowledge that their end-of-life wishes will be honored. Often, the greatest spiritual comfort offered by caregivers or family comes from active listening and meaningful presence by sitting and hold their hands and knowing that they are not abandoned and alone.

Spiritual healing may also come from life review, as patients are offered an opportunity to reminisce about their lives, reflect on their accomplishments, reflect on their misgivings, and forgive themselves and others for their imperfections. Indeed, such spiritual care conveys that even in the shadow of death, there can be discovery, insight, the completion of relationships, the experience of love of self and others, and the transcendence of emotional and spiritual pain. Often, patients with AIDS, by their example, teach nurses, family, and others how to transcend suffering and how to die with grace and dignity.

ADVANCED CARE PLANNING

Advanced planning is another important issue related to end-of-life care for patients with HIV/AIDS. According to Ferris and colleagues,[98] health care providers can assist patients and families by (*1*) discussing the benefits from health care and social support programs; unemployment insurance, worker's compensation, pension plans, insurance, and union or association benefits; (2) emphasizing the importance of organizing information and documents so that they are easily located and accessible; (3) suggesting that financial matters be in order such as power of attorney on bank accounts, credit cards, property, legal claims, and income tax preparation; (*4*) discussing advance directives or power of attorney for care and treatment, as well as decisions related to the chosen setting for dying; and (5) discussing the patient's wishes regarding their death such as whom does the patient want at the bedside; what rituals are important to the dying patient; does the patient wish an autopsy; what arrangements does the patient want regarding the funeral services and burial; and where should donations in remembrance be sent? It is important to realize that these issues should be discussed at relevant stages in the person's illness and in a manner that is respectful to the patient's wishes and strengths and which promotes the patient's sense of control over their life and death.

Health care providers must also understand the concept of competency, which is a "state in which the person is capable of taking legal acts, consenting or refusing treatment, writing a will or power of attorney."[98] In assessing the patient's competency, the health provider must question whether the decision maker knows the nature and effect of the decision to be made and understands the consequences of his or her actions, and determine if the decision is consistent with an individual's life history, lifestyle, previous actions, and best interests.[98]

When an individual is competent, and in anticipation of the future loss of competency, he or she may initiate advance directives such as a living will and/or the designation of a health care proxy who will carry out the patient's health care wishes or make health care decisions in the advent that the patient becomes incompetent. The patient may also give an individual the power of attorney with regard to financial matters and care or treatment issues. Advanced directives include the patient's decisions regarding such life-sustaining treatments as cardiopulmonary resuscitation, use of vasoactive drips to sustain blood pressure and heart rate, dialysis, artificial nutrition and hydration, and the initiation or withdrawal of ventilatory support. The signing of advance directives must be witnessed by two individuals who are not related to the patient or involved in the patient's treatment. Individuals who are mentally competent can revoke at any time their advance directives. If a patient is deemed mentally incompetent, state statutes may allow the court to designate a surrogate decision maker for the patient.

PALLIATIVE CARE THROUGH THE DYING TRAJECTORY

Death from AIDS is usually due to multiple causes, including chronic infections, malignancies, neurological disease, malnutrition, and multisystem failure.[99] However, even for patients with HIV/AIDS for whom death appears to be imminent, spontaneous recovery with survival of several more weeks or months is possible. The terminal stage is often marked by periods of increasing weight loss and deteriorating physical and cognitive functioning.[27] The general rule related to mortality is that the greater the cumulative number of opportunistic infections, illnesses, complications, and/or deviance of serologic or immunologic markers in terms of norms, the less the survival time.[24] Survival time is also decreased by psychosocial factors such as a decrease in physical and emotional support as demands increase for the caregivers, feelings of hopelessness by the patient, and older age (greater than 39 years).[100] In the terminal stage of HIV disease, decisions related to prevention, diagnosis, and treatment pose ethical and clinical issues for both patients and their health care providers as they must decide on the value and frequency of laboratory monitoring, use of invasive procedures, use of antiretroviral and prophylactic measures, and patients' participation in clinical trails.[24]

The dying process for patients with advanced AIDS is commonly marked by increasingly severe physical deterioration leaving the patient bedbound, experiencing wasting, dyspnea at rest, and pressure ulcers. Ultimately, patients become dependent on others for care. Febrile states and changes in mental status often occur as death becomes more imminent. Maintaining the comfort and dignity of the patients becomes a nursing priority. Symptomatic treatments, including pain management, should be continued throughout the dying process, since even obtunded patients may feel pain and other symptoms.

The end of life is an important time for individuals to accept their own shortcomings and limitations, and differences with significant others so that death may be accepted without physical, psychosocial, and spiritual anguish.[29] Through an interdisciplinary approach to care, health professionals can assist patients in reducing their internal conflicts, such as fears about the loss of control; promote the patient's sense of identity; support the patient in maintaining important interpersonal relationships; and encourage patients to identify and attempt to reach meaningful though limited goals.

Members of the palliative care team can provide much needed assistance to patients and their families by encouraging patients and loved ones to express their fears and end-of-life wishes. Encouraging patients and families to express such feelings as "I love you," "I forgive you," "Forgive me—I am sorry," "Thank you," and "Good-bye" is important to the completion of relationships.[101] Peaceful death can also occur as families give the patient permission to die, and assure them that they will be remembered.[3]

LOSS, GRIEF, AND BEREAVEMENT FOR PERSONS WITH HIV/AIDS AND THEIR SURVIVORS

Throughout the illness trajectory, patients with HIV disease experience many losses, such as a sense of loss of identity as they assume the identity of a patient with AIDS; loss of control over health and function; loss of roles as the illness progresses; loss of body image due to skin lesions, changes in weight, and wasting; loss of sexual freedom because of the need to change sexual behaviors to maintain health and prevent transmission to others; loss of financial security through possible discrimination and increasing physical disability; and loss of relationships through possible abandonment, self-induced isolation, and the multiple deaths of others from the disease.[102]

Each occurrence of illness heightens the patient's awareness of their mortality and provides an opportunity for health professionals to respond to cues of the patients in addressing their concerns and approaching the subject of dying and death. Given that grief is the emotional response to loss, patients dying from AIDS may also manifest the signs of grief, which include feelings of sadness, anger, self-reproach, anxiety, loneliness, fatigue, shock, yearning, relief, and numbness; physical sensations such as hollowness in the stomach, tightness in the chest, oversensitivity to noise, dry mouth, muscle weakness, and loss of coordination; cognitions of disbelief, confusion; and behavior disturbances in appetite, sleep, social withdrawal, loss of interest in activities, and restless overactivity.[103]

Upon the death of the patient, the patient's family and significant others enter a state of bereavement, or a state of having suffered a loss, which is often a long-term process of adapting to life without the deceased.[103] As had the patient, family and significant others may experience the signs of grief, which may also include a sense of presence of the deceased, paranormal experiences or hallucinations, dreams of the deceased, a desire to have cherish objects of the deceased, and to visit places frequented by the deceased. The work of grief is a dynamic process that is not time-limited and predictable.[104] It may be that one never "gets over" the loss, but rather finds a place for it in their life and creates through memory a new relationship with their loved one.

Families, and partners of patients with AIDS may experience disenfranchised grief, defined as the grief that persons experience when they incur a loss that is not openly acknowledged, publicly mourned, or socially supported.[105] Support is not only important in assisting families in the tasks of grieving, but is also important for nurses who have established valued relationships with their patients. Indeed, disenfranchised grief may also be experienced by nurses who do not allow themselves to acknowledge their patient's death as a personal loss, or who are not acknowledged by others, such as the patient's family or even professional colleagues for having suffered a loss.

For all individuals who have experienced a loss, Worden[106] has identified the tasks of grieving as (*1*) accepting the reality of the death; (*2*) experiencing the pain of grief; (*3*) adjusting to a changed physical, emotional, and social environment in which the deceased is missing; (*4*) and finding an appropriate emotional place for the person who died in the emotional life of the bereaved. To facilitate each of Worden's tasks, Mallinson[102] recommends the following nursing interventions:

- Accept the reality of death by speaking of the loss, and facilitating emotional expression
- Work through the pain of grief by exploring the meaning of the grief experience
- Adjust to the environment without the deceased by acknowledging anniversaries and the experience of loss during holidays and birthdays; helping the bereaved to problem solve and recognize their own abilities to conduct their daily lives
- Emotionally relocate the deceased and move on with life by encouraging socialization through formal and informal avenues.

The complications of AIDS-related grief often comes from the secrecy and social stigma associated with the disease.[107] Reluctance to contact family and friends can restrict the normal support systems available for the bereaved.

In addition to a possible lack of social support, the death of patients with AIDS may result in complicated grief for the bereaved, given that death occurs after lengthy illness, and the relationships may have been ambivalent. Through truthful and culturally sensitive communication, health professionals can offer families support in their grief and promote trust that their needs are understood and validated. Further bereavement and related nursing interventions are discussed in Chapter 25.

CONCLUSION

The care of patients with HIV/AIDS requires both active treatment and palliative care throughout the disease trajectory to relieve the suffering associated with opportunistic infections and malignancies. With up-to-date knowledge regarding HIV disease, including changes in epidemiology, diagnostic testing, treatment options, and available resources, nurses can offer effective and compassionate care to patients, alleviating physical, emotional, social, and spiritual suffering at all stages of HIV disease. Patients can maintain a sense of control and dignity until death, by establishing a partnership with their health care professionals in planning and implementing their health care, as well as through advanced care planning to insure that their end-of-life preferences and wishes are honored. The control of pain and symptoms associated with HIV/AIDS enables the patient and family to expend their energies on spiritual and emotional healing, and the possibility for personal growth and transcendence even as death approaches. Palliative care offers a comprehensive approach to address the physical, emotional, social, and spiritual needs of individuals with incurable progressive illness throughout the illness trajectory until death. Palliative care therefore preserves a person's quality of life by protecting their self-integrity, reducing a perceived helplessness, and lessening the threat of exhaustion of coping resources.[108] Through effective and compassionate nursing care, patients with can achieve a sense of inner well-being even at death, with the potential to make the transition from life as profound, intimate, and precious an experience as their birth.[101]

REFERENCES

1. George, R. J. (1991). Palliation in AIDS: Where do we draw the line? Genitourinary Med 67: 85–86.

2. Knaus, W. et al. (1995). A controlled trial to improve care for seriously ill hospitalized patients. JAMA 274: 1591–1598.

3. O'Neill, J. and Alexander, C. (1997). Palliative medicine and HIV/AIDS. HIV/AIDS Management in Office Practice 24: 607–615.

4. Centers for Disease Control and Prevention (1999). HIV/AIDS Surveillance Report 10: 1–43.

5. Flaskerud, J. H. and Ungvarski, P. (1999). HIV/AIDS: A Guide to Primary Care Management. W. B. Saunders Co., Philadelphia.

6. Mann, J. and Tarantola, D. (1996). AIDS in the World II: Global dimensions, social roots, and responses. New York: Oxford University Press.

7. Goldstone, I. (1992). Trends in hospital utilization in AIDS care 1987–1991: Implications for palliative care. J Palliat Care 8: 22–29.

8. Sherman, D. W. and Ouellette, S. (1999). Moving beyond fear: Lessons learned through a longitudinal review of the literature regarding health care providers and the care of people with HIV/AIDS. In HIV/AIDS Update Nursing Clinics of North America (D. W. Sherman, ed.), pp. 1–48. Philadelphia: W. B. Saunders Co.

9. Centers for Disease Control and Prevention (1999). HIV/AIDS Surveillance Supplemental Rep 5:1–8.

10. Denning, P., Ward, J., Chu, S., et al. (1996). Current trends in AIDS incidence among young men who have sex with men, United States

(abstract TuC2405). Presented at XIth International Conference on AIDS, Vancouver, British Columbia.

11. Ropka, M. E. and Williams, A. B., eds. (1998). HIV Nursing and Symptom Management. Jones & Bartlett Publishers, Sudbury, MA.

12. Andrews, L. (1998). The pathogenesis of HIV infection. In HIV Nursing and Symptom Management (M. E. Ropka and A. B. Williams, eds.), pp. 3–35. Jones & Bartlett Publishers, Sudbury, MA.

13. Melroe, N. H., Stawarz, K. E., and Simpson, J. (1997). HIV RNA quantitation: Marker of HIV infection. J Assoc Nurses AIDS Care 8:31–38.

14. Kirton, C. A., Ferri, R. S., and Eleftherakis, V. (1999). Primary care and case management of persons with HIV/AIDS. In HIV/AIDS Update (D. W. Sherman, ed.), pp. 71–93. Nurs Clin N Am, W. B. Saunders Co., Philadelphia.

15. Ferri, R. (1998). Treating HIV infection. Clin Advisor 1: 30–36.

16. Foley, F. J., Flannery, J., Graydon, D., Flintoft, G., and Cook, D. (1995). J Palliat Care 11: 19–22.

17. Gerard, L., Flandre, P., Raguin, G., Le Gall, J. R., Vilde, J. L., and Leport, C. (1996). Life expectancy in hospitalized patients with AIDS: Prognostic factors on admission. J Palliat Care 12: 26–30.

18. Butters, E., Webb, D., Hearn, J., and Higginson, I. (1996). Prospective audit of eight HIV/AIDS community palliative care services. International Conference on AIDS 11(2): 223 (abstract no. TH.B. 190). Unique Identifier: AIDSLINE MED/96924269.

19. Malcolm, J. and Dobson, P. (1994). Palliative care of AIDS: The last month of life. Annual Conference of the Australias Society of HIV Medicine 6: 266.

20. Barnes, R., Barrett, C., Weintraub, S., and Holowacz, G. (1993). Hospital response to psycho-social needs of AIDS inpatients. J Palliat Care 9: 22–28.

21. Bloomer, S. (1998). Palliative care. J Assoc Nurses AIDS Care 9: 45–47.

22. Malcolm, J.A. (1993). What is the best model for AIDS palliative care? Annual Conference of the Australias Society of HIV Medicine 5: 60 (abstract no. Spa1). Unique Identifier: AIDSLINE ASHM5/94349010.

23. Walsh, T. D. (1991). An overview of palliative care in cancer and AIDS. Oncology 6: 7–11.

24. Kemp, C. and Stepp, L. (1995). Palliative care for patients with acquired immunodeficiency syndrome. Am J Hospice Palliat Care 9: 14–27.

25. Higginson, I. (1993). Palliative care: A review of past changes and future trends. J Public Health Med 15: 3–8.

26. Sherman, D. W. (in press). Palliative care: Addressing the physical, emotional, social and spiritual needs of persons with HIV/AIDS. In Pocket Guide to HIV/AIDS Nursing (D. Talotta, K. Zwolski, and C. Kirton, eds.), W. B. Saunders Co., Philadelphia.

27. Glare, P. A. (1994). Palliative care in acquired immunodeficiency syndrome (AIDS): Problems and practicalities. Ann Acad Med 23: 235–243.

28. Post, L. and Dubler, N. (1997). Palliative care: A bioethical definition, principles, and clinical guidelines. Bioethics Forum 13: 17–24.

29. Bone, R. (1995). Hospice and palliative care. Disease-a-Month 61: 773–825.

30. Last Acts Palliative Care Task Force (1997). Palliative Care Core Precepts. Princeton, NJ: Last Acts Palliative Care Task Force.

31. Grothe, T. M. and Brody, R. V. (1995). Palliative care for HIV disease. J Palliat Care 11: 48–49.

32. Fraser, J. (1995). Sharing the challenge: The integration of cancer and AIDS. Journal of Palliative Care 11: 23–25.

33. Malcolm, J. A. and Sutherland, D. C. (1992). AIDS palliative care demands a new model. Medical Journal of Australia 157(10), 572–573.

34. Bloom, J. A. and Flannery, J. (1989). Problems in an AIDS hospice setting. International Conference on AIDS 414 (abstract no. W.B.P. 378). Unique Identifier: AIDSLINE ICA5/00210489.

35. O'Keefe, E. A. and Wood, R. (1996). Quality of life in HIV infection. Scan J Gastroenterol 31: 30–32.

36. Ragsdale, D. and Morrow, J. (1992). Quality of life as a function of HIV classification. Nursing Research 39: 355–359.

37. Ragsdale, K., Kortarba, J., and Morrow, J. (1992). Quality of life of hospitalized persons with AIDS. Image 24: 259–265.

38. Nichel, J., Salsberry, P., Caswell, R., Keller, M., Long, T., and O'Connell, M. (1996). Quality of life in nurse case management of persons with AIDS receiving home care. Res Nurs Health 19: 91–99.

39. Baigis-Smith, J., Gordon, D., McGuire, D. B., and Nanda, J. (1995). Healthcare needs of HIV-infected persons in hospital, outpatient, home, and long-term care settings. J Assoc Nurses AIDS Care 6: 21–33.

40. Greenspan, J. S. and Greenspan, D. (1997). Oral complications of HIV infection. In The Medical Management of AIDS (M. A. Sande and P. A. Volberding, eds.), pp. 224–240. Philadelphia: W.B. Saunders Co.

41. Rene, E. and Roze, C. (1991). Diagnosis and treatment of gastrointestinal infections in AIDS. In Gastrointestional and Nutritional Manifestations of AIDS (D. Kotler, ed.), pp. 65–92. New York: Raven.

42. Aron, J. (1994). Optimization of nutritional support in HIV disease. In Nutrition and AIDS (R. R. Watson, ed.), pp. 215–233. CRC Press, Boca Raton, FL.

43. Freeman, E. M. and MacIntyre, R. C. (1999). Evaluating alternative treatments for HIV infection. In HIV/AIDS Update (D. W. Sherman, ed.), pp. 147–162. Nurs Clin North Am, W. B. Saunders Co., Philadelphia.

44. Semba, R., Graham, P., and Caiaffa, J. (1994). Maternal vitamin A deficiency and mother-to-child transmission of HIV-1. Lancet 343: 1593–1597.

45. Nieman, D. (1996). Exercise immunology: Practical applications. Int J Sports Med 18: 91–100.

46. LaPerriere, A., Klimas, N., and Fletcher, M., et al. (1997). Change in CD4+ cell enumeration following aerobic exercise training in HIV-1 disease: Possible mechanisms and practical applications. Int J Sports Med 18: 56–61.

47. Centers for Disease Control and Prevention (1996). Physical Activity and Health: A Report of the Surgeon General 45: 591–592.

48. Ironson, G., Field, T., Scafidi, F., et al. (1996). Massage therapy is associated with enhancement of the immune system's cytotoxic capacity. Int J Neurosci 84: 205–217.

49. Sherman, D. W. and Kirton, C. (1998). Hazardous terrain and over the edge: The survival of HIV-positive heterosexual minority men. J Assoc Nurses in AIDS Care 9: 23–34.

50. Eller, L. S. (1995). Effects of two cognitive-behavioral interventions on immunity and symptoms in persons with HIV. Ann Behav Med 17: 339–344.

51. Remien, R. H., Rabkin, J. G., and Williams, J. B. W. (1992). Coping strategies and health beliefs of AIDS longterm survivors. Psychol Health 6: 335–345.

52. Casey, K. (1997). Malnutrition associated with HIV/AIDS. Part one: Definition and scope, epidemiology, and pathophysiology. J Assoc Nurses AIDS Care 8: 24–34.

53. Sherman, D. W. and Kirton, C. A. (1999). Relapse to unsafe sex among HIV-positive heterosexual men. Appl Nurs Res 12: 91–100.

54. Kaplan, J., Masur, H. and Holmes, K. (1995). USPHS/IDSA guidelines for the pre-opportunistic infections in persons infected with human immunodeficiency virus: Introduction. Clin Infect Dis 21: 1–S11.

55. Porche, D. (1999). State of the art: Antiretroviral and prophylatic treatments in HIV/AIDS. In HIV/AIDS Update Nursing Clinics of North America, (D. W. Sherman, ed.), pp. 95–112. W. B. Saunders Co., Philadelphia.

56. World Health CME (1999). Highlights from the 6th conference on retroviruses and opportunistic infections. HIV Frontline Fax Newsletter 2: 1–5.

57. Von Gunten, C. F., Martinez, J., Neely, K. J., and Von Roenn, J. H. (1995). AIDS and palliative medicine: Medical treatment issues. J Palliat Care 11: 5–9.

58. Institutional AIDS Society (2000). Antiretroviral therapy in adults: Updated Recommendations. JAMA 283: 381–390.

59. Hammer, S. M. (1999). Strategies for treatment and management of antiretroviral failures. Improving the Management of HIV Disease 7: 12–16.

60. Klaus, B. D. and Grodesky, M. J. (1999). Update from the 6th conference on retroviruses and opportunistic infections. Nurse Practitioner 24: 117–121.

61. Hilts, A. E. and Fish, D. N. (1998). Antiretroviral dosing in patients with organ dysfunction. AIDS Reader 8: 179–184.

62. Condra, J. H. and Ernini, E. A. (1997). Preventing HIV-1 drug resistance. Science Medicine 4: 17–25.

63. Haynes, R. B., Taylor, D. W., and Sackett, D. L. (1979). Compliance in Health Care. Baltimore: Johns Hopkins University Press.

64. Williams, A. B. (1999). Adherence to highly active antiretroviral therapy. In HIV/AIDS Update Nursing Clinics of North America, (D. W. Sherman, ed.), pp. 113–127. Philadelphia: W. B. Saunders Co.

65. Chesney, M. (1997). Adherence to HIV/AIDS treatment. In Program of Adherence to New HIV Therapies: A Research Conference. Office of AIDS Research, Washington, DC: National Institutes of Health.

66. Meichenbaum, D. and Turk, C. (1987). Facilitating Treatment Adherence: Practitioner's Guidebook. New York: Plenum.

67. Haynes, R. B., McKibbon, K. A., and Kanani, R. (1996). Systematic review of randomized trials of interventions to assist patients to follow prescriptions for medications. Lancet 348: 383–389.

68. Newshan, G. and Sherman, D. W. Palliative care: Pain and symptom management in persons with HIV/AIDS. In HIV/AIDS Update (D. W. Sherman, ed.), pp. 131–145. Nursing Clinics of North America, Philadelphia: W. B. Saunders Co.

69. Singer, E. J., Zorialla, C., Fay-Chandon, B., Chi, D., Syndulko, K. and Tourtellotte, W. W. (1993). Painful symptoms reported in ambulant HIV-infected men in a longitudinal study. Pain 54: 15–19.

70. Breitbart, W. and McDonald, M. (1996). Pharmacologic pain management in HIV/AIDS. J Int Assoc Physicians in AIDS Care 7: 17–26.

71. Shofferman, J. and Brody, R. (1990). Pain in far advanced AIDS. In Advances in Pain Research and Therapy (K. M. Foley et al., eds.). Vol. 16, pp. 379–386. Raven Press, New York.

72. Breitbart, W., Passik, S., Rosenfeld, B., McDonald, M., Thaler, H., and Portenoy H. (1994). Undertreatment of pain in AIDS. (Abstract) American Pain Society, 13th Annual Meeting, Miami, Nov 10–14.

73. Cleeland, C. S. Gonin, R., Hatfield, A. K., Edmonson, J. H., Blum, R. H., Stewart, J. A. and Pandya, K. J. (1994). Pain and its treatment in outpatients with metastatic cancer: The eastern cooperative group's cooperative study. N Engl J Medicine 300: 592–596.

74. American Pain Society (1992). Principles of analgesic use in the treatment of acute pain and cancer pain (3rd ed.) Skokie, IL.: American Pain Society.

75. Jacox, A., Carr, D., Payne, R., Berde, C. B. and Breitbart, W. (1994). Clinical Practice Guideline Number 9: Management of Cancer Pain. Washington, DC: U. S. Department of Health and Human Services, Public Health Service, Agency for Health Care Policy and Research (Pub. No. 94-0592), pp. 139–141.

76. Hughes, A. M. (1999). HIV-related pain. Am J Nurs 99: 20.

77. Fantoni, M., Ricci, F., Del Borgo, C., Izzi, I., Damiano, F., Moscati, A., Marasca, G., Bevilacqua, N., and Del Forno, A. (1997). Multicentre study on the prevalence of symptoms and somatic treatment in HIV infection. Central Italy PRESINT Group. J Palliat Care 13: 9–13.

78. Singh, S., Fermie, P., and Peters, W. (1992). Symptom control for individuals with advanced HIV infection in a subacute residential unit: Which symptoms need palliating? International Conference on AIDS 8: 428 (abstract).

79. Holzemer, W., Henry, S. and Reilly, C. (1998). Assessing and managing pain in AIDS care: The patient perspective. J Assoc Nurses AIDS Care 9: 22–30.

80. Reiter, G. and Kudler, N. (1996). Palliative care and HIV. Part II: Systemic manifestations and late stage illness. AIDS Clin Care 8: 27–30.

81. Avis, N., Smith, K. and Mayer, K. (1996). The relationship among CD4, hemoglobin, symptoms, and quality of life domains in a cohort of HIV-positive men. International Conference on AIDS 11:116 (abstract).

82. Greene, K. B., Berger, J., Reeves, C., Moffat, A., Standish, L. J., and Calabrese, C. (1999). Most frequently used alternative and complementary therapies and activities by participants in the AMCOA study. J Assoc Nurses AIDS Care 10: 60–73.

83. Brashers, D. E., Neidig, J. L., Reynolds, N. R. and Haas, S. M. (1998). Uncertainty in illness across the HIV/AIDS trajectory. J Assoc Nurses AIDS Care 9: 66–77.

84. Grassi, L. and Sighinolfi, L. (1996). Psychosocial correlates of quality of life in patients with HIV infection. AIDS Patient Care and STDs 10: 296–299.

85. Butters, E., Higginson, I. and George, R. (1993). Palliative care needs of patients referred to two HIV/AIDS community teams. International Conference on AIDS, 9(1), 522 (abstract no. PO-B34-2322). Unique Identifier: AIDSLINE ICA9/93335959.

86. Friedland, J., Renwick, R. and McColl, M. (1996). Coping and social support as determinants of quality of life in HIV/AIDS. AIDS Care 8: 15–31.

87. Sherman, D. W. (1998). Reciprocal suffering: The need to improve family caregiver's quality of life through palliative care. J Palliat Med 1: 357–366.

88. Atkinson, J. H. and Grant, I. (1994). Natural history of neuropsychiatric manifestations of HIV disease. Psychiatric Clin North Am 17: 33.

89. McEnany, G. W., Hughes, A. M., and Lee, K.A. (1996). Depression and HIV. Nurs Clin North Am 31: 57–80.

90. Flaskerud, J. H. and Miller, E. (1999). Psychosocial and neuropsychiatric dysfunction. In HIV/AIDS: A Guide to Primary Care Management (J. H. Flaskerud and P. Ungvarski, eds.), pp. 225–291. Philadelphia: W.B. Saunders Co.

91. Camacho, L. M., Brown, B. S., and Simpson, D. (1996). Psychological dysfunction and HIV/AIDS risk behavior. J Acquired Immune Defic Syndr Hum Retrovirol 11: 198–202.

92. Capaldini, L. (1997). HIV disease: Psychosocial issues and psychiatric complications. In The Medical Management of AIDS (M. S. Sande and P. A. Volberding, eds.), pp. 217–238. W. B. Saunders Co., Philadelphia.

93. Chesney, M. A., Folkman, S., and Chambers, D. (1996). Coping Effectiveness training decreases distress in men living with HIV/AIDS. International Conference on AIDS 11: 50.

94. Kinara, M. (1996). Transcendental meditation: A coping mechanism for HIV-positive people. International Conference on AIDS 11: 421.

95. Lee, S. T. (1996). Holistic approach with spiritual support enhance people with HIV/AIDS. International Conference on AIDS 11: 423.

96. Mellors, M., Riley, T., and Erlen, J. (1997). HIV, self-transcendence and quality of life. J Assoc Nurses AIDS Care 8: 59–69.

97. Elkins, D., Hedstrom, L. J., Hughes, L., Leaf, J. A., and Saunders, C. (1998). Towards a humanistic-phenomenological spirituality. J Humanistic Psychol 28: 5–18.

98. Ferris, F., Flannery, J., McNeal, H., Morissette, M., Cameron, R. and Bally, G. (1995). Palliative care: A comprehensive guide for the care of persons with HIV disease. Mount Sinai Hospital/Casey House Hospice, Ontario, Canada.

99. Wood, C., Whittet, S., and Bradbeer, C. (1997). ABC of palliative care. BMJ 315: 1433–1436.

100. Goldstone, I., Kuhl, D., Johnson, A., Le, R., and McCleod, A. (1995). Patterns of care in advanced HIV disease in a tertiary treatment centre. AIDS Care 7: 47–56.

101. Byock, I. (1997). Dying Well: The Prospect for Growth at the End of Life. Riverhead Books, New York.

102. Welsby, P., Richardson, A., and Brettle, R. (1998). AIDS: Aspects in adults. In Oxford Textbook of Palliative Medicine (2nd ed., D. Doyle, G. Hanks, and N. MacDonald, eds.), pp. 1121–1148. Oxford: Oxford University Press.

103. Rando, T. (1984). Grief, Dying, and Death: Clinical Interventions for Caregivers. Champaign, IL: Research Press Co.

104. Mallinson, R. K. (1999). Grief work of HIV-positive persons and their survivors. In HIV/AIDS Update Nursing Clinics of North America; (D. W. Sherman, ed.), pp. 163–177. Philadelphia: W. B. Saunders Co.

105. Doka, K. (1989). Disenfranchised Grief: Recognizing the Hidden Sorrow. Lexington, MA: Lexington Books.

106. Worden, J. (1991). Grief Counseling and Grief Therapy: A Handbook for the Mental Health Practitioner. New York: Springer Publications.

107. Maxwell, N. (1996). Responses to loss and bereavement in HIV. Prof Nurse 12: 21–24.

108. Bayes, R. (1997). A way to screen for suffering in palliative care. J Palliat Care 13: 22–26.

109. Centers for Disease Control and Prevention (1999). Guidelines for the Prevention of Opportunistic Infections in Persons with Human Immunodeficiency Virus, Morbidity and Mortality Weekly Report 48 (RR-10): 40–43.

Part VI

End-of-Life Care Across Settings

37 Improving the Quality of Care Across All Settings

MARILYN BOOKBINDER

A humane system of care is one that people can trust to serve them well as they die, even if their needs and beliefs call for a departure from typical practices. It honors and protects those who are dying, conveys by word and action that dignity resides in people, not physical attributes—and helps people to preserve their integrity while coping with unavoidable physical insults and losses. Such reliably excellent and respectful care at the end of life is an attainable goal, but realizing it will require many changes in attitudes, policies, and actions. System changes—not just changes in individuals' beliefs and actions—are necessary.[1]

One system that can address health and end-of-life care is the inclusion of quality methodologies designed to improve education, streamline health care bureaucracies, help measure costs, and even address how people feel about their jobs. Whether your organization is a Joint Commission on Accreditation of Hospitals Organization (JCAHO) accredited one and mandated to use a quality improvement (QI) methodology or not, a planned change approach is needed to achieve positive outcomes and cultivate an infrastructure that maintains optimal standards of care for those at the end of life.

This chapter provides perspectives on QI-based initiatives in U.S. health care organizations across settings and populations, and discusses their impact on patient, professional, and system outcomes in palliative care. Principles of QI and structural, process, and outcome approaches to conducting QI studies are introduced. A case example of a pathway for the end of life, that is now being tested, and that is used to establish the linkages between QI principles and practice to improve end-of-life care is presented. The chapter closes by showcasing nurses within interdisciplinary teams who are providing leadership in the field of palliative care.

THE TERMINOLOGY TURMOIL

Quality improvement is increasingly commonplace in the lexicon of industry and government health care systems in the United States. Typically, QI is used to describe a process of improving things. Although the terms used vary, distinct vocabulary, tools, and techniques used to conduct QI studies are the same. Other labels include continuous quality improvement (CQI), total quality management (TQM), total quality systems (TQS), quality systems improvement (QSI), total quality (TQ), and performance improvement (PI).[2,3]

Because consensus regarding these terms is unlikely, it is recommended that each organization define a methodology and terms that apply across the board and be consistent in their use. This will encourage users of QI to read beyond labels and to examine the meaning behind concepts and the value of teamwork in achieving goals. For the purposes of this chapter, quality improvement is defined generically as the label for the philosophy driving a systematic approach to improving clinical practice, systems, issues, education, and research.

QUALITY IMPROVEMENT IN HEALTHCARE

What Is Quality Improvement?

As a philosophy, QI is broadly defined as "a commitment and approach used to continuously improve every process in every part of an organization, with the intent to exceed customer expectations and outcomes."[4] As a management approach, QI is a way of doing business: a way to stimulate employees to become part of the solution by improving the ways care is delivered, identifying the root causes of problems in systems, designing innovative products and services, and evaluating and continuously improve.[5]

The concepts of QI go back to the 1920s with pioneers in the field such as Deming, Shewhart, Juran, and Ishikawa. W. Edwards Deming, an American engineer and statistician, most widely known for his efforts to assist Japan in its quest for quality after World War II,[2] was all but unknown in his own country (U.S.) until the 1980s. In fact, the Deming prize, Japan's highest award for industrial productivity and quality, was first awarded to an American company, the Florida Electric and Light Company, in 1989. To date, no healthcare organizations have received the Deming prize. Joseph Juran, also involved in the Japanese quality transition in the 1940s and 1950s, added the concepts of planning and control to the quality process and addressed the "costs" of poor quality, which includes wasted effort, extra expense, and defects. Readers wanting more detail about the rationale and statistical methods behind quality improvement philosophy and methods are referred to the writings of Deming[6] and others.[7,8]

Although Deming's quality method has been used extensively in industry with much success, it has only been adapted to education and health care since the early 1990s. The U.S. Health Care Reform Act of 1992[9] fueled the need for QI methods and better control over inconsistencies in services. Effects of the reform include (*1*) increased managed care contracts in health systems and reductions in reimbursement; (*2*) reorganization and downsizing of hospitals and staff; (*3*) cross training and the development of multi-purpose personnel; (*4*) shorter hospital stays for patients, and (*5*) a shift in the provision of services from hospital care to ambulatory and home care.

Table 37–1 describes six key principles of QI, based on the doctrines of W. Edwards Deming. These principles are being applied to a QI project to improve end-of-life care at Continuum's Beth Israel Medical Center (BIMC) in New York City.[10] At BIMC, chart reviews of inpatient deaths and other sources of data provided evidence that end-of-life care could be improved. The purpose of the one-year pilot study, funded by a New York State Quality Measurement grant, is to create a benchmark for the care of the imminently dying inpatient.

The QI process begins and ends with

Table 37–1. Principles of Quality and Application for Improving End-of-Life Care

Principle	Discussion	Application
1. Customer-driven	The focus is on customers, both internal and external and understanding them. Teams strive to achieve products/services to better meet needs and exceed expectations of customers.	Chart reviews of patient deaths reveal areas to improve: Documentation re: advanced directive discussions, symptom management effectiveness, spiritual and psychosocial care, treatment decisions in last 48 hours of life Focus groups with caregivers reveal need for better communication with health professionals about patient's progress
2. System optimization and alignment	Organizations/teams are systems of interdependent parts, with the same mission and goals for customers. Optimizing performance of the entire system means aligning the processes, technology, people, values, and policies to support team efforts to continually improve.	Hospital wide multidisciplinary CQI Team is formed to reduce variation in EOL care with a three standardized tools that provide guidelines for care (carepath), documentation, and physician orders Ongoing resources from Pain and Palliative Care available to pilot unit staff (1 advanced practice nurse)
3. Continual improvement: and innovation	Focus shifts to processes of care and using a systematic and scientific approach. Methods seek to reduce and control unnecessary process variation and improve outcomes.	Flowcharting and brainstorming techniques help identify current activities and unit norms for EOL care re: establishing goals of care, advanced directives respecting patient and family preferences barriers to implementing goals of project
4. Continual learning	Resources are available to develop a culture in which people seek to learn from each other and access new sources of evidence. Feedback mechanisms support the use of evidence to drive improvements.	Extensive literature searches and team expertise guide development of clinical tools and educational materials. Team members receive education re: issues in EOL care, viewing of Educational Program for End-of-Life Care (EPEC). Adult learning principles guide sequencing and content of educational sessions for unit staff:, e.g., physiology of dying.
5. Management through knowledge	Decision-making is based on knowledge, confirmed with facts about what is "best practice," and guided by statistical thinking.	Team uses FOCUS-PDCA methodology to structure study processes. Content experts in EOL, measurement, outcomes, and QI guide sampling, selected outcome measures, and graphic display of data
6. Collaboration and mutual respect	Organizations/teams engage everyone in the process of improvement and in the discovery of new knowledge and innovations. Mutual respect for the dignity, knowledge, and potential, contributions of others is valued by members.	Team forms subcommittees to develop materials in four areas based on expertise and interest: Carepath development, flow sheet, MD orders Implementation (timeline for phases of planning, launching, roll out, evaluation, dissemination, and decisions to adopt practice changes) Education (staff, patient and family) Outcomes (patient, family, staff knowledge, process audit of new tools)

customers, determining their needs, and creating products that meet or exceed their expectations. To achieve the necessary improvement, multidisciplinary teams are needed to break down barriers between disciplines and departments, promote collaboration and mutual respect among health care workers, and encourage participation from frontline staff. In the BIMC pilot study, to determine the causes of variation in end of life (EOL) care processes while developing realistic solutions, a 28-member team was formed to involve staff integral to the EOL process on five pilot units: oncology, geriatrics, hospice, medical intensive care, and step-down unit. Early in the study, QI techniques of brainstorming and flowcharting were used to identify health system barriers and to identify possible strategies for dealing with them.

QI teams use a systematic, scientific approach and statistical methods to study problems and make decisions. This paradigm encourages an environment of life-long learning and promotes a team approach to identifying and developing the "best practices." The BIMC project identified a critical need for multidisciplinary education and teambuilding. For example, monthly QI meetings included a segment of the American Medical Association's Education for Physicians on End-of-Life Care[11] training program. Discussions, led by Russell K. Portenoy, M.D, a co-investigator for the AMA project and chairperson of the QI Team, provided team members fundamental information about the components of good end-of-life care, as well as opportunities to voice their own ideas and concerns.

The QI Team worked in four subcommittees over a five-month period to reach the implementation schedule of the project. One subcommittee developed the Palliative Care for Advanced Disease pathway (PCAD), which has three parts: a multidisciplinary care path, a flow sheet for daily documentation of care, and a physician's order sheet, that includes suggested medications for treating 15 of the most prevalent symptoms at end of life. The other three subcommittees addressed (*1*) education of nurses, physicians; other staff, patients, and families; (2) a timeline and detailed plan for implementation; education, and evaluation of PCAD; and (3) tools and methods for evaluating patient, family, staff, and system outcomes of the project.

Effectiveness of Quality Improvement

While many organizations have embraced the notion of using QI to improve cost and quality outcomes, the U.S. experience is relatively new. In fact, a national survey of U.S. hospitals in 1993 found that 69 percent had adopted or were beginning to implement some form of QI program. Seventy-five percent of hospitals adopting QI had done so within the previous two years,[12] studying administrative issues, such as patient scheduling, record keeping, and billing, rather than clinical practice.

One study provides evidence that quality and outcomes of care can be improved and certain efficiencies achieved through the application of QI. A review of the literature from 1991 through 1997 revealed 42 single-site and 13 multi-site QI studies for examination.[13] Of the 42 single-site studies, nearly 60 percent focused on two major areas: streamlining surgical or medical procedures and reducing length of stay. Thirteen studies addressed overuse of services (i.e., provision of health services when the risks outweigh the benefits); three looked at underuse (i.e., failure to provide health services when benefits exceed risks); and 23 evaluated misuse (i.e., appropriate health services selected but poorly provided). Only two studies used randomized design, while most used weaker designs, such as pre-post observation.

Of the thirteen multi-site studies, seven addressed misuse of services (i.e., focusing on improving care without questioning the amount of care provided); four focused on appropriateness of care in terms of underuse (e.g., pediatric immunizations rates, use of guidelines); and two examined overuse of services (e.g., length of stay). Only one multi-site study used a randomized design. Although some study outcomes included standards for better pain management, none addressed the application of QI in palliative care or, specifically, end-of-life care.

Given the emphasis in health care on using QI to improve quality and cost in health care, nurses can expect to see increases in accountability in the following areas: performance monitoring; participation in multidisciplinary team meetings; education in quality improvement; implementation of process improvement approaches; use of flowcharts and other tools and techniques for data gathering; restructuring of work flow patterns and removal of barriers to patient care; development and use of quality indicators; and focus on patient and caregiver outcomes.

Quality Improvement in Palliative Care

The World Health Organization defines palliative care as the "the active total care of patients whose disease is not responsive to curative treatment . . . when control of pain, of other symptoms and of psychological, social and spiritual problems is paramount."[14] Palliative care is often referred to as *supportive care* or *comfort care* that seeks to prevent, relieve, alleviate, lessen, or soothe the symptoms of disease without effecting a cure.

A valuable resource for those working in end-of-life care is the landmark report published by a committee of the Institute of Medicine (IOM), "Approaching Death: Improving Care at End of Life."[1] The committee of twelve experts in medical and nursing care for chronically ill and severely ill patients summarized four areas of improvement: the state-of-the-knowledge in EOL care, evaluation methods for measuring outcomes, factors impeding high-quality care, and steps toward agreement on what constitutes "appropriate care" at end of life. The four major findings, suggest starting points for QI work: patient care, organizations, education and research;

- Too many people suffer endlessly at the end of life, both from errors of omission—

when caregivers fail to provide palliative and supportive care known to be effective—and from errors of commission—when caregivers do what is known to be ineffective and even harmful.
- Legal, organizational, and economical obstacles conspire to obstruct reliably excellent care at the end of life.
- The education and training of physicians and other health care professionals fail to provide them with knowledge, skills, and attitudes required to care well for the dying patient.
- Current knowledge and understanding are inadequate to guide and support consistent practice of evidence-based medicine at the end of life.

STRUCTURES FOR QI AND END-OF-LIFE CARE

QI Methodologies Provide Structures

Various methodologies can be used as structural elements in a framework designed to support an end-of-life care program. Such structures also help to explain the interrelationship of parts. One type of structure, a systematic methodology, organizes and guides the activities of people performing QI; and a second type assures the validity and appropriateness of a study to improve end-of-life care.

A systematic methodology is needed to conduct a QI study and various models exist, some of them widely recognized in healthcare. Others have been designed specifically for particular institutions' QI Departments. Although QI models may vary, all of them support QI as an unceasing, organization-wide effort that focuses on improving processes of work. They are not intended for policing or blaming people for errors after the fact. Systematic methodologies provide the infrastructure needed to carry out a study that may span a period of years to reach targeted goals.

Ruskin writes "Quality is never an accident. Quality is always the result of intelligent effort, intent, and vigilance to make a superior thing."[15] One frequently used methodology designed to support "intelligent effort" is the FOCUS-PDCA cycle,[7,16,17] which illustrates the BIMC team's application of each step in the cycle (see Appendix A). The details and application of the FOCUS-PDCA cycle and tools and techniques for conducting QI studies have been described elsewhere.[15,18,19]

The FOCUS-PDCA methodology is briefly described below using the BIMC example. Its first five steps are aimed at team building, clarifying the nature and scope of the improvement needed, and gathering information about the culture and setting in which the study will be done.

FOCUS
- *Find a process to improve.* The focus for the BIMC study was care of imminently dying inpatients on the five hospital units known to have the highest volume of patient deaths. Chart reviews of patient deaths identified the need for the study.
- *Organize to improve a process.* A 28-member QI team spanned departments and disciplines to address end of life issues, such as ethics, social work, chaplains, pharmacists, nurses, and physicians.
- *Clarify what is known.* Flowcharts were used to map the ideal process of care and increase dialogue among the team about "why" the care varies. The Team's four subcommittees on care path development; implementation, education, and evaluation searched internal and external sources for evidence and rationale in end of life care.
- *Understand variation.* Brainstorming techniques helped the team elicit reasons for variations in the care process and identify potential barriers. An Ishikawa diagram (to display cause and effect) was used to show the barriers: materials, methods, people, and equipment categories were used. Subcommittees considered the barriers when planning and developing elements of the program.
- *Select a process improvement.* Four subcommittees of the QI team developed evidence-based interventions, including the three-part Palliative Care for Advanced Disease (PCAD) care path, educational materials, and appropriate tools to measure professional, patient and family, and system outcomes. This step starts the PDCA cycle.

The PDCA Cycle: Plan/Do/Check/Act. The Shewhart Cycle[6,7] constitutes the evaluation aspect of the study and it is repeated until the team reaches its goals. The implementation of these steps during the BIMC pilot follows:

- *Plan.* In this step, a timeline of activities for the one-year pilot prepared administration, team members, and others with direction, goals, and resources. The sample timeline in Appendix A illustrates the various phases involved in launching a project: the planning phase, roll out or introduction phase, implementation, evaluation, and dissemination and reporting. The study design is created. This includes determination of sample size and selection, what data will be collected and by whom, what tools will be used and when they will be applied, what training will be conducted and by whom, and who will perform data analysis. Table 37–2 outlines principles for assuring the quality of data.
- *Do.* The interventions are implemented and data collection begins. In the BIMC study several pre-measures were obtained, including baseline knowledge, using the Palliative Care Quiz for Nurses,[20] chart reviews, and focus groups with staff to obtain baseline data.
- *Check.* The results of data collection are analyzed by the team and next steps formulated. The BIMC group used the findings from the knowledge pretest to identify areas for continuing education. Through consensus, members agreed that knowledge items answered incorrectly by >15% of staff would be targeted for continued education.
- *Act.* Action plans are developed. The BIMC Team gave feedback to the QI Team, Pilot Units, and the Hospital QI Department in a quarterly report. Staff requested education in "the physiology of dying."

Standards of Care Provide Structure

Quality care begins in clinical settings with well-defined standards of care that are accepted by professionals as authoritative. Such standards represent acknowledged conditions against which comparisons are made and levels of excellence are judged. They serve to establish consistency, expectations, and patterns for practice. They articulate what health care professionals do, which they serve, and they define what clinical services and resources are needed. Standards also provide a framework against

Table 37–2. Principles of Assuring the Quality of Data

Principle	Key point
Validity/reliability	Accuracy and consistency in data collection
Completeness	Measurement system includes a policy for missing data and timeliness of collection
Sampling method	Sample size determined by power analysis to assure representativeness of population
Outlier cases	Measurements systems make efforts to validate or correct outliers
Data specification	Standardized definitions and terminology for transmission/ use of data across departments
Internal standards	Pre-specified data quality standards tailored for individual performance measures
External standards	Commitment to implementing data sets, codes, methodologies developed by accrediting bodies, e.g., government, professional organizations, for data use across health care systems
Auditability	Data are traceable to the individual case level
Monitoring process	Ongoing data measurement process in place based on pre-specified standards
Documentation	Data standards and findings are recorded and available for review
Feedback	Performance systems regularly provide summary reports on data quality to organization leadership
Education	Performance systems provide support, through education, on-site-visits, guidelines to ensure quality data
Accountability	Measurement systems are responsible for data quality and dissemination to participating members

which quality of care can be measured and constantly improved.

In QI, the term *benchmark* is used to refer to "the search for the best practices that consistently produce best-in-the-world results"[7]—the gold standard. Standards of care,[21] guidelines,[22,23,24,25] position papers,[26,27,28,29,30] principles of professional practice,[31,32,33,34] and research models for end-of-life care[35,36] are increasingly becoming available to improve appropriateness, effectiveness, and cost-effectiveness of care.

If explicit, guidelines can describe appropriate management of specific symptoms and at the same time provide a basis for assessment, treatment, and possible outcomes. However, if the evidence is weak, as is the case for much of end-of-life care, guidelines or standards need to be supported with recommendations made through consensus.[1]

PROCESSES FOR QI AND END-OF-LIFE CARE

Answering the question "What are the processes for giving care to a dying patient?" can generate many ideas for a QI study." *Process* refers to the series of activities or functions that bring about a result. Nurses' contributions are critical in the processes of assessment, diagnosis, treatment, and evaluation of patients. Pain, dyspnea, agitation, nausea, diarrhea, and constipation are some important symptoms leading to nursing interventions that can reduce the suffering of dying patients.

To meet the health care reform challenges of high quality at lower cost, there has been an explosion of tools designed to reduce variability in the processes of care. Critical pathways and algorithms are two types of tools that provide useful strategies for nurses to monitor and manage the processes of patient care. These tools define desired patient outcomes for specific medical conditions and delineate the optimal sequence and timing of interventions to be performed by healthcare professionals.

Clinical Pathways

In the QI context, *pathway* refers to clinical approaches or critical paths that form a structured, multidisciplinary action plan that defines the key events, activities, and expected outcomes of care for each discipline during each day of care. Pathways delineate the optimal sequence and timing of interventions.[37] The goal of using a pathway is to "reduce variation" in services and practices, thus reducing costs.[38,39,40,41,42] Table 37–3 shows a six-step process for developing pathways. Table 37–4 lists commonly used elements of care and interventions.[39] In bringing these aspects of QI into action to improve end-of-life

Table 37–3. The Six-Step Process for Developing a Care Path

1. Identify high volume, high priority case types, review medical records, review and evaluate current literature to characterize the specific problems, average length of stay, critical events, and practical outcomes
2. Write the critical path, defining the sequence and timing of functions to be performed by physicians, nurses, and other staff
3. Have nurses, physicians, and other disciplines involved in the process, review the plan of care
4. Revise the pathway until consensus on care components is reached
5. Pilot-test the pathway and revise as needed
6. Incorporate pathway patient management into quality improvement programs, which include monitoring, and evaluating patient care outcomes

Described by Janken et al., 1999.[37]

Table 37–4. Routine Elements of Care Paths

1. Physical elements
2. Medications
3. Nutrition and dietary
4. Vital signs, intake and output, weight
5. Comfort assessment
6. Safety and activity
7. Diagnostic lab work
8. Intravenous use
9. Transfusions
10. Diagnostic tests
11. Psychosocial and Spiritual needs
12. Referrals and Consultations
13. Patient and Family Counseling and Education

care, the BIMC QI Team pilot-tested the pathway in oncology, geriatrics, and the hospice setting.

Pilot-Test of a Pathway to Improve End-of-Life Care. The entire QI Team at BIMC designed an evidenced-based PCAD pathway consisting of three parts: (*1*) a Care Path—the interdisciplinary plan of care; (*2*) a Daily Patient Care Flow Sheet for documentation of assessments and interventions (including automatic referrals to Social Work and Chaplaincy); and (*3*) a standardized Physician Order Sheet with suggestions for medical management of fifteen symptoms prevalent at the end of life (see Appendix A). This three-part pathway was designed to guide interdisciplinary management of the imminently dying inpatient once the patient's primary physician has ordered PCAD (see Table 37–5).

Implementation of PCAD in daily care on three units has confirmed the enormous complexity of predicting the timing of a patient's death.[44] Although "imminently dying" was defined for the study as "hours to two weeks until death," nurses and physicians reported discomfort about making this decision. Assessment of each patient PCAD for eligibility during daily morning report or at weekly discharge planning rounds is based on the answer to the question, "Whose death would not surprise you this admission?"[45] Designated nurse leaders on each unit serve as the liaison between staff and primary physicians to request a patient's enrollment into PCAD. During the three-month start-up period of the pilot-study, multidisciplinary teams reported that their greatest difficulty was identifying patients who were imminently dying. As patients were identified by nurses as candidates, barriers to implementing PCAD began to surface: Patients and families wanted "everything done" to continue curative treatment; a physician evaluated a patient as "fragile" and unable to hear "bad news;" a patient's physical status changed dramatically in 24 hours, from dying to "rallying" and preparing for discharge; and a house staff physician felt that he was already prescribing PCAD and could not see the benefit of enrollment.

Table 37–5. Goals of the Palliative Care for Advanced Disease (PCAD) Pathway

1. Respect patient autonomy, values, decisions
2. Continually clarify goals of care
3. Minimize symptom distress at end of life
4. Optimize appropriate supportive interventions and consultations
5. Reduce unnecessary interventions
6. Support families by coordinating services
7. Eliminate unnecessary regulations
8. Provide bereavement services for families and staff or
9. Facilitate the transition to alternate care settings, such as hospice, when appropriate

Several positive outcomes of using PCAD have been identified thus far. These include: (*1*) a heightened awareness by staff of the disease trajectory (such as initial diagnosis, curative treatment, life-prolonging treatment, palliative care, symptomatic palliative care, and care of the imminently dying) and patient wishes for this admission; (*2*) increased discussions about the goals of care and the rationale for treatment orders; and (*3*) development of a systematic process for recognizing patient's needing referral to Hospice and to Pain Medicine and Palliative Care for symptom management and family support following discharge.

Debriefing sessions with staff after a patient dies are also an important aspect of the PCAD process. At these sessions, staff members are encouraged to discuss their satisfaction or dissatisfaction with the experience of the PCAD pathway. Such questions as "Were the patient's wishes honored?" "Were unnecessary tests/procedures performed?" "Did the patient have a peaceful death?" "What is the family's likelihood for complicated grieving and the need for follow-up?" generate much dialogue and opportunity for teaching and grief resolution. Overall, staff has expressed appreciation for the opportunity to talk about experiences of patient care and the personal involvement in caring for a patient and family that they may have known over several admissions. Another positive outcome for unit nurses relates to using the PCAD Daily Flow Sheet. Staffs report that it provides them with an easy and comprehensive system for documenting the assessment and intervention of key elements in end-of-life care: comfort; physical, psychosocial, and spiritual care; and patient and family support.

QI Team members have identified areas for improvement while implementing PCAD: (*1*) definition and measurement of the concept of "comfort"; (*2*) identifying the best forum for educating voluntary physician staff, who have less unit/hospital involvement than staff physicians; (*3*) documentation of spiritual care and issues; (*4*) systematic identification of families at risk for complicated grieving; and (*5*) resources about local bereavement services and education for families.

Early results of the pilot study suggest that PCAD is a means for: (*1*) increasing multidisciplinary team discussions of patients' goals of care during hospitalization; (*2*) reducing the variation in the documentation of care of imminently dying patients, placing emphasis on comfort, patient and family wishes, closure for caregivers; (*3*) increasing staff awareness of patients who are imminently dying or in need of palliative care services, long-term care, and hospice; and (*4*) identifying areas in end-of-life care for continual improvement in organizational systems, education, practice, and evaluation.

Algorithms and Standardized Orders

Algorithms have also become popular tools designed to deliver consistent, timely care, especially symptom management at end of life. Figure 37–1 shows one example of an algorithm developed at Dartmouth-Hitchcock Medical Center, Lebanon, NH,[46] to improve the management of dyspnea. The tool offers clinicians a methodology for assessing the symptom and its etiology, directing treatment options, and establishing guidelines for pharmacological and non-pharmacological interventions.

The Providence Hospice, Yakima, WA is a model program of QI thinking applied in daily practice and service. A pocketsize handbook of standing orders and algorithms, "Symptom Management Algorithms for Palliative Care,"[47] is available for clinicians. The symptom management algorithms allow for a team approach involving the referring physician, medical director, nurse, pharmacist, patient, and family caregivers. QI results have been positive thus far. In one study, use of an algorithm reduced the turnaround time of medication delivery to home hospice patients, from 24–48 hours to less than 2 hours. Other topics in the handbook include algorithms for pain, and other distressing symptoms, e.g., mucositis, anxiety, and terminal agitation.

OUTCOMES FOR QI AND END-OF-LIFE CARE

Federal and state governments, private purchasers, physicians, nurses, insurers, labor unions, health plans, hospitals, and accreditation organizations, among others, have begun to address some of the significant quality problems in the U.S. health care systems (www.ahcpr.gov/qual)[48] by improving the ability to measure and report the quality of care being delivered. Such reporting prompts a closer look at provider and health care practices, both as feedback for clinicians, and as publicly available scorecards for consumer evaluation. Two approaches are described for measuring outcomes in palliative care improvement efforts: using a single indicator of a quality of service or using multiple measures.

QI Indicators: Measures of Organizational Performance

A clinical indicator is defined as a quantitative measure that can be used as a guide to monitor and evaluate the quality of important patient care and support service activities.[8,49] Indicators that directly affect quality services include such factors as timeliness, efficiency, appropriateness, accessibility, continuity, privacy and confidentiality, participation of patients and families, and safety and supportiveness of the care environment. Although they are not direct measures of quality, indicators serve as "screens" or "flags" that direct attention to specific performance issues that should be targets for ongoing investigation within an organization.

For institutions that have had a JCAHO survey within the last decade, it is clear that there has been a shift in focus of performance from competence and skills ("Is the organization able to provide quality services?") to productivity and outcomes ("To what extent does the organization provide quality services?"). For example, rather than focusing on whether the institution has a pain management program, surveyors might evaluate whether pain standards have been implemented and if they have had an effect on patients satisfaction with pain management or patient understanding of side effects associated with specific analgesics.

Indicators reflect a performance measure composed of competence and productivity.[4] Competence means that individuals or the organization have the ability (e.g., education, behavioral skills) to provide quality services; productivity means those abilities are translated into actions that achieve quality outcomes. Indicators also reveal deviations from the norm and may warn of impending problems. The amount and types of resources and expertise available on QI teams will influence the indicators selected to assess quality care. Indicators of care at the end of life, for example, may require a single item measure, multiple items with a summary score, or multiple tools. Indicators are expressed as an event or ratio (percentage) and can be categorized into structure, process, or outcome indicators that are clinical, professional, or administrative in scope. Three examples are provided below.

- *Structural indicators* are derived from written standards of care and need to be in concert with the mission, philosophy, goals, and policies of a department or unit. Structure standards measure whether the rules are being followed. For example, a policy may read that all patients admitted to the hospital require discussion and documentation about advanced directives within 48 hours of admission. A structural indicator might read:

$$\frac{\text{Number of records with discussion/ documentation of advanced directives}}{\text{Number of patients who were admitted to the oncology unit}}$$

A structural indicator used frequently in a rapidly changing health care job market relates to competence. This indicator might require that all staff working on a geriatrics unit pass a written exam and demonstrate behavioral competencies related to end-of life care, including pain management (see Appendix A for sample knowledge quiz in palliative care). For this indicator, a threshold is determined, e.g., 90% on the written exam and three return demonstrations in the use of the pathway, for what constitutes successful completion in education in end-of-life care.

- *Process indicators* measure a specific aspect of nursing practice that is critical to patient outcomes. Examples of process indicators might include screening, assessments, and management of complications. These indicators describe "How care is to be delivered and recorded." Sometimes it may be difficult to separate process indicators from outcome indicators. For example, if an improvement study is directed toward reducing discomfort related to noisy respirations (death rattle) in dying patients, the indicator might involve the process of assessment of respirations, obtaining an order, and giving appropriate medication. The indicator might read:

$$\frac{\text{Time medication given to time of relief from noisy respirations (in min.)}}{\text{The total time patient experienced noisy respirations (in min.)}}$$

- *Outcome indicators*[49] measure what does or does not happen to the patient after something is or is not done. More recently, QI teams have strengthened outcome indicators by using research instruments when available. Tools with validity and reliability, for which benchmarking data exist, have a greater potential to predict outcomes and improve practices. For example, an outcome of implementing a multidisciplinary pathway to improve care

Evaluate dyspnea severity &/or category

Initial Steps

1. Increase air movement over patient's face (fan, open window)
2. Reassurance/pursed lip breathing/massage/distraction/sit upright
3. Assess, if appropriate; cyanosis, pulse oximetry, ABG's, Hgb
4. Consider consulting Palliative Care Team (PCT)

Mild Dyspnea (1) →

Anxiolytic: Lorazepam 0.5–1.0 mg IV/PO
Evaluate peak effect at 15 min IV/2 hour PO, then titrate if necessary. Evaluate for RTC dosing.

Moderate Dyspnea (2) →

Anxiolytic: As above, except, Lorazepam 1–2 mg IV/PO

Opioid: If not on,
STAT MSO4 5 mg IV bolus, then increase each dose by 100% q3–5 min until relief
If on,
Increase opioid dose by 50–100%, in addition to analgesic dose

Extreme Dyspnea (3) →

Anxiolytic: as above

Secretions: Atropine 1.0 mg IV & .6–1.0 q20 min use with caution in patients with tachy arrhythmias and/or CHF
Transderm Scop. strip 1.5 mg patch q72h

Opioid: If not on,
STAT MSO4 5 mg IV bolus, then increase each dose by 100% q3–5 min until relief
If on,
STAT 25% PO MSO4 dose IV bolus then increase each dose by 100% q3–5 min until relief, and/or 5–10 mg nebulized morphine with 5 ml saline.

Progressive Dyspnea (A) →

Anxiolytic: as above

Secretions: Atropine 0.4–0.8 mg IV q2–4h
Transderm Scop. strip 1.5 mg patch q72h

Opioid: If not on,
Start at 50–100%, increase q4h, then increase dose by 100% q3–4 min until relief. May require >200–400% increase

If on,
STAT MSO4 5 mg IV bolus, then increase each dose by 100% q3–5 min until relief

Consider: Steroids, Radiation, Diuretics, Antibiotics, Nebulized morphine, PCT consult

Sudden Dyspnea (B) →

Anxiolytic: as above

Secretions: Atropine 0.8–1.0 mg q1–2h & prn
Transderm Scop. strip 1.5 mg patch q72h

Opioid: If not on,
STAT MSO4 5 mg IV & repeat & repeat q5–10 min until settled, the MSO4 by PO/ PR/5C q4h/prn

If on,
STAT MSO4 or Dilaudid1x-of-PO 1x-of-PO dose by SC. Repeat q5–10 min until relief, then titrate.

Treatment Options for specific causes of dyspnea

Hypoxia
- Assess if patient is CO2: Commence oxygen and titrate to relief 24% via mask if COPD with CO2 retention
- If gas exchange very poor consider measures for failed or inappropriate treatment

Ventricular Failure
- Loop diuretic (furosemide)
- other therapy as indicated

Tracheal or SVC obstruction
- Give glucocorticoids IV/PO
- If airway obstruction: arrange for stent insertion or laser if patient able to tolerate bronchoscopy
- If SVC obstruction, add loop diuretic
- Arrange for urgent radiotherapy if tumor is radiosensitive and previously untreated

Pleural air or fluid due to:
1. pneumothorax; intercostal drainage
2. effusion: aspirate
3. pleurisy: intercostal block

Pulmonary embolism
- heparin/warfarin/urokinase

Pericardial effusion
- pericardial paracentesis under ECO control

Lymphangitic spread of cancer

Reactive airways:
- Bronchodilators, if severe deliver via nebulizer
- Consider steroids

Cough:
- • Secretions: Anticioane and prevent

7/8/98

Fig. 37–1. Algorithm designed to improve the management of dyspnea. (Developed at Dartmouth-Hitchcock Medical Center, Lebanon, NH, 1998, used with permission.)

MARY HITCHCOCK MEMORIAL HOSPITAL
Lebanon, NH
Last Breaths (Resource #)
DOCTOR'S ORDERs
DATE/TIME: ____________

Draft

1. **Evaluate severity of dyspnea:** (see reverse side for scale description)

0	1	2	3	4	5	6	7	8	9	10
no dyspnea		mild dyspnea			moderate dyspnea				extreme dyspnea	

2. **Useful nonpharmacological methods to reduce dyspnea**
   - ❑ Positioning (sit, lean forward, elevate head)
   - ❑ Direct fan toward patient
   - ❑ Breathing strategies (Pursed lip breathing)
   - ❑ Guided imagery, desensitization
   - ❑ Reassurance
   - ❑ Nasal cannula (c O2 ______
   - ❑ Mask (c O2 ______

3. **Medication Categories**

Medication Categories	Dose	Route	Frequency
EXPECTORANTS			
❑ Glycerol Bualacolate	______	______	______
MUCOLYTIC AGENTS			
❑ Acetylcysteine (Mucomyst)	______	______	______
OPIOIDS (BE SURE TO FOLLOW-UP WITH BOWEL ORDERS WHEN PRESCRIBING OPIOIDS)			
❑ Morphine Sulfate	______	______	______
SEDATIVES/ANXIOLYTICS			
❑ Diazepam (Valium)	______	______	______
❑ Lorazepam (Ativan)	______	______	______
❑ Midazolam (Versed)	______	______	______
❑ Promethazine (Phenergan)	______	______	______
❑ Chlorpromazine (Thorazine)	______	______	______
STEROIDS			
❑ Prednisone	______	______	______
❑ Dexamethasone (Decadron)	______	______	______
❑ ______	______	______	______
ANTIMUSCARINICS			
❑ Atropine	______	______	______
❑ Scopalamine patch	______	______	______
❑ Levsin	______	______	______
DIURETICS			
❑ Furosemide (Lasix)	______	______	______
❑ Bumelanide (Bumex)	______	______	______
COUGH SUPPRESSANTS			
❑ Benzonate (Tessalon)	______	______	______
❑ Codeine	______	______	______
NEUROLEPTICS			
❑ Haloperidol (Haldol)	______	______	______
INHALED MEDS (nebulizer for patients with COPD and hypercapnia should be air and not oxygen)			
❑ Morphine	______	______	______
❑ Lidocaine	______	______	______
❑ Saline	______	______	______
BRONCHODILATORS			
❑ Albuterol	______	______	______

______ / ______ / ______
Physician Signature — RN Signature — Secretary Signature

Print Physician Name: ______ Beeper Number: ______

DYSPNEA SCALE

MILD DYSPNEA *(1–3)*
Usually can sit and lie quietly
May be intermittent or persistent
Worsens with exertion
No or mild anxiety during SOB
Breathing not observed as laboured
No cyanosis

MODERATE DYSPNEA (4–7)
Usually persistent
May be new or chronic
SOB worsens if walk or exert; settles partially with rest
Pause while talking q30 sec
Breathing mildly laboured
Cyanosis usual

EXTREME DYSPNEA (8–10)
Agonizing air hunger
Talk only 2–3 words between gasps for air
Very frightened
Exhausted—tries to sit and lean forward, falls back
Total concentration on breathing
Cyanosis usual
+/− resp. congestion
+/− confusion
Maybe cold, clammy

PROGRESSIVE DYSPNEA (A)
Often acute on chronic
Worsening over few days/wks
Anxiety present
Often awaken suddenly with SOB.
+/− cyanosis
+/− onset confusion
Laboured breathing awake & asleep
Pause while talking q15 sec
Cough often present

SUDDEN DYSPNEA (B)
Sudden onset (min. to few hrs.)
High anxiety & fear
Agitation with very laboured respirations
Pause while talking

+/− resp. congestion
~+/− acute chest pain
+/− diaphoresis
+/− confusion

Use incremental titration until, when asked, "Is your breathing easy now?" the patient replies, "Yes."

MEDICATION CATEGORIES	DOSE	ROUTE	FREQUENCY
Acetylcysteine (Mucomyst)	10% 2–20 ml	nebulizer	QID
Albuterol (Proventil, ventolin)	1–2 puffs	MDI	QID
Atropine	0.4–1.0 mg	PO/SC	Q4-12H
Benzonate (Tessalon)	100 mg	PO	Q4-6H
Butemide (Bumex)	0.5–2.0 mg	IV	prn
Chlorpromazine (Thorazine)	25–100 mg	PO	Q4-6H/prn
Codeine	30 mg	PO	Q3-4H
Dexamethasone (Decadron)	1–4mg	PO	QID
Diazepam (Valium)	2–10 mg	FO	prn
Furosemide (Lasix)	20–80 mg	IV	prn
Glycerol guaiacolate	5 ml	PO	Q4H
Haloperidol (Haldol)	.5–30 mg	IV	!6H
Levsin			
Lidocaine 2%	2.5–5 ml	nebulizer	Q6H prn
Lorazepam (Ativan)	1–2 mg	PO	Q8H/prn
Metaproterenol (Alupent)	20 mg	PO	Q6-8H
Midazolam (Versed)	1–10 mg	IV	Q10min
Morphine	5–10 mg	nebulizer	Q4H or 4 hourly prn
Morphine Sulfate	5–10 mg (initial bolus)	1V	Q15 min
	2.5–5 mg/hr (infusion), or		
	5–10 mg, or	PO	Q4H
	2–5 mg	SC	Q4H
Prednisone	10–15 mg	PO	~ TID
Promethazine (Phenergan)	25–50 mg	PO	Q4–6H/prn
Saline	5 ml	nebulizer	Q4H or 4 hourly prn
Scopalamine	1.5 mg	patch	Q72H
Theophylline	100 200 mg	PO	Q6H

Fig. 37–1. *(Continued)*

of dying patients might be to achieve family satisfaction with care at 90% very satisfied, using a 0 to 5 scale (0 = very dissatisfied to 5 = very satisfied). Using one of the items related to satisfaction with care in a standardized tool, an outcome indicator might read:

$$\frac{\text{Number of families scoring very satisfied with care}}{\text{Number of families completing satisfaction survey}}$$

Models and Domains to Assess End-of-Life Care

Organizations have shifted their focus from examining the documentation of processes of care to measuring outcomes of care and learning which treatment works best, under what conditions, by which individuals, and at what cost. Although no tested methods currently exist to measure the quality of care at the end of life,[34] efforts are underway to address this need. Results of a controlled trial, the SUPPORT study, support the deficiencies in care, citing the frequency of aggressive medical treatment at end of life (deaths occurring in the ICU) and the lack of adequate symptom management (conscious patients with moderate to severe pain).[50]

Figure 37–2 presents a model used by the BIMC Department of Pain Medicine and Palliative Care for outcomes research in the medically ill. The model illustrates the feedback loop between outcomes and health care. Outcomes research requires ongoing data collection and analysis that feeds into the modification of guidelines for clinical practice, resulting in improved patient, caregiver, professional, and systems outcomes, including costs.[35]

Table 37–6. Areas for Improving Quality Care at the End of Life

1. Physical and emotional symptoms
2. Support of function and autonomy
3. Advance planning
4. Aggressive care near death, including preferences about site of death, CPR, and hospitalization
5. Patient and family satisfaction
6. Global quality of life
7. Family burden
8. Survival time
9. Provider continuity and skill
10. Bereavement

Recommended by the American Geriatrics Society, 1996.[40]

The American Geriatrics Society proposes ten domains to measure performance and assess quality at end of life[34] (see Table 37–6). Organizations using the Clinical Value Compass[7] approach to achieve quality and evaluate outcomes use four broad domains that can be applied to end-of-life care: (*1*) clinical outcomes, e.g. pain, dyspnea; (*2*) functional health status, e.g., communication with family; (*3*) satisfaction, e.g., perceived symptom relief; and (*4*) costs, e.g., caregiver out-of-pocket expenses, inpatient charges.

Outcome Measures to Assess the End of Life

Joan Teno, M.D., of the Center for Gerontology and Health Care Research at Brown University, together with faculty and staff at the Center to Improve Care of the Dying (1998), has assembled a comprehensive annotated bibliography of instruments to measure the quality of care at the end of life. The Toolkit of Instruments to Measure End-of-Life Care (TIME) includes a Patient Evaluation, After Death Chart Review, and After Death Caregiver Interview.[52] Additional outcome measures suggested for improving end-of-life care are shown in Table 37–7. A review of the current literature related to each tool in the kit can be found at http://www.gwu.edu.

Donabedian[53] stated that "achieving and producing health and satisfaction, as defined for its individual members is the ultimate validator of the quality of care." There has been limited research to date in examining satisfaction among terminally ill patients and families. Yet, for most dying patients, satisfaction may be the most important outcome variable for themselves and their families.

Professor Irene J. Higginson, Ph.D., a leading researcher for more than fifteen years has been using the audit cycle, a feedback process similar to QI methods, to improve outcomes in palliative care. Currently at King's College School of Medicine and Dentistry and

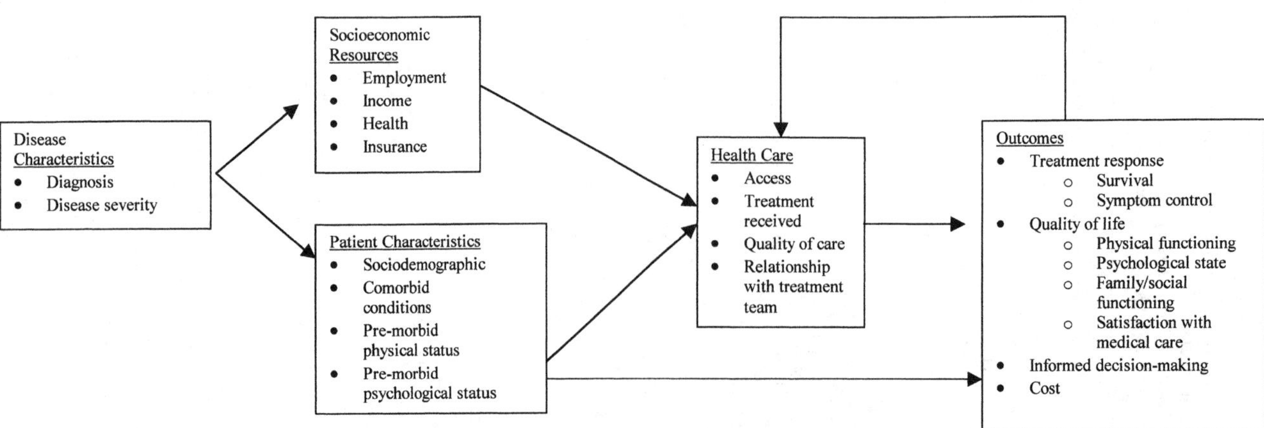

Fig. 37–2. Model of outcomes research in the medically ill. (From Kornblith, 1999, with permission.)

Table 37–7. Executive Summary of the Toolkit of Instruments to Measure End of Life Care (TIME)

Chart review instrument, surrogate questionnaires, patient questionnaires
Measuring quality of life
Examining advance care planning
Instruments to assess pain and other symptoms
Instruments to assess depression and other emotional symptoms
Instruments to assess functional status
Instrument to assess survival time and aggressiveness of care
Instruments to assess continuity of care
Instruments to assess spirituality
Bibliography of instruments to assess grief
Bibliography of instruments to assess caregiver and family experience
Instruments to assess patient and family member satisfaction with the quality of care

J. Teno, MD Center To Improve Care of the Dying http://www.gwu.edu/~cicd/

St. Christopher's Hospice in London, England, she notes the difficulties in obtaining outcome information, such as quality of life, from the weakest group of patients.[54,55,56] She supports the need to test the use of proxies to obtain this important information. One tool currently available for clinicians used to measure the quality of life for patients with terminal illness is the Missoula-VITAS quality of life index.[57]

Measures of family satisfaction in palliative care like the FAMCARE scale[58,59,60] are also available. FAMCARE is based on qualitative research that asks family members to list indicators of quality of palliative care from the patient's perspective and their own. A similar instrument, the National Hospice Organization Family Satisfaction Survey,[61] is an 11-item survey that asks about satisfaction with aspects of hospice care.

SUMMARY

Nurses are poised to have pivotal roles in improving the quality of care of the dying in the decade ahead. As nurses, we need to continue to learn what works and does not work for patients and families in our practice settings and stay active in developing and testing QI models, tools, and interventions toward better end-of-life care. Nurses are providing leadership in areas of clinical practice[62,63,64,65,66,67,68,69] education,[70,71] and research.[72,73,74,75,76,77] Nurses are testing interventions for improved symptom management,[78,79,80] developing models for assuring "best practices" using research,[81,82,83,84] and integrating QI methods into palliative care curriculums in nurses' education.[85,86] Nurses will need to strengthen their involvement in national and international efforts that educate professionals and consumers and influence health care policy in end-of-life care issues.

To survive, healthcare systems must be able to change and improve.[7] If the quality of end-of-life care is to improve, nurses will need to have expert knowledge about making change: how to encourage it, and how to manage and evaluate it within and across organizations and settings. This knowledge needs to be coupled with the methods and "know-how" to produce change. QI methods and tools are a powerful means for designing and testing strategies to improve end-of-life care.

REFERENCES

1. Institute of Medicine. In M. J. Field & C. K. Cassel (eds). Approaching Death: Improving Care at the End of Life. Committee on Care at the end of life, Division of Health Care Services, Institute of Medicine. Washington DC: National Academy Press, 1997.

2. Walton, M. The Deming Management Method. Putnam: NY, 1986.

3. George, S. & Weimerskirch, A. Total Quality Management: Strategies and Techniques Proven at Today's Most Successful Companies, 2nd Ed. John Wiley & Sons: New York, 1998.

4. Schroeder, P. Improving quality and performance: Concepts, programs, and techniques. St. Louis: C.V. Mosby, 1994.

5. Batalden, P, & Staltz, PK. A framework for the continued improvement of health care. The Joint Commission Journal on Quality Improvement 1993;9:425–447.

6. Deming, WE. Out of the Crisis. Cambridge: Massachusetts Institute of Technology Center For Advanced Engineering Study, 1986.

7. Nelsen, EC, Batalden, PB, & Ryer, JC. (Eds). Joint Commission Clinical Improvement Action Guide. Oakbrook Terrace: Ill. The Joint Accreditation of Healthcare Organizations, 1998.

8. Joint Commission on Accreditation of Hospitals Organization (JCAHO). http://www.jcaho.org/, 1999.

9. Coile RC Jr. Health care:top 10 trends for the "era of health reform". Hosp Strategy Rep 1993;5:3–8.

10. Portenoy, RK, Wollner, D, & Bookbinder, M et al. Developing a benchmark for the care of the imminently dying inpatient. New York State Department of Health Quality Measurement Grant, 1999–2000.

11. American Medical Association (AMA). Education for Physician's on End-of-Life Care (EPEC). http://www.ama-assn.org, 1999.

12. Barsness, ZI, Shortell, RR, Gillies, et al. The Quality March Hospitals and Health Networks. December, 1993;5:52–55.

13. Shortell, S, Bennett, C. & Byck, GR. Assessing the impact of continuous quality improvement on clinical practice: What it will take to accelerate progress? The Milbank Quarterly 1998; 76:593–624.

14. World Health Organization: Cancer Pain Relief and Palliative Care. Geneva: WHO, 1989.

15. American Hospital Corporation. FOCUS - PDCA Methodology. Sponsored by Medical Risk Management Associates, LLC.HRM Consulting and Software Development Specialists. http://www.sentinel-event.com/focus-pdca_index.htm, 1989.

16. Channing L. Bete. Co., Inc. Performance Improvement: A health-care staff handbook, South Deerfield, MA, 1999.

17. Executive Learning, Inc. Continual improvement principles: An introduction to concepts and tools for healthcare leaders, Brentwood, TN 1993.

18. Bookbinder, M. Research dissemination: The practitioner's perspective. In E. Dunn, P. Norton, M. Stewart, F. Tudiver, & M. Bass. (Eds). Disseminating research/changing practice. Research methods for primary care. Vol. 6. (pp. 186–198) Sage: Newbury Park, 1994.

19. Bookbinder, M, Kiss, M, Coyle, N, Brown, M., Gianella, A. & Thaler, H. Improving pain management practices. In D. McGuire, C.Yarbro, & B. Ferrell (Eds.), Cancer Pain Management (2nd Edition, pp. 321–361). Jones and Bartlett: Boston, 1995.

20. Ross, M. et al. The palliative care quiz for nurses. The Journal of Advanced Nursing 1996; 23:128–137.

21. National Hospice Organization, National

Council for Hospice and Specialists in Palliative Care Services. Making palliative care better: Quality improvement, multi professional audit and standards. Arlington,VA 1997.

22. American Association of Colleges of Nursing (AACN). Peaceful death: Recommended competencies and curricular, Guidelines for end-of-life nursing care. Washington DC, 1998.

23. National Hospice Organization, Working Party on Clinical Guidelines in End-of-Life Care. Changing gears: Guidelines for managing care in the last days of life in adults. Arlington, VA 1997.

24. American Medical Association: Council on Scientific Affairs. Good care of the dying patient. JAMA 1996;275:474–478.

25. Cherny, N, Coyle, N, & Foley, K. Guidelines in the care of the dying cancer patient. Hematology/Oncology Clinics of North America 1996;10:261–287.

26. American Academy of Pain Medicine (AAPM). Position Statement: Quality care at the end-of-life. Greenview: IL 1998.

27. American Society of Pain Management Nurses (ASPMN). Position Statement: End-of-life care. Pensacola,Fl 1998.

28. American Nurses' Association (ANA). Position Paper: Foregoing Nutrition and Hydration, http://www.nursingworld.org/readroom/position/ethics/etnutr.htm, 1992.

29. American Nurses' Association (ANA). Position Paper: Promotion of Comfort and Relief of Pain in Dying Patients. http://www.nursingworld.org/readroom/position/ethics/etnutr.htm,1992.

30. Oncology Nursing Society (ONS). Oncology Nursing Society and Association of Oncology Social Work joint position paper on end-of life care. Oncology Nursing Forum 26, 1999.

31. Cassel, CK, & Foley, K. Principles for care of patients at the end-of-life: An emerging consensus among the specialties of medicine. Milbank Memorial Fund: NY, 1999.

32. American Association of Critical-Care Nurses (AACCN). Designing an agenda for the nursing profession on End of Life Care. Report of the Nursing Leadership Consortium Workshop on End-of-Life Care. http://prc.coh.org.

33. Canadian Palliative Care Association. Palliative Care: Towards a Consensus in Standardized Principles of Practice, 1995.

34. American Geriatrics Society (AGS). (1996). Measuring quality of care at end-of-life: A statement of principles. NY, http://www.american-geriatrics.org/positionpapers/quality.html, 1996.

35. Kornblith, A. Outcomes research in palliative care. Newsletter: Department of Pain Medicine and Palliative Care 2:1–2. Beth Israel Medical Center, New York, NY, 1999.

36. Byock, IR. Integrating palliation into end-of-life care. Innovations in Breast Cancer Care 1998;4:18–21.

37. Janken, JK, Grubbs, JH, & Haldeman, K. Toward a research-based critical pathway: A case study. On-Line Journal of Knowledge Synthesis for Nursing. Clinical Column, Document Number 1C, 1999.

38. Association of Community Cancer Centers. Oncology Critical Pathways. Rockville, MD, 1998.

39. Blancett, S. S., & Flarey, D. L. Health Care Outcomes: Collaborative, Path-Based Approaches. Aspen Publishers: MD, 1998.

40. National Hospice Organization. A pathway for patients and families facing terminal illness. Arlington, VA, 1997.

41. Gordon, DB. Critical pathways: A road to institutionalizing pain management. Journal of Pain and Symptom Management 1996;11:252–259.

42. Zander, K. CareMaps.® The core of cost/quality care. The New Definition 1991;6:1–3.

43. Continuum Health Partners, Inc., Beth Israel Medical Center, Department of Pain Medicine and Palliative Care. Palliative Care for Advanced Disease (PCAD) Care Path. (CQI Team on End-of-Life Care), NY. http://www.stoppain.org, 1999.

44. Pirovano, M, Maltoni, M, Nanni, O, Marinari, M., Indelli, M, Zaninetta, G, Petrella, V, Barni, S, Zecca, E, Scarpi, E, Labianca, R, Amadori, D, & Luporini, G. A new palliative prognostic score: A first step for the staging of terminally ill cancer patients. Journal of Pain and Symptom Management, 1999:17:231–247.

45. Lynne, J. Personal communication with Russell K. Portenoy, MD, April, 25, 1999.

46. Dartmouth-Hitchcock Medical Center: Hematology/Oncology Group. A dyspnea algorithm. Lebanon: NH, 1998.

47. Wrede-Seaman, L. Symptom Management Algorithms: A Handbook for Palliative Care. Yakima: Intellicard. http://www.Intelli-card.com, 1999.

48. Agency for Healthcare Research and Quality (AHRQ). http://www.ahcpr.gov/qual/

49. Kirk, R. Managing Outcomes, Process, and Cost in a Managed Care Environment. Gaithersburg: MD Aspen Publishers, 1997.

50. SUPPORT Principal Investigators. A controlled trial to improve care for seriously ill hospitalized patients: The Study to Understand Prognoses and Preferences for Outcomes and Risks of Treatments (SUPPORT). JAMA 1995;274:1591–1598.

52. Teno, J. Center to Improve Care of the Dying. Toolkit of instruments to measure end-of-life. http://www.gwu.edu/ 1998.

53. Donabedian A. Evaluating the quality of medical care. Milbank Memorial Fund Quarterly 1996;44:166–203.

54. Innovations in End-of-Life Care. Measuring the Quality of Care in Palliative Care Services: An Interview with Irene Higginson, PhD. http://www2.edc.org/lastacts/featureinn.asp, 1999.

55. Higginson, I (ed.). Clinical Audit in Palliative Care. Oxford: Radcliffe, 1993.

56. Higginson IJ, Hearn J, Webb D. (1996). Audit in palliative care: Does practice change? European Journal of Cancer Care 4:233–236.

57. Byock, IR. & Merriman, MP. Measuring quality of life for patients with terminal illness: the Missoula-VITA quality of life index. Palliative Medicine 1998;12:231–244.

58. Kristjanson, LJ. Indicators of quality of palliative care from a family perspective. Journal of Palliative Care 1986;2:7–19.

59. Kristjanson, LJ. Quality of terminal care: Salient indicators identified by families. Journal of Palliative Care 1989;5:21–30.

60. Kristjanson, L. J. Validity and reliability testing of the FAMCARE scale: Measuring family satisfaction with advanced cancer care. Social Science Medicine 1993;36:693–701.

61. National Hospice Organization. Family Satisfaction Survey. Arlington:VA, 1996.

62. Schwarz, J.K. Assisted dying and nursing practice. Image: Journal of Nursing Scholarship 1999;31:367–373.

63. Lewis, AE. Reducing burnout: Development of an oncology staff bereavement program. Oncology Nursing Forum 1999;26:1065–1069.

64. Ferrell, BR., Whedon, M.B. & Rollins, B. Pain, quality assessment, and quality improvement. Journal of Care Quality Care 1995;9:69–85.

65. Rabinowitz, R. et al. End-of-life Decision-Making. Innovations in Breast Cancer Care 1998;4:1–35.

66. Haisfield-Wolfe, ME. End-of-life care: Evolution of the nurses' role. Oncology Nursing Forum 1996;23:931–935.

67. Brant, JM. The art of palliative care: Living with hope, dying with dignity. Oncology Nursing Forum 1998;25:995–1004.

68. Stanley, K. End-of-life care: Where are we headed? What do we want? Who will decide? Innovations in Breast Cancer Care 1998;4:3–12.

69. McCaffery, M. & Pasero, C. Pain: Clinical Manual (2nd ed.). Mosby Inc.,1999.

70. Hainsworth, DS. The effect of death education on attitudes of hospital nurses toward care of the dying. Oncology Nursing Forum 1996;23:963–967.

71. Ferrell, BR, Virani, R, & Grant, M. HOPE: Home care outreach for palliative care education, Cancer Pract 1998;6:79–85.

72. Bookbinder, M, Coyle, N, Kiss, M, Thaler, H, Brown, M, Gianella, A, Goldstein, ML., Derby, S, & Portenoy, R. Implementing national standards for cancer pain management: Program model and evaluation. Journal of Pain and Symptom Management 1996;12:334–347.

73. Matzo LaPorte, M, & Emmanuel, EJ. Oncology nurses practices of assisted suicide and patient-requested euthanasia. Oncology Nursing Forum, 1997;24:1725–1732.

74. Ferrell, B, Virani, R., Grant, M., Coyne, P., & Uman, G. Beyond the Supreme Court Decision: Nursing Perspectives on end-of-life care. Oncology Nursing Forum, 2000;27:445–455.

75. Murphy, P. Kreling, B, Kathryn, E, Stevens, M, Lynne, J, & Dulac, J. Description of the SUPPORT intervention. J Am Geriatr Soc 2000;48: S54-S161.

76. Schwarz, J.K. Assisted dying and nursing practice. Image: Journal of Nursing Scholarship, 1999;31:367–373.

77. Kirchhoff, K.T. & Beckstrand, R.L. Critical care nurses perceptions of obstacles and help-

ful behaviors in providing end-of-life care to dying patients. American Journal of Critical Care 2000; 9:96–105.

78. Wickham, RS Managing dyspnea in cancer patients. Developments in Supportive Cancer Care 1998;2:33–40.

79. Elshamy, M. & Whedon, MB Symptoms and care during the last 48 hours of life. Quality of Life: A, Nursing Challenge Quality Assessment 1997;5:21–29.

80. Hospice Nurses' Association (HNA). Hospice and palliative care clinical practice protocol: Dyspnea. Pittsburgh, PA 1996.

81. Bookbinder, M., Goldstein, M.L., Derby, S., Racolin, A., Holritz, K., Berenson, S., Altilio, T., Gianella, A., Rizzo, J., Byrnes, M., & Kiss, M. The research connection to quality in the 21st century. Part I. In S. M. Hubbard, M. Goodman, & M. T. Knobf (Eds.), Oncology Nursing: Patient Treatment and Support. 3:1–15, 1997.

82. Bookbinder, M., Goldstein, M.L., Derby, S., Racolin, A., Holritz, K., Berenson, S., Altilio, T., Gianella, A., Rizzo, J., Byrnes, M., & Kiss, M. The research connection to quality in the 21st century: Part II: . In S. M. Hubbard, M. Goodman, & M. T. Knobf (Eds.), Oncology Nursing: Patient Treatment and Support 1997;4:1–14.

83. Miaskowski, C., & Donovan, M. Implementation of the American Pain Society quality assurance standards for relief of acute pain and cancer pain in oncology nursing practice. Oncology Nursing Forum, 1992;19:411–415.

84. Bookbinder, M. & Whedon, M. QUEST for pain relief. Proceedings from the 25th Oncology Nursing Congress. San Antonio, TX, 2000.

85. Ferrell, B., Grant, M., Virani, R., & Marugg. End-Of-Life Care Content Guideline. City of Hope National Medical Center. Duarte, CA. http://prc.coh.org, 1999.

86. Ferrell, B., Virani, R., & Grant, M. Analysis of end-of-life content in nursing textbooks. Oncology Nursing Forum, 1999;26:869–876.

APPENIDX A

Sample CQI Study Proposal to Improve End-of-life Care Using FOCUS –PDCA

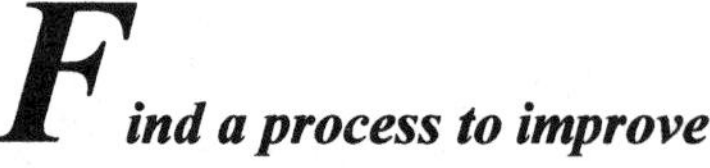

Find a process to improve

Set the boundaries be defining the beginning and end points of the process

Opportunity statement
An opportunity exists to improve EOL care for the imminently dying inpatient
(Name the process)
Beginning with a physicians' order for the Palliative Care for Advanced Disease care path ending with death or discharge to homecare, hospice, or residential facility)
(Set boundaries)
This effort should improve patient comfort and family satisfaction with EOL care
(Name outcome measure)
for hospitalized oncology, geriatric, hospice, and intensive care unit patients.
(Name the customers)

The process is important to work on now because good EOL care is an institutional priority, no benchmarks are currently available in the US, and no standard approach is used at BIMC to assess and treat patients who are imminently dying. *(State significance)*

Organize to improve the process

Form a multidisciplinary CQI team; establish roles, rules, and meeting times.

Multidisciplinary Team (22 members)
Department of Pain Medicine and Palliative Care
MDs, Nurses, Social Work, Psychologist, Chaplain
Hospital Departments
Ethics
Pediatrics
Social Work
Chaplain
Nutrition
Quality Improvement
Pharmacy
Outcomes Measurement (Research Grants and Contracts)
Pilot Units (Oncology, Geriatrics, Intensive Care, Hospice)
MDs, Nurse Managers, Case Managers, Clinical Nurse Specialists

Clarify what is known

FLOWCHART OF PALLIATIVE CARE FOR ADVANCED DISEASE (PCAD) CARE PATH

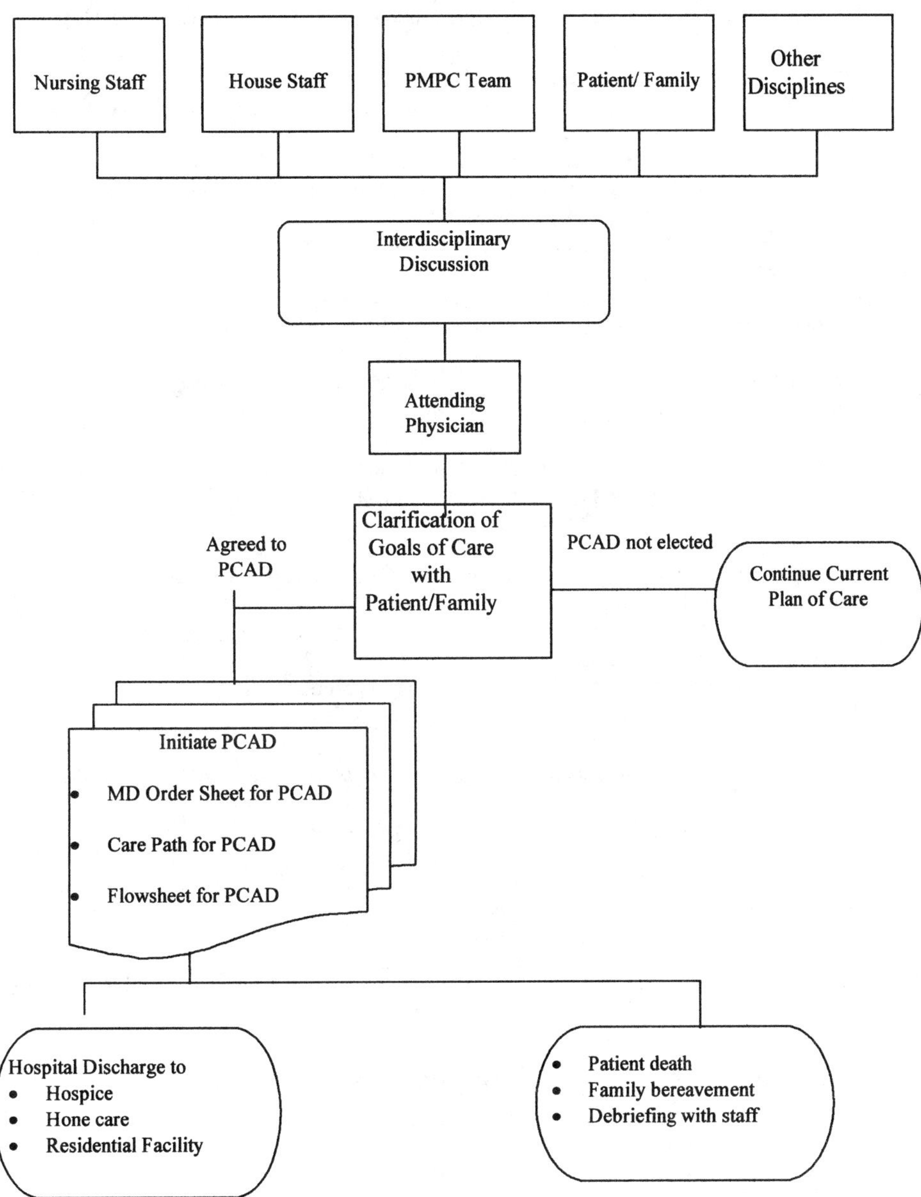

Understand the variation

Brainstorm with those at the grass roots level about why the process varies. Categorize sources of variation by people, materials, methods, and equipment. Display data using a cause and effect diagram.

Brainstorming Session with CQI Team on End-of-life (EOL) Care
Question: What barriers could be encountered in implementing an EOL Pathway at BIMC?

EOL awareness/ discomfort/readiness
- What is "end of life care?" –when is treatment palliative vs. life ending? How do we choose?
- Patient, family, readiness/awareness of dying
- Physician, family, patient willingness to acknowledge that death is imminent
- Issues of truth telling: family may not know status of patient prior to the pathway
- Physician discomfort with stopping treatment
- Medical uncertainty about when to stop treatment

Team communication
- Physician and nurse discomfort in discussing change in treatment strategy
- Is it the physician's decision alone? The heath care team as a whole needs to be acknowledged in decision.
- Definition of terms. Need to define who the team is. May need a new paradigm
- Nurses' comfort-may be put in the middle of team/family attending and decisions

Unit Resistance
- Resistance of unit teams. May see this project as "another thing to do"
- Large-scale resistance. Some may not see that there is something to "fix."
- Organizational pressure to discharge quickly.

Knowledge deficit
- Assumptions about pastoral care (patient, family, staff) and what the experience will be.
- Knowledge deficit about medical and nursing interventions
- How to implement the care path: and encourage people to speak up front rather than later
- Large cultural diversity at BIMC
- Education needed about biomedical analysis and ethical problems
- Physician/patient and physician/family communication skills

Cause and Effect (Ishikawa) Diagram (Barriers to implementing PCAD) Themes above

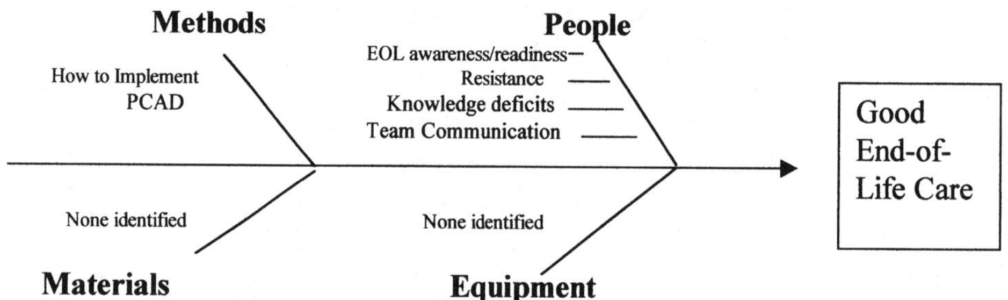

Select the process improvement

Describe the new intervention in detail. Palliative Care for Advanced Disease (PCAD) Pathway: Care Path, Flow sheet, and Physicians' Order Sheet **(see next pages)**

BETH ISRAEL HEALTH CARE SYSTEM ☐ **PETRIE DIVISION** ☐ **NORTH DIVISION** ☐ **KINGS HWY DIVISION**

Care Path: ***PALLIATIVE CARE for ADVANCED DISEASE***	**PRE-ADMISSION CONSIDERATION/ ADMISSION CRITERIA** ☐ **Disease at Advanced Stage – limited life expectancy** ☐ **HCP: Agent**__________ ☐ **DNR** ☐ **Primary Caregiver**__________ ☐ **Next of Kin**__________	**DISCHARGE OUTCOMES** ☐ **Discharge to Community:** __ **Hospice** __ **Home Care** __ **Alternate Care Facility** __**Home** **or** ☐ **Patient expired/Bereavement resources provided to family**	STAMP ADDRESSOGRAPH NAME OF SERVICE/ATTENDING/ HOUSE MD:

PLAN	**START DATE:**	**ONGOING DAYS:**
TREATMENT/INTERVENTIONS/ ASSESSMENTS	1) CLARIFY GOALS OF PALLIATIVE CARE FOR ADVANCED DISEASE (PCAD) WITH PATIENT AND/OR FAMILY 2) FACILITATE DISCUSSION & DOCUMENTATION OF ADVANCE DIRECTIVES: Identify designated individuals & roles in decision-making: 1) Health Care Agent 3) Primary Care Giver 2) Durable Power of Attorney 4) Next-of-kin Identify patient/family preferences regarding: • Health Care Proxy • Resuscitation status/DNR • Living Will 3) INITIATE PHYSICIAN ORDER SHEET/REVIEW DAILY 4) COMFORT ASSESSMENT to include • Pain and symptom management needs • Psychosocial coping , anticipatory grieving, and social/cultural needs • Spiritual issues and distress 5) VS – None unless useful in promoting pt/family comfort 6) ASSESS FOR AND PROVIDE ENVIRONMENT CONDUCIVE TO MEET PATIENT & FAMILY NEEDS	REPEAT CARE PATH DAILY DOCUMENT IN: DAILY PATIENT CARE FLOW SHEET PROGRESS NOTES
PAIN MANAGEMENT	1) ASSESS PAIN Q 4 HR and evaluate within 1 hr post intervention. Complete pain assessment scale. Anticipate pain needs.	
TESTS/PROCEDURES	1) USUALLY UNNECESSARY for patient/family comfort (All lab work and diagnostic work is discouraged)	
MEDICATIONS	1) Medication regimen focus is the RELIEF OF DISTRESSING SYMPTOMS.	
FLUIDS/NUTRITION	1) DIET: Selective diet with no restrictions • Nutrition to be guided by patient's choice of time, place, quantities and type of food desired. Family may provide food. • Educate family in nutritional needs of dying patient 2) IVs for symptom management only 3) TRANSFUSIONS for symptom relief only 4) INTAKE AND OUTPUT – consider goals of care relative to patient comfort 5) WEIGHTS – consider risks/benefits relative to patient comfort	

ACTIVITY	1) ACTIVITY DETERMINED BY PATIENT'S PREFERENCES AND ABILITY. Patient determines participation in ADLs, i.e.,turning and positioning, bathing, transfers	REPEAT CARE PATH DAILY DOCUMENT IN: DAILY PATIENT CARE FLOW SHEET PROGRESS NOTES
CONSULTS	1) INITIATE referrals to institutional specialists to optimize comfort and enhance Quality of Life (QOL) only.	
PSYCHOSOCIAL NEEDS	1) PSYCHOSOCIAL COMFORT ASSESSMENT of: • Patient • Primary caregiver • Grieving process of patient & family 2) PSYCHOSOCIAL SUPPORT: Referral to Social Work • Offer emotional support • Support verbalization and anticipatory grieving • Encourage family caring activities as appropriate/individualized to family situation and culture • Facilitate verbal and tactile communication • Assist family with nutrition, transportation, child care, financial, funeral issues • Assess bereavement needs	
SPIRITUAL NEEDS	1) SPIRITUAL COMFORT ASSESSMENT • Spiritual supports • Spiritual needs and/or distress 2) SPIRITUAL SUPPORT: Referral to Chaplain • Provide opportunity for expression of beliefs, fears, and hopes • Provide access to religious resources • Facilitate religious practices	
PATIENT/FAMILY EDUCATION	1) ASSESS NEEDS AND PROVIDE EDUCATION REGARDING: • Goals of Palliative Care for Advanced Disease • Physical and psychosocial needs during the dying process • Coping techniques/Relaxation techniques • Bereavement process and resources	
DISCHARGE PLANNING	1) FOR DISCHARGE TO COMMUNITY: Referral to Pain Medicine & Palliative Care/ Hospice/Home Care/Social Work as needed. 2) AT TIME OF DEATH: • Post Mortem care observing cultural and religious practices and preferences • Provide for care of patient's possessions as per family wishes • Bereavement support for family and staff	

This document is to be used as a guideline only. Each case should be evaluated and treated individually based upon clinical findings.

Beth Israel Health Care System

Palliative Care for Advanced Disease

DAILY PATIENT CARE FLOW SHEET

ADDRESSOGRAPH

DATE:

☐ **DNR**	☐ **NO DNR**	☐ **HCP**	☐ **NO HCP**	**HCP AGENT:**	**CAREGIVER:**

COMFORT ASSESSMENT: Comfort Level Patient states or appears to be

1. Always comfortable 2. Usually comfortable 3. Sometimes comfortable 4. Seldom comfortable 5. Never comfortable

TIME (per MD order)													
PATIENT Comfort Level (Indicate number)													
VITAL SIGNS ONLY AS ORDERED	T												
	P												
	R												
	BP												

PAIN		
TIME		
LOCATION		
PAIN RATING		
RELIEF/SEDATION		

PAIN/RELIEF SCALE KEY

NONE ←→ WORST

0 1 2 3 4 5 6 7 8 9 10

COMPLETE RELIEF — NO RELIEF

SEDATION SCALE

0 Alert
1 Awake but drowsy
2 Drowsy/Easily awakened
3 Sleeping/Easily awakened
4 Sleeping/Difficult to awaken
5 Unarousable

*See Progress Note A = Assessment I = Intervention Check mark = present or done ► Needs MD Order

		Time			
EYES	A	Moist/Clear			
		Inflamed			
		Dry/Crusted			
	I	Routine Care			
		► Artificial tears			
		► Oint/Lubricant			
LIPS	A	Smooth/moist			
		Dry/Cracked			
		Ulcerated			
	I	Routine Care			
		Topical Lubricant			
MOUTH	A	Moist			
		Dry			
		Coated			
		Stomatitis			
	I	Routine Care			
		► Artificial Saliva			
		► Magic Wash			
		Meds as ordered			

		Time			
BREATHING	A	Rate: Normal			
		Rapid			
		Slow			
		Rhythm: Reg			
		Irregular			
		Depth: Normal			
		Shallow			
		Labored			
		Secretions: None			
		Mild			
		Copious			
		Breath sounds:			
		Clear			
		Diminished			
		Absent			
		Crackles			
		Wheeze			
		Dyspnea			
	I	None			
		Reposition			
		► O2 via__@__lpm			
		Suctioning q____			
		Trach Care			
		Elevate HOB			
		Fan			
		Meds as ordered			

		Time			
NUTRITION	A	Full meal			
		> 50%			
		< 50%			
		Refused			
		Nausea/vomiting			
		NPO			
		Dysphagia			
	I	Diet as tolerated			
		NG/G tube			
		Enteral feeding			
		Feeding set changed			
		Residual vol-cc's			
		Placement check			
		Meds as ordered			
IV LINES	A	IV site			
		No S&S infil/phleb			
		Dry & intact			
	I	IV Dsg change			
		IV Tubing change			
		See progress note			
		Cap Change			
		Huber needle change			

		Time			
MOBILITY	A	Bedbound			
		OOB Chair			
		Amb w Assist			
		OOB ad lib			
		BR Privileges			
	I	T&P per pt comfort			
		ROM q _____			
		Assistive Device			
		► Ted Stocking(s)			
		Side Rails Up			
ELIMINATION	A	Voiding qs			
		Anuria			
		Incontinent Urine			
		Bowel Movement			
		Incontinent feces			
		Diarrhea			
		Constipation			
	I	►Foley Catheter			
		Texas Catheter			
		Inc't Pads			
		►Enema			
		Meds as ordered			
SKIN	A	Normal/Intact			
		Feverish			
		Diaphoretic			
		Pressure Ulcer Stg ___			
		Ostomy site D/I			
		Edema			
		Pruritis			
		Cool/Mottled			
WOUND CARE	I	Site			
		Dressing _______			
		Dry & Intact			
		Drain			
		Drainage _______			
		Odor			
		Ostomy site care			
		Tube site care			

		Time			
SLEEP	A	Normal			
		Interrupted Cycle			
		Insomnia			
	I	Modify Environment			
		Relaxation			
		Meds as order			
PSYCHOSOCIAL	A	Awake/alert			
		Responds to voice			
		Resp to tactile stim			
		Unresponsive			
		Oriented			
		Confused			
		Hallucinating			
		Calm			
		Anxiety			
		Agitated			
		Depression			
		Spiritual distress			
	I	Emotional support			
		Verbal/tactile stimulation			
		SocialWorker visit			
		Chaplain visit			

		Time			
FAMILY	A	Engaged w pt			
		Coping w loss			
		Distressed			
	I	Goals of care reviewed			
		Encourage verbal & non-verbal communication w pt			
		Family Meeting			
		Bereavement support			
MISCELLANEOUS		AM Care			
		PM Care			
		PresUlcer Prev Plan			
		Fall Prev Plan			
		Precautions:			
		Isolation:			
		Siderails Up			
		ID Bracelet			
		Allergy Bracelet			
		DNR Bracelet			
		Post Mortem care			

Comments/Progress Notes

PATIENT/FAMILY EDUCATION: ☐ See IPFER

PCAD Care Path: ☐ **Initiated** ☐ **Reviewed/Continue With Plan Of Care** ☐ **Revised (See Progress Note)**

OTHER NURSING DOCUMENTATION:
☐ I & O SHEET ☐ RESTRAINT FLOW SHEET ☐ NEURO-ASSESSMENT ☐ OTHER ___________

SIGNATURE/TITLE	DATE	SHIFT	INITIALS	SIGNATURE/TITLE	DATE	SHIFT	INITIALS
1.				6.			
2.				7.			
3.				8.			
4.				9.			
5.				10.			

Beth Israel Health Care System

DOCTOR'S ORDER SHEET
PALLIATIVE CARE FOR ADVANCED DISEASE

ADMISSION HT_________ ADMISSION WEIGHT________

ADDRESSOGRAPH AREA

ORDERS OTHER THAN MEDICATION/INFUSION	MEDICATION/INFUSION (Specify route & directions)
1 Primary Diagnosis:	1. Assess patient for the following symptoms: Anxiety & Insomnia, Hiccups, Confusion/Agitation, Nausea/Vomiting, Constipation, Pain, Depressed Mood, Pruritis, Diarrhea, Stomatitis, Dyspnea, Terminal Secretions (Noisy Respirations), Fever. *See reverse side for suggestions for Pain Management and Symptom Control*
2 Activate PCAD Pathway	
3 Anticipated time on PCAD Pathway ___ hours ___days ___weeks ___unknown	
4 Allergies:	
5 Diet: ☐ No restrictions (food may be provided by caregiver) ☐ NPO ☐ Other:	
6 Activity: ☐ OOB as tolerated ☐ OOB with assistance	
7 Vital Signs: ☐ Discontinue ☐ Daily ☐ q shift ☐ q ___hours	2. DISCONTINUE ALL PREVIOUS MED ORDERS
	3. ORDERS:
8 Comfort Assessment: ☐q __ hr ☐q 2 hr ☐q 4 hr ☐q shift	
9 Weight: ☐ None ☐ q ____ day(s)	
10 I & O: ☐ None ☐ q ________	
11 Visiting: ☐ Open visiting, nurse-restrictions apply ☐ Per routine policy ☐ Other:	
12 DNR ☐ Yes ☐ No	
13 PCAD Care Path will include (specify if otherwise): Psychosocial Care – Social Work Referral Spiritual Care – Chaplaincy Referral	
14 Consults: ☐ Pain Medicine & Palliative Care Consult ☐ Ethics Consult ☐ Hospice Consult ☐ Other:	
15 Labs: ☐ Discontinue all previous standing orders ☐ Continue previous lab orders ☐ Other labs:	
16 Oxygen Therapy: ______L/min via___________	
17 Other orders:	

DATE TIME NURSE'S SIGNATURE PRESCRIBER'S SIGNATURE ID# DATE TIME CLERK

The following are medications for consideration in treating pain and symptoms of patients on PCAD:

PAIN MANAGEMENT

For Opioid Naïve Patient:

Morphine Sulfate 15 mg po or 5 mg SQ/IV.
Repeat q 1 hr until pain relief is adequate. Begin Morphine Sulfate 30 mg po or 10 mg SQ/IV q 4 hr ATC or begin IV Morphine Sulfate Basal infusion at 2 mg per hour and 2 mg SQ/IV q 1 hr prn.

For Opioid-Treated Patient:

If pain uncontrolled, increase fixed schedule dose by 50%.

Many non-opioid analgesics are available and should be considered after opioid therapy has been optimized. If pain remains uncontrolled, consider consult to Department of Pain Medicine and Palliative Care (Beeper #6702).

ANXIETY & INSOMNIA

Lorazepam 0.5mg po/SQ/IV BID-TIDq HS for anxiety.
Temazepam 15 – 30 mg po q HS for anxiety/ insomnia.
Clonazepam 0.5 – 2 mg po BID-TID for anxiety/myoclonus.

CONFUSION/AGITATION

Haloperidol 0.5 mg po/SQ/IV. Repeat q 30 minutes until symptom intensity declines.
Haloperidol 0.5 – 5 mg po/SQ/IV q 4 hr prn.

CONSTIPATION

Lactulose 30 ml q 2 hr prn until constipation relieved. When symptom improves, begin Lactulose 30 ml q 12 hr.
Warm Fleets Enema TIW prn

To prevent constipation:
Senokot 1 – 2 tabs po BID and
Colace 1 – 2 tabs po BID.

SYMPTOMS OF DEPRESSION

If anticipated survival is in weeks:

Begin SSRI, e.g., Paroxetine 20 mg po daily, and titrate to effect.

If anticipated survival is in days:

Methylphenidate 2.5 mg po q morning and at noon and escalate daily to 5 – 10 mg po q morning and at noon or Pemoline 18.75 mg po q morning and at noon and escalate daily to 37.5 mg po q morning and at noon.
Higher doses may be needed.

Consider Liaison Psychiatry consultation

DIARRHEA

Loperamide 4 mg po q 4 hr prn

DYSPNEA

For Opioid Naïve Patient:

Morphine Sulfate 5 – 15 mg po or 2 – 5 mg SQ/IV. Repeat q 1 hr, if needed. When symptom is improved, begin Morphine Sulfate 30 mg po or 10 mg SQ/IV q 4 hr ATC; or begin Morphine Sulfate Basal infusion at 2 mg per hour and 2 mg SQ/IV q 1 hr prn.

For Opioid-Treated Patient:

If dyspnea uncontrolled, increase fixed schedule dose by 50%.
If breathlessness continues, add Lorazepam 0.5mg po or SQ/IV prn. Repeat q 60 minutes if needed until symptom intensity declines, then begin 1 mg po/SQ/IV q 3 hr.

Additional therapies may include:
Dexamethasone 16 mg po/IV, followed by 4 mg po/IV q 6 hr
Albuterol 2.5 mg via nebulization q 4 hr prn if wheezing present

FEVER

Acetaminophen 650 mg po/PR q 4 hr prn, and/or
Dexamethasone 1.0 mg po/SQ/IV q 12 hr prn

HICCUPS

Chlorpromazine 10 – 25 mg po/IM TID prn
Haloperidol 0.5 – 2 mg po/SQ/IV TID – QID

INTRACTABLE SYMPTOMS, MANAGEMENT OF

Consider referral to Department of Pain Medicine & Palliative Care (Beeper # 6702).

IV HYDRATION

Consider decreasing IV rate to 0.5 – 1 liter/24 hr

NAUSEA/VOMITING

Metoclopromide 10 mg po/IV q 4 hr prn, or
Prochlorperazine 10 mg po/IV q 4 hr or 25 mg PR q 8 hr prn with or without Dexamethasone 4 mg po/IV PB q 6 hr

PRURITIS

Diphenhydramine 25 – 50 mg po/IV q 12 hr
Hydrocortisone 1 % cream to affected areas q 6 hr
Dexamethasone 1.0 mg po daily alone or in combination with above

STOMATITIS

Viscous lidocaine 2 % to painful areas prn
Clotrimazole 10 mg troche 5 times daily
Nystatin S & S q 6 hr prn
Magic Mouthwash prn

TERMINAL SECRETIONS (NOISY RESPIRATIONS)

Scopolamine patches 1.5 – 3 mg 72 hr, or
Scopolamine 0.4 mg SQ q 4 – 6 hr

PLAN-DO-CHECK- ACT (the Shewhart cycle)

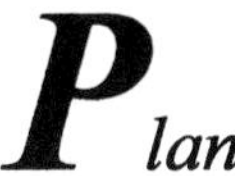

Create a timeline of resources, activities, training, and target dates. Develop a data collection plan, the tools for measuring outcomes, and thresholds for determining when targets have been met.

Timeline for One-Year Pilot CQI EOL Project

Phase 0 – Planning

Jan – June	Formalize CQI Team for the Development of a Clinical Pathway
	Clarify knowledge of processes: review literature and existing data sources, conduct brainstorming, flowcharting with pilot units
	Evaluate and synthesize literature, tools, other data gathered
	Identify content for Care Path
	Develop and pilot audit tool for chart reviews
	Create database, codebook, scoring guidelines for data entry
	Identify Patient Outcome Assessment Tools
	Identify Family Outcome Assessment Tools
	Identify Staff Assessment Tools
	Refine study tools/procedures
	Develop staff education
	Develop caregiver educational materials
June 21	Medical Records Review
Aug 2	Tools Committee Review
July 3	Committee on Scientific OSA Application & Approval

Phase I – Launching the project

August 2 Meet with Hospital Leadership – Introduction to Palliative Care for Advanced Disease Care Path

- PCAD Care Path, MD Orders, and Flow sheet
- Timeline for Education/Evaluation

August 11 Introduction of PCAD Care Path to Medical Staff

Phase II – Unit Implementation and Education of PCAD Care Path

	Cohort 1
• Meet with Unit Leaders of Pilot Units	June 21
• Pre-test	August 23-25
• Unit Leadership Team Meeting	TBS
• Introduction of PCAD Care Path to Unit Staff	August 31 - September 1
• In-service of Unit Staff	September 1 September 2 September 3
• Rollout of Care Path	September 6
• Brainstorming – Educational Needs	October 11
• Educational Series	September – February
• Focus Groups	October & January
• Feedback/Closure/ Continuation	March
• Post-test	March

Phase III — Evaluation

	Chart Reviews using Chart Audit Tool (CAT) (Total =330)
June – Aug	• 20 Retrospective audits for 5 pilot units (Total = 100)
Sept '99 –	• 20 Retrospective audits for 2 control units (Total = 40)
	• 10 During Implementation audits for 5 pilot units (Total = 50)
Mar'20	• 20 Post Implementation audits for 5 pilot units (Total = 100)
	• 20 Post Implementation audits for 2 control units (Total = 40)
	Each patient on PCAD Care Path as admitted
Sept '99 – Mar'20	Tool – Teno's After death (interview or mailed survey)
Dates TBD	Staff Survey Post-tests (Four mos. post initiation of PCAD) Tool - Palliative Care Quiz
Sept '99 –	Process Audits (PAT) Ongoing throughout time patient on PCAD Care Path
Mar'20	
Sept '99 –	Brainstorming sessions and focus groups with staff to identify education
Mar'20	1 – 2 months after each unit begins PCAD

Phase IV – Reporting

April 15, Report to Grant Agency, Hospital, and unit staff

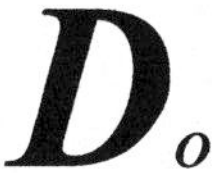

Collect data and monitor the intervention until fully implemented.

Palliative Care Quiz for Nurses (PCQN)

Background Information:
Department/ Service
1. Nursing
2. Medicine
3. Surgery
4. Critical Care
5. Social work
6. Pharmacy
7. Chaplaincy
8. Other (describe)___________

Unit ____________________

Age ____

Sex
1. Male
2. Female

Years of experience in discipline
1. 0-5
2. 6-10
3. >10

Educational preparation
1. HS diploma
2. Associate degree
3. Baccalaureate degree
4. Masters' degree
5. Post graduate degree

Previous education/ training in Palliative Care
1. No
2. Yes (describe)_________________________

4/98 The 20-item survey below is used with permission. Ross, M. M., McDonald,B., & McGuinness, J. (1996). The palliative care quiz for nurses (PCQN): the development of an instrument to measure nurses' knowledge of palliative care. *Journal of Advanced Nursing*, 23:125-137.

Please circle your response to the items below using the following key:
T=True F= False DK= Don't Know

1.Palliative care is appropriate only in situations where there is evidence of a downhill trajectory or deterioration.	T	F	DK
2.Morphine is the standard used to compare the analgesic effect of other opioids.	T	F	DK
3.The extent of the disease determines the method of pain treatment.	T	F	DK
4.Adjuvant therapies are important in managing pain.	T	F	DK
5.It is crucial for family members to remain at the bedside until death occurs.	T	F	DK
6.During the last days of life, the drowsiness associated with electrolyte imbalance may decrease the need for sedation.	T	F	DK
7.Drug addiction is a major problem when morphine is used on a long-term basis for the management of pain.	T	F	DK
8.Individuals who are taking opioids should follow a bowel regime.	T	F	DK
9.The provision of palliative care requires emotional detachment.	T	F	DK
10.During the terminal stages of an illness, drugs that can cause respiratory depression are appropriate for the treatment of severe dyspnea.	T	F	DK
11.Men generally reconcile their grief more quickly than woman.	T	F	DK
12.The philosophy of palliative care is compatible with that of aggressive treatment.	T	F	DK
13.The use of placebos is appropriate in the treatment of some types of cancer pain.	T	F	DK
14.In high doses, codeine causes more nausea and vomiting than morphine.	T	F	DK
15.Suffering and physical pain are synonymous.	T	F	DK
16.Demerol is not an effective analgesic in the control of chronic pain.	T	F	DK
17.The accumulation of losses renders burnout inevitable for those who seek work in palliative care.	T	F	DK
18.Manifestations of chronic pain are different from those of acute pain.	T	F	DK
19.The loss of a distant or problematic relationship is easier to resolve than the loss of one that is close or intimate.	T	F	DK
20.The pain threshold is lowered by anxiety or fatigue.	T	F	DK

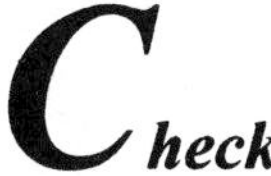

Check

Analyze findings, graph results, and evaluate reasons for variations. If targets are reached, set a date to stop or decrease the frequency of monitoring. Summarize what was learned.

Sample: Results of Palliative Care Knowledge Quiz, Pre-Implementation of PCAD

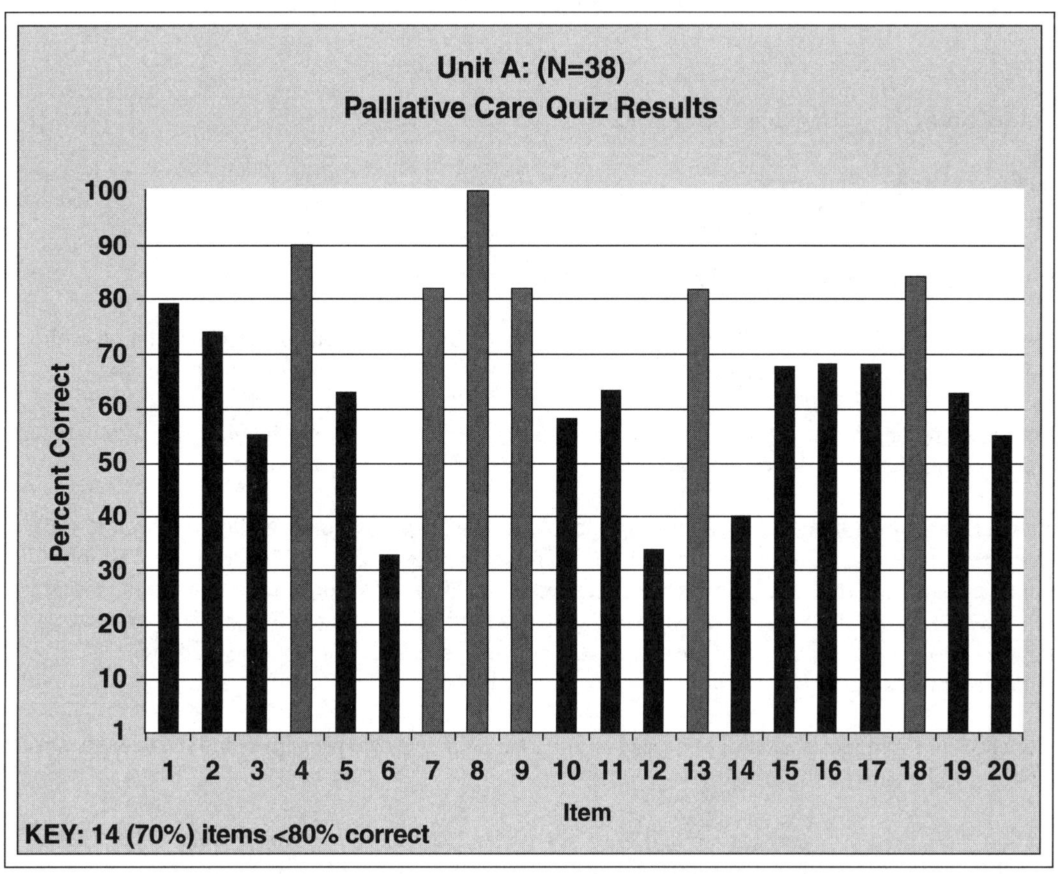

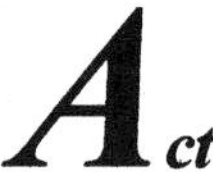

ct

Act on what is learned and determine next steps. If successful, act to hold the gain achieved and work at making the intervention a part of standard operating procedure.. If not successful, analyze the sources of failure, design new solutions and repeat the PDCA cycle.

Sample: Quarterly Reporting Form

Beth Israel Medical Center
Pain Medicine and Palliative Care
Quality Improvement Study Report

Title of Study: Improving End-of-Life Care

Date(s) of study:
1st Quarter X 2nd Quarter__ 3rd Quarter__ 4th Quarter __

Interdisciplinary Team: See listing of CQI Team members.

Sample: The Palliative Care Knowledge Quiz was given to all nursing staff pre implementation of the Palliative Care for Advanced Disease (PCAD) Care Path on three of five planned units thus far.

Findings: In this quarter, we report on the results of knowledge surveys. A total of 90 staff from three units has completed the survey thus far. Analyses have been completed on Unit A.

Analysis/interpretation: Unit A, above, is used to describe the process of providing feedback to staff. The threshold for competency was set for 80%. In fourteen of twenty items (70%) are targeted for improvement. No formal education has been given thus far. This data will be used to a) measure change pre and post an educational series and use of the PCAD in practice, b) determine levels of competency and targeted areas for continued education, and c) to stimulate discussion and dialogue with the multidisciplinary team.

Conclusion: Continued education is needed to integrate palliative care principles into the mainstream of daily clinical practice.

Action Plan: **Step 1:** In-services are scheduled in Quarter 2, 2000. All survey answers will be shared. The Pain Medicine and Palliative Care team will lead a discussion, supported by research results, about the 14 items for which staff answered <80% correctly. Three content areas were identified: end-of-life issues, pain treatment and side effects, and philosophy of palliative care.
Step 2: Based on the dialogue and discussion, subsequent in-services using case-based teaching, will be scheduled. A post-test survey is planned following 6 months of implementation PCAD on each unit.

Follow-up plan: We will report progress at monthly CQI Team meetings. Next report will include chart audit results.

38 Long-Term Care

SARAH A. WILSON

Well, my mom was dying of cancer. Her days in the hospital were used up. We couldn't manage her at home because she was on pain medicine, feeding and everything. We couldn't find a hospice that was available, so she came here to the nursing home to die.

—A daughter

Quality end-of-life care in nursing homes is becoming more important as the number of older adults increases and managed care continues to minimize hospital stays. Nursing home residents are sicker today and have different care needs. Although nursing homes were not established as sites for terminal care, they are becoming the place where many people do die. Statistics on the place of death tell us little about the environment where someone lived and died. This chapter addresses nursing homes, the environment of nursing homes, the staff, the care of dying residents, and model programs to support dying residents.

The terms *institutional care* and *long-term care* have been used interchangeably in reference to nursing home care, although neither is synonymous with *nursing home care.*[1] *Long-term care* refers to a continuum of services addressing the health, personal care, and social service needs for persons who need help with activities of daily living due to some functional impairment.[2] Services may be provided in the home, community, or a nursing home.

Before the late 1970s, nursing homes were the primary source of care for persons needing long-term care that could not be provided by families. Nursing homes have been described as the offspring of the almshouse and boarding house and the stepchild of the hospital.[3] In the mid-nineteenth century, older people who were poor, sick or disabled, and without family support had few options other than the almshouse.[4] Private homes for the aged emerged as an alternative to public almshouses after the passage of the Social Security Act in the 1930s. Women who were caring for their ill family members at home took in other patients to help pay the bills. From these small homes, proprietary nursing homes evolved. When nurses were added to the staff, the homes were referred to as nursing homes, a term that continues to be used today.[5]

Growth of Nursing Homes

The growth of nursing homes from the 1930s to the 1960s was related to six key factors.[3] First, Old Age Assistance allowed a portion of the elderly to directly purchase services. Second, payments were made directly to facilities for the care of older adults, easing the state's financial obligations and creating a source of payment for care. Third, construction loans and loan guarantees were available through the federal Hill–Burton Act, the Small Business Administration, and the Federal Housing Authority. Fourth, the Kerr–Mills Program extended financial participation to medically indigent older adults. Fifth, the American Association of Nursing Homes became a strong lobby for those with interests in the new industry. Sixth, the federal government began in a limited way to develop some standards for nursing homes. The growth of nursing homes occurred largely by chance; however, with the passage of Medicare and Medicaid in 1965, nursing homes became an industry.

Nursing homes continue to be a growing industry as people are living longer with more complex health problems. Currently there are nearly 17,000 nursing homes with 1.5 million occupied beds,[6] almost triple the number of acute care hospitals and double the number of acute care hospital beds.[5,6] Data from the Agency for Health Care Policy Research (AHCPR) indicate that nursing homes increased by 20% between 1987 and 1996.[7,8] Most of this increase was associated with the growth of for-profit, or proprietary, nursing homes. Approximately 80% of nursing homes fall into this category.[7] Nursing homes are licensed or certified to designate the level of care provided and method of reimbursement. Skilled nursing facilities (SNFs) are those certified for Medicare funding. Medicare provides for up to 150 days of skilled care in a nursing home after a three-day hospitalization. However, reimbursement for nursing home care by Medicare is restricted by narrowly defining what is "skilled" and by limiting the duration of the "skilled" benefit. The cost of nursing home care, averaging $37,000 a year, is beyond the means of most Americans.[9] Federal and state Medicaid programs cover approximately 50% of the cost for nursing home care.[9] Rates for Medicaid reimbursement vary considerably from state to state. Most elderly who need nursing home care for more than a few weeks spend or liquidate all their resources to qualify for Medicaid. Reimbursement for nursing homes will continue to be an issue with our changing population demographics.

Population Demographics and Nursing Homes

The population of the United States increased 5.1% in the last decade of the twentieth century. One of the most significant developments was the growth of the older population.[10] The number of people over 65 in the year 1900 was 1.3 million, by the year 2000 it is projected that this number will increase to 35 million.[11] The fastest growing age group in the United States is people aged 85 and over. In the twenty-first century the increase in the elderly population and rapid growth of those over 85 will have a major effect on health care in terms of services needed, the delivery of health care, and education of health care providers. Older persons have more health problems, use more health services, and are hospitalized more often for longer lengths of stay than younger persons.

The figure of 5% is most often cited for the proportion of older adults living in nursing homes. However, this is misleading, as the use of nursing homes increases with age. For older adults age 75–84 the rate is 7%, and for those age 75–84 the rate increases to 20%.[12] The characteristics and needs of nursing home residents have changed with the implementation of the prospective payment system for Medicare. Nursing homes are experiencing changes in the reasons for admissions and discharges. For example, the intensity of care has increased as more people enter nursing homes as a result of early hospital discharge. Some people are entering nursing homes for a relatively short stay and rehabilitation, others are being discharged home, and still others are being transferred to hospitals in the final stages of life and ultimately die there.

Persons who live to age 65 have more than a 40% chance of living in a nursing home before they die.[12] This probability affects millions of lives. Death occurs more frequently among older adults in institutions than at home among family and friends. A widespread belief is that the majority of older people die in hospitals. In fact, the older people are, the more likely they are to die in nursing homes.[13] Data from the National Center for Health Statistics (NCHS) for 1992 show that fewer than half the deaths of people age 65 and over occurred in hospitals.[14] Deaths in hospitals decrease after age 84 and steadily increase in nursing homes after age 65.[13,14] Although nursing homes were not established as places for terminal care, they are increasingly becoming such facilities.

Regulation of Nursing Homes

Nursing homes are highly regulated. The number of rules and regulations have led some to compare the regulations to those of nuclear power plants. The nursing home population is viewed as a population of vulnerable adults who need protection, which, in combination with the history of patient abuse by some providers, has led to a strong tradition of regulation by federal and state governments. Most of the effort in quality assessment has been directed toward detecting problems; less has been devoted to assessing and acknowledging good care.[3]

The response of the industry to regulations has been reactive rather than proactive. Almost two decades ago, concern with the quality of care in nursing homes led Congress to commission the Institute of Medicine (IOM) to study nursing homes. The recommendations of the IOM Committee on Nursing Home Regulation, as well as many consumer advocacy groups, led Congress to enact major reforms in nursing home regulations as part of the Omnibus Budget Reconciliation Act of 1987 (OBRA 87).[15] The intent of OBRA was to improve the quality of care through establishing a single set of certification conditions for all nursing homes.[16] Also, these regulations addressed residents' care, rights, and quality of life. A key aspect of OBRA 87 was that residents have the right to be free of physical and chemical restraints. Also, the emphasis of regulations shifted toward addressing outcomes of care. The Minimum Data Set (MDS), a standardized interdisciplinary assessment tool, was mandated for residents within the first 14 days after admission and whenever there was a significant change in a resident's condition.

Some improvements have been noted in nursing homes since OBRA 87 was implemented.[16,17] The focus on resident's rights and the empowerment of residents in care decisions have been identified as one of the most significant accomplishments of OBRA.[16] Perhaps most significant, there has been an overall reduction in the use of both physical and chemical restraints. Nevertheless, a number of individual facilities still fail to promote a reduction in restraint use.[10] More work needs to be done to improve quality of care in all nursing homes.

Although OBRA was enacted in 1987, it was implemented in an incremental way. Regulations were first issued in 1990, but the final regulations for certification and enforcement of nursing facilities were not issued until November 1994.[10] It is significant that OBRA included no provisions for improving reimbursement to increase staffing.

Accreditation

Nursing homes may apply for voluntary accreditation by the Joint Commission on Accreditation of Healthcare Organizations (JCAHO), an organization created for the accreditation of hospitals but expanded to include home health agencies and nursing homes, among other health care institutions. The facility pays a fee for the inspection to determine if JCAHO standards are being followed. According to JCAHO, approximately 17% of 16,000 nursing homes are accredited.[18] Some nursing homes that seek JCAHO accreditation believe that it adds to a facility's credibility and makes it more marketable to the consumer. In addition, accreditation may make the facility eligible for research grants and training for medical students and residents.

In summary, growth in nursing homes has been proportionate with the increasing elderly population and the need for long-term care services will continue to increase as the population ages. Palliative care is an important component of nursing home care. Along with understanding the structure of nursing homes, it is important to consider the sociocultural environment of these institutions.

SOCIOCULTURAL ENVIRONMENT OF NURSING HOMES

The sociocultural environment of long-term care differs from that of hospitals. Whereas hospitals must always have physicians present, nursing homes are required only to have physician services available as needed, 7 days a week, 24 hours a day. A medical director, full-time or part-time, is responsible for coordinating and directing resident services.

Physician Involvement

Physician visits to residents in nursing homes are often limited to once every 30 days. Federal regulations require physicians to make at least one visit every 60 days to nursing home residents, in contrast to the acute care environment, where physicians usually see patients every day. The nurse in the nursing home is responsible for communicating any changes in a resident's condition to the physician. If the physician does not respond in a timely manner, the medical director intervenes.

Length of Stay

The length of stay is either short-term or long-term.[5] In most nursing homes length of stay varies, although there is greater movement of residents into and out of nursing homes as a result of early hospital discharges. The short-term resident is usually someone under 75 years of age who stays in the nursing home for 4–6 weeks for rehabilitation after an acute illness such as a stroke or hip replacement. The long-term resident is usually older than 75 and has numerous chronic diseases and functional and cognitive impairments. Almost half (47.7%) of all nursing home residents have some form of dementia.[19] The 1995 National Nursing Home Study indicated the typical resident is a female, 75 years old and older, who needs assistance with one or more activities of daily living and instrumental activities of daily living.[6] The long-term resident is much more likely to die in the nursing home or hospital. Compared to previous years, the current nursing home resident is older, frailer, and needs more specialized care.[6] Patients in acute care settings have shorter lengths of stay and may be younger or older adults.

Nursing Home Staff

Nursing homes and hospitals differ in the type of staff employed and in staffing patterns. The acute care hospital has a higher ratio of professional staff to patients than the nursing home. Nursing assistants, the primary caregivers in nursing homes, spend the most time with residents and constitute more than 40% of a nursing home's full-time equivalent (FTE) employees. In comparison, registered nurses (RNs) constitute only 7% of the FTE employees.[20] Licensed practical nurses (LPNs) constitute only 10% of the nursing home's FTE employees.[20] Many nursing homes do not have an RN on duty 24 hours a day. Only 7% of all employed RNs were working in nursing homes or other extended care facilities in 1992.[20] The National League for Nursing (NLN) reported survey results that project only 3% of new RNs will work in long-term care.[21]

The educational level and preparation of staff in the two types of institutions also differ. The LPN program may be completed in 12–24 months and is limited in the amount of educational content devoted to geriatrics, palliative care, and death and dying. Most nursing assistants have not completed high school, work for low pay, and receive few benefits. The work assigned to nursing assistants is often difficult and stressful, and there is little recognition of their contribution to resident care. The salary level for nurses and nursing assistants is lower in nursing homes than in hospitals.[22] The IOM committee strongly supports the need to increase the number of professional nurses in nursing homes, noting that there is a clear connection between the RN to resident ratio and the quality of nursing care provided.[10]

The use of geriatric nurse practitioners (GNPs) and clinical nurse specialists (CNSs) in nursing homes has improved resident outcomes and quality of care.[3] Studies have demonstrated that the use of GNPs and CNSs has decreased unnecessary hospitalizations, improved assessments of residents, and decreased urinary incontinence.[23] Cost savings result from the use of GNPs and CNSs because of the decrease in hospitalization.

Public Expectations

The public and the family of nursing home residents may have unrealistic expectations. It is a difficult decision for families to decide on nursing placement. Families expect the same type of care to be provided in the nursing home that was provided in the home. For example, families may believe a physician will visit every day instead of once a month. The media reinforces negative images of nursing homes. Cases of abuse and poor management receive more attention in the media than positive images of nursing homes.

The sociocultural environment of nursing homes differs from other health care institutions: the average length of stay is longer, physicians visit less frequently, the primary care providers are nursing assistants, and RNs constitute a small portion of the home's FTE employees. Many residents will spend their final days in the nursing home.

STUDIES OF DEATH AND DYING IN NURSING HOMES

Early studies of death and dying focused on hospitals as the place of death. The attitudes of hospital staff toward dying patients, the stresses encountered by nurses in caring for dying patients and families, and communication with dying patients and families were described in these studies.[24–27] More recent studies of death and dying have focused on other settings, including nursing homes.

Studies of death and dying in nursing homes have examined predictors of bereavement outcomes, family perceptions of care, and the educational needs of staff. In a study of adult children whose parents died in a nursing home, Pruchno[28] reported that family members who had negative experiences with the nursing home were sadder and had less comfort in memories. Hanson, Danis and Garrett[29] interviewed family members to describe their perceptions of end-of-life care. Families were asked to make positive or negative comments about any aspect of terminal care. Comments related to hospice care were the most positive, and comments related to nursing home care were the most negative, frequently mentioning poorly trained staff. Several families questioned if suffering was increased because of problems with the quality of care. Maccabee[30] interviewed family members whose relative was transferred from a palliative care unit to a nursing home. Family members believed the nursing home staff was not qualified to provide palliative care, and as a result that the quality of end-of-life care was less. Wilson and Daley,[31] as a part of larger study of death and dying in nursing homes, interviewed family members whose relatives died in nursing homes. Family members described caring behaviors of staff that were helpful to them. The primary concerns expressed by these family members were lack of spiritual care in some facilities and not being present when their relative died because they were not notified in time by the nursing home staff.

Studies have identified the educational need of staff in nursing homes.[31–33] Wilson and Daley conducted focus group interviews in 11 nursing homes with 155 participants.[34] Staff identified the need for education about pain management and comfort measures, grief management, communication skills, and spiritual care. Ersek, Kraybill, and Hansberry[33] reported findings similar to Daley and Wilson in their preliminary studies of educational needs of staff providing end-of-life care in nursing homes. Gibbs[35] reported that nurses in nursing homes were less likely to have continuing education courses about pain management and palliative care than nurses in acute care settings.

Problems with pain management in nursing homes have been documented in other studies.[36–38] Pain is often untreated in the nursing home population. Closs[39] described pain as a neglected phenomenon in the elderly. Nurses tend to overestimate mild pain and underestimate severe pain in the elderly.[40]

In summary, studies of death and dying in nursing homes have described family perceptions of care, the educational needs of staff in providing end-of-life care, and problems with pain management. Further study needs to be done to learn more about dying in long-term care facilities. The Institute on Medicine recommends that studies of end-of-life care in nursing homes include: how well informed residents and families are about who is responsible for care and what they can expect; how resident and family preferences are assessed and determined; what practice guidelines and protocols are used to guide care; how the quality of care provided to dying residents is evaluated; the adequacy of physician and nursing support for dying residents; what palliative care expertise is available to guide care; and whether dying residents are segregated from other residents.[10] Clearly, the nursing home is an environment where end-of-life care research is needed.[41]

Many nursing homes are apprehensive about participating in research studies because of the costs involved, both monetary as well as staff time required. Studies are needed to address issues of protection of study subjects, since many elderly persons in nursing homes are unable to give informed consent. It is important that the researchers clearly explain the purpose(s) of the research and its objectives, the potential benefits to the nursing home, the time and costs involved, and the amount of staff involvement necessary. Researchers should meet with nursing home administration and staff during the course of the study to explain study progress and discuss any problems. They should also meet with family members to explain the research project. At the completion of the study, the researchers should provide feedback to the nursing home, and personnel may be invited to participate in a conference at which the study results are discussed.

CARING FOR DYING RESIDENTS

A number of issues relate to providing quality end-of-life care in the nursing home environment. Nursing home staff, especially RNs, can make significant contributions to enhance terminal residents' quality of life.

Advance Directives: Where Are the Letters of Preference?

Nursing home residents have the right to participate in decisions about their care, including end-of-life care. Passage of the federal Patient Self-Determination Act (PSDA) in 1990 required all health care agencies that receive federal funding to recognize advance directives.[42] The purpose of the PSDA was to encourage greater awareness and use of advance directives. The OBRA 87 regulations emphasized that residents have the right to self-determination, including the right to participate in care planning and the right to refuse treatments. Residents are usually informed of their rights, including the right to advance directives, at the time of admission to the nursing home, a stressful time for both resident and family members. A completed form for advance directives is then filed in the resident's record. The National Medical Expenditure Survey[19] of 1996 reported that only 58% of nursing home residents had some type of advance directive.

Most nursing homes have policies regarding advance directives. However, as Wilson and Daley[34] reported, the nursing staff was often confused regarding advance directives. Staff were not sure where the advance directive was located in the resident's record, if it was current, or if any changes had been made. This becomes a problem when a resident's condition changes. Nurses, especially those on the night shift, might be unfamiliar with the resident or family and were reluctant to call the family. Administrative groups clearly described policies and procedures for advance directives and were unaware of any confusion on the part of staff.

Studies have shown that many of the elderly welcome the opportunity to discuss advance directives and treatment options with health professionals.[43] Before doing so, professional staff need to determine that the elderly person is competent to complete an advance directive. If the person is not competent, a health care agent may be designated. The resident should also understand that in the case of incapacitation, decisions will be made by proxy. Terms used in advanced directives should be explained, and residents and family members should be informed that advance directives may be changed at any time. It may be helpful to ask what residents' goals are for health care treatment and how they wish to live out the remainder of their lives. Proxy health care agents should be informed of their obligation to approximate the residents' wishes as much as possible. Advance directives should be reviewed with the resident or proxy health care agent at regular intervals and always when there is a change in condition. It may be helpful to designate a time for this, such as at the care planning conference.

Ethical Issues

Autonomy is based on the assumption that an individual is the best judge of what is in his or her best interest. Nursing homes have been criticized as dehumanizing and promoting dependence. Semradek and Gamroth[44] believe that when autonomy is discussed in relation to nursing homes, autonomy is more than choice; it gives meaning to one's life. Autonomy is being able to direct and influence others in decisions regarding daily living situations. The routines, regulations, and restricted opportunities in nursing homes have been described as enemies of autonomy and the regimentation contributes to a "loss of control." Most nursing homes were designed based on a hospital or medical model of care, which focuses on routines and tasks. The medical model tends to foster a paternalistic approach of "we know what is best." The physical environment of the nursing home also limits autonomy. Space is limited, with most residents sharing a room and toilet facilities that restrict privacy and space for personal possessions. Residents may also wander in and out of others' rooms. The environment could be more individualized by using personal furnishings and creating a home-like common area, such as a dining room. All nursing home residents should have private rooms.

Autonomy is further restricted in nursing homes by limiting residents' ability to make choices and by failing to provide a range of choices. It is important that nursing home staff know and respect the residents' values. Conflict can occur when staff have differing values, which can affect decisions about starting or withholding treatment.

One of the most difficult and sometimes controversial areas involves decisions regarding food and hydration. Food in all societies is part of the ongoing cycle of daily interaction and activity around which much of family life is organized and is symbolic of life and caring. Families may continue to try to feed their relatives when they are no longer able to eat. Nursing home staff can assist families by explaining that it is normal to lose appetite at the end of life and that the body only takes in what it needs. Trying to force someone to eat may cause more harm than good. Families should understand that there is a risk of aspiration as a person gets weaker. Nursing staff may encourage families to offer small amounts of liquids, ice chips, or Popsicles.

Providing nutritional support and hydration through intravenous or enteral routes should be discussed with residents and family members as part of health care decisions. The courts have recognized artificial nutrition as medical treatment that can be refused like any other medical treatment.[45] Unwanted nutrition and hydration through intravenous or enteral routes may be associated with an increase in medical complications and a reduction in the quality of life.[43] In a study of the appropriate use of nutrition and hydration for terminal residents on a comfort unit of a long-term care facility, McCann[46] reported that residents generally did not experience hunger, and those who did needed only a small amount of food to alleviate hunger. Complaints of thirst and dry mouth were relieved by mouth care, sips of liquids, and lubricants. When some residents ate to please their families, they experienced abdominal discomfort.

The following case illustrates some of the ethical issues in nursing homes.

Case Study: Ethical Issues at the End of Life

Ed Walker, an 86-year-old male, was discharged from the hospital and admitted to Springdale Nursing Home three days ago. Prior to his hospital admission, Ed was living at home and was in relatively good health. He enjoyed visiting with friends, going to sports events, and reading the paper. Ed has one adult son who either called or saw his father every day. When the son was visiting, Ed experienced difficulty with speech and left sided weakness. The son called 911 and Ed was hospitalized. He suffered an infarct of the right middle cerebral artery. After seven days, Ed failed to improve and was unresponsive to noxious stimuli. His prognosis is poor. Ed is a full code because his son believed his father would want everything done. A nasogastric (NG) tube was inserted with difficulty, using a scope for insertion. Ed is restrained to prevent him from pulling out the NG tube. The physician indicated that the code status and NG tube need to be addressed with the son. The nurses at Springdale questioned why Ed is a full code and if the NG tube should be continued.

What are the issues in this case? Who should be involved in making decisions? Why might this be difficult for the son to decide? What would Ed want done? What are the options, and what are the benefits or consequences of these options? Would the American Nurses Association (ANA) Code of Ethics be useful in making a decision? What are the roles of the nurse and physician in this case? Should anyone else be involved? What can be learned from this case?

Pain Management

One of the major themes reported in the IOM's study on improving care at the end of life was that too many people suffer from pain that could be prevented or relieved with the use of existing knowledge and therapies.[38] The primary concern of bereaved family members in studies of death and dying in nursing homes was that their relative be comfortable.[29,31,34] Issues of pain management in nursing homes are discussed below, and a comprehensive discussion of pain management may be found in Chapters 5 and 6.

The nursing home environment has some barriers to pain management particularly in that there is little direct physician contact. Physicians are dependent on nurses to assess and report pain and may be unaware of measures that can be used to control pain in nursing homes. For example, some physicians are unaware that morphine can be given intravenously in many nursing homes. In addition, LPNs receive little education in pain management. Nursing homes have an extreme concern about state and federal regulations and have few protocols for pain management. Pain management is further complicated by the large number of cognitively impaired residents who are unable to communicate if they are in pain.

Considerable variation exists in how pain is managed in nursing homes.[34] Nursing homes that have a designated group or team to deal with pain management naturally have a greater understanding of pain and how to mange it. In a series of focus group interviews with nurses and nursing assistants, nurses expressed concern about "addiction" and "giving too much medication."[34] Nurses also indicated they had difficulty communicating with physicians and were unsure how to approach physicians. Nursing assistants requested more knowledge about comfort measures and what conditions to report to nurses.

Daley and Wilson[34] developed a continuing education program to address the learning needs of nursing home staff. One of the content areas dealt with how to communicate with physicians. Nurses were provided with a guide for telephoning physicians about pain that covered how to prepare for the telephone call and what assessment data to report. Steps in preparing to make the call included stating the purpose of the call, enumerating goals for the resident, and defining what they would like to have happen. Assessment data included location, intensity, and quality of pain; what made it better or worse; what medications had been tried, etc. Nurses were encouraged to develop a standard form to record information. Six to eight weeks after the continuing education program, participants were asked to describe how they used information from the course. Nurses indicated that they were more comfortable talking to physicians on the phone and used a more assertive approach. Others developed a training program for other staff on comfort measures. Nursing assistants increased their knowledge of what information to report to nurses. Becauase nursing assistants spend the most time in direct care activities, it is important to include them in efforts to promote comfort. Providing the nursing home staff with an educational program on pain management had a positive impact on its practice.

Providing Support to Dying Residents and Their Families

Nursing home staff may provide support to dying residents and their families in coping with the eventual loss of the family member. It is important that nurses be able to communicate openly with families, explain changes in condition, and answer questions honestly. Listening is an important communicative skill. Active listening is usually more helpful than judging or giving advice. Effective active listening skills include being able to convey that you want to listen, that want to be helpful, and that you accept the other's feelings. When communication is a concern for staff, it may be helpful to role-play some representative situations. For example, role-playing can teach what to say on the telephone when informing a family member their relative is dying and how to help families decide about options.

Families have identified a number of caring behaviors of nursing staff that helped them cope with the eventual loss of their relative.[31] It was important to families for staff to take the time to come to residents' rooms and ask how they were doing. Families also identified that listening to the family's concerns and getting answers to their questions were helpful. Staff also demonstrated concern for families in other ways, such as asking if they would like a cup of coffee or getting a comfortable chair for a family member. Families appreciated the fact that the staff respected their privacy and seemed to know when they wanted to be left alone.

It is important for families to understand the dying process. Staff may explain signs and symptoms of approaching death to families and keep them informed of what is changing and why. If the family is not present, they should be kept informed by telephone. Family decisions, such as being present at the time of death or not being present, should be respected. Every effort should be made to notify families early enough that they may be present at the time of death, if that is their wish. Families may be encouraged to reminisce together. They may participate in providing care by holding a hand or giving a back rub. Staff should remind families that even though the family member cannot respond, the sound of familiar voices may be a source of comfort.

There are some barriers to providing support for dying residents and families in the nursing home environment. The lack of privacy in most nursing homes is a problem, and it is often difficult to find a private area to talk to families and residents. One social worker commented that "dying is almost a public spectacle in the nursing home." Another barrier is the lack of staff time to spend with dying residents and families, as the staffing patterns of most nursing homes do not take into account labor intensive care at the end of life.

Providing Spiritual Support

An important component of palliative care is spiritual support. Spirituality is often associated with religion, but the two are not identical. Religion is a means of expressing spirituality and refers to feelings, beliefs, and behaviors associated with a faith community. Spiritual needs include the need to see one's self as a person of worth and value, to love and be loved, and to have meaning and purpose in life.[47] Spiritual support is an integral part of supportive care. The search for meaning or spiritual comfort at the end of life is often guided by religious or philosophical beliefs. Spiritual well being in relation to the end of life has been described as "meaningful existence, ability to find meaning in daily experience, ability to transcend physical discomfort, and readiness for death."[48] Families and residents may fear the future and have questions about life in general. Residents are usually asked about their religious affiliation and the name of their clergy at the time of admission to most nursing homes, but unfortunately, this may be the only time spirituality is mentioned. Spiritual needs vary and can change at the end of life.

Private, religiously affiliated nursing homes usually have pastoral care available and most have a room that is designated as a chapel, and many nursing homes have funeral and memorial services for residents. Nonprivate nursing homes usually attempt to make arrangements for pastoral care through volunteer clergy in the community. Some have been successful with these arrangements, but some nursing home staff have stated that it is difficult to find clergy when you need them.

Meeting the spiritual needs of dying residents and their families has been identified as an educational need of nursing home staff.[34] Staff often are aware of spiritual needs but are unsure of what to do or say and what would be considered acceptable to their facilities in meeting spiritual needs. Staff may use a number of interventions to provide spiritual care including praying with the resident and family, reading the Bible or other religious works, singing hymns, and providing therapeutic presence, all of which may help decrease the loneliness and separation persons are experiencing. When a resident is expressing a spiritual need, the following matrix[47] (Table 38–1) may be useful in responding or making suggestions.

With proper staff education and training, most barriers to providing spiritual support in nursing homes can be eliminated. Continuing education programs need to be developed to address staff needs for education on spirituality. Staff need to know the facility's policies regarding spiritual care. Many nursing homes do not have a space designated as a meditation room or chapel. It is important for families and residents to have a private, quiet area where they can meditate. If pastoral care is not available in the nursing home, it may be arranged by contacting local clergy or lay leaders in the community.

Providing Support for Staff

Nursing staff develop an attachment to residents that may be defined as a strong emotional bond and connectedness that develops between residents and staff over time.[34] Attachment is fostered by staff efforts to treat residents as "family." The nursing home *is* home for many residents, as some live there for years, so much so that staff often experience feelings of loss and sadness when a resident dies.

Staff members need to be able to talk about their feelings of loss when a resident dies. Nursing home administrators are often unaware of the intensity of staff feelings toward residents, and hence it is important that staff be given time to talk about the loss of a resident and what it means to them. As one staff member commented, "I get on the bus and go home, I don't have anyone to talk to about it."

Nursing homes need to develop programs to assist staff in coping with the loss of a resident. Allowing staff time to talk about a resident at staff meetings, sharing memories of a resident, and planning a memorial for residents who

Table 38–1. Spiritual Needs: Example of Needs and Suggested Responses

Need	Danger Sign	Response	Suggestions
A. Person of worth	Person says, "I can't even get dressed." "I have made a mess of my life." or example of person who arranges to get ignored	"God loves you." "I like you just the way you are."	Address residents with their names to confirm value and worth. Spend time. Find tasks the resident can do.
B. Love and be loved	People who are lonely	Express your feelings to resident.	Help them recall memories of being loved.
C. Meaning and purpose	Not being able to do what they used to "Why am I still here?"	Convey that resident did and does make a difference. "You have let me journey with you." Part of the gift I get is letting me take care of you and experience you as a person."	Assist them with other meaningful activities: journaling, assisting other residents, praying for others.

have died may be helpful. Other staff members should acknowledge that the loss must be difficult when they know a particular staff member was close to a certain resident.

The loss of a resident may also be stressful for other nursing home residents. Residents develop friendships with other residents over time; they may have shared a room with the resident or sat next to the resident for meals. The death may remind residents of their own mortality. Residents may want to attend the funeral of the deceased resident, or the nursing home may have a memorial service or time of remembrance. Staff should acknowledge the loss and what it means to other residents.

In summary, the nursing home environment influences the care of residents at the end of life. Nursing home staff need to be comfortable talking with residents and families about death and dying. Knowledge of pain management is as important in nursing homes as it is in other settings. Families should be included in the care of dying residents, and their need for privacy should be respected. Some nursing homes have developed innovative programs to meet the needs of dying residents and the staff who care for them.

MODEL PROGRAMS TO PROVIDE SUPPORT TO DYING RESIDENTS

A number of nursing homes around the United States have developed model programs to provide support to dying residents and their families. Some of these programs deal with the specific problems of a subset: of those nursing home residents who are near death. Several of these programs are described below.

Abides Ministry

Abides Ministry addresses a variety of the needs of dying residents. It is a model program developed by Luther Manor, a long-term care facility in Milwaukee, Wis. The program was initiated when a group of nurses began talking about how important it was to sit with residents who were dying. Members consist of staff who volunteer after-hours, residents at Luther Manor, and others from the community who want to be present for those who would otherwise die alone.

Abides has developed a training manual. Prospective members are screened to be sure they are not bringing personal agendas to the bedsides of a dying residents. New group members are paired with a "buddy" to ensure that another Abider is present the first time he or she sits with a dying resident. Quarterly meetings are held to share concerns, and members stay in close contact to help one another through the loss of a resident.

The Abiders try to anticipate the needs and wishes of dying residents. Abiders sit with a resident and read Bible passages, sings hymns, or most often just hold a resident's hand. Abiders stay with the dying resident 24 hours a day. They also provide relief for family members.

The Abiders program won a national award for innovation from the American Association of Homes and Services for Aging. The program chaplain has met with other area chaplains to set up similar programs and has received requests from other groups across the country on how to start similar programs. This is an example of a successful program that was initiated as a result of staff nurses talking about the needs of dying residents. The Abider's program was developed in a long-term care setting, but it could be adapted to other settings with few modifications.

Hospice Care in Nursing Homes

Several nursing homes have contracts with hospices for services. Because the nursing home is considered the residents' home, they may be eligible for Medicare hospice benefits under home care. The hospice staff is responsible for the plan of care, and any changes in the treatment plan must be discussed with and approved by the hospice case manager. The hospice nurse visits the nursing home, arranges the assessment of the resident, and schedules nursing assistance to provide personal care. The resident is provided with services that would otherwise not be available.

Coordinating hospice care in a nursing home requires good communication between the nursing home staff and hospice staff. Some nursing home staff members sometimes see the hospice staff as outsiders. Nursing home staff frequently believe that they know the resident best because they interact and care for the resident every day, whereas hospice staff members may see the resident only two or three times a week. Although hospice care is a benefit to residents, some question why special services are available to one group of residents and not all residents.

Hospice Households for Persons with End-Stage Dementia

The hospice households project for persons with end-stage dementia is an example of an innovative approach that applies hospice concepts in nursing homes.[50,51,52] Persons with end-stage dementia do not meet the traditional requirements for hospice care, which are typically someone with a diagnosis of cancer and a limited life expectancy, usually six months or less. Persons with end-stage dementia may reside in a nursing home for ten years or more. The care of persons with end-stage dementia differs from the care of persons with end-stage cancer in that the course of cancer is more predictable. Persons with cancer often have problems with pain, nausea, vomiting, and breathing. These problems are less common in persons with end-stage dementia. The person with end-stage dementia is unable to communicate needs and has severe impairments in cognitive and social abilities. Careful assessment is essential to determine possible causes of discomfort in persons with end-stage dementia.

Five hospice households were developed in three nursing homes for residents with end-stage dementia. The project was guided by the following research question: What is the effect of hospice-oriented care on comfort, physical complications, and behaviors associated with dementia for nursing home residents with a dementing illness?

Residents were eligible to participate in the study if they had a diagnosis of irreversible dementia, had a score on the Short Portable Mental Status Questionnaire[53] that indicated severe cognitive impairment, were unable to participate in group programming for persons with dementia, had a functional behavior profile score of less than 40, and had advance directives that requested no cardiopulmonary resuscitation (CPR) be initiated. The researchers met with family members to explain the study and asked for permission for the relative to participate. Residents who met the criteria for participating in the study were assigned to a treatment group or control group. The treatment group received the intervention and were part of the hospice households.

The hospice households were clustered on six to eight bed areas on units that had 22–44 beds. The intention was not to isolate residents on a distant unit. The households were made as home-like as possible by using colorful afghans, pillows, home furniture, and plants. Pictures and biographical sketches of each resident whose guardian consented were displayed in the room. Each facility provided a lounge for the project. Residents ate their meals in the lounge, which became a center for activities.

Case managers for the project were selected by the director of nursing in each facility. The case manager led the interdisciplinary team at the facility and assisted with developing and implementing individualized care plans. Case managers received formal classes in hospice care, care planning, assessment techniques, and case management from the researchers. In addition, an all-day conference was held for all staff involved in the project. Classes focused on hospice concepts, dementia, treatment of behaviors associated with dementia, and activity programming, as well as family and spiritual care. The conference generated interest and enthusiasm for the project.

Five main programs goals were identified that are consistent with hospice goals: comfort, quality of life, dignity, support for family, and support for the staff. The goal for comfort was that staff be able to tell when a resident was experiencing discomfort and when a resident was not. Staff used physical and behavioral assessment skills to recognize discomfort. When a resident displayed a change in behavior, he or she was evaluated for signs of constipation and for signs and symptoms of common infections, such as urinary tract infection using a leukocyte esterase dipstick. Urinary tract infections were common. If the cause for discomfort was not clearly identified, a behavioral intervention, such as distraction, quiet time in the resident's room, or music therapy, was initiated. All residents had orders for Tylenol as needed. If the resident displayed behavior such as agitation or perseverance and behavioral interventions were not effective, nurses were instructed to administer Tylenol rather than a chemical restraint.

To promote the goal of quality of life, each resident had a schedule of activities that balanced sensory calming and sensory stimulating activities. Staff had identified that residents often received too much stimulation from the environment.

The goal of human dignity was enhanced by treating all residents in a kind and caring manner and respecting resident choices when possible. A written care plan was developed for each resident to aid communication. Interventions were developed to include the goal of the family being an integral part of care planning. Families were surveyed at regular intervals to determine their satisfaction with care. A bulletin board was hung for families to share information, and a periodic family night was held that focused on friendship and support. The final program goal was that staff have an understanding of behaviors associated with dementia and receive support from one another. Staff participated in educational programs, and every effort was made to assure that the project had sufficient staff to achieve its goals.

This project demonstrated that hospice concepts may be incorporated into the care of persons with end-stage dementia with little additional cost to the facility. The facilities that participated in the project did not require any additional staff. A statistically significant difference in levels of discomfort was established between the treatment and control group, and behaviors associated with dementia were lessened in the treatment group, although this difference was not large enough to be statistically significant. Staff reported increased job satisfaction as a result of participating the project.[50–52,54] The following is a case example from this project.[54]

Case Study: End-Stage Dementia in a Hospice Environment

Mrs. Williams was an 88-year-old widow who had been living at Riverview Nursing Home for four years. She had one adult child, Jean. Mrs. Williams remained in her home after the death of her husband. Jean visited daily and began to notice some changes in her mother that were of concern. Mrs. Williams neglected her personal hygiene, was forgetful, could not recall the names of friends, and unintentionally left the stove on. Jean decided her mother needed to be in a supervised environment. Mrs. Williams adjusted to the nursing home, but over time her condition deteriorated to the point that she was confused, not able to communicate with intelligible speech, and became incontinent. She was not able to participate in group activities and spent most of her time wandering up and down the halls. The nursing home staff noticed Mrs. Williams had repetitive behavior such as holding one arm up and repeating one-syllable words (e.g., "put, put, put"). Her verbalizations became more intense as she became more agitated. One of the staff suggested Mrs. Williams be considered for admission to a new unit for Alzheimer's residents that was incorporating hospice concepts in care. The approach to care was explained to Jean and she agreed to her mother's participation in this program. The nurse and nursing assistants (CNA) who worked with Mrs. Williams discussed her behavior and explored ways to decrease her agitation. They discovered consistent caregivers were able to notice changes that might otherwise be overlooked. When Mrs. Williams was agitated they took her to a quieter environment and her agitation decreased; the "put" sounds diminished. Sometimes they assisted her in going to her room or a lounge. The CNA often took her to a window where they could watch the birds. The CNA often talked about the birds and noticed that Mrs. Williams followed commands with her eyes. One day, to the CNA's surprise, Mrs. Williams pointed to a bird and said, "Look!" This was the first time the staff had any idea that Mrs. Williams could speak. A human connection had been established. After that Mrs. Williams uttered a few words that had some meaning for the staff. Mrs. Williams did well on this unit until she started getting weaker and refused to eat. Her temperatures were high and she was diagnosed with pneumonia. The nurse discussed treatment options with Jean. She explained that Mrs. Williams could be transferred to the hospital or remain in the nursing home. The nurse reassured Jean that if Mrs. Williams remained at Riverview every effort would be made to keep her comfortable and she would receive oral antibiotics and medications for fever and discomfort. Jean did not want to have her mother experience the stress of relocation and new caregivers. After meeting with the physician, nurse, and chaplain, Jean decided to keep her mother at the nursing home. Jean commented, "This is her home, this is where she would want to be." Mrs. Williams was provided with comfort measures and given oral antibiotics until she could no longer swallow. A CNA spent time sitting with Mrs. Williams, holding her hand and was with her when she died.

The nursing staff provided a caring environment for Mrs. Williams and her daughter, Jean, and supported Jean's decision to have her mother remain in the nursing home. Relocating Mrs. Williams to a hospital would have been stressful for both her and her daughter. The nursing home staff provided comfort measures through the use of analgesics and antipyretics as well as the presence of a caring staff. Mrs. Williams was a special person that the staff came to know and appreciate.[54]

In summary, nursing homes can develop innovative programs to address quality-of-life issues. Many of these programs may be implemented without increasing costs. Nursing home staff should be consulted about ways to make changes in the environment. Other recommendations for change are discussed in the following section.

RECOMMENDATIONS FOR CHANGE

The quality of life in nursing homes can be enhanced by implementing the following changes. (*1*) Reimbursement needs to be addressed to improve staff ratios. (2) More professional staff is needed. (3) The environment needs to be adapted to improve quality of life and human dignity. (*4*) Nursing homes benefit from incorporating palliative care concepts.

Reimbursement

Reimbursement and regulations in nursing homes are often impediments to quality end-of-life care. Policy makers and the public need to be educated about the cost of nursing home care. Reimbursement should change from an emphasis on procedures to a focus on continuing comfort measures and palliation. Nursing homes receive most of their revenue from private-pay residents and Medicaid. Medicaid rates need to be increased to reflect the labor-intensive nature of long-term care. The IOM[10] recommends that additional research projects on the use of financial and other resources to improve quality of care and outcomes in nursing homes be funded. An issue closely related to reimbursement is the number and type of staff in nursing homes.

Nursing Home Staff

The relationship between the ratio of RNs to residents and quality of care has been clearly established in nursing homes.[10,20,22,23] Considering the projected growth in the elderly population, the need for RNs in nursing homes is expected to increase. In addition, nursing home residents will be sicker as a result of shorter hospital stays. A major barrier to increased staffing in nursing homes are the fiscal limits of government support. RN salaries are lower in nursing homes than in hospitals, and vacancy rates are higher.[10] In general, RNs working in nursing homes suffer from a lack of prestige in the health care system. The majority of RNs in nursing homes are associate degree graduates who have limited education in the areas of geriatric and palliative care. Nursing homes are starting to use advance practice nurses to deal with the complex needs of older adults. Advance practice nurses, geriatric nurse practitioners, and clinical specialists in geriatrics can improve outcomes and contribute to the quality of care.[10,12] Nursing education programs need to incorporate palliative care training.

Nursing assistants provide the most direct care for residents and have the least amount of training. Their work is often difficult, with few rewards: salaries are low, and there are few benefits. The care provided by nursing assistants is important to residents' quality of life, yet they are often paid little more than minimum wage. Interaction with professional staff is limited due to the demands of their work. Nursing assistants should be provided with training for their jobs, and salaries should be increased. Efforts need to be made to include nursing assistants as part of the team.

Adapting the Environment

The environment of nursing homes needs to be changed to promote resident autonomy and quality of life. Most residents would prefer a single room with some space for personal belongings. Nursing homes should be designed to accommodate residents. Common areas, such as the dining room and lounge, need to be more home-like, with separate conversational areas. Space should be designated for a meditation room to allow residents and families a quiet place.

Incorporating Palliative Care Concepts

Palliative care concepts should be an integral part of nursing home care. The emphasis of care should be directed toward the quality of life at the end of life. Both the resident and family should participate in care planning. The nursing home environment should be a therapeutic milieu that addresses the physical, psychological, social, and spiritual needs of all residents. Research by nurses is needed to improve end-of-life care in nursing homes. As Moody[55] states, "negligible research has been done on the care of elderly residents who are nearing death in nursing homes and who would benefit from a palliative care approach." Nurses can make a difference.

REFERENCES

1. Miller CA. Nursing Care of Older Adults: Theory & Practice. Philadelphia: Lippincott, 1999.
2. Kane RA. Ethical themes in long-term care. In: Katz PR, Kane RL, Mezey MD, eds. Quality Care in Geriatric Settings New York: Springer, 1995:130–148.
3. Kane RL. The evolution of the American nursing home. In: Binstock RH, Cluff LE, Von Mering O, eds. The Future of Long-Term Care: Social and Policy Issues. Baltimore: John Hopkins University Press, 1996:145–168.
4. Holstein M, Cole TR. The evolution of long-term care in America. In: Binstock RH, Cluff LE, Von Mering O, eds. The Future of Long-Term Care: Social and Policy Issues. Baltimore: Johns Hopkins University Press, 1996:19–48.
5. Ignatavicius DD. Introduction to Long-Term Care Nursing: Principles and Practice. Philadelphia: F. A. Davis, 1998.
6. National Center for Health Statistics. 1995 National Nursing Home Survey. Advance Date No. 280. Hyattsville, Md: Public Health Service, 1997.
7. Agency for Health Care Policy and Research (AHCPR). Nursing Home Update–1996: Medical Expenditure Panel Survey Highlights No. 2. AHCPR Publication No. 97–0036. Maryland: AHCPR.
8. Agency for Health Care Policy and Research (AHCPR). Nursing Home Update–1996: Medical Expenditure Panel Survey Research Findings No. 4. AHCPR Publication No. 98–0006. Maryland: AHCPR.
9. Meiners MR. The financing and organization of long-term care. In: Binstock RH, Cluff LE, Von Mering O, eds. The Future of Long-Term Care: Social and Policy Issues. Baltimore: Johns Hopkins University Press, 1996:191–214.
10. Institute of Medicine. Nursing Staff in Hospitals and Nursing Homes: Is it Adequate? Washington, DC: Academy Press, 1996.
11. U.S. Census Bureau (1999). Statistical Abstracts of the United States: 1999. 119th ed. Department of Commerce, Washington, D.C.
12. Kane RL, Ouslander JG, Abrass IB, eds. Essentials of Clinical Geriatrics. New York: McGraw-Hill, 1994.
13. Alliance for Aging Research. Seven Deathly Myths: Uncovering the Facts About the High Costs of the Last Year of Life. Washington, DC: Alliance for Aging Research, 1998.
14. National Center for Health Statistics. Vital Statistics of the United States, 1992. Vol. II, Mortality Part A. Washington, DC: U.S. Public Health Service.
15. Institute of Medicine (IOM). Improving the Quality of Care in Nursing Homes. Washington, DC: National Academy Press, 1986.
16. Marek KD, Rantz MJ, Fagin CM, Krecki JW. OBRA '87: Has it resulted in better quality care? Journal of Gerontological Nursing, 1996; 122(10):28–36.
17. Cotton P. Nursing home research focus on outcomes may mean playing catch up with regulations. Journal of the American Medical Association 1993;269:2337–2338.
18. Joint Commission on Accreditation of Healthcare Organizations (JCAHO). Personal communication: Long-Term Care Accreditation Program, September 14, 1999.
19. Agency for Health Care Policy Research. New MEPS data show changing nursing home market. Research Activities 1998;217:4–5.
20. Mass M, Buckwalter K, Specht J. Nursing staff and quality of care in nursing homes. In Institute of Medicine. Nursing Staff in Hospitals and Nursing Homes: Is it Adequate? Washington, DC: Academy Press, 361–425.
21. National League for Nursing. Only 3% of nurses are working in long-term care facilities. Contemporary Long-Term Care, 1989;12:5.
22. Johnson J, McKeen-Cowles C, Simmons SJ. Quality of care and staff in nursing homes. In Institute of Medicine. Nursing Staff in Hospitals and Nursing Homes: Is it Adequate? Washington, DC: Academy Press, 426–452.
23. Mezey MD, Lynaugh JE. The teaching nursing home program: A lesson in quality. Geriatric Nursing 1991:76–77.
24. Germain C. Cancer Unit: An Ethnography. Wakefield, Mass., Nursing Resources, 1979.
25. Glaser BG, Strauss AL. A time for dying. Chicago: Aldine, 1968.
26. Mumma CM, Benoliel JQ. Care, cure, and hospital dying trajectories. Omega 1984;85: 275–288.
27. Sundnow D. Passing On: The Social Organization of Dying. Englewood Cliffs, New Jersey: Prentice-Hall, 1967.
28. Pruchno RA, Moss MS, Burant CJ, Schinfeld S. Death of an institutionalized parent: Predictors of bereavement. Omega 1995;31:99–119.
29. Hanson LG, Danis M, Garrett J. What is wrong with end-of-life care? Opinions of bereaved family members. Journal of the American Geriatric Society 1997;45:1339–1344.
30. Maccabee J. The effect of a transfer from a palliative care unit to nursing homes: Are patients and relatives needs being met? Journal of Palliative Medicine 1994;8:211–214.
31. Wilson SA, Daley BJ. Family perspectives of dying in long-term care. Journal of Gerontological Nursing 1099;25(11):19–25.
32. Daley BJ, Wilson SA. Needs assessment in long-term care facilities: Linking research and continuing education. The Journal of Continuing Education in the Health Professions 1999;19: 111–121.
33. Ersek M, Krayabill BM, Hansberry J. Investigating the educational needs of licensed nursing staff and certified nursing assistants in nursing homes regarding end-of-life care. American Journal of Hospice and Palliative Care 1999;16(4): 573–582.
34. Wilson SA, Daley BJ. Attachment/detachment: Forces influencing care of the dying in long-term care. Journal of Palliative Medicine 1998;1:21–34.
35. Gibbs G. Nurses in private nursing homes: A study of their knowledge and attitudes to pain management in palliative care. Palliative Medicine 1995;9:117–124.
36. Ferrell BA, Ferrell BR, Osterweil D. Pain in the nursing home. Journal of the American Geriatric Society 1990;38:409–414.
37. Ferrell BA. Pain evaluation and management in the nursing home. Annals of Internal Medicine 1995;123:681–687.
38. Institute of Medicine. Approaching death: Improving care at the end-of-life. Washington, DC: National Academy, 1997.
39. Closs SJ. Pain in elderly patients: A neglected phenomenon? Journal of Advanced Nursing 1994;19:1072–1081.
40. Bergh I, Sjostrom B. A comparative study of nurses' and elderly patients' ratings of pain and pain tolerance. Journal of Gerontological Nursing 1999;25:30–36.
41. Ouslander JG, Osterweil D, Morely J. Medical care in the nursing home. New York: McGraw Hill, 1991.
42. Rantz MJ, Zwygart-Stauffacher M. Nursing homes and the chronically ill resident: Policy and issues. In: Swanson EA, Tripp-Reimer T, eds. Advances in Gerontological Nursing: Chronic Illness and Older Adult. New York: Springer, 1997: 179–195.
43. Miller T. Advance directives: Moving from theory to practice. In: Katz PR, Kane RL, Mezey MD, eds. Quality Care in Geriatric Settings. New York: Springer 1995:68–86.
44. Semradek J, Gamroth L. Prologue to the future. In: Gamroth LM, Semradek J, Tornquist EM, eds. Enhancing Autonomy in Long-Term Care: Concepts and Strategies. New York: Springer, 1995:207–218.
45. Barnes A. Legal and ethical issues. In: Kovack CR, ed. Late-Stage Dementia Care: A Basic Guide. Washington, DC: Taylor & Francis, 1997: 207–220.
46. McCann RM, Hall WJ, Groth-Juncker A. Comfort care for terminally ill patients: The ap-

propriate use of nutrition and hydration. Journal of the American Medical Association 1994;26: 1263–1266.

47. Weinrich C. Spiritual needs of the dying. In: Wilson SA, Daley BJ, eds. Fostering Humane Care of Dying Persons in Long-Term Care: A Guidebook for Staff Development Instructors. Milwaukee: Marquette University Press, 1997:28–36.

48. Stewert A. Quality of life. Paper prepared for Conference on Measuring Care at the End-of-Life, August 27–28, 1996.

49. Baurer F. A comfort to the dying. Milwaukee Journal Sentinel, March 13, 1999:3b.

50. Kovach CR, Wilson SA, Noonan PE. The effects of hospice interventions on behaviors, discomfort, and physical complication of end-stage dementia nursing home residents. American Journal of Alzheimer's Disease 1996:7–15.

51. Wilson SA, Kovach CR, Stearns S. Hospice concepts in the care for persons with end-stage dementia. Geriatric Nursing 1996;17:6–10.

52. Kovach CR ed. Late-stage demential care: A basic guide. Washington: Taylor & Francis.

53. Folstein MF, Folstein SE, McHugh PR. Mini-mental state: A practical guide for grading the cognitive state of patients for the clinician. Journal of Psychiatric Research 1975;129(3): 180–198.

54. Wilson SA. Palliative care for late-stage dementia. In: Kovach CR, ed. Late-stage dementia care: A basic guide. Washington, DC: Taylor & Francis, 1997:13–23.

55. Moody LE. Living longer, dying longer: Nursing's opportunity to make a difference. Nursing Outlook 1999;47:41–42.

39 Home Care

PAULA MILONE-NUZZO
and RUTH McCORKLE

When my husband died from lung cancer, nursing care in our home allowed us to remain as a family. I'll always be grateful for his nurses. . . . Looking back on this experience, I have peace knowing that my husband was able to spend his last months of life in comfort. With the skills the nurses taught me, I was able to keep him home until he died. He wanted that and that was my gift to him.

—Spouse caregiver

Originally, palliative care in home care nursing was linked to situations in which patients were clearly near the end of life. The contemporary philosophy of palliative care had its beginnings in Great Britain in 1967, when Dame Cicely Saunders founded St. Christopher's Hospice. Home and respite care continue to be a major component of that program. Palliative care, by definition, focuses on the multidimensional aspects of patients and families, including physical, psychological, social, spiritual, and interpersonal components of care. These components of care need to be instituted throughout all phases of the illness trajectory and not only at the point when patients qualify for hospice services. Palliative care also needs to be given across a variety of settings and not be limited to in-patient units.

The primary purpose of palliative care is to enhance the quality and meaning of life and death for both patients and loved ones. To date, health professionals have not utilized the potential of palliative care to maximize the quality of life of patients in their homes. In this chapter we discuss home care as an environment that provides unique opportunities to promote palliative care for patients and families throughout their illnesses. The chapter gives background information on what home care is, its historical roots, the types of providers available to give services, the regulatory policies controlling its use, examples of models of palliative home care programs, and recommendations to professionals for facilitating the use of home care in palliative care, concluding with a case study illustrating key elements of palliative care provision in the home.

Historical Perspective on Home Care Nursing

The period spanning the middle of the twentieth century, during which patients were routinely cared for in acute care hospitals, may turn out to have been but a brief period in medical history. Before that time patients were cared for primarily at home by their families. Today social and economic forces are interacting to avoid hospitalization if possible and to return patients home quickly if hospitalized. Although at face value these changes seem positive, they have highlighted gaps and deficiencies in the current health care delivery system.

Scientific advances have allowed us to keep patients with diseases such as cancer alive increasingly longer despite complex and chronic health problems. The burden of their care usually falls on families, who often are not adequately prepared to handle the physically and emotionally demanding needs for care that are inherent in chronic and progressive illnesses. In addition, family members often become primary care providers within the context of other demands, such as employment outside the home and competing family roles. The necessity among most of the nation's family members to assume employment outside the home and to alter those arrangements when faced with a sick relative has created an as yet immeasurable strain on physical, emotional, and financial resources. The increasing responsibilities of the family in providing care in the face of limited external support and the consequences of that caregiving for patient and family raise important challenges for clinicians.[1]

The origins of home care are found in the practice of visiting nursing, which had its beginnings in the United States in the late 1800s. The modern concept of providing nursing care in the home was established by William Rathbone of Liverpool, England, in 1859. Mr. Rathbone, a wealthy businessman and philanthropist, set up a system of visiting nursing after a personal experience when nurses cared for his wife at home before her death. In 1859, with the help of Florence Nightingale, he started a school to train visiting nurses at the Liverpool Infirmary, the graduates of which focused on helping the "sick poor" in their homes.[2]

As in England, caring for the ill in their homes in the United States focused, from its inception, on the poor. In the nineteenth century dismal living and working conditions, particularly in the cities, gave rise to problems with hygiene and increases in various diseases. Like most city dwellers, the urban poor usually chose to stay at home during illnesses, relying on traditional healing methods. Most of the sick were sick at home. Compared to the upper and middle class who received frequent visits from the family physician, either in their homes or in the hospital pay wards, treatment of the sick poor seemed careless at best. Visiting nurse associations (VNAs) in the United States were established by groups of people who wanted to assist the poor to improve their health. During 1885 and 1886 visiting nurse services developed in Buffalo, New York, Boston, and Philadelphia focused on caring for the middle-class sick as well as the sick poor.[2]

In the late 1800s, visiting nurse agencies grew in number, mostly appearing in the large cities of the country. In the early 1900s, the Metropolitan Life Insurance Company began the first insurance-based program for home care. Their success at saving money with home care to policyholders during times of illness was the foundation for the current system of health care for the ill in their homes. By 1916, the Metropolitan Life Insurance Company made visiting nurse services available to its 10.5 million industrial policy holders in over 2000 cities.

During World War II, as physicians made fewer home visits and focused instead on patients who came to their offices and were admitted to hospitals, the home care movement grew, with nurses providing most of the health and illness care in the home.

Up until the mid-1960s, not-for-profit VNAs were developed in major cities, small towns, and counties throughout the United States. Under their auspices, nurses focused on providing health services to women and infants and illness care to the poor in their homes, while most acute care was provided to patients in hospitals.

The face of home care in the United States changed dramatically with the passage of an amendment to the Social Security Act that enacted Medicare in 1965. Home care changed from almost exclusively care for well mothers and children and the sick poor to a program focused on care of the sick elderly in their homes. In 1967 there were 1,753 home care agencies, a large percentage of which were not-for-profit VNAs. In 1998, more than 30 years later, there were 9,655 home care agencies, with the largest percentage of agencies represented by the proprietary sector.[3] Not only did the types of agencies change, the acuity of patients increased and the development of technology allowed for the delivery of highly complex care in the home setting. The structural changes in the health care delivery system associated with the passage of the Medicare legislation in 1965 provided the foundation for the contemporary practice of home care nursing in the United States.

In the early 1980s, to curb the increasing hospital costs incurred by the Medicare program and the increasing number of elderly patients needing hospitalization, diagnostic-related groupings (DRGs) were phased in over a four-year period in hospitals nationwide. Two results of the implementation of the DRG system were a decrease in patient lengths of stay in the hospital and an increase in the use of home care services to these patients. Also, because Medicare did not cover hospitalization for some conditions, many patients were not admitted to a hospital, and the needed care was, therefore, provided in the home by a home care agency. Following the federal government's lead with the Medicare program, Medicaid programs were established for the economically underprivileged and administered individually by the states and private insurance companies. Other payers who covered home health services also began restricting payments for hospitalizations, thus increasing the need for home care services. The result was that home care became the fastest growing segment of the health care delivery system.[4] Heart disease and respiratory diseases were the most common diagnoses of patients seen in the home.

The 1990s brought a new challenge in the form of managed care to health care in general and home care specifically in the United States. The most significant impact of managed care on home care was a decline in the number of visits allowed per patient per episode of illness. The result was a decline in the amount of home care patients received with a resultant stabilization of the rapid growth in the home care delivery system. The American Balanced Budget Act of 1997 (PL 105-33) mandates the implementation of a prospective payment system for home care for Medicare beneficiaries. In this system home care agencies receive a designated dollar amount per episode of illness to provide care for a Medicare patient based on the patient's admitting diagnosis and other factors related to physical status. Just as the DRG system caused a significant decline in the number of hospital beds in 1980s, it is anticipated that prospective payment for home care will result in significant shrinkage of the home health care industry due to patients receiving fewer visits per episode of illness.

DEFINITION OF HOME CARE NURSING

Home care, home health care, and home care nursing can be confusing terms, both to providers and consumers because they are often used interchangably. Numerous definitions of home care have been provided by the many professional and trade associations (National Association for Home Care, Consumer's Union, American Hospital Association, American Medical Association, Health Care Financing Administration, etc.) that address home care issues. Common to all the definitions is the recognition that home care is care of the sick in the home by professionals and paraprofessionals with the goal to improve health and quality of life. *Home care nursing* is defined here as,

> . . . the provision of nursing care to acute and chronically ill patients of all ages in their home while integrating community health nursing principles that focus on the environmental, psychosocial, economic, cultural, and personal health factors affecting an individual's and family's health status.[5]

HOME CARE UTILIZATION IN THE UNITED STATES

Home care is a diverse industry providing a broad scope of care to patients of all ages. In 1998 it was estimated that more than 8 million people received home care services for acute illness, long-term health conditions, permanent disability, and terminal illness.[3] Although home care is provided to a large number of people, it still represents a very small percentage of national health care expenditures. While hospital care consumed 40% and physician services 22%, home care represented only 3% of the total national health expenditure in 1996,[3] demonstrating the cost-efficient nature of home care practice.

The majority of patients (67.5%) who received home care were discharged primarily to urban home care agencies.[6] As the reimbursement for home care visits decreases and the cost of home visiting in rural areas increases because of increased travel time, many rural home care agencies have been forced to close, limiting access to home care for the population in the region.

The demographic picture of home health care recipients shows a predominately female (66.8%) and white (65.5%) population. The majority (72.4%) of home care patients are 65 years of age and over, although home care is provided to patients of all ages, from birth to death. The most common primary diagnosis for home care patients is diseases of the circulatory system, most often heart disease. Other common primary diagnoses of patients receiving home care are diseases of the musculoskeletal system and connective tissue, diabetes mellitus, diseases of the respiratory system, injury, and poisoning. A primary diagnosis of malignant neoplasm represents only 4.7% of home health care patients, while it accounts for 58.3% of all patients in hospice.[6] Clearly, non-hospice home care has not been used adequately as an integral part of care for cancer patients and families as they endure the physical and emotional demands of complex cancer treatments and move across the acute, chronic, and terminal phases of their disease. This is an ideal context in which the need for palliative care should drive an increased use of home care services.

TYPES OF HOME CARE PROVIDERS

Home care providers are traditionally characterized as either formal or informal caregivers. Informal caregivers are those family members and friends who provide care in the home and are unpaid. It is estimated that almost three-quarters of the elderly with multiple comorbidities and severe disabilities who receive home care rely on family members or other sources of unpaid assistance. More than 75% of those providing informal home care are female, and nearly 33% are more than 65 years of age. Eighty percent of informal caregivers provide assistance four hours per day, seven days per week.[3] The type of care provided by informal caregivers ranges from routine custodial care, such as bathing, to sophisticated skilled care, including tracheostomy care and intravenous medication administration. Informal caregivers assume a considerable physiological, psychological, and economic burden in the care of their significant other in the home. When layered on top of existing responsibilities, caregiver tasks compete for time, energy, and attention. As a result, caregivers frequently describe themselves as emotionally and physically drained.[7] Perceptions of family members regarding the magnitude of the caregiving burden change over time and with the length of the caregiving episode. Chan and Chang[7] found that caregivers with a longer duration of caregiving appeared to handle the caregiver tasks with less difficulty, suggesting that skill in managing the caregiver role increases with time.[7] The economic cost of providing informal care in the home also places a significant burden on caregivers. With the shift toward community-based care, a number of costs have shifted to the patient and caregiver. Out-of-pocket financial expenditures include medications, transportation, home medical equipment, supplies, and respite services.[8] These costs are non-reimbursable and often invisible but are very real to families who are trying to provide care on a fixed income.

Formal caregivers are those professionals and paraprofessionals who are compensated for the in-home care they provide. In 1998 an estimated 662,000 persons were employed in home health agencies. In home care, nurses represent 36% of the formal caregivers providing care to patients in Medicare-certified home care agencies. Home health aides also represent a large proportion of the formal caregivers in home care, accounting for 33% of the full-time equivalents in home care.[9] The professionals and paraprofessionals who represent the range of home care providers in home health agencies are described in Table 39–1.

REIMBURSEMENT MECHANISMS

Home health services are reimbursed by both commercial and government third-party payers as well as by private individuals. Government third-party payers include Medicare, Medicaid, CHAMPUS, and the Veterans Administration system. These government programs have specific requirements that must be met for the coverage of services. Commercial third-party payers include insurance companies, health maintenance organizations (HMOs), preferred provider organizations (PPOs), and case management programs. Commercial insurers often allow for more flexibility in their requirements than Medicare. For example, the home care nurse may negotiate with an insurance company to obtain needed services for the patient on the basis of the cost-effectiveness of the home care plan, even though that service may not be routinely covered.

Medicare

Medicare is a federal insurance program for the elderly (65 and over), the permanently disabled, and persons with end-stage renal disease in the United States and is the single largest payer for home health services. To be eligible for this program, an individual or spouse must have paid Social Security. Medicare is a federal program, and as such the benefits are the same from state to state. The Health Care Financing Administration (HCFA), a department in the federal government, regulates payments for services under Medicare. The rules developed by HCFA that guide the Medicare program are detailed in the Health Insurance Manual-11 (HIM–11).

Table 39–1. Types of Providers in Home Care

Type of Provider	Role and Responsibilities
Nurses:	
• Registered Nurses	Deliver skilled care to patients in the home. Considered the coordinator of care.
• Licensed Practical Nurses	Deliver routine care to patients under the direction of a Registered Nurse.
• Advanced Practice Nurses	Coordinate total patient care to complex patients, supervise other nurses in difficult cases related to their speciality, develop special programs, and negotiate for reimbursement of services. Teach patients and caregivers special skills and knowledge.
Therapists	
• Physical Therapists	Deliver skilled care that includes assessment for assistive devices in the home. Perform therapy procedures with the patient and teach the patient and family to assist in treatment. Assist patient to improve mobility.
• Occupational Therapists	Focus on improving physical, mental and social functioning. Rehabilitation of the upper body and improvement of fine motor ability.
• Speech Therapist	Rehabilitation of patients with speech and swallowing problems.
• Respiratory Therapists	Provide support to patients using respiratory home medical equipment such as ventilators. Perform professional respiratory therapy treatments.
Other Clinical Staff	
• Social Workers	Help patients and families identify needs and refer to community agencies. Assist with applications for community based services and provide financial assistance information.
• Dieticians	Provide diet counseling to patients with special nutritional needs. Direct service of a dietician is not a reimburseable service in home care.
Para-professionals	
• Home Health Aides	Perform personal care, basic nursing tasks (as opposed to skilled), and incidental homemaking.
• Homemakers	Perform housekeeping and chores to ensure a safe and healthy home care environment.

HCFA contracts with insurance companies called fiscal intermediaries (FIs) to process Medicare claims that are submitted from home care agencies.

There are five criteria a patient must meet in order for home care services to be reimbursed by Medicare. The five criteria are summarized in Table 39–2.

Medicare is the main payer of hospice services in the United States under the Medicare Hospice Benefit, which Congress first enacted as part of Medicare Part A in 1982 under the Tax Equity and Fiscal Responsibility Act (TEFRA; P.L. 97–248). The law was in effect from 1983 to 1986, when Congress made hospice a permanent part of the Medicare program.[10] The impetus behind Medicare's hospice benefit came from the recognition that the regulations and restrictions for traditional Medicare are not well suited to meet the needs of terminally ill patients.

Medicare hospice was designed primarily as a home care benefit that included an array of services that assist care providers in the clinical management of the terminally ill in the home.[5] However, the regulations for hospice care also require home care providers to have in-patient hospice beds available for terminally ill patients who are unable to remain in their homes. Recognizing that hospice is a philosophy of care rather than a place for care, it seems appropriate that hospice care is given in a variety of settings.

In order for a patient to elect the Hospice Medicare benefit, the patient must waive the traditional Medicare benefit. By electing the Hospice Medicare benefit, the patient is acknowledging the terminal nature of the illness and opting no longer to have curative treatment. For a full description of the Hospice Medicare benefit and a discussion of the criteria for admission into the hospice program, see chapter 2.

Medicaid

Medicaid is an assistance program for the poor, some disabled persons, and children. Unlike Medicare, Medicaid is jointly sponsored by the federal government and the individual states. Therefore, Medicaid coverage varies from state to state. These differences can often be dramatic and in some cases dependent on the state's financial solvency. Eligibility for Medicaid is based on income and assets and is not contingent on any previous payments to the federal or state governments.

Unlike the requirements of the Medicare program, Medicaid covers both skilled and unskilled care in the home and usually does not require that the recipient be homebound. To qualify for the home care benefits under Medicaid, patients must meet income eligibility requirements, have a plan of care signed by a physician, and the plan of care must be reviewed by a physician every 60 days.

Table 39–2. Criteria for Home Care Reimbursement under Medicare

Criterion	Description
Homebound	A patient is considered homebound if absences from the home are rare and of short duration and attributable to the need to receive medical treatments.
Completed plan of care	A plan of care for home care services must be completed on Health Care Financing Administration (HCFA) forms 485, 486, and 487. The plan of care must be signed by a physician.
Skilled service	Medicare defines a skilled service as one provided by a Registered Nurse, Physical Therapist or Speech Therapist. Skilled nursing services include skilled observation and assessment, teaching, direct care and management and evaluation of the plan of care.
Intermittent and part-time	Part-time means that skilled care and home health aide services combined may not exceed 8 hours per day or 28 hours per week. Intermittent means that skilled care is provided or needed on fewer than 7 days per week or less than 8 hours of each day for periods of 21 days or less with extensions for exceptional circumstances.
Reasonable and necessary	The services provided must be reasonable for the patient given the diagnosis and necessary to assist the patient to achieve the expected outcomes.

Commercial Insurance

Many commercial insurance companies are involved in health insurance for individuals or groups. These local or national companies often write policies that include a home care benefit. Commercial insurers often cover the same services covered by Medicare in addition to preventive, private duty, and supportive services, such as a home health aide or homemaker. Commercial insurance companies cover patients of all ages, including Medicare patients with supplemental insurance policies that cover health care expenditures not reimbursed by Medicare.

Commercial insurance often includes a maximum lifetime benefit as part of the policy. The high cost of high-technology care forces a growing number of patients to reach this maximum rather quickly and face the loss of coverage. This has resulted in the development of case management programs administered by insurance companies. The case manager projects the long-term needs and costs of care for the patient and develops a plan with the patient to meet those needs in a cost-efficient manner. Consideration is given to the life expectancy of the patient in relationship to the maximum lifetime benefit.

Unlike the Medicare program, in which negotiation for services is not an option, it may be important for home care nurses to identify the needed services for a patient with a commercial insurance plan and intervene to obtain funding for those services. When working with an insurance case manager, the home care nurse must be specific about the services the patient will need, the overall cost of those services, and the expected outcome related to the services requested. The more precisely the home care nurse can portray the impact of the care plan on the patient outcomes with objective data, the more inclined the case manager will be to authorize services. Insurance companies are very concerned with the satisfaction of their enrollees. Patients and families should be empowered to make their voices heard about the services they need to remain safe in the home. If out-of-network services or special pricing is negotiated with the insurance case manager, written documentation of the agreement should be included in the patient's record. Ideally, the patient should be given a copy of this agreement in the event any disputes over payment occur.

The Home Health–Hospice Connection

In order for a patient to receive the full array of hospice services under Medicare, the care must be provided by a certified hospice provider. Home care agencies that are not certified hospice providers must refer their terminally ill patients to an agency that carries the certification in order to be reimbursed. This regulation affects clinical care in several ways. Home care nurses have a long history of developing strong and intimate bonds with patients and families.[11] As patients progress toward the terminal phase of their illnesses, it is very difficult, emotionally, for home care nurses to refer their patients to hospice providers. At times, it is equally as difficult for a family to accept the referral, knowing that they will have to give up "their nurse." The home care nurse and the family may believe that the relationship that has developed among the patient, the family, and the home care nurse is more important than any additional benefits the hospice might bring.

The greater flexibility in traditional Medicare regulations that came with the resolution of the Duggan vs. Bohan case[12] in 1988 has allowed nonhospice home care agencies to provide extended nursing and home health aide services for patients in the terminal phase of illness. In this legal case, a group of home care agencies challenged the HCFA regarding their strict interpretation of the Medicare regulation on patient qualifications for part-time intermittent care. The suit was won by the home care agencies, requiring HCFA to be more generous in interpreting Medicare regulations. Although families may feel that they are getting sufficient home care, they are not able to take advantage of the prescription drug components of the hospice benefit, which may result in significant financial burden. They also usually do not receive the supportive services, such as pastoral care and bereavement follow-up, that are integral to the hospice program. Because the emotional impact of the patient's death is unknown at the time when the patient makes the decision to forego a hospice referral, it is impossible to predict the significance of a service such as bereavement follow-up. Because both the non-hospice home health agency and the hospice provider offer important services, especially nursing care to patients at the end of life, strengthening mechanisms that facilitate transitions between these two types of services is essential. See chapter 2 for a comprehensive discussion of the hospice admission criteria, including the certification by the physician of a terminal diagnosis and the sixth-month rule.

CANCER AS A PROTOTYPE FOR HOME CARE USE IN PALLIATIVE CARE

Over the years cancer has shifted from a terminal illness to a chronic disease. Even patients with advanced disease and guarded prognoses initially may be treated as if their disease is curable rather than progressive and terminal. Because the philosophical underpinnings and goals of curative and palliative treatments are quite different, approaching an individual who has advanced disease with a curative stance may have long-term negative effects on physical, social, and emotional functions that ultimately affect the individual's quality of life. Characteristics of advanced cancer that require aggressive intervention, often delayed due to an initial flight into curative treatment, include multiple physical needs, intense emotional distress manifested by anxiety and depression, and the complex needs of both patients and families, requiring coordinated ongoing care. Recognizing that palliative care is needed early on and that one of the most efficient ways of monitoring patients' needs is to coordinate the overall plan of management with home care nursing is an important option for decreasing fragmentation and promoting continuity.

Needs of Cancer Patients

Because of the growing trend to discharge hospitalized patients early, the increasing use of ambulatory care services, and the increasing use of complex therapies, the need for ongoing monitoring and instruction of patients and families has never been greater. Family members, often without the assistance of any formal home care services, are assuming primary responsibility for the care of patients at home.[13,14,15,16] This demand on families is not new, although the caregiver role has changed dramatically from promoting convalescence to providing high technology care and psychological support in the home. Members of a patient's family are of vital importance in meeting the patient's physical and psychosocial needs and accomplishing treatment goals.[17,18] The burden of caring for patients with a diagnosis of cancer, however, may adversely affect families who lack adequate resources or who are insufficiently prepared for this new, complex role. There is mounting evidence that changes in family roles and the burden placed on family caregivers may have negative effects on the quality of life of both cancer patients and their caregivers,[16] particularly during advanced stages of cancer.

Research to identify patient-defined home care needs is limited. Evidence suggests, however, that both patients and their families benefit from home care services directed at physical and psychological concerns. One pilot study identified pain, sleep, and elimination management as major patient needs. Wellisch and his colleagues[19] investigated the types and frequency of problems experienced by two separate groups of seriously ill cancer patients and their families in their homes in the Los Angeles area and explored the types of interventions that helped to reduce the problems. The five most frequent problem categories identified included somatic side effects, including pain; patient mood disturbance; equipment/technology problems; family relationship impairment; and patient cognitive impairment. Interventions reported to be effective included reinforcement to the patient and family, no intervention, and counseling and emotional support. They noted that patients with cognitive deficits had special needs, and their family members were at high risk for ongoing problems.[20]

In Pennsylvania, Houts and colleagues[21] found that the unmet needs of patients with cancer included assistance with emotional problems, transportation, finances, and interactions with medical staff. Wingate and Lackey[22] identified the needs of patients and primary caregivers in the home and compared the priorities between the two. Both identified their psychological distress as their highest priority. For patients, physical and informational needs were next. For caregivers, household management needs, which included direct patient care, were second, followed by informational needs. McCorkle and colleagues[23] enrolled 233 cancer patients in a study designed to follow them over six months post-hospitalization. Half the sample were newly diagnosed ($n = 115$); the other half had had their cancers for more than a year. Patients were discharged with a range of complex problems, including unrelieved symptoms (pain, fatigue, dyspnea, poor appetite), wound care, feeding devices, elimination devices, intravenous medication administration, and other highly technical procedures, such as tracheostomies. The majority of these patients were not referred to formal home care services for monitoring, despite their ongoing needs, primarily because they were under 65 years of age.

Needs of Caregivers

A number of studies have identified the needs of patients and family members providing care to patients with cancer. A study by Grobe and colleagues[24] identified methods of education that were provided for 87 patients in the advanced stages of cancer and their homebound caregivers. This study revealed that families perceived that little, if any, education was provided to them. Hinds[25] conducted a study examining the perceived needs of 83 family caregivers. Findings indicated that family members felt inadequately prepared to provide care for their sick relatives in the home and identified numerous informational and skill deficits. Siegel and colleagues[26,27] divided caregiving tasks into categories of personal care, instrumental tasks, and transportation. Each of these areas was associated with greater demands as patients' physiological factors worsened or if their caregivers associated their care with a high level of burden.

Oberst and colleagues[28] assessed the demands on cancer caregivers, including their perceptions of providing care in the home environment. Caregivers reported that the majority of their time was spent providing transportation, giving emotional support, and maintaining the household. More than one-third of the caregivers reported a lack of assistance from health professionals in providing care. In addition, demands on the caregivers escalated as the treatment regimen progressed. Another study lends support to the sense of isolation and the stressful nature of caregiving in that 85% of a sample of cancer caregivers failed to utilize available resources to assist them in caregiving activities. In addition, 77% of the caregivers reported increased stress, and 28% required medication to help them cope with the burden associated with caregiving.[29] These accounts present persuasive documentation that caring for a person with cancer is a stressful experience and can have major emotional and physical consequences for caregivers. In their review of caregiver research, Sales, Schultz and Biegel[30] concluded that a significant number of cancer caregivers exhibit psychological distress and physical symptoms. Predictors of distress included a number of illness-related variables, including more advanced stages of cancer, disability, and complex care needs. Given and colleagues[31,32] reported that patients' symptoms and symptom distress, mobility, and dependency for instrumental activities were linked to significant burdens in family caregivers.

In general, the literature on the needs of cancer patients and caregivers of cancer patients highlights (*1*) that patients are increasingly being treated in ambulatory clinics and have ongoing, unmet complex care needs; (2) that caregivers are assuming more and more responsibility for monitoring patients' status and providing direct care in the home; (3) that caregivers have a high proportion of unmet needs; (4) that the caregiving experience encompasses both positive and negative elements; and, (5) that the conceptualization of caregiver burden is positively linked to negative reactions to caregiving.

MODELS OF PALLIATIVE HOME CARE PROGRAMS

A number of studies have proved useful as models for palliative home care. Both patients and their caregivers have served as subjects of these studies. Some of the more important of these are discussed below.

Patient Programs

Hinton[33] questioned whether home care can maintain an acceptable quality of life for patients with terminal cancer and their relatives. He defined quality-of-life outcomes to include mood, attitude to condition, perceived help, and preferred place of care. The study included 77 randomly selected patients followed by the hospice palliative home care service at St. Christopher's Hospice in England. Overall, the results were extremely positive. Patients' physical symptoms were tolerable, caregivers' depression and anxiety were limited, and the majority of care provided in the home (90%) was complemented by hospitalizations for one to three days (30%) or longer (41%). Treatment was usually praised by relatives, and at follow-up relatives approved where patients had received care and died. In countries other than the United States, home care is an integral part of well planned palliative care, and a number of palliative home care programs have demonstrated positive patient and caregiver outcomes.

The most recognized model of palliative home care was developed at St. Christopher's Hospice, yet programs in other countries have been equally committed, including programs in Canada,[34] Sweden,[35] and Italy.[36,37] These programs included hospice-like services, but, more importantly, they were targeted at symptom management and not limited to imminent dying and death. They also encompassed the care of the patient and the family and facilitated transitions from hospitals to homes. In our opinion, the main reasons they have been successful have been not only the commitment and passion of nurses, but also the involvement of physicians who recognize their interdiscplinary role in the palliative care component of patients' diseases and the government reimbursement systems.

In the United States, some attempts have been made by other than traditional home health agencies to integrate palliative care into home nursing care. Martinson's[38,39] seminal study of facilitating the management and death of children in rural Minnesota after discharge from an urban medical center demonstrated that families wanted and assumed the responsibility to provide necessary care with supervision of the specialty nurses from the medical center. Much of the teaching and instruction was provided to families over the telephone.

Yates and his colleagues[40] designed a study to compare two groups of patients with advanced cancer who were treated in rural Vermont through the Vermont Regional Cancer Center and the University of Vermont. The patients were paired based on population density, distance from the medical center, socioeconomic status, local medical facilities, referral patterns, and local social service resources. The groups were divided into intensive and nonintensive groups. The intensive group received regular home visits by nurse practitioners, and the nonintensive group was not visited by nurses. Both groups received the same multidisciplinary care from the cancer center and monitoring of cancer status through the ambulatory cancer clinic. A total of 199 patients (98 in the intensive group and 101 in the nonintensive group) were followed, and at the end of the four-year study 139 patients had died. The results were very positive in demonstrating that patients in the intensive group fared better overall than those in the nonintensive group. They demonstrated less need for medical care at the cancer center and greater independence over the course of the study than those in the nonintensive group. Most striking, the home nursing interventions improved individual patient pain management. The authors found that physicians often prescribed pain medications without follow-up monitoring of patient status, whereas the home nurses were vigilant in monitoring patients' comfort. The nurses also improved patient and family negotiations for available community resources. Although the study failed to show a survival difference between the two groups, the researchers did demonstrate cost-effective outcomes. The study demonstrated a decrease in the overall cost of care by facilitating a greater number of home deaths in the intensive group. They concluded that cost savings occurred without sacrifice of patient well-being and with concomitant advantages in patient pain management.

In a state-wide study of home care utilization patterns among cancer patients in Illinois, physicians were found, in general, to be the primary source of patient referral to home health services. More than two-thirds of the sample were referred to home services for the purpose of monitoring health status, more often for post-surgical than post-medical treatment effects.[41] Oncology clinical nurse specialists served as consultants to staff nurses in home health agencies in rural Illinois. Both staff and patients reported satisfaction with this model of care delivery. The clinical specialists spent a majority of their time teaching the nurses specific skills and were readily available by telephone to both staff and patients.

McCorkle has designed a number of studies to test the role of the advanced practice nurse on patient outcomes in home nursing care. In 1986, McCorkle and her colleagues[42,43] completed a randomized controlled trial to assess the effects of home nursing care on either an oncology home care group (OHC) that received care from home care nurses, a standard home care group (SHC) that received care from oncology home care nurses, or an office care group (OC) that received whatever care they needed except home care. Patients with lung cancer entered the study two months after diagnosis and were followed for six months. Participants experienced significant differences in symptom distress and functional abilities. The two home nursing care groups remained less distressed and more independent six weeks longer than the office care group. These results suggested that home nursing care assisted patients in minimizing distress from symptoms and maintaining their independence longer, in comparison to patients who received no home nursing care.

Subsequently, McCorkle and her colleagues followed patients who were discharged from seven hospitals with complex care problems requiring home care services. The patients numbered 233, with eight different solid tumors, and 103 caregivers were recruited for the study and followed for three months. Although all these patients could have benefitted from home care, only about half were referred to home care. Patients receiving home care demonstrated improvement in their symptoms, function, and mental health status compared with patients who did not receive home care. Results provided insight into the home care needs of patients with cancer and their families and aided in identifying interventions that may help patients deal with specific problems related to cancer and treatment effects.[23]

McCorkle and colleagues[44] conducted a secondary analysis to test the effects of oncology home care for terminally ill lung cancer patients on spousal distress during the bereavement period. Forty-six lung cancer patients and spouse dyads were entered into the study two months after diagnosis and remained until the spouse's death. Follow-up continued for 25 months after the death. Advanced practice nurses developed "Oncology transition services" to assist dying patients and their families through the living-dying transition.[45] The intervention consisted of personalized care in the home which focused on advanced symptom management. The nurse served as central coordinator for care and 24 hour access was provided. Psychological distress was the primary outcome variable.[44] This was significantly lower among the spouses cared for in the oncology home care group and was sustained over time. Findings suggested that the bereaved's psychological distress was positively influenced by the nursing interventions provided during the terminal phase of illness. This study also supports the notion that nursing interventions that incorporate caregivers into a patient's care should be operationalized and linked with specific outcomes in future studies.[44]

In another study, McCorkle and colleagues[46] tested the effect of a standardized nursing intervention protocol (SNIP) on post-surgical cancer patients' outcomes. This study was intended to compare the length of survival of post-surgical cancer patients who received specialized home care intervention by advanced practice nurses (APNs) after their surgery to the length of survival of those who received the usual follow-up care in ambulatory settings. The patients numbered 190 (50.7%) in the intervention group and 185 (49.3%) in the usual care group. Both groups were equivalent on all variables except stage at diagnosis: the intervention group contained patients with more late stage cancers. Patients in the control group received standard post-operative care in the hospital and routine follow-up in outpatient surgical clinics upon discharge. The home care intervention was intended to enhance recovery from surgery and to improve quality of life outcomes. The intervention was developed as a protocol that consisted of standard assessment and management guidelines, doses of content, and schedules of contacts. APNs followed specific guidelines to assess and monitor the physical, emotional, and functional status of patients; provided direct care when needed; assisted in obtaining services or other resources from the community; and provided teaching, counseling, and support during the recovery period. Nurses also functioned as liaisons to health care settings and providers, as well as to patients and families in the provision of technical and psychological support.

By the end of November 1996, 93 (24.8%) patients had died. Of these, 41 (44%) were from the intervention group and 52 (56%) from the usual care group. For all patients who died, causes of death were documented. Cancer was listed either as the primary or secondary cause on all death certificates. Other causes listed were pulmonary embolus, heart failure, sepsis, and cardiac arrest. Patients receiving the home care intervention had a longer length of survival than the control group. During the first three months after discharge, a total of eight patients in the control group died, and one patient from the intervention group died. The intervention, occurring over a period of four weeks immediately after surgery and hospitalization, corresponded to a period when the difference in mortality rate between the intervention and control groups was the largest. The combination of physical care and psychosocial support during the acute postoperative period addressed two critical issues. The first was to assist patients and families during the period of transition from hospital to home and to offer education, guidance, and reassurance during high psychological distress and uncertainty. The second was to monitor patients' physical status and offset potential lethal complications that are most prevalent in the acute postoperative period. This study supports the importance of such nursing interventions during the critical diagnostic and surgical treatment phases and is clearly defined within the realm of palliative care, since many of these patients were diagnosed as late-stage.[46]

As part of an earlier study, Jepson, McCorkle, Adler, Nuamah, and Lusk[47] examined changes in the psychosocial status of caregivers of postsurgical cancer patients at the patients' discharge and over time. Within a week after being discharged from the hospital, patients were randomly assigned to either the treatment or control condition. Patients in the treatment group received the SNIP over a four-week period between discharge and the end of three months. The intervention was provided by APNs and consisted of three home visits and six telephone calls. The nursing interventions included problem assessment; monitoring of the patient's condition; symptom management; and teaching caregivers how to problem solve, administer medications, and provide self-care behaviors. Psychosocial status was measured using the Caregiver Reaction Assessment.[32] Overall, caregiver's psychosocial status improved from baseline to three months and stabilized thereafter; however, among caregivers with physical problems, the psychosocial status of those in the treatment group declined over time compared to those in the control group. The researchers concluded that caregivers of cancer patients who have their own physical problems are at risk for psychologic morbidity as they assume the caregiving role.[47]

Naylor and colleagues[48] studied the effects of comprehensive discharge planning and home visitation by APNs with a population of elderly patients hospitalized for specific medical and surgical problems, including heart disease, orthopedic procedures, and bowel surgery. The intervention group received standardized comprehensive discharge planning specific for elderly persons at high risk of poor postdischarge outcomes and APN home visits and telephone calls. The intervention benefitted from the clinical experience of APNs and their abilities in communicating, coordinating, and collaborating with physicians. Outcomes included hospitalization rates, days in the hospital, time to first readmission, functional status, level of depression, patient satisfaction with care, and overall cost of postindex hospitalization health services. Patients in the intervention group were less likely to be readmitted to the hospital, experienced fewer days in the hospital, and had a longer time to the first hospital readmission for any reason. Functional status scores for both groups were improved over baseline, as were mean depression scores. Patients in both groups were satisfied with their care. Overall costs for postindex hospitalization health services for the intervention group were half that of the control group. The results of this study indicate that a comprehensive intervention including home care by an APN has a significant positive effect on patient outcomes and the cost of care for high-risk elderly patients.

Caregiver Programs

Two unique programs have been developed to teach caregivers direct care responsibilities for patients in the home. Both programs have had positive outcomes for patients and caregivers.

Ferrell and colleagues[49] examined the impact of cancer pain education on family caregivers of elderly cancer patients. Fifty family caregivers of elderly patients who were at home and experiencing cancer related pain were recruited for participation in this quasiexperimental study. Caregiver outcomes examined included quality of life, knowledge about pain, and caregiver burden. Findings demonstrated the significant burden to caregivers associated with pain management, particularly in the psychological realm. The pain education program proved efficacious in improving caregiver knowledge and quality of life. This study highlights, as do many nursing studies, interventions that teach caregivers to become proficient in the physical aspects of patient care. As demonstrated, this type of intervention often indirectly improves the caregiver's well being.

A second study included testing a psychoeducational curriculum intervention developed by Barg and colleagues.[50] The structured education intervention consisted of six to eight hours of intense educational, skills training, and communication enhancing strategies, with the intent to assist caregivers in being more prepared to care for patients at home. Caregivers reported they were more informed about cancer, its treatment, and symptom control. Part of the content, which focused on expected psychological reactions to cancer and to caregiving, helped normalize distressing emotions that were being experienced by patients and caregivers. These experiences provided a great source of relief for the caregivers. Despite a clear program description and the delineation of measurable outcomes, the researchers reported that a lack of willingness by many cancer caregivers to attend group meetings posed a major obstacle to obtaining a large number of participants. Group-style interventions clearly lend themselves to the study of a self-selected sample. In fact, caregivers who attend groups may possibly be those who are least in need of intervention, since they demonstrate an ability to utilize social support and/or have respite care available, making group attendance feasible. Alternative, individualized strategies are needed to assist caregivers who are unable to participate in groups.

RECOMMENDATIONS FOR FACILITATING THE USE OF HOME CARE NURSING IN PALLIATIVE CARE

Home care nursing is a logical component of effective palliative care, but, for a number of reasons, it has been underutilized. Patients who need palliative care have complex and often challenging physical and psychological problems. Palliative care for specific types of diseases requires knowledgeable and competent clinicians. It is common for many of the professional staff nurses in home care agencies to lack the knowledge and expertise to manage patients' symptoms and to teach caregivers the skills they need to manage the day-to-day problems they encounter in caregiving. Yet, because of the barriers described to receiving hospice care, home care nurses have to provide much of the palliative care in the community. In addition, for palliative care to be successful in the home, physicians must work collaboratively with nurses and be available to solve problems as they arise. It is often easier for physicians to admit patients to the hospital than to work with home care nurses to keep patients at home.

The state of the science in home care was reviewed for this chapter. Results from these studies have not been systematically incorporated into clinical practice where services are reimbursed. However, we identified critical factors in these studies that, if adopted, could become the basis of successful home care palliative nursing. These include the following:

1. Staff nurses who are responsible for direct patient care in the home must have contact and access to APNs with specialized knowledge and skills related to the disease-specific needs of patients. The term *advanced practice nurse* is defined as a professional nurse who has graduated from a master's program in a specialty field such as an oncology advanced practice program, including clinical nurse specialists and nurse practitioners. To assist the staff nurse in dealing with the complexity of palliative care, either a palliative care physician or an APN should serve as a supervisor/consultant to the team and be directly involved in clinical decisions. There may be fewer opportunities for APNs than needed working directly in home care agencies because of the perception that they are too costly to employ. As agencies move to prospective payment and greater efficiency, the role of the APN will factor more prominently in home care agencies. APNs may also work independently and provide care to a group of patients, such as case managers from an ambulatory clinic. As a result of the Balanced Budget Act of 1997 (PL 105-55), APNs, specifically clinical nurse specialists and nurse practitioners, practicing in any setting can be directly reimbursed at 85% of the physician fee schedule for services provided to Medicare beneficiaries. In home care, this change has the potential to facilitate access to care for patients who do not have access to a home care agency or other primary care provider, specifically those in rural and underserved areas.
2. Because of the barriers to entering hospice care, home care nurses should become knowledgeable and highly skilled in providing palliative care to patients. This will require not only the development of skills in a new area of clinical expertise but also a paradigm shift in the way home care nurses view the episode of care for home care patients. Home care has traditionally been viewed as a component of the long-term care delivery system. Although the number of home visits per episode of illness has decreased significantly, home visits tend to be spread out over a greater period of time, usually a 60-day certification period. For patients requiring palliation, home care may need to be very intensive over a relatively short period of time. In this model, the home care nurse can assist the patient and family in methods of managing symptoms and coping with the caregiving role. In the long term, as the patient's disease progresses, the patient and caregivers will need "booster" visits, but the majority of visits and care may be given in short periods of time, when the patient and caregivers are most in need. Telephone visits to provide care has been shown to be an effective strategy for chronic illnesses in which the needs are for support and education.
3. Patients are usually hospitalized when symptoms get out of control. When patients are hospitalized, comprehensive discharge planning and follow-up by skilled palliative care nurses is needed to ensure that the plan is implemented, evaluated, and revised as needed. These nurses may be based in a variety of settings, such as home care agencies, clinics, and private offices. The complexity of symptom management following hospitalization may require the advanced skills of an APN to provide consultation to the palliative care team or to implement a plan of care with a patient and family.
4. Patients who have complex problems and receive home care nursing need family caregivers who have been taught skills to provide care. In the event these caregivers are ill themselves, additional or complementary services need to be provided to help with the patients' care. APNs providing home care for ill patients should conduct ongoing assessments of family caregivers, including their health and demands made upon them. Standardized educational programs to teach family caregivers skills to provide care are needed and should be a part of routine home nursing care.
5. The use of innovative models must be considered as a strategy for providing care to patients and families. Telephone visits

have been shown to be a very effective strategy to help families cope with the caregiver role. Under prospective payment for home care, home care providers are no longer constrained by the per-visit method of reimbursement, and telephone visits can be integrated into the plan of care. Telehealth programs have also been used effectively with populations of patients at home. As the technology becomes less expensive, increased opportunity to implement these strategies will occur.

6. Palliative home care should be provided by professionals from multiple disciplines, and physicians must be an integral part of program management. The multidisciplinary care provided by therapists, nurses, paraprofessionals, and physicians is essential to the development of positive outcomes. Physicians, as members of the multidisiciplinary team, must work in collaboration with other professionals to provide comprehensive care to patients and families. Collaboratively, the team determines the amount of care needed, the most appropriate setting for care, and the type of interventions required to improve the quality of life.

Case Study: A Dyad Study of Mr. And Mrs. Rizzi

A growing number of cancer patients are being discharged from the hospital following surgery or other cancer treatments to be cared for at home by spouses who have chronic illnesses themselves. Mr. S. Rizzi, a 68-year-old Italian retiree, and his wife, Mrs. T. Rizzi, age 64, are good examples. Mr. Rizzi was diagnosed with Stage IIIA non–small cell lung cancer following five months of chest and shoulder pain, fatigue, dyspnea, weight loss, and persistent cough. Despite his medical history, he was physically active until these symptoms, along with his cancer treatment, constrained him. For 50 years before diagnosis, Mr. Rizzi smoked two packs of cigarettes a day. He also had a history of hypertension, osteoarthritis, and a healing duodenal ulcer.

Mrs. Rizzi was a part-time beautician who identified herself as her husband's primary caregiver despite her own comorbidities of hypertension, osteoarthritis, and diabetes. These conditions required regular medical management and caused some physical discomfort and loss of mobility. Mr. Rizzi's treatment included a right upper lobectomy that required chest drainage tubes and subsequent radiation therapy and chemotherapy. He was discharged from the hospital ten days after surgery. Like many postsurgical patients, Mr. Rizzi went home to be cared for by his wife.

At discharge, Mr. Rizzi's medical care included wound care at the drain site for postsurgical chest tubes and management of symptoms from the disease and from treatment. He was concerned about his ability to recover and anticipated postoperative pain and loss of his independent, active lifestyle. Despite her own chronic illnesses, Mrs. Rizzi reported her overall health as good and considered herself fit to provide home care. She was determined to help her husband with the physical and emotional needs associated with cancer and its treatment. Mrs. Rizzi was unsure of her ability to manage her husband's physical care and doubted her ability to distinguish normal postoperative recovery from more serious complications. She was apprehensive about her new role as manager of the family finances and worried about their ability to pay their bills now that physical limitations prevented part-time employment.

Mr Rizzi was referred for home care at discharge to the local VNA. This VNA was unique in having an oncology APN on staff to consult with the staff nurses on their cases. Mr. Rizzi's initial assessment visit was conducted within 24 hours following discharge from the hospital. The staff nurse learned that Mr. Rizzi needed wound care and symptom management related to pain control and bowel regimen. She also conducted a family assessment and learned that Mrs. Rizzi had concerns about her role as caregiver. Recognizing the acuity of the problems identified, and after consultation with an APN, the home care nurse scheduled the Rizzis for daily home visits for a week to address the clinical problems of Mr. Rizzi and provide education to Mrs. Rizzi in the caregiver role. Because maintaining the comfort of her husband was her primary concern, the home care nurse taught Mrs. Rizzi about pain management with medications and alternative comfort measures, such as massage, heat and cold applications, and guided imagery. In addition, the nurse referred the Rizzi's to the VNA social worker to assist in dealing with the financial issues associated with Mr. Rizzi's illness. Following the week of intensive home care visits by the nurse, she instituted telephone visits every other day for two weeks, followed by weekly telephone calls. Mrs. Rizzi used the telephone calls to discuss changes in her husband's clinical situation and receive advice on how to manage minor clinical problems. They were also a welcome source of support for Mrs. Rizzi as the complexity of the caregiving role increased. As the care of Mr. Rizzi became more complex, the home care nurse spent a great deal of time convincing Mrs. Rizzi that she was doing a good job.

One of the critical factors in Mrs. Rizzi's ability to perform the role of caregiver was the stability of her own health. Given her comorbidities, Mrs. Rizzi might have fallen ill herself under the additional burden of the caregiver role. Instead, the home care nurse coached Mrs. Rizzi to pay special attention to her own health during these stressful times. On each visit and telephone call, the home care nurse inquired about Mrs. Rizzi's health, making sure she kept her primary care provider appointments and adhered to her medical regime. Opportunities for respite were arranged so that Mrs. Rizzi could go to get her hair fixed and retain some normalcy in her activities.

As Mr. Rizzi became more ill, Mrs. Rizzi consulted the home care nurse about a hospice referral. The home care nurse consulted with the physician, who agreed that Mr. Rizzi had a prognosis of less than 6 months and was a good candidate for hospice care. Because the VNA did not have a certified hospice program, the home care nurse referred the Rizzis to the local hospice provider in their community. Although it was difficult to discharge the Rizzis from the home care agency, at the hospice, Mr. and Mrs. Rizzi took advantage of the pastoral care services, art therapy program, and the additional resources available under Medicare, such as prescription drug coverage for medications related to the terminal illness. The hospice nurse provided the majority of direct care, with consultation with their APN on the team when Mr. Rizzi's pain became unmanageable. Mr. Rizzi died at home following a two-month service from hospice. The hospice nurse also visited Mrs. Rizzi twice after Mr. Rizzi's death.

CONCLUSION

For palliative care to be a viable component of the service provided by home care agencies, changes are needed in both the structure of home care and the mechanisms for reimbursement. The regulations for the provision of home care under Medicare must be substantively modified to allow increased access to palliative care. Under the current regulations, the physician is the only provider who has the ability to order and supervise a home plan of care through home care agencies. The literature is consistent in its description of the positive role APNs play in supporting both the patient and family caregivers in the home, yet APNs are not given the authority to direct patient care through home care agencies for patients needing palliation. Exceptions do exist through hospital-based programs. For example, Memorial Sloan Kettering Cancer Center has a successful hospital based supportive care program that provides palliative care in the home for patients. This program is directed by an APN, and services are billed through the outpatient service. Regulations that support the critical role APNs play in the clinical management of patients at home who require palliative care and that legitimize the APN's ability to order and supervise the plan of care are essential. The few successful models in hospital-based and ambulatory clinics should be implemented in home care agencies.

Additionally, the historical structure of Medicare reimbursement is a disincentive for the use of APNs in home care agencies. As defined by Medicare, nursing home visits are reimbursed the same regardless of the preparation of the provider. For example, a home care agency receives the exact same dollar amount for a home visit provided by an LPN, an RN with a bachelor's degree, or an APN. Medicare regulations must be modified to reimburse home care agencies at a higher rate for care provided by APNs, consistent with their expertise and impact on patient care outcomes. In so doing, an incentive will be created to include APNs as part of the team in home care agencies.

The earlier case study had a successful outcome even though the current home care delivery system is fragmented. The need for palliative care to be integrated into both home care as well as hospice care is essential for the provision of a continuum of care to patients at the end of life. For these changes to be integrated into the care delivery system, regulations need to be changed to allow home care nurses to provide end-of-life care in situations in which hospice care is unavailable, or at the request of the patient or family.

In summary, home care is an important component of palliative care. Clinical and regulatory barriers have forced palliative care in the home to be provided by certified hospices at the end of life. Structural changes in home care are needed to fully integrate palliative care into the home care delivery system. Additionally, the role of APNs must be fully developed and reimbursement mechanisms established to integrate palliative care into home care for both patients and home caregivers.

REFERENCES

1. Sarna L, McCorkle R. Burden of care and lung cancer. Cancer Practice 1996; 4(5):245–251.
2. Clemon-Stone S, Eigsti DG, McGuire SL. Comprehensive Community Health Nursing, 4th ed. St. Louis: Mosby, 1995.
3. National Association for Home Care. Basic Statistics About Home Care. Washington, DC: 1999.
4. Seeber S, Baird SB. The impact of health care changes on home health. Seminars in Oncology Nursing 1996; 12(3):179–187.
5. Humphrey C, Milone-Nuzzo P. Manual of Home Nursing Orientation. Gaithersburg, Maryland: Aspen 1996.
6. Haupt B. An overview of home health and hospice care patients. 1996 Home and Hospice Care Survey (297). Washington, DC: Department of Health and Human Services, National Center for Health Statistics, 1998.
7. Chan C, Chang A. Managing caregiver tasks among family caregivers in cancer patients in Hong Kong. Journal of Advanced Practice Nursing 1999; 29(2): 484–489.
8. McEnroe L. Role of the oncology nurse in home care: Family centered practice. Seminars in Oncology Nursing 1996; 12(3): 188–192.
9. United States Department of Labor, Bureau of Labor Statistics. National Industry-Occupation Employment Data. 1999.
10. United States House of Representatives. Committee on Ways and Means, 1998 Green Book. Washington, DC: 105th Cong, 2nd sess. 1998.
11. Christakis N, Escarce J. Survival of medicare patients after enrollment in hospice programs. New England Journal of Medicine 1996; 335: 172–178.
12. Dombi W. Home care and the law. Caring 1991; 10 (9):1.
13. Cawley MM, Gerdts EK. Establishing a cancer caregivers program: An interdisciplinary approach. Cancer Nursing 1988; 11: 267–273.
14. Conkling VK. Continuity of care issues for cancer patients and families. Cancer 1989; 64: 290–294.
15. McCorkle R, Given B. Meeting the challenge of caring for chronically ill adults. In: Chin P., ed., Health Policy: Who Cares? Kansas City, MO: American Academy of Nursing, 1991:2–7.
16. McCorkle R, Yost LS, Jepson C, Malone D, Baird S, Lusk E. A cancer experience: Relationship of patient psychosocial responses to caregiver burden over time. PsychoOncology 1993; 2: 21–32.
17. Ganz PA. Current issues in cancer rehabilitation. Cancer 1990; 65: 742–751.
18. Mor V, Guadagnoli E, Wool M. An examination of the concrete service needs of advanced cancer patients. Journal of Psychosocial Oncology 1987; 5: 1–17.
19. Googe MC, Varrichio C. A pilot investigation of home health care needs of cancer patients and their families. Oncology Nursing Forum 1981; 8: 24–28.
20. Wellisch D, Fawzy F, Landsverk J, Pasnau R, Wocott D. Evaluation of psychosocial problems of the home-bound cancer patient: The relationship of disease and sociodemographic variables of patients to family problems. Journal of Psychosocial Oncology 1983; 1(3): 1–15.
21. Houts PS, Nezu AM, Nezu CM, Bucher JA. The prepared family caregiver: A problem-solving approach to family caregiver education. Patient Education & Counseling 1996; 27(1): 63–73.
22. Wingate A, Lackey N. A description of the needs of noninstitutionalized cancer patients and their primary caregivers. Cancer Risk 1989; 12: 216–225.
23. McCorkle R, Jepson C, Malone D, Lusk E, Braitman L, Buhler-Wilkerson K, Daly J. The impact of post-hospital home care on patients with cancer. Research in Nursing and Health 1994; 17: 243–251.
24. Grobe ME, Istrup SM, Ahmann EL. Skills needed by family caregivers to maintain the care of an advanced cancer patient. Cancer Nursing 1980; 4: 371–375.
25. Hinds C. The need of families who care for patients with cancer at home: Are we meeting them? Journal of Advanced Practice Nursing 1985; 10: 575–581.
26. Siegel K, Raveis VH, Houts P, Mor V. Caregiver burden and unmet patient needs. Cancer 1991a; 68: 1131–1140.
27. Siegel K, Raveis VH, Mor V, Houts P. The relationship of spousal caregiver burden to patient disease and treatment related conditions. Annals of Oncology 1991b; 2: 511–516.
28. Oberst MT, Gass KA, Ward SE. Caregiving demands and appraisal of stress among family caregivers. Cancer Nursing 1989; 12: 209–215.
29. Perry GR, Roades de Menses M. Cancer patients at home. Needs and coping styles of primary caregivers. Home Healthcare Nurse 1989; 7: 27–30.

30. Sales E, Schultz R, Biegel D. Predictors of strain in families of cancer patients: A review of the literature. Journal of Psychosocial Oncology 1990; 10: 1–26.

31. Given B, Helms CW, Stommel M, Devoss DN. Determinants of family caregivers reaction: New and recurrent cancer. Cancer Practice 1997; 5: 17–24.

32. Given CW, Given B, Stommel M, Collins C, King S, Franklin S. The caregiver reactions assessment (CRA) for caregivers to persons with chronic physical and mental impairments. Research in Nursing and Health 1992; 39: 271–283.

33. Hinton J. Can home care maintain an acceptable quality of life for patients with terminal cancer and their relatives? Palliative Medicine 1992; 8: 183–196.

34. McWhinny IR, Bass MJ, Orr V. Factors associated with the location of death (home or hospital) of patients referred to a palliative care team. Canadian Medical Association Journal 1995; 152 (3): 361–367.

35. Axelsson B, Sjoden P. Quality of life of cancer patients and their spouses in palliative home care. Palliative Medicine 1998; 12: 29–39.

36. Perusseli C, Marinari M, Brivio B, Castaganni G, Cavana M, Centrone G, Magni C, Merlini M. Evaluating a home palliative care service: Development of indicators for a continuous quality improvement program. Journal of Palliative Care 1997; 13(3): 34–42.

37. Constantini M, Camoirano E, Madeddu L, Bruzzi P, Verganelli E, Henriquet F. Palliative home care and place of death among cancer patients: A population based study. Palliative Medicine 7(4) 323–331, 1993.

38. Martinson I. Why don't we let them die at home? RN 1976; 39: 58–65.

39. Martinson I, Armstrong G, Geis O, Anglim M, Gronseth E, McInnis H, Kersey J, Nesbit M. Home care for children dying of cancer. Pediatrics 1978; 62: 106–111.

40. Yates J, McKegney P, Kun L. A comparative study of home nursing care of patients with advanced cancer. Proceedings of the American Cancer Society Third National Conference on Human Values and Cancer: Recommendations for Facilitating the Use of Home Care in Palliative Care. Washington, DC: American Cancer Society 1981.

41. Oleske D, Hauck W, Heide E. Characteristics of cancer patient referrals to home care: A regional perspective. American Journal of Public Health 1983; 73: 678–682.

42. McCorkle R, Benoliel JQ, Georgiadou F, Donaldson G, Moinpour C, Godell B. A randomized clinical trial of home nursing care for lung cancer patients. Cancer 1989; 64: 1375–1382.

43. McCorkle R, Benoliel JQ, Georgiadou F. The effects of home care on patients' symptoms, hospitalizations and complications. In Key Aspects of Comfort: Management of Pain, Fatigue and Nausea. New York: Springer 1989.

44. McCorkle R, Nuahmah I, Robinson L, Lev E, Benoliel J. The effects of home nursing care for patients during terminal illness on the bereaved psychological distress. Nursing Research 1998; 47 (1): 2–10.

45. Tornberg MJ, McGrath BB, Benoliel JQ. Oncology transition service: Partnerships of nurses and families. Cancer Nursing 1984; 7(2):131–137.

46. McCorkle R, Strumpf NE, Nuamah IF, Adler DC, Cooley ME, Jepson C, Lusk EJ, Torosian M. A specialized home care intervention improves survival among elderly of post-surgical cancer patients. JAGS (In press) December 2000.

47. Jepson C, McCorkle R, Adler D, Nuamah I, Lusk E. Effects of home care on caregiver's psychosocial status. Image: Journal of Nursing Scholarship 1999; 31(2): 115–120.

48. Naylor M, Brooten D, Campbell R, Jacobson B, Mezey M, Pauly M, Schwartz JS. Comprehensive discharge planning and home follow-up of hospitalized elders. JAMA 1999; 281 (7): 613–620.

49. Ferrell BR, Grant M, Chan J, Ahn C, Ferrell BA. The impact of cancer pain education on family caregivers of elderly patients. Oncology Nursing Forum 1995; 22(8): 1211–1218.

50. Barg F, Cooley M, Pasacreta JV, Senay B, McCorkle R. Development of a self administered psychosocial cancer screening tool. Cancer Practice 1994; 2(4): 288–296.

51. Wong ST. Reimbursement to advanced practice nurses (APN) through medicare. Image: Journal of Nursing 1999; 31(2): 167–174.

40 Pediatric Care: The Hospice Perspective

LIZABETH H. SUMNER

> *I try to put up a face in front of him because I don't want him to know that I'm crying, that I'm sad or anything, because he's very much like myself, you know. And he will tell you how he feels. He can remember since he was small I was working, and I always had my hair fixed, my face, my make-up, and things like that. I try to keep it up, you know, put on a face. But, I'm bleeding inside.*
>
> —Mother

Perhaps a simple children's book on the life cycle of nature, *Lifetimes*, illustrates it best:

> There are lots of living things in our world. Each one has its own special lifetime. All around us, everywhere beginnings and endings are going on around us all the time. So, no matter how long they are, or how short, lifetimes are really all the same. They have beginnings and endings and there is *living* in between.[1]

Although much has been written about end-of-life care for adults, far less emphasis has been placed on the needs of dying infants and children. The ongoing painful dilemmas and struggles for families with infants and children who are dying remain hidden from society's view. Yet the demands and challenges of caring for a dying child are being addressed within hospitals and homes on a daily basis. Individuals committed to children with life-threatening illnesses and a modest number of hospice programs are making a difference, finding ways to significantly impact the imbalance. The irony for pediatric caregivers is that "end-of-life care" is often necessary at the very beginning of a child's life. Nurses can be instrumental in blending this contradiction into a realistic and compassionate framework for care of children and families dealing with terminal illnesses.

The ultimate goal is not only to promote excellent end-of-life care for these children but also to elevate their status in a health care delivery model. Appropriate hospice care will bring them into the sunlight to be cherished among the living, where they will be removed from the isolating experiences of their dying. Improving quality of life for even a brief life can benefit the patient and all those affected by the death of a young child. Such a powerful wave goes beyond those most obviously affected, the parents and siblings. The rippling effect extends to grandparents, other relatives, teachers, school friends, family friends and neighbors, as well as the many health care professionals involved in their care and treatment. Each of these may also be deeply influenced by the child's illness and subsequent death. Compared to a terminally ill adult, the comparatively larger number of people affected by a child's illness or impending death is significant. Few, if any, have had any previous experience with the death of a child. Typically, multiple physicians, care providers, suppliers, school professionals, and a variety of family members are involved with these children. Each has unique needs and roles in the child's experience. In addition, knowledge and skills regarding both palliative care and curative care are essential to guide families through this transition in the focus of care.[2]

Hospice care for children has not been well integrated into the existing national guidelines and regulatory standards. When this eventually takes place, the outcome will be a heightened visibility, credibility, and accountability for hospices, allowing home health programs and hospitals to adequately serve dying infants, children, and their families. The National Hospice and Palliative Care Organization (NHPCO) and Children's Hospice International (CHI) trends reveal disheartening underutilization of hospice services for pediatric patients and related health care practitioners. The 1998 CHI survey reported that less than 1% of children needing hospice care receive it.[3] Most state hospice organizations do not delineate which programs even serve children. The NHPCO is currently revising its "Hospice Standards of Practice" in an effort to integrate pediatrics into those guidelines. CHI publishes "Standards of Hospice Care." However, the standards are rarely put into practice at the predominantly adult patient organizations[4] (see Table 40–1). The result is an ongoing struggle for professional staff in pediatric care *and* for families, both of whom are dealing with end-of-life issues, unprepared for the journey they are on together. Calls for help and consultation come on a weekly basis to the author from health care professionals expressing concern and inadequacy regarding their ability to meet the demands and challenges of these young patients, their families, the schools they are connected to, and the increasing complexity of their care.

Adult focused programs and staff are typically unprepared to respond to the infrequent pediatric referrals and also lack connections to pediatric providers to assist them in providing safe, appropriate hospice care. Treating children as small adults can be risky and is mis-

Table 40–1. Children's Hospice International Standards of Hospice Care for Children

Access to Care

Principle

Children with life-threatening, terminal illnesses and their families have special needs. Hospice services for children and their families offer developmentally appropriate palliative and supportive care to any child with a life-threatening condition in any appropriate setting. Children are admitted to hospice services without regard for diagnosis, gender, race, creed, handicap, age or ability to pay.

Standards

A.C.1. Hospice care services are accessible to children and their families in a setting that is desired and/or appropriate for their needs.

A.C.2. The hospice team is available to provide continuity of care to children and their families in the home and/or in an institutional setting.

A.C.3. The hospice program has eligibility admission criteria for the children and families they serve. Care plans are developed which take into consideration the child's prognosis, and the child and family's needs and desires for hospice services. Admission to the hospice care service does not preclude the child and family from treatment choices or hopeful, supportive therapies.

A.C.4. The hospice program provides information to the community and referral sources about the services that are offered, who qualifies, and how services may be obtained and reimbursed.

Child and Family as a Unit of Care

Principle

Hospice programs provide family-centered care to enhance the quality of life for the child and family as defined by each child-and-family unit. It includes the child and family in the decision making process about services and treatment choices to the fullest degree that is possible and desired.

Standards

C.F.U.1. The unit of care is the child and family. Hospice provides family-centered care. The family is defined as the relatives and/or other significant persons who provide physical, psychological, social and/or spiritual support for the child.

C.F.U.2. The hospice program recognizes the unique, personal values and beliefs of all children and families. The hospice respects and maintains, as possible, the wishes and dignity of every child and his or her family.

C.F.U.3. The hospice program encourages that children and their families participate in decisions regarding care, including discontinuation of hospice care at any time, and maintains documentation related to consent, advance directives, treatments, and alternative choices of care.

C.F.U.4. The hospice program provides care that considers each child's growth, development and stage of family life cycle. Children's interests and needs are solicited and considered, but are not limited to those related to their illness and disability.

C.F.U.5. The hospice team seeks to assist each child and family to enjoy life as they are able, and to continue in their customary life-style, functioning and roles as much as possible, especially helping the child to live as normal a life as is possible.

Policies and Procedures

Principle

The hospice program offers services that are accountable to and appropriate for the children and families it serves.

Standards

P.P.1. The hospice program establishes and maintains accurate and adequate policies and procedures to assure that the hospice is accountable to children, their families, and the communities they serve.

P.P.2. The hospice agency is in compliance with all local, state and federal laws and regulations which govern the appropriate delivery of hospice care services.

P.P.3. The hospice program provides a clear and accessible grievance procedure to families outlining how to voice complaints or concerns about services and care without jeopardizing services.

Interdisciplinary Team Services

Principle

Seriously ill children with life-threatening conditions and/or facing terminal stages of an illness and their families have a variety of needs that require a collaborative and cooperative effort from practitioners of many disciplines, working together as an interdisciplinary team of qualified professionals and volunteers.

Standards

I.T.1. The hospice program provides care to the child and family by utilizing a core interdisciplinary team which may include: the child, the family and/or significant others, physicians, nurses, social workers, clergy and volunteers.

I.T.2. Representatives of other appropriate disciplines are involved in the team as needed, i.e., physical therapy, occupational therapy, speech therapy, nutritional consultation, art therapy, music therapy. The team might also include psychologists, child life specialists, teachers, recreation therapists, play therapists, home health aides, nursing assistants, and other specialists or services as needed.

I.T.3. The hospice core team meets on a regular basis and an integrated plan of care is developed, implemented and maintained for every child and family.

Source: Children's Hospice International. Reprinted with permission.

guided for the patient, the family, and the staff.

The NHPCO has developed four end result patient/family outcomes it requests that hospice programs use to measure their own effectiveness. These outcomes create goals to which all care and interventions should be based, thus creating opportunities for patients and families to achieve optimum care. The outcome measures are: (*1*) safe dying, (*2*) comfortable dying, (*3*) self-determined life closure, and (*4*) effective grieving.[5] Although these outcome measures were not specifically intended for the hospice *pediatric* population, they remain highly relevant and are intended to apply to the patient and caregiving family. Hospice programs are encouraged to use these measures as the foundation for the philosophy and clinical practice behind their service delivery. For example, dying children frequently have specific goals and ideas about what should be directed toward self-determined life closure (e.g., reaching a milestone of completing a grade level, celebrating a holiday/birthday early, a desire regarding place of death expressed by child and/or parent). The many ways in which the child and parents desire to remain in control over several aspects of their lives can be woven into interventions so that each feels successful.

Table 40–2. 1996 Top Causes of Death by Age in San Diego County, California

Cause	Number of Deaths	Cause	Number of Deaths
<1 Year		**5–14 Years**	
Certain conditions originating in the perinatal period	113	Unintentional injury	19
Congenital abnormalities	69	Neoplasms malignant	13
Symptoms, signs, and ill-defined conditions	23	Nervous system and sense organs diseases	5
Respiratory system diseases	6	Congenital abnormalities	2
Infectious and parasitic diseases	4	Homicide	4
Heart disease	2	Respiratory system diseases	3
Nervous system and sense organs diseases	10	Suicide	2
Unintentional injury	3	Heart disease	3
Homicide	4	Other circulatory system disease	3
Digestive system diseases	3	Digestive system diseases	1
Total <1 year	243	Total 5–14 years	58
1–4 Years		**15–24 Years**	
Unintentional injury	9	Unintentional injury	103
Congenital abnormalities	11	Homicide	35
Homicide	7	Suicide	40
Neoplasms malignant	5	Neoplasms malignant	22
Nervous system and sense organs diseases	4	Heart disease	12
Respiratory system diseases	4	Nervous system and sense organs diseases	6
Infectious and parasitic diseases	2	AIDS	1
Heart disease	1	Symptoms, signs, and ill-defined conditions	9
Endocrine, nutritional and metabolic diseases and immunity disorders	3	Infectious and parasitic diseases	1
Symptoms, signs, and ill-defined conditions	3	Congenitial abnormalities	6
Total 1–4 years	53	Endocrine, nutritional, and metabolic diseases and immunity disorders	2
		Total 15–24 years	253
		Grand Total 0–24 years	607

Source: Death Certificate Records, Health and Human Services Agency, County of San Diego 1996 (Health Status of San Diego County Report 1997), San Diego, California.

THE UNDERUTILIZATION OF HOSPICE FOR INFANTS AND CHILDREN

A review of local (San Diego County, CA; see Table 40–2) and national (U.S.; see Table 40–3) death statistics illustrates the potential diagnoses considered appropriate for pediatric hospice care. Traditionally, cancer diagnoses have dominated the list of relevant diseases for hospice eligibility. Data related to the neonatal and infant (less than age 1) age group were compelling. Causes of death in this category include prematurity, genetic/chromosomal anomalies, hydroencephaly, anencephaly, severe cardiac anomalies, cerebral palsy, gastroschisis, rare syndromes, etc., many of which were expected to be life-limiting in nature. Until recently, most pediatric patients served by hospices had predominantly cancer diagnoses, congenital anomalies, or Acquired Immunodeficiency syndrome. National data, however, indicate other diagnoses that threaten life, including heart diseases, central nervous system, degenerative disorders, mucopolysacchariduria, degenerative neuromuscular disorders, cystic fibrosis, liver and heart failure, and death as a result of trauma (e.g., drowning, motor vehicle accident, etc).[6] At San Diego Hospice, the ratio of cancer to noncancer diagnoses referrals has shifted to reflect improved access to families by identifying more underserved groups by diagnosis and age. A greater number of children with noncancer diagnoses are now referred (Fig. 40–1).

These less "traditional" patients include: children being discontinued from ventilators following a motor vehicle accident or in the perinatal period who are not expected to survive; withdrawal of aggressive care at any age; drowning accident victims who have not died immediately; chronically ill children with a progressive decline; babies who are "born dying," that is, transferred from a neonatal intensive care unit to home or inpatient hospice care; and rare and unusual syndromes.

In addition to the above underserved pediatric patients, some circumstances also lead to other categories of underserved children, including those without insurance coverage for hospice care, uncertain prognosis, chronically ill deteriorating children, children cared for by unprepared adult hospice staff, home health patients undertreated for holistic needs, and children of adult hospice patients (see Table 40–4). Increased outreach to the health care specialists who work with these groups has resulted in increased referrals and utilization for

Table 40–3. Fifteen* Leading Causes of Death Among Children Aged 1–14, United States, 1994†

Rank	Cause of Death	Number of Deaths	Death Rate per 100,000 Population	Percent of Total Deaths
	All causes	15,264	27.5	100.0
1	Accidents	6,025	10.9	39.5
2	Cancer	1,571	2.9	10.3
3	Congenital anomalies	1,148	2.0	7.5
4	Homicide	1,045	1.9	6.8
5	Heart diseases	612	1.1	4.0
6	HIV infection	381	0.7	2.5
7	Cerebral palsy	344	0.6	2.3
8	Suicide	322	0.7	2.1
9	Pneumonia and influenza	281	0.5	1.8
10	Benign neoplasm	180	0.3	1.2
11	Chronic obstructive pulmonary disease	171	0.3	1.1
12	Septicemia	142	0.2	0.9
12	Diseases of infancy	142	0.2	0.9
13	Viral diseases	137	0.2	0.9
14	Cerebrovascular diseases	128	0.2	0.8
	All others	2,635		17.3

*Two diseases received the ranking of 12; septicemia and diseases of infancy have the same number of deaths and the same death rate.
†Age-adjusted to the 1970 US standard population.
Data source: Vital Statistics of the United States, 1997.

consultation/collaboration. The development of the perinatal hospice component has created the opportunity for families to access hospice care during a pregnancy that is anticipated to have a fatal outcome for the baby at, or soon after birth (see Table 40–5).

BARRIERS TO ACCESSING HOSPICE CARE

Barriers for the pediatric population differ from those for adult patients because the patients are young children or infants. Society's belief that "children shouldn't die," along with denial of the process, make end-of-life care a distant and mysterious concept. Within the health care profession, a profound silence of discomfort and denial exists regarding babies and children dying. In some cases the health care professional's own attitudes and denial become the greatest barrier to their patients'/families' ability to access additional options for expert palliative care and support services. In effect, this denies families the possibility of an informed decision regarding the range of choices available during the child's illness. Excellence in end-of-life care as part of the *continuum* of clinical expertise should be readily available for families who may transition or alternate their focus of care from a strictly cura-

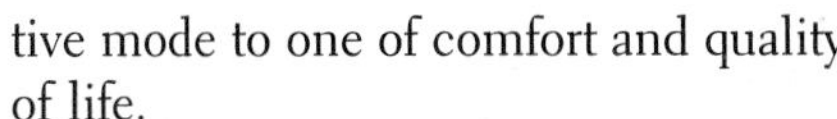

tive mode to one of comfort and quality of life.

The original hospice demonstration project in the 1980s was designed as a Medicare program for older adults with cancer as the "typical" disease process. The constantly changing continuum of needs in the pediatric population, from birth through 21+ years (including diagnoses, variable prognoses, developmental issues and needs, and varying family situations), has made it difficult to "fit into" the adult oriented guidelines for admission and standards of care. These only increase the barriers to access to appropriate care for the dying child and their support system.

Personal Issues and Biases

Nurses may experience emotional turmoil over their young patients' declining conditions and poor prognoses. The professional role of the nurse may quickly give way to the perspective of a parent, mother, or father toward the child. Expressions of transference may emerge and become problematic to the parents, the child, the nurse, or other team members. In programs where nurses are not clinically trained or emotionally prepared to manage pediatric patients, many issues can emerge

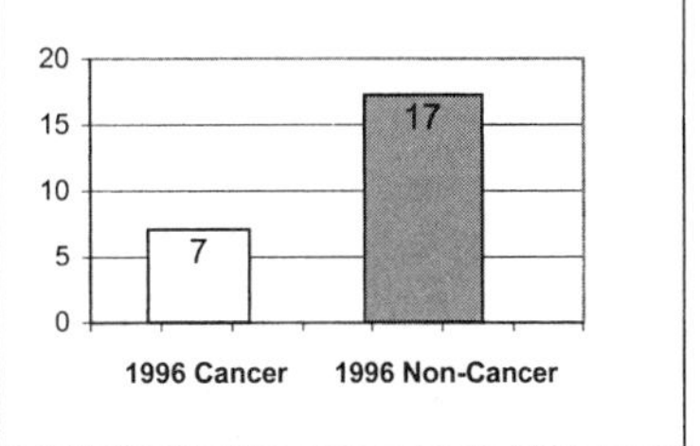

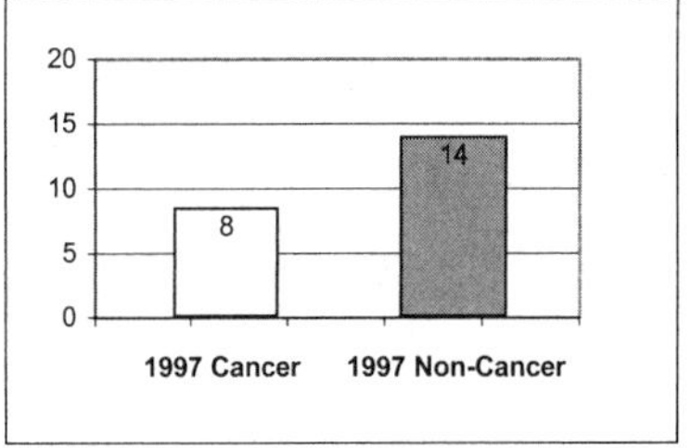

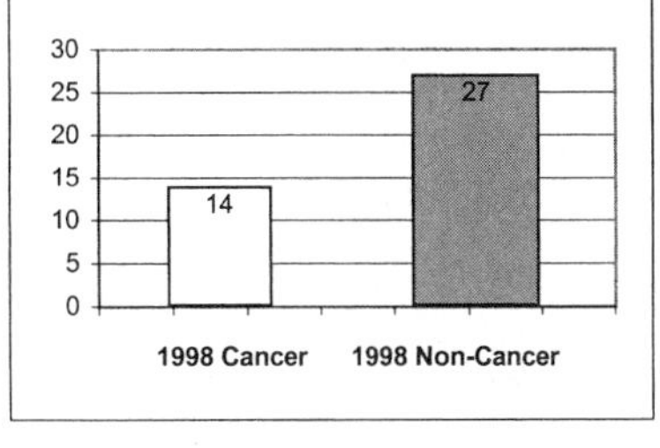

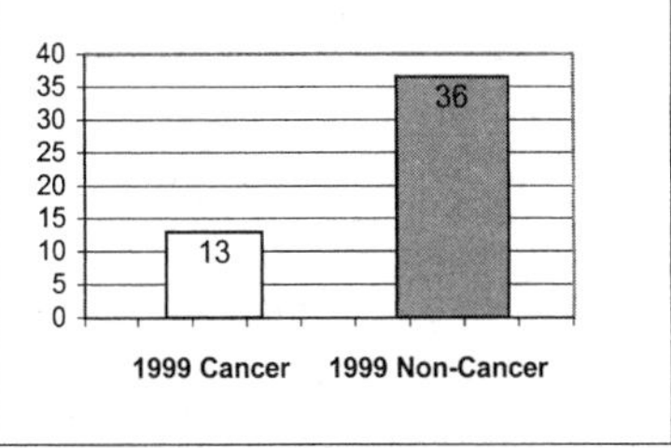

Fig. 40–1. Summary statistics for San Diego Hospice Children's Program: cancer and non-cancer diagnoses, 1996–1999.

Table 40–4. Children's Program of San Diego Hospice

Pediatric Hospice Patients	Children of Adult Hospice Patients	Community Outreach and Education
• Serving infants, children and adolescents, young adults. 0–21 years of age. • "Early Intervention Program": Perinatal Hospice. Support to families during the pregnancy through birth. Their babies have life-threatening conditions. • Includes extended support system of patient—outreach to classroom, faculty, school. • Adults 21+ case by case based on circumstances.	• Counseling, resources and consultation available for children in the adult San Diego Hospice patients families. • For children experiencing the life threatening illness of a parent, grandparent, or other relatives. Guidance and education for adults who care for them. • Children's books, therapeutic games and activities • Play therapy. • Art therapy • Memory making/keepsake activities.	• Creating a bridge between hospice, the school community and families. • Individualized presentations or training based on a specific situation or a general request to support the students/faculty. • Collaboration with school nurses, teachers, counselors, school psychologists and other faculty on issues related to children experiencing loss, grief, serious illness—their own or a loved one. • Provide resources and access to materials on the needs and concerns of children experiencing serious illness, loss and grief.

through their anguish. Previous losses of a similar nature, unresolved grief issues, conflicting beliefs regarding "supportive care only" interventions, and insecurities and self-doubt are all common, even within the hospice setting. The "if it were *my* child" frame of thinking can even be imposed upon parents who are already desperately struggling with their child's condition and the future that lies ahead for them. Personal and ethical dilemmas can emerge regarding withdrawal of aggressive care or nutritional support. Ethics consultations can bring an invaluable contribution to the decision-making process and often raise the option of a hospice consult or referral to hospice care.

Professional Issues

Nurses may lack pediatric physical assessment and symptom management skills, as well as knowledge of the diverse disease processes and developmental stages and related needs essential to care for neonatal and pediatric patients. Those with a background in aggressive and curative care may find it difficult to support a family in transition to a palliative focus of care. A struggle for control may erupt between the family, the staff, and the child. By continually asking "Whose need is this meeting?" one can maintain focus on the patient's care.

Most nursing education programs include little or no emphasis on care of dying children and their families, death and dying issues, grief and loss (professional and family), perinatal death, or hospice care. A recent study was conducted to determine the amount and types of content regarding pain and end-of-life care included in major nursing textbooks. Three of the 50 books reviewed were pediatric texts. Of those, only two had chapters on end-of-life care for this population. The findings revealed that textbooks had limited content regarding end-of-life care in general, with the pediatric subtopic being an even smaller percentage.[7]

This explains why many nurses lack a foundation for care of pediatric patients at the end of life. In addition, there may be limited access to pediatric experienced staff of all disciplines to train or offer clinical support to the hospice staff.

Table 40–5. Early Intervention Program at San Diego Hospice: Perinatal Hospice

- Create a birthing plan with parents and other health care providers that may include: the family's preference on interventions for the baby at birth, and options for the San Diego Hospice team's involvement with the family.
- Assist parents in identifying resources, psychosocial and spiritual counseling to help their family cope during the pregnancy and after the birth of the baby.
- Address the emotional needs and concerns of other children in the family.
- Provide guidance and encouragement in finding hope and comfort amidst the family's anguish and grief.
- Support the needs of the baby and family if hospitalized and assist the inpatient staff in coordinating a plan of care, including discharge planning, if appropriate.
- Assist in creating ways to celebrate and welcome the baby to the family in the hospital or at home.
- Assist in creating special keepsakes, rituals and treasures prior to and after the baby's birth (for example, a memory box, handprints of baby and family members, photographs, locks of hair, etc.)
- Provide referrals to support groups and resource materials provide by various community organizations and San Diego Hospice.
- Help in planning final arrangements, memorial services and good-byes at the hospital or at home, as appropriate.
- Provide bereavement support for all family members and other caregivers for a minimum of 18 months after baby dies.

Source: San Diego Hospice Children's Program.

Uncertainty in Determining the Child's Prognosis

State and federal regulations and standards governing hospice care and the clinical guidelines for ongoing appropriateness (Medicare and Medicaid) did not address pediatric patients when they were developed. Determining the required six months or less prognosis is extremely difficult for pediatric physicians because of the wide variability of prognoses in children, often varying from days, weeks, or months to years. Referral to hospice care by physicians also may represent to them "giving up" on their young patients. The requirement to certify that the child will be dead in six months is often perceived as a direct assault on the practice of physicians. Parents may still wish to continue active treatment, which may in fact prolong their child's life to some extent, but typically are not ready to "give up everything". Parents should not be forced to give up all treatment in order to avail themselves of help and guidance to actually *make* the transition to comfort care.

Payor or insurance providers may impose restrictions that deny access to hospice care for patients continuing curative treatment, and this is particularly problematic for children and parents. Parents and/or the child may want to pursue options that "buy more time," even if the goal is clearly palliative care, in order to be together longer. These families are not just "waiting longer for death" but intentionally trying to maximize the "living time" they have left. The resiliency of children is often astounding in the face of information that says they should have only hours or days to live. This has led to more pediatric hospice patients being discharged from the program. They have converted to a chronically ill child on a very different illness trajectory. These children are referred to as our "graduates" and the event is celebrated with the famly. Adult programs are penalized for patients who do not die fast enough, and the pediatric population is even more difficult to predict. Frequent case review and discussions with parents, physicians, the hospice team, and, if possible, the child, ensure that everyone has the same goals and perceptions of the child's condition and appropriateness of care.

Reimbursement Issues

The cost of caring for this population is often a barrier to pursuing a pediatric hospice program. Pediatric hospice care typically requires longer, more frequent home visits; more coordination of care with multiple physicians, other providers, and insurance companies; visits to schools by members of the team on behalf of the sick child or siblings; and hiring or access to pediatric experienced nurses, social workers, and aides. Ongoing therapies for palliation of distressing symptoms continues longer, typically, for children than adults, including blood transfusions, antibiotics, chemotherapy, and enteral and gavage feedings. The cost and responsibility for covering these therapies may be an additional factor to providers in deciding whether to serve children.

Insurance coverage may be inadequate or nonexistent for hospice services. Many states have waiver programs that provide nursing shift care in lieu of hospitalization or for respite care, but these programs also make the child and family ineligible to receive hospice care, creating an unacceptable conflict of needs. Many programs must raise additional funds to offset the expense of the staff-intensive support required for these families. The caseloads for staff managing this population typically are smaller than in adult hospice programs because of the increased time needed for coordination and care, especially if nurses do their own admissions. Traditional measures of productivity are impacted by these factors as well. The norms for practice with the neonatal and pediatric population stands apart from adult hospice care. Play and settling-in time are inherent to interactions with children, which starkly contrast with the direct care approach for adults.

Lack of Knowledge and Awareness of What Hospice Care Is: Successful Strategies

Physicians and nurses dealing with neonatal and pediatric patients may be completely unaware of the option of hospice/palliative care, how to access it, and the appropriate conditions or diseases for eligibility. In reality, pediatric programs are starting from the ground level, trying to educate and build bridges with "hospice-naïve" health care professionals to insure optimal end-of-life care for infants and children. For many clinical areas in pediatrics, death is an infrequent event; staff may not be particularly adept at managing the needs of dying children and their families from lack of familiarity and experience. In intensive care settings, a change in focus to comfort care seems for many completely contradictory to their "culture of high-tech."

Opportunities for families to receive hospice care begin when a relationship can be developed between a unit or department (e.g., neonatal intensive care unit, pediatric intensive care unit, hematology/oncology, labor and delivery, etc.) and the hospice team. Learning the needs and unique issues of each setting facilitates a customized approach to the specific populations served and the professional trust and accountability that are essential components for success. Discussing how to make referrals, adopting techniques for introducing the concept of hospice care to families and staff, exchanging expertise and resources, and providing in-service programs and educational opportunities are all methods to create a partnership between two specialties. This type of partnership can greatly influence the quality of life for patients, their families, and staff.

Participating in community based programs (e.g., Fetal Infant Mortality Review, perinatal nurse groups), coalitions regarding children's health care issues, collaborations on grief and loss of children, and presenting cases at grand rounds and professional meetings are all excellent ways to connect with other providers and develop vital linkages for a thriving pediatric hospice program. Some clinical areas allow a hospice team member to attend patient conferences and rounds to provide input to the team as part of case reviews, or even to be an observer in identifying potential patients. Participating in the "informational only," or evaluation, visit with the child, parents, and staff can provide an excellent opportunity for modeling, learning the language of hospice care, and learning how to explain hospice services and roles. Trust is transferred between inpatient and hospice staff from seeing, hearing, and experiencing what the other has to offer. The patients and families become more confident if they sense the confidence in those who make the referral. Many years of experience have revealed a higher level of expected accountability and responsiveness expected from pediatric caregivers regarding their patients when they are referred to hospice than for typical adult hospice care. Once trust and accountability have been established, they can form a strong and lasting foundation that can be passed on to new members as they join the hospice team. The need for ongoing, honest, and open communication between the two groups is critical.

Myths About Hospice Care for Children

Dispelling myths about hospice care can be helpful in creating an appropriate message about end-of-life or palliative care for pediatric patients. Many misconceptions need to be addressed, such as hospice care equals death; hospice care means giving up; hospice care means no more hope; hospice care means letting go or failure. It is important to clarify the scope and intent of hospice and palliative care and to address false perceptions when developing any collaborative relationship. If healthcare professionals do not have a clear and factual understanding about what hospice care is and is not, they will pass incorrect perceptions on to each other and to families. In no other area of health care is it more important for parents to know what we do and do not do. They must be aware of the following:

1. The team does *not* come in and force discussions on death and dying.
2. The hospice team does not insist that families be in complete acceptance of the terminality of their child's condition.
3. No one comes into their home and takes over or interferes with their sense of normalcy.
4. The team does not decide what happens when.
5. Team members do not get in between parents and their child.
6. Team members do not challenge or judge the family's belief system.
7. Team members do not discipline the child or children, but only set reasonable limits with parental input.

Each of these issues should be discussed during interactions with patients and families. Parents are entitled to be told these things to dispel the unspoken or as yet unarticulated fears they may have concerning hospice care. The hospice team can make this difficult transition somewhat easier for parents by addressing what parents may fear the team *might* do with, for, or to their child or to them.

Competition Between Home Health and Hospice Programs

Terminal nursing care and pain management programs are incorrectly equated with the interdisciplinary, holistic approach to end-of-life care that hospice programs can provide. The collaborative model of the interdisciplinary hospice team weaves a stronger, broader safety net of support and care around the family, enhancing their ability to meet the extraordinary challenge of a life-threatening illness.

Agencies are challenged with the moral responsibility to make the right decision for the dying child and his or her family, informing them of *all* relevant options to best meet the needs of the child. It may be in the child's best interest for a home care agency to refer the child to another, more appropriately qualified provider, such as a hospice program, if the program is better equipped to provide end-of-life care for the child. The multidimensional experience of a terminal illness requires attention to all aspects of the child's, parents', and siblings' needs, including spiritual, physical, and emotional, and psychosocial needs. An individual nurse may feel overwhelmed by the enormous burden of trying to meet all those needs alone or may experience intense frustration and helplessness in not being able to do so at all within the limitations of traditional home health care. Difficulties can also arise when a referral to hospice care is offered but refused by families based on unfamiliarity and perhaps dependency on the home health care nurse.

Possible solutions to this situation might be a joint case conference to discuss the family's issues and concerns or making a few joint, overlapping visits to transfer trust and to ease the often well established relationships to the hospice team. These may be unreimbursed visits, but they may create an openness between the two programs and increase referrals. These visits may require discussions with the parents regarding their fears and concerns and how their needs might be met.

Staffing Issues

Many hospices are not staffed with nurses who are comfortable dealing with babies, young children, and adolescents who are dying or with the unique issues of the parents' and/or extended family. Because the family's outlook is greatly influenced by the personalities and reactions of the staff, a special degree of confidence and caring is required.[8] Staffing after hours poses a particular challenge, and sometimes a hardship, on the agency and its staff. Adult care staff may be unwilling or incapable of caring for pediatric patients. The most serious outcome would be added stress and uncertainty imposed by the very experts from whom families are seeking refuge and comfort. Partnering with pediatric staff to train other staff, as well as thorough reporting to the after-hours staff are helpful actions. Anticipation of needs and problems with a plan for appropriate treatment can minimize and even prevent symptom crises.

Cultural Issues

Various cultures approach the child with a terminal illness differently. This involves decision making, communication, openness with the patient, the role of the parents in protecting the child from the truth about his or her condition, the role religion or faith plays in health care issues, and determination of who can translate for the family respectfully. Language barriers and lack of translation options can create great obstacles to providing adequate care. For example, parents may direct staff not to address the dying process with the child so as not to discourage the child. They may believe that in saying "it" aloud, it will cause it to come to pass. Or simply speaking of death may be too direct within the context of their culture. Hope is often intertwined in cultural issues and in the expression of that culture within the experience of serious illness. For some families this may necessitate frequent and ongoing reteaching and subsequent validation that a plan for collaborative care has been respected.

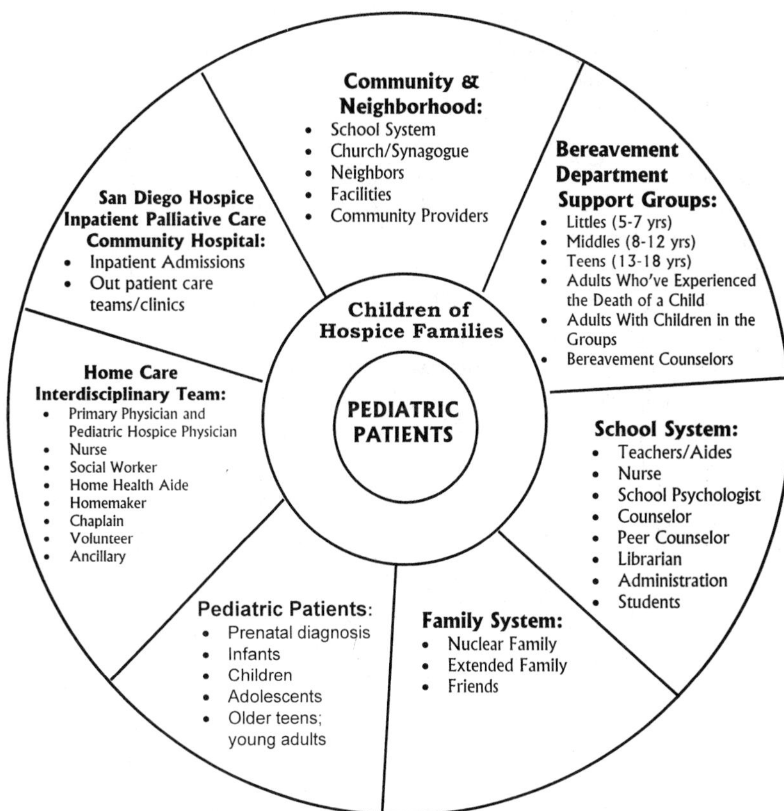

Fig. 40–2. A model for a hospice children's program that originated with the San Diego Hospice and has been adopted by many other institutions.

STRETCHING THE BOUNDARIES OF HOSPICE CARE: A MODEL FOR A COMPREHENSIVE PROGRAM FOR INFANTS AND CHILDREN

Since 1987 San Diego Hospice has been serving pediatric patients and striving to integrate pediatrics into the mainstream of the hospice culture and industry. What began as an informal relationship with a hospice staff nurse and the nurses and doctors at Children's Hospital evolved into "the team," a model for other programs across the country. Through many twists and turns, a vision emerged to seek to broaden the continuum of services for children at San Diego Hospice. The focus shifted from serving only a narrow target of sick and dying children to serving *all* children under the umbrella of care. This meant adding a component of specialized support and clinical intervention for the children of adult hospice patients (Fig. 40–2 and Table 40–6).

Children's Program social workers and, as appropriate, a chaplain, work directly with children who have a loved one, such as a parent, grandparent, aunt, or uncle, dying. Their interventions include opportunities for play and art therapy; rituals and keepsake activities for themselves or the family; therapeutic games; and storybooks on coping with feelings and illness, grief and loss, death and dying, the life cycle of nature, funerals, etc. For this new approach, the entire Children's Program considers the focus of care not to be the "patient and family," but the patient (adult or pediatric), family, and *school.*

The team extends the circle of care to involve the child or childrens' school in its web of support for the family. Typically (with parental permission), the social worker will confer or even meet with the teacher, school counselor, or nurse to include them in the plan of care. The primary hospice team, focused on the adult patient, is kept abreast of their involvement and goals. The aim is to facilitate more involvement of the child in the illness experience *before* the death occurs, maximizing their support systems as well as their ability to cope with the death when it does occur. A great deal can be done to better prepare children for the death and loss of a loved

Table 40–6. San Diego Hospice Children's Program: Children in Families of Adult Hospice Patients Served by the Children's Program

1998		1999	
Total by Relationship to Patient		Total by Relationship to Patient	
Children	74	Children	96
Grandchildren	110	Grandchildren	140
Great Grandchildren	0	Great Grandchildren	7
Nephew/Niece	3	Nephew/Niece	4
Other	7	Other	29
TOTAL	194	TOTAL	276

one by early intervention. Besides anticipatory grieving, many practical issues, fears, and concerns emerge for the children and their caregivers. In addition, the team provides adult caregivers with strategies and education regarding children's needs during the loved one's illness and in bereavement.

Families are never fully prepared for a child to be gone from their lives. The hospice professional can take steps to assist them down the long road of bereavement by helping them create tangible reminders of and treasures from their child's life, no matter how short or long it is. San Diego Hospice has developed a lengthy profile of activities and rituals for families to consider performing while a child is sick. For example, families might create a memory box with the child of special things that remind the child of favorite activities, trips, people, accomplishments—anything that helps to celebrate the child's life. Letters and journals can also be created by parents, the sick child, and siblings and friends. The most popular activity with families is doing handprints. This is done by making handprints of the baby or child, along with parents, siblings, etc., using tempera or poster paint to create a unique family portrait. Ear prints can be taken of a baby with anomalies of the extremities and as another way of preserving something physical of the child. An "All About Me Booklet" can be created over time through regular visits of a volunteer or family member, capturing the child's identity before and after the illness and his or her role as part of a family. Schoolmates can send notebooks or letters back and forth to stay connected, and later these can become lovely remembrances of friendships.

The possibilities are endless, and these tangible keepsakes may help siblings and parents stay better connected to memories and significant events as they pass through developmental milestones over the years. These physical tokens may help relatives find their way back to special memories and events concerning their loved one. These treasures may help them survive their experience a bit more whole, having a toolbox to help them integrate this tremendous loss into their being and may help them create a sense of meaning about the experience over time.

These additional components were added to the Children's Program to meet the needs identified by both the agency and community. The adult hospice patient referrals have been positively influenced by the availability of additional help, specifically for the children in the adult patient families. The number of these children served by the Children's Program continues to increase dramatically (see Table 40–6).

Local schools began to seek support, training, resources, and family intervention from this team. The next component added to the program became a commitment to assist and support the school community, in confronting the illness, death, grief, and loss experiences of their students, families, faculty, and community members.

The first priority was to develop a staffing model for a mixed pediatric patient population. Hospice Board and Administrative support enhanced resources for a growing census and expanded focus. Critical to preserving the stability and integrity of the program was maintaining consistent staff focused on the needs of children, pediatric patient care, and program development. Requiring staff to work on both adult care and children on a constant basis had led to high staff turnover. While creating problems, these changes were essential in order to increase the visibility and credibility of the program within the community. These changes provided the optimal continuity of care desired by families, staff, and referral sources. It enhanced the ability of the program to meet the enormous demands of educating the hospice-naïve health care professionals throughout the community.

The Children's Program next partnered with the local children's hospital and healthcare center to become the hospice provider for their entire system. Adding a pediatrician as the children's program medical director has also been highly valuable. This role includes building physician relationships in various specialty areas, consulting on potential patients, physician education, identifying potential research, and enhancing clinical practice by hospice nurses.

OVERVIEW OF NURSING CARE ISSUES FOR PEDIATRIC HOSPICE CARE

Nursing responsibilities when caring for a dying infant or child are extensive. An awareness of "total suffering" requires the nurse understand the interconnectedness of the four aspects of the experience of illness and suffering: physical, emotional/psychological, spiritual, and social. Each component greatly affects the others. In the words of Attig, "Suffering is the experience of brokenness. Illness unravels the pattern that belongs uniquely to each child, interrupting the ongoing stories of children's lives."[9] Nurses must assess for imbalances and indications of suffering in each of these areas in order to appropriately intervene. Without physical comfort, a child has little energy to be "present" to those around him or her and engage in meaningful exchanges. Management of symptoms in children requires the same degree of diligence and aggressive intervention as that used for adult patients.

Symptoms in children are generally similar to those in adults. However, discomfort/seizure management, pain in nonverbal patients, and feeding issues are more common. The age and developmental level of the child directly influence the selection of pain assessment tools, intervention strategies, route of medication, and type of medication. Many excellent resources are available to nurses for gaining competence in pain and symptom management for children. In addition, families require practical help, information, explanations, and support.[10,11,12] Attention must be paid to the practical issues of preparing for pediatric-appropriate supplies, medications, formulas, feeding tubes, medical equipment, documentation, and teaching tools for parents and children. A gently written, parent-friendly handout on the signs and symptoms of approaching death is an invaluable tool.

Interaction with School

To provide education, support, and resources to classmates, teachers, other parents, etc., the team goes to the school of the sick child. The bridge developed between the hospice and schools has been a successful addition to the program. This came about in response to an ongoing need identified by the school community to support children during life's challenging experiences.

For example, a child with astrocytoma was still attending school while having intermittent, recurrent seizures despite aggressive pharmacological intervention to control them. The hospice team and supervisor, parents, teachers, school administrator, school nurse, and classroom aide attended a conference at the school to create a plan to respond to her seizures. The need for proper documentation regarding her resuscitation status and hospice involvement had to be kept on hand and accessible in the event of a crisis, since the district was legally required to call 911 despite the parents' wishes. Issues for the other students were addressed and recommendations were made. The emotional reactions of all involved were discussed, and support was offered.

Another example involved a severely disabled child who strongly desired to remain at school as long as possible. A similar conference was held, but with the child in attendance as well. A plan was made among all participants for the hospice staff to visit the patient at school occasionally. Again, a contingency plan was made in the event of an emergency so that the patient's and parents' wishes could be honored. In both situations the schools were amazed at the collaborative effort and concern demonstrated by the hospice team. To them, it seemed extraordinary. When the object of care is a child, a family, *and* a school, this is the expected standard of excellence.

Support for Siblings

Two unique areas of concern when dealing with a pediatric population are the issues of the parents and those of the siblings. Siblings require explanations along the way and opportunities to be included, not excluded, from these experiences that affect the entire family. Siblings relish the chance to be helpers to nurses and parents as a way to feel important and contribute to the tasks at hand. Helping serves to validate their relationship with the sick child, diminish their feelings of helplessness, and may well affect how they integrate the loss over time.

As mentioned earlier for the children of adult patients, in the same way for siblings, the goal for siblings of terminally ill children is to enhance their feelings of involvement to the greatest degree possible while the sibling is alive in order to facilitate a healthy grieving process. The attempt to assist in achieving "effective grieving" for the sibling must begin when the sick child is diagnosed, because the family is changed profoundly from that moment on.

Strategies for including siblings in care may be as simple as the nurse including the siblings in her visit, asking to see their rooms or favorite toys, or reading a story together. Joint visits with a social worker are highly effective in spreading the attention and interventions among the sick child, siblings, and parents. It is important to repeatedly evaluate the well child's level of understanding about the sibling's condition. Family meetings are also a good setting in which to discuss how everyone is doing, including the patient, how they each perceive the situation, how their needs are (or are not) being met, and how their fears and concerns can be addressed. With parents' permission, an occasional small treat for the sibling is a simple gesture that may help make the well children feel special and included. Hospice volunteers make an excellent addition to the team for the specific role of being available to the sibling for a picnic, playing outside, reading, or a specific project or memory-making activity. Of these, the primary activity of the San Diego Hospice Children's Team is handprinting with the whole family. The sick baby or child is handprinted and the rest of the family's handprints are placed around the child's. The activity lifts the family from focusing on the tasks of the illness to a playful yet reverent level. Subsequently, the print becomes a treasure for the family. The same activity can be done with children of a dying adult as a keepsake for the children. Siblings may wish to have their own set of prints as well. Parents and children are also given "memory boxes" to store treasures in.

Support for Parents

To counterbalance the overwhelming sense of powerlessness and helplessness parents frequently feel, nurses can assist in identifying ways in which they can feel more in control. For example, with ongoing preparation for anticipated changes in the child's condition, a nurse can have medications in the home or instructions written for who and when to call for assistance.

Typically, parents of dying children have two overriding concerns: a fear of a sudden or acute increase in pain that they will be unable to manage, especially as death approaches; and fear of a crisis situation or unexpected change in condition, including how and when death may occur. It is critical to address these issues on an ongoing basis.

The need to feel a sense of control is also relevant to the sick child, who may be fearful from experiencing so many physical and emotional changes. Nurses can assist parents in methods of helping their child gain control over aspects of his or her experience, retain choices regarding care, and feel comfortable with a daily routine, all of which have great affirmational value. Managing medication regimens and symptoms is a daunting task for parents, having enormous impact on the family.[13] Nurses should consider the overall responsibilities of parents for managing care as well as maintaining family routines when planning medication and treatment regimens with the physician.

PRESERVING HOPE IN THE MIDST OF SERIOUS ILLNESS

A common characteristic of pediatric patients and their families is a prevailing sense of hope, evidenced in their language and decision making. It is important to preserve and nurture hope during all stages of the child's life-threatening illness. No matter how grim the situation, one should always strive to deal with matters in a positive yet realistic manner. The focus of hope inevitably must change over time, for example, from hope for cure, to hope for a longer remission than the previous, to hope that the child can continue to be cared for at home, to hope that the child will die without pain. Hope has a powerful and practical place within these families. With the presence of hope, parents speak of being able to continue their caregiving responsibilities, having the strength to put one foot in front of the other, and being able to carry on in their day-to-day existence. Without hope, the burden of the child's impending death would be utterly paralyzing. Hope offers opportunities for growth for the child and family. Examples of a child's hopes are a wish to return to school once more, to celebrate an important birthday, or to reach a significant milestone or rite of passage. Other expressions of hope include planning for a visit from grandparents, having friends gathered together, or even gaining the understanding that their loved ones will, indeed, survive after they die.

One young boy desperately wanted to be "normal" by continuing to play soccer despite his frail condition. After his blood transfusions, he was able to get out on the field and marvel at his own achievement. He touched many around him. This was a way for him to feel like he was still *living* with an illness and not just dying from it. Over time, his goals began to change as the benefits from transfusions became negligible and it became more difficult for him to recover from the activity. He, his father, and the medical team needed assistance from the hospice team to make the transition in his care plan to reduce and finally eliminate the ineffectual blood transfusions. It was an important lesson for many on the changing meaning, purpose, and role the therapies had for the child, his father, and his physicians. The hospice team was able to facilitate that discussion, thus enabling forward movement.

HOSPICE CARE FOR INFANTS

When a dying child is an infant, the need for hope is similar, but time constraints are severe. Parents may need support and encouragement to consider going home with their baby to have the opportunity to "welcome baby home." They may be offered a selection of "keepsake" activities to consider in order to preserve the presence of their little one's life and record the connectedness they had for such a brief period. For them, it may be a simultaneous greeting and farewell. Strengthening this experience may help diminish long-term psychological implications for parents and siblings.

Baby Angel was born with trisomy 18 and not expected to live more than a few days at most. Upon that determination, the neonatal intensive care unit (NICU) social worker referred the family to San Diego Hospice. The team went to the hospital to meet with the young parents, who were weighted down with grief, their dreams and hopes shattered as the new reality for their baby was sinking in. The option of home hospice care seemed overwhelming while still adjusting to the news of their child's impending demise. To ease the potential transition to home care, the parents and their infant were transferred to the Inpatient Hospice Care Center. Angel died within hours of her arrival, with her parents around her. The staff, unaccustomed to the needs of such parents, wondered why she was transferred at all. Was it "inappropriate" and a waste of effort? According to the parents, it was abundantly clear that it had been worth it and had allowed them to truly feel like parents in a peaceful environment. Compared to the crowded, public, hectic environment of the NICU, they felt peace in the hospice setting. They expressed tremendous gratitude for the efforts made on behalf of Angel's brief life.

In another case, Baby Joseph was born with hypoplastic left ventricle and was, again, not expected to survive more than a few days. His parents were determined to take him home with them for whatever time they could manage and were eager to plan and fulfill this hope. The team worked quickly with the NICU team to arrange for his discharge and to be met at home by a pediatric hospice nurse and social worker. At home they were admitted to the hospice program and settled in as family gathered to be with Joseph. Together, they created the opportunity to welcome Joseph into the family and into their home. Joseph kept them awake a lot with typical new baby needs. He died quietly in the early morning hours of the following day. Although to many it seemed tragic, his parents were grateful that they had been able to truly *be* parents for one day. In those hours they were able to etch some precious yet ordinary memories like other parents have and experience the normal stresses as well as provide the comfort all babies need.

The implications for staff in caring for dying infants and children are enormous. Some are more suited for this field than others. Key personal attributes of those identified as successful in this role include a high tolerance for ambiguity and flexibility; an appreciation for individual differences; good external support networks; a realistic awareness of personal limits; a joy for life in general; a sense of humor; an open communication style; a tendency to value self-awareness as an asset; empathy; and a willingness to learn continually. Being able to function in a self-directed mode facilitates using one's own resourcefulness to meet the challenges of an ever-fluctuating schedule.

Perhaps the most basic necessary characteristic is a comfort with death. Only by coming to terms with one's own thoughts and feelings about death is it possible to adapt philosophically to working with children who will die.[14] Swanson-Kaufmann[15] developed a model of caring for nurses dealing with perinatal loss. She states that fundamental to caring is understanding the personal meanings of the loss; resonating emotionally with the mother's feelings; offering realistic support, nurturance, and protection; facilitating the expression of grief; and helping maintain her faith in her capacity to come through her loss a functioning, whole person.[15] These also apply to the baby's fathter.

PERINATAL HOSPICE: THE EARLY INTERVENTION PROGRAM

In response to a need identified by the community, specifically parents, an innovative addition to the Children's Program was developed as an extension of existing hospice care. This new program grew out of the existing population of newborns with limited life expectancy described as "babies born dying."

Mothers and parents were coming directly to the hospice for help out of desperation, facing a prenatal diagnosis of a devastating nature for their unborn baby. These parents had decided to continue the pregnancy and treasure their child's life for as long as they could, yet they lacked any ongoing support. Their message was clear: "Finally, someone will just accept our decision and help our family deal with this experience. We don't want to just sit back and wait for our baby's death." Hospice professionals are trained to utilize an individualized approach to assist patients and families in dealing with life threatening illnesses and their decisions concerning that experience. This unique group of parents faced the daunting challenge of anticipating and preparing for the birth *and* death of their baby simultaneously. What they are given, with the help of this unique program, is the opportunity to feel some level of control by making plans based on their individual needs for supporting themselves, their other children, the grandparents, and friends.

The Early Intervention Program provides support to expectant parents through counseling and spiritual guidance for the entirety of the pregnancy, starting prior to and continuing after the delivery. Parents are advised of ways to create a personalized birthing plan that addresses their wishes for themselves and the care of their baby once born. The plan may include specific instructions and preferences for the labor and delivery staff, such as keepsakes and rituals they may wish to create or perform. Some parents await a definitive diagnosis after the baby is born to decide the extent of care to be provided.

The parents' goals and plans are discussed in collaboration with their physician. The physician is kept up to date regarding their psychological state and the development of their birthing plan. Prenatal nursing care is not a part of this program. These women continue their prenatal care under their physician's guidance. The pediatric hospice nurse is involved in educating the parents on the diagnosis, helping them understand what to expect, planning for the possibility of home care, and helping siblings understand the baby's condition.

Perhaps as a reaction to the lack of responsiveness by the health care system and society in general toward perinatal loss, these parents have found ways to support each other. They have truly disenfranchised grief, one not recognized as equal to the grief experienced with other types of death. The Internet is rich with amazing and profoundly intimate resources and ideas, shared experiences, practical help, opportunities to gain support, and even memorials to lost children. These parents have discovered help from within their isolation from others like themselves. Hospice professionals can gain valuable insight from their perspectives and excellent ideas on ways to improve support for these parents.

Initial feedback from the hospice bereavement counselors who work with these parents has highlighted the potential and anticipated impact of the perinatal hospice service. The bereaved parents who received help through the Early Intervention Program demonstrated the following: They were more emotionally and spiritually prepared for their infant's death; less intense despair/sadness; better marital relationship communication and support, less "raw" intense emotions such as anger, rage and uncertainty regarding the cause of death. The parents without hospice care during pregnancy and after birth seemed to demonstrate a more intense grieving experience, whereas the others expressed a sense of gratitude and peace surrounding the brief life of their child. Parents have told us themselves that they are able to be fully present for their baby when he/she is born due to the planning and guidance beforehand. It also allowed them to maximize the limited time to truly celebrate and welcome the baby before they had to say goodbye—an essential ingredient to their healing process.

Over time, the keepsakes accumulated during the pregnancy and birth—photographs and other objects can assist young siblings and parents to integrate the loss of the child into their family experience. Before delivery, a family picture can be taken with the family gathered closely around the mother, all hands placed gently on her abdomen. Because the baby may die in utero or at birth, this earlier image may be helpful in recording and preserving his or her presence in their lives. The team provides paint, poster board, and a memory box, then assists in obtaining handprints of the baby as well as of the entire family at the hospital to create another "family portrait." Because almost all NICUs and labor/delivery areas have developed procedures and activities for the experience of infant death, the hospice team works with the inpatient staff as a bridge of continuity in the parents' experience. Planning the "who, what, when, and where" for the delivery and beyond is important. If this information is not shared with the hospital staff, time may be lost and opportunities missed forever for some critical experiences for the family.

Making both the pregnancy and the death more real helps reduce denial of the loss. Mourning the dead child is facilitated by visual reminders over which families can grieve.[16] The social worker can provide parents with ideas for memorial services or assistance with final arrangements. The chaplain can assist them in personalizing these arrangements, helping to create the theme that reflects their beliefs and desires, and even helping to facilitate their wishes. Even a brief life is mourned for a very long time. Seeds for more "effective grieving" may be planted for the long journey ahead to recovery and healing.

ACCULTURATING AN AGENCY TO A PROGRAM TO SERVE CHILDREN

Integrating the Children's Program into the culture and values of San Diego Hospice is a goal in progress. Similarly, efforts continue on a national level to integrate pediatrics into the NHPCO's infrastructure and scope. Internal education and ongoing discussions were the first steps toward creating awareness of the service needs related to this unique population. Just as hospices initially had to confront issues of discomfort, fear, and personal barriers when caring for AIDS patients, the same must be done regarding pediatric patients. Admitting dying infants and children into programs poses an equally challenging situation for both clinical and nonclinical staff. The challenge is to "normalize" children as part of who is served by hospice care providers. As an industry, hospice and palliative care must commit to serving dying patients across the entire life span so that all families may receive this help as they face end-of-life care. Only then will it become integrated into more individual programs.

Ongoing efforts are needed for addressing the ethical issues related to removing life support, discontinuing aggressive care with a dying child, maintaining confidentiality, and incorporating the child or sibling's school into the plan of care. Prospective hospice employees, both clinical and nonclinical, are informed that infants, children, and young parents are part of the continuum of care. A detailed description of pediatric hospice care during staff interviews and hiring constitutes "informed consent" that the prospective employee acknowledges that these issues will be encountered within the agency. From the education committee to new hire orientation, and from the ethics committee to business development and marketing, the message is reiterated that children are part of the organizational mission and service population in a variety of ways. If left as the responsibility solely of the Children's Program staff, the potential may be diminished to truly foster an emphasis on children's issues in agency philosophy and practice.

Perhaps with this model as an example, other hospice programs and providers will examine how they might better address the needs of children and enhance their capacity to integrate the very young into their existing services. There is much to be done to support these families and advance the quality of end-of-life care for infants and children. Each step toward increasing awareness regarding these issues is a step forward on behalf of the children who are dying without access to all the resources available to them and their loved ones.

Nurses who choose to care for dying infants and children and their families need a significant support system themselves in order to maintain the difficult and delicate task of balancing perspectives. However, in doing so, nurses receive a spiritual treasure that only comes from experience with these children, parents, siblings, and others around them—heightened awareness of how very precious life is. Families share their wisdom from their tragedy, urging others to make the most of each moment in their own lives with their own loved ones. The courage and strength observed in families on this pilgrimage is humbling and strengthening at once. The staff of the Children's Program cherish and are grateful for the opportunity to be eyewitnesses to one of life's most intimate and powerful experiences.

Attempts to enhance end-of-life care for infants and children are gaining momentum, as evidenced by recent efforts to create a demonstration project with the Health Care Finance Administration, CHI, and NHPCO. Their effort aims to redesign the model of hospice care to more appropriately meet the needs of young patients and families. It will allow hospices to care for them through a model that begins at diagnosis of a terminal condition and continues through bereavement for the family. Through a collaborative effort with leaders in hospice care, pediatric hospice care, children's health care, and various branches of government, plans are moving forward for appropriations and site applications for the demonstration project.

The Children's International Project on Palliative/Hospice Services (ChiPPS) is an international work group led by Marcia Levetown, M.D. It represents the work of international experts and leaders in the field of pediatric hospice care who are developing a variety of research plans and identifying "best practice" examples and models of care for a compendium of resources to assist hospice programs more quickly to develop services for infants and children.

Hospice care for infants, children, and those around them focuses on living as fully and as normally as possible within the context, limitations, and opportunities that come with life-threatening illnesses. It seeks to provide children and their families with the means and opportunities to achieve self-directed life closure in a manner that is theirs to define. Pediatric hospice care aims to raise the consciousness of our society that claims to value children as a treasured resource. If this is so, then we must treasure them and honor them, in sickness and in health, in living and dying, until death do they part from us.

REFERENCES

1. Mellonie B, Ingpen R. Lifetimes: A Beautiful Way to Explain Death to Children. Toronto: Bantam, 1983.

2. Stevens M, Jones P, O'Riordan E. Family Responses When a Child With Cancer is in Palliative Care. Journal of Palliative Care 1996; 12: 51–55.

3. CHI 1998 Survey. Hospice Care for Children. Executive Summary Report, Alexandria, VA, June 1999.

4. "Hospice Standards of Practice: Draft", National Hospice Organization; Standards and Accreditation Committee, Alexandria, VA, July, 1999.

5. Ryndes, T. A Pathway for Patients and Families Facing Terminal Illness. Standards and Accreditation Committee; National Hospice Organization. Alexandria, VA, 1997.

6. Kaye P. Notes on Symptom Control in Hospice and Palliative Care. Essex, CT: Hospice Education Institute, 1994: 67–70.

7. Ferrell B, Virani R, Grant M. Analysis of End of Life Content in Nursing Textbooks. Oncology Nursing Forum 1999; 26:869–876.

8. Doyle D, Hanks GWC, McDonald N. Psychological Adaptation of the Dying Child. In: Oxford Textbook of Palliative Medicine: Oxford: 1993; 699–707.

9. Attig T. Beyond Pain: The Existential of Children. Journal of Palliative Care 1996; 12:20–23.

10. Jordan-Marsh MA, Sutters K, Sumner L. Pediatric Pain Management. In: Comprehensive Pain Management in Terminal Illness. 1996; 62–93.

11. Quick Reference Guide. Acute Pain Management in Infants, Children and Adolescents; Operative and Medical Procedures. Quick Reference Guide for Clinicians. Rockville, Maryland: Agency for Health Care Policy and Research, US Department of Health and Human Services, 1993.

12. Doyle D, Hanks GWC, MacDonald N, eds. Pain Control. In: Oxford Textbook of Palliative Medicine: Oxford: 1993: 681–698.

13. Ferrell BR, Rhiner M, Shapiro B, et al. The Family Experience of Cancer and Pain Management in Children. Cancer Practice 1994; 2: 441–446.

14. Doyle D, Hanks GWC, MacDonald N. Psychological Adaptation of the Dying Child. In: Oxford Textbook of Palliative Medicine 1993; 699–707.

15. Swanson-Kauffman K. "Caring in the instance of unexpected early pregnancy loss." Top Clin Nursing 1986; 8:37–46.

16. Leon IG. Perinatal Loss: A Critique of Current Hospital Practices. Clinical Pediatrics 1992; 366–374.

41 Pediatric Care: The Inpatient/ICU Perspective

MARCIA LEVETOWN

We always knew "Jorge" would die. I dreamed he would die in the Butterfly Room and so did he. Thank you—it was just as I imagined.

—Mother of 15-year-old with end-stage renal disease who died of sudden brain hemorrhage

Awful, gross—It's the worst thing in the world, having a child with cancer. The 20 months before her being diagnosed with cancer, I was in the hospital with blood clots . . . so my family went through entire craziness during that period. But at least from my point of view it was happening to me and not to my child. It's much worse when it's my child, and when she's in agony we're all in agony, and it's been terrible.

—A mother

Palliative care is comprehensive, interdisciplinary care focusing primarily on promoting quality of life for patients living with a life-threatening illness and their families.[1] It can and should occur from the earliest recognition of a life-threatening condition and can be concurrent with efforts to prolong life.[2,3] It is as applicable in the intensive care unit (ICU) setting as it is in the home. This is a critically important issue for children who die, since the vast majority of childhood deaths occur in an ICU setting. In fact, Wanzer and colleagues state:

> As sickness progresses toward death, measures to minimize suffering should be intensified. Dying patients may require palliative care of an intensity that rivals that of curative efforts. Even though aggressive curative techniques are no longer indicated, professionals and families are still called on to use intensive measures—extreme responsibility, extraordinary sensitivity, and heroic compassion.[4]

More than 55,000 children die annually in the United States.[5] Infants (<1 year of age) die primarily of congenital defects and prematurity; however, sudden infant death syndrome (SIDS) and trauma (including accidents and homicide) account for 11% of infant deaths. For children (age 1 year–19 years), 88% of deaths are the result of trauma, while the remaining 12% are comprised primarily of cancer, congenital anomalies, and heart disease. Trauma occurs in previously healthy children who are suddenly injured, and, in most cases, the initial use of all resuscitative measures is called for. In addition, some previously healthy children become suddenly ill from an overwhelming illness, such as a viral cardiomyopathy. Thus, the vast majority of children who die are appropriately cared for at least initially in the ICU setting, and most of those who die of these conditions currently die there as well. Even children with chronic illnesses and anticipated deaths often die in the ICU, though this may be less due to need or preferability than lack of alternatives or effective advance planning. In fact, 4.6% of pediatric ICU admissions end in death.[6–8]

However, few ICUs are places that one would choose to die. Most children and adults, when asked, prefer to die at home.[9,10] ICUs are not "homey."

There are a lot of rules that keep the ICU safe and efficient; these same rules may interfere with simultaneous visits from extended family and friends as a child's life draws to a close. ICUs are in the business of saving lives; scrupulous attention to communication, symptom control, and grief management have not been a traditional focus of training for personnel or health care delivery.[11] Yet, children and neonates will continue to die in ICUs. There are ways to meet these patients' and their families' needs for a peaceful, family-centered death even in these circumstances.

While individuals and families differ in the details and nuances of what their conception of a good death is, common themes emerge. Just as with adults, chronically ill children's biggest fears are abandonment by their medical caregivers and families.[12] It is often observed that children will endure treatments they no longer value to protect and not disappoint their parents and doctors. However, children also have needs and priorities in their final days and months that are determined to a large extent by their developmental maturity. For infants, this includes the physical presence of their family. The smell and feel of familiar people provide essential comfort. For toddlers, routines and familiar people and objects assume great importance; for older children, social contacts; and for teens, the ideal of having left a legacy and peer support are critical. The common ICU policy of limiting visitation can interfere with these aspects of achieving a "good death."

Most children and their families want as much honest, clearly and empathically communicated information regarding prognosis as they can get, beginning as early as possible in the course of illness, followed by regular updates as the prognosis changes. This allows rational decisions to be made based on the facts and on the values of the child and his or her family. Patients and families need to understand the anticipated disease trajectory and its associated symptoms and feel confident that they can manage them. They need to understand realistic options for medical care goals and the projected benefits and burdens of each option. They need to feel that have done everything that is "appropriate"; that they have been good, brave, and loving parents; and that the child has "been a fighter." They need to know what care venues are available to them and how to access them to avoid recurrent, nonbeneficial ICU admissions in the setting of chronic illness. Children with terminal conditions and their families often want spiritual consultation and guidance; it is very hard to understand why so tragic a thing as a child's death has to occur. Above all, children and their families want to feel valued as individuals, with the awesomeness of the impending death duly noted and the opportunity for closure and growth at the end of life to be realized to the greatest extent possible.[12–15] If these things are done well, more children with chronic, life-threatening conditions will have the opportunity to die outside the ICU, in a setting they or their family prefer. Avoidable ICU deaths are very taxing to the patient and family as well as the ICU personnel, who often begin to ask, "Are we doing this *to* the child or *for* him?"

Nevertheless, since a large proportion of children who die do die of acute conditions in the ICU, consideration of palliative care issues must be a part of the care plan.[16,17] The remainder of this chapter delineates the topics to be considered, explicates concrete suggestions for implementation, and provides case examples in a university hospital system that has instituted some of these strategies in the care of infants and children.

COMMUNICATION

Clear, honest, open communication is as critical a factor in the care of terminally ill infants and children as is any other factor. It may be even more significant because of the sensitivity required to assess the cognitive development of young patients. Some of the factors involved in achieving good communication during the terminal illnesses of children are covered in the following sections.

Preparation and Adherence to Advance Directives

Families and children need, and usually want, honest information with which to make good decisions regarding the goals of medical care. Children have a right to be offered information about their treatment options and the associated benefits and burdens.[4,18,19] This information must be presented in a manner consistent with the child's developmental capacity. Ideally, a patient with a chronic, progressive, and ultimately fatal illness would be provided information gradually and recurrently, in an outpatient setting, tailored to the child's particular condition and the family's value system, orchestrated by a longstanding primary care physician.[20–22]

Most state advance directive laws do not specifically mention children. However, while there is no mandate to address the issues of prognosis or future anticipatable medical interventions and their expected benefits and burdens for chronically ill children, the intent of advance directives applies equally to children with decision-making capacity as it does to adults.

Unfortunately, even when advance directives have been thoughtfully crafted and executed, there are rarely mechanisms in place to honor these decisions. In addition, parents may feel too guilty and too unprepared to follow through with their decisions to limit medical intervention. All too often, when the child begins to have the predicted deterioration, symptoms are inadequately controlled because no palliative care plan is in place and the patient appears in the emergency room in extremis.

On arrival at the emergency room, the family is often asked: "Do you want us to do 'everything'?" *Everything* is not further explained, so there is no reasonable answer but "Yes!" However, *everything* to the child and his or her family may mean everything to make the child comfortable, whereas to the physician it may mean everything to prolong survival, regardless of the extent of suffering. Assumptions should not be made; clarification of ambiguous terms must be accomplished to ensure that the care rendered is the care desired.[23] In addition, if the child's symptoms are aggressively controlled in the emergency room, more rational decision making can take place. The family could, for example, choose to have the child intubated for respiratory distress or to accept comfort management outside the ICU if extended survival is unduly burdensome for the child as an individual.

Moreover, many families harbor significant misconceptions regarding the outcomes of life-sustaining treatments. In particular, the misperceptions of a high likelihood of survival following CPR and the lack of awareness of the potential to develop significant disability after cardiac arrest have been documented;[24,25] the impact of accurate information on the increased likelihood to forgo CPR has also been proven.[26–28] Children have a particularly poor outcome from true cardiac arrest.[29–32] In the absence of intoxication and congenital heart disease, primary cardiac causes of arrest are exceedingly rare. Children have very healthy hearts. Thus, if cardiac arrest has occurred, it indicates that there is severe multi-organ dysfunction or that there has been a prolonged hypoxemia; neither of these underlying causes of arrest are amenable to medical treatment. Resuscitation in these settings does not commonly lead to intact survival. However, this is not the message that families understand when they are asked, "Do you want us to restart his heart?".

Similarly, seemingly benign comments, such as "He is stable," can be misinterpreted by families of dying children to mean "He is going to be all right." "She has gained weight" may mean the child's condition is worsening if the infant has heart failure but is universally interpreted as good news by parents. It is critical that members of the health care team communicate effectively with each other and that they give clear and consistent messages to the family. Participation of the bedside nurse in daily rounds and in family meetings makes this process smoother. The information that nurses gather from patients and parents at the bedside is critically important to the entire team in understanding what the patient and family already know, what questions they have, and what further explanations or discussions are needed. In addition, there is a need for excellent communication between nurses at shift change about what the family has been told and what they seem to understand. Parents often call at night to check on their children and get confused by conflicting messages.

It is important to realize that the role of parents as protectors is threatened by the possibility of the death of their child; this occasionally renders them unable to acknowledge or notice the suffering involved in the ongoing attempts to prolong life. For this reason, whenever possible, the knowing child (who may be as young as 3 years if he or she has been chronically ill)[12] should have a voice in the discussion of the goals of medical intervention.[16,33] In addition, the issues of parental guilt ("I can't let my child go—it would mean I failed as a parent") and family suffering should be frankly discussed. Reassuring parents that letting go is a loving decision has been helpful in the author's experience.

When discussing the choice to forgo life-sustaining medical intervention, the topic of current burdens of therapy as well as the probability of the hoped-for benefits must be clearly explained. Ineffective therapies must not be offered, and common misperceptions about the effectiveness of CPR must be proactively addressed. The proposal to forgo further attempts to prolong life should be presented as a recommendation, not a choice for the family to make alone. The benefits of stopping life-sustaining treatments can be presented as the benefit of dying at home, where possible, or, more commonly, increasing the chances of dying in the hospital at a time when the family is all there together to support the child and each other instead of at some unpredictable time in the middle of the night with no one around. Presenting the option inaccurately as "stopping care" is, not surprisingly, usually rejected. Patients and families fear abandonment above all else.[34,35] One of the most damaging sentences uttered in the context of irreversible illness is "There is nothing more that we can do." Above all, it is patently untrue. Despite our inability to cure or prolong life at all times, we *always* have something to offer, even if it is only ourselves.[36] Most important are the promises to care; to aggressively control symptoms; to be available; to assist (as a multidisciplinary team) in the arrangement of visits of family and friends; to facilitate the observation of important rituals; to provide spiritual guidance (when desired); and to transfer to alternate settings (according to the patient's and family's wishes).[37] The family may also need assistance with funeral arrangements and may benefit from bereavement follow-up.

Time-Limited Trials

Once the child is in the ICU receiving life-sustaining care, it is helpful to review the patient's progress continuously, monitoring the "big picture" of whether the patient is progressing along the hoped-for trajectory of illness or whether he or she is deteriorating despite the best medical management. Daily updates of this clinical information provided to the patient (when possible and appropriate) and the family can facilitate reasonable decision making, thereby avoiding burdensome and unhelpful care and diminishing the element of surprise on the day the patient dies.

Breaking Bad News: The Nurse's Role

While breaking bad news is difficult and stressful for everyone, being uninformed is even more stressful for patients and families. One of the most common complaints of patients and families is the lack of accurate and clearly communicated information.[38–43] Accompanying comments indicate a willingness and desire to receive bad news as long as it is empathically communicated. The diagnosis and prognosis associated with chronic conditions often provide confirmation of what was already suspected, thus frequently resulting in relief and reduction of anxiety. Reactions to bad news in the setting of an acute event are much more dramatic. In either case, accurate information allows a shifting of the goals of medical intervention and allows planning for family and friends to gather in a timely fashion to honor the dying child. Effective and compassionate communication may even allow the child to be discharged from the ICU, when desired, to die at home, or to die in a more private area of the hospital.[1,37,44]

Sometimes, in response to our own pain, medical caregivers communicate the news of a bad prognosis in a brief encounter and may use technical terms to "soften" the blow, or avoid the conversation altogether or wait until the child is unconscious.[21,45] Research on breaking bad news does not support these techniques.[46,47] Suggestions for breaking bad news in a way that leaves the child and family, as well as the medical caregivers, more satisfied include:

1. Provide a "warning shot" or an introductory sentence before presenting the distressing information: "I am sorry that I have some bad news to tell you."
2. Provide an opportunity for supportive friends or family to be present when the information is shared: "Would you like to call someone to be with you when we talk?"
3. Tell the news in a private setting, with the physician, nurse, and social worker present. Bring the family (generally parents without the child first, depending on relationships and preferences) to a private conference room rather than speaking to them in the waiting room or the hall. Bring tissues. If appropriate and desired by the family, assist them in telling their children (patient and siblings) afterwards.
4. Sit down near the family, not across a table. Do not stand. Children and families want to be on an even plane with their caregivers. Look the family members in the eye to engender trust. Ask them to tell

you about their child and about any consistent values of the child and about the things that give him or her pleasure. Ask how much they want to know about his or her medical condition and prognosis. Ask them what they understand is happening. Clarify misconceptions, particularly about the cause of the problem and attempt to assuage any guilt that may derive from having an inherited or developmental problem ("You did not wish for your child to have this") or from trauma or other causes. Then, let them know this news is difficult for you as well. Nurses can help guide the physician to present the truth in a jargon-free manner that is consonant with the family's educational level, sophistication, and stated desire for knowledge. Ask the family to explain what they understood was said. Clarify misconceptions. Then, solicit additional questions.

5. Be unhurried. If there is only a limited time available for the physician, let the family know: "I'm sorry the doctor only has 15 minutes now, but I will stay with you and answer any questions I can and the doctor will be back later this afternoon to answer anything I can't and to update you." Don't look at your watch. Have the charge nurse or another nurse care for your patients while you sit with the family. Remind the other team members to give their beepers to someone else during the family meeting, when possible; otherwise, switch the beepers to vibrate mode.
6. Ideally, members of the multidisciplinary team participate as full members during the family conference.[48] The bedside nurse, chaplain, and social worker benefit from hearing the physician–family interaction. They can solicit questions, clarify misconceptions during the meeting and after the physician leaves, and address other facets of the patient's situation that the conversation with the physician evokes. Team members can also give the physician feedback regarding his or her communication with the patient and family, such as words they did not understand, and can help the physician address any unresolved issues at the next meeting. This technique requires interdisciplinary respect and cooperation, which are essential to successful, comprehensive end-of-life care; it prevents divisive misunderstandings between disciplines regarding suspected coercion or other undesirable communication.
7. Bring trainees to the family meeting. This allows the assigned nursing or medical student and resident to learn from directly observing the interdisciplinary critical care team, as well as the patient and family responses. It keeps trainees informed so that unnecessary and often damaging miscommunications do not occur. Trainees often get lost in the minutiae of the patients' laboratory values and vital signs and may unwittingly provide contradictory information to the family. However, do not overwhelm the family with white coats—have trainees take turns in attending family meetings.
8. Be specific. The physician should present the options, include a description of life-sustaining treatments, the child's current status, the chance of survival, the probability of full recovery (and the probability of significant disability), and the possible effects of the child's long-term survival on the family.[21] Recommendations for the next step should be presented, based on the team's experience and on the goals and values of the patient, as well as the observations of patient and family members during the meeting and the hospitalization overall. Be sure to explain the benefits and burdens (including prolongation of suffering) of each potential care plan, the potential reversibility or irreversibility of the conditions being treated, the time frame for reevaluation, the projected future quality of life, and the comfort measures available if the ICU interventions are curtailed or discontinued. Give reassurances that, if life-sustaining medical interventions are discontinued, the child will continue to receive attentive care for the relief of symptoms; describe the procedures to be undertaken, including the opportunities to observe important customs and rituals and the visitation allowances.[16]

Avoidance of the topic of a poor prognosis and the performance of "slow codes" are ethically unjustifiable actions.[49,122] They deprive the family and patient of the potential for peaceful and final goodbyes, a commonly lamented missed opportunity.

AGGRESSIVE SYMPTOM MANAGEMENT

The symptoms most commonly suffered by dying children are poorly documented but include pain, seizures, problems with secretion control, dyspnea, vomiting;[50] perceptions of isolation and abandonment;[12] existential pain ("What did my existence mean to the world?"[51]); relational pain ("I was mean to my brother and I need to say I'm sorry"); and spiritual pain ("What could I have done to deserve this?"). The SUPPORT (Study to Understand Prognoses and Preferences for Outcomes and Risks of Treatment) trial demonstrated that current adult ICU practice does not address these issues adequately;[52,53] it is unlikely that pediatric and neonatal ICUs do any better. In fact, a recent paper[123] demonstrates that even the most respected institutions frequently fail to effectively manage pain. When attended to by a skilled multidisciplinary team focusing on these issues as primary concerns, these symptoms are usually successfully addressed. (For explanations of the management of these issues, the reader is referred to *The Oxford Textbook of Palliative Medicine* by Doyle, Hanks, and MacDonald, New York: Oxford University Press, 1998.) A few overarching principles deserve further mention, however.

Pain

Pain is a subjective phenomenon. It is not measured by vital signs, presence or absence of sleep, blood or imaging tests, or the size of an incision. Pain severity is most accurately assessed when measured by patient self-report.[54–56] Several tools exist to facilitate child pain self-report, including visual analogue scale (a 10-cm. line with anchors "no pain = 0 and the worst pain you can imagine = 10. Mark the amount of pain you are experiencing"); the categorical scale (no pain, a little pain, medium pain, and very, very bad pain); and the numerical scale ("0–5, 5 is the worst pain you can imagine"). Children <7 years of age respond well to the faces scale (categorical, with face cartoons to illustrate), the best validated being the Bieri scale,[57] which has too many choices for very young children. Other options include the Oucher scale,[58] Eland color tool,[59] and Wong–Baker faces scales,[60] among others.[61] Of course, when children are sedated or unable to communicate because of developmental immaturity, caregivers need to interpret the child's pain. Primary nursing assignments facilitate this assessment. Parents also are important resources for pain assessment.

The severity of reported pain dictates the category of pain relievers needed to relieve the pain, irrespective of etiology. For example, according to the World Health Organization (WHO) pain management guidelines for children, severe pain, regardless of etiology, demands prompt treatment with a "strong opioid," such as morphine, hydromorphone (dilaudid), fentanyl, or methadone.[56]

Dying adult patients often have pain. The occurrence of pain is not well documented in the terminally ill pediatric patient, but suspicion of pain must remain high, and presumptive treatment should occur if there are indications it is present. Where possible, each pain needs to be categorized not only by severity, but also by character (burning, gnawing, throbbing, sharp, crampy), location and radiation, duration, continuous or intermittent nature, and precipitating and relieving factors. The quality and timing of the pain suggest the etiology of the pain and dictate the most efficacious treatment. This ideal is very difficult to achieve in young or developmentally disabled children and in sedated or intubated patients. An empiric judgment of the etiology and physiology of the pain often dictates the choice of intervention in the ICU setting.

Constipation, a common problem in the ICU setting, may present with intermittent, poorly localized, crampy abdominal pain. Treatment with opioids would not be as beneficial as a heating pad and a laxative or, when needed, an enema. Burning pain in a patient who received neurotoxic chemotherapy is a sign of neuropathic pain, that is, pain related to nerve injury. This pain is best treated with "adjuvant pain relievers" (medications most often used for other purposes, but which are effective in the relief of certain types of pain), such as tricyclic antidepressants and anticonvulsants in addition to "traditional" pain-relieving agents. Unfortunately, in the ICU setting, some adjuvants may not be of benefit, as they must be given for at least one week to achieve effectiveness. Thus, depending on the patient's circumstance, the best pain management may be the use of nonpharmacologic techniques and aggressive use of traditional pain relievers, including opioids.

Concerns about addiction, a psychological phenomenon of craving a drug despite harm to oneself (which has been shown to be vanishingly rare in the medical use of opioids), are inappropriate in the ICU. "As needed" or PRN medications should be ordered for the alleviation of the expected side effects of opioids, such as nausea, pruritus, urinary retention, and somnolence (when it is undesirable). Constipation is a predictable side effect that does not resolve, but it is less of an issue in a child who is expected to die within 24 hours, as do most ICU patients undergoing the withdrawal or withholding of life-sustaining medical intervention.[53] Changing the specific opioid used[62] may also be considered for the management of refractory opioid-induced side effects when the child's expected survival is longer. Alternative routes of pain relief, such as epidurals for children who are excessively somnolent or who become delirious with systemically administered opioids, may be of benefit in some cases.

Respiratory depression in the face of pain is an uncommon occurrence, despite aggressive use of opioids for pain relief.[63,64] Irregular breathing caused by pain can often be smoothed and become more effective for gas exchange when pain is relieved. Pupillary size can help in the assessment of the opioid titration of preverbal or nonverbal patients (personal observation).

Pain can be treated effectively only if the results of the intervention are reassessed at the appropriate interval, based on the pharmacokinetics of the medication and route used.[54,56] If pain relief is not achieved, an additional intervention should be undertaken immediately, *not* at the next timed dosage. For instance, if the patient reports severe pain (a score of 10/10) and morphine is administered intravenously, the child should be reassessed in 15 minutes. If the report remains the same ("severe pain, pain scale score 8/10"), an additional dose of morphine should be administered *immediately*. This process should continue until the child is comfortable. *There is no maximum dose of opioids. The proper dose is the dose that controls the pain.* The goal is not to sedate the child unless the child desires this; the goal is to relieve the pain. On occasion, pain can be relieved only with aggressive analgesia and sedation.[65]

Medication for consistent pain should be administered on a schedule, around the clock or by constant infusion (not PRN, or "as needed"). Additionally, medication for "breakthrough" pain (pain occurring despite the regular administration of medication) should be prescribed. The reader is referred to the Agency for Health Care Policy and Research (AHCPR) guidelines for pain management,[55] available from the U.S. federal government online, as well as other standard pain references[66,67] and to chapter 6 on pain management in this text. Successful pain management cannot occur unless pain is regarded as a priority, pain is regularly assessed and reassessed, and pain scale scores are documented routinely.[68]

Dyspnea

Often children or their families prefer to forgo mechanical ventilation if there is no reasonable expectation of improvement or cure, with the exception of some patients with neuromuscular disorders who are still young and intellectually intact. When the choice is to discontinue or not initiate mechanical ventilation, scrupulous attention to the management of dyspnea must be explained and promised to the child (if capable of participating) and the family, and the promise must be realized. The idea that there may be a trade-off between relief of dyspnea and sedation, or even a slightly earlier death, must also be broached and preferences elicited. Most families express preferences for enhanced comfort even in the face of a potentially foreshortened survival. However, this is not a foregone conclusion and, as has been previously reported,[69] occasionally patients are much less distressed than anticipated and are able to enjoy a few hours or even days with carefully titrated opioids, as needed.

In the few studies reviewing duration of survival related to the administration of morphine during withdrawal of mechanical ventilation, however, patients of all ages actually survive *longer* when liberal doses of morphine are used to ease the dyspnea.[64,69,70] The goals of care must be clear in everyone's mind prior to proceeding, lest the tragedy of perceptions of wrongdoing plague survivors.[71]

Dyspnea is a symptom that is even more distressing than pain to experience or witness. It is difficult to control and requires intensive hands-on management and reassessment. Several nonpharmacologic approaches can be helpful, such as sitting the child upright, having a parent or other close family member or friend present, saying soothing words, and touching the child. In addition, having a small fan blowing air across the child's face has been found to be helpful in the hospice setting.

There are no published data on the treatment of dyspnea in children; the few small controlled studies done support the use of opioids as the pharmacologic agents of choice in the management of dyspnea.[72] Clinical experience has shown efficacy of opioids in alleviating dyspnea as well.[73,74] The dose of opioids that is optimal is the dose that effectively relieves the dyspnea. This dose must be established by titration to clinical effect. Again, there is no maximal dose.

Various recommendations for the pharmacologic management of dyspnea exist.[70,73–75] Regardless of the protocol used, it is imperative that the child be continuously observed and repeatedly treated until symptom relief is achieved. The dose should be rapidly and aggressively escalated if ineffective. The author's preference is to use intravenous preparations in the setting of extubation to gain rapid control. For example, if the child is receiving 5 mg. of morphine intravenously per hour, the bolus dose would be 5 mg. if dyspnea occurred at extubation. If the initial dose is totally ineffective, the next dose should be 50% to 100% higher, 7.5 to 10 mg. If, 5 minutes later, the patient is still *in extremis*, the next dose would be 50%–100% higher. Often, children respond to these first few doses and the dyspnea is controlled without loss of consciousness. The expected response to opioids is gradual slowing of respirations to a more normal level; respirations do not suddenly cease unexpectedly. Reversal with naloxone or other opioid antagonists should rarely, if ever, be undertaken. The recommended procedure, when done, is to dilute the naloxone 1:10 and administer very slowly, repeating as needed.

Benzodiazepines alleviate the breathlessness associated with anxiety but not the sensation of dyspnea itself. Administration of diuretics to children with pulmonary edema, withholding intravenous fluids or enteral feedings, or adding anticholinergic agents may decrease excess secretions. Thorough suctioning of endotracheal tubes prior to extubation of mechanically ventilated children is very helpful as well.

Terminal Sedation

Occasionally, a technique known as terminal sedation is necessary to control symptoms, most often pain, dyspnea, and intractable seizures. At least within the palliative care community, terminal sedation has become a generally accepted plan of care for adults in the case of otherwise uncontrollable symptoms, though somewhat more reluctantly so for children who, cannot always independently consent in advance.[65] Although considered an "acceptable and justifiable form of euthanasia or physician-assisted suicide" (PAS) by some,[76–78] others see terminal sedation as the extension of the tenet that, above all, the health care provider's duty is to relieve suffering. The intention is not to bring about the demise of the child (as in the case of PAS and euthanasia),[79,80] but rather to control the symptom, even at risk of death (principle of double effect).

Regardless of the philosophical underpinnings that lead to the practice, terminal sedation is widely regarded as the only humane solution to an otherwise uncontrollable and severely distressing problem. It is only undertaken after all other attempts at symptom control have failed and with the full agreement of the child and family.[65] Full explanations of the inability to reverse the underlying process must precede this decision. Some practitioners also utilize barbiturates for the management of terminal dyspnea and pain.[75] Barbiturates are particularly helpful in relieving labored or agonal respirations.

Unfortunately, significant discomfort and uncertainty on the part of many critical care practitioners impede the availability of these therapeutic strategies. Clinicians fear being perceived as the proximate cause of death due to the administration of opioids,[69] despite numerous well-known ethical opinions that the relief of symptoms is the primary obligation to the dying patient. Critical care nurses giving opioids to terminally ill patients withdrawn from mechanical ventilation reported that they believed they were engaging in euthanasia.[81] On the other hand, the administration of neuromuscular blocking agents can constitute euthanasia, impedes the ability to assess dyspnea, and should be avoided whenever possible.[82]

Extubation Technique

Prior to extubation, engaging in family-centered rituals is important (see case examples below). This allows unhurried family time while the child is still pink and breathing. As the family is approaching readiness to extubate, they should be informed about what they can expect after extubation, making this difficult time easier. ("He may turn blue; we will treat this with morphine and oxygen if he looks uncomfortable. He may not breathe at all or may breathe comfortably for some time. I do not know how long he will live, but I expect it will be on the order of (minutes, hours, days). I will stay with you until he is comfortable.") Positive thoughts about extubation are important to share as well. ("This will be the first time you see your daughter's beautiful face without tape and a tube interfering"; "I am giving you back your son as a child, not as a patient"; "You can hear his voice for the first time in a while", depending on the age and circumstances of the child.)

The author's practice, both as an intensivist and as a palliative care physician tending primarily to pediatric ICU patients, is to avoid "terminal weaning," or the gradual decrease of mechanical ventilation support. Terminal weaning allows the child to be dyspneic as well as to have the discomfort of being intubated until he or she becomes unconscious, either from sedatives or carbon dioxide narcosis. Continued intubation also masks the severity of the child's distress and may lead to inadvertent undermedication; it is critical to constantly assess discomfort and take steps to alleviate it, whether this consists of the simple act of having a loved one stroke the child's hand, giving reassurances of love, or rapidly increasing dosages of opioids or other interventions. The policy of decreasing supplemental oxygen in hypoxic children puts them at increased risk of discomfort. On the other hand, nonhypoxic children do not require the inconvenience and discomfort of supplemental oxygen. Another reason to prefer rapid extubation is that the tape and endotracheal tube create physical barriers between the child and family, who otherwise may feel more freedom to ply the child with kisses, indicating continued love and devotion, attending the devastating symptom of perceived abandonment.

Children with significant central nervous system compromise may have noisy respirations due to floppy pharyngeal soft tissues. The family needs to be made aware of this possibility *prior* to extubation. Management strategies include repositioning, discontinuation of intravenous fluid or enteral intake, administration of anticholinergic medications, aggressive suctioning of artificial airways prior to removal, or placement of a nasal trumpet. The latter, however, creates a physical wedge between the child and family and should be avoided when possible.

CHILD PREFERENCES AND CRITICAL CARE PRACTICES OF WITHHOLDING OR WITHDRAWING MEDICAL INTERVENTIONS

Physician indoctrination of the imperative to preserve life at all costs must not override patients' values. Most studies indicate that, in practice, the justification for forgoing life-sustaining medical intervention (LSMI) in ICUs, whether the patient is a child[8] or an adult,[48] is physician assessment of poor prognosis for survival, rather than quality of life considerations.[83–88] Reassessing the goals of treatment only when the child is dying deprives the patient of choices that the child and family may make earlier to enhance the quality of life rather than extend the duration of life.[16,40] Children who cannot be cured and their families often have preferences regarding medical interventions. Their opinions are not knowable by the medical team a priori; they must be actively solicited.[89–93] In addition, the child's perceptions of discomfort relative to various medical interventions may be very different than medical caregivers' perceptions. In fact, regardless of the presence of a terminal prognosis, patients and their surrogates have the right to forgo LSMI.[94–96]

Thus, the current practice of withholding discussions regarding burdens and benefits of ongoing LSMI is insupportable. Refusing to honor a child's or surrogates' requests to stop LSMI until the child is certain to die is even worse.[97–99] Patient suffering must play a much more prominent role in the decision making process if "good deaths" are to be attained for a higher proportion of patients.[48,100] On the other hand, physicians' personal biases regarding quality of life and economic motivations for the withdrawal of LSMI should not play any role in the decision to forgo treatment.[89,101]

Finally, it has been shown that physicians' practices in withdrawing medical interventions are more determined by personal idiosyncrasy[89,102] and fears of litigation or accusation of wrongdoing than by the patient's comfort.[103,104] In several studies, vasopressors were withheld first, oxygen next, and mechanical ventilation next. However, oxygen supplementation and extubation may be preferred and more comfortable. In addition, withholding antibiotics and allowing the peaceful death associated with sepsis may be the most humane option available for some children. In other cases, forgoing nutrition may ease nausea, and forgoing hydration may decrease the discomfort of renal failure or congestive heart failure.[105,106] Obviously, much depends on the child's symptoms and clinical situation and the child's and family's values and preferences. Effecting a philosophical change among medical decision-makers to proactively solicit children's and families' perspectives may be accomplished by educational intervention, although it is likely that cultural changes within institutions may have more promise.[44]

Review of the Patient Care Plan

After it has been determined that the child and family no longer subscribe to the goal of prolongation of life, because either the burdens are too great or the effort is "futile," the care plan must be reviewed in detail. The likely mechanisms of death must be determined and plans to ameliorate associated symptoms of these mechanisms should be made. It is not uncommon for the child to have several potential mechanisms for death; often, one route can be anticipated to be the most comfortable, such as dying from hyperkalemia or sepsis as opposed to hypoxemia. In this case, kayexalate or dialysis as well as antibiotics should be discontinued, and oxygen, by nasal cannula or "blow-by," if possible, should be continued.

Anticipation of likely symptoms and care plans that address them proactively are essential.[107] For instance, if the child is likely to have seizures but cannot swallow, rectal or parenteral, rapid-onset anticonvulsants should be written as a p.r.n. order. Developmentally appropriate explanations about the possible course of events should be given to the child and family unless they refuse this information. It is unwise to predict an exact time of death, but approximations (with significant margin for error) are very helpful for the family to arrange for the child's other loved ones and friends to visit before or be present at death.

All interventions that either interfere with comfort or that do not enhance it should be discontinued. For instance, laboratory tests are not designed to enhance comfort. Sometimes in clinical practice, laboratory parameters, such as platelet counts, are monitored to prevent symptoms such as bleeding from arising. However, it is just as efficacious and less intrusive to monitor the patient for clinical bleeding and treat if and when it arises, if desired. Medications that do not enhance comfort, often including antibiotics, should be considered for discontinuation. Even feeding and intravenous fluids may interfere with comfort if the child has pulmonary edema, heart failure, or renal failure; a decrease in or cessation of these therapies may enhance the child's comfort.

Monitors, such as pulse oximeters, cardiorespiratory monitors, and the like should be removed; they create physical barriers to the closeness of loved ones with the child, distract them from attending to the child with their color displays and flashing lights, create distressing alarms that all have agreed not to respond to, and create a reason for the health care team not to enter the room. Visitation restrictions and many of the usual rules should be reconsidered. Maximization of holding the child or even allowing the family members to climb in bed with the child should be facilitated. Letting the family bathe the child and dress him or her in clothing of the family's choice is often helpful. Other special requests should be honored if at all possible.

Transfer to Alternative Care Settings

When children are acknowledged to be dying, it is common for large numbers of loved ones to gather. They need to support the child, parents, siblings, and each other. Sometimes they may desire to perform rituals that may be difficult to accommodate in the ICU setting. Thus, consideration for transfer to an alternate care setting should be made. If the child is anticipated to live for a few days once ICU interventions are discontinued, referral to hospice in the home care setting should be considered. Usually a one- to two-day stay in the hospital to ensure "stability" and to provide family caregiver teaching is needed. Alternatively, if the child will have significant distress in his or her final days, or the child and/or family prefer to stay in the hospital, admission to the floor, or preferably a palliative care unit, may be the best plan.[1,37,101,102] As large a room as is needed to accommodate the child and his or her loved ones should be provided, if possible.

The Butterfly Room

At the University of Texas Medical Branch at Galveston, we have created an alternative care unit for children with life-threatening conditions called the Butterfly Room.[108] It is a home-like setting distinctly different from any other room in the hospital, with carpeting, wallpaper with butterflies, a kitchenette, TV, Nintendo and VCR, pull-out sofa beds and chairs, padded window seats overlooking the Gulf of Mexico, and storage, as well as a place for the child to sleep. It is as large as two semiprivate rooms and is designed to accommodate the entire family.

One use of the room is for ICU patients who are expected to die within minutes to days following extubation, and who are thus generally not candidates for transfer home. After consultation with the family, it is our practice to review the medical orders and discontinue all laboratory tests, all invasive equipment (extra intravenous sites, nasogastric tubes, urinary catheters, etc.), all monitors (including the recording of vital signs, fluid balance, and weights), and all medications other than those contributing to the comfort of the patient. Orders not to resuscitate are written with the family's agreement. The child, who is still being mechanically ventilated, with vasopressors infusing as needed, is then moved from the ICU to the Butterfly Room. Resuscitative medications, such as atropine and epinephrine, are brought in the elevator for unstable patients to ensure that the family will have a chance for final togetherness, but these medications have never been used. Cardiopulmonary resuscitation beyond these medications would not be done, however.

In the Butterfly Room, the child's loved ones are invited to sit in a rocking chair, or, in the case of an older child, they are invited to sit on a couch and hold the child. Even young siblings participate in this activity. Usually, each family member in turn will whisper loving thoughts and memories to the dying child. Numerous photographs are taken in most cases. The family is offered the opportunity to bathe the child, make handprints and footprints, and dress the child in clothing of their choice. Other rituals specific to the family or their heritage may be undertaken. Once these events have taken place, with the family's acknowledgment of readiness, the child is extubated. Morphine, benzodiazepines, and blow-by oxygen are immediately available. The multidisciplinary hospice team, including a spiritual leader of the family's choosing, if desired, a social worker, a child life therapist for siblings, and the nurse and physician remain either in the room or close by, often mingling among the distressed relatives and listening to their concerns, as well as attending to the patient's symptoms.

CONSIDERATION OF SUFFERING AND FUTURE QUALITY OF LIFE

It has been documented that, against the legal and ethical principles currently in place, physicians often refuse requests to forgo life-sustaining treatment.[95] Since discontinuation of LSMI often leads to the patient's death, this action must be undertaken with caution, ensuring that the child is not making decisions on the basis of depression or the family making decisions based on exhaustion or financial pressures. However, refusal of LSMI may well represent the child's and family's assessment of future quality of life, often based on the experience of lived, progressive disability and chronic illness, or on long-held values.

Surrogates' (or parents') duties are to act on the *child's* wishes and in his or her best interests.[91–94,109–112] This role is often not clear and requires explanation. Surrogates, in the author's experience, more often request prolongation of a child's death due to guilt and fear, rather than discontinuation of LSMI too prematurely. Thus, overriding requests to terminate LSMI must also be done with significant forethought and analysis. In addition, the motivation for requests to continue LSMI in the face of an extremely small likelihood of survival, or very large chance of a significantly poor quality of life, must be explored fully. Issues of guilt ("What do you think caused his problems? You were away at work when the accident happened?") and loss ("Tell me about what has happened to your family as a result of your child's condition?" "It sounds like you've been through a lot. I wish I could make your child healthy and make it all OK again but unfortunately, there are limits to what medicine can do. The best we can reasonably hope for, medically, is. . . . Does that change your perspective on treatment options? Our recommendations, based on all you've told us and our assessment of your child's condition is. . . ."). Eliciting and demonstrating respect for the family's and child's (where applicable) values can be helpful in resolving these dilemmas.

Notification of Death

Unless there are extremely extenuating circumstances, even if the death is expected, most experts strongly encourage that the notification of death be done in person. ("Mrs. Smith, I am afraid I have some bad news. Could you come in to discuss it?") Empathy can be more easily expressed in person by sitting close at the time of the discussion, perhaps even giving the bereaved a hug, or shedding a genuine tear. These small tokens of warmth and understanding help the family to know that the medical team cared about the child as a person. Additionally, insistence that the family come in allows them to see the dead child, which facilitates the acceptance of the fact that death has occurred and allows the family to participate in important rituals, such as bathing the dead, sometimes assisting in the removal of equipment, or sitting vigil as some cultures require. These efforts result in improved bereavement outcomes, particularly for siblings, who often imagine the child has not actually died.

Bereavement Follow-Up

Studies have repeatedly shown an increased mortality rate of surviving spouses in the year following death.[113–115] No similar studies of bereaved parents or siblings have been done, though the divorce rate in the first year after a child's death is higher than the national average. (Over the long term, however, the proportion returns to the national average of 50%.) It is not known what interventions are most effective for bereaved parents. Some lessons may derive from studies of bereaved spouses.

A simple strategy of routinely sending a bereavement card two weeks following the death of a hospitalized patient was investigated. One year later, the bereaved survivors could consistently and without warning retrieve the card, indicating the importance to them of such a gesture. Remarks of survivors of patients who had died in the emergency room included, "At least I know my husband died among caring people."[116] Attending the deceased's funeral is an even more powerful demonstration of caring and may provide relief for the medical caregiver as well.[117]

If an autopsy was performed, families need a face-to-face appointment (autopsy conference) with the treating physician to explain the autopsy findings in understandable terms. Often, this explanation gives the bereaved family a profound sense of peace by affirming the cause of death, affirming the irreversibility of the problems, or determining a cause of death that was unknown antemortem. It is particularly important to rule out heritable conditions that may affect surviving or future siblings. This process has even been found to improve adaptation to loss. The autopsy visit also allows monitoring of the family's grieving process and provides the opportunity for referral to counseling, if needed, for pathologic grief reactions. In the absence of a face-to-face session, families consenting to an autopsy often complain that they had no follow-up and express anger and suspicion about the motivations for the autopsy. This post-death conference is also helpful for families who did not consent to autopsy, to answer questions and monitor for adaptive grieving. Referrals can be made for families needing counseling or other assistance.

A memorial service may also be offered. This may take several forms; two are particularly suggested for the ICU. Some children's families who have either come to the ICU recurrently, or others who have particularly bonded with the staff due to a child's prolonged stay or for other reasons, may be invited back to the unit with the families of a few other children who have died within the last month or six weeks for a ceremony of sharing. The family may bring a picture of the child, and the family and staff can exchange memories of the child. Songs may be sung, poems may be read, and prayers may be shared. Gratitude and admiration may be exchanged. In addition, all families bereaved of children could be invited to a group memorial service conducted on an annual or more frequent basis.

Grief of Medical Caregivers

Not only do children suffer and families and loved ones grieve, but we as medical caregivers grieve for our patients, their families, and ourselves. We are exposed to pain and grief both vicariously and in empathy and are forced to confront the certainty of our own and our fellow humans' mortality on a daily basis. In caring for dying children, we are threatened by the reality that our own children, too, could die. The ability to share these feelings in a supportive environment, without sanction, and the ability to take leave to attend funerals can assist in increased job satisfaction and retention of highly skilled critical care personnel. It can also help reinforce the humanity that makes us optimal medical caregivers.

Palliative Care for All Patients

The focus on prevention of suffering and on the person as a whole should not be reserved solely for the dying child. All children, from clinic patients to ICU patients to dying children, should have access to the best that medicine has to offer. As a wise man stated very long ago, "The medical care provider's duty is to cure sometimes, to relieve often, and to comfort always."[118]

TEACHING END-OF-LIFE CARE

Once palliative care philosophy and methods are embraced, they should extend beyond the ICU. Ongoing efforts to teach the principles and practice of palliative medicine must occur to ensure that our trainees are as capable as possible of carrying on the tradition of humane and person-centered end-of-life care. Several courses are described in the literature and could easily be adapted for use in other settings.[118–121]

RECOMMENDATIONS FOR IMPLEMENTATION

Improved end-of-life care begins with more highly focused attention on the individual child and his or her preferences and values. Pediatric and neonatal ICU practitioners are the caregivers for the vast majority of children who die; thus, they must have expertise in palliative care. Some recommendations to enhance end-of-life care in the pediatric and neonatal ICU setting are:

- Admission procedures should include a values history; solicitation of any advance directives for older, chronically ill children; and discussion of expressed preferences in light of the child's current situation. This should not be reserved only for imminently dying children. Waiting until that time only increases the chances that the child's preferences will never be known and the family's guilt will be unnecessarily increased in the event they are later called upon to consent to the withdrawal of life-sustaining medical intervention. Good coordination with primary care providers and specialists who care for chronically ill children is helpful.
- Attention to pain and the relief of other symptoms, both during procedures and more generally, must become a priority for all children. This can be accomplished only with training and appropriate documentation procedures, as well as emphasis by supervisors and attending physicians.
- Improved communication techniques must be employed that allow children or their surrogates to understand their options in a supportive and unbiased way. Guilt, missed opportunities, love, and existential and spiritual issues should be included in these discussions. Again, training must be developed and carried out. The importance of these issues must be emphasized, demonstrated, and reflected in the practices of the opinion leaders within the unit.
- Cooperation, respect, and regular interdisciplinary rounds among the disciplines of nursing, medicine, social work, pastoral care, and, possibly, palliative care (and others as indicated, such as pharmacy, occupational therapy, physical therapy, child life) will enhance the larger understanding of the child and his or her needs and facilitate the team's ability to assist the child with the accomplishment of his or her goals.
- Establishment of a bereavement follow-up program, including the mailing of bereavement cards, autopsy debriefing or post-death sessions, "sharing sessions," and memorial services will improve the bereavement outcome for surviving loved ones and ICU staff.
- Excused paid absences for funeral attendance and staff support sessions will prevent burnout and turnover and allow the retention of the ideals and values that brought each staff member to the healing professions.

SUMMARY

Infants die primarily of congenital defects, prematurity, and SIDS. Children older than one year of age die primarily from trauma, thus predisposing them to die in ICU settings. The principles of palliative care must be applied to all children, even those whose fate is to die in the ICU. Our challenge, as practitioners of neonatal and pediatric critical care medicine, is to provide each of these children a "good death." This can be achieved by intensive attention to the child's and family's perspectives and goals, communication within the team and with the child and his or her loved ones, dedication to the meticulous management of symptoms, particularly during procedures—the most common source of discomfort in ill children—and effective bereavement follow-up.

Case Study: F. L., a Near-Drowning Victim

F. L., a 14-year-old Pakistani boy suffered a near-drowning episode that compromised his central respiratory drive mechanism and left him neurologically devastated. His family was informed that life-sustaining medical interventions were futile. They agreed to move him to the Butterfly Room to achieve a family-centered death. Orders not to resuscitate were written in a clear and detailed manner. All laboratory analyses were discontinued, and all monitors were removed. Medications were reviewed and all were discontinued. Morphine and lorazepam were added for the management of dyspnea, I.V. fluids were discontinued, and scopolamine was administered for terminal secretions. One intravenous catheter was left intact, but all other invasive monitors, such as nasogastric tubes, urinary and arterial catheters, etc., were removed. During his transfer from the ICU to the Butterfly Room, he remained mechanically ventilated.

Although F. L. had a small family, he belonged to a close-knit community. Thirty people of all ages came to be with him on his final day of life. They encircled the boy's bed, chanting but not touching him. After approximately 30 minutes, they approached the team and announced their readiness for the discontinuation of mechanical ventilation. One caregiver stated that she was unfamiliar with Pakistani traditions and customs, but had not observed anyone touching F. L. She suggested that if touching was allowable and desirable for them, they were welcome to do so. The whole tenor of the group changed, with the circle drawing nearer the bed and men openly grieving and weeping, holding the boy and their wives, as well as each other. People stroked F. L.'s face and body. After an hour, they again informed the team that they were now ready to have the mechanical ventilation discontinued.

F. L. was suctioned and extubated and needed little pharmacologic intervention.

His loved ones chanted from the moment the endotracheal tube was removed. Each visitor, in turn, put small amounts of holy water in his mouth. Although the water bubbled out of his nose, a caregiver wiped it away, giving "permission" for the next person to engage in the ritual. After 27 minutes of nonstop chanting, F. L. died. A peaceful hush fell over the room, and all eyes turned to the same window leading to the outside.

Case Study: L. F., a Newborn with Hypoplastic Left Heart Syndrome

L. F., a newborn, was diagnosed with hypoplastic left heart syndrome. After a full explanation of the surgical options, the family opted for palliative care. The mother preferred never to see the baby again, because she feared bonding with her child. The baby was in the ICU but, because of her parents' decision, was not receiving ICU interventions. The parents were approached about the Butterfly Program, providing surrogate parents and moving the baby to the Butterfly Room; they agreed. They decided to visit the baby the next day. She was wearing normal baby clothes, being cared for and appearing like any other baby. When they saw that the baby did not need highly skilled care, they felt that they could care for her themselves at home with the help of the Butterfly Program. The next day, the parents took their daughter home. L. F. lived well there and visited many churches for blessings, went to numerous restaurants, had house guests, received several hospice visits, and was asymptomatic until her final day at two weeks of age, when she began to vomit and become intermittently cyanotic. The Butterfly Team (nurse, social worker, and physician) was summoned to the home. Additional explanations of what was happening and assurances of the child's comfort were provided. The baby received one dose of morphine, but the family assessed that she did not need more. She died in her mother's arms eight hours after the first cyanotic episode.

Case Study: G. G., a Seven-Day-Old Infant with Anuria

G. G., a seven-day-old male infant, was anuric and referred from a hospital located three and one-half hours away by ground transport from the tertiary care hospital. Diagnostic studies showed complete absence of a urinary collecting system and hypoplastic lungs. He underwent intubation for acidosis and respiratory insufficiency while the implications of the findings were communicated to his parents.

G. G.'s seven-yr-old brother had begged his parents for a new baby, resulting in G. G.'s birth. He had seen "his baby" for a total of 20 minutes; now the baby was far away and dying. It was unlikely that G. G. could live long enough to be transported home without life support. The extended family and friends were unable to arrange transportation to the hospital in a timely manner. In addition, they preferred G. G. to die at home, if at all possible.

The ICU social worker arranged for Medicaid to cover the ambulance expenses of transporting the intubated patient to his home. The Butterfly Team arranged for the ambulance to be met at the house by a local hospice team, which had orders to extubate on arrival and had medications for dyspnea. The baby was taken to the living room, where his brother and family awaited him. His brother was the first person to hold him. A peaceful 3 hours were spent, and the baby died at home with minimal symptoms.

Case Study: E. C., a Seven-Month-Old Infant with Severe Neurologic Compromise

E. C., a seven-month-old infant, had a rare chromosomal anomaly resulting in severe neurologic compromise. He had unrelenting gastroesophageal reflux, causing recurrent pneumonia and ICU admissions, and constant sensations of choking, according to his parents. His family agreed to a fundoplication to enhance his daily comfort rather than to extend his life. The family realized that he would not live very long because, during his entire lifetime, he had spent a total of seven weeks out of the hospital.

Five days postoperatively, the fundoplication dehisced, and E. C. developed peritonitis. The family interpreted this as a sign to stop interfering with their son's dying process. They accepted antibiotics but refused further surgery. After two days, they chose to take him home. Within 2 hours, he was on a commercial jet to his home, an 8-hour drive away. A hospice team met the family on the tarmac and drove behind them with medications. He arrived safely home and spent three days with his family, with frequent visits from the hospice team to ensure his and his family's comfort. He is buried on the family property with a ring of evergreens surrounding his grave. His older sister wrote a poem about him. The family adopted a needy Mexican infant 2 years later. They are doing well.

Case Study: D. C., a Five-Week-Old Infant with Intraventricular Hemorrhages

D. C. was born after a 25-week gestation to a 41-year-old mother who had cervical incompetence. The mother underwent a tubal ligation at the time of D. C.'s birth. Her first child was born at 30-weeks gestation and had done well. Both parents were schoolteachers of young, disabled children.

D. C. suffered bilateral grade IV intraventricular hemorrhages early in his course. His parents did not understand the implications of this initially, and he continued an unstable course, with the development of severe bronchopulmonary dysplasia and frequent desaturation episodes. He also developed hydrocephalus. The prognosis became clear to the parents when D. C. was five weeks old; they requested discontinuation of his life support. He was transported to the Butterfly Room and intubated. The family requested a rabbi and support from the Butterfly Team.

No one in his family had ever held D. C. because the referring neonatal team had felt that he was "too unstable." When his mother held him to her chest and stroked her son for the first time, he became pink and his heart rate decreased from 180 to 140 beats per minute. The infant's 20-month-old brother sat with him and had photographs taken. D. C. remained stable.

After some time, a conversation with the parents and aunts confirmed that they were making the decision to stop life support out of love for their child and concern for his suffering, that they had been good parents to him, and that their other son would always be a brother. The rabbi affirmed that their religion supported their decision. A description of what might happen postextubation was offered. The family understood and requested that the ventilator be discontinued. The mother held her son without the impediment of medical equipment, crying quietly to herself and rocking him with her husband, son, and sisters at her side until D. C.'s death 26 minutes later.

Over the ensuing months, the family frequently called the Butterfly Program social worker for counseling, and occasionally they met for lunch. They have been lost to long-term follow-up.

Case Study: K. D., a Child with Multisystem Organ Dysfunction

K. D., a two-and-one-half-year-old boy, had one of 20 world-reported cases of a syndrome that caused multisystem organ dysfunction, primarily liver and digestive, as well as bone marrow. For most of his life, K. D. was hospitalized an average of two to three days per month for diarrheal or infectious episodes. He was extremely small for his age (one medical student estimated he was six months old on his last admission) but was alert, interactive, and able to talk, although assessed to be "delayed." He enjoyed music and playing "air guitar." His family loved him dearly and had made many sacrifices to ensure his well being. His mother, the main wage earner, quit her job, and her husband became the sole source of family income. The family had to move to a new neighborhood.

During his last 2 months, K. D. was continuously hospitalized for severe diarrhea. After one month, K. D. began to require ICU interventions for sepsis episodes. After four episodes in the ICU over the course of three weeks, his parents approached the ICU team because they felt that K. D., who was intubated for fungal sepsis and general debility, was not going to get better; they requested comfort measures only. They felt that their boy was not benefiting from life-sustaining medical interventions. This was difficult for his medical care team to accept.

K. D. and his family were moved to the Butterfly Room, where they were joined by an extended family and a circle of friends, a total of 45 people. All monitors were discontinued, and all laboratory testing was discontinued. The desired limitations of medical interventions were documented in the chart.

A discussion with the extended family affirmed that the decisions made for K. D. were loving decisions. Their chaplain visited and affirmed their choices and the support of the church. Then, a discussion of what K. D. might look like after extubation, the uncertain time course to death, methods of controlling symptoms, and the principle of double effect were explained. Handprints and footprints of K. D. were made, his mother and father bathed him, and he was dressed in an outfit that the family had brought from home.

K. D. was held by everyone in a rocking chair; some people, such as his seven-year-old sister, needed to hold K. D. several times before they were ready. The family took as much time as they needed while the Butterfly team (nurse, social worker, child life specialist, and physician) circulated among the group, listening with empathy and encouraging communication. The family was reluctantly ready to stop the ventilator after four hours of rocking. As usual, the care team stayed with the family.

K. D. turned immediately cyanotic and was gasping postextubation; 100% blow-by was administered as well as 0.1 mg./kg. IV of morphine. After five uncomfortable minutes and no effect on his breathing effort, 0.2 mg./kg. of morphine was given. Again, 5 minutes passed with no change; the morphine was again doubled. This process continued until K. D. relaxed and seemed no longer to be dyspneic. He remained cyanotic, which, despite forewarning, was upsetting to his family. He died two and one-half hours postextubation.

Bereavement follow-up included attendance at K. D.'s visitation and funeral by members of the care team; a truckload of clothing, paper goods, and shelf food, as well as Christmas presents, donated by a local service group; phone calls and mailings; and an invitations to a yearly memorial service, as well as support groups. Three years later, the family is doing well.

REFERENCES

1. Billings JA. What is palliative care? Journal of Palliative Medicine 1998;1:73–81.

2. Institute of Medicine. Approaching Death: Improving Care at the End of Life. Washington, DC: National Academy Press, 1997.

3. Association for Children with Life-Threatening or Terminal Conditions and Their Families, Royal College of Paediatrics and Child Health. A Guide to the Development of Children's Palliative Care Services. London: Royal College of Paediatrics and Child Health, 1997.

4. Wanzer SH, Federman DD, Adelstein SJ, et al. The physician's responsibility toward hopelessly ill patients: A second look. N Engl J Med 320:844–849.

5. Guyer B, Hoyert DL, Martin JA, et al. Annual summary of vital statistics—1998. Pediatrics 1999;104(6):1229–1246.

6. Prendergast TJ, Luce JM. A national survey of withdrawal of life support from critically ill patients. Abstr. Am J Respir Crit Care Med 1996; 153: A360.

7. Koch KA, Rodeffer HD, Wears RL. Changing patterns of terminal care management in an intensive care unit. Crit Care Med 1994;22:233–243.

8. Levetown M, Pollack MM, Cuerdon TT, et al. Limitations and withdrawals of medical intervention in pediatric critical care. JAMA 1994; 272:1271–1275.

9. Gallup Organization. Knowledge and Attitudes Related to Hospice Care. Arlington, Va.: National Hospice Organization 1996.

10. The George H. Gallup International Institute. Spiritual Beliefs and the Dying Process: A Report on a National Survey Conducted for the Nathan Cummings Foundation and the Fetzer Institute, www.ncf.org/reports/rpt-fetzer-contents.html.

11. Cullen EJ, Lawless ST, Nadkarni VM, et al. Evaluation of a pediatric intensive care residency curriculum. Crit Care Med 1997;25:1898–1903.

12. Bluebond-Langner M. The Private Worlds of Dying Children. Princeton, New Jersey: Princeton University Press, 1978.

13. Webb M. The Good Death: The New American Search to Reshape the End of Life. New York: Bantam Books, 1997.

14. Byock I. Dying Well: The Prospect for Growth at the End of Life. New York: Riverhead Books.

15. Goldman A. Care of the Dying Child. New York: Oxford University Press, 1994.

16. Levetown M. Ethical aspects of pediatric palliative care. J Palliat Care 1996;12:35–39.

17. Phipps EJ, Cooper MR, Greenstein S. The last days of life: A retrospective study of when resuscitation decisions are made. Family Systems Medicine 1993;11:83–88.

18. Committee on Bioethics, Committee on Hospital Care, American Academy of Pediatrics. Palliative Care for Children. Pediatrics, August 2000 (In Press).

19. United Nations Children's Fund. First Call for Children: World Declaration and Plan of Action from the World Summit for Children, and Convention on the Rights of the Child. New York: UNICEF, December, 1990.

20. Hofmann JC, Wenger NS, Davis RB, et al. Patient preferences for communication with physicians about end-of-life decisions. Ann Intern Med 1997;127:1–12.

21. Johnston SC, Pfeifer MP, McNutt R. The discussion about advance directives: Patient and physician opinions regarding when and how it should be conducted. Arch Intern Med 1995;155: 1025–1030.

22. Gordon M. Decisions and care at the end of life. Lancet 1995;346:163–166.

23. Tolle SW. Care of the dying: Clinical and financial lessons from the Oregon experience. Ann Intern Med 1995;128:567–568.

24. FitzGerald JD, Wenger NS, Califf RM, et al. Functional status among survivors of in-hospital cardiopulmonary resuscitation. Arch Intern Med 1996;156:72–76.

25. Diem SJ, Lantos JD, Tulsky JA. Cardiopulmonary resuscitation on television: Miracles and misinformation. N Engl J Med 1996;334: 1604–1605.

26. Murphy DJ, Burrows D, Santilli S, et al. The influence of the probability of survival on patients' preferences regarding cardiopulmonary resuscitation. N Engl J Med 1994;330:545–549.

27. O'Brien LA, Grisso JA, Maislin G, et al. Nursing home residents' preferences for life-sustaining treatment. JAMA 1995;274:1775–1779.

28. Bruce-Jones PNE. Resuscitation decisions in the elderly: A discussion of current thinking. J Med Ethics 1996;22:286–291.

29. Sichting K, Berens R. Outcomes following resuscitations at Children's Hospital of Wisconsin. Crit Care Med 1997;25(1):A61.

30. Lantos JD, Miles SH, Silverstein MD, Stocking CB. Survival after cardiopulmonary resuscitation in babies of very low birth weight. N Engl J Med 1998;318(2):91–95.

31. Torres A, Pickert CB, Firestone J, et al. Long-term functional outcome of in-patient pediatric cardiopulmonary resuscitation. Pediatr Emerg Care 1997;13(6):369–373.

32. Schindler MB, Bohn D, Cox PN, et al. Outcome of out-of-hospital cardiac or respiratory arrest in children. N Engl J Med 1996;335(20): 1473–1479.

33. Wier R. Affirming the decisions adolescents make about life and death. Hastings Cent Rep 1997;27:29–40.

34. Quill TE. Nonabandonment: A central obligation for physicians. Ann Intern Med 1995; 122:368–374.

35. Pellegrino ED. Nonabandonment: An old obligation revisited. N Engl J Med 1995;122: 377–378.

36. Lynch J. Regaining compassion. JAMA 1998;279:1422.

37. Miller FG, Fins JJ. A proposal to restructure hospital care for dying patients. N Engl J Med 1996;334:1740–1742.

38. McSkimming S, Hodges M, Super A, et al. The experience of life-threatening illness: Patients' and their loved ones' perspectives. Journal of Palliative Medicine 1999;2(2):173–184.

39. Greisinger AJ, Lorimor RJ, Aday LA, et al. Terminally ill cancer patients: Their most important concerns. Cancer Practice 1997;5(3):147–154.

40. Nitschke R, Humphrey GB, Sexauer CL, et al. Therapeutic choices made by patients with end-stage cancer. J Pediatr 1982;101(3):471–476.

41. Vohra S, Camfield P, Camfield C. Assessing communication after the death of a child. The Canadian Journal of Paediatrics 1994;1(7): 208–211.

42. Adams DW, Deveau EJ. Helping dying adolescents: Needs and responses. In: Corr CA and McNeil JN, eds. Adolescence and Death. New York: Springer 1986:76–96.

43. Vernick J, Daron M. Who's afraid of death on a leukemia ward? Amer J Dis Child 1965; 109:393–397.

44. Solomon MZ. The enormity of the task: SUPPORT and changing practice. Hastings Center Report Special Supplement 1995;25: S28–S32.

45. The Society of Critical Care Medicine Ethics Committee. Attitudes of critical care medicine professionals concerning forgoing life-sustaining treatments. Crit Care Med 1992;20:320–326.

46. Division of Mental Health, World Health Organization. Communicating Bad News. Geneva, Switzerland: Behavioural Science Learning Module, 1993.

47. Lo B. Caring for patients with life-threatening or terminal illness. In: Lipkin M, Putnam SM, and Lazare A, eds. The Medical Interview; Clinical Care, Education and Research. New York: Springer, 1995:303–315.

48. Keenan SP, Busche KD, Chen LM, et al. A retrospective review of a large cohort of patients undergoing the process of withholding or withdrawal of life support. Crit Care Med 1997;25: 1324–1331.

49. Gazelle G. The slow code—Should anyone rush to its defense? N Engl J Med 1998;338: 467–469.

50. Hunt AM. A survey of signs, symptoms and symptom control in 30 terminally ill children. Dev Med Child Neurol 1990;32:341–346.

51. Attig T. Beyond suffering: The existential suffering of children. J Pall Care 1996;12:20–23.

52. Lynn J, Teno JM, Phillips RS, et al. Perceptions by family members of the dying experience of older and seriously ill patients. Ann Intern Med 1997;126:97–106.

53. The SUPPORT Principal Investigators. A controlled trial to improve care for seriously ill hospitalized patients: The study to understand prognoses and preferences for outcomes and risks of treatment (SUPPORT). JAMA 1995;274:1591–1598.

54. American Pain Society Quality of Care Committee. Quality improvement guidelines for the treatment of acute pain and cancer. JAMA 1995;274:1874–1880.

55. Carr DB, Jacox AK, Chapman CR, et al. Acute pain management: Operative or medical procedures and trauma, clinical practice guideline. In: AHCPR Publication No. 92–0032. Rockville, Maryland: US Public Health Service, Agency for Health Care Policy and Research, 1992.

56. World Health Organization and International Association for the Study of Pain. Cancer Pain Relief and Palliative Care in Children. Geneva: 1998.

57. Bieri D, Reeve RA, Champion GD, et al. The faces pain scale for the self-assessment of pain experiences by children: Development, initial validation and preliminary investigation for ratio scale properties. Pain 1990;41:139–150.

58. Beyer JE, Villarruel AM, Denyes M. The Oucher: Technical Report and User's Manual. Bethesda, MD: Association for the Care of Children's Health, 1995.

59. Eland JM. Minimizing pain associated with prekindergarten intramuscular injections. Issues Compr Pediatr Nurs 1981;5:361–372.

60. Wong DL, Baker CM. Pain in children: Comparison of assessment scales. Pediatr Nurs 1998;14:9–17.

61. McGrath PA. Pain in children: Nature, assessment and treatment. New York: Guilford Publishing, 1998.

62. de Stouz ND, Bruera E, Suarez-Almazor M. Opioid rotation for toxicity reduction in terminal cancer patients. J Pain Symptom Manage 1995;10:378–384.

63. Citron ML, Johnson-Early A, Fossieck BE Jr., et al. Safety and efficacy of continuous morphine for severe cancer pain. Am J Med 1984;77: 199–204.

64. Partridge JC, Wall SN. Analgesia for dying infants whose life support is withdrawn or withheld. Pediatrics 1997;99:76–79.

65. Kenny NP, Frager G. Refractory symptoms and terminal sedation of children: Ethical and practical management. J Pall Care 1996;12: 40–45.

66. The Textbook of Pain, 3d ed. Wall PD, Melzack R, eds. New York: Churchill Livingstone, 1994.

67. Schechter NL, Berde CB, Yaster M. Pain in infants, children and adolescents. Baltimore: Williams and Wilkins, 1993.

68. Walco GA, Cassidy RC, Schechter NL. Pain, hurt and harm: The ethics of pediatric pain control. N Engl J Med 1994;331(8):541–544.

69. Daly BJ, Thomas D, Dyer MA. Procedures used in withdrawal of mechanical ventilation. Am J Crit Care 1996;5:331–338.

70. Wilson WC, Smedira NG, Fink C, et al. Ordering and administration of sedatives and analgesics during the withholding and withdrawal of life support from critically ill patients. JAMA 1992; 267:949–953.

71. Campi CW. When dying is as hard as birth. The New York Times, Jan. 5, 1998.

72. Bruera E, Macmillan K, Pither J, et al. Effects of morphine on the dyspnea of terminal cancer patients. J Pain Symptom Manage 1990;5: 341–344.

73. Campbell ML. Managing terminal dyspnea: Caring for the patient who refuses intubation or ventilation. Dimens Crit Care Nurs 1996;15:4–11.

74. Cohen MH, Anderson AJ, Krasnow SH, et al. Continuous intravenous infusion of morphine for severe dyspnea. South Med J 1991;84: 229–234.

75. Truog RD, Berde CB, Mitchell C, Grier HE. Barbiturates in the care of the terminally ill. N Engl J Med 1992;327:1678–1682.

76. Billings JA, Block SD. Slow euthanasia. J Palliat Care 1996;2:21–30.

77. Quill TE, Lo B, Brock DW. Palliative care options of last resort: A comparison of voluntarily stopping eating and drinking, terminal sedation, PAS, and voluntary, active euthanasia. JAMA 1997;78:2099–2104.

78. Quill TE, Dresser R, Brock DW. The rule of double effect—A critique of its role in end-of-life decision making. N Engl J Med 1997;37: 1768–1771.

79. Mount B. Morphine drips, terminal sedation and slow euthanasia: Definitions and facts, not anecdotes. J Palliat Care 1996;2:31–37.

80. Roy DJ. On the ethics of euthanasia. J Palliat Care 1996;12:3–5.

81. Asch DA. The role of critical care nurses in euthanasia and assisted suicide. N Engl J Med 1996;334:1374–1379.

82. Rushton CH, Terry PB. Neuromuscular blockade and ventilator withdrawal: Ethical controversies. Am J Crit Care 1995;4:112–115.

83. Liben S. Pediatric palliative medicine: Obstacles to overcome. J Pall Care 1996; 2:24–28.

84. Smedira NG, Evans BH, Grais LS, et al. Withholding and withdrawal of life support from the critically ill. N Engl J Med 1990;322:309–315.

85. Stinson R, Stinson P. The Long Dying of Baby Andrew. Boston: Little, Brown, 1983.

86. Lantos JD, Tyson TE, Allen A, et al. Withholding and withdrawing life-sustaining treatment in neonatal intensive care: Issues for the 1990's. Arch Dis Child 1994;71:F218–F223.

87. Luce JM. Withholding and withdrawal of life support: Ethical, legal and clinical aspects. New Horiz 1997;5:30–37.

88. Solomon MZ, O'Donnell L, Jennings B, et al. Decisions near the end of life: Professional views on life-sustaining treatment. Am J Public Health 1993;83(1):14–23.

89. Susman EJ, Hersh SP, Nannis ED, et al. Conceptions of cancer; the perspectives of child and adolescent patients and their families. J Pediatr Psychol 1982;7(3):253–261.

90. Freyer DR. Children with cancer: Special considerations in the discontinuation of life-sustaining treatment. Med Pediatr Oncol 1992;20: 136–142.

91. Doyal L, Henning P. Stopping treatment for end-stage renal failure: The rights of children and adolescents. Pediatr Nephrol 1994;8:768–791.

92. Committee on Bioethics, American Academy of Pediatrics. Informed consent, parental permission and assent in pediatric practice. Pediatrics 1995;95(2):314–317.

93. Committee on Bioethics, American Academy of Pediatrics. Guidelines on forgoing life-sustaining medical treatment. Pediatrics 1994; 93(3):532–536.

94. President's Commission for the Study of Ethical Problems in Medicine and Biomedical and Behavioral Research. Deciding to Forgo Life-Sustaining Treatment: Ethical, Medical and Legal Issues in Treatment Decisions. Washington, DC: US Government Printing Office, 1983.

95. The Hastings Center. Guidelines on the Termination of Life-Sustaining Treatment and the Care of the Dying. Bloomington, Indiana: Indiana University Press, 1987.

96. Council on Ethical and Judicial Affairs, American Medical Association. Withholding or withdrawing life-prolonging medical treatment. In Code of Medical Ethics, Current Opinions. Chicago: American Medical Association, 1992.

97. Asch DA, Hansen-Flaschen J, Lanken PN. Decisions to limit or continue life-sustaining treatment by critical care physicians in the United States: Conflicts between physicians' practices and patients' wishes. Am J Respir Crit Care Med 1995; 151:288–292.

98. Nelson LJ. Forgoing treatment of critically ill newborns and the legal legacy of Baby Doe. Clinical Ethics Report 1992;6(2):1–6.

99. Traugott I, Alpers A. In their own hands: Adolescents' refusals of medical treatment. Arch Pediatr Adolesc Med 1997;151:922–927.

100. Battle CU. Beyond the nursery door: Our obligation to the survivors of technology. Clin Perinatol 1987;14(2):417–427.

101. Luce JM. Making decisions about the forgoing of life-sustaining therapy. Am J Respir Crit Care Med 1997;156:1715–1718.

102. Randolph AG, Zollo MB, Wigton RS, et al. Factors explaining variability among caregivers in the intent to restrict life-support interventions in a pediatric intensive care unit. Crit Care Med 1997;25:435–439.

103. Alpert HR, Emanuel L. Comparing utilization of life-sustaining treatment with patient and public preferences. J Gen Intern Med 1998; 13:175–181.

104. Christakis NA, Asch DA. Biases in how physicians choose to withdraw life support. Lancet 1993;342:642–646.

105. Nelson LJ, Rushton CH, Cranford RE, et al. Forgoing medically provided nutrition and hydration in pediatric patients. J Law Med Ethics 1995;23:33–46.

106. Levetown M, Carter MA. Child-centred care in terminal illness: An ethical framework. In: Doyle D, Hanks GWC, and MacDonald N, eds. Oxford Textbook of Palliative Medicine, 2nd ed. Oxford: Oxford University Press, 1998.

107. Horsburgh CR Jr. Healing by design. N Engl J Med 1995;333:735–740.

108. Levetown M. Different and needing to be more available. Hospice Magazine 1995; Winter: 15–36.

109. Leikin S. The role of adolescents in decisions concerning their cancer therapy. Cancer 1993;71(10):3342–3346.

110. King NMP, Cross AW. Children as decision-makers: Guidelines for pediatricians. J Pediatr 1989;115(1):10–16.

111. Leikin S. A proposal concerning decisions to forgo life-sustaining treatment for young people. J Pediatr 1989;115(1):17–22.

112. Grisso T, Vierling L. Minors' consent to treatment: A developmental perspective. Professional Psychology 1978;9(3):412–427.

113. Helsing KJ, Szklo M. Mortality after bereavement. Am J Epidemiol 1981;114:41–52.

114. Clayton PJ. Mortality and morbidity in the first year of widowhood. Arch Gen Psychiatry 1974;30:747–750.

115. Parkes CM, Brown RJ. Health after bereavement: A controlled study of young Boston widows and widowers. Psychosom Med 1972;34: 449–461.

116. Tolle SW, Bascom PB, Hickam DH, et al. Communication between physicians and surviving spouses following patient deaths. J Gen Intern Med 1986;1:309–314.

117. Irvine P. The attending at the funeral. N Engl J Med 1985;312:1704–1705.

118. Anonymous. 16th century aphorism, quoted from MacDonald N. The interface between oncology and palliative medicine. In: Oxford Textbook of Palliative Medicine, 2nd ed. Oxford: Oxford University Press, Oxford 1998: Section 2.1, 11.

119. Goldschmidt RH, Hess PA. Telling the patient the diagnosis is cancer: A teaching module. Fam Med 1987;19:302–304.

120. Wolraich M, Albanese M, Reiter-Thayer S, et al. Teaching pediatric residents to provide emotion-laden information. J Med Educ 1981;56: 438–440.

121. Gordon GH, Tolle SW. Discussing life-sustaining treatment: A teaching program for residents. Arch Intern Med 1991;151:567–570.

122. Billings JA, Block SD. Opportunity to present our observations and opinions on slow euthanasia (letter). J Palliat Care 1997;13:55–56.

123. Wolfe J, Grier HE, Klan N, Levin SB, et al. Symptoms and suffering at the end of life in children with cancer. N Engl J Med 2000;342: 326–333.

42 Hospital Care

MARIE BAKITAS WHEDON

We all felt guilty about bringing Dad into the hospital near the end, but we just couldn't do it at home anymore. He was incontinent, his pain was out of control, and we were just at wit's end. The staff on the oncology unit were great. They managed his symptoms and we were able to just be with Dad. We could be his kids, not his nurses. I think it made all the difference.

—Family member commenting on hospital death[1]

At the turn of the twentieth century the cause, age, and place of death were very different than what is reality at the turn of the new millennium. Table 42–1 compares some characteristics of dying between 1900 and 1990. Chronic illness and longer life are the legacy of this century. The hospital is a common location for a good portion of end-of-life (EOL) care in contemporary times, despite Americans' stated preference for death at home.[2] Approximately 73% of all 1994 U.S. deaths occurred in people age 65 and older—the population insured by Medicare.[3] An analysis of the experience of dying in Medicare recipients (based on claims data between 1995–1996) demonstrated that the incidence of dying in hospital varies, but in some regions of the United States it approaches 50% (see Figure 42-1.)[4] An additional 25%–35% of the nation's elderly die in nursing homes.[2,3] Although a percentage of patients experience their final admission in the critical care unit, by and large hospital deaths occur in a noncritical care unit[4] and are likely anticipated for hours or days before death actually occurs.[5]

Several investigators have described the quality of dying in the acute care hospital.[6–9] Each reports that patients experience pain, dyspnea, anxiety, and other distressing symptoms up until the time of death. Table 42–2 summarizes selected findings of the well-known Study to Understand Prognoses and Preferences for Outcomes and Risks of Treatments (SUPPORT). This multi-hospital, two-phase investigation attempted to alter the quality of the hospitalized adult, end-of-life experience by "reducing the frequency of a mechanically supported, painful, and prolonged process of dying" by increasing communication and improving the provision of information necessary for decision-making among patient, family, and their health care providers.[5] The discouraging outcomes from SUPPORT and other studies cannot be explained by providers' lack of awareness or inability to relieve symptoms. Many studies in the area of pain management demonstrate that effective methods exist to relieve cancer pain in 90% of patients.[10] It is also not the case that acute care hospitals employ unskilled, insensitive personnel who allow suffering to occur. Rather, the issue appears largely one of system design. Inpatients are cared for in a system that is designed to provide acute, episodic interventions for patients with reversible disorders.

This philosophy is exemplified by hospital policies that require all persons having patient contact to be certified in the provision of cardiopulmonary resuscitation (CPR) in order to rescue any patient who experiences cessation of respiration and/or heartbeat. The application of this death-reversing intervention is applied to all hospitalized inpatients unless specifically ordered to the contrary. Clearly, in such institutions, patients who are dying are viewed as exceptions who require special additional thought, paperwork, and attention to receive a different sort of care.

Implementing other tenets of palliative and hospice type care may not be consistent with standard hospital policy. For instance, having family, friends, pets, and familiar items in the immediate patient environment often requires special exceptions or violations of standard hospital protocols. In many institutions, beloved pets, home audio equipment used for listening to special music, or multiple significant others sitting around-the-clock vigils are considered contrary to standard hospital infection control, electrical use rules, and security policies. As stated by Berwick on the nature of system improvement: "Every system is perfectly designed to get the results it gets."[11] In the case of end-of-life care, it is hard to imagine how hospital-based end-of-life care could occur any differently than it does. A change in the quantity and quality of deaths in hospital will only come about as a result of fundamental system reform and redesign.[12,13]

This situation ought not be viewed as discouraging, but rather a call to action, particularly for nurses. Because people are admitted to hospitals primarily to receive nursing care, much of the care and the system that patients experience can be influenced by *nurses* at all organizational levels. (Most other care, such as physician consultation, diagnostic tests, and pharmaceutical treatments are available in outpatient or home settings). The information contained in

Table 42–1. Comparison of Characteristics of Dying and Death (1900 vs1990)*

	1900	1990
Life expectancy	50	75.8
Cause of death	Infectious disease (e.g. influenza, tuberculosis, diptheria)	Heart disease, cancer, stroke
Location of death	Home	Hospital/nursing home

*Institute of Medicine. *Approaching Death: Improving Care at the End of Life.* Washington, DC, National Academy Press 1997.

this chapter is usable by all hospital-based nurses, including the senior nursing leader, clinical nurse specialists, nurse managers, educators, quality improvement nurses, and especially the nurses on the front line at the bedside. Nurses can define, direct, and lead multidisciplinary and interdisciplinary teamwork and modify efforts at multiple levels of the hospital care system in efforts to improve this complex care process.[14,15]

This chapter outlines how nurses and others can take a leadership role in improving the quality of end-of-life care in acute care hospitals. Some improvements may result from using specific "quality improvement" methods, while other improvements may not employ this specific process. A brief description of a specific continuous quality improvement process, as it applies to hospital-based EOL care, opens the discussion. (Although a step-by-step primer on the process of "quality improvement" is beyond the scope of this chapter, a detailed discussion is found in Chapter 37; other excellent sources are available.[16]) Discussion then focuses on methods to reduce hospital admissions at the end of life. Individual and multihospital innovations to improve hospital-based EOL care are described. Examples from hospitals that have used the approach of developing critical pathways and protocols and new services to improve care, such as palliative care consulting teams and inpatient palliative care units, are included. In closing, economic issues that influence the quality and quantity of hospital-based EOL care, educational endeavors, research, resources, and future directions complete the discussion.

HOSPITAL EOL CARE AS A PROCESS

Case Study: Emma

Emma, a 72-year-old retired teacher and grandmother who lived alone in a small town was found by her family, conscious but moaning in extreme pain on the floor of her apartment (3 P.M. Thursday). She indicated that she had fallen multiple times in the past four days (not reported to family) and was not able to get up after the latest fall, which is why she contacted family. She was brought via ambulance to the emergency room of a teaching hospital. Upon initial assessment by the emergency room staff she was found to be alert, febrile, and unable to answer questions due to exquisite pain she exhibited by moaning and calling out wherever she was touched. Minimal available medical history included hepatic cirrhosis (no ETOH for past 15 years) and heart disease. Diagnostic tests were performed and she was admitted to a medical unit (at 5 P.M.) for further evaluation. Family were present and were distressed, as were nursing staff, due to the patient's obvious discomfort, exhibited by continuous groaning and calling out that was audible throughout the medical unit and was escalating. She was suspected to be septic from an unknown source (possible urinary) and to have head trauma and fractures from her falls. The nurses contacted the admitting medical team multiple times for pain medication, but the MDs were reluctant for fear of masking symptoms of unknown medical problems. At 11 P.M. the patient was transferred to an intensive care unit for her high acuity nursing care, although there was a DNR order in place. The patient eventually received a small dose of analgesic. She died in the ICU bed from overwhelming sepsis (+ blood and urinary sources) at 9 A.M. Friday morning.

Case Study: Professor L.

Prof. L., 72, a lanky retired scientist was found to have advanced pancreatic cancer following a biopsy done to diagnose the source of his painless jaundice. Within 2 weeks, he met simultaneously with the oncologist and palliative care nurse practitioner to discuss treatment options. He decided to undergo a Phase II research treatment, as he understood his prognosis was poor, and he wished to take a chance and contribute to science. He also enrolled in a palliative care program that provided for information about cancer, symptom control, and advanced care planning. Implanted port placement, needed for the study drug, was scheduled for after the Christmas holidays at his request. On admission to the same-day surgery program midafternoon, his wife called the physician, who contacted the nurse practitioner (NP) to assess the patient, as his wife was worried about her husband's ability to tolerate the ride home late in the day following the procedure and then to return in the early morning for a baseline ultrasound requiring him to be NPO through the night. The NP met with the wife, assessed the patient following the procedure, and concurred that his condition had worsened since his last appointment, as evidenced by increased jaundice, weight loss, and general deterioration. Together with the oncologist, an overnight observation admission was planned. The liver ultrasound in the morning revealed rapidly progressive disease that had essentially replaced his liver, and his liver function tests had quadrupled over the past two weeks. The patient and wife decided, with the advice of the oncology team, not to pursue the investigational treatment and to focus solely on symptom management. He requested to go home that afternoon with hospice care. Throughout the ordeal, the patient had minimal pain, which was relieved by oxycodone, and he remained functional. Most of the arrangements with the hospice care provider focused on establishing a safe environment for the patient to move around in a weakened state. Three days later, during the night, the patient started to bleed from his GI tract, and his wife called an ambulance, as she was unable to cope with the distress of this type of death at home. Within hours, he died comfortably in the hospital, cared for by nurses specially trained in palliative care. The following day, the palliative care NP contacted the wife to offer condolences and ask if she needed any resources, mailed a

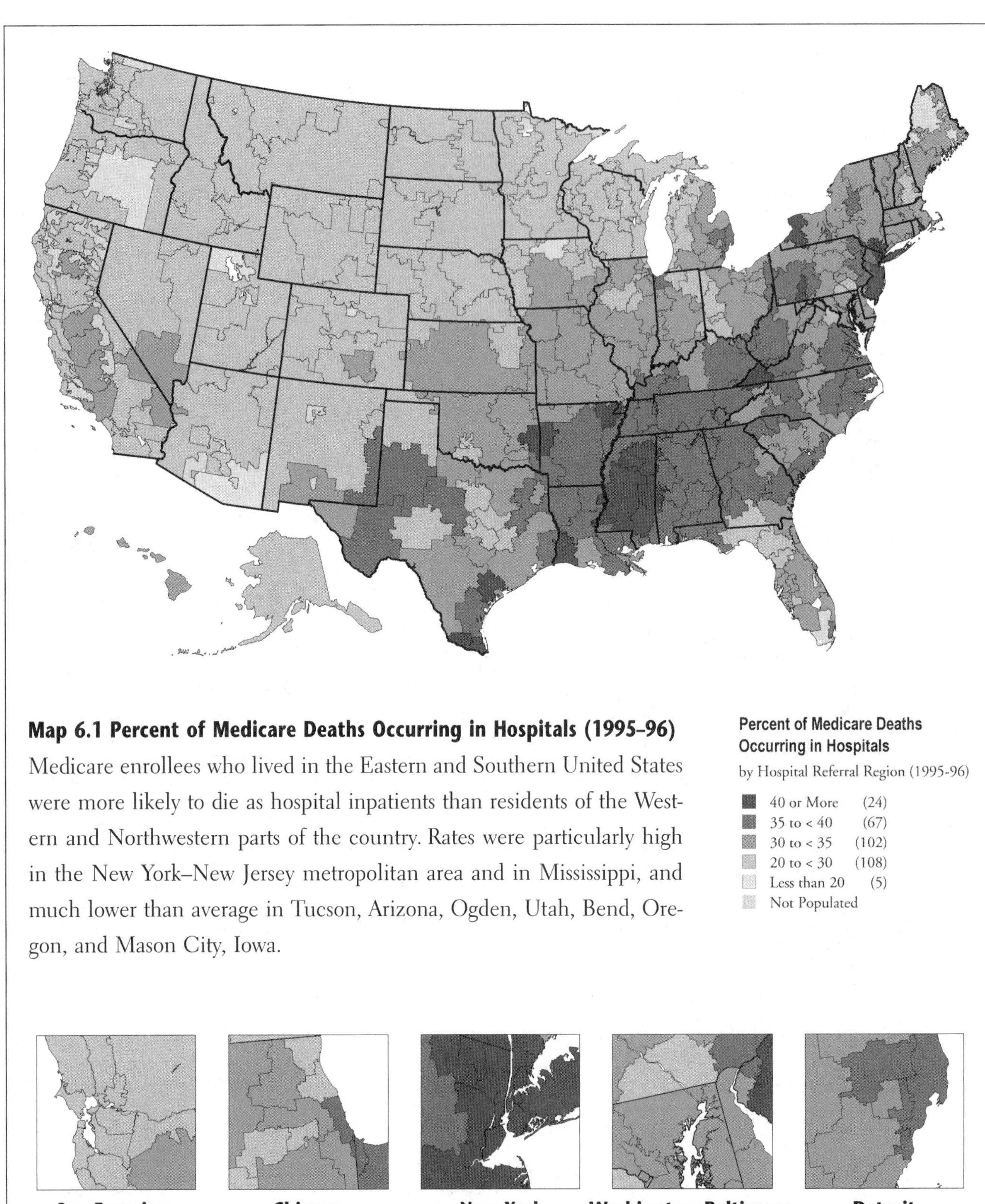

Fig. 42–1. Dartmouth Atlas Map of Incidence of Death in Hospital. From Wennberg JE, Cooper MM, eds. The Quality of Care in the United States: A Report on the Medicare Program/Dartmouth Atlas of Health. Chicago: AHA Press, 1999. Reprinted by permission.

Table 42–2. Selected Results from the Study to Understand Prognoses and Preferences for Outcomes and Risks of Treatments (SUPPORT)*

Study Aims:

To document and influence: patterns of communication (patient/family/health care team), frequency of aggressive treatment, characteristics of hospital death

Methods:

Two phase study in 5 academic medical centers
Phase I: 2-year prospective observational study (n = 4301)
Phase II: 2-year controlled clinical trial with intervention group (n = 2652) and control group (n = 2152)

Intervention:

A specially trained nurse had multiple contacts with patient/family/health care team to facilitate communications and to provide physicians with accurate information about patients prognoses and preferences for care.

Main Results:

There were no differences between the control group and the intervention group on the measures of the study which included:
Communication between physician and patients (discussions of CPR preferences)
Number of days spent in an ICU receiving mechanical ventilation and in coma
Level of pain reported by patient
Use of hospital resources
Further based on interviews with 3357 survivors:
40% of patients died in severe pain
55% were conscious
63% had difficulty tolerating symptoms

*SUPPORT Principal Investigators. A controlled trial to improve care for seriously ill hospitalized patients. The study to understand prognoses and preferences for outcomes and risks of treatments (SUPPORT). *JAMA* 1995; 274: 1591–1598
*Lynn J, Teno JM, Phillips, R. Wu AW, Desbiens N, Harrold J, Claessens M, Wenger, Kreling B, Connors. A for the SUPPORT Investigators. Perceptions of family members of the dying experience of older and seriously ill patients. *Ann Intern Med* 1997; 126: 97–106.

sympathy card, and put her on a list of those to be offered bereavement services in the ensuing weeks.

Both cases illustrate ways in which EOL care occurs in hospitals. Table 42–3 outlines a high-level process of care that illustrates hospital-based EOL care similar to the events of the first case. Areas for improvement (some of which are illustrated by the second case) are suggested adjacent to the process steps. These cases serve as a basis for the remaining discussion, which describes ways that hospitals can create care systems that result in improved EOL outcomes for patients requiring hospital-based care.

CLINICAL QUALITY IMPROVEMENT STRATEGIES: A BRIEF SYNOPSIS OF METHODS AND MEASURES

Quality improvement strategies have been successfully integrated in many sites of health care delivery. One clinical improvement methodology widely employed specifically in hospitals is called Plan Do Study Act (PDSA)[17] (see Chapter 37). Briefly, using this methodology, a core process in need of improvement is identified (e.g., caring for the hospitalized dying patient, as depicted in Table 42–3). A team is formed, pertinent literature is reviewed, and the improvement is planned, implemented (do), results of the change are analyzed (study), and finally a decision is made to adopt the change with or without modifications (act).

Although this system has many similarities to the research process, it differs in a number of important ways. First, unlike the research process, the intervention is not held constant for the duration of the study. Rather, if an intervention can be improved or should be otherwise changed during the test, it is. Also, improvements are meant to be tested in small numbers, and turnaround of data collection and analysis is much more rapid than what is expected in research.[16,17]

A similar but related process for improving EOL care in the United Kingdom is the clinical audit,[18,19] another formalized system of systematically assessing the quality of care a service is delivering. The clinical audit is described as similar to performing one cycle of a larger quality improvement project. Other similarities between quality improvement and audits are that they are used in small samples, use a standardized measure, and include the provision of continuous feedback to practitioners so that practice improvement can be ongoing. A clinical audit might focus on a subset of the entire process of care, such as access to care or bereavement. The reader is referred to an in depth overview of clinical audit by expert Irene Higginson, Ph.D.[18]

To know if one has arrived, one must first decide where he or she is going. In quality improvement, determining measures of success is a vital step before attempting to implement any change. Beyond simply determining if something in the practice environment has changed, the question to be answered is "How will you know if the change is an improvement?"[17] A multidisciplinary team must prospectively agree on what the clinically relevant desired outcomes are and on ways to measure success (or failure). For instance, is evidence of improved documentation of pain to be considered a successful proxy measure of improvement in pain assessment, or

Table 42–3. Process of Care for Seriously Ill Hospitalized Patient at the End of Life with Suggestions for Improvements

Current Process of Care	Possible Areas of Improvement
Symptomatic seriously ill patient admitted to emergency department (ED)	Prospective symptom management to avoid hospitalization Advance care planning communicated to care team
Work up by ED staff	Direct admission of symptomatic/ respite patients
Admission to medical unit	Availability of palliative care unit/consult team
Diagnostic work-up continues with medical house staff	Minimize/standardize diagnostics to focus on ones that will contribute to comfort
MD(s) notified	MD aware and guiding admission process
Initial plan of care determined	Plan of care states palliative care goals/ advance care planning /patient preferences
Treatment is implemented/ symptoms managed	Palliative care pathway and or standardized symptom assessment
Team acknowledges that patient is dying	Patient's prognosis and preferences guide palliative care plan from time of admission
DNR status determined	This step implemented upon admission and plan of care also includes patient's care preferences in addition to DNR order
Comfort measures implemented	Appropriate comfort care measures implemented at admission
Patient dies in hospital	Patient dies in preferred site of death Bereavement care offered to family following death

is patient interview about how often their pain was assessed the target?

The Clinical Values Compass is one method to measure outcomes.[17] It has four points, like a compass, and each considers a different but important domain in assessing outcomes: functional, clinical, satisfaction (the extent to which care meets expectations), and costs (resource utilization). Given the different philosophies and missions in hospitals, a balanced approach in measuring outcomes recognizes that change can affect multiple domains simultaneously. Hence, as a change is being assessed, it is important to determine if a positive change in one outcome results in adverse effects in another. For instance, in evaluating a change, a reduction in costs may be realized, but the team may be concerned if there is a concurrent decrease in measures of patient, family, and/or staff satisfaction. (See values compass in Figure 42–2.) Multiple measures and methods can be applied to each domain.

One of the benefits of doing quality improvement in hospitals is that most have readily available and often computerized systems in which some relevant data may be collected. Measures such as length of stay by unit, number of deaths by unit, diagnostic-related grouping (DRG) codes, diagnoses, and charge data on patients who have died are some examples of such data. Some institutions have easily obtainable qualitative clinical data, such as pain intensity measures from a vital signs documentation sheet (e.g., some institutions document pain on a bedside graph along with temperature, pulse, etc., a practice known as "pain the fifth vital sign"). An institutional CPR committee may keep data on the number of do-not-resuscitate (DNR) orders written and how often resuscitation occurs relative to the number of hospital deaths. Pharmacy information systems may be able to provide figures of opioid usage or other pharmaceutical interventions that may indicate appropriate symptom management. Pastoral care department figures can indicate the numbers of EOL patients served. Ethics committees may also have consultant data available that relate to difficulties they see in EOL care. Most institutions have some sort of patient satisfaction survey that can indicate adequacy of symptom management or respect for patients' rights. Many of these are important indirect measures of those system-wide improvements that should be designed or of how an improvement project might be influencing care.

For instance, in one academic hospital, an analysis of DNR orders revealed some important issues. Data readily

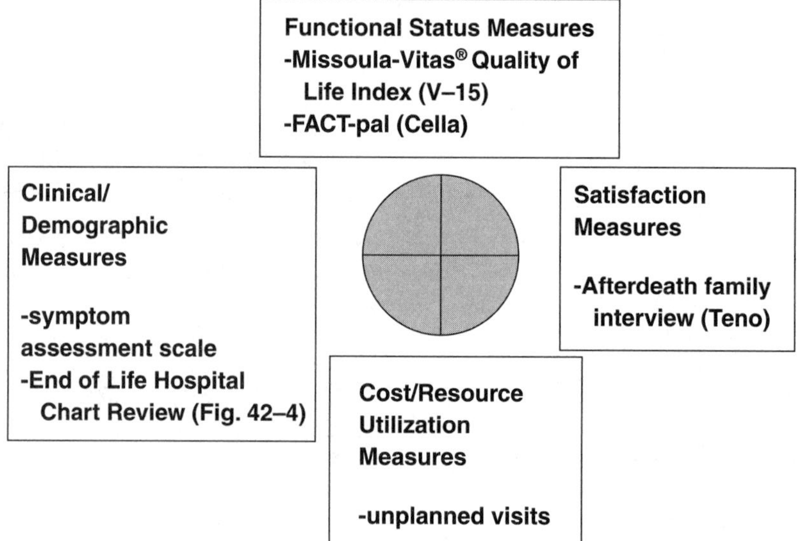

Fig. 42–2. This clinical values compass lists examples of measures under each domain that may be used in evaluating a project to improve palliative care. Information on each of these tools can be found on the website listed in referenced 20.

available from the CPR committee showed that in one year slightly more than 400 deaths occurred, and in that same year 900 DNR orders were written.[20] Most patients with DNR orders were discharged to home. Most patients who died had DNR orders, but a third of the patients who died with DNR orders had been in the hospital less than 48 hours. These types of data can inform an improvement team about populations of patients who might benefit from palliative care services. Questions asked by improvement teams from the above data included: "For what reasons are patients with DNR orders being admitted only to die within 48 hours? What manner of home care services were available to (nontrauma) patients who died in the hospital within 48 hours? What forces might influence why patients died in the hospital rather than at home (or in a nursing home)? How can expert palliative care be provided when hospital staff have little time to get to know patients and their families prior to the patient's death?"

In addition to available hospital clinical data, the focus group is another methodology increasingly used in health care systems to evaluate consumer satisfaction and perception of services. A focus group can provide greater depth of information than most quantitative surveys; further, it can serve as the background in developing relevant quantitative surveys. One academic teaching hospital supplemented available clinical data about pain and dyspnea management at the end of life with information from a focus group consisting of the surviving family members. Specifically, next of kin were asked about their perception of symptom management for pain and dyspnea, followed by a more open-ended discussion of EOL care in the hospital in general.[1] From this analysis, important information was gained regarding symptom management as perceived by the family, and key quality characteristics of good EOL care in general were identified. Following this, a brief quantitative survey was constructed (Appendix A) to gain input from a broader group of survivors on these points and to monitor evidence of change as improvement strategies were implemented. Table 42–4 lists some additional outcomes of multiple quality improvement projects from an institution that relied primarily on available clinical data sources.

Table 42–4. Examples of Ideas Generated and Implemented to Improve EOL Care From Multiple Improvement Projects in an Academic Medical Center*

1. Contact between oncology fellow/nurse practitioner on call and emergency department (ED) staff facilitates EOL patients admitting process through ED.
2. Improvements in DNR notification in medical record and communications.
3. Standardized pain and symptom assessment and management for oncology patients via inservices, critical pathway, standard physician order sheets (including pain assessment, standardized equianalgesia, dyspnea, opioid-induced constipation).
4. Implementation of "5th Vital Sign" on inpatient oncology and medical units.
5. Palliative care/comfort measures inpatient orders and clinical pathway designed, piloted, revised, and implemented.
6. Implementation of case management role to foster continuity and efficiency of care for complex patient populations.
7. Created pocket card for house staff to improve process of patient pronouncement of death.
8. Implemented bereavement process for families of all patients who die in hospital including letter of condolence to family, resources for bereavement, delayed billing, prestamped cards for staff to send to families, and a script for staff to make bereavement calls.
9. Standardized process for home DNR bracelet.
10. Poor prognosis patients (lung, advanced GI, and metastatic breast) identified at diagnosis and introduced to palliative care support services and resources.

*The improvements were a result of the work of several DHMC CQI teams between 1994–1999.
Improvement team work received funding from the following sources:
Mayday Fund-Dartmouth Demonstration Project to Improve Post Operative Pain (Whedon, Marrin, Mroz, Ahles).
The Kornfeld Foundation (Goodlin, Whedon, Ahles).
The Soros Foundation Project on Death in America (Goodlin)
DHMC Support for attendance at the Institute for Health Care Improvement (Mills, Whedon, Bedell, Avery)
Robert Wood Johnson-Project ENABLE (Greenberg, Stevens, Ahles, Whedon, Skalla)

Increasing efforts to define clinically useful measures of end-of-life care have produced a ready resource for clinicians and quality improvement initiatives called the Toolkit of Instruments to Measure End-of-Life Care (TIME).[16,21] Multiple foundations concerned with improving care of seriously ill and end-of-life patients sponsored this endeavor to catalog and evaluate the "state of the science" of measurement in this area, resulting in the Toolkit project.[21] It continues to evolve as measurement tools are added, analyzed for reliability and validity, and used in clinical practice. Teno[21] states in the introduction to the Toolkit Website (http://www.chcr.brown.edu/pcoc/toolkit.htm):

> A fundamental barrier in the quality of care at the end of life is the lack of measurement tools. These measurement tools should identify opportunities for improving medical care, examining the impact of interventions or demonstration programs, and holding institutions accountable for their quality of care. The ultimate objective of the proposed research is to develop patient focused and family-centered survey instruments that address the needs and concerns of patients and their families, as defined by them.

The Website provides information and multiple sample tools in each of 10 domains of end-of-life care:

- Quality of life
- Pain and other symptoms
- Depression and other emotional symptoms
- Functional status
- Survival time and aggressiveness of care
- Advance care planning
- Continuity of care
- Spirituality
- Grief and family experience
- Patient centered reports and rankings on quality of care.

Family as proxy for quality of care is the target of an after-death interview used to question the experience of end-of-life care.[22] It is significant that many of these tools to measure end-of-life care are directed at adults; as yet there are few measures that specifically address the needs of dying children.

One of the most important issues in measuring quality of care and improvement in end of life care is to begin *somewhere*. It is easy to become overwhelmed by a sense of too much to do and not knowing where to begin. A team can quickly lose heart and motivation if the task seems impossible. Energy draining activities of quality improvement teams include: developing a tool rather than using an available measure that is "good enough," and creating measurement schemes that require a lot of additional time or personnel to complete. The reader is referred to Nelson et al.,[23] which addresses the latter issue in depth and describes strategies for incorporating measurement into daily clinical practice. Another efficient and very practical tool used in hospitals for a relevant retrospective chart review of deaths in hospitals that can quickly "screen" the state of care is shown in Figure 42–3. It lends itself to use by students or staff as it requires minimal training and takes approximately 20 minutes per chart to complete. It has been used to screen hundreds of charts in multiple agencies to ascertain quality of care at the end of life. In New Hampshire it was voluntarily completed on approximately 20 deaths/agency in 60 agencies across the state, including acute care hospitals. The data from this retrospective statewide chart review served as the basis for a Robert Wood Johnson–funded statewide project on improving advance care planning.[24]

The remaining discussion follows a typical process of care (Table 42–3), covering prehospital care, in-hospital care, and posthospital care, and describes areas of improvement that are ripe for ideas as well as examples of improvement ideas that have been used.

IMPROVING NONHOSPITAL SYSTEMS OF CARE TO AVOID HOSPITALIZED DEATH

Perhaps one of the first and most important ways to improve hospital-based

End of Life Hospital Chart Review

I. *Photocopy administrative data sheets for name, diagnosis, age, length of stay, contact/next of kin information, insurance, and attending MD.*

Patient Name________________________ **Medical Record #**____________

II. *Information should be obtained from (a.) orders throughout the patient's stay, (b.) progress notes on the first day of admission, the day of death and the day before, and (c.) any formal advance directives.*

1. Were any formal advance directives mentioned (ie Living Will, Durable Power of Attorney for Health Care)? **YES**_____ **NO** ______ (Check One)

   If yes, is the actual document located in the chart? **YES**______ **NO** _______

2. Date of first formal advance directive chart documentation: ___/___/___

3. Were any of the following noted?:

_____ Do Not Resuscitate (DNR) ___/___/___ (first date)
_____ Do Not Intubate (DNI) or other instruction for partial life support (i.e. "no pressors") ___/___/___ (first date)
_____ Comfort measures only ___/___/___ (first date)
_____ CPR tried ____/___/___ (first date)
Comments on planning ________________________________

4. ICU
___ Was ICU used? Admit date ___/___/___ and discharge date ___/___/___
___ Was patient in an ICU at the time of death or within the last 2 days?
___ Was discharge from ICU in the last 2 days due to expecting death?

5. Discharge Plans

___ Death intended to be in this program in the last 2 days?
___ Hospice discussed with patient or family?
___ Use of Hospice intended?
___ Hospice used?
days of hospice care______ Any inpatient?______ (# of days) DON'T KNOW
Comments on care near death? ______________________________

S:\BREAKTHR\EOL\COORD\JLCHAR~1.DOC
PAGE 1 of 2

End of Life Hospital Chart Review Medical Record # ________________

Refer to progress notes and orders for the day of death and the day before.

6. Was patient comatose throughout?_______**YES** (If YES, skip table and go to Q 7). **NO** (If NO, complete table using √)

Symptom/ Problem	Assessed?	Problem for patient?	Plan of treatment documented?	Monitor or follow-up of treatment plan?	Effective?
Pain/ discomfort					
Anxiety					
Confusion/ Delirium					
Agitation/ restlessness					
Shortness of breath					
Decubitus ulcers					
Spiritual issues					
Other ______					
Other ______					
Other ______					

7. **Treatments Administered (Check for YES)**
___ antibiotics
___ family issues and support noted before death
___ family issues and support noted after death
___ chaplaincy involvement
___ chemotherapy - drugs used: ____________________________
explicit focus on palliation (not life prolonging) Yes ___ No ___
___ enteral tube (NG/peg/G)
___ foley catheter
___ intravenous medication
___ intubation
___ narcotics (total dose, last full calendar day before death: ___________)
___ physical restraints (type: vest ____ wrist _____ ankles _____)
___ surgery in the OR (type: ___________________________)
___ ventilator (dates) from ___/___/___ to ___/___/___

8. **Diagnostics (Check for YES)**
___ A line
___ blood draws
___ Swan
___ x-rays
___ weight

9. **Autopsy (Check One)**
_____ Completed
_____ Not Mentioned
_____ Mentioned but Declined

PAGE 2 of 2

Fig. 42–3. End of life hospital chart review. © 1997 Center to Improve Care of the Dying.

EOL care is to develop other infrastructures of care outside the hospital so that other alternatives exist. Alternatives such as home hospice care or skilled hospice care within assisted living, free-standing hospices, or specially designated areas in nursing homes or rehabilitation facilities[25] can provide expert palliative and hospice care at the EOL. Many areas of the country lack these sorts of options, however. For instance, in some rural areas health care services, such as visiting nurses or home care, are sparse or unprepared to care for people who require intensive EOL care.[26] Some visiting nurse and home care agencies may see so few symptomatic persons at the EOL that it is difficult to maintain adequate palliative care and hospice expertise in these home health nurses and assistive personnel.

The lack of hospice and palliative care expertise outside the hospital can be compounded by another very real problem: reimbursement for out-of-hospital EOL care. This problem must be viewed in the context of the Medicare hospice benefit, which provides a standard per diem rate of $97.11 for routine home care; $566.82/day or $23.62/hr for continuous care during a crisis to maintain a patient at home; $100.46/day for up to 5 days of respite care; and $432.01/day for hospital, skilled, or freestanding inpatient hospice care for symptom management (1999). These amounts are intended to cover all care needs, including nursing, home health aides, other discipline visits, pharmaceuticals, and medical equipment. For many patients eligible for Medicare hospice care, effective palliative interventions for symptom management (such as radiation therapy, chemotherapy, higher priced supportive care medications for nausea and pain) may be too costly, given the reimbursement rate. Hence, patients who could otherwise benefit from hospice care are delayed in accessing the benefit until all of the aforementioned palliative treatments have been applied. It is therefore not an issue of patient identification but more one of finance that is responsible for late hospice referrals. Quality improvement efforts directed at improving EOL care by encouraging earlier referrals to the Medicare hospice benefit but that ignore the financial issues will likely fail. Agencies that place patients on the benefit despite ongoing expensive treatments will likely find themselves in a state of financial instability.

Another barrier that must be overcome in order to realize lower in-hospital death rates is that of home care provision in the current culture of single-parent and two-parent working families. Currently, 75% of women work outside the home, yet they are often the ones called upon to provide care for ailing family members.[27] When patients are enrolled in the Medicare hospice benefit, it is assumed that a family member or other person will be with the patient every day[28] and that hospice staff will visit intermittently. For symptomatic or very ill patients, this means that a family member may need to take a leave of absence or risk jeopardizing employment in order to provide adequate coverage for home care. Many families report the severe financial burden of providing care to a family member for an extended period at the EOL from out-of-pocket medical expenses as well as the lost income from both the patient and the caregiver.[29] In the absence of any other solution, the hospital may be the only source of family respite. Quality improvement teams may find foundational support in this area from the Last Acts Workplace Task Force, the report of an employer survey and a set of model activities designed to help caregivers and their families with ill or dependent relatives in need of workplace supports.[30]

An intermediate step in preventing hospital admissions altogether is to develope a system that allows for early identification of patients who are palliative care and/or hospice care eligible and to identify the long-term plan for EOL care. This early identification can take place at the beginning of the disease trajectory or at the point of a hospital admission. Putting prospective screening mechanisms in place can reduce the number and type of hospital admissions for palliative care. For instance, consider the situation of discharging a patient with adequate relief of pain without a long-term plan for dealing with worsening disease and increased pain. In this case, neglecting the bigger problem of long-term pain management only postpones the problem until a later date, when pain is likely to increase and the only available solution will be readmission. In addition to creating a long-term plan for already hospitalized patients, pre-hospitalization programs that identify elders at home or in nursing homes who do not wish to have their conditions treated in a hospital can preclude undesired admissions.

The Patient Self-Determination Act of 1991 requires that all institutions, including hospitals, receiving Medicare or Medicaid funding provide written information to patients about their rights to make decisions to accept or refuse medical care.[31] Further, it stipulates that mechanisms known as advance directives (ADs), including living wills and appointment of a health care proxy, may be used to provide for substituted judgment in the event of patients' inability to speak for themselves regarding their wishes about health care decisions. On the surface, this legislation appears to be an infrastructure evolution and process-of-care change that ought to improve EOL care in hospitals. Theoretically, patients outline their preferences for accepting or refusing treatments and provide a mandate to guide all health care providers as they provide care. For several reasons, however, this legislation has had little impact, for the most part, in defining the type of care received by hospitalized patients.[32] Not all patients actually choose to complete these documents, the documents apply only when the patients are incapacitated, they may not be specific enough to address the situation in which patients find themselves, when they do exist the health care provider may not be aware of them,[5] or the health care proxy may not interpret them as the patient intended.[33] This lack of respect for patients' preferences is illustrated in the process of care diagram (Table 42–3). In the case of

Emma, presented earlier in this chapter, no evidence of advance care planning existed, nor were efforts made by the team to determine the existence of documents or proxy decision-makers who might have voiced Emma's preferences for care.

Recent research and improvement efforts have attempted to study this phenomenon and improve the availability of such information and the consistency between patient's stated preferences and the actual care administered.[16,34] Incorporating such endeavors into quality improvement activities has the potential to influence hospital based EOL care.[35] An encouraging finding in one chart review of deaths of hospitalized patients indicated an increased implementation of comfort care in patients at the end of life in the minority of patients who had specified a proxy decision-maker compared to those who did not.[36]

Innovative approaches to avoiding unnecessary hospitalization or other undesired care at the end of life are being tested through the Robert Wood Johnson Initiative on Improving Care at the End of Life. (See Last Acts Website, www.edc.org/lastacts/, for a full description of this program and the specific projects of the grantees.) These organizations, through demonstration projects, are testing strategies designed to move the knowledge and decision making about palliative care options earlier in the course of illness than is currently the norm. Four comprehensive cancer centers are attempting to integrate palliative care options and approaches at the time of diagnosis of life threatening, poor prognosis cancers such as of the lung. One example, Project ENABLE (Educate, Nurture, Advise Before Life Ends), identifies and enrolls all patients with incurable lung cancer, advanced gastrointestinal malignancies, and metastatic or recurrent breast cancers at the time of diagnosis into a program that emphasizes palliative care options. The program provides for nurse coordination, prospective standardized symptom assessment, and an educational curriculum that focuses on topics of empowerment for patient and family decision making and communication.[37] Unlike the nurse coordinator of the SUPPORT study, these advanced practice nurses (and nurse practitioners) are members of the oncology care team and provide nonthreatening, expert intervention that has prospectively garnered the support and sanction of the care team. This collaborative approach emphasizes shared ownership of the process and, to date, seems to influence and shape the care trajectory for this population.[38] The case of Professor L. is one example of a prospective identification system that is readily able to respond when a patient's condition deteriorates.

In some areas of the United States, such as New York State, the issue of managing patients at home who are dying and do not want to be resuscitated occurs through the use of home labeling systems, such as "DNR bracelet," sticker, or forms. Specific details can be obtained in a 138-page report that details the results of a national survey conducted in 1999 of state laws and protocols providing for DNR orders effective in nonhospital settings.[39] In New Hampshire, before DNR bracelet for home use were adopted, emergency medical technicians were required to begin resuscitation and transport the patient to a hospital, even when it was clear that this was not the patient's wish. Often, despite teaching, the family faced with a dying loved one paniced as breathing became labored, heart rate slowed or stopped, or bleeding ensued. Even if documents such as living wills and durable powers of attorney for health care were produced, this did not release the emergency medical technicians of the responsibilities of response. In conjunction with New Hampshire Emergency Medical Services, a procedure was developed for outpatients and pre-hospital care to indicate patient preferences for no emergency care when cardiopulmonary arrest occured outside the hospital.[40] The DNR bracelet, which looks similar to a typical green hospital bracelet—except it is blue—can be obtained from a local hospital upon the completion of specific paper work. In the event of cardiopulmonary arrest at home or in an emergency department, this releases the responders from providing emergency care other than comfort care, symptom relief, and family support.

Finally, despite the development of nonhospital sites of EOL care, one analysis concluded that the main impetus behind hospital death is the number of hospital beds available in a referral area.[41] This study suggests that regardless of the availability of out-of-hospital alternatives, hospital deaths will continue at a higher rate in areas that have abundant hospital beds available than in those with fewer. Since that report was published, another study from Oregon, which has had the lowest in-hospital death rate in the United States (31%), has identified factors that facilitate arrangements for death to occur outside the hospital.[42] Many of the factors already mentioned were found to be significant in the Oregon study, as evidenced by the following quote: "For Oregon, it seems that economic forces and trends, coupled with an array of end-of-life resources, foster an environment in which patients and families more often obtain care during the lasts days of life in the setting they prefer."[42]

INITIATIVES TO IMPROVE EOL CARE IN HOSPITALS

As stated earlier, nurses are situated at the forefront of improving the quality of care in hospitals, because nurses provide the majority of care patients receive. Efforts to improve pain management,[43] especially in cancer, provided early leadership in the initiative to improve EOL care in hospitals. Besides creating a foundation for easing the pain associated with EOL care in hospitals, the process used to improve pain management by creating small and large multidisciplinary changes can be applied to EOL institutional efforts. The *Wisconsin Resource Manual for Improvement* reviews the process of quality improvement;[44] the City of Hope Pain Resource Center[45] provides articles and tools for pain management, many of which also are useful for palliative care; and an institutional assessment of the quality of pain management[46] can be easily adapted to help a project team think more broadly about palliative care and symptoms in addition to pain.[47] The programs described below are examples of how many of these ideas have been developed into improvement initiatives for EOL care in hospitals.

Institute for Healthcare Improvement (IHI)

In 1997 a quality improvement organization known as IHI adopted betterment of EOL care in hospitals and other parts of the health care system as a major thrust. Table 42–5 shows the organization and backbone of the initiative. The results of the initiative are fully elaborated in a manual.[16] In brief, the organization provided quality improvement assistance to organizations, and the resulting methods and results constitute a wide variety of outcomes to which almost any hospital or health care agency might aspire. To assist groups in getting started, a table (Table 42–6) focusing on four major issues in EOL care was distributed to ecourage organizations to compare their problems and issues, called "current practice," with what were proposed as "best" and "optimum" practices. Another aspect of the table consisted of examples of specific, measurable target outcomes that a group might choose to adopt.[48] The four selected areas resulted from brainstorming by the planning group, who were all nationally recognized leaders and clinicians in EOL care. They concluded that the following four areas are most in need of attention and amenable to change:

- improving the management of pain and other symptoms
- continuity of care
- advance directives
- family support

Each institution sent a team of at least two or more members representing the key disciplines implementing change in their organizations (nurses, physicians, chaplains, social workers, administrators, etc.) involved in to a series of three meetings between July 1997 and July 1998. Steps to ensure support from senior lead-

Table 42–5. Structure of The Institute for Healthcare Improvement (IHI) Collaborative: Improving Care at the End of Life*

The Institute for Healthcare Improvement (IHI) is a Boston-based, independent, non-profit organization working since 1991 to accelerate improvement in health care systems in the United States, Canada, and Europe by fostering collaboration, rather than competition, among health care organizations.

IHI provides bridges connecting people and organizations that are committed to real health care reform and who believe they can accomplish more by working together than they can separately.

Background

Study after study finds that patients, families, doctors, and other professionals want the same qualities of care at the end of life: Dignity, comfort, communication, and the company of loved ones. Yet time and again we seem trapped in desperate struggles and wasted energies that help no one. Rational, respectful care at the end of life is possible; now we need to assure it.

Participants

Since July 1997, 48 organizations from throughout the United States and Canada have been working intensively to improve the quality of care at the end of life while also reducing unwanted, non-beneficial care.

Overall Goals

Reduce incidence of severe pain by 25 percent.

Increase by 35 percent the number of patients who have made their wishes known about end-of-life care.

Reduce by 50 percent the number of patients with transfers in the last two weeks of life.

Areas of Focus

Collaborative teams are focusing on the following areas for improving care at the end of life:

- Pain management and palliative care.
- Advance care planning for end of life.
- Optimizing transfers among care settings.
- Family support.

Key Changes

Successful interventions that improve care at the end of life for patients and their families include:

- Instituting pain and symptom management protocols.
- Initiating advanced care planning discussions within 24 hours of admission and documenting the plan in a patient's chart. If this is not done, someone other than the patient's physician initiates advanced care planning within 36 hours of admission.
- Increasing 24-hour access to staff, using pagers and other communication devices to decrease hospital emergency room utilization.
- Using a "pull-system"—one-to-one case finding in the hospital to arrange early admission of target patients to palliative and hospice care.
- Beginning bereavement assistance and support for the family and friends before patients die.

Chair

Joanne Lynn, MD
President, Center for Improving Care of the Dying
George Washington University
Washington, DC

*From Web site: IHI (See Appendix B.)

Table 42–6. Recommendations for Areas of Focus and Targets for Improvement in Health Care Agencies Involved in IHI Collaborative

Current	Best Practices	Optimum Practice	Proposed Targets (for your Population)
Pain/Symptoms			
• Most often not assessed/monitored. • Routinely treated with predictably inadequate treatment (e.g., drugs and dosages). • Usually treated only after established, rather than preventively. • Gaps and delays in treatment are agonizing and commonplace. • Major symptoms are treatable: pain, dyspnea, depression, anxiety (also nausea, itching, insomnia). • No one held accountable for shortcomings. • Patients and families expect severe symptoms.	• 100% assessment on regular, recurrent basis, e.g., "5th Vital Sign" or item in nursing home quarterly review. • WHO/APS/AHCPR guidelines for cancer pain. • Low rate of use of opioids for breakthrough pain; all opioids on regular dosing. • Patients or families in control of dose timing. • Coverage doses travel with patient to procedures or during transfers. • Serious symptoms considered appropriate for emergency response (stat page, rapid home visit, calling on back-up provider). • Performance routinely reviewed and shortcomings addressed. • Patients and families expect comfort.	• 100% assessment of pain, depression, dyspnea, and anxiety on appropriate schedule (admission, change in status, and periodically). • Use of all appropriate modalities, often on time limited trials—including opioids, biofeedback, hypnosis, steroids, neuroablative procedures, stimulants, etc. Severe symptoms always have appropriately aggressive response. • Ready availability of skilled consultants in all settings (including ICU, hospital, nursing home, and home). • Patient and family have expectations of competence, control, comfort; and are enabled to be active participants in deciding and providing care. • Patient never left suffering due to relocation. • Emergency response "on call" for serious symptoms in any setting. • Routine care review and routine system feedback for quality improvement, public eduation and accreditation.	1. 100% compliance with recurrent assessment protocol. 2. Guarantee initial assessment of serious pain or dyspnea within 5 minutes in hospital, 15 minutes in nursing home or at home, and initial intervention within 15 minutes in hospital and 1 hour in nursing home or at home. 3. All patients have pain <5 (of 10) in last 2 days of life (by patient or family report). 4. Reduce by 50% the number of patients who report pain >5 (of 10) in any time period or episode of care. 5. All cancer patients with pain >5 (of ten) on appropriate opioids, and all patients with >5 (of ten) are on appropriate analgesics. 6. All patients at risk of severe dyspnea have "stand by" plans and needed skills/supplies in place (also advanced care planning goal). 7. Resource people with proven skills in chronic pain management and in management of neuropsychiatric complications of serious illness (depression, psychosis, delirium, anxiety, seizures) are readily available to every patient regardless of setting or insurance. 8. Eliminate times when patient or family reports pain being overwhelming or out of control. 9. Reduce "prn" for breakthrough pain to less than 20% of opioid use. 10. All patients/families understand the patient's symptoms and management and can adjust medications within agreed range. 11. All patients with signs of depression have a trial of drug treatment. 12. Individual and regular shortcomings noted and reviewed in Incident Reports, M&M conferences, QI committee and credentials review.

(*continued*)

Table 42–6. Recommendations for Areas of Focus and Targets for Improvement in Health Care Agencies Involved in IHI Collaborative (*Continued*)

Current	Best Practices	Optimum Practice	Proposed Targets (for your Population)
Continuity/Transfers			
• Seriously ill persons have no one who stays with them throughout. • Transfers between settings are dictated mostly by utilization and financing issues for the care system, not patient or family preferences. • Transfers among professionals are dictated by professional convenience. • Most patients change settings and/or caregivers multiple times in the last few weeks of life. • The fact and the expectation of discontuity precludes intimacy, empathy, promise-making, and trust. • Many transfers lose settled care plans, treatment schedules, and understanding. • Frequent transfers mean no one is held accountable for the overall course—or even for there being a standard for a good course. • Transfer to hospice or nursing home is especially discontinuous, and transfer by EMS is routinely maximally life-extending.	• Hospice usually ensures continuity in all settings, once enrolled. • Some nursing homes have developed capacity to care for seriously ill resident on-site, including a "hospice-like" mode. • Some special "advanced illness" programs coordinate all care out of one office and keep one nurse/social worker/physician in charge of care throughout. • Some programs have coordinated records available at all sites electronically, or by having the patient carry the record, or both. • Some nursing home or home care agencies have arranged for special direct hospital or hospice admission to avoid trauma in ambulances and ERs. • Some states and regions have developed accord on orders that reshape EMS services.	• People dying with cancer, advanced old age, or dementia virtually always die where they live. Services should be mobilized to these settings. • People dying with strokes and organ system failures die at home (or nursing home) or in a hospital, but in either case under the care of those who know them and with appropriate services. • Utilization-induced transfer should almost never happen in the last two days of life. • Switching key personnel while a patient is in any one setting should be uncommon, viewed as unfortunate, and should be the subject of careful planning to support patient and family. • Patients dying in ICU, ER, or busy ward settings should have available more family-attentive settings for temporary use.	1. For cancer patients >50% are in hospice >4 weeks and <20% are in hospice for <2 weeks. 2. >60% of those living at home with established fatal disease should die there, with good care. 3. <10% of deaths have change of setting in last 2 days. 4. 90% of families can name the one or two care providers who (together) were constant over the period when their family member was very ill. 5. >80% of those living in nursing homes should die there, with good care. 6. >80% of dying persons who have available an integrated care system should get all services from that system. 7. >50% of deaths from CHF, COPD, cirrhosis, and stroke have >4 weeks in hospice or another special end-of-life program. 8. Serious errors in transfer yield adverse events for all participants: review, payment penalty, QI efforts. 9. DNR orders established in one setting are transferred to another (and confirmed when appropriate) all of the time. 10. <10% of deaths have change of physician in last 2 days. 11. Written oral care plan moves with or ahead of patient for every change of care setting. 12. 90% of families feel that they knew who was "in charge" and how to reach that person at all times.
Advance Care Planning			
• Very little attention is paid to overall future course—not discussed, articulated, planned for. • Most people are not even asked to name a surrogate, even when who that would be is quite unclear. • Among persons who have very little chance of surviving CPR and substantial chances of cardiopulmonary arrest, few have discussions	• Regularly offering formal written planning opportunities, e.g., Vermont Ethics Network form. • Area-wide advance planning • Emergency kit of drugs and other paraphernalia at home, appropriate to family training and professional availability. • Emergency response team to go to home for pain,	• Likely course, including urgent complications and major decision points, is articulated for all chronically ill patients. • "Last phase of life" is noted, negotiated, and shared—among providers, patient and family—for >80% of dying. • Plans are written and discussed for likely "urgent complications" and for	1. CPR is attempted at death for <3% of patients who are known to be in the "last phase of life." 2. Decrease unplanned admissions by 50%. 3. A written care plan documents priorities and plans or >80% of "last phase of life" patients. 4. An appropriate surrogate is known (and documented if necessary) for 80% of those in the "last phase of life."

(*continued*)

Table 42–6. Recommendations for Areas of Focus and Targets for Improvement in Health Care Agencies Involved in IHI Collaborative (*Continued*)

Current	Best Practices	Optimum Practice	Proposed Targets (for your Population)
about DNR, even when put at special risk by being in hospital. • Most legal advance directives are too non-specific, unavailable, or inapplicable to direct care, yet patients think they have solved their problems by filling them out. • Almost no care planning deals with the specific drugs, skills, or procedures needed to allow the patient's preferences to be effected. • Some specific documented patient preferences are thoughtlessly abrogated.	dyspnea, seizures, family crisis, etc. • Formatted advance planning discussions (Emanuel, Emanuel).	prolonged incompetence for every "last phase of life" • Plans made in one setting or or by one set of providers working with patient and family are honored and confirmed, as appropriate, throughout care system. • Plans for urgent complications are translated into specific service needs (e.g., drugs, oxygen, etc.) and these are put in place in the appropriate settings. • CPR is allowed with strong patient/family preference, but is very rare. • Patients and families are not browbeaten into acquiescence with caregivers, nor are they brutalized by having to review painful decisions too often.	5. 90% of those who die in the system, of chronic disease, are identified as dying 2 months earlier, and 50% are identified 1 year earlier. 6. Patients and families are aware of eventual fatal nature of disease for >75% of those so identified. 7. >80% of patients in families know what to do for worsening pain, dyspnea, or for cardiac arrest and know the signs of impending death and what to do. 8. Plans for after death (who should come to share that time, funeral, burial, family support) are made and documented for >50%. 9. ER and 911 use declines by 50% in a target population. 10. 80% of "last phase of life" patients at home have plans documented to shape 911/EMS response appropriately.
Support of Family and of Meaningfulness			
• Families are excluded or ignored, granted only the role of veto in care planning. • Families do not know prognosis, uncertainties, desirable timing of behaviors, who to turn to for counsel, or what is reasonably expected of them. • Many opportunities to complete relationship (human or transcendent) are not taken. • Many patients or families do not have opportunity to attend to religious/spiritual issues, or meaningful rituals. • Most families have no follow-up in bereavement. • Many dissatisfied or guilt-ridden families are never heard, and some have lives blighted by their experience. • Families and patients have little practice at leave-taking.	• Care in hospice routinely includes family, spiritual concerns. • Hospice and home care agencies sometimes provide brochures and counseling about what to expect and how one might respond. • Hospice and some individual programs routinely follow families in bereavement, providing or referring to services as appropriate. • Some care providers insist upon enabling family cohesion and rearrangement, spiritual search for meaning and culturally meaningful rituals. • Some care settings help patients and families "rehearse" for dying by practicing leave-taking and imagining the time after.	• Center the experience in terms of spirituality and meaning, rather than medical and physiological issues. • Make human relationships and spiritual issues the central concern and thus professional caregiver habits are always. subservient. • Use episodes of serious illness as "dress rehearsals" for eventual death. • Create rituals that mark stages and ensure reassurance. • Always follow up with family—explain, reassure, counsel. • Learn how to provide care that is death accepting/enhancing life prolonging and physiology restoring.	1. Have >90% of families report that they would want to be cared for in this way if ever they were similarly sick. 2. Have >90% of families report that they cannot recall: • a time when they were kept "in the dark" • a cruel or uncaring remark from acaregiver • a "put down" of their beliefs or practices or views. 3. All bereaved families get at least one follow-up call from a doctor or nurse who can answer "medical" questions and check for seriously dysfunctional grief. 4. Double the rate at which patients and families agree that "the last few weeks or months were especially meaningful." 5. For chronic organ system failure, develop a care pattern in which 80% of staff and of patients/families feel that staff are pleased and supportive of survival (in an exacerbation) and also supportive of a good dying. 6. Have >90% of families report that: • Their loved one was given tender care • The family's emotional state was noticed and responded to. • Caregiver said or did something especially meaningful.

Ref: Lynn, Teno, Phillips, Wu, Desbiens, Harrold, Clessens, Wenger, Kreling, Connors, 1997.
Used with permission J. Lynn, MD, IHI chair.

ers of each organization were considered vital at the outset. Teams were provided with large-group didactic content and written materials. They also participated in concentrated, small-group meetings to identify what they would do upon return to their institutions. Regular progress reports were sent to IHI, monthly conference calls were held, and online discussions were conducted to support the teams and offer advice if particular barriers or issues developed. These teams were successful in achieving many of their goals from, improving pain relief and dyspnea, reducing hospitalizations, improving advance care planning, to implementing bereavement services. The experiences of these organizations provide a wealth of practical advice and methods for accomplishing quality improvement in many areas and settings of care and are available on the IHI website and in print.

Table 42–7. The United Hospital Fund's Hospital Palliative Care Initiative: What the Hospitals Learned: Observations and Insights

Areas for improvement in current hospital practice

Clinical staff training and skills development
Greater attention to patients' spiritual needs
Better communication among caregivers, patients, and families

Necessary institutional commitments to change New York City hospitals

Expanding the acute care mission
Communicating the commitment of hospital leaders
Redefining professional roles and lines of authority
Creating a palliative care infrastructure
Finding the necessary resources

Source: Data from ref # 49, The Challenge of Caring for Patients near the End of Life: Findings from the Hospital Palliative Care Initiative.

United Hospital Fund's Hospital Palliative Care Initiative

This multiyear, multihospital research and demonstration initiative sought to improve the quality of hospital care for persons at the EOL. In the first phase of the initiative, 12 hospitals received grants to analyze the institutional, professional, fiscal, and regulatory forces shaping EOL care. In the second phase, two-year program grants were awarded to the following five New York City hospitals to seek specific goals:

1. Beth Israel Medical Center—To develop an array of new palliative care service delivery and education activities, including the creation of a new position, medical director for palliative care.
2. The Brooklyn Hospital Center—To create a new position of palliative care expert, with responsibility and authority to facilitate the coordinated delivery of palliative care services to a select group of patients and their families.
3. Montefiore Medical Center—To evaluate and improve physician practice patterns concerning EOL care by using evaluative feedback for a one-year period, focused on five areas of EOL care.
4. The Mount Sinai Medical Center—To create a comprehensive new supportive care service to provide coordinated palliative care services across a range of settings.
5. Saint Vincent's Hospital and Medical Center—To create a new palliative care consulting team to build on the existing outpatient supportive care service and expand them to include physician and psychiatric expertise for a select group of patients and their families in both the inpatient and outpatient settings.

Although not all are specifically using quality improvement methods, the outcomes and products to improve palliative care that evolved from these projects can inform other hospitals wishing to replicate their successes.[49] Table 42–7 summarizes the major areas of learning reported by hospitals in the study.

Veterans Health Administration Initiatives

The Department of Veterans Affairs (VA) health care system has shown leadership in improving EOL care in their hospitals in multiple initiatives that have been designed and/or implemented since the early 1990s. In 1992, Secretary Jesse Brown mandated that VA hospitals establish hospice consultation teams to respond to the complex palliative care needs of patients with advanced disease. The VA provided training for team members during 1992 and 1993. One team reported success in pain and cost reduction while also undertaking significant institution-wide improvements through education of nurses and house staff and making pain management resources available.[50]

In 1997 the Veterans Health Administration (VHA) began an intensive, system-wide, continuous quality improvement (CQI) initiative to improve pain management. This endeavor resulted from a 1997 survey that found both acute and chronic pain management services to be inconsistent, inaccessible, and nonuniform throughout the system. Two major thrusts formed the basis of the initiative: issuing a system-wide mandate and forming a permanent National Pain Advisory Committee to provide direction and encouragement to the development of the program. Thus, this initiative incorporated two essential elements found in all successful system-wide improvement strategies: an influential champion at the highest level of the organization and a mandate for organizational commitment to this activity. The charge document offered a variety of suggestions for system improvement: making pain more visible by enhancing current measurement and reporting methods (using the 5th Vital Sign approach in all patient contacts in the system); increasing access to pain therapy and increasing professional education about pain; adopting the Agency for Health Care Policy and Research and American Pain Society standards for pain management; pursuing research on pain therapies for veterans; distributing and sharing pain management protocols via a central clearinghouse; and exploring methods to maintain cost-effective pain therapy.

Also in 1997, the Department of Veterans Affairs incorporated a palliative care measure in the performance criteria of its regional directors. In this program, performance of the directors is evaluated based on the number of charts that contain information about veterans' preferences regarding various palliative care indicators.[51] Faculty leadership is another important thrust of the VA. In 1998 the Robert Wood Johnson Foundation Last Acts program awarded a two-year grant to promote development of 30 faculty fellows from VA-affiliated internal medicine training programs. Their goal was to develop curricula to train residents in the care of dying patients, to integrate relevant content into the curricula of residency training programs, and to add internal medicine faculty leaders and innovators to the field of palliative medicine. All of these initiatives attack the need for improvement on multiple fronts and create a momentum in the Veterans Administration system that can set an example for other large hospital-based systems of care.

PALLIATIVE CARE PATHWAYS AND STANDARD ORDERS

Reducing variation is a major strategy used by quality improvement leaders. *Variation* refers to the fluctuations in a process that can result in delays or unpredictable outcomes.[52] As described earlier, a patient with a serious illness who is experiencing an acute crisis may follow many different paths (see Table 42–4). Numerous institutions have studied their current process of care and have created clinical pathways that can help standardize procedures and reduce the variation of care experienced by terminally ill or symptomatic EOL patients as they traverse the complex health care system.[53,54,55] Usual components include attention to patient symptoms as well as family needs at system entry and throughout the course of stay until discharge. Time frames designed to address needs help in monitoring progress and tracking outcomes that have been met, as well as those that continue to need attention. Although published guidelines and standards may offer similar suggestions, the road map format of clinical pathways identifies practical and accountable mechanisms to keep patient care moving in the direction of specific identified outcomes. Some paths allow

Dartmouth Hitchcock Medical Center

Comfort Measures
Physician Orders

Date ______ **Time** ______ **Attending Physician** ______________________

_____ **DISCONTINUE ALL PREVIOUS ORDERS**

NEW ORDERS:
Activity: ___ OOB as tolerated ___ OOB with assistance ___ Bedrest
Hunger: ___Diet as tolerated ___ NPO ___ Other______________________
Thirst: ___PO Fluids as tol. **IV Fluids:** ___ No IVF ___Yes________________
Dyspnea: _____O2 prn for patient comfort _____ No Oxygen _____ Fan at bedside
Elimination: ___Insert Foley Catheter prn ___ Narcotic Bowel Orders (see NBO form)
Oral Care per nursing standards
Skin Care per nursing standards
Monitoring:
Vital Signs: ___No ___ Yes - specify _____________
Weight: ___No weights ___ Yes - specify _____________
Labs: ___No lab draws ___ Yes labs - specify________________
Psychosocial Consults:
___ Palliative Care ___ CRC ___ Social Work ___ Pastoral Care

Previous Adverse Drug Reactions ____________________

Medication for Symptom Management (Routine & PRN)
Pain - Scheduled:
Pain - Breakthrough:
Anxiety/Depression:
Dyspnea: (Consider nebulized morphine)
Agitation:
Sleep Disturbance:
Pruritus:
Fever: (Consider rectal route)
Nausea/Vomiting:
Constipation:
Diarrhea:
Other Orders:

MD Signature______________________ **Print**______________ **Beeper**________

Comfort Measures Standards
Standards based on concepts from **Oxford Textbook of Palliative Medicine**

DISCONTINUE ALL PREVIOUS ORDERS- All previous orders should be assessed for relation to comfort management.

Activity: Goal is patient comfort
The nurse will maintain activity based on patient's preference.

Hunger: Goal is to respond to patient's hunger, not maintain a "normal nutritional intake."

Thirst: Goal is to respond to patient's thirst which is best accomplished by PO fluids, sips, ice chips per patient desires verses IV hydration.

IV Fluids: Small volume of fluid may assist with medication metabolism and delirium verses over hydration which may lead to discomfort from edema, pulmonary and gastric secretions, and urinary incontinence.

Dyspnea: Respond to the patient's perception of breathlessness verses "numerical abnormalities" i.e. pulse oximetry.
Interventions for dyspnea include oxygen, opioids, antianxiety agents, steroids, decrease in IV fluids, and atropine to decrease secretions.
O2 Therapy prn for patient comfort – nasal cannula or mask as needed.
Fans at Bedside – Fans are available for patient comfort and are often more effective for perception of breathlessness than other interventions.
Consider Nebulized Morphine – on or off protocol.

Elimination: Focus on managing distress from bowel or bladder incontinence.
Insert Foley Catheter prn – per patient comfort and desire
Consider MHO diarrhea management algorithm and constipation standard care plan.

Oral Care per nursing standards: studies show dry mouth is the most common and distressing symptom in conscious patients at end of life.
Ice chips and sips of fluid prn
Mouth care q 2 hours and prn – sponge oral mucosa and apply lubricant to lips and oral mucosa
Consider MHO mouth care algorithm guidelines.

Skin Care per nursing standards:
Incontinent care every 2 hours and prn
Pressure Sore Prevention Measures: per DHMC skin care guidelines.

Monitoring The focus of monitoring is on the patient's responses to comfort measures.

Psychosocial Consults Goal is to supply resources and support through the dying process

Medication for Symptom Management (Routine & PRN)
Pain Management- scheduled and breakthrough: consider IV/SQ/rectal analgesics
Depression Management: evaluate for antidepressants or methylphenidate
Dyspnea Management: consider nebulized morphine, atropine for secretions
Anxiety/Agitation Management: consider lorazepam (Ativan) or haloperidol (Haldol)
Sleep Disturbance Management: consider diphenhydramine (Benadryl)
Pruritus Management: consider diphenhydramine (Benadryl) PO/IV
Fever Management: consider acetaminophen (Tylenol) PO/ rectal
Nausea/Vomiting Management: consider prochlorperazine (Compazine), 5-HT3 antagonist PO/IV
Constipation Management: consider NBO order sheet
Diarrhea Management: consider Lomotil or loperamide (Imodium)

Fig. 42–4. Comfort Measures Physician Orders sheet (**left**) with guidelines for care as reference for house staff education on the back (**right**).

for documentation of variation from the designated path. Analysis of several instances of variation might alert a care team of a potential system "defect" in need of improvement.

Many institutions have implemented standard orders or evidence-based algorithms to guide various aspects of care pertinent to end-of-life situations. Some of these include limitations of certain types of therapies such as cardiopulmonary resuscitation and blood pressure medications. Additionally, preprinted order sheets that outline management of symptoms and side effects, such as nausea, constipation and pain, are making it easier for physicians and trainees to reproduce comprehensive plans that do not vary because of individual opinion. These order forms can be valuable teaching tools in a setting of regularly changing care providers. Figure 42–4A shows a sample order sheet, and Figure 42–4B shows the companion guidelines printed on the reverse for patients who are hospitalized and have a palliative focus of care. Certainly, important considerations in the development of such "recipes" for care include having broad, multidisciplinary, evidence-based input. The process of producing such documents is also potentially a care consensus and learning environment for many teams.

PALLIATIVE CARE CONSULTANCY TEAMS

A growing literature summarizes the development within hospitals of palliative care teams formed to offer specialized consultation and expertise to all health care providers. Dunlop published a manual in 1990 and a second edition in 1998 describing the experience in England.[56,57] He described the movement as one that tries to take the hospice philosophy of care and bring it into the hospital using a consultancy team. More recently, U.S. and Canadian hospital-based teams have described their experiences.[58–60] Among the components of successful teams are a multidisciplinary approach, strong nursing leadership, physician and nonphysician referral, rapid response to requested consultation, around the clock referral service, and ability to follow patients through all care settings.[14]

From a quality improvement perspective, these teams can be effective in modeling behaviors that are supportive of appropriate hospital-based EOL care, but they should also recommend infrastructure changes as part of their approach to consultation. For assessment of care and processes to improve, demographic statistics about the location and nature of regular consultations is needed. For instance, if a particular unit or care provider has regular difficulty managing patients with dyspnea, targeted educational approaches and treatment algorithms or standardized orders may help achieve consistent and long-lasting change. Theoretically, a consultancy team could "put itself out of business" with such an approach. However, teams to date have not reported the need to dissolve as an outcome of implementing system changes.

INPATIENT HOSPICE AND PALLIATIVE CARE UNITS IN GENERAL HOSPITALS

Some hospitals, faced with the problem of providing high quality EOL care in the acute hospital, have found the development of a specialized unit to be the solution. In the United Kingdom these units have been developed from preexisting oncology units, as part of another unit, or sometimes in a separate building that is distinct but near the hospital it serves.[57] U.S. hospitals have varying amounts of experience with opening specialized units for the care of patients with EOL, hospice, or palliative care needs.[57,61,62,63] This in-hospital approach has some general benefits and burdens.[14] Some of the benefits include:

- Patients requiring palliative care have a familiar place to go during the exacerbations and remissions that come with progressive disease.
- Unit staff and policies are under the control and financing of experts trained as a team who are skillful at difficult care and communications.
- Patients may get palliative care earlier if other care teams see the advantages of this approach and trust patients will receive good care.
- Providers who follow their patients on these units (if allowed) can learn valuable lessons about palliative care that can be carried forward to future patients. These future patients may not require admission to the palliative care unit for some types of care.

Some of the disadvantages of creating a distinct unit include:

- It can prevent others from learning valuable palliative care techniques if the principles are seen as "specialized" and are secluded in one area.
- Care providers may come to rely on this expertise instead of learning palliative care techniques themselves.
- If unit transfer includes a transfer of doctors to a palliative care specialist, patients and families may feel abandoned by their prior team in the final hours.
- Hospice providers fear the loss of the hospice philosophy when a palliative care unit is in the context of the general hospital.

Some mature palliative care programs have been able to provide a trinity of services,[14] including a consultancy team, an inpatient palliative care/hospice unit, and a home care program, all under the jurisdiction of a single hospital system. This full-service approach can ease transitions among different levels of care and has the potential to be the optimum in seamless care for patients at the EOL. Such programs can serve as models and can set a standard for other programs to aim for.

A major consideration in the utilization of such services, regardless of how broadly based, is the barrier to care presented by not recognizing that a patient may be dying. Many studies now document health care providers' inaccuracy in predicting prognosis.[2,5,13] As a result, many patients who could benefit from palliative care and hospice services are denied admission. A comprehensive discussion on the reasons for inaccuracy of prognosis is beyond the scope of this chapter, although it remains a major issue that must be addressed within any institution wishing to develop specialty palliative care services. Hospice programs are very familiar with such issues, and palliative care programs would be wise to review lessons learned in providing hospice care earlier in the disease trajectory for patients in need.

HOSPITAL-BASED BEREAVEMENT PROGRAMS AND SERVICES

Improving the quality of EOL care in hospitals does not end with the development of mechanisms to ensure peaceful, pain-free patient death. Although accomplishing this goal is surely a comfort to family and friends, the aftermath for survivors is considered an important final step in the process of EOL care. Which families are most in need of specific services? Identifying families at the greatest risk has been the topic of palliative care research, particularly in evaluating the quality of palliative care services.[64]

Bereavement services for survivors are an important part of the total care plan following the patient's death (see Chapter 25). Adverse physical and psychological outcomes of unsupported grief are known to occur during the bereavement period. Because of this, bereavement services are a typical component of the services offered to families when patients die as part of a hospice program. Because only 10% of all deaths in the United States have Hospice involvement in EOL care, a large portion of families must rely on follow-up offered by other care providers. Few hospitals routinely offer bereavement services to families following patient deaths in hospital.[65] Evaluating survivors during the bereavement period serves two main purposes in quality improvement: (*1*) Development of these services by hospitals can address currently unmet needs of survivors, who usually need to discuss their own needs for information and support in order to cope with the loss. (*2*) This is a time when hospitals can learn more about the effectiveness of their provision of EOL care from the families' perspectives, both what went well and what can be improved.

For instance, during a focus group of bereaved family members it was found that although the family was quite satisfied with pain management, breathing changes and dyspnea were not anticipated and were very distressing.[1] Another institution determined from a bereavement survey that the institution needed to make improvements in the areas of respecting patient privacy and dignity, family communications, emergency care, advanced directives, and bereavement support.[65]

Following evaluation, hospitals can develop a project to improve and standardize bereavement care and would be well advised to consult with a local hospice program to collaborate on how this might occur. Instituting some very simple, standardized responses to death can vastly improve family satisfaction with care. These actions might include sending a note of sympathy or establishing some other contact from a staff member, mailing a list of local bereavement resources or a pamphlet, and using a prescribed timing to mail the hospital bill.

MEDICAL AND NURSING EDUCATION AS A MEANS TO IMPROVE EOL CARE IN HOSPITALS

The majority of medical, nursing, and other health care disciplines receive training for practice in hospitals. And, until recently, with the shift to ambulatory care, the majority of medical and nursing student education was provided in the hospital setting. From the perspective of EOL care, most hospitals were not models for teaching this skill. The following is one of several comments made by family members about the insensitive way the act of "pronouncing" the death of their loved one was handled by house staff:

> I was holding his hand when he stopped breathing. I called the nurse who called the doctor. He went over and looked at him lying in the bed, listened for a heartbeat with his stethescope and said "He's dead," and walked out of the room. That's it, not "I'm sorry," no "Is there anything we can do?" just "he's dead." It was painful—and made us think that the staff didn't care.

It is not surprising that this death occurred at the beginning of July, when staff began their first rotations directly out of medical school. A study by Ferris and colleagues[66] showed how little attention EOL care has been given in medical school. A small survey of medical interns revealed significant concern and fear over providing these services with no or little supervision. It is unclear why this activity, unlike other experiences that are subject to the traditional "see one, do one, teach one" supervisory principle of medical education was ignored. One resident surveyed explained that the pronouncing experience was not one that was perceived as causing harm when performed by the inexperienced. Another stated "I felt really inadequate, I had absolutely no idea what to do when the nurse called me to pronounce this patient who I never met—my first night on call. I was never taught the steps, how long should I listen to the chest to be sure there was no heartbeat, what, if anything else, I should do, what should I say to the family. Thankfully, the death coordinator was there to help me fill out the paperwork." Conversely, in states where nurses are allowed to pronounce deaths, some course work exists to teach a process that gives attention to the family.

Clearly, such a predictable and easily defined process is amenable to quality improvement if it is identified as an educational priority for an institution or health care provider. A sample pocket card developed from multiple data sources of such a project is shown in Figure 42–5. This is printed internally on brightly colored stock on a standard laser printer so that it can be easily modified and so that quantities are readily available. A similar card was developed by others. Part of a multimedia packet for resident education, it is called the Art of Compassionate Death Notification.[67] Other components of this comprehensive program include a facilitator's guide, manuals for learners, and videos demonstrating communication skills.

Dartmouth-Hitchcock Medical Center

Quick reference card for: PRONOUNCEMENT OF DEATH

When you are called to pronounce a patient:

- *• **Recognize the extreme emotional significance of the actual pronouncement of death to family members in room.**
- *• Establish eye contact with family members(s) present.
- *• Introduce self to family.
- Examine patient for absence of breath sounds and heart sounds.
- Note time of death.
- After confirmation of death, verbally acknowledge patient's death to family.
- *• Communicate condolences verbally (i.e., "I'm sorry for your loss.") or non-verbally.
- Determine legal next-of-kin from chart face sheet.
- Ask legal next-of-kin about autopsy, organ donation, funeral home name (family can call it in later).
- Nurse/secretary will contact Deceased Patient Coordinator (beeper #9399) to help complete the paper work (3 forms).
- Notify attending MD of death.

***DHMC study (Mills, Whedon, et al 1998) revealed these steps were often omitted from the pronouncement process.**

© DHMC End of Life Project 7-7-98

Fig. 42–5. Pronouncement card used as a reference at the time of death. © 1998 DHMC End of Life Project.

The problem is further compounded by the lack of EOL care coverage in student curricula[68] and major textbooks.[69,70] These sources have been analyzed and have been found sorely lacking in the content that would inform students about the basics of EOL symptom management, decision-making, and critical communication skills. Neither textbooks nor clinical experiences are effective in providing critical guidance to health professionals in how to provide effective EOL care. In response, funding is becoming available to study the issue and develop solutions to remedy it.[71,72,73]

Chapter 49 discusses the topic in detail. For the purposes of this chapter, it is important to remember to involve students in the process of change. Improvements in hospitals should address the learning environments of students. Specific ideas for improving the interface between education and quality improvement of hospital-based EOL care include:

- Arrange for clinician role models to provide lectures to students and faculty.
- Assist with curriculum review of current EOL care training.
- Change elective coursework and clinical work in hospice and palliative care to required, and include these subjects in other mandatory clinical assignments.
- Use texts that contain clinically relevant palliative care content.
- Include content on ambulatory-based symptom management and decision making that defines patient preferences for care.
- Encourage students to describe evidence-based approaches to palliative care and to challenge their mentors about approaches and interventions that increase the burden of care without clear patient benefit.
- Encourage students to learn from staff role models appropriate ways of communicating bad news and of presenting options that respect patient preferences and values.
- Identify opportunities for undergraduate or graduate fellowships in palliative care.
- As part of quality improvement teams, offer students opportunities to become data collectors from patients, charts, and staff.

ECONOMIC ISSUES IN IMPROVING HOSPITAL BASED EOL CARE

The use of the DRG system has played a role in the current provision of EOL care. The prospective payment system of Medicare was one of the first economic stimuli that began to shift EOL care out of hospitals. Simultaneously, the Medicare hospice benefit was instituted, which reconfigured financing for Hospice care (described earlier) and reimbursed some home care, acute care, and specialized units in nursing homes.[25]

The Health Care Financing Administration (HCFA) uses DRG codes for defining Medicare reimbursement, although at present limited mechanisms exist to obtain reimbursement for various types of palliative care in hospitals under Medicare. In response to this limitation, in October 1996 a trial of using the v code 66.7 was initiated as a mechanism to collect data about palliative care being provided in hospitals.[74] At present, this code does not elicit reimbursement but allows for data to be collected about the current nature of palliative care.

Some professionals and administrators may see development of palliative care services as a way to save money as less invasive procedures and tests are recommended compared to more expensive aggressive care. Although palliative care may be economical in terms of dollars and reduced suffering, this has not been demonstrated. It would seem that providing less unwanted care would result in fewer intensive care unit stays and costly, invasive procedures, but this will be difficult to document.

Although there is a bias against hospital death, as hospital care is associated with high-tech interventions, there are times when dying in the hospital allows for a more comfortable death than at home. In any case, valid reimbursed hospital admissions for palliative care may be difficult to obtain within the current DRG codes. In the best case, the palliative care DRG would remedy this. However, some oppose the creation of a new DRG because the assignment of the code may only describe what is currently being done, which may not be adequate and hence not reflect what state of the art palliative care could achieve.

Managed care can influence the quality of end-of-life care in hospitals in both positive and negative ways. Patients in a managed care plan need approvals and are carefully observed so that they do not spend unnecessary days in the hospital. This approach can be quite restrictive when extra planning time to assure patient comfort is restricted. On the other hand, several features of managed care make it a potentially positive force for improvement.[75] Anthem Blue Cross and Blue Shield of New Hampshire–Matthew Thornton Health Plan has implemented an innovative approach (Fig. 42–6). In response to two letters complaining of frustrations regarding pain management and reimbursement issues concerning care of dying family members, the director of medical management and the clinical quality improvement coordinator (both nurses) redesigned the plan's hospice benefit.[76] Their aim, methods, and outcomes are shown in Figure 42–6. Their standards of pain and hospice care were sent to all providers, and a monitoring system was implemented to ensure adherence and to provide for review of situations that were outside the scope of of the guidelines. This use of quality improvement methodology outside the hospital to simplify care and hold providers and insurers accountable for a predetermined standard of EOL care proved successful. The approach ultimately benefited plan members by increasing access to appropriate levels of EOL care (including hospital-based, when appropriate).

Another effort to evaluate how health plans and systems provide end of life care consists of a strategy to measure and compare outcomes across organizations. Funded by the Robert Wood Johnson Foundation in 1997, the Foundation for Accountability (FACCT) assembled an expert panel of EOL clinicians, quality improvement specialists, research scientists, and health plan administrators and held focus groups of high-risk patients to develop a strategy to measure the quality of EOL care in health plans. The intent was to allow for comparisons of plan performance and to help health plans set goals for quality improvement

Aims

- To ensure that all members/families have access to quality end-of-life care and verbalize satisfaction with that care.
- To provide dignity, respect, support, effective pain control, and guidance to our terminally ill members and their families at the end-of-life.
- To improve benefit design and ensure that hospice members receive optimal health care services in a timely, consistent, and comprehensive manner.

Program Components

- Precertification for all Hospice Services.
- Hospice certified case managers.
- Pain management guidelines.
- Contracted Hospice levels of care.
- Standards of practice for home health, hospice care and infusion therapy.
- Outcome measures of satisfaction and clinical quality.

Improvement Methods

- Early recognition of those members who need end-of-life care.
- Provider education regarding the importance of early referral to Hospice Case Management.
- Utilize ICD-9, CPT Codes, and pharmaceutical data to identify members who may need the service.
- Implement pt/family questionnaire data collection tool specific to hospice issues.

Desired Outcomes

- Process outcomes of education and guideline development (achieved).
- Compliance with increased ALOS > 50 days on Hospice case management benefit.
- 95% caregivers express needs met by redesigned specialty case management.
- 95% caregivers felt pain management strategies explained at end-of-life (post-death questionnaire).

Fig. 42–6. Blue Cross Blue Shield of New Hampshire Quality Improvement Project to Improve Members EOL Care.

activities at the EOL.[77] The report summarizes distinctions between measures for public accountability and quality improvement, consumer opinion about what is important at the EOL, and important measures and reporting categories for capturing plan performance in eight areas of care within three major categories: steps to good care, results of care, and experience and satisfaction with care. In addition, practical advice about the measurement process and additional areas of needed research are described.[77]

RESOURCES AND RESEARCH TO ASSIST WITH IMPROVING EOL CARE IN HOSPITALS

The good news is that there is a growing foundation of resources to assist the clinician or team wishing to apply a quality improvement process to hospital-based EOL care. However, such abundance may overwhelm the beginning clinician, quality improvement personnel, or project team. A mantra from an unknown source on the cover of one quality improvement manual lends heart—"We cannot do everything at once, but we must do something at once."[44] A few key sources provide major overviews of projects, groups, and contacts. Palliative care as a developing specialty lacks an adequate evidence base.[78] However, as more research findings become available, the rapid-cycle improvement infrastructure is one way to quickly test and translate findings into clinical practice. Although funding mechanisms exist for research, fewer funding opportunities exist for quality improvement.

An example of funding for quality improvement is the Oncology Nursing Foundation Clinical Scholars Program. The goal of this program is to link research and practice in areas where there is a growing evidence base, such as fatigue and pain management. The 1998 Clinical Scholars Program in pain management specifically addressed several important aspects of improving EOL care as research findings were put into practice.[79] These projects covered standardized pain screening and assessment in both inpatient and outpatient settings, education about high-tech pain procedures to improve care in a hospice converting to a palliative care unit, improvement of assessment and management of neuropathic pain, and understanding the experience of bone pain in patients with multiple myeloma since the advent of pamidronate.

FUTURE DIRECTIONS

The first and biggest step in improving EOL care is to reduce the number of unnecessary in-hospital deaths. As death in hospitals will never be completely eliminated, the second biggest improvement will come as a result of improved communication among the health team, patient, and family. Strategies can be put into place to identify the goals of hospital care and implement a prompt, effective, holistic plan to meet predetermined values and preferences.

A number of features of hospitals actually make it easier to employ successful full scale improvements, such as the amount of readily available data and regulatory efforts like those of the Joint Commission on Accreditation of Healthcare Organizations (JCAHO). Innovations such as consultation teams, units, and pathways have already begun to provide successful models for improvement.

Sometimes a disadvantage can really be an advantage. For example, the perceived endless paperwork, rigidity, and regulations common to hospitals may be among the biggest advantages to making improvements in hospital-based EOL care. Extensive and readily accessible databases of variables that reflect the quality of EOL care are available and are the positive side of monumental documentation requirements. Because of this accessibility, the study of the quality of EOL care in hospitals and some areas of quality improvement have been brought to light relatively rapidly, plans for change have been implemented, and results have been monitored. In the context of hospital oversight and regulation, medical professionals have much more control over hospital operations than can ever be expected in the community or home. Improvement of pain relief in hospitals is likely to experience a boon under the newly created pain management standards from the JCAHO.

Quality improvement in hospitals has the potential to provide a significant foundation on which to build a larger health care system and culture of humane care at the EOL. Dr. Christine Cassel provides a simple guideline for success in the preface to the National Academy of Sciences Institute of Medicine report entitled *Approaching Death: Improving Care at the End of Life*[2]:

> When medicine can no longer promise an extension of life, people should not fear that their dying will be marked by neglect, care inconsistent with their wishes, or preventable pain and other distress. They should be able to expect the health care system to assure reliable, effective, and humane care giving. If we can fulfill that expectation, then public trust will be strengthened.

The author acknowledges Joanne Lynn, M.D., M.S., M.A., Polly Campion, R.N., and Marilyn Bedell, R.N. for thoughtful insights and review during manuscript development, and Daphne Ellis for assistance with manuscript preparation.

REFERENCES

1. Mulrooney T, Whedon M, Bedell A. Focus group of family members after death of a loved one in the hospital. Part of IHI project. Also published as an abstract not selected for presentation at the 1999 ONS congress. Unpublished data. Dartmouth Hitchcock Medical Center.

2. Institute of Medicine. Approaching Death: Improving Care at the End of Life. Washington, DC: National Academy Press, 1997.

3. Brock DB, Foley DJ. Demography and epidemiology of dying in the U.S. with emphasis on deaths of older persons. The Hospice Journal 13 (1/2):49–60.

4. Wennberg JE, Cooper MM, eds. The Quality of Care in the United States: A Report on the Medicare Program/The Dartmouth Atlas of Health. Chicago: AHA Press, 1999.

5. The SUPPORT Principal Investigators. A controlled trial to improve care for seriously ill hospitalized patients. The study to understand prognoses and preferences for outcomes and risks of treatments (SUPPORT). JAMA 1995;274:1591–1598.

6. Elshamy M, Whedon MB. Symptoms and

care during the last 48 hours of life. Quality of Life: A Nursing Challenge. Quality Assessment 1997;5(2):21–29.

7. Goodlin SJ, Winzelberg GS, Teno J, Whedon MB, Lynn J. Death in the hospital. Arch of Intern Med 1998;158 (July 27:)1570–1572.

8. Lynn J, Teno JM, Phillips R, Wu AW, Desbiens N, Harrold J, Claessens M, Wenger, Kreling B, Connors. A for the SUPPORT Investigators. Perceptions of family members of the dying experience of older and seriously ill patients. Ann Intern Med 1997;126:97–106.

9. Seale C, Cartwright A. The Year Before Death. Aldershot, Hants, England: Ashgate Publishing, 1994.

10. Agency for Health Care Policy and Research. Clinical Practice Guideline: Management of Cancer Pain. (AHCPR Publication No. 94–0592). Rockville, MD: U.S. Department of Health and Human Services, Public Health Services, Agency for Health Care Policy and Research, 1994.

11. Berwick DM. A primer on leading the improvement of systems. Br Med J 1996; 312(7031):619–622.

12. Miller FG, Fins JJ. A proposal to restructure hospital care for dying patients. NEJM 1996;334:1740–1742.

13. Solomon MZ. The enormity of the task: SUPPORT and changing practice. Special Supplement, Hastings Center Report 25, no 6: S28–S32.

14. Krammer LM, Muir JC, Gooding-Kellar, N, Williams MB, von Gunten CF. Palliative care and oncology: Opportunities for oncology nursing. Oncology Nursing Updates: Patient Treatment and Support 1999;6(3):1–12.

15. Weggel JM. Palliative care: New challenges for advanced practice nursing. The Hospice Journal 1997;12(1):43–56.

16. Lynn J, Schuster JL. Improving Care for the End of Life: A Sourcebook for Health Care Managers and Clinicians. New York: Oxford University Press 2000.

17. Nelson EC, Batalden PC, Ryer JC, eds. Joint Commission Clinical Improvement Action Guide. Oakbrook, IL: Joint Commission on Accreditation in Healthcare Organizations, 1998.

18. Higginson I. Clinical and organizational audit in palliative care. In: Doyle et al., eds. Oxford Textbook of Palliative Medicine, 2nd ed. Oxford: Oxford University Press, 1998: 67–81.

19. Higginson I. Measuring quality of care in palliative care services: An interview with Irene Higginson, Ph.D., innovations in end-of-life care. An international journal and on-line forum of leaders in end-of-life care, 2000;2(1): http://www2.edc.org/lastacts/featureinn.asp.

20. Personal communication, J. Boehm, May 5, 1999:1997 Unpublished CPR Committee Data, Dartmouth-Hitchcock Medical Center;.

21. Teno J. Executive summary of the first conference on making a tool kit of instruments to measure end of life care (TIME). http://www.chcr.brown.edu/pcoc/toolkit.htm 1999.

22. Teno JM. Putting the patient and family voice back into measuring the quality of care for the dying. Hospice Journal 1999;14:167–176.

23. Nelson EC, Splaine, ME, Batalden, Plume SK. Building measurement and data collection into medical practice. Ann Intern Med 1998;128:460–466.

24. LaFrance S. Death in New Hampshire: A Review of Medical Charts, New Hampshire Partnership for End-of-life Care Final Report. Available from the Foundation for Healthy Communities, Concord, NH, or Website www.fhconline.org 1999.

25. Castle NG, Mor V, Banaszak-Holl J. Special care hospice units in nursing homes. Hospice Journal 1997;2(3):59–69.

26. Ferrell BR, Virani R, Grant M. HOPE: Home care outreach for palliative care education. Cancer Practice 1998;6(2):79–85.

27. Emanuel EJ, Fairclough DL, Slutsman J, Alpert H, Baldwin D, Emanuel LL. Assistance from family members, friends, paid care givers, and volunteers in the care of terminally ill patients. NEJM 1999;341:956–963.

28. Medicare Hospice Benefit. Patient Guide 2000.

29. Covinsky KE, Goldman L, Cook EF, et al. The impact of serious illness on patients' families. JAMA 1994;272:1839–1844.

30. Weinberg M. Research findings from studies with companies and caregivers. Last Acts; Robert Wood Johnson Foundation, 1999.

31. Position statement on nursing and the self-determination act. Washington, DC: American Nurses Association, 1991.

32. Teno JM, Licks S, Lynn J, et al. Do advance directives provide instructions that direct care? JAGS 1997;45:508–512.

33. Sulmasy DP, Terry PB, Weisman CS, et al. The accuracy of substituted judgments in patients with terminal diagnoses. Ann Intern Med 1998;128:621–629.

34. Hammes BJ, Rooney BL. Death and end-of-life planning in one Midwestern community. Ann Intern Med 1998;158: 383–390.

35. Lynn J, Schall MW, Milne C, Nolan K, Kabcenell A. Qualty improvements in end of life care: Insights from two collaboratives. J on Qual Improvement 2000;26(5):254–267.

36. Fins JJ, Miller FG, Acres CA, Bacchetta MD, Huzzard LL, Rapkin BD. End-of-life decision-making in the hospital: Current practice and future prospects. J Pain Symp Mgmt 1999;17: 6–15.

37. Daubenspeck, M. At last. . . . Dartmouth Medicine 2000; Winter: 33–39, 53.

38. Skalla K, Kane N, Roy G. Project ENABLE. Personal communications and unpublished data, 2000.

39. Commission on Legal Problems of the Elderly. Survey of State EMS–DNR Laws and Protocols. Contact abaelderly@abanet.org to obtain the full report. ($15 fee.)

40. New Hampshire pre-hospital do not resuscitate program physician guidelines. Written by the Bureau of Emergency Medical Services, New Hampshire Chapter of American College of Emergency Physicians, and the Emergency Medical Directors Advisory Board. 1999.

41. Pritchard RS, Fisher ES, Teno JM, Sharp SM, Reding DJ, Knaus WA, et al. Influence of patient preferences and local health system characteristics on the place of death. J Am Geriatr Soc 1998;46;1242–1250.

42. Tolle SW, Rosenfeld AG, Tilden VP, Park Y. Oregon's low in-hospital death rates: What determines where people die and satisfaction with decisions on place of death? Ann Intern Med 1999;130:681–685.

43. Bookbinder M, Kiss M, Coyle N, Brown MH, Gianella A, Thaler HT. Improving pain management practices. In: McGuire DB, Yarbro CH, Ferrell BR, eds. Cancer pain management, 2nd ed. Boston: Jones and Bartlett, 1995:321–345.

44. Gordon DB, Dahl JL, Stevenson KK. Building an institutional commitment to pain management. In: Wisconsin Resource Manual for Improvement, 2nd ed. Madison WI: UW Board of Regents, 2000.

45. City of Hope Pain Resource Center: 626-359-8111, ext. 3829, or http://prc.coh.org

46. McCaffrey M, Pasero, C. Building institutional commitment to improving pain management. In: Pain Clinical Manual, 2nd ed. St. Louis, MO: Mosby 1999.

47. Ferrell BR, Whedon MB, Rollins B. Pain, quality assessment, and quality improvement. Journal of Nursing Care Quality 1999;9(3):69–85.

48. Lynn J, Kabcenell A. Breakthrough Series, Improving Care at the End of Life, Virginia: Institute for Healthcare Improvement, 1997.

49. United Hospital Fund. The Challenge of Caring for Patients near the End of Life: Findings from the Hospital Palliative Care Initiative Paper Series. $15 available from (888) 291-4161 or United Hospital Fund, c/o W&C, 100 Newfield Avenue, Edison, NJ 08837. 1998.

50. Abrahm JL, Callahan J, Rossetti K, Pierre L. The impact of a hospice consultation team on the care of veterans with advanced cancer. Journal of Pain and Symptom Management 1996; 12(1):23–31.

51. Hume M. Improving care at the end-of-life. The Quality Letter for Healthcare Leaders 1998;10(10):2–10.

52. Berwick DM. Controlling variation in health care: A consultation from Walter Shewhart. Med Care 1991;29:1212–25.

53. Stair J. Oncology critical pathways: palliative care: A model example from the Moses Cone Health System. Oncology 1998;14(2):26–30.

54. Du Pen S, Du Pen AR, Polissar N, Hansberry,J Kraybill BM, Stillman M, Panke J, Everly R, Syrjala K. Implementing guidelines for cancer pain management : Results of a randomized controlled clinical trial. J Clin Onc 1999;17(1):361–370.

55. Manning C, Lands R, Jones M. The team approach to pain management: A critical pathway. Oncology Pain Management, A supplement to Oncology Issues. Rockville MD: ACCC, 1999.

56. Dunlop RJ, Hockley JM. Terminal Care Support Teams. New York: Oxford University Press, 1990.

57. Dunlop RJ, Hockley JM. Hospital-Based Palliative Care Teams: The Hospital-Hospice interface. 2nd ed. New York: Oxford University Press 1998.

58. Bascom PB. A hospital-based comfort care team: Consultation for seriously ill and dying patients. American Journal of Hospice and Palliative Care 1997;57–60.

59. Weissman DE. Consultation in palliative medicine. Arch Intern Med 1997;157:733–737.

60. O'Neill, WM, O'Connor P, Latimer EJ. Hospital palliative care services: Three models in three countries. J Pain Symptom Management 1992;7:406–413.

61. Kellar N, Martinez J, Finis, Bolger A, von Gunten CF. Characterization of an acute inpatient hospice palliative care unit in a U.S. teaching hospital. JONA 1996;26(3):16–20.

62. www. stoppain.org

63. http://www.palliative.org

64. Kelly B, Edwards P, Synott R, Neil C. Baillie R, Battistutta D. Predictors of bereavement outcomes for family carers of cancer patients. Psychooncology 1999;8:237–49.

65. Billings JA, Kolton E. Family satisfaction and bereavement care following death in the hospital. J Pall Med 1999;2:33–49.

66. Ferris TGG, Hallward JA, Ronan L, Billings JA. When the patient dies: A survey of medical housestaff about care after death. J Pall Med 1998;(1)3:231–239.

67. www.gundluth.org/eolprograms

68. Stoehr PJ. The inadequacy of death and palliative care education in the Northeastern University Baccalaureat Nursing Program. Boston: Northeastern University School of Nursing (unpublished undergraduate project), 1999.

69. Ferrell BR, Virani R, Grant M. Analysis of end of life content in nursing textbooks. Oncology Nursing Forum. 1999;26(5):869–876.

70. Carron AT, Lynn J, Keaney P. End-of-life care in medical textbooks. Ann Intern Med 1999; 130:82–86.

71. Ferrell BR, Grant M, Virani R. Strengthening nursing education to improve end-of-life care. Nursing Outlook 1999;47(6):252–256.

72. American Medical Association. The Education for Physicians on End-of-Life Care (EPEC) Project. Chicago: American Medical Association, 1997.

73. Matzo M. What is care of the dying patient: An educational program for the associate degree nurse? http://mancstra.tec. nh.us/deathcare/about.html. 2000.

74. Capello CF, Meier DE; Cassel CK. Payment code for hospital-based palliative care: Help or hindrance? J Pall Med 1998;1(2):155–160.

75. RWJ Task Force. Meeting the Challenge: Improving End-Of-Life Care in Managed care: Access, Accountability, and Cost. (A Report of the National Task Force on End-of-Life Care in Managed Care-prepared under a grant from the Robert Wood Johnson Foundation by The Center for Applied Ethics and Professional. Practice, Education Development Center, Inc; Newton, MA, 1999.)

76. Montana J, Duffy M. NH Blue Cross Blue Shield Report on Insurer's Redesign Hospice Benefit to Improve EOL Care. Presented at RWJ Grantees meeting, Tucson, AZ, 1999.

77. Yurk R, Lansky D, Bethell C. Care at the End of Life: Assessing the Quality of Care for Patients and Families. Portland, OR: FACCT-The Foundation for Accountability, 1999.

78. Robbins M. Evaluating Palliative Care: Establishing the Evidence Base. Oxford: Oxford University Press, 1998.

79. Bookbinder M, Whedon M. QUEST for pain relief: Building "Best Practices" ONF 2000 27(2):335, abstract #118.

APPENDIX A: DARTMOUTH–HITCHCOCK MEDICAL CENTER CARE AT THE END OF LIFE QUESTIONNAIRE

Please answer the following questions about your loved one's care during their last hospitalization by putting a check mark next to the response which best describes your opinion. If the question is about something that did not apply to your loved one's last hospitalization, please check the "Does not apply" option. Feel free to use the "Comments" section to give details about your experience that would help us understand your response.

Questions #1-5 are about the care your loved one and your family received.

1. The staff providing care did so in a thoughtful and sensitive manner.

   _____ Strongly agree _____ Agree _____ Disagree _____ Strongly disagree
   _____ Does not apply

   Comments: ____

2. We felt that the doctors and nurses did all they could to carry out the wishes of our loved one and family.

   _____ Strongly agree _____ Agree _____ Disagree _____ Strongly disagree
   _____ Does not apply

   Comments: ____

3. We had enough privacy and space to comfortably stay with our loved one during the last hours of life.

   _____ Strongly agree _____ Agree _____ Disagree _____ Strongly disagree
   _____ Does not apply

   Comments: ____

4. Staff helped to meet our family's needs in a caring and sensitive manner at the time of death.

   _____ Strongly agree _____ Agree _____ Disagree _____ Strongly disagree
   _____ Does not apply

   Comments: ____

5. We felt supported after our loved one's death.

   _____ Strongly agree _____ Agree _____ Disagree _____ Strongly disagree
   _____ Does not apply

   Comments: ____

Questions #6-8 are about pain control. If your loved one did not experience pain during their last hospitalization, please skip to question #9.

6. Our loved one's pain was well controlled prior to their death.

   _____ Strongly agree _____ Agree _____ Disagree _____ Strongly disagree
   _____ Does not apply

   Comments: ____

7. The staff responded quickly to our loved one's needs for pain relief.

   _____ Strongly agree _____ Agree _____ Disagree _____ Strongly disagree
   _____ Does not apply

   Comments: ____

8. There was an acceptable balance between pain relief and side effects of the medication such as drowsiness and/or confusion.

   _____ Strongly agree _____ Agree _____ Disagree _____ Strongly disagree
   _____ Does not apply

   Comments: ____

Questions #9- 10 are about breathing difficulties. If your loved one did not have breathing difficulties during their last hospitalization, please skip to question #11.

9. We were satisfied with the care provided for our loved one's breathing difficulty.

____ Strongly agree ____ Agree ____ Disagree ____ Strongly disagree
____ Does not apply

Comments: ________________________________

10. We received enough information about changes in breathing to understand what was happening.

____ Strongly agree ____ Agree ____ Disagree ____ Strongly disagree
____ Does not apply

Comments: ________________________________

Questions #11-15 are about communication.

11. We felt there was good communication between:

The doctors at Mary Hitchcock Memorial Hospital and us.

____ Strongly agree ____ Agree ____ Disagree ____ Strongly disagree
____ Does not apply

The nurses at Mary Hitchcock Memorial Hospital and us.

____ Strongly agree ____ Agree ____ Disagree ____ Strongly disagree
____ Does not apply

The doctors and nurses at Mary Hitchcock Memorial Hospital.

____ Strongly agree ____ Agree ____ Disagree ____ Strongly disagree
____ Does not apply

The doctors at Mary Hitchcock Memorial Hospital and our loved one's local doctor.

____ Strongly agree ____ Agree ____ Disagree ____ Strongly disagree
____ Does not apply

Comments: ________________________________

12. We received consistent information about our loved one's condition *(reason for hospitalization)* and what to expect.

____ Strongly agree ____ Agree ____ Disagree ____ Strongly disagree
____ Does not apply

Comments: ________________________________

13. We felt well informed about what was happening during the last hospitalization prior to death.

____ Strongly agree ____ Agree ____ Disagree ____ Strongly disagree
____ Does not apply

Comments: ________________________________

14. We received the information we needed to move forward with funeral arrangements.

____ Strongly agree ____ Agree ____ Disagree ____ Strongly disagree
____ Does not apply

Comments: ________________________________

15. Overall, how would you rate the care that your loved one and your family received during their last hospitalization? (1 = the worst possible care and 10 = the best possible care). Please circle one.

1 2 3 4 5 6 7 8 9 10

Please feel free to share any additional comments you may have regarding your loved one's care prior to death. Also, please comment if you have suggestions on how we might improve care to future patients in the hospital who are at their end of life.

APPENDIX B: TABLE OF RESOURCES TO HELP GET STARTED IN EOL HOSPITAL QI

Books

Nelson EC, Batalden PC, Ryer JC (eds). Joint Commission Clinical Improvement Action Guide. Oakbrook IL: Joint Commission on Accreditation in Healthcare Organizations 1998.

This manual provides practical advice and worksheets on how to approach institutional quality improvement using the PDCA worksheet.

Institute of Medicine. Approaching Death: Improving Care at the End of Life. Washington, DC: National Academy Press 1997.

The IOM report contains an appendix (C) pp: 327–357 summarizing examples of initiatives to improve EOL care that use QI approaches.

Lynn J, Schuster JL, The Center to Improve Care of the Dying. Improving Care for the End of Life: A Sourcebook for Health Care Managers and Clinicians. New York: Oxford University Press 2000.

This manual summarizes outcomes of a national quality improvement efforts in end of life care of 48 agencies using the Institute of Healthcare Improvement "Breakthrough Series" method that was conducted between July 1997–98.

The Wisconsin Resource Manual for Improvement. Building an Institutional Commitment to Pain Management. Wisconsin Cancer Pain Initiative 1996.

This "how-to" manual presents suggestions for improvement of pain management practices in institutions with an extensive listing of measurement tools, protocols, policies, and other documents and strategies useful to creating infrastructure change.

Websites with Specific Reference to EOL Quality Improvement

www.abcd-caring.com
Americans for Better Care of the Dying, (ABCD)
4125 Albemarle St. NW, Suite 210
Washington DC 20016

www.edc.org/lastacts/
RWJ Last Acts web sites also contain information and links to many other sites that have specific information about quality improvement efforts that are ongoing in EOL care:(e.g. *Innovations in End-of-Life Care-An on line journal and forum for leaders in end-of-life care* published as part of Last Acts, an initiative funded by Robert Wood Johnson Foundation).

www.ihi.org/
Institute for Healthcare Improvement website describes the collaborative on improving care at the end of life.

www.chcr.brown.edu/pcoc/toolkit.htm
This website contains extensive information on measures to evaluate end-of-life care. (The Toolkit or TIME)

www.growthhouse.org
Growth House is a website dedicated entirely to end of life care and it contains a subsection specifically on "Quality Improvement" that allows links to some of the sources mentioned above as well as others. Multiple listings (links) are available.

www.facct.org
The organization for accountability. White paper on measures and accountability standards for health plans at end of life.

www.uhfnyc.org/initiat/initiat.htm
United Hospital Fund
This site describes the work of the United Hospital Fund on EOL care and QI activities.
The 12 Phase I hospitals were Bellevue Hospital Center, Beth Israel Medical Center, The Brooklyn Hospital Center, Elmhurst Hospital Center, Long Island Jewish Medical Center, Lutheran Medical Center, Montefiore Medical Center, The Mount Sinai Medical Center, The New York Hospital, St. Joseph's Hospital, Saint Vincent's Hospital and Medical Center, and Staten Island University Hospital.
The Challenge of Caring for Patients near the End of Life: Findings from the Hospital Palliative Care Initiative Paper Series, 64 pp., $15, ISBN 1-881277-37-2. March 1998

www.aacn.nche.edu/deathfin.htm
End of Life Nursing Education Consortium (ELNEC)
This site contains educational standards and recommended competencies and curricular guidelines for nurses to help educators include EOL content in nursing curriculum. Project of the American Association of Colleges of Nursing (AACN) and City of Hope Medical Center.

43 The Intensive Care Unit

KATHLEEN PUNTILLO and DAPHNE STANNARD

You're prepared for the worst, but hoping for the best.
—Family member of a critically ill patient[1]

An intensive care unit (ICU) is, by tradition, the setting where the most aggressive care is rendered to hospitalized patients. Patients are admitted to an ICU so that health professionals can perform minute-to-minute titration of care. The primary goals of this aggressive care are patient resuscitation, stabilization, and recovery from the acute phase of an illness or injury. However, many patients die in ICUs. The hospital mortality rate for cancer patients admitted to ICUs is 42%,[2] and the overall mortality rates in ICUs in the United States are estimated to be as high as 69%, depending on the preadmission severity of illness.[3] In one study involving three ICUs, patients who died after life support was removed most frequently had diagnoses of sepsis and postcardiac arrest.[4] Of those patients with cancer admitted to ICUs, bone marrow transplant patients had the highest mortality (57%).[2]

Deaths in an ICU can come at high cost in terms of pain, suffering, loss of human dignity, and finances.[5] In regard to the latter, numerous costly technological and human resources are used to provide aggressive care, although the dispersion of these resources is not uniform. Indeed, 50% of resources consumed in an ICU are used for 10% of the critically ill patients. For example, the use of laboratory tests and radiologic examinations during the last 48 hours of life substantially affects the cost of care in an ICU.[6] Decisions about the use of such diagnostic and aggressive treatment interventions are, logically, predicated upon health professionals' beliefs that they are doing what is best for the patient and the patient's family. However, 70% of patients who use the greatest amount of resources ultimately die in the ICU.[7,8]

In the high-technology environment of an ICU, it may be difficult for health professionals and families of dying patients to acknowledge that there are limits to the effectiveness of medical care. However, in an ICU outcomes study of 402 patients, the criterion of "potentially ineffective care," defined as resource use in the upper 25th percentile and survival for less than 100 days after discharge, was ascribed to 13% of the patients.[9] It is important to focus on providing the type of care that is appropriate for the individual patient and the patient's family, be it aggressive life-saving care or palliative end-of-life care. This chapter discusses the provision of palliative care in intensive care units. Specifically, challenges and barriers to providing such care in ICUs are described and recommendations offered for the provision of symptom assessment and management. Current issues related to withholding and withdrawing life-sustaining therapies are covered. Finally, recommendations are offered for attending to the needs of families as well as health care providers who care for ICU patients at the end of life.

THE LIMITATIONS OF END-OF-LIFE CARE IN ICUs

Although many deaths occur in ICUs, an ICU is rarely the place that one would choose to die.[10] Health professionals in ICUs, frequently uncertain about whether a patient will live or die, are caught between the opposing goals of preserving life and preparing the patient and family for death. It is important for professionals to realize that a patient's death is not necessarily an indication of ineffective care.[9] Yet, there are serious limitations to the care provided to seriously ill and dying patients and their families. Communication between physicians and patients may be poor; physicians often may not implement patients' refusals of interventions; patients may be overly optimistic about the outcomes of cardiopulmonary resuscitation (CPR); and many hospitalized patients die in moderate to severe pain and with other troubling symptoms.[11–13]

In a recent study, more than 5000 seriously ill hospitalized patients or their family members were asked questions about the patients' pain.[14] Almost one-half of these patients had pain during their last three days, and almost 15% had pain that was moderately or extremely severe and occurred at least half of the time. Of those with pain, 15% were dissatisfied with its control. Other distressing symptoms, such as fatigue, dyspnea, and dysphoria, have been reported by seriously ill and elderly hospitalized patients and their family members.[13] While patients with colon cancer had the most pain, many of the patients reporting pain had diagnoses that were not surgery- or cancer-related (e.g., chronic obstructive pulmonary disease or congestive heart failure). These findings stress the importance of attending to the assessment and management of pain and other symptoms in *all* ICU patients.

PLANNING PALLIATIVE CARE FOR ICU PATIENTS

All critically ill patients should receive aggressive care.[10] The goals of this care may vary, from the prolongation of life to the provision of a peaceful death. Providing comfort to patients should accompany all care, even during aggressive attempts to prolong life. However, when a patient is not expected to survive, the focus shifts to an emphasis on palliative care.

It is often extremely difficult in an ICU to determine the appropriate time for a change of focus in care. A transition period occurs during which the health professionals, the patient's family, and sometimes the patient recognize the appropriateness of withdrawing and/or withholding treatments and begin to make preparations for death. The time from ICU admission to decisions about withdrawing care varies, often according to the patient's diagnosis. For example, for patients with neurosurgical or neurologic conditions, the decisions clustered around two to three days postadmission, while decisions regarding patients with respiratory failure clustered around 22 days postadmission.[4]

The transition period (i.e., the time from decision to death) may be a matter of minutes or hours, as in the case of a patient who sustained massive motor vehicle injuries; or it may be a matter of weeks, as in the case of a post–bone marrow transplant patient with multiple negative sequelae while in the ICU. Median times to death following withholding or withdrawal of life support have been documented to be from one minute to 11 days[15,16] for adults and 12 hours to 14 days for children.[17] Clearly, this time difference must be recognized as a factor that can influence the experience of a patient's family members. When patients rapidly approach death, their family members may not have had time to overcome the shock of the trauma and adjust to the possibility of death. On the other hand, when death is prolonged, family frustration and fatigue may be part of their experience. Health professionals who are sensitive to these different experiences can individualize their approaches and interventions for family members.

However, this aggressive care-to-death-preparation transition period has not been well operationalized. Children who die in ICUs often do so after physician determination that death is imminent and after care has been restricted.[18] The restrictions are usually equally divided among withholding resuscitation, limiting medical interventions in addition to withholding resuscitation, and withdrawing medical interventions.[18,19] In a retrospective study of 300 pediatric patient deaths, the most common mode of death was active withdrawal of support.[20] Usually physicians raise the issue of restricting care (76% of the time), but sometimes it is the family that initiates these discussions (16% of the time).[18] The unique interdependence between a child and family makes it essential and justifiable for the family to participate in treatment-related decisions[21] during the transition period and throughout the dying process.

The transition period is clearly uncomfortable for many health care professionals. In fact, when scenarios concerning end-of-life decision-making in the absence of patient or family input were presented to over 1300 ICU staff, respondents were very confident of their choices less than 30% of the time.[22] Physicians were more confident than nurses, who were more confident than housestaff. Although some guidelines exist to assist ICU professionals through the processes of maintaining, limiting, or stopping life-sustaining treatments;[23] there are no well tested standards to assist in the decision-making process. It is important, therefore, for ICU professionals to consider the following when caring for any patient at risk for not surviving their ICU course:

1. Identify and communicate the goals of care for the patient at least once a day. Ascertain if the patient has developed an advanced directive, if a family member has durable power of attorney, and if the patient has communicated a preference about CPR. Research has shown that almost half of 960 seriously ill patients who wanted CPR withheld did not have a do not resuscitate (DNR) order written during their hospitalization, and almost one third died before discharge.[11]
2. Outline the steps that need to be taken in order to accomplish the goals of care, and evaluate their effectiveness. It is important to realize that technology should not drive the goals of care.[21] Instead, technology should be used when necessary to *accomplish* the goals, and its use should be minimized when the primary goal is achievement of a peaceful death.
3. Use a multidisciplinary team approach to decision-making regarding transition to end-of-life care. All team members, including the patient's family, should reach a consensus, sometimes through negotiation, that the withdrawal of life support and a peaceful death are the appropriate patient outcomes.[24,25] Family involvement is never so important as when the dying person is a child.
4. Develop and communicate to professionals and family the palliative care plan, and identify the best person(s) for implementing the various actions in the plan. End-of-life treatment decisions are particularly complex when the dying patient is an infant or child.[23] De Groot-Bollujt and Mourik[26] provide specific suggestions for involving a child's family member(s) in the dying process. These include offering them opportunities to participate in preparing the child to die and even holding the child during the dying process.
5. Developing a plan of care can include enlisting the assistance of in-hospital palliative care staff and/or hospice services. Whenever feasible and desired by the family, consideration should be given to transferring the adult or pediatric patient from the ICU to in-hospital support care services, such as those at Detroit Receiving Hospital.[27] Or, when possible and desired, patients may be able to be transferred to the home or to community hospice services. A major focus in any palliative care plan is on providing optimal symptom management.

SYMPTOM ASSESSMENT AND MANAGEMENT: AN ESSENTIAL COMPONENT OF PALLIATIVE CARE

Pain Assessment

While pain is one of the most prevalent and distressing symptoms of seriously ill patients dying in large teaching hospitals,[11,13] pain research focusing on these patients is scant. Advances that have been made in the assessment of pain in other critically ill patient populations can be applied to dying patients. For patients who are able to self-report, research has shown that many who are critically ill are able to use simple tools to communicate their pain, even when mechanically ventilated.[28,29] Simple numeric or word rating scales, word quality scales, and body outline diagrams can be offered to patients who are able to point to words, numbers, and figures.[30] It is important to determine the quality, timing, and location of pain whenever possible so that treatment may be guided by accurate information rather than assumptions. For example, intermittent, poorly localized, crampy abdominal pain may be related to constipation, and burning pain may be a sign of neuropathic pain.[10] The specificity of the pain presentation will guide the selection of optimal treatment interventions.

Often, critically ill patients are unable to self-report because of their disease process, technological treatment interventions (such as mechanical ventilation), or even because of the effects of medications (such as opioids or benzodiazepines). As to the latter, the use of benzodiazepine infusions may make patients too sedated to respond to pain, although pain may still be present. On the other hand, the use of the anesthetic agent propofol or neuromuscular blocking agents (NMBAs), such as vecuronium, limits or entirely masks the patient's ability to express or show any behavioral signs of pain. It is essential that clinicians understand that propofol and NMBAs have no analgesic properties, even though visible signs of pain disappear during their use. When these agents are used, they must be accompanied by infusions of analgesics, sedatives, or both. In these situations, the nurse can enlist the assistance of family members or friends in their evaluation of the patient's discomfort. The nurse can ask them about any chronic pain experienced by the patient or methods used by the patient at home to decrease pain or stress. This information can then be incorporated into the patient's care plan.

When patients are unable to self-report, the nurse can use a structured, systematic method of pain assessment that includes observation of behavioral and physiologic signs of pain.[31,32] In fact, ICU physicians and nurses report that they are more apt to use patient behaviors and physiological signs than to use patients' own reports.[33] While it is important to stress that these measures are only proxies for the patient's subjective reports, frequently they are the only measures available. As another proxy measure, nurses can use their imaginations to identify possible sources of pain by asking the question "If I were this patient and had intact sensations, what might be making me uncomfortable?" Even when patients are not exhibiting behavioral or physiologic signs of pain, it does not mean that the patient is pain-free.

Recently, investigators assessed the comfort of 31 adult patients undergoing terminal weaning from mechanical ventilation by using behavior observation and physiologic measures.[34] Moderate correlations ($r = .60$; $p < .001$) found between the Bizek Agitation Scale (BAS)[35] and the previously validated COMFORT scale[36] suggest that these observational measures may be able to evaluate responses to pain, distress, and/or agitation in certain dying ICU patients. Correlations between electroencephalogram (EEG)-derived data, obtained through the use of a cerebral function monitor,[37] and the BAS and COMFORT scales were $r = .53$ and $r = .58$, respectively ($p < .001$). Findings from this study about behavior and physiological measures are preliminary at best. EEG data were derived from only 11 of the 31 patients because the others had global anoxic encephalopathy. Furthermore, the specific origin or cause of "discomfort" (i.e., pain, dysphoria, etc.) cannot be determined from these global measures. However, the findings show promise of the clinical usefulness of "comfort" assessment measures that can assist clinicians to assess pain and the effectiveness of treatment interventions at the end of life.

Procedural Pain

Before and during the transition from aggressive care to end-of-life care, critically ill patients undergo many diagnostic and treatment procedures. Many of these, such as central, arterial, and peripheral line placements, nasogastric tube placements,[38] chest tube removal, and endotracheal suctioning[39] are very painful and may be the primary cause of suffering at the end of life.[38] Other procedures that may be unnecessary, painful, and unpleasant include frequent vital sign assessment, frequent turning, wound debridements, frequent dressing changes, and the use of sequential compression devices.[40] Nurses can act as "gatekeepers" by evaluating the appropriateness of procedures being planned for patients, especially after a decision has been made to end life support, and they can advocate for their omission. Helping patients avoid iatrogenic suffering is a fundamental part of palliative care.[38] The most important procedures for patients to experience at the end of life are those that promote comfort. Yet, when necessary procedures must be performed, the nurse can facilitate pain management before and during procedures.

Pharmacologic Management of Pain

Numerous categories of analgesics and types of modalities exist for administration to critically ill patients. As in all situations, selection of analgesics should depend on the specific pain mechanism, and selection of the route and modality should be matched to their predictability of effectiveness. While no comprehensive survey of pain management techniques used for dying ICU patients has been reported, intravenously (IV) administered opioids appear to be the most common analgesic intervention. Use of a continuous infusion of an opioid allows for titration of the drug to a level of analgesic effectiveness and for maintenance of steady plasma levels within a therapeutic range. This method can help minimize respiratory depression and oversedation if those are concerns for specific patients. A goal in the use of continuous opioid infusions is to achieve a minimum effective analgesic concentration (MEAC). With MEAC, an opioid plasma level that provides adequate pain relief for a particular individual is achieved and maintained.[41] Stevens and Edwards[41] recommend steps to achieve MEAC through front-loading the opioid to analgesia and making a determination about the continuous infusion rate. Health care professionals can consider the administration of intermittent opioid boluses for breakthrough pain (see Table 43–1).

Clearly, concerns about patients becoming tolerant of or dependent on opioids are mislaid during terminal care. What *is* important is that professionals recognize the development of tolerance, which is the need for larger doses of opioid analgesics in order to achieve the original effect[42] and to increase the dosage as necessary. There is no ceiling effect from opioids; thus, the dose can be increased until the desired effect is reached. If it is the family's wish to have the opioid infusion decreased in a sedated patient in order for that patient to be able to participate in end-of-life decision making, this must be done slowly and carefully. Opioid dependent patients are at high risk of developing withdrawal symptoms,[42] which would seriously increase their discomfort. In this situation, physical dependence can be addressed by gradually lowering the opioid dose while carefully assessing for signs of pain or withdrawal.

Titration of analgesics to achieve the desired effect is one of the most challenging and important contributions that ICU nurses can make to the comfort care of dying patients. The desired effect can often be described as use of the least amount of medication necessary to achieve the greatest comfort along with the optimum level of tranquil awareness.

In ICU settings, concern may arise that administering analgesics in the amounts necessary to provide comfort may "cause" death. It is essential that ICU health professionals understand the "double effect" principle. In brief, the double effect principle states that administering analgesics to dying patients in the amounts necessary to decrease pain and suffering, although it may have the unintended consequence of hastening death, is a good, ethically sound way to treat a dying patient.[43] This principle, framed in ethics, provides support to such an action when the clinician's moral intent is directed primarily at alleviating suffering rather than intending to kill. In a recently completed survey of 906 critical care nurses in the United States, almost all respondents (98%)

Table 43–1. Pharmacological Symptom Management*

Symptom	Drug Type Most Frequently Used	Method of Administration	Usual Dose†
Pain	Opioids (e.g., morphine, fentanyl, hydrocodone, methadone)	Continuous IV infusions with use of intermittent boluses for procedure-related pain or during treatment withdrawal	Continuous infusion: 1–10 mg/hour morphine equivalents Bolus: 1–5 mg IV morphine equivalent slow push; titrate to effect
Anxiety/ Agitation	Benzodiazepines (e.g., lorazepam, midazolam)	Same as opioids	Continuous midazolam infusion: 2–25 mg/hour or titrate to effect. Bolus midazolam: 5–10 mg IV to augment continuous infusion Continuous lorazepam infusion: 1–5 mg/hour or titrate to effect. Bolus lorazepam: 1–10 mg IV every 6 to 8 hours to augment continuous infusion
	Haloperidol	IV boluses	Bolus: 0.5–10 mg IV
	Propofol	Continuous IV infusion	Continuous: 50–300 mg/hour
Dyspnea	Oxygen	Multiple methods e.g., nasal cannula, mask, ventilator	Concentration as needed
	Opioids e.g., morphine	Continuous IV infusion and/or IV bolus; or per nebulizer	See above for IV doses Per nebulizer: 2.5 mg in 3 cc NaCl (preservative free) or sterile water every 4 hours
	Benzodiazepines	See above	See above
	Bronchodilators, e.g., alupent	Per nebulizer	Alupent: 2.5 ml 0.4–0.6% solution
	Diuretics, e.g., lasix	IV bolus, slow push	Bolus lasix: 20–40 mg IV
	Anticholinergic, e.g., atropine	Per nebulizer	Atropine: 0.025 mg/kg diluted with 3–5 ml saline 3 or 4 times daily. Doses not to exceed 2.5 mg.

*References: Govoni LE, Hayes JE. *Drugs and nursing implications.* Norwalk: Appleton & Lange.
Harvey MA. Managing agitation in critically ill patients. *American Journal of Critical Care* 1996; 5(1), 7–16.
Kuebler KK. *Dyspnea.* Pittsburgh, PA: Hospice and Palliative Nurses Association, 1996.
†Drug doses are general recommendations. Dosing should be individualized to a particular patient. Under usual circumstances, start with low doses, wait for effect, and titrate to desired effect.

agreed or strongly agreed with the double effect principle.[44]

Nonpharmacological Management of Pain

Numerous therapies can be used by critical care nurses to augment the administration of medications to promote patient comfort. They include the use of patient-preferred music and appropriate use of cold, heat, and massage.[45] It is important, however, to consider that massage may increase the patient's discomfort, as noted by non-ICU patients interviewed by Donovan and colleagues.[46] Information, especially about expected sensations, has been shown to decrease the pain intensity or distress related to procedures performed on patients.[47] Even during occasions when the cognitive status of a somnolent ICU patient is uncertain, the patient can be provided information about activities being done to and around them. Family members can be encouraged to assist with the provision of comfort measures and may welcome this way of participating in care and decreasing their sense of helplessness. Family involvement is discussed in further detail in a later section of this chapter.

ANALGESIA DURING WITHDRAWAL FROM LIFE SUPPORT

During patient withdrawal from life support, continuous opioid infusions are frequently used, with morphine being the most frequently used.[48,49] Additional boluses can be used as necessary. Morphine provides analgesia and sedation as well as pulmonary vasodilation, which can decrease dyspnea by decreasing venous return to the heart. It is recommended that a morphine infusion be readily available before the procedure is initiated so as to avoid delay in beginning its administration. Morphine administration, either by bolus injection or infusion, should precede the withdrawal process in most patients and should continue throughout and after the procedure in order to ensure a comfortable death. Patients receiving an opioid other than morphine, such as hydromorphone or fentanyl, could continue to receive that opioid during withdrawal. Opioid infusion rates should be adjusted in response to signs of distress, such as tachycardia, tachypnea, restlessness, or grimacing. The recommended doses and rates of opioid infusions are those that are needed to provide comfort. Dosing can vary widely, especially if the patient is "opioid-naïve" as opposed to having received opioids for a period of time. Cumulative morphine doses from one to 70 mg/hour have been reported to be used for terminal weaning.[34,48–50]

ANXIETY AND DISTRESS

An important part of palliative care in the ICU is assessment and treatment of anxiety and distress. There are many reasons for a dying patient to feel anxious and/or distressed. In fact, both anxiety and depression have been associated with increased pain and increased levels of dissatisfaction with pain control in seriously ill patients.[13] What is unclear is whether pain worsens distress, whether pain increases as a response to distress, or both.[13] However, assessment of anxiety and distress provides the practitioner with information that can guide the use of specific interventions.

Simple numeric rating scales for anxiety and distress can be used with patients who can self-report to identify how much the patient is psychologically bothered. Critical care clinicians and patients are quite familiar with the use of the 0–10 numeric rating scales (NRSs) for pain. Anxiety or distress word anchors can be substituted for pain word anchors so that NRSs also can be used to quantify the degree of anxiety or distress.

Common behavioral or physiological signs of anxiety include trembling, restlessness, sweating, tachycardia, tachypnea, difficulty sleeping, and irritability.[40] The Bizek Agitation Scale (BAS)[35] is a simple method for assessment of distressing behavioral responses in nonverbal patients. With this scale, an observable action is scored numerically according to the following: 1 = no agitation; 2 = agitated to noxious stimulus only; 3 = agitated to verbal/tactile stimulus; 4 = agitated at times without stimulus; 5 = very agitated without stimulus. This scale can be printed on the patient flowsheet or on a separate form and used as a bedside assessment tool. Nurses can plan periodic and simultaneous assessments of pain using pain rating scales and agitation using scales such as the BAS. The frequency with which the scales are used will depend on the patient's condition and the schedule for evaluating treatment interventions.

Pharmacological Management of Anxiety

Along with opioids, other categories of sedating drugs are frequently used in ICUs, especially when patients are being mechanically ventilated.[45] The appropriate pharmacological agent to control agitation and anxiety is selected according to the desired effect. For example, uncomplicated anxiety is best treated with benzodiazepines (BZDs), while paranoia, panic, and fear accompanied by delusions and hallucinations may require the addition of antipsychotic agents.

BZDs are excellent agents for anxiolysis, but they possess no analgesic or psychologic properties. Concomitant use of BZDs, opioids, and certain neuroleptic agents may relieve anxiety-provoking symptoms through a synergistic action.[51,52] When used together, these drugs can be administered in lower doses less frequently, have fewer side effects, and can decrease or delay development of tolerance or dependence through the use of smaller doses of each drug. At lower doses, BZDs reduce anxiety without causing central nervous system (CNS) sedation or a decrease in cognitive or motor function. With increasing dosages, inhibition of motor and cognitive functions as well as CNS depression does occur. Sufficiently high doses can induce hypnosis and coma.[53]

The most frequently used BZDs in critical care are midazolam and lorazepam. When used as a continuous infusion, the dose of midazolam can be

1–2 mg/hour for mild sedation or as high as 25 mg/hour for severe agitation if the patient is mechanically ventilated (see Table 43–1). If the degree of sedation is not adequate, the serum level of midazolam can be raised by 1–3 small bolus IV injections while simultaneously increasing the infusion rate.[54]

Lorazepam gives effective sedation and anxiety relief over a longer period than does midazolam. Cardiovascular and respiratory effects occur less frequently with this drug than with other BZDs. It may also act synergistically with haloperidol, a neuroleptic agent discussed below. Lorazepam can be administered intravenously, intramuscularly, or orally. IV doses may be 1–10 mg every 6 to 8 hours. In the critical care setting it can also be administered as an infusion at 1–5 mg/hour and titrated to clinical effect.[54]

As with opioids, tolerance to BZD effects can develop in critically ill patients receiving midazolam infusions.[55] In addition, BZD dependence can occur, evidenced by symptoms such as increased levels of anxiety and insomnia, as well as profound responses such as psychomotor agitation with muscle twitching, sweating, and seizures.[56] BZDs are sometimes used in conjunction with opioids to provide patient comfort during withdrawal from life support.[49,57]

Haloperidol is a frequently used neuroleptic for critically ill patients and can be administered in boluses of .5 to 10 mg IV.[54] This drug has few cardiovascular effects unless given rapidly; then vasodilation and hypotension may occur. Haloperidol does not depress respirations but, rather, has a calming effect on agitated, disoriented patients, making them more manageable without causing excessive sedation. Once a drug dosage has been established, it should not be necessary to increase the dose to obtain the same effect over time, since tolerance should not occur.

Propofol is a highly lipophilic IV sedative/hypnotic agent that has a very rapid onset of action and short duration. It is indicated for use in the ICU to control agitation and the stress response in patients who are mechanically ventilated and/or for patients who require deep sedation for procedures.[58] However, it must be remembered that propofol has no analgesic properties and must always be used in conjunction with analgesics whenever the patient might experience pain. During initial use of propofol, a drop in systolic blood pressure, mean arterial blood pressure, and heart rate may occur in patients with fluid deficits and in those receiving opioids. The rapid offset of clinical effect of propofol renders it a valuable sedative agent in the critical care environment. Continuous infusion doses may range from 50–300 mg/hour[54] (see Table 43–1). The short effective half-life of propofol allows rapid clinical evaluation of the patient's level of consciousness and determination of the minimum dose required for effective sedation. This may make it a useful drug during situations in which intermittent interaction with professionals and family members is desired.

Nonpharmacological Interventions for Anxiety and Distress

Numerous interventions exist that may promote tranquility and sedation in a critical care environment.[45] These include control of environmental noise and the use of clocks, calendars, and personal articles, such as pictures from home. Music therapy can be used to decrease anxiety and pain as well as promote sleep. Imagery and relaxation techniques also provide a means of distraction for patients and help to alleviate anxiety.[54,59]

The act of physically caring for a patient and providing gentle touch is a major source of comfort for patients in critical care. Taking the time to provide simple measures such as a back rubs and massages, repositioning the patient, smoothing bed linen wrinkles, removing foreign objects from the bed, providing mouth and eye care, and taping tubes to maintain patency and inhibit pulling, are all effective in promoting comfort and decreasing anxiety.[54,60] Family member participation in caregiving activities, such as bathing, massages, and back rubs, can have a powerful calming effect on patients and promote sleep and psychological integrity.

For alert patients, increasing opportunities for control is a strategy that can reduce the sense of helplessness that often accompanies patients who are critically ill. This sense of control can be promoted by allowing alert patients to make decisions about the timing of interventions. Facilitating contact and communication with clergy, psychologists, or psychiatrists, when appropriate, can help to alleviate the distress experienced by both patients and families.

OTHER SYMPTOMS: DYSPNEA AND FATIGUE

Dyspnea was one of the major symptoms reported by patients or their family members in a sample of hospitalized seriously ill patients.[13] There are a number of etiologies for dyspnea, including pulmonary or cardiac disease, as well as anxiety, fear, and depression.[61] In addition, pharmacologic and nonpharmacologic conditions can be both the causes of and treatments for dyspnea.[62] For example, dyspnea can increase when patients are receiving adrenergic agonists (e.g., Metaproterenol or albuterol) and theophylline, because these drugs can cause severe agitation, anxiety, and tremor.[63] On the other hand, morphine can directly improve dyspnea by decreasing cardiac preload, and benzodiazepines can indirectly improve dyspnea through their anxiolytic effects. Combined use of opioids and benzodiazepines may sometimes be more beneficial than use of either one alone. The choice of dosing should be based on individual patient assessment and evaluation of patient response. Bronchodilators, diuretics, and anticholinergics also may be considered for treatment of dyspnea. (See Table 43–1 for dosing suggestions.) Of course, administration of oxygen can lead to improved patient comfort.

Being in a stifling ICU room surrounded by machines can enhance the feeling of shortness of breath. Placing the patient in a position of comfort (e.g., sitting upright) can help to relieve dyspnea, while use of a bedside fan can provide a cool breeze and make breathing easier. Repeated reassurance is an effective intervention for dyspnea when the patient trusts the professional staff.[64] This reassurance can be more effective if team members give consistent explanations. Alert dyspneic patients can obtain comfort from knowing that they will not be left alone and from being provided some degree of control in their care.

Fatigue at the end of life was reported by almost 80% of more than 3000 patients or their surrogates in a study of seriously ill hospitalized patients.[13] When cure is no longer the goal in a patient's plan of care, the critical care nurse can help to control the patient's environment and promote sleep by implementing a rest-activity schedule for the patient and his or her family.[65] The nurse can cluster care activities, use "do not disturb" signs on patients' doors, consider using a tape recorder with patient-preferred music, and turn down or off monitor alarms in order to promote a sleep environment for the patient. Whenever possible, and when it is in the patient's best interest, transfer from ICU to a less intensive and quieter environment may promote rest and improve patient and family comfort.

ICU nurses play a major role in alleviating pain, anxiety, distress, dyspnea, fatigue, and other symptoms experienced by patients at the end of life. Nurses are the health care providers constantly at the bedside. Thus, they can assess the presence of these symptoms, advocate for effective pharmacologic therapy, use additional nursing comfort measures, and provide for continuity of therapy. Symptom management is a special contribution that ICU nurses can make to their patients at the end of life.

END-OF-LIFE PRACTICE ISSUES: WITHHOLDING AND WITHDRAWING LIFE-SUSTAINING THERAPIES

Limiting life-sustaining care in an ICU is becoming more common. It is estimated that withholding or withdrawing life support precedes 40%–60% of deaths in ICUs.[15,66] In two university-affiliated ICUs, 90% of 200 patients who died did so following a decision to limit therapy during 1992 and 1993.[15] Only 51% of 224 patients died in the same units in 1987 and 1988 after similar decisions were made to limit therapy.[16] Few ICU patients are competent to make treatment decisions,[15] so these decisions must be made on the patients' behalf by surrogates and/or the health care team. It is essential that patients' living wills or advance directives provide the direction for decisions related to treatment withholding or withdrawal. Nevertheless, it may take as many as four or more family meetings before a consensus can be reached about withdrawal of life support.[4] Decisions to limit treatment are made based on assessments of the patients' prognoses and wishes and on moral, legal, and, less often, economic criteria.[67] The decisions are often related to the patients' poor prognoses, concern about patients' suffering, and concern about the patients' quality of life.[4]

The President's Commission for the Study of Ethical Problems in Medicine and Biomedical and Behavioral Research[68] supported the right of a competent patient to refuse life-sustaining and life-prolonging therapy. The Commission also noted that there is no moral difference between withholding and withdrawing therapy. A number of critical care–related professional organizations[69–71] have published position papers in support of the patient's autonomy regarding withholding and withdrawal decisions. In contrast to the perspectives of these organizations, however, some physicians (26% of 271 survey respondents) drew a moral distinction between the withholding and withdrawal of mechanical ventilators,[57] finding withholding more acceptable than withdrawal. This finding demonstrates the continuing angst of health professionals who work in the traditionally "life-saving setting" of an ICU.

When a decision to forgo life-saving therapy is made in an ICU, ventilator, oxygen, and vasopressors are the most frequent therapies to be withdrawn or withheld.[4,67] The following discussion focuses on the withdrawal of ventilator therapy.

It is important to understand the methods by which mechanical ventilation may be removed. Indeed, the primary goal during this process should be to assure that patients and family members are as comfortable as possible, both psychologically and physically. Ventilator removal is indicated when the informed patient requests its withdrawal, when interventions to save the patient's life are deemed to be futile, and/or in order to reduce a terminally ill patient's pain and suffering.[48]

Two primary methods of mechanical ventilation removal exist. The first method is described as terminal weaning. With this method, physicians or other members of the ICU team (e.g., respiratory therapists or nurses) gradually withdraw ventilator assistance. This is done by decreasing the amount of inspired oxygen, decreasing the ventilator rate and mode, removal of positive end expiratory pressure (PEEP), or a combination of these maneuvers. The second method is a more abrupt removal of the patient from ventilator assistance by extubation. Debates continue as to which of these methods is optimal for the patient. Each method has been argued to be more comfortable for the patient than the other.[57] Some health care professionals[72–74] object to termination of life support by extubation, explaining that this method frequently causes marked respiratory distress that is disturbing to the patient and family. Instead, they argue for rapid terminal weaning, in that it is deliberate and ethically proper and causes less suffering than gradual terminal weaning or extubation.

Studies that provide clinical guidance for ventilator withdrawal are few.[73] A small group of adult patients ($n = 42$) underwent withdrawal as part of a treatment limitation plan.[75] Clinical data were collected from their medical records, including the specific method of ventilator withdrawal. The vast majority died after having ET (endotracheal) tubes and mechanical support removed (n = 28; 85%); 10 died with artificial airways in place but mechanical support removed; and 4 died after gradual removal of airway and/or mechanical support. The majority of the patients (88%) received morphine during withdrawal. At some time during the withdrawal process, 64% of the patients exhibited at least one sign of distress, most often labored breathing or upper airway noise. The investigators noted that their data suggest that little is gained by gradual withdrawal of respiratory support.

Recently, investigators evaluated responses of 31 adult patients to rapid terminal weaning from mechanical ventilation.[34] Using both observational and physiological measures, they determined that the predominantly comatose patients in their sample remained comfortable with use of low doses of morphine and benzodiazepines. A larger, randomized clinical trial of various methods of withdrawal may help to determine if one method is more efficacious than another.

Recommendations regarding specific procedures for withdrawal are available.[34,40,48,49] Regardless of the method used, the critical care nurse plays a major role during the decision and implementation of withdrawal of patients from mechanical ventilation.[49] However, in a recent study,[4] nursing staff was involved in conversations with physicians, patients, and families about withdrawal of life support only 16% of the time. Increased nursing involvement can help provide optimal care to these patients. Specifically, the nurse can ensure that a rationale for and all elements of the plan have been adequately discussed among the team, patient, and family. She or he can see that adequate time is given to families and their support persons, such as clergy, for them to reach as good a resolution as possible. The family will need reassurance that they and the patient will not be left alone and that the patient will be kept comfortable with the use of medications and other measures. As discussed earlier, opioids, alone or in combination with BZDs, are used during withdrawal to ensure that patients are provided the optimal degree of comfort. In a sample of 44 ICU patients,[50] physicians ordered opioids and BZDs to decrease pain in 88% of patients and to decrease anxiety in 85% of patients. They ordered these drugs to decrease air hunger in 76% and to comfort families in 82%. An associated, but not exclusive, goal of hastening death was a motivation in the ordering of drugs for 39% of the patients.[50]

Although the use of paralytic agents during ventilator withdrawal has been reported by up to 10% of 211 physicians,[57] this practice should *never* occur. The use of paralytics such as Vecuronium or Acuronium makes it almost impossible to assess patient comfort; while appearing comfortable, patients may be experiencing pain, respiratory distress, or severe anxiety. Their use prevents the struggling and gasping that may be associated with dying, but not the patient's suffering.[76] The horror of such a death can only be imagined.

CARE FOR THE FAMILY OF THE DYING ICU PATIENT

Although the focus of care in many critical care areas is on the critically ill patient, nurses and other clinicians with family care skills realize that comprehensive patient care includes care of the patient's family. A reciprocal and all-important relationship exists between the family and the critically ill patient. A change in one affects the other. Classic and contemporary research that describes the anticipatory and acute grief reactions experienced by family members when their loved one is dying accent this powerful reciprocal relationship.[77–80] Therefore, no discussion of palliative care in the ICU is complete without also discussing care of the dying patient's family. *Family* is defined as any significant other who participates in the care and well-being of the patient.

The clinical course of any given critically ill dying patient can vary tremendously, ranging from a rapid unfolding over several hours to a gradual unfolding over several days, weeks, or even months. How a family copes, of course, is also highly variable. Caring for families at any point along the dying trajectory, however, encompasses three major areas: access, information and support, and involvement in caregiving activities.

Access

A crucial aspect of family care is ensuring that a family can be with their critically ill loved one. Yet, historically, critical care settings have severely restricted family access. Commonly cited rationales to limit family access include concerns regarding space limitations, patient stability, infection, rest, and privacy; the effect of visitation on the family; and clinicians' performance abilities. Some of these concerns have merit. With regard to space limitations, for example, most ICUs were designed for efficient use of life-saving machinery and staff and were not designed for end-of-life vigils by large, extended families. As such, ensuring that all interested family members have access to their loved one's bedside can present challenges to the often already narrow confines of the ICU.

Many ICUs around the world routinely limit visitors to two at any one time.[81,82] Space limitations in critical care areas are real. However, family members of dying loved ones should be allowed more liberal access (both in visiting time and number of visitors allowed). Patients are confronting what may be the most difficult of life's passages, and they therefore may need support from their family members.

In terms of patient-related issues, numerous studies have investigated family visitation and found no adverse effects on patient stability or infection.[83–93] These concerns, however, are typically moot regarding the dying patient. Other studies have examined the effect of visitation on the family and found no negative consequences.[94–96] Because children as young as five years old have been reported to have an accurate concept of death,[97] their visitation needs also should be considered when a family member is dying. With proper preparation and debriefing, children can visit a critically ill family member in the ICU without ill effects.[98]

Finally, caring for the critically ill dying patient and her or his family can call forth feelings of failure for clinicians bent on cure and force healthcare providers to reflect on their own mortality. Although these feelings can affect clinicians' performance abilities, typically restricting family access relates to healthcare providers' clinical competence while performing life-saving measures.[99] As such, this concern is also moot when caring for dying patients and their families. The emotional burden for healthcare providers when providing palliative care is discussed later in this chapter.

Information and Support

Information has been identified as a crucial component in families' coping and satisfaction in critical care settings.[100–102] Support, in the form of nurses' caring behaviors and interactions, is enormously influential in shaping the critical care experience for both patients and their families.[1,99,103–107] In the context of caring for a critically ill dying patient, however, nurses and physicians alike have reported high stress related to "death-telling," or notifying family members of the patient's death or terminal prognosis.[108–111] These same studies point to the fact that few health care providers feel they have the skills and knowledge necessary to counsel families effectively during this emotionally charged time. The ethical principle of honesty and truth-telling collides with the limits of knowledge precisely when there is clinical ambiguity and also with the suffering imposed on a family having to face the hard truth. Compassionate truth-telling requires dialogue and relationship, timing, and attunement,[112] all of which are relational aspects that are too frequently overlooked in the frantic pace of the ICU. Perhaps this helps to explain why a recent survey of relatives of ICU patients who had died expressed dissatisfaction with the information conveyed to them by health care providers.[113] The educational implications for clinicians are addressed later in this chapter.

Some hospitals have created multidisciplinary teams of helping professionals to work with hopelessly ill patients and their families in an effort to meet patients' and families' physical, informational, and psychosocial needs.[114,115] Such teams usually include a nurse, physician, chaplain, and social worker. Working in concert with the nurses and physicians at the bedside, these multidisciplinary teams can more fully concentrate on end-of-life issues so that, theoretically, no patient or family needs go unmet during this time.

Finally, because feelings of grief in surviving family members are still commonly unresolved at one year following a loved one's death, many critical care units across the life span have organized bereavement follow-up programs.[116–119] These programs typically involve contacting the surviving family (by phone and/or mail) monthly for some period of time and at the one-year anniversary of the loved one's death. In addition to remembering and supporting the surviving family, these programs have also been shown to help health care providers cope with the loss as well.

Involvement in Caregiving Activities

Few interventional studies have examined the effect of family involvement on adult critically ill patients and their families, although expert nursing behaviors in caring for the dying patient's family include encouraging family participation in patient care.[1,120,121] Family involvement in caregiving can range from minor activities, such as assisting with oral care or rubbing the dying patient's feet, to major activities, such as assisting with postmortem care. This involvement may help family members work through their grief by demonstrating their love in caring and comforting ways. Being involved in meaningful caregiving activities can make a family member feel useful rather than useless and helpful rather than helpless.

Although physical death occurs in the dying patient, the social level of death is felt in the patient's surviving family. Because the memory of death lingers at the family level long after the physical death has occurred, involving family members who are interested in participating in their loved one's care may go far in providing closure, comfort, and connection. Unfortunately, many critical care nurses still feel that families should provide a supportive, although nonparticipative, role in the provision of care for their loved ones.[122,123] Nurses' facilitation of family involvement in their dying loved one's care is a practical family intervention that should be more widely employed if the most humane and comprehensive palliative care is desired.

CARE FOR THE HEALTH CARE PROVIDER ATTENDING THE DYING ICU PATIENT AND FAMILY

Numerous studies have described the tension between the cure-oriented critical care setting and palliative care.[1,99,124,125] The bedside health care provider, typically a nurse, often feels caught among differing perceptions held by physicians and family members concerning patient progress and treatment goals. Facilitating and coordinating dialogue and consensus among these groups as well as caring for the dying patient and family can be physically and emotionally exhausting. When the dying process is prolonged, the patient's nurse can become frustrated and fatigued. Although health care providers often cope with this stress by emotionally disengaging themselves from the charged atmosphere, emotional distancing has been shown to hamper skill acquisition and the development of involvement skills.[1,103] Involvement skills are the cluster of skills that enable a nurse, the patient, and the family to establish a relationship. Two strategies are summarized below to help healthcare providers sustain their caring practices and extend their involvement skills, namely, sharing narratives and death education.

Sharing Narratives

Debriefing, either formally or informally, has been used effectively in many settings to discuss and process critical incidents; analyze health care providers' performance in terms of skill, knowledge, and efficiency; and learn, both personally and institutionally, from mistakes and system breakdown.[99,126,127] Informally sharing stories or narratives of practice can be used to achieve the same goals, but formal story telling from practice enables clinicians to (*1*) increase their skill in recognizing patient and family concerns; (*2*) learn to communicate more effectively with patients, families, and other health care providers; (*3*) reflect on ethical comportment and engaged clinical reasoning; and (*4*) articulate clinical knowledge development.[103,128]

Creating the interpersonal and institutional space in which to both tell and actively listen to stories from practice also enables health care providers to share the skills of involvement and sustaining strategies. These understandings can provide clinicians with guidance—and in some cases, corrective action—to intervene in ways that are true to the patient's condition and to the patient's and family's best interests.[112] Through reflection and dialogue with others, nurses and other health care providers can pool their collective wisdom and extend their abilities to care for dying patients and their families.

Death Education

Closely coupled with sharing clinical narratives is the use of seminars and other reflective exercises aimed at preparing nurses and other health care providers for the care of dying patients and their families. Death education often consists of both didactic and experiential classes. Participants in these classes are encouraged to reflect on and share their own perceptions and anxieties about death as well as their attitudes toward care of the dying patient and family. This approach has been used with varying degrees of success with nurses, nursing students, and physicians.[129–131] Because many healthcare providers feel uneasy and ill-prepared to effectively care for terminally ill patients and their families, this is a promising strategy that deserves more implementation and research.

Case Study: A "Good Death" in the ICU

In this clinical incident,[1] a critical care nurse described a 70-year-old patient who was admitted to the ICU with end-stage liver failure. The patient's son was an ICU nurse himself and was the patient's primary caregiver at home. The nurse described how her relationship with the patient's son developed:

NURSE: [The patient] had diabetes, hepatitis C of unknown etiology, and end-stage liver failure. And the [patient's] son would go to the library and pull up articles on hepatitis C and hepatorenal syndrome. You know, he wanted her started on CVVH (Continuous Veno-Venous Hemofiltration) because somebody else was on it and because [the therapy] was a kind of hope. The son was with [the patient] when she was on the ward, too, and he pretty much called the shots, or that's the impression I got from the floor nurses. And I guess some nurses in the ICU might have felt that way about him, too, but this was his mom, and I guess I can understand his wanting to be involved. That's the only mother he has. Anyway, I guess I don't feel threatened by family members who need to be involved. . . . Over the next 3 weeks, I [involved the son in her care]—he was like my extra pair of hands. I mean, he takes care of her at home and he's a nurse. So, why ignore that part of him—that is him. He takes care of her, she wants him there, she was calmer when he was there, and he wants to help. He helped me turn her, he gave her back rubs, he was just there. And I passed that on from shift to shift. I said, "He wants to help. Let him. Why go look for somebody else when somebody who wants to help is right here?" Being involved gave him a sense of helping and doing something [for his mother]. If everything works out, he'll be caring for her at home. He needs to know what her skin looks like. . . . Another thing about that family, I always take it as a compliment when a family feels they can leave when I'm taking care of their family member.

INTERVIEWER: And why is that?

NURSE: Because I think that means that they trust me and that it's OK for them to leave. Even after nights and nights of staying with his mother, [the son] was still able to go out and take a break for himself. He knew I would call him on his cellular phone if anything came up. . . . But it was a pretty hopeless situation. She was evaluated for a liver transplant but was not a candidate because of her age and her diabetes. . . . It just got to a point where it looked like [the patient] was suffering so much. She just got more and more bloated, she was like twice the size she normally was. So, we ended up withdrawing support late in the shift. They were short the next shift, so I stayed over with the patient and family for another four hours just to kind of finish up with them. I didn't want them to have yet a new face [work with them] for the last hour or two of her life. Nobody who had been following this patient was back on nights and there were no other co-primaries coming on. And it wasn't that big of a deal, but I guess it was for them. About a week and a half later, the [patient's family] came in and brought me this humongous cake and two dozen roses! So, it was really a good experience because, even though it was a sad outcome, they felt supported and that was pretty much the only goal I had for them.

This clinical incident illustrates the three major aspects of caring for families of dying patients, namely, access, information and support, and involvement in caregiving activities. The nurse in this situation tailored her family care to match what was both required and desired by the patient's son. Because the son was a nurse himself, he researched his mother's condition extensively and suggested different treatment modalities. Rather than being threatened by the son's interest, the nurse understood and supported him. The nurse ensured that the son had liberal access to his critically ill mother and encouraged hands-on involvement in his mother's care.

The nurse developed a trusting relationship with the son, which enabled him to leave his mother's bedside with confidence, knowing that he would be called regarding any changes in her status. This trusting relationship also helped, no doubt, when discussions concerning his mother's prognosis arose. Because the son trusted the nurse, one can imagine, for example, that he actively listened when the nurse pointed out his mother's bloated condition while they were bathing her together. These daily, often mundane, encounters helped to forge the nurse–son relationship, from which both drew immense satisfaction.

Once the decision was made to withdraw life support, the nurse stayed past her shift to continue her work with the grieving son. The nurse "stayed over" out of respect for the relationship that had developed but also to provide the son with a "familiar face" during the uncharted and emotionally charged death of his mother. As this nurse was bearing witness to the death in particular ways shaped by the nurse–family relationship, a new person would not have been able to enter the situation and support the son in the same way. The nurse responded to the ethical responsibility of maintaining a relationship with the patient's family and, in so doing, facilitated the son's closure with this major family event.

SUMMARY

As noted by Todres and colleagues,[23] "there is not one best way to die." We believe, however, that a pain-free, ethically intact, and dignified death is the right of all ICU patients. Research to date has offered little guidance for managing the issues that surround ICU patient deaths.[25] However, Chapple[25] has presented important goals to consider during an ICU patient's dying process. The goals are to: (*1*) honor the patient's life, (*2*) assure that the patient and the patient's family are not abandoned, (*3*) provide a sense of moral stability, and (*4*) ensure the patient's safety and comfort. ICU nurses are privileged to be able to strive toward the accomplishment of these goals.

REFERENCES

1. Stannard D. Reclaiming the house: An interpretive study of nurse-family interactions and activities in critical care. Unpublished Ph.D. dissertation, University of California at San Francisco. San Francisco, 1997.

2. Groeger JS, Lemeshow S, Price K, Nierman DM, White P, Klar J, Granovsky S, Horak D, Kish SK. Multicenter outcome study of cancer patients admitted to the intensive care unit: A probability of mortality model. J Clin Onc 1998;761–770.

3. Knaus WA, Wagner DP, Zimmerman JE, et al. Variations in mortality and length of stay in intensive care units. Ann Intern Med 1993; 118(10):753–761.

4. Keenan SP, Busche KD, Chen LM, McCarthy L, Inman KJ, Sibbald WJ. A retrospective review of a large cohort of patients undergoing the process of withholding or withdrawal of life support. Crit Care Med 1997;25(8):1324–1331.

5. Schapira DV, Studnicki J, Bradham DD, Wolff P, Jarrett A. Intensive care, survival, and expense of treating critically ill cancer patients. JAMA 1993;269(6):783–786.

6. Bamburger PK, Maniscalco-Theberge ME, Pearl RH, Jaques DP. Death and dollars: The cost of dying in the surgical intensive care unit. J Trauma 1996;40(1):39–41.

7. Oye RK, Bellamy PE. Patterns of resource consumption in medical intensive care. Chest 1991;99:685.

8. Zook CJ, Moore FD. High-cost users of medical care. N Engl J Med 1980;302:996.

9. Esserman L, Belkora J, Lenert L. Potentially ineffective care: A new outcome to assess the limits of critical care. JAMA 1995;274(19):1544–1551.

10. Levetown M. Palliative care in the intensive care unit. New Horizons 1998;6(4):383–397.

11. The SUPPORT Principal Investigators. A controlled trial to improve care for seriously ill hospitalized patients: The study to understand prognoses and preferences for outcomes and risks of treatments (SUPPORT). JAMA 1995;274(20): 1591–1598.

12. Lo B. Improving care near the end of life: Why is it so hard? JAMA 1995;274(20):1634–1636.

13. Lynn J, Teno JM, Phillips RS, Wu AW, Desbiens N, Harrold J, Claessens MT, Wenger N, Kreling B, Connors AF Jr. Perceptions by family members of the dying experience of older and seriously ill patients. Ann Intern Med 1997;126: 97–106.

14. Desbiens NA, Wu AW, Broste SK, Wenger NS, Connors AF Jr., Lynn J, Yasui Y, Phillips RS, Fulkerson W. Pain and satisfaction with pain control in seriously ill hospitalized adults: Findings from the SUPPORT research investigations. Crit Care Med 1996;24:1953–1961.

15. Prendergast TJ, Luce JM. Increasing incidence of withholding and withdrawal of life support from the critically ill. Am J Respir Crit Care Med 1997;155:15–20.

16. Smedira NG, Evans BH, Grais LS, Cohen NH, Lo B, Cooke M, Schecter WP, Fink C, Epstein-Jaffe E, May C, Luce JM. Withholding and withdrawal of life support from the critically ill. N Engl J Med 1990;322(5):309–315.

17. Anderson B, McCall E, Leversha A, Webster L. A review of children's dying in a paediatric intensive care unit. New Zealand Med J 1994;107(985):345–347.

18. Levetown M, Pollack MM, Cuerdon TT, Ruttimann UE, Glover JJ. Limitations and withdrawals of medical intervention in pediatric critical care. JAMA 1994;272(16):1271–1275.

19. Balfour-Lynn IM, Tasker RC. Futility and death in paediatric medical intensive care. J Med Ethics 1996;22:279–281.

20. Vernon DD, Dean JM, Timmons OD, Banner W, Allen-Webb EM. Modes of death in the pediatric intensive care unit: Withdrawal and limitation of supportive care. Crit Care Med 1993; 21(11):1798–1802.

21. Task Force on Ethics, Society of Critical Care Medicine. Consensus report on the ethics of foregoing life-sustaining treatments in the critically ill. Crit Care Med 1990;18(12):1435–1439.

22. Walter SD, Cook DJ, Guyatt GH, Spanier A, Jaeschke R, Todd TR, Streiner DL. Confidence in life-support decisions in the intensive care unit: A survey of healthcare workers. Crit Care Med 1998;26(1):44–49.

23. Todres ID, Armstrong A, Lally P, Cassem EH. Negotiating end-of-life issues. New Horizons 1998;6(4):374–382.

24. Danis M, Federman D, Fins JJ, Fox E, Kastenbaum B, Lanken PN, Long K, Lowenstein E, Lynn J, Rouse F, Tulsky J. Incorporating palliative care into critical care education: Principles, challenges, and opportunities. Crit Care Med 1999;27:2005–13.

25. Chapple HS. Changing the game in the intensive care unit: Letting nature take its course. Critical Care Nurse 1999;19(3):25–34.

26. DeGroot-Bollujt W, Mourik M. Bereavement: Role of the nurse in the care of terminally ill and dying children in the pediatric intensive care unit. Crit Care Med 1993;21(9):S391.

27. Campbell M, Frank RR. Experience with an end-of-life practice at a university hospital. Crit Care Med 1997;25(1):197–202.

28. Puntillo K, Weiss SJ. Pain: Its mediators and associated morbidity in critically ill cardiovascular surgical patients. Nurs Res 1994;43:31–36.

29. Puntillo KA. Dimensions of procedural pain and its analgesic management in critically ill surgical patients. Am J Crit Care 1994;3(2): 116–122.

30. Puntillo KA, Wilkie DJ. Assessment of pain in the critically ill. In: Puntillo KA, ed. Pain in the Critically Ill. Gaithersberg, MD: Aspen, 1991.

31. Puntillo K, Miaskowski C, Kehrle K, Stannard D, Gleeson S, Nye P. Relationship between behavioral and physiological indicators of pain, critical care patients' self-reports of pain, and opioid administration. Crit Care Med 1997;25: 1159–1166.

32. Stannard D, Puntillo K, Miaskowski C, Gleeson S, Kehrle K, Nye P. Clinical judgment and management of postoperative pain in critical care patients. Am J Crit Care 1996;5:433–441.

33. Puntillo K, Schell H, Cohen N. Assessing pain in intensive care unit (ICU) patients: The state of practitioners' knowledge. Proceedings of the 9th World Congress on Pain, Vienna, Austria, August 22–27, 1999.

34. Campbell ML, Bizek KS, Thill M. Patient responses during rapid terminal weaning from mechanical ventilation: A prospective study. Crit Care Med 1999;27(1):73–77.

35. Bizek KS. Optimizing sedation in critically ill, mechanically ventilated patients. Critical Care Nursing Clinics of North America 1995;7(2): 315–325.

36. Ambuel B, Hamlett KW, Marx CM, et al. Assessing distress in pediatric intensive care environments: The COMFORT scale. J Pediatr Psych 1992;17:95–109.

37. Aspect Medical Systems. The Aspect A-1000 Bispectral (BIS) Index Manual. Natick, MA: Aspect Medical Systems, 1996.

38. Morrison RS, Ahronheim JC, Morrison GR, Darling E, Baskin SA, Morris J, Choi C, Meier DE. Pain and discomfort associated with common hospital procedures and experiences. J Pain Symptom Manage 1998;15:91–101.

39. Puntillo K. Dimensions of procedural pain and its analgesic management in critically ill surgical patients. Am J Crit Care 1994;3:116–122.

40. Campbell ML. Foregoing Life-Sustaining Therapy. Aliso Viejo, CA: AACN Critical Care Publication, 1998.

41. Stevens DS, Edwards WT. Management of pain in the critically ill. Journal of Intensive Care Medicine 1990;5:258–291.

42. American Pain Society. Principles of analgesic use in the treatment of acute pain and cancer pain, (4th ed.). Glenview, IL: American Pain Society, 1999.

43. Fohr SA. The double effect of pain medication: Separating myth from reality. J Palliat Med 1998;1(4):315–328.

44. Puntillo KA, Benner P, Drought T, Drew B, Stotts N, Stannard D, Rushton C, Scanlon C, White C. End-of-life issues in intensive care units: A national random survey of nurses' knowledge and beliefs. (In review).

45. Puntillo KA, Casella V. Pain, analgesia, and sedation. In: Kinney MR, Dunbar SB, Brooks-Bruns J, Molter N, Vitello-Ciccui J, eds. AACN Clinical Reference for Critical Care Nursing, 4th ed. St. Louis: Mosby, 1998.

46. Donovan M, Dillon P, McGuire L. Incidence and characteristics of pain in a sample of medical–surgical inpatients. Pain 1987;30(1):69–78.

47. Johnson JE. Effects of accurate expectations about sensations on the sensory and distress components of pain. J Pers Soc Psychol 1973; 27:61–275.

48. Campbell ML, Carlson RW. Terminal weaning from mechanical ventilation: Ethical and practical considerations for patient management. Am J Crit Care 1992;1(3):52–56.

49. Daly BJ, Newlon B, Montenegro HD, Langdon T. Withdrawal of mechanical ventilation: Ethical principles and guidelines from terminal weaning. Am J Crit Care 1993;2(3):217–223.

50. Wilson WC, Smedira NG, Fink C, McDowell JA, Luce JM. Ordering and administration of sedatives and analgesics during the withholding and withdrawal of life support from critically ill patients. JAMA 1992;267(7):949–953.

51. Guerrero M. Combined pharmacotherapy of anxiety. In: Bone R, ed. Recognition, Assessment, & Treatment of Anxiety in the Critical Care Patient. Proceedings of a consensus conference. Yardley, PA: The Medicine Group, Inc., 1994.

52. Vinik HR, Kissin I. Sedation in the ICU. Intensive Care Med 1991;17:S20–S23.

53. Shelly MP, Sultan MA, Bodenham A, Park GR. Midazolam infusions critically ill patients. Eur J Anaesthesiol 1991;8:21–27.

54. Harvey MA. Managing agitation in critically ill patients. Am J Crit Care 1996;5(1):7–16

55. Miller LG, Greenblatt DJ, Roy RB, Summer WR, Shader RI. Chronic benzodiazepine administration.II. Discontinuation syndrome is associated with upregulation of gamma-aminobutyric acid receptor complex binding a function. J Pharmacol Exp Ther 1988;246:177–182.

56. Mets B, Horsell A, Linton DM. Midazolam-induced benzodiazepine withdrawal syndrome. Anaesthesia 1991;46:28–29.

57. Faber-Langendoen K. The clinical management of dying patients receiving mechanical ventilation. Chest 1994;106(3):880–888.

58. Covington H. Use of propofol for sedation in the ICU. Critical Care Nurse 1998;18(4): 34–39.

59. Fontaine DK. Recognition, assessment, and treatment of anxiety in the critical care setting. Critical Care Nurse (suppl) 1994;August: 7–10.

60. Halloran T, Pohlman AS. Managing sedation in the critically ill patient. Critical Care Nurse (suppl) 1995;August:1–4.

61. Hospice Nurses Association. Dyspnea. Pittsburgh, PA: Hospice Nurses Association, 1996.

62. Puntillo KA. The role of critical care nurses in providing and managing end-of-life care. In: Curtis R, Rubenfield G, eds. The Transition from Cure to Comfort: Managing Death in the Intensive Care Unit. New York: Oxford University Press 2001:149–164.

63. Storey P. Symptom control in advanced cancer. Semin Oncol 1994;21:748–753.

64. Kaye P. Symptom control in hospice and palliative care. Essex, CT: Hospice Education Institute, 1990.

65. Sheehan DC, Forman WB. Symptomatic management of the older person with cancer. Clin Geriatr Med 1997;13:203–219.

66. Prendergast TJ, Claessens MT, Luce JM. A national survey of end-of-life care for critically ill patients. Am J Respir Crit Care Med 1998; 158:1163–1167.

67. Carton RW. Defining the limits of treatment: When may it be withheld or withdrawn? Journal of Critical Illness 1991;6(2):138–147.

68. President's Commission for the Study of Ethical Problems in Medicine and Biomedical and Behavioral Research. Deciding to Forgo Life-Sustaining Treatment: A Report on Ethical, Medical and Legal Issues in Treatment Decisions. Washington, DC:US Government Printing Office, 1983.

69. American Association of Critical Care Nurses. Withholding and/or Withdrawing Life-Sustaining Treatment. Newport Beach, CA: 1990. Position statement.

70. Task Force on Ethics, Society of Critical Care Medicine. Consensus report on the ethics of forgoing life-sustaining treatments in the critically ill. Crit Care Med 1990;18(12):1435–1439.

71. Medical Section, American Lung Association. Withholding and withdrawing life-sustaining therapy. Am Rev Respir Dis 1991;144:726–731.

72. Gilligan T, Raffin TA. How to withdraw mechanical ventilation: More studies are needed. Am J Crit Care 1996;5(5):323–325.

73. Gilligan T, Raffin TA. Rapid withdrawal of support. Chest 1995;108(5):1407–1408.

74. Krishna G, Raffin TA. Terminal weaning from mechanical ventilation. Crit Care Med 1999; 27(1):9–10.

75. Daly BJ, Thomas D, Dyer MA. Procedures used in withdrawal of mechanical ventilation. Am J Crit Care 1996;5(5):331–338.

76. Rushton, CH, Terry PB. Neuromuscular blockade and ventilator withdrawal: Ethical controversies. Am J Crit Care 1995;4(2):112–115.

77. Friedman SB, Chodoff P, Mason JW, Hamburg DA. Behavioral observations on parents anticipating the death of their child. Pediatrics 1963;32:616–625.

78. Lindemann E. Symptomatology and management of acute grief. Am J Psychiatry 1944; 101:141–148.

79. Sheagren TG, Puppala BL, Mangurten HH. Grief reaction to sudden unexpected cardiorespiratory arrest in a normal newborn nursery. Clin Pediatr 1987;26(7):369–371.

80. Vance JC, Foster WJ, Najman JM, Embelton G, Thearle MJ, Hodgen FM. Early parental responses to sudden infant death, stillbirth or neonatal death. Med J Aust 1991;155:292–297.

81. Miranda DR, Ryan DW, Schaufeli WB, Fidler V. Organisation and management of intensive care: A prospective study in 12 European countries. Update in Intensive Care and Emergency Medicine 1998;29:5–269.

82. Younger SJ, Coulton C, Welton R, Juknialis B, Jackson DL. ICU visiting policies. Crit Care Med 1984;12(7):606–608.

83. Ballard JL, Maloney M, Shank M, Hollister L. Sibling visits to a newborn intensive care unit: Implications for siblings, parents, and infants. Child Psychiatry Hum Dev 1984;14(4):203–214.

84. Bay EJ, Kupferschmidt B, Opperwall BJ, Speer J. Effect of the family visit on the patient's mental status. Focus on Critical Care 1988;15(1): 10–16.

85. Kleman M, Bickert A, Karpinski A, Wantz D, Jacobsen B, Lowery B, Menapace F. Physiologic responses of coronary care patients to visiting. J Cardiovasc Nurs 1993;7(3):52–62.

86. Kowba MD, Schwirian PM. Direct sibling contact and bacterial colonization in newborns. J Obstet Gynecol Neonatal Nurs 1985; 14(5):412–417.

87. Lazure LLA, Baun MM. Increasing patient control of family visiting in the coronary care unit. Am J Crit Care 1995;4(2):157–164.

88. Oehler JM, Vileisis RA. Effect of early sibling visitation in an intensive care nursery. J Dev Behav Pediatr 1990;11(1):7–12.

89. Prins MM. The effect of family visits on intracranial pressure. West J Nurs Res 1989;11(3): 281–297.

90. Schulte DA, Burrell LO, Gueldner SH, Bramlett MH, Fuszard B, Stone SK, Dudley WN. Pilot study of the relationship between heart rate and ectopy and unrestricted vs. restricted visiting hours in the coronary care unit. Am J Crit Care 1993;2(2):134–136.

91. Simpson T, Shaver J. Cardiovascular responses to family visits in coronary care patients. Heart Lung 1990;19(4):344–351.

92. Solheim K, Spellacy C. Sibling visitation: Effects on newborn infection rates. J Obstet Gynecol Neonatal Nurs 1988;17(1):43–48.

93. Umphenour JH. Bacterial colonization in neonates with sibling visitation. J Obstet Gynecol Neonatal Nurs 1980;9(2):73–75.

94. Paludetto R, Faggiano-Perfetto M, Asprea AM, Curtis MD, Margara-Paludetto P. Reactions of sixty parents allowed unrestricted contact with infants in a neonatal intensive care unit. Early Hum Dev 1981;5:401–409.

95. Schwab F, Tolbert B, Bagnato S, Maisels MJ. Sibling visitation in a neonatal intensive care unit. Pediatrics 1983;71(5):835–838.

96. Yu YH, Jamieson J, Astbury J. Parents' reactions to unrestricted parental contact with infants in the intensive care nursery. Med J Aust 1981;1:294–296.

97. Mahon MM. Children's concept of death and sibling death from trauma. J Pediatr Nurs 1993;8(5):335–344.

98. Nicholson AC, Titler M, Montgomery LA, Kleiber C, Craft MJ, Halm M, Buckwalter K, Johnson S. Effects of child visitation in adult critical care units: A pilot study. Heart Lung 1993; 22(1):36–45.

99. Benner P, Hooper-Kyriakidis P, Stannard D. Clinical Wisdom and Interventions in Critical Care: A Thinking-in-Action Approach. Philadelphia, PA: W. B. Saunders, 1999.

100. Doerr BC, Jones JW. Effect of family preparation on the stated anxiety level of the CCU patient. Nurs Res 1979;28(5):315–316.

101. Nyamathi AM. Perceptions of factors influencing the coping of wives of myocardial infarction patients. J Cardiovasc Nurs 1988;2(4): 65–76.

102. Zawatski E, Katz B, Krekeler K. Perceived needs and satisfaction with nursing care by spouses of patients in the coronary care unit. Percept Mot Skills 1979;49:170.

103. Benner P, Tanner CA, Chesla CA. Expertise in Nursing Practice: Caring, Clinical Judgment, and Ethics. New York: Springer, 1996.

104. Burfitt SN, Greiner DS, Miers LJ, Kinney MR, Branyon ME. Professional nurse caring as perceived by critically ill patients: A phenomenologic study. Am J Crit Care 1993;2:489–499.

105. Chesla, CA. Reconciling technologic and family care in critical-care nursing. Image J Nurs Sch 1996;28(3):199–203.

106. Holland C, Cason CL, Prater LR. Patients' recollections of critical care. Dimensions of Critical Care Nursing 1997;16(3):132–141.

107. Warren NA. Perceived needs of the family members in the critical care waiting room. Critical Care Nursing Quarterly 1994;16(3):56–63.

108. Greenberg LW, Ochsenschlager D, Cohen GJ, Einhorn AH, O'Donnell R. Counseling parents of a child dead on arrival: A survey of emergency departments. Am J Emerg Med 1993;11(3): 225–229.

109. Field D. Nurses' accounts of nursing the terminally ill on a coronary care unit. Intensive Care Nursing 1989;5:114–122.

110. Swisher LA, Nieman LZ, Nilsen GJ, Spivey WH. Death notification in the emergency department: A survey of residents and attending physicians. Ann Emerg Med 1993;22(8):1319–1323.

111. Tinsley ES, Baldwin AS, Steeves RH, Himel HN, Edlich RF. Surgeons', nurses' and bereaved families' attitudes toward dying in the burn centre. Burns 1994;20(1):79–82.

112. Benner P. A dialogue between virtue ethics and care ethics. Theor Med 1997;18:47–61.

113. Malacrida R, Bettelini CM, Degrate A, Martinez M, Badia F, Piazza J, Vizzardi N, Wullschleger R, Rapin CH. Reasons for dissatisfaction: A survey of relatives of intensive care patients who died. Crit Care Med 1998;26(7): 1187–1193.

114. Frank RR, Campbell ML. Caring for terminally ill patients: One hospital's team approach. Journal of Critical Illness 1999;14(1): 51–55.

115. Field BE, Devich LE, Carlson RW. Impact of a comprehensive care team on management of hopelessly ill patients with multiple organ failure. Chest 1989;96(2):353–356.

116. Coolican MB, Pearce T. After care bereavement program. Critical Care Nursing Clinics of North America 1995;7(3):519–527.

117. Hodge DS, Graham PL. A hospital-based neonatal intensive care unit bereavement follow-up program: An evaluation of its effectiveness. J Perinatol 1988;8(3):247–252.

118. Jackson I. Bereavement follow-up service in intensive care. Intensive and Critical Care Nursing 1992;8:163–168.

119. Nesbit MJ, Hill M, Peterson N. A comprehensive pediatric bereavement program: The patterns of your life. Critical Care Nursing Quarterly 1997;20(2):48–62.

120. Degner LF, Gow CM, Thompson LA. Critical nursing behaviors in care for the dying. Cancer Nurs 1991;14(5):246–253.

121. McClement SE, Degner LF. Expert nursing behaviors in care of the dying adult in the intensive care unit. Heart Lung 24:408–419.

122. Hickey M, Lewandowski L. Critical care nurses' role with families: A descriptive study. Heart Lung 1988;17(6):670–676.

123. Warren N. Bereavement care in the critical care setting. Critical Care Nursing Quarterly 1997;20(2):42–47.

124. Chambliss DF. Beyond Caring: Hospitals, Nurses, and the Social Organization of Ethics. Chicago: University of Chicago Press, 1996.

125. Muller JH, Koenig BA. On the boundary of life and death: The definition of dying by medical residents. In: Lock M, Gordon DR, eds. Biomedicine Examined. Boston: Kluwer Academic, 1988.

126. Faulkner SC. Mobile extracorporeal membrane oxygenation. Critical Care Nursing Clinics of North America 1995;7(2):259–266.

127. Isaak C, Paterson BL. Critical care nurses' lived experience of unsuccessful resuscitation. West J Nurs Res 1996;18(6):688–702.

128. Benner P, Stannard D, Hooper PL. A "thinking-in-action" approach to teaching clinical judgment: A classroom innovation for acute care advanced practice nurses. Advanced Practice Nursing Quarterly 1996;1(4):70–77.

129. Berman S, Villarreal S. Use of a seminar as an aid in helping interns care for dying children and their families. Clin Pediatr 1983;22(3): 175–179.

130. Degner LF, Gow CM. Preparing nurses for care of the dying: A longitudinal study. Cancer Nurs 1988;11(3):160–169.

131. Hainsworth DS. The effect of death education on attitudes of hospital nurses toward care of the dying. Oncol Nurs Forum 1996;23(6): 963–967.

44 The Outpatient Setting

ANNA R. DU PEN and
JEANNE ROBISON

I'm so afraid. Every time the pain comes back I am reminded of how bad it can get . . . and I'm so afraid of dying alone and in pain.
—Marianne, 41, breast cancer patient

Individuals with chronic and terminal illnesses receive the majority of their care in the outpatient clinic or office setting.[1–4] In these settings, significant long-term relationships develop among providers, patients, and families.[5] As patients move toward the end of life, visits to the clinic provide an excellent opportunity to assess the patient and family's needs, desires, struggles, and fears.

The months or years spent providing and receiving care in an outpatient setting are fundamental to establishing trust between the care team and the patient. This trusting relationship is vital both early in the disease continuum and at the end of life. Personnel at all levels of care within the outpatient setting get to know patients and participate at some level in their care. Unlike in an acute care setting, patients and families have time scheduled with physicians and staff to address their needs. This allows families to avoid the frustration of waiting in a hospital room trying to connect with a physician or nurse to raise issues or ask questions. The patient and family's questions are answered and processed at one visit, and further clarifying questions and detailed responses can ensue at the next office visit. In most cases, an outpatient setting is more intimate and less crisis-driven than a hospital setting.

There is generally a certain structure to the clinic visit that can lend itself to the integration of palliative care. In addition to taking a history, performing a physical exam, and reviewing medication history, a discussion about advanced directives can be effectively integrated into the routine. Treatment plans can be discussed and negotiated with the patient. An assessment of pain and symptoms can be done at the time vital signs are taken or during phone triage. In addition, the recently drafted pain-related standards for outpatient care of the Joint Commission on Accreditation of Health Care Organizations (JCAHO) can assist in incorporating pain and symptom management in the routine documentation of outpatient care.

CHALLENGES IN OUTPATIENT CARE

A number of challenges associated with the outpatient setting exist. The absence of a strong nursing presence is arguably the most critical barrier to the successful integration of palliative care. For example, ideally, in an outpatient oncology practice, registered nurses would be on staff to administer chemotherapy, to provide patient teaching, and to staff phone triage systems.[6,7] Assistive personnel are generally utilized for nonnursing duties, such as cleaning equipment, stocking, setting up exam rooms, and scheduling.[8] However, with shrinking resources available in all spheres of health care, the use of nonlicensed personnel is expanding, and this trend is not likely to reverse.

While it is generally considered preferable for licensed personnel to be responsible for duties such as medication administration and phone triage, many outpatient settings employ medical assistants or administrative assistants to collect intake data, take vital signs, and answer telephone calls. Some offices have no registered nurse at all in the outpatient setting, causing patients to have to wait for a chance to speak with the doctor before any assistance or suggestions can be offered. This may result in considerable delay in addressing symptom management issues and is clearly less than optimal.

Managed care has played a role in further splintering outpatient care in some medical centers. For example, with a reduction in reimbursement for chemotherapy, patients may be required to receive their treatment at an infusion center far from the cancer center together with patients receiving antibiotic therapy, inhalation therapy, etc. Although this is a more cost-efficient way to provide parenteral therapy, it offers less continuity of care over time than does having outpatient cancer center nurses provide all care, from diagnosis through active treatment and on to palliative care.

While registered nurses in office settings increasingly are being replaced by nonlicensed personnel, the increase in the use of nurse practitioners as physician extenders in outpatient care is a positive development.[9–11] These advanced practice nurses can enable same-day office visits for emergencies or symptoms that require acute management.[9,12] Many clinics use nurse practitioner to take histories and perform physical exams for routine admissions to the hospital, while the physician sees patients in the clinic. A new and growing specialty group of acute care nurse practitioners sees very ill or unstable patients in the hospital, again working closely with the physician to balance outpatient and inpatient services. They often facilitate discussions of end-of-life care for patients with life-threatening illnesses and maintain a high level of expertise in pain and symptom management (Fig. 44–1).

One challenge facing advanced practice nurses is that some states limit their prescriptive authority.[13] In these states, advanced practice nurses, trained and skilled in palliative care management, can assess pain, address symptoms, and develop treatment plans but cannot prescribe to the most potent medications. This limits patients' access to pain and symptom management and creates a cumbersome process for refilling pain medications and addressing needs for antianxiety agents. These practitioners often become experts at the optimal use of nonsteroidal antiinflammatory drugs, co-analgesic agents (such as the tricyclic antidepressants and anticonvulsants), antiemetics, bowel care agents, and a host of other pharmacologic therapies.

Several states do allow nurse practitioners full prescriptive authority,[14] which improves access to palliative care.[15] They are able to see patients with pain or symptom problems on the same day and prescribe therapy without a physician being present. Patients do not have to wait to receive a written prescription from a physician or travel to an emergency room to be seen by physicians not familiar with their cases.

Finally, another significant challenge in the outpatient setting is managing the increasingly burdensome gatekeeper role.[16] Before a chronically ill patient can be discharged from an acute care setting, arrangements for extended care or home nursing must be made by a hospital discharge planning team. Once this plan of care is established, the outpatient team must coordinate and facilitate the patient's care plan. This can be an overwhelming burden on outpatient nurses, who must constantly field phone calls and faxes, fill out disability or family leave paperwork, and communicate with caregivers in the community.[17] Balancing the phone calls that urgently need attention with those of a more bureaucratic nature is a significant problem in many practices. Keeping track of what is happening with outpatients is difficult in the best staffed clinics and may be overlooked entirely in poorly staffed settings. Return visits to the clinic are vital for evaluating treatment outcomes, assessing ongoing needs of patients, and effective management of available resources. If clients are unable to travel to the clinic, visits to a nursing home or house calls by a physician or nurse practitioner can be helpful.

The two major benefits of the outpatient setting include a more intimate, structured environment and more time to develop long-term relationships. However, the setting also has disadvantages: fewer registered nurses, the increased burden of gatekeeping, and poor access in busy outpatient practices. Providing quality palliative care in the outpatient setting requires creativity and commitment to meeting these challenges.

CRITICAL BUILDING BLOCKS FOR OUTPATIENT PALLIATIVE CARE

A number of critical elements provide an excellent framework for integrating basic palliative care concepts into almost any outpatient setting. Improving provider accessibility to patients and caregivers, promoting active listening by all staff, providing a sense of control, and continuously assessing psychological and spiritual distress are the building blocks to successful outpatient palliative care.[18–20]

Accessibility

In the outpatient setting, accessibility is critical to the palliative care of patients. Having 24-hour support available to patients and their caregivers helps reduce anxiety and, when necessary, facilitates identification of after-hours problems that need immediate attention, such as escalating pain or shortness of breath.[21] Accessibility is not, of course, only an after-hours issue. A well organized phone triage system is necessary to provide access during regular clinic hours.[22] The clerk or other nonlicensed personnel who answers the phone should receive very clear instructions on how to distinguish problems that need immediate attention (e.g., billing questions or insurance issues receive call backs; pain, shortness of breath, changes in level of consciousness require a nurse or physician to take the call, etc.). These criteria should be agreed upon by all and followed consistently. Calls that require high-level triage should be handled by trained nurses armed with protocols and standing orders that have been approved by the patient's physician. The triage system should include procedures for bringing patients into the clinic for same-day evaluation or for admission to the hospital.[7] Such a system has three main benefits:[23] (*1*) the patient sees the nurse as a qualified member of the team who is available and ready to assist; (2) the patient and family caregivers become more confident in making adjustments to medications for pain or symptom management, and (3) telephoning allows the nurse to reassess, reassure, and reinforce the teaching that has taken place (Fig. 44–2).

Advanced practice nurses clearly improve accessibility for patients undergoing palliative care management.[9] Many nurse practitioners share being on call with physicians, thereby alleviating some of the workload that 24-hour accessibility requires. Flexible scheduling of advanced practice nurses can allow for "same day work-ins," nursing home visits, or home visits, as circumstances require.

Active Listening

Active listening is a key element to effective communication among patients, the outpatient care team, and the patients' families.[24] This component of palliative care helps to support patients and families who feel physically and emotionally isolated or overwhelmed by a terminal illness.[25] Active listening also leads to more efficient use of time and a stronger relationship with the client,[20] which is important in the outpatient setting, both during face-to-face interactions as well as over the telephone. Therapeutic communication involves watch-

Pain and Symptom Management
Waiting Room Checklist

Patient Name: ____________________
Date: ____________

(circle one)

Since you saw your doctor last have you had any "new" pain or symptoms? Yes No

The level of pain is described on a 0 to 10 scale where 0 is no pain and 10 is the worst pain you can imagine. Please circle the number that best indicates the level of pain you have had over the last 24 hours:

0 1 2 3 4 5 6 7 8 9 10

No Pain **Mild** **Discomforting** **Distressing** **Horrible** **Excruciating**

Check the box beside all of the below words that describe your pain

❑ aching ❑ burning ❑ shooting ❑ throbbing

❑ tender ❑ sharp ❑ stabbing ❑ cramping

Please indicate which symptoms you are currently experiencing:

	No	Yes	If yes, is the symptom ✓ Mild	✓ Moderate	✓ Severe	If yes, how long has it been
Nausea						
Hard/infrequent bowel movements						
Drowsiness						
Shortness of Breath						
Dry Mouth						
Feeling Very Tired						
Stomachache after my pills						
Muscle jerking/twitching						
Bad dreams or "seeing things" that are not there						

(circle one)

Are you having any problems with your medications? Yes No

Is there anything that you feel is a priority to discuss at today's clinic appointment? (if yes, please indicate what)

____

____

____

Fig. 44–1. Patient waiting room checklist for pain and symptom assessment. The questions relate to pain and any side effects of analgesics—information that can facilitate discussions of symptom management.

Phone Triage Tools

Patient name ______________________________ **Date** __________

Pain/Symptom Phone Assessment

Location: ________________
Intensity (now) - ___/10
Is this a new pain? Yes No
Other Pain Descriptors: (circle) continuous pain, intermittent spikes of pain, pain changes all the time, dull, sharp, radiating, aching, burning, shooting
What pain medicine is ordered? ______________________________
What pain medicine is patient actually taking? ______________________
Side effects (constipation, dry mouth, drowsiness, confusion, nausea, vomit)

Treatment Plan

- ❏ Make appointment to come in: __________________________
- ❏ Increase/decrease scheduled/prn opioid dose ________________
- ❏ Change opioid ________________ ❏ Change route
- ❏ Reinforce: take meds on schedule, use prn meds, report unrelieved pain, refills
- ❏ Add tricyclic antidepressant / anticonvulsant: ________________
- ❏ Add NSAID:
- ❏ Add non-drug intervention: (circle) heat, cold, massage, distraction, relaxation, TENS
- ❏ Treat side effects: (circle) constipation, dry mouth, drowsiness, confusion, nausea
- ❏ Referrals: (circle) social work, psychiatry, physical therapy, anesthesia, radiation

Notes: ____

____

Next follow up (phone _________ , visit _________)

Signature ______________________________ Date _________

Fig. 44–2. Phone triage tools. Concise assessment and treatment progress note designed for telephone interview for triage of pain and symptoms.

ing for nonverbal clues, showing empathy, and assessing the patient and family's knowledge base.[26] In the outpatient setting staff become more familiar with the patient and family over months and perhaps years, which makes the process of listening actively and with empathy easier. This ability and opportunity to make assessments over a long time period is unique to the outpatient setting.[27]

Helpful tools for opening dialogues with patients include open-ended questions, such as "Tell me how your pain has been this past week," or "You look really tired today, what has your week been like?"[28] When a formerly hopeful patient with a "fighter" attitude responds with "I don't think I can do this anymore," the active listener understands that a transition is occurring. Time must be set aside for this patient, either immediately or with a plan for a follow-up phone call or family conference. Time spent proactively facilitating these transitions will almost always save crisis-induced time spent later in the patient's course.

Another critical component of active listening involves identifying barriers to effective palliative care. The classic example of a barrier to care is the fear of opioid addiction. A clinic nurse often first identifies the patient's or family members concern about taking opioids. It is important to discuss this attitudinal barrier early and frequently. Another barrier to pain management at the end of life is the belief that using pain medications hastens death. Because of this belief, family members may resist optimizing opioids and adjuvants at the end of life. In addition to verbal instructions at the time of the clinic visits, written materials on the rationale and role of symptom management in end-of-life care can be extremely helpful.

Another issue that is frequently present and often requires active facilitation by clinic staff is the social context of care. The cost of care is an increasing concern and is an area that patients and families are frequently uncomfortable discussing. This often results in conflicts that are identified only late in the course of care. Distressing issues may arise surrounding long-term care and, particularly, the distribution of financial support and caregiving responsibilities among family members. Whenever possible, prompt initiation of family conferences or referrals to social workers are advisable.

Providing a Sense of Control

Helping the chronically and terminally ill patient regain a sense of control is a key element in managing the helplessness many patients experience.[29] Within the acute and long-term care settings, "power symbols" exist that shift the locus of control away from the patient.[30] These symbols include the sea of white coats, high tech equipment, hospital beds that place patients below their professional caregivers, and a general lack of privacy. Interventions that can promote a sense of control in the outpatient setting include allowing patients to remain dressed during most office calls, at least until an exam is required; reducing the clinical, white coat formality; and providing a safe, nonthreatening, private place for meetings with patients and their families. These accommodations return a sense of control and dignity to the patient with a terminal illness and promote health and well being.[18]

Tuning In to Distress

Psychological and spiritual health are often profoundly affected by life-threatening illness. In fact, patients with chronic and terminal illnesses display a high incidence of frank psychiatric morbidity, documented in several studies to range from 40%–53%.[31,32] Common psychiatric diagnoses among the terminally ill include delirium, amnesia, major depression, and anxiety.[32] However, many patients with significant symptoms of anxiety, depression, and anger do not qualify as having a major psychiatric illness. These symptoms have been described throughout the palliative care literature as distress.[19,32,33] Identifying distress early in the palliative care continuum allows for early intervention, prevention of comorbid psychological problems, and improved quality of life.

Easy-to-use, inexpensive, brief, noninvasive, and generally well accepted self-reporting questionnaires can be used in the outpatient settings.[34,35] Two good examples are the Hospital Anxiety and Depression Scale (HAD)[36] and the Distress Thermometer.[35] The HAD consists of 14 questions to which the client answers yes or no. This tool omits somatic complaints and focuses on questions that can help differentiate anxiety and depression. Despite its title, it has also been successfully used in the outpatient setting.[34]

The Distress Thermometer has been tested in men with prostate cancer.[35] It consists of a visual analogue scale made to look like a thermometer, with the bottom of the thermometer reading 1, or no distress; 5 being moderate distress, and 10 (at the top of the thermometer) being extreme distress. Distress is defined in a generic sense of unpleasant stress. This is a simple scale that can be used at the beginning of each office visit or on a regular basis (e.g., quarterly). Responses can be used to open discussions of the symptoms of distress being experienced by a client in the outpatient setting (e.g., "I see that you're feeling a moderate amount of distress. Can we talk about what you're feeling?").

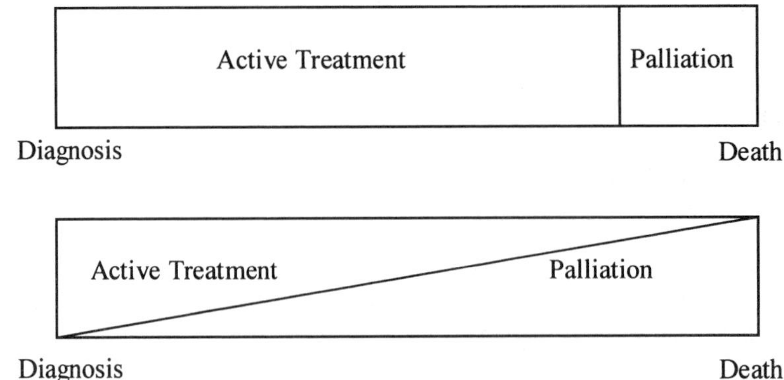

Fig. 44–3. Active treatment versus palliative care depicted in a mutually exclusive "old" model and an integrated "new" model.

Spiritual distress can be equally devastating to the patient and family. Hearing "What did I do to deserve this?" and "How could God let this happen to my husband?" from a patient or family member are cues that spiritual support is needed. Some health care systems have chaplains available in the outpatient setting. Many churches and synagogues provide outreach ministries to the gravely ill. Other nontraditional spiritual support may include meditation or rituals to explore the meaning of events. Whenever possible, the clinic should be given a list of resources for community spiritual support.

INTEGRATING PALLIATIVE CARE INTO OUTPATIENT CARE

A combination of philosophical mission, strategic planning, and bottom line pragmatism are necessary to integrate palliative care successfully into the current outpatient medical model (Fig. 44–3). The philosophical mission must come from the institution and the strategic planning from administration, but the practical, day-to-day implementation occurs in the clinical practice at the hands of nurses and physicians. Integrating palliative care must begin at the initial and continue in the ongoing evaluation and management process.

Assessment

Assessment of the patient and families' goals and preferences begins during the initial meeting. In most outpatient settings a baseline history, a physical exam, X-rays, and laboratory tests should accompany a review of preventive, general, or specialty health care needs during the first few office visits. A routine evaluation of current health needs and preventive health issues can be followed by a review of end-of-life care preferences. If such a discussion is delayed and occurs during a later or exacerbated illness, the patient and family are much more likely to fear that death is imminent or that the doctor is "holding something back." This makes it much more difficult for all involved to reach clarity on the patient's goals. A sample clinic conversation is shown in Table 44–1.

Table 44–1. Sample Dialogue for Opening Advanced Directive Discussion

Nurse: Mrs. Jones, have you thought about what you want us to do if your heart stops?
Mrs. Jones: Oh goodness, no. I'm healthy as can be.
Nurse: Do you have a living will?
Mrs. Jones: No. I don't like to think about that sort of thing.
Nurse: It's true that most healthy people don't want to talk about dying, but we need to discuss all aspects of your health care, including end-of-life care, so that we'll be able to do the best job possible of treating you and at the same time respecting your wishes.

Table 44–2. Sample Dialogue for Goal-Oriented Pain Assessment

Nurse: Mr. Edwards, in addition to treating your disease, we also want to be successful at relieving your symptoms. What's your pain level today on the 0 to 10 scale?
Mr. Edwards: Oh, don't worry about my pain—it's only about a 6 today.
Nurse: You mentioned that your pain is 6 out of 10, but I see that you haven't been taking as much pain medicine as the doctor has ordered for you. What level of pain relief would be your goal?
Mr. Edwards: Well, it would be nice to be down around a 4, but the medicine is so darn expensive that I try not to use it unless it gets pretty bad.
Nurse: I see . . . your goal would be to get the pain down to a 4 or so if the cost factor wasn't there . . . is that right? Well, let's ask Dr. Jones if there is a less expensive drug that would work for you. We could also check to see if the drug company has a program to help out with the cost of medication.

If the patient already has a life threatening diagnosis, it is appropriate early on to establish a routine for assessing pain, fatigue, nausea, and other physical, psychological, and functional parameters. It is critically important to establish a standard approach to assessing the palliative care needs of the patient and family in the outpatient setting. To save time and obtain preliminary information, patients may be given a standard form to fill out before the exam. This can also help narrow down the priority issues for the visit. Increasingly, electronic forms are being used that may be accessed through a waiting room kiosk or even over the internet from the patient's home.

Patients and their families should be educated early about the importance of symptom assessment and reporting as well as evaluation of treatment efficacy and side effects. Establishing the patient and family as part of the team will improve outcomes. As always, the patient's goals of care become the central focus for facilitating optimized palliative care. A sample dialogue is shown in Table 44–2.

Reassessment of pain and symptoms should occur with new or continuing problems and with a resaonable frequency and method. For example, a patient with pain of 7 on a scale of 10 is seen in the office for opioid titration. An explicit follow-up assessment plan should be established *before* the patient leaves the clinic. Either a clinic nurse should telephone the patient in a day or two, or alternately, the patient or a family member should call the office nurse if the pain level does not drop below 4 within a day or two. Patient instructions should include specifics, such as "Call the clinic if you go three days or more without having a bowel movement," or "Call the clinic tomorrow if the antinausea medicine is not working." These instructions can be incorporated into a standard handout for patients and then individualized as needed (see Table 44–3).

Because it is clear that some patients and family members are hesitant to "bother" the clinic with phone calls, it is often desirable for the reassessment phone call to be initiated by the clinic. These reassessment, or "check back," calls can be done by a trained medical assistant or other nonlicensed personnel (see Table 44–4).

An organized reminder system for callbacks should be instituted. One method is to route a copy of the patient's last waiting room checklist (Fig. 44–1) or "Things to Report to the Clinic" sheet to a medical assistant or clerk for follow up. As with the phone triage criteria, the caller must be given clear criteria for what to do with the information obtained (e.g., document resolved problems vs. report unresolved problems to the provider).

Criteria for further follow up can be established such that unresolved symptoms identified by the office nurse or medical assistant at phone triage lead to notification of the physician and further revision of the treatment plan. For example, any new problems should be triaged by a registered nurse or physician. Phone triage notes can be designed for easy completion with "check-off boxes" and "circle the symptom"–type documentation. (see Figure 44–2).

Patients who have a knowledge

Table 44–3. Reminder List

__ Any new pain
__ Pain that is constantly above a 5 on a 0–10 scale, even with your pain medicine
__ Severe episodes of pain, even with your pain medicine
__ Stools that are hard and difficult to pass, or if you are moving your bowels only every 2nd or 3rd day or less
__ Feeling very drowsy after taking your medicine
__ Having bad dreams or "seeing things"
__ Nausea, vomiting, or stomachache after taking your medicine
__ Muscle twitching or jerking
__ Other: 1) <u>Call the clinic tomorrow if the nausea medicine is not working</u>
2) <u>Call the clinic tomorrow if the pain is still > 4/10</u>

Other Issues Important to Discuss with the Doctor or Nurse

__ Not having enough instruction on how to take your medicines
__ Not being able to afford your medicines
__ Worries about taking pain medicine

Table 44–4. Sample Dialogue for "Check-Back" Calls

Examples of Call-Back Scripts for Follow-up on Clinic Visits

Mrs. Edwards, this is Jesse from Dr. Jones' office. I'm calling to check back on Mr. Edwards' constipation since we increased his stool softeners. Has he had a normal bowel movement today?
Mr. Smith, this is Jesse from Dr. Jones' office. I'm calling to check back on your nausea. Is that antinausea medicine working for you?

deficit about their medications or treatment regimen may require a follow-up call from a registered nurse or pharmacist.

New or escalating symptoms require timely response. A reasonable time frame should be set for follow-up of new problems. Ideally, the patient should be seen within 12 hours of the onset of new symptoms—essentially, the same day, if possible. This is particularly true for patients with significant symptom management issues, for whom trips to the emergency room or urgent care center would be extremely tiring would result in the patient being evaluated without all pertinent data available. Any patient with significant new or escalating symptoms who is seen in an emergency room should be seen back in the outpatient setting within 24 to 48 hours. If the patient receives home care or is involved with a hospice, an initial evaluation can be done at home, with phone contact with the clinic. If home care or hospice care are not in place, an escalation of symptom management problems is often a very good indication to initiate these resources. Home visits or nursing home visits by a physician or nurse practitioner may be necessary for patient's unable to travel to a clinic.

Evaluation and Management

At its core, the outpatient setting is concerned with evaluation and management (E & M). The E & M codes drive reimbursement and consequently dictate documentation requirements. The "evaluate and treat" construct is deeply entrenched in the traditional medical model. Both the reimbursement driven E & M process and the traditional medical model do not always support palliative care. In fact, one of the most persistent problems in palliative care is the "hospice as last resort" assumption of some providers, causing referrals from the outpatient setting to a home care agency within the last days of life and virtually never before suspension of active treatment. This late utilization of home health resources is further complicated by the "crackdown" on Medicare fraud in home health care and has resulted in drastically reduced home stays across the country. Some providers also worry that hospice care will "take over" and that the patient will therefore not have access to appropriate medical oversight. In such cases the provider essentially "loses" a patient and family with whom they have developed a relationship during long-term treatment. In some cases, this concern results in an "us or them" mentality in which everyone loses.

Fortunately, many clinicians reject the stark line drawn between active treatment and palliative care and successfully merge the concepts in outpatient care. Conceptually, this model was described by the World Health Organization.[37]

The "old" model depicts health care system involvement starting from diagnosis with active treatment and then abruptly, shortly before death, switching to a purely palliative model. The "new" model depicts the health care system using active and palliative care concurrently, with a primarily active treatment focus at diagnosis, integration along the trajectory, and primarily a palliative focus at death.

Take, as an example, an elderly gentleman with metastatic prostate cancer who has begun hospice care and has developed 9 on a scale of 10 pain in his back that shoots down his legs. His opioid therapy has been increased aggressively over the past week, and he is now somnolent between periods of extreme pain. His wife also notices he needs more help getting out of bed because his legs "won't hold him up." He and his wife explain that their goals are to keep his pain under control and keep him as functional as possible. This patient may benefit dramatically from steroids and radiation to reduce pain and save the functions of his lower extremities, bowel, and bladder, even though he is receiving hospice care. In such situations, a very clear understanding of the patient and family's goals of care, well defined and known to both outpatient providers and home care or hospice care providers, will facilitate the best possible outcomes.

Treatment algorithms or protocols can promote efficiency in the clinic and enhance outcomes. These tools can be successfully put into place and implemented both by clinic nurses and home care or hospice care nurses. One such algorithm was used in outpatient oncology with resulting improved pain management.[38] The Cancer Pain Algorithm is a decision tree model for pain treatment developed as a practical interpretation of the Agency for Health Care Policy and Research Guidelines for Cancer Pain Management. The algorithm consists of a bulleted set of analgesic "guiding principles" for use with opioids, nonsteroidal anti-inflammatory drugs, tricyclic antidepressants, anticonvulsants, and drug side effects. For example, the statement "titrate to efficacy or side effects" is an underlying principle throughout the algorithm. Drug choice decisions depend on pain assessment data. The flow chart then directs the oncology nurse or oncologist to side effect protocols, equianalgesic conversion charts, and a primer for intractable pain.

Figure 44–4 represents the high level algorithm decision-making flow. Etiology and location correlate the pain with its known tumor or treatment-related source, or indicate the need for further diagnostic work-up. Pain intensity is based on self-report on a scale from 0–10, where 0 is no pain and 10 is the worst pain imaginable. Pain character is divided into nociceptive versus neuropathic components. The character of the pain is the primary variable to direct the choice of nonopioid or coanalgesic therapies. The frequency and method of reassessment is outlined for the practitioner based on the results of the last pain assessment contact. An algorithm reference tool contains drug-specific content such as titration parameters and side effect protocols and a number of highly specific flow charts. The algorithm process is intended as a team effort, relying on the physician/clinic nurse/home care nurse/family caregiver network as a cohesive outpatient unit, all applying the principles of the algorithm as they relate to the individual patient.

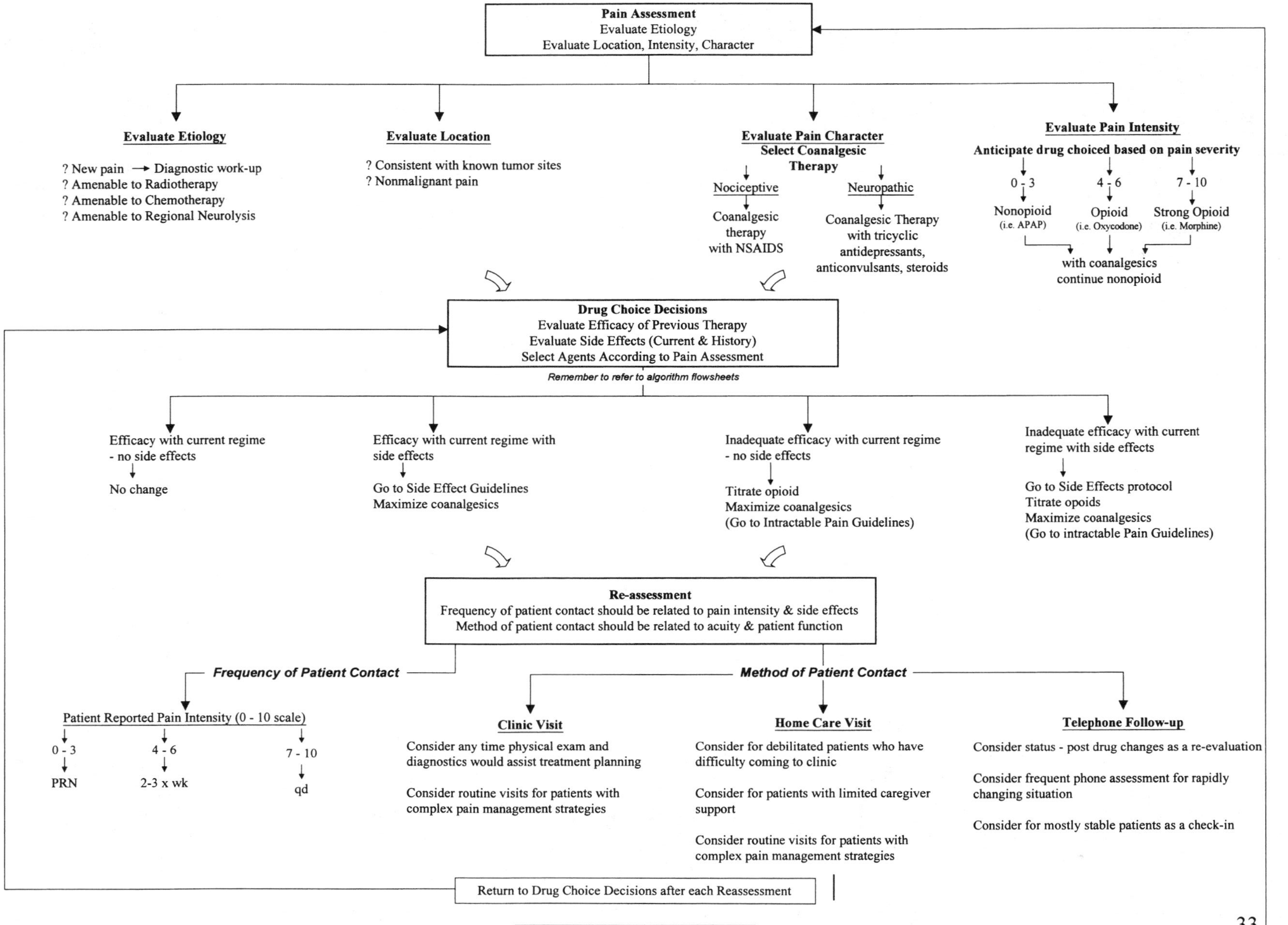

Fig. 44–4. Du Pen Cancer Pain Algorithm. An algorithm designed to aid decision making in outpatient management of cancer pain. Use of this algorithm in clinical trials showed a significant ($p < .02$) reduction from usual pain levels.

Another concept now being used in outpatient care is that of the primary nurse "navigator." The navigator takes the concept of case manager a step further, in the sense of acting as a "learned guide" rather than a plan "manager." The navigator is responsible for tracking the course of the patient's care through the myriad of services. A treatment plan becomes the "road atlas," and the nurse navigator steers the patient's care to the key stops along the highway. These stops may be follow-up diagnostic studies, interdisciplinary consultations, hospice referrals, or a variety of other patient-specific services. This model works well for outpatient services that, in general, are disconnected one from another and that might be overlooked under strained resources. The navigator works from critical pathways, or algorithms, and updates the physician weekly.

THE THREE C'S OF OUTPATIENT PALLIATIVE CARE: COOPERATION, COMMUNICATION, AND CLOSURE

At the heart of palliative care in the outpatient setting are the three concepts of cooperation, communication, and closure. The concepts of cooperation and communication are woven throughout this chapter. The outpatient setting is the site of cooperation among patient, family, and outpatient staff. This cooperation then expands to the agencies within the community caring for the patient. This may include home health care nurses, long-term care staff, local pharmacists, neighbors and friends of the client, and the local church. The physician and advanced practice nurses cooperate to provide easy access to care. The specialist and primary care physician, who both often monitor the patient in the outpatient setting, cooperate. Care in the outpatient setting is not provided in isolation, but by a well coordinated and dedicated community team.

At the heart of this cooperation is good communication. Communication begins with active listening, fostered in the outpatient setting. Efficient and accurate documentation of patient teaching, phone calls, and interventions is the key to continuity of care. A variety of tools have been developed for use in the outpatient setting to improve this communication.

Not yet addressed, but also important in the outpatient setting, is closure. Bereavement is an issue for nurses, physicians, and staff in the outpatient setting.[39] As patients become sicker and eventually homebound, the outpatient staff is no longer able to see the patients, despite being in close contact with family and home care staff over the phone. In many cases, this early separation from the patient complicates the ability of the outpatient staff to come to closure with what often has been a long-term relationship with the patient. This abrupt loss of connection can be a significant source of bereavement for staff.

Outpatient nurses may have had years to assess the family or caregivers' previous experiences with death, the support available, and the coping resources of those who have suffered the loss.[39] This familiarity with the family or caregiver helps the nurse in the outpatient setting better to support grieving loved ones.

Often, family members or caregivers will be drawn back to the outpatient setting to say final goodbyes or give gifts of thanks to staff who have become as close as family to the patient and caregivers. Staff should be prepared for this visit by being informed of patient's deaths. Work should stop for a moment to embrace the returning family members and give them time to tell the story of the death and share feelings of grief and joyful memories of the deceased.[40] Gifts or pictures brought by the family should be accepted graciously. Many offices take time out each month to send cards to families of patients who have died.

Staff of the outpatient clinic, the front desk receptionist, the medical assistant, the nurse, and the physician may experience grief after the loss of a patient. Often, staff require support through the death of patients dear to them. It is important to allow for special opportunities to celebrate the life and mourn the death of these patients. Attending funerals, keeping scrapbooks, and having occasional symbolic tributes to patients can help staff through the grieving process. Occasionally, it may be helpful to provide staff professional counseling or to send them on a retreat, where feelings regarding death and loss can be shared. Caregivers as well as family and friends need closure when death comes. In the outpatient setting this affords all who have experienced the loss support on the journey toward healing.

SUMMARY

The outpatient setting has both advantages and disadvantages. As more and more patients with end-stage disease choose to remain in their homes, the outpatient clinic has become the main point of contact for care and coordination of resources. The outpatient clinic staff act as gatekeepers, maintaining checks and balances on the home health care system or the long-term care facility. Relationships are develop over many years, creating a sense of trust that fosters the holistic care that is at the heart of palliative medicine.

Strategies for providing palliative care in this setting apply to all diseases. The concepts of active listening, promoting patient control, assessing for distress, and promoting access to care all improve the delivery of palliative care in the outpatient clinic. The use of nurse-staffed phone triage systems, nurse practitioners, and tools for assessing palliative care needs benefit both the terminally ill patient and the patient with advanced chronic disease. Care algorithms and critical pathways assist staff in implementing research-based interventions to prevent suffering and promote quality of life. Finally, the three C's of outpatient palliative care emphasize the necessity of coordination, communication, and closure.

There is perhaps a fourth quality needed when caring for chronically or terminally ill clients in the outpatient setting—commitment. Through a commitment to alleviate suffering and promote quality of life, caregivers in the outpatient setting assist patients in finding physical, psychological, and spiritual wellness, even at the end of the disease trajectory.

REFERENCES

1. Burda D. Growth in outpatient care reflected in managers' compensation—study. Modern Healthcare 1993;23(20):58.

2. Gardner J. VA revamp emphasizes move to outpatient care. Modern Healthcare 1995; 25(22):8.

3. Japsen B. Special report. Another year of major growth in outpatient care. Post-acute care. Modern Healthcare 1998;28(21):58–62, 64–66, 68–72.

4. Wodinsky HB, Sone M, Kerr IG. Outpatient palliative pain control. Dimensions in Health Services 1998;65(3):10,15–17.

5. Schulmeister L. Trends in health care delivery: Their impact on oncology nurses in the office setting. In: Baird SB, Hartigan K, Holton-Smith D. eds. The Role of the Oncology Nurse in the Office Setting. Columbus, Ohio: Adria, 1987: 25–31.

6. Harris MG, et al. Changing the role of the nurse in the hematology-oncology outpatient setting. Oncology Nursing Forum 1991;18(1):43–46.

7. Stacey D. et al. Telephone triage: An important role for oncology nurses. Cancer Oncology Nursing Journal 1997;7(3):178–179.

8. Medvec BR, Pelusi JL, Camp-Sorrell D, Kleinschmidt P, Krebs L, Mooney K. Assistive personnel: Their use in cancer care—An oncology nursing society position paper. Oncology Nursing Society 1996;23(4):647–651.

9. Kinney AY, Hawkins R, Hudmon KS. A descriptive study of the role of the oncology nurse practitioner. Oncology Nursing Forum 1997; 24(5):811–820.

10. Kovner C, et al. Practice and employment trends among nurse practitioners in New York State. Journal of New York State Nurses Association 1997;28(4):4–8.

11. Pitts J, et al. The use of nurse practitioners in pediatric institutions. Journal of Pediatric Health Care 1998;12(2):67–72.

12. Mason DJ, et al. Managed care organizations' arrangements with nurse practitioners. Nursing Economics 1997;15(6):306–314.

13. Straub P, Geller JM. Restrictive practice environment and nurse practitioners' prescriptive authority. J Am Nurse Pract 1997;9(1):9–15.

14. McDermott KC. Prescriptive authority for advanced practice nurses: current and future perspecitves. Oncology Nursing Forum 1995;22(8 Suppl):25–30.

15. Hamric AB, Worley D, Lindebak S, Jaubert S. Outcomes associated with advanced nursing practice prescriptive authority. Journal of the American Academy of Nurse Practitioners 1998;10(3):113–118.

16. Young GP, Lowe RA. Adverse outcomes of managed care gatekeeping. Academy of Emergency Medicine 1997;4(12):1129–1136.

17. Halm EA, Causino N, Blumenthal D. Is gatekeeping better than traditional care? A survey of physicians'attitudes. Journal of the American Medical Association 1997;278(20):1677–1681.

18. Fryback PB, Reinert BR. Facilitating health in people with terminal diagnoses by encouraging a sense of control. Medical Surgical Nursing 1993;2(3):197–201.

19. Jacobsen PB, Brietbach W. Psychosocial aspects of palliative care. Cancer Control 1996; 3:214–222.

20. Straka DA. Are you listening? Have you heard? Advanced Practice Nursing Quarterly 1997;3(2):80–81.

21. Brown C. Health care system changes and nursing. ABNF Journal 1994;5(2):41–42.

22. Fawcett SD. Telephone triage: An important role for oncology nurses. Cancer Oncology Nursing Journal 1997;7(3):178–179.

23. Hartigan K. Administrative issues for the oncology nurse in the office setting. In: Baird SB, Hartigan K, Holton-Smith D. eds. The Role of the Oncology Nurse in the Office Setting. Columbus, Ohio: Adria, 1987:25–31.

24. Srnka QM, Ryan MR. Active listening: A key to effective communication. Am Pharm 1993; NS33(9):43–46.

25. Rydholm L. Patient-focused care in parish nursing. Holist Nurs Practice 1997;11(3): 47–60.

26. Willen J. The skills of listening. A review of helpful communication techniques. Am J Hosp Care 1986;3(4):39–41.

27. Stoner C. Practice issues for the oncology nurse in the office setting. In: Baird SB, Hartigan K, Holton-Smith D. eds. The Role of the Oncology Nurse in the Office Setting. Columbus, Ohio: Adria, 1987:17–24.

28. Holton-Smith D, Benson J. Providing patient and educational support in the oncology office setting. In Baird SB, Hartigan K, Holton–Smith D, eds. The Role of the Oncology Nurse in the Office Setting. Columbus, Ohio: Adria, 1987: 25–31.

29. Aasen, N. Interventions to facilitate personal control. Journal of Gerontologic Nursing 1987;13(6):21.

30. Ebersol P, Hess P. Crisis and stress management. In: Toward Healthy Aging. Fifth Ed. St. Louis: Mosby, 1998:676–701.

31. Derogatis LR, Morrow GR, Fetting J, Penman D, Piassetsky S, Schmale AM, et al. The prevelance of psychiatric disorders among cancer patients. JAMA 1983;249–751:751–757.

32. Minagawa H, Uchitomi Y, Vamawaki S, Ishitahi K. Psychiatric morbidity in terminally ill cancer patients. A prospective study. Cancer 1996; 78(5):1131–1137.

33. Cleary JF, Carbone PP. Palliative medicine in the elderly. Cancer 1997;80:1335–1347.

34. Moorey S, et al. The factor structure and factor stability of the Hospital Anxiety and Depression Scale in patients with cancer. British Journal of Psychiatry 1991;158:255–259.

35. Roth AJ, Kornblith AB, Batel-Copel L, Peabody E, Scher HI, Holland JC. Rapid screening for psychologic distress in men with prostate carcinoma. A pilot study. Cancer 1998;82: 1904–1908.

36. Zigmond AS, Snaith RP. The hospital anxiety and depression scale. Act Psychiatrica Scandinavica 1983;67:361–370.

37. World Health Organization. Cancer Pain Relief and Palliative Care, 2nd ed. Geneva: World Health Organization, 1995.

38. Du Pen SL, Du Pen AR, Polissar N, Hansberry J, Miller-Kraybill B, Stillman M, Panke J, Everly R, Syrjala K. Implementing guidelines for cancer pain management: Results of a randomized controlled clinical trial. Journal of Clinical Oncology 1999;17(1):361–370.

39. Martocchio B. Grief and bereavement, healing through hurt. Nursing Clinics of North America 1985;20(2):327–341.

40. Dufault KJ, Martocchio BC. Breavement: The price of loving. In: Dimond M, ed. Advances in Geriatric and Long Term Nursing Care. Villanova, Pennsylvania: Pro Scientia Inc., 1982.

45 Rehabilitation

KATHLEEN MICHAEL

I want to do as much as I can for as long as I can. I want to continue being myself.

—Rehabilitation patient

Even when it is not reasonable to expect cure or reversal of disease processes, or to restore a previous level of functionality and independence, a rehabilitative approach to nursing care improves the quality of the experience of life's completion. Rehabilitation nursing interventions are designed with the knowledge that life always has an end and that every day counts. With respect for each unique patient, rehabilitation nurses address palliative and end-of-life care with concern for preserving hope, human dignity, and autonomy. They involve social, spiritual, and functional support systems. They help patients and families make the most of each day in spite of the disease trajectory. The language of rehabilitation nursing is a language shared with those who practice palliative care.

Rehabilitation nurses work with the concepts of independence and interdependence, self-care, coping, access, and quality of life, skillfully weaving them into the assessment, planning, implementation, and evaluation of nursing care.[1] While the focus is on function, acceptance of varieties of life experiences, including those at life's end, is fundamental to this practice.

REHABILITATION NURSING

Rehabilitation nursing concerns itself with "adaptation of the whole being to a new life"[2] and may be envisioned as a logical and essential component in the health process across the continuum of life.[1] As life proceeds to its end, adaptation to a new state allows a being to remain whole: to interact with the environment, to experience human relationships, and to achieve personally meaningful goals. Rehabilitation nurses find themselves at work in every phase of growth, development, and dying as individuals strive to adapt.

Persons with incurable progressive diseases are cared for in various venues of rehabilitation nursing. Whether patient-, provider-, or setting-centered, the merging of rehabilitation and palliative nursing principles is evident.

Acute comprehensive inpatient rehabilitation units are set up in such a way that complex medical–surgical issues may be managed concurrently with the functional processes of comprehensive rehabilitation. For example, patients with metastatic cancer affecting their bones may have significant care needs related to mobility and the activities of daily living that would be well-addressed in an inpatient rehabilitation setting.

For many patients with terminal illnesses, the transition to an acute rehabilitation unit represents a crucial point in their health care experience. It is a time when the future begins to come into focus and goals are defined based on the likely disease process. Sometimes a stay on an inpatient rehabilitation unit makes it possible for patients to return to a home setting because of the gains in independent function that may be realized. Patients and family members may begin to face limited prognoses, decline in abilities, and changes in roles. Through an interdisciplinary therapeutic process, care needs are clarified, and skills and adaptational strategies are taught to patients and those who will care for them outside of the hospital.

Long-term care settings, such as skilled nursing facilities, are often places where lives are completed. *Geriatric facilities* focus on the care needs of aging persons, often requiring specialized rehabilitation interventions. In both of these settings, rehabilitation nurses may plan and direct care activities, and ensure that patient and family concerns are kept in the forefront. Optimizing function and self-care as well as addressing physical care issues occur in this setting.

Subacute rehabilitation facilities provide additional therapy activities, such as physical, occupational, and speech therapy, based on patient need, endurance, and tolerance. The pacing and amount of therapy is gauged according to individualized goals. Again, the aim is to facilitate improved physical function and to achieve as much independence as possible, even when the disease process moves the patient toward death. For example, patients with advanced disease who are too frail to participate in a full acute rehabilitation program may benefit from the slower paced rehabilitation of a subacute setting.

Hospice settings may also benefit from a rehabilitative approach to end-of-life care. Careful planning of care to take into account limitations yet promote function and autonomy is a key factor in smoothing the transition to an inevitable death. Rehabilitative techniques and strategies make it easier for caregivers to manage increasing deficits, thereby protecting patient comfort and dignity through the dying process.

Pediatric rehabilitation focuses on guiding the development of children to minimize disability and handicap that may result from physical or cognitive impairment. Situations exist in pediatric rehabilitation in which palliative care comes into play, and efforts are directed toward enhancing the normal function of both the patient and family through the course of disease. For example, family members of a child with progressive neuromuscular disease may learn how to use adaptive devices to position the child in a wheelchair for comfort and social interaction as well as for physiological function.

In the *insurance industry* and *managed care systems*, rehabilitation nurses have the opportunity to advocate for the needs of persons with disease or disability and to reduce barriers to their access to care and resources. Near the end of a terminal disease course, planning and resource management are essential to ensure optimal care without undue economic and emotional burdens to families.

Care of dying patients occurs frequently at *home*. Successful end-of-life care at home is the preference of many patients and families. Such care depends on skillful and compassionate guidance, keen assessment, and creative problem solving. Rehabilitation nursing is well suited to this charge. *Community health systems* benefit from input from rehabilitation professionals, as they design services to meet changing demographic trends, such as the aging of the American population or the increasing numbers of persons living with disease and disability in the community.

Case Management is an expanding practice area for rehabilitation nurses, usually with multidisciplinary relationships.[1] Because palliative care needs are unique to individuals and require coordination of care across disciplines, usual patterns of delivery and resource use are not always appropriate. The implementation of care pathways in palliative care requires careful and compassionate guidance and evaluation, tailored to meet individual strengths, abilities, needs, and preferences.[3,4]

REHABILITATION NURSING AND PALLIATIVE CARE

A need clearly exists for rehabilitation nursing presence in the arena of palliative care. If future health care services are to center on needs, preferences, and informed consent of patients and families in our society, less emphasis will be placed on cure, illness, paternalism, and prescription. More attention will be paid to self-care and client participation, holistic wellness, primary care and prevention, and the quality attributes of care as defined by the consumer.[1]

Patient- and family-centered care is clearly appropriate for the unique experience of dying. Understanding and designing interventions relative to the ecological balance of life and death make it possible to guide health policy and resource allocation in ways that support care across the continuum. Permitting a kind of wellness to exist even at the point of death, such as the experience of a "good death," fits with the rehabilitation philosophy. Many rehabilitation nursing actions center around prevention of complications, which remains appropriate at the end of life. Finally, rehabilitation has long been concerned with understanding and measuring quality of life, whether related to physical, psychosocial, or spiritual domains.

The real value of a rehabilitative approach to the nursing care of persons with declining health states lies in the foundations of rehabilitation nursing practice. Rehabilitation nurses

- attend to the full range of human experiences and responses to health and illness
- deal with families coping with lifelong issues
- provide a holistic approach to care
- facilitate team dynamics and integration
- educate patients and their families to help them control and manage a wide range of challenges associated with chronic illness or disability
- form partnerships with patients and other health care providers to attain the best possible outcomes.[5]

The hallmark of rehabilitation is interdisciplinary collaboration. This potentiates the value of rehabilitation nursing interventions and assures that patient needs are addressed from a variety of perspectives. Typically, the rehabilitation team consists of physicians with specialized training in physical medicine and rehabilitation; rehabilitation nurses; physical, occupational, speech, respiratory, and recreation therapists; exercise physiologists; dietitians; social workers; and others as required to address particular needs (see Table 45–1). Effective teamwork requires mutual understanding and synchrony of the roles and responsibilities of each member. When the rehabilitation team works in synergy, it serves patients and families across the continuum of care.

CONCEPTUAL FRAMEWORK

A common view holds that rehabilitation has a place somewhere between curative and palliative care.[6] Rehabilitation seems not really to fit with curative processes, in which care issues resolve with specific treatments and patients' levels of function and independence ultimately return to normal. Nor does rehabilitation seem in keeping with the irrevocable progress toward death, because rehabilitation implies a return to a previous way of living through adaptation. However, rehabilitation is relevant at each point of the continuum, from wellness to death. In wellness, the concern is to prevent health problems and reduce factors that might lead to illness and disability. At the end of life, the concern is to promote autonomy and dignity by enhancing function and independence as much as possible.

To conceptualize how rehabilitation nursing fits with care at the end of life, it is helpful to consider a diagrammatic representation (Fig. 45–1). In this diagram, curative and palliative care are pictured as opposing triangles. Rehabilitation fills in across the field. At all points in the continuum, there is a place for rehabilitation. In fact, at the transition point between curative and palliative care, rehabilitation may find its greatest impact.

REHABILITATION PRINCIPLES APPLIED TO PALLIATIVE CARE

The rehabilitation of patients with palliative care needs should begin as early as possible. As soon as functional deficits

Table 45–1. Roles of Interdisciplinary Rehabilitation Team Members

Physiatrists	Direct the rehabilitation team in providing comprehensive, integrated, patient-centered care
Rehabilitation nurses	Address physical care needs, such as mobility, daily living skills, bowel and bladder care, skin care, medications, and pain management and coordinate the overall rehabilitation process.
Physical therapists	Address strength, endurance, mobility, activity level, equipment needs, range of motion, balance and stability, and education about ongoing exercise programs to facilitate independent function.
Occupational therapists	Address energy conservation needs, upper extremity strength and function, self-care and home management skills, need for assistive devices, perceptual evaluation and guidance, and education for adaptation needs.
Speech/language pathologists	Address expressive and receptive communication needs as well as eating and swallowing issues.
Social workers	Address home care and extended care needs, provide patient and family with counseling and resources.
Rehabilitation psychologists	Address complex emotional and psychological needs of patients and families, guide the team in psychosocial care, and provide comprehensive psychological testing.
Vocational counselors	Address concerns and options related to school or work.
Recreation therapists	Address adaptation of leisure skills, recreational activities, socialization, stress management, establishment of therapeutic environment, and enhancement of normalization.

are observed or anticipated, appropriate consultation with members of the rehabilitation team should be initiated. Certain diagnoses should trigger mobilization of the rehabilitation team. In particular, rehabilitation consultation should be considered for patients with diagnoses such as progressive neuromuscular diseases; malignancies affecting the brain, spinal cord, or skeletal system; organ failure; and many other conditions that result in functional impairments. The goals of rehabilitation are to prevent secondary disability, to enhance the functions of both affected and unaffected systems, and to help patients adapt to their physical and social environments by means of physical restoration and adaptive devices.[7] Rehabilitation nursing strategies focus on

- caring for whole persons in their social and physical environments
- preventing secondary disability
- enhancing function of both affected and unaffected systems
- facilitating use of adaptive strategies
- promoting quality of life.

To illustrate rehabilitation strategies as they may be applied in actual palliative nursing care situations, some case studies are offered for contrast and comparison. The stories serve to illuminate the role of rehabilitation nursing in palliative care and represent issues shared by many rehabilitation patients.

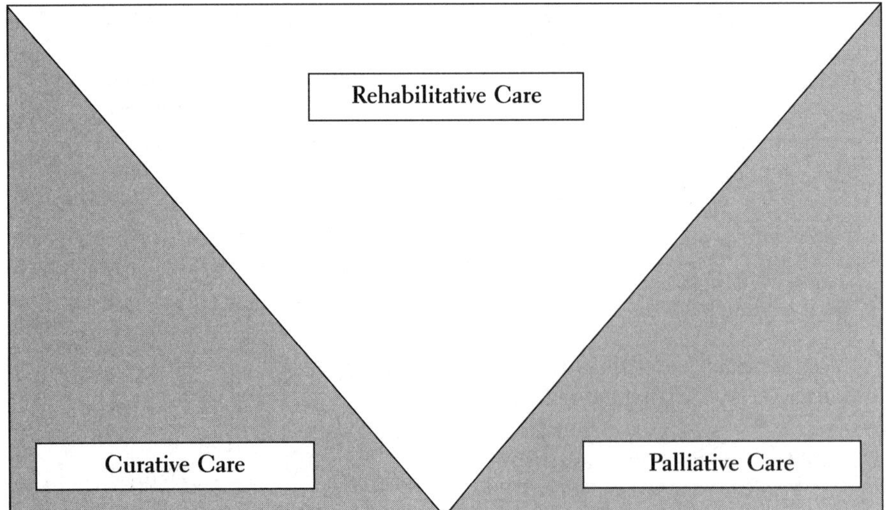

Fig. 45–1. A conceptual framework for curative, palliative, and rehabilitative care.

CARING FOR WHOLE PERSONS IN THEIR SOCIAL AND PHYSICAL ENVIRONMENTS

Knowing something about each person as a unique individual is extremely important to the rehabilitation process. While it may be evident to rehabilitation professionals that certain goals and interventions will suit a patient's needs, it is even more important to find congruence with the patient's own goals and values.

Case Study: Edna, A Patient with Chronic Obstructive Pulmonary Disease

With a history of rapidly worsening chronic obstructive pulmonary disease, 60-year-old Edna Van Wert (pseudonym) was faced with few options. As every breath became a struggle, she wondered how she could go on with her life and whether it was worth continuing the fight. She had lost so much of what was important to her: mobility, independence, and social relationships. Now she found herself homebound, exhausted, and unable to carry on even a telephone conversation with the friends and family she so cherished.

After much consultation and deliberation, she agreed that lung transplantation was the only course of treatment that would afford her the function and independence she believed made her life worthwhile. She received the transplanted lungs after a relatively short wait, but her expectations of returning to wellness were not to be fulfilled. Edna began an extraordinarily complicated postoperative course, a journey that would lead her to a life's end on which she had not planned.

Initially, Edna required prolonged ventilatory support. She struggled with infection and rejection of her new lungs. She experienced shock, sepsis, distress; her records thickened with stories of heroics and near misses, of technology, of miracles, of persistent argument with fate. She had established with her family that she would want everything possible done to preserve her life, and thus the critical balancing act went on for months. Just as her condition seemed to be stabilizing, she had a massive stroke involving the left brain, resulting in dense right-side hemiplegia and loss of speech/language function.

She was admitted to the inpatient rehabilitation medicine service to focus on mobility, self-care, and speech functions in order to help her to return home to her family. She progressed very slowly, with numerous complications arising related to her pulmonary status, immunosuppression, and cardiovascular deterioration.

A second stroke left her with even more limited language and cognitive functions. She required maximum assistance for all activities of daily living, and she ceased to make progress toward her rehabilitation goals. Her pulmonary function declined. Her family recognized that they would not be able to meet her care needs at home. Further evaluation of her lungs revealed that she had developed a lymphoma, for which (in her case) no treatment could be offered. Her prognosis plummeted, with the likelihood of death in a matter of weeks.

The focus of her rehabilitation care shifted. No longer would it be reasonable to expect her to reach the level of independence she would need to achieve to return home. A rigorous exercise program would not change the trajectory of her disease, and in fact might sap her energies and contribute to more frustration and discomfort.

The occurrence of the fatal malignancy made it clear that the quality of her remaining time would be the priority. She spent the last of her days in the hospital and died six months after receiving the lung transplantation.

By talking with family and friends, the rehabilitation team learned that Ms. Van Wert was strong-willed, stubborn, difficult, but deeply loved. She was seen as the matriarch of the family. For most of her adult life, she had balanced her responsibilities as a single parent with her work as a postal clerk. She was characterized as determined and cantankerous, impatient, critical, and quick to frustrate. Her family was close and extremely important to her. She had a wide circle of friends. Her four sons took turns visiting her in the hospital and sincerely wanted to bring her back home again.

With these facts in mind, the rehabilitation team designed communications and interventions that took into account the personal traits and values that were particular to Edna Van Wert. They knew that she would have difficulty tolerating frustration. They knew that she would need to feel in control as much as possible. They also knew that involvement of her family and friends would be essential. They anticipated the effects of prolonged stress on the family and recognized the profound loss they would sustain as her life concluded.

Rehabilitation nursing actions focused first on communication. Because of her dense aphasia, she was unable to verbalize her thoughts or feelings. Instead, she perseverated on one word, growing increasingly agitated when people were unable to understand her. A speech therapist set up nonverbal methods of communication, such as picture boards. As the nursing staff worked with Edna Van Wert, they tuned into behavioral cues and expressions. Family members also helped in the interpretation of her attempts to communicate. Strategies for communication included

- direct eye contact
- relaxed, unhurried approach
- slow, distinct phrases in normal tone of voice
- one thought presented at a time
- time allowed to process information
- gestures to convey and clarify meaning.

Efforts were directed toward maintaining her comfort and dignity. Whenever possible, she was supported in making her own choices. Occupational and physical therapies concentrated on interventions that would promote her autonomy. Functional activities, such as dressing, grooming, and eating, allowed her opportunities to exercise her independence. Access to her physical environment was accomplished through the use of adaptive devices and wheelchair mobility skills. As her condition deteriorated, it was more difficult to ascertain her desires. Inclusion of family members became more important, both for carrying out her wishes as they knew them and for giving the family the active role in her care that they wanted.

Throughout the course of Edna Van Wert's final illness, spiritual and psychosocial support were priorities. With her ability to communicate so severely impaired, her needs for support might have been misunderstood or overlooked. She was suddenly unable to serve as the source of stability and strength for her family, and roles and expectations were greatly changed. The rehabilitation nurses, the psychologist, the social worker, and the chaplain worked together to counsel and care for both patient and family.

When death came to Edna Van Wert, the family described a mixture of feelings of relief, sorrow, and satisfaction. Through their sadness, they recognized the efforts of the rehabilitation team to preserve Edna Van Wert's uniqueness and integrity as a human being. Thus they would remember her.

PREVENTING SECONDARY DISABILITY

Whatever the disease process, persons in declining states of health are at risk for developing unnecessary complications. Even at the end of life, complications can be prevented, thereby enhancing comfort, function, independence, and dignity. Treatment of one body system must not compromise another.[7] For example, patients who are bed-bound are at risk for developing muscular, vascular, integumentary, and neurological compromise, which could result in secondary disability.

Case Study: Joseph, a Patient with Amytrophic Lateral Sclerosis

Joseph Brown knew his days were numbered, irrevocably ticking away with the advance of amyotrophic lateral sclerosis. Bit by bit, his body functions eroded. Weakness began in his lower extremities, then spread to his trunk and upper extremities. He was troubled with spasticity, which soon made ambulation nearly impossible. He depended on his wife to help him with all of his daily living activities but continued to get out each day in his electric wheelchair to work with the city government on disability policies. When he went on a ventilator to support his breathing, he likened his health to driving an old truck down a mountain road: no way to stop, no way to turn around, nothing to do but drive on home.

As Mr. Brown's disease progressed, he was at risk for the development of secondary disabilities. Concerns included the potential development of edema, contractures, and skin breakdown. Mr. Brown lacked the normal muscular activity that would promote vascular return, and he developed significant edema in his extremities. Knowing that "edema is glue" when it comes to function, rehabilitation nursing actions included range of motion exercises and management of dependent edema with compression and elevation.[7]

Spasticity complicated the positioning of Mr. Brown's limbs. It was important to avoid shortened positions that favored the flexors, because that allowed contractures to occur. Contractures further limited his mobility and function, so he and his wife were taught a stretching program as well as the use of positioning devices and splints to maintain joints in neutral alignment.

Because of his impaired mobility, Mr. Brown was at risk for developing skin breakdown. He enjoyed spending a lot of time in his wheelchair. Although his sensation was basically intact, he was not able to react to the message of skin pressure and change his position. Mr. Brown learned how to shift his weight in the wheelchair, either by side-to-side shifts or tilt-backs. A small timer helped remind him of pressure releases every 15 minutes when he was in his chair. In addition, a special wheelchair cushion protected bony prominences with gel pads.

ENHANCING FUNCTION OF BOTH AFFECTED AND UNAFFECTED SYSTEMS

A chief concern in rehabilitative care is enhancing the function of both affected and unaffected body systems, thereby helping patients to be as healthy and independent as possible. In palliative care, many care issues involve the interconnections of body systems and the need to enlist one function to serve for another.

Case Study: Paul, a Patient with Metastatic Prostate Cancer

Paul O'Neill had been a successful attorney for thirty years. A burly, loud-spoken Irishman, he prided himself on bringing life and laughter everywhere he went. Although diagnosed and treated for prostate cancer, he never slowed the hectic pace of his law practice or his busy social calendar. In fact, he had little time to pay attention to the ominous symptoms that were developing that indicated the advance of his disease.

When he sought medical attention at last, the cancer had metastasized to his spine, resulting in partial paralysis and bowel and bladder impairment. Orthopedic spine surgeons attempted to relieve pressure on his spinal cord in the hope of restoring motor and sensory function. However, when they performed the surgery, they found the cancer had spread extensively, and they were unable to improve significantly his spinal cord function. Radiation followed, but it had little effect on the spreading cancer.

Paul O'Neill was stunned. He could not believe the turn his life had taken. Suddenly, nothing seemed to work. He had to depend on others for the first time in his life. He felt like some kind of freak, unable to move his legs or even manage normal bodily functions. His bulky frame became a heavy burden as he tried to relearn life from a wheelchair. He wrestled with the unfairness of the situation, finally promising himself that he would "go out in style." He wanted to go home as soon as possible so as not to waste his precious remaining time.

Paul O'Neill spent twelve days on the inpatient rehabilitation unit, then transitioned to home with continued therapies and nursing care. Two months later, at home with his family present, Paul O'Neill died.

In Mr. O'Neill's case, several body systems were at risk for complications, although not all were directly affected by the disease process. Mobility was a critical concern. Bowel and bladder management also presented challenges. His neurologic deficits and rapidly progressing disease, combined with his size and the need to learn new skills from a wheelchair, placed him at risk for developing contractures, skin breakdown, and deep vein thrombosis. Problems with bowel and bladder function put him at risk for developing constipation, distention, and infection. He experienced severe demoralization. In keeping with his wishes, rehabilitation nursing staff designed a plan for Mr. O'Neill and his family to follow at home. Priority rehabilitation nursing issues included

- managing fatigue related to advancing disease
- pain control
- promoting mobility and independence
- managing neurogenic bowel and bladder
- alleviating social isolation related to the effects of terminal illness
- anticipatory grieving and spiritual care.

Managing Fatigue Related to Advancing Disease

The rehabilitation team planned care to protect Mr. O'Neill's periods of rest through the day. They knew that his therapy would be more effective and his ability to carry over new learning of functional activities would be better when he was in a rested state. His sleep–wake cycle was restored as quickly as possible. Occupational therapists taught him strategies for energy conservation in his activities of daily living, including the use of adaptive devices, planning, and pacing.

Pain Control

Mr. O'Neill initially described his pain as always with him, dull and relentless, and wearing him down. Rehabilitation nurses evaluated his responses to different medications and dosage schedules as well as to nonmedication pain control interventions, such as positioning and relaxation. The most effective method of pain control for Mr. O'Neill was scheduled doses of long-acting morphine, coupled with short-acting doses for break-through or procedural pain. This method of pain management is frequently used in rehabilitation settings because it does not allow pain to become established and because the patient does not have to experience a certain level of pain and then wait for relief. It also minimizes sedative effects. With his pain under better control, Mr. O'Neill was able to actively participate in his own care and make deliberate decisions about his goals.

Promoting Mobility and Independence

Bed Positioning. Positioning and supporting the body in such a way that function is preserved and complications prevented are important considerations in mobility. As Paul O'Neill's disease progressed and he experienced increasing weakness and fatigue, he spent more and more time in bed. The education of the patient and family focused on the techniques of bed mobility and specific precautions to prevent complications.

Supine lying was minimized because of Mr. O'Neill's high risk for sacral skin breakdown. Even with a pressure-reducing mattress, back-lying time needed to be restricted. Shearing is a force generated when the skin does not move as one with the structures beneath it. Stretching and breakage of capillaries and subcutaneous tissues contributes to the potential for deep skin breakdown. To reduce shearing forces, the bed was placed in reverse Trendelenburg position to raise the head, rather than cranking up just the head of the bed. Draw sheets were used to move Mr. O'Neill, again to prevent shearing.

Positioning lower extremities is important in preventing the development of such complications as foot drop, skin breakdown, contractures, and deep vein thrombosis. When supine, care should be taken to support the feet in neutral position. This can be accomplished by using a footboard or box at the end of the bed or by the application of splints. Derotational splints were placed on Mr. O'Neill's lower legs to keep his hips in alignment, to prevent foot-drop contractures, and to reduce the risk of heel breakdown. Range of motion exercises were performed at least twice daily.

When side-lying, pillows were employed to cushion bony prominences and maintain neutral joint position. His uppermost leg was brought forward and the lower leg straightened to minimize hip flexion contractures. Frequently overlooked as a positioning choice, prone lying offers advantages not only of skin pressure relief and reduction in hip flexion contractures but also in promoting greater oxygen exchange.[8] Mr. O'Neill's bed position was alternated between back, both sides, and prone at least every two hours.

Sitting. There are many physiologic benefits of upright posture. Blood pressure, digestive and bowel functions, oxygenation, and perception are geared toward being upright. Weight bearing helps to avert skeletal muscle atrophy. Sitting, standing, and walking provide for changes in scenery and enhance the ability to socialize. This was an important consideration for Mr. O'Neill, who experienced emotional distress at the social isolation his illness imposed.

It is important to choose seating that supports the patient, avoiding surfaces that place pressure on bony prominences. A seat that is angled back slightly helps keep the patient from sliding forward. Placing the feet on footrests or a small box or stool may add comfort, as may supporting the arms on pillows or on a table in front of the patient. Sitting time should be limited, based on patient comfort, endurance, and skin tolerance. Mr. O'Neill followed a sitting schedule that increased by 15 minutes a day until he was able to tolerate about two hours of being up. That was enough time to carry out many of his personal activities, yet not so much as to overly tire him.

Planning for Mr. O'Neill's return home involved careful assessment of his equipment needs. Physical and occupational therapists conducted a home evaluation to determine how he would manage mobility and self-care activities and what equipment would be appropriate there. Family members practiced using equipment and devices under the guidance of the rehabilitation team. The objective was to simplify the care as much as possible while still supporting Mr. O'Neill's active participation in his daily activities.

Examples of home care equipment often used include commodes, wheelchairs, sliding boards, Hoyer lifts, and adaptive devices, such as reachers, dressing sticks, long-handled sponges, tub/shower benches, hospital beds, and pressure-relieving mattresses. Examples of home modifications might include affixing handrails and grab bars, widening doors, using raised toilet seats, and installing stair lifts and ramps.

Management of Neurogenic Bowel and Bladder

For Mr. O'Neill, the loss of bowel and bladder function was especially distressing. It placed him in a position of dependence and impinged on his privacy. It reinforced his feelings of isolation and being different. The focus of rehabilitation nursing interventions was to mimic the normal physiologic rhythms of bowel and bladder elimination. By helping Mr. O'Neill gain control of his body functions, nursing staff hoped to promote his confidence, dignity, and feelings of self-worth.

Bowel regulation and continence were achieved by implementing a classic bowel program routine. Mr. O'Neill was especially prone to constipation due to immobility and the effects of pain medications. The first intervention was to modify his diet to include more fiber and fluids. He also took stool softener medication twice daily. His bowel program occurred after breakfast each morning, to take advantage of the gastro-colic reflex. He was assisted to sit upright on a commode chair. A rectal suppository was inserted, with digital stimulation at 15-minute intervals to accomplish bowel evacuation. The patient and his wife were taught how to manage this program at home. Although reluctant at first, Mr. O'Neill became resigned to the necessity of this bowel program and worked it into his morning routine. His wife, eager to help in any way she could, also learned the techniques. Once a regular pattern of elimination was established, Mr. O'Neill no longer experienced incontinence.

For bladder management, nursing staff implemented a program of void trials and intermittent catheterization. The patient learned to manage his own fluid intake and catheterize himself at four-hour intervals, thereby preventing overdistension or incontinence. However, as his disease progressed, he opted for an indwelling urinary catheter because it was easier for him to manage. There is a continuous need to evaluate and individualize rehabilitation goals and to alter goals as patients experience more advanced disease.

Alleviating Social Isolation Related to the Effects of Terminal Illness

With a history of active social involvement, Mr. O'Neill had great difficulty with the limitations his disease imposed on his energy level and his ability to remain functional. He did not want others to see him as incapacitated in any way. He did not want to be embarrassed by his failing body. The rehabilitation team concentrated on solving the physical problems that could be solved. A recreation therapist assessed his leisure and avocational interests and prescribed therapeutic activities that would help build his confidence in social situations. Together, the team helped him learn to navigate around architectural barriers and helped him practice new skills successfully from a wheelchair.

Anticipatory Grieving and Spiritual Care

Mr. O'Neill concentrated on making plans and settling financial matters in preparation for his death. He continued to set goals for himself and to maintain hope, but the nature of his goals shifted. Initially, he was concerned with not becoming a burden to his family and focused on his physical functioning. As his mobility and endurance flagged and he had to rely more on others for assistance with basic care needs, he began to change his goals. Some of his stoicism fell away. He revealed his feelings more readily and described the evolution of his emotions. Now the focus became his relationships: an upcoming wedding anniversary, a son's graduation from law school. Rehabilitation nurses, home care nurses, a psychologist, and a social worker supported the patient and his family as they began to grieve over the past that would never return and the future that was not to be. Pastoral care was a significant part of the process, as Mr. O'Neill struggled with spiritual questions and sought a peaceful understanding of what was happening to him. The rehabilitation team endeavored to help the patient live all the days of his life by helping body and soul continue to function.

FACILITATING USE OF ADAPTIVE STRATEGIES

The ability of patients to continue to participate actively in living their lives has much to do with successful adaptation to changes in function. Even at the end of life, patients' capacity to adapt remains. Everyday activities may become very difficult to perform with advancing disease. But rehabilitation nursing actions that promote communication, the use of appropriate tools and equipment, family participation, and modifications to the environment all enhance the process of adaptation.

Communication

Opening the doors to communication is the most important rehabilitation nursing intervention. By removing functional barriers to speech, by teaching and supporting compensatory strategies, and by allowing safe opportunities for patients and families to discuss difficult issues around death and dying, rehabilitation nurses perform a critical function in the adaptation process.

Tools and Equipment

Many adaptive devices are available to patients and families that enhance functional ability and independence. Rehabilitation offers the chance to analyze tasks with new eyes and solve problems with creativity and individuality. Examples of useful tools to assist patients in being as independent as possible include reachers and dressing aids such as sock-starters, elastic shoe laces, and dressing sticks. For some patients, adapted eating utensils increase independence and thereby support nutritional intake. Modifications to clothing may permit more efficient toileting and hygiene, conserving both energy and dignity

Family Participation

As illustrated in the previous case studies, the involvement of family and friends brings multifaceted benefits. Because of the social nature of humankind, the presence and involvement of family and friends has great importance at the end of life. Family members may seek involvement in the caring activities as an expression of feelings of closeness and love. They may try to find understanding, resolution, or closure of past issues. For the person at the end of life, the presence of family, friends, and even pets may be a powerful affirmation of the continuity of life.

Modifications to Environment

Rehabilitation professionals are keenly aware of the effect the environment of care has on function, independence, and well-being. The physical arrangement of furnishings can be instrumental not only in promoting patient access to the environment but also in the ease with which others care for him or her. The environment can be made into a powerful tool for orientation, for spatial perception, and for preserving a territorial sense of self.

Light has a strong effect not only on visual perception but also on mood and feelings of well-being. Light may be a helpful tool in maintaining day–night rhythms and in orienting patients to time and place.[9] Sound is also an important environmental variable. For example, music has been implicated as a therapeutic intervention in both rehabilitation and palliative care.[10]

PROMOTING QUALITY AT THE END OF LIFE

The concept of quality of life is linked to function and independence. Patients often describe their satisfaction with life in terms of what they are able to do. Rehabilitation focuses on the essential components of mobility, self-care, cognition, and social interaction that define what people can do.

Case Study: Louise, a Patient with a Malignant Brain Tumor

Forty-two-year-old Louise Nichols had just started her own consulting business when she began to experience headaches and visual disturbances. At first she attributed her symptoms to the long hours and stress related to building her business, but when she experienced weakness of her left side, she knew that something more serious was happening.

She had a glioblastoma multiforme growing deep in her brain. Surgery was performed to debulk the tumor, but in a matter of weeks it was clear that the mass was growing rapidly. A course of radiation was completed to no avail. Her function continued to decline, and it seemed that every body system was affected by the advancing malignancy. Now her left side was densely paralyzed, she had difficulty swallowing and speaking, and her thinking processes became muddled.

Her family was in turmoil. On one hand, they resented the disruption her sudden illness imposed on their previously ordered lives. On the other hand, they wanted to care for her and make sure that her remaining time was the best that it could be. As they watched her decline day by day, ambiguities in their relationships surfaced, and conflicts about what would define quality of life emerged.

Rehabilitation's part in promoting quality of life at the end of life is severalfold. Rehabilitation is a goal-directed process. Realistic, attainable goals based on the patient's own definition of quality of life drive the actions of the team. In the area of physical care, rehabilitation strategies support energy conservation, sequencing and pacing, maintaining normal routines, and accessing the environment. Beyond that, rehabilitation nurses facilitate effective communication and problem solving with patients and families. They offer acceptance and support through difficult decision making and help mobilize concrete resources.

When rehabilitation nurses approach care, it is with the goal of enhancing function and independence. In Louise Nichols' case, the brain tumor created deficits in mobility, cognition, and perception. Also, more subtle issues greatly influenced the quality of her remaining time. It was important to understand how the patient would define the quality of her own life and to direct actions toward protecting those elements.

Promoting Dignity, Self-Image, and Participation

Ms. Nichols' concept of quality of life was evident in how she participated in her care and the decisions that she made about her course of treatment. The rehabilitation team learned that Ms. Nichols' mother had died several years before of a similar brain tumor. Caring for her mother had solidified her beliefs about not wishing to burden others. Part of Ms. Nichols' definition of quality of life was that she would not be dependent on others.

Ms. Nichols prided herself on being industrious and self-sufficient. To her, the ability to take care of herself was a sign of success. Rehabilitation nurses and therapists focused on helping to manage symptoms of advancing disease so that she would be able to do as much for herself as possible. This included adaptive techniques for daily living skills, for pain management, for eating, for dressing, for grooming, and for bowel and bladder management. Even with her physical and cognitive decline, retaining her normal routines helped to allay some feelings of helplessness and to promote a positive self-image.

Control, Hope, and Reality

As her illness progressed, Ms. Nichols felt she was losing control. It became difficult for her to remember things, and expressing herself became more laborious and frustrating. She slept frequently and seemed disconnected from external events. Her family understood her usual desire for control and made many attempts to include her in conversations and support her in making choices.

At first, her concept of hope was tied to the idea of cure. Radiation therapy represented the chance of cure. When that was completed without appreciable change in her tumor, some of her feelings of hopefulness slipped away. She sank into a depression. Her family was alarmed: her psychologic well-being was a critical component in her own definition of quality of life. Treating her depression became a priority issue for the rehabilitation team. Through a combination of rehabilitation, psychological counseling, and antidepressant medications, her dark mood slowly lifted. Hope seemed to return in a different form, less connected to a cure and more a part of her interactions with her daughter and sister.

Family Support

Another significant area that related to quality of life for Ms. Nichols had to do with social well-being. She struggled with the idea of becoming a burden to her family and realized that she was losing control over what was happening to her. Her relationships with others were complex, and now they were challenged even further. At the same time, her family members wrestled with memories of the mother's death and feared the responsibilities for care that might be thrust upon them.

The rehabilitation team tried to help the patient and her family work through their thoughts, feelings, and fears and helped them to find ways to express them. The team arranged several family conferences to discuss not only the care issues but also the changes in family roles and structure. Whenever possible, the team found answers to the family's questions and made great efforts to keep communications open. Creating safe opportunities for family members to express their ambivalence and conflict helped move them toward acceptance. The family was able to prepare in concrete ways for the outcome they both welcomed and dreaded.

UNDERSTANDING OUTCOMES

In rehabilitation, there is a strong emphasis on the measurement of patient outcomes. Since the 1950s, many functional assessment instruments have been developed and used to help quantify the changes that occur in patients as a result of care and recovery. Some instruments to measure functional and physical outcomes are applicable, as well, to the assessment of patients in the last month of life.

More than a dozen functional outcome measurement tools are in common use in rehabilitation settings in the United States and Canada (see Table 45–2). Measurement of self-care and mobility are central to rehabilitation,[1] but the functions and behaviors required to lead a meaningful life are much broader. They may include cognitive, emotional, perceptual, social, and vocational function measurements as well.

Table 45–2. Measures of Functional Outcomes

Barthel Index[15] (Mahoney 1958)
Dartmouth COOP Functional Health Assessment Charts[16]
Edmonton Functional Assessment Tool[17]
Functional Activities Questionnaire[18,19]
Functional Independence Measure[13]
Functional Status Index[20,21]
Index of Independence in Activities of Daily Living (ADL)[22,23]
Kenny Self-Care Evaluation[24,25]
Lambeth Disability Screening Questionnaire[26]
Medical Outcomes Study Physical Functioning Measure[27]
Physical Self-Maintenance Scale[28]
PULSES Profile[29]
Rapid Disability Rating Scale[11]
Self-Evaluation of Life Function Scale[30]
Stanford Health Assessment Questionnaire[31]

For measuring function in the final 30 days of life, three scales may be particularly useful. The Rapid Disability Rating Scale (RDRS-2)[11] broadly includes items related to the activities of daily living, mental capacity, dietary changes, continence, medications, and confinement to bed. The Health Assessment Questionnaire (HAQ)[12] is a widely used instrument that summarizes the patients' areas of major difficulty. The Functional Independence Measure (FIM)[13,14] is an ordinal scale that quantifies 18 areas of physical and cognitive function in terms of burden of care. These scales are appropriate to palliative care because they focus on specific aspects of function that relate to patients' independence. The scales may be used to determine whether interventions at the end of life serve to foster independence and function for as long as possible.

There is also strong interest in the field of rehabilitation to measure patient perceptions of quality of life. When the measured domains are considered, the connection between rehabilitation and end-of life care becomes evident. Most of the measurements of quality of life have to do with physical, cognitive, social and spiritual function, the chief concerns of the rehabilitation practitioner (see Table 45–3).

Outcome measurements can reveal much about the quality of life experienced by persons near the end of life. For example, by assessing at intervals, it is possible to determine how much function patients retain as they approach death. By identifying and measuring differences in this experience, it is possible to determine the essential interventions and care activities that contribute to the highest levels of functional independence up to the end of life. Further research is needed to

- Establish norms and indications for the application of rehabilitation in palliative care
- Determine the cost-effectiveness of rehabilitation interventions
- Determine optimal time frames for providing rehabilitation services after the onset of disease
- Define variables having the greatest impact on patient outcomes.

CONCLUSION

Rehabilitation nursing approaches have value in palliative care. Regardless of the disease trajectory, nurses can do something more to preserve function and independence and positively affect perceptions of quality of life, even at its end. Rehabilitation nurses facilitate holistic care of persons in their social and physical environments. They direct actions toward preventing secondary disability and enhancing both affected and unaffected body systems. They foster the use of adaptive strategies and techniques to optimize autonomy. Rehabilitation nurses' deliberate focus on function, independence, dignity, and the preservation of hope makes a fitting, meaningful contribution to care at the end of life.

Table 45–3. Examples of Quality-of-Life Measure

Name of Instrument	Domains Measured
CARES-SF[32]	Rehabilitation and quality of life for patients with cancer
Chronic Respiratory Disease Questionnaire[33]	Measuring outcomes of clinical trials for patients with COPD
City of Hope Quality of Life, Cancer Patient Version[34]	Physical well-being, psychological well-being, and spiritual well-being
COOP Charts[35]	Screen patients in an outpatient setting
Daily Diary Card-QOL[36]	Changes in quality of life related to symptoms induced by chemotherapy
EORTC QOL-30[37]	Physical function, role function, cognitive function, emotional function, social function, symptoms, and financial impact
EuroQol Quality of Life Scale[38]	Mobility, self-care, role (or main) activity, family and leisure activities, pain and mood
FACT-G[39]	Patients undergoing cancer treatment
FAHI[40]	HIV-positive patients
Ferrans and Powers Quality of Life Index[41]	Satisfaction with and importance of multiple domains
FLIC[42]	Physical/occupational function, psychological state, sociability, and somatic discomfort
HIV Overview of Problems Evaluation Systems (HOPES)[32]	Rehabilitation and quality of life for patients with HIV
Hospice Quality of Life Index—Revised[43]	Physical, psychological, spiritual, social, and financial well-being
McGill Quality of Life Questionnaire[44]	Quality of life at the end of life
Medical Outcomes Study, Short Form Health Survey[45]	Physical functioning, role limitations, bodily pain, social functioning, mental health, vitality, and general health perceptions
National Hospice Study Quality of Life Scale [46]	Quality of life at end of life
Nottingham Health Profile[47]	Physical, social, and emotional health problems and their impact on functioning
Painter (unpublished)	Number of "good days" in the last week of life
Perceived Quality of Life Scale[26]	Health status and satisfaction with functioning
Quality of Life Index[48]	General physical condition, important human activities, and general quality of life
Quality of Life for Respiratory Illness Questionnaire[49]	Chronic nonspecific lung disease
Quality of Well-Being scale[50]	Mobility, physical activity, social activity, and 27 symptoms
SELF Scale[30]	Persons age 60 and older
Sickness Impact Profile[51]	How an illness affects a person's behavior
Southwest Oncology Group Quality of Life Questionnaire[52]	Function, symptoms, and global quality of life measures
Spitzer QL-Index[53]	Activity level, social support, and mental well-being
VITAS Quality of Life Index[54]	Symptoms, function, interpersonal domains, well-being, and transcendence

REFERENCES

1. Hoeman SP. Rehabilitation Nursing: Process and Application. 2nd ed. St. Louis: Mosby, 1996.
2. Stryker RP. Rehabilitative Aspects of Acute and Chronic Nursing Care, 2d ed. Philadelphia: Saunders, 1977.
3. Fletcher D. CARF . . . the Rehabilitation Accreditation Commission. 1997;68:46.
4. Maloof M. The 1989 CARF nursing standards: Guidelines for implementation. Commission of Accreditation of Rehabilitation Facilities. Rehabil Nurs 1989;14:134.
5. Joint Committee on Rehabilitation Nursing Practice, American Nurses' Association, Association of Rehabilitation Nurses. Rehabilitation Nursing: Scope of Practice: Process and Outcome Criteria for Selected Diagnoses. Kansas City, Mo: American Nurses' Association, 1988.
6. Fox E. Predominance of the curative model of medical care. A residual problem. JAMA 1997;278:761.
7. Hansen ST, Swiontkowski MF. Orthopaedic Trauma Protocols. New York: Raven Press, 1993.
8. Ciesla ND. Chest physical therapy for patients in the intensive care unit. Phys Ther 1996; 76:609.
9. Stewart KT, Hayes BC, Eastman CI. Light treatment for NASA shiftworkers. Chronobiol Int 1995;12:141.
10. Rykov M, Salmon D. Bibliography for music therapy in palliative care, 1963–1997. Am J Hosp Palliat Care 1998;15:174.
11. Linn MW, Linn BS. The rapid disability rating scale-2. J Am Geriatr Soc 1982;30:378.
12. Steen VD, Medsger TA, Jr. The value of the Health Assessment Questionnaire and special patient-generated scales to demonstrate change in systemic sclerosis patients over time. Arthritis Rheum 1997;40:1984.
13. Granger CV, Brownscheidle CM. Outcome measurement in medical rehabilitation. Int J Technol Assess Health Care 1995;11:262.
14. Stineman MG, Shea JA, Jette A, Tassoni CJ, Ottenbacher KJ, Fiedler R, Granger CV. The Functional Independence Measure: Tests of scaling assumptions, structure, and reliability across 20 diverse impairment categories. Arch Phys Med Rehabil 1996;77:1101.
15. Jacelon CS. The Barthel Index and other indices of functional ability. Rehabil Nurs 1986; 11:9.
16. Nelson EC, Kirk JW, Bise BW, Chapman RJ, Hale FA, Stamps PL, Wasson JH. The Cooperative Information Project: Part 1: A sentinal practice network for service and research in primary care. J Fam Pract 1981;13:641.
17. Kaasa T, Loomis J, Gillis K, Bruera E,

Hanson J. The Edmonton Functional Assessment Tool: Preliminary development and evaluation for use in palliative care. J Pain Symptom Manage 1997;13:10.

18. Pfeffer RI, Kurosaki TT, Harrah CH, Jr., Chance JM, Filos S. Measurement of functional activities in older adults in the community. J Gerontol 1982;37:323.

19. Pfeffer RI, Kurosaki TT, Chance JM, Filos S, Bates D. Use of the mental function index in older adults. Reliability, validity, and measurement of change over time. Am J Epidemiol 1984; 120:922.

20. Jette AM, Deniston OL. Inter-observer reliability of a functional status assessment instrument. J Chronic Dis 1978;31:573.

21. Jette AM. Functional capacity evaluation: An empirical approach. Arch Phys Med Rehabil 1980;61:85.

22. Katz S, Akpom CA. A measure of primary sociobiological functions. Int J Health Serv 1976; 6:493.

23. Brorsson B, Asberg KH. Katz index of independence in ADL. Reliability and validity in short-term care. Scand J Rehabil Med 1984;16: 125.

24. Schoening HA, Anderegg L, Bergstrom D, Fonda M, Steinke N, Ulrich P. Numerical scoring of self-care status of patients. Arch Phys Med Rehabil 1965;46:689.

25. Schoening HA, Iversen IA. Numerical scoring of self-care status: A study of the Kenny self-care evaluation. Arch Phys Med Rehabil 1968; 49:221.

26. Patrick DL, Darby SC, Green S, Horton G, Locker D, Wiggins RD. Screening for disability in the inner city. J Epidemiol Community Health 1981;35:65.

27. Stewart AL, Hays RD, Ware JE, Jr. The MOS short-form general health survey. Reliability and validity in a patient population. Med Care 1988;26:724.

28. Lawton MP, Brody EM. Assessment of older people: Self-maintaining and instrumental activities of daily living. Gerontologist 1969;9:179.

29. Moskowitz E. PULSES profile in retrospect. Arch Phys Med Rehabil 1985;66:647.

30. Linn MW, Linn BS. Self-evaluation of life function (self) scale: A short, comprehensive self-report of health for elderly adults. J Gerontol 1984;39:603.

31. Fries JF, Spitz PW, Young DY. The dimensions of health outcomes: The health assessment questionnaire, disability and pain scales. J Rheumatol 1982;9:789.

32. Schag CA, Ganz PA, Heinrich RL. Cancer Rehabilitation Evaluation System—short form (CARES-SF). A cancer specific rehabilitation and quality of life instrument. Cancer 1991;68:1406.

33. Guyatt GH, Berman LB, Townsend M, Pugsley SO, Chambers LW. A measure of quality of life for clinical trials in chronic lung disease. Thorax 1987;42:773.

34. Ferrell BR, Dow KH, Grant M. Measurement of the quality of life in cancer survivors. Qual Life Res 1995;4:523.

35. Larson CO, Hays RD, Nelson EC. Do the pictures influence scores on the Dartmouth COOP Charts? Qual Life Res 1992;1:247.

36. Gower NH, Rudd RM, Ruiz de Elvira MC, Spiro SG, James LE, Harper PG, Souhami RL. Assessment of 'quality of life' using a daily diary card in a randomised trial of chemotherapy in small-cell lung cancer. Ann Oncol 1995;6: 575.

37. Aaronson NK, Ahmedzai S, Bergman B, Bullinger M, Cull A, Duez NJ, Filiberti A, Flechtner H, Fleishman SB, de Haes JC, et al. The European Organization for Research and Treatment of Cancer QLQ-C30: A quality-of-life instrument for use in international clinical trials in oncology. J Natl Cancer Inst 1993;85:365.

38. Myers C, Wilks D. Comparison of Euroqol EQ-5D and SF-36 in patients with chronic fatigue syndrome. Qual Life Res 1999;8:9.

39. Cella DF, Tulsky DS, Gray G, Sarafian B, Linn E, Bonomi A, Silberman M, Yellen SB, Winicour P, Brannon J, et al. The Functional Assessment of Cancer Therapy scale: Development and validation of the general measure. J Clin Oncol 1993;11:570.

40. Cella DF. Quality of life outcomes: Measurement and validation. Oncology (Huntingt) 1996;10:233.

41. Ferrans CE, Powers MJ. Quality of life index: Development and psychometric properties. ANS Adv Nurs Sci 1985;8:15.

42. Finkelstein DM, Cassileth BR, Bonomi PD, Ruckdeschel JC, Ezdinli EZ, Wolter JM. A pilot study of the Functional Living Index–Cancer (FLIC) Scale for the assessment of quality of life for metastatic lung cancer patients. An Eastern Cooperative Oncology Group study. Am J Clin Oncol 1988;11:630.

43. McMillan SC, Mahon M. Measuring quality of life in hospice patients using a newly developed Hospice Quality of Life Index. Qual Life Res 1994;3:437.

44. Cohen SR, Mount BM, Strobel MG, Bui F. The McGill Quality of Life Questionnaire: A measure of quality of life appropriate for people with advanced disease. A preliminary study of validity and acceptability. Palliat Med 1995;9:207.

45. Ware JE, Jr, Sherbourne CD. The MOS 36-item short-form health survey (SF-36). I. Conceptual framework and item selection. Med Care 1992;30:473.

46. Greer DS, Mor V. An overview of National Hospice Study findings. J Chronic Dis 1986; 39:5.

47. Hunt SM, McKenna SP, McEwen J, Williams J, Papp E. The Nottingham Health Profile: Subjective health status and medical consultations. Soc Sci Med [A] 1981;15:221.

48. Padilla GV, Presant C, Grant MM, Metter G, Lipsett J, Heide F. Quality of life index for patients with cancer. Res Nurs Health 1983;6: 117.

49. Maille AR, Koning CJ, Zwinderman AH, Willems LN, Dijkman JH, Kaptein AA. The development of the 'Quality-of-life for Respiratory Illness Questionnaire (QOL-RIQ)': A disease-specific quality-of-life questionnaire for patients with mild to moderate chronic non-specific lung disease. Respir Med 1997;91:297.

50. Kaplan RM, Ganiats TG, Sieber WJ, Anderson JP. The Quality of Well-Being Scale: Critical similarities and differences with SF-36. Int J Qual Health Care 1998;10:509.

51. Bergner M, Bobbitt RA, Pollard WE, Martin DP, Gilson BS. The sickness impact profile: Validation of a health status measure. Med Care 1976;14:57.

52. Moinpour CM, Hayden KA, Thompson IM, Feigl P, Metch B. Quality of life assessment in Southwest Oncology Group trials. Oncology (Huntingt) 1990;4:79.

53. Spitzer WO, Dobson AJ, Hall J, Chesterman E, Levi J, Shepherd R, Battista RN, Catchlove BR. Measuring the quality of life of cancer patients: A concise QL-index for use by physicians. J Chronic Dis 1981;34:585.

54. Byock IR, Merriman MP. Measuring quality of life for patients with terminal illness: The Missoula-VITAS quality of life index. Palliat Med 1998;12:231.

SUGGESTED READINGS

Association of Rehabilitation Nurses. *Rehabilitation Nursing.* (published bimonthly) Glenview, IL.

Association of Rehabilitation Nurses (1998) *Position statements* [online]. Available: http://www.rehabnurse.org/resources/frame/poststlt.htm. (July 19, 1999).

Davis MC. The rehabilitation nurse's role in spiritual care. *Rehabilitation Nursing* 1994;19: 298–301.

Dodds TA, Martin DP, Stolov WC, et al. A validation of the Functional Independence Measurement and its performance among rehabilitation inpatients. *Arch Phys Med Rehabil* 1993; 74:531–S36.

Edelman CL, Mandle CL. *Health promotion throughout the lifespan* (3rd ed.) St. Louis: Mosby Year Book, 1994.

Field MJ, Cassel CK, eds. *Approaching death: Improving care at the end of life.* Washington, DC: National Academy Press 1997.

Frank C, Hobbs N, Stewart G. Rehabilitation on palliative care units. *Journal of Palliative Care* 1998;14(2):50–53.

Glick OJ. Interventions related to activity and movement. *Nursing Clinics of North America* 1992;27:541–568.

Granger CV, Gresham GE, eds. *Functional assessment in rehabilitation medicine.* Baltimore, Maryland: Williams and Wilkins 1984:99–121.

Haase JE, Britt T, Coward DD, Leidy NK, Penn PE. Simultaneous concept analysis of spiritual perspective, hope, acceptance and self-transcendence. *Image* 1992;24:141–147.

Herzog JA. Deep vein thrombosis in the rehabilitative client: Diagnostic tools, prevention, and treatment modalities. *Rehabilitation Nursing* 1993;18:8–11.

Hoeman SP. Pediatric rehabilitation nursing. In: Molnar G, ed., *Pediatric rehabilitation* (2nd ed.) Baltimore: Williams and Wilkins, 1992.

Kottke SJ, Stillwell GK, Lehman JS. *Krusen's handbook of physical medicine and rehabilitation* (4th ed.). Philadelphia: W. B. Saunders, 1990.

Krieger, Di Meo E. Rx for spiritual distress, *Rehabilitation Nursing* 1991;54:22–24.

O'Brien T, Welsh J, Dunn F. ABC of palliative care: Non-malignant conditions. *BMJ* 1998; 316:7127,286–289.

O'Neill B, Fallon M. ABC of palliative care: principles of palliative care and pain control. *BMJ* 1997;315:7111, 801–804.

O'Neill B, Rodway A. ABC of palliative care: Care in the community. *BMJ* 1998;316:7128, 373–377.

O'Young B, Young MA, Stiens SA. *PM&R Secrets*. Philadephia: Hanley & Belfus, Inc, 1997.

Rehabilitation Nursing Foundation. *Rehabilitation nursing. Concepts and practice—A core curriculum* (3rd ed.). Glenview, IL: Author, 1993.

Rehabilitation Nursing Foundation. *Application of rehabilitation concepts to nursing practice.* Glenview, IL: Author (independent study program), 1995.

Rehabilitation Nursing Foundation. *Advanced practice nursing in rehabilitation: A core curriculum.* Glenview, IL: Author, 1997.

Roberts KT, Messenger TC. Helping older adults find serenity. Are there potential nursing interventions that may help older adults reach a serene state? *Geriatric Nursing* 1993;14:317–322.

Rubin M. The physiology of bedrest. *American Journal of Nursing* 1988;88:50.

Watson PG. The optimal functioning plan: A key element in cancer rehabilitation. *Cancer Nursing* 1992;15:254–263.

Wood C, Whittet S, Bradbeer C. ABC of palliative care: HIV infection and AIDS. *BMJ* 1997; 315:1433–1436.

RESOURCES

American Academy of Physical Medicine and Rehabilitation (AAPM&R)
One IBM Plaza, Suite 2500
Chicago, IL 60611
http://www.aapmr.org

American Congress of Rehabilitation Medicine (ACRM)
4700 W. Lake Avenue
Glenview, IL 60025
http://www.acrm.org

Americans with Disabilities Act (ADA)
United States Department of Justice
http://www.usdoj.gov/crt/ada/adahome1.htm

Association of Rehabilitation Nurses (ARN)
4700 W. Lake Avenue
Glenview, IL 60025–1485
http://www.rehabnurse.org

Commission for the Accreditation of Rehabilitation Facilities (CARF)
4891 E. Grant Road
Tucson, AZ 85712
http://www.carf.org

National Rehabilitation Association
633 S. Washington St.
Alexandria, VA 22314
http://www.nationalrehab.org

Rehabilitation Foundation, Inc.
http://www.rfi.org

Part VII

Special Issues for the Nurse in End-of-Life Care

46 The Nurse's Role: The World of Palliative Care Nursing

MARY L. S. VACHON

It's such a fine line between trying to be emphatic and care about them and also not take it home to your own life. It seems like you have to do something to kind of separate yourself from it.

—Home care nurse

Palliative care has traditionally been thought to begin at the time when active treatment aimed at curing the disease or prolonging life has ceased to be effective. More recent definitions see palliative care as extending across the illness continuum.[1,2]

Leaders in end-of-life care recently developed a set of precepts for palliative care under the auspices of the Robert Wood Johnson Foundation's Last Acts Campaign:

> Palliative care refers to the comprehensive management of the physical, psychological, social, spiritual and existential needs of patients, in particular those with incurable, progressive illnesses. Palliative care affirms life and regards dying as a natural process that is a profoundly personal experience for the individual and family. The goal of palliative care is to achieve the best possible quality of life through relief of suffering, control of symptoms and restoration of functional capacity while remaining sensitive to personal, cultural and religious values, beliefs and practices.[3]

This chapter will discuss the world of the palliative care nurse from the above perspective, and the nurses who work with patients with a variety of illnesses, including cancer, AIDS, motor neurone disease, end stage cardiac or respiratory disease, and other life-threatening illnesses. This care occurs in many settings, including acute care hospitals, the community, chronic care hospitals, nursing homes, hospices, clinics, and other settings.

The term *palliative care* will refer to the attempt to provide care that recognizes the need for the comprehensive management of the physical, psychological, social, spiritual, and existential needs of patients and families facing incurable, progressive illnesses. The use of the term will not be limited to integrated palliative care teams or units. It is recognized that the ideals of palliative care or of hospice care are not always met in the reality of today's health care environment.

The term *hospice* has sometimes been used interchangeably with the term *palliative care*, but more recently the terms have come to have different meanings (Table 46–1). In the United Kingdom, a hospice is a building where dying persons are cared for, but many of these people are discharged home and followed by home care teams.[2] In Canada, hospices are often community-based, volunteer-driven programs providing care in the home. Such programs may or may not have physicians affiliated with them.

In the United States, the term *hospice* refers to a specific programmatic model for delivering palliative care. Hospice care, therefore constitutes a subset of palliative care. Hospice care is a discrete program that assumes case-management responsibilities for all care related to a person's advanced, life-limiting illness, including support for the family through the dying experience and during their bereavement.[4] Hospice has and will continue to represent the epitome of palliative care.[4] However, hospices currently serve only 23% of Americans in their dying days (50% of those dying from cancer) and serves them for decreasing lengths of time.[5] The median length of stay in a hospice has recently decreased from 29 days to 25 days.[6] Five percent of people referred to a hospice in the United States die within the first two days of admission to the program, and 15% survive longer than 6 months.[7] It is estimated that in Canada 10% of those who need palliative care receive it.[9] The population served by hospices is still primarily white adults with cancer.[4]

The Medicare Hospice Benefit in the United States limits care to those with a prognosis of six months or less if the disease runs its normal course and the patient must be willing to forgo further treatment.[9] This six-month time frame is arbitrary and is a reflection of neither patient preference nor medical necessity. Studies suggest that health care professionals believe the optimal referral time is three months prior to death, but one month is more common.[10] Referral to hospice is also limited by the difficulty physicians have in predicting death. In a recent study of terminally ill cancer patients, physicians were found to correctly predict life expectancy to within one month in 25% of terminal patients. Twenty-three percent of patients lived longer than predicted and physicians overestimated survival in 52% of the cases. Of patients whom oncologists predicted would live between two and six months, one-third survived less than two months.[11] Other factors interfering with patients being referred to hospice programs include:

Table 46–1. Common Terms Encountered by the Palliative Care Nurse

Term	Definition
Chronic Bereavement	Being exposed to constant losses, or to several losses simultaneously. Chronic bereavement involves anticipatory grief, unresolved grief, and chronic grief.[105] Chronic bereavement includes multiple loss syndrome.
Chronic Grief	The accumulation of unresolved grief because of the lack of time to finish grieving for one loss before another occurs.
Compassion Fatigue	Identical to secondary traumatic stress disorder and the equivalent of post traumatic stress disorder.[100]
End-of-Life Care	Extending the concepts of hospice and palliative care to patients with chronic, life-threatening illness who may have one to two years to live. This might involve those with chronic cardiac or respiratory diseases, or those with advanced Alzheimer's disease.
Hardiness	A personality characteristic consisting of three characteristics-commitment, control and challenge.[56,57]
Hospice	The definition differs across countries. It may involve inpatient and/or community care. Hospice care assumes case management responsibilities for all care related to a person's advanced, life-limiting illness, including support for the family through the dying experience and during their bereavement.[4] Hospice constitutes a subset of palliative care.
Medicare Hospice Benefit	In the United States, limits care to those with a prognosis of six months or less if the disease runs its normal course and the patient must be willing to forgo further treatment.[10]
MediCaring Project	Extending the hospice concept to a larger population with a wider array of services over a longer time. The model will be tested in patients with congestive heart failure and chronic obstructive pulmonary disease with an estimated life expectancy of 1–2 years.[18]
Multiple Loss Syndrome	The effects of chronic, anticipatory, and unresolved grief, as well as the compounding effects of experiencing several episodes of grief concurrently.[105]
Palliative Care	The comprehensive management of the physical, psychological, social, spiritual and existential needs of patients, in particular those with incurable, progressive illnesses.[3]
Secondary Traumatic Stress (STS), or Compassion Stress	The natural consequent behaviors and emotions resulting from knowing about a traumatizing event experienced by a significant other-the stress resulting from helping or wanting to help a traumatized or suffering person.[100]
Secondary Traumatic Stress Disorder	A more severe manifestation of STS. A "syndrome of symptoms nearly identical to PTSD (post-traumatic stress disorder), except that exposure to knowledge about a traumatizing event experienced by a significant other is associated with the set of STSD symptoms, and PTSD symptoms are directly connected to the sufferer, the person experiencing the primary traumatic stress"[100]
Sense of Coherence	"A global orientation that expresses the extent to which one has a pervasive, enduring though dynamic feeling of confidence that one's internal and external environments are predictable and that there is a high probability that things will work out as well as can reasonably be expected"[60]

clients' wanting to remain under the care of physicians and nurses who have given care throughout the continuum of illness, patient resistance, concerns about home care capability or someone dying in the house, and the inability of physicians to communicate a prognosis until it is obvious the patient is near the end.[10,12,13]

The philosophy of end-of-life care once unique to hospice settings is slowly becoming part of mainstream medicine,[12,13,14,15] as was the intention of early hospice leaders. The models of integration vary considerably. In the United States, palliative care is sometimes seen as an alternative to hospice care. In some settings a palliative care service may be identical to that of a hospice, while in another setting, it may be composed of just one team member—a physician, or an advanced practice nurse, or it may be composed of a small team.[4] Much of what is called palliative care is simply not authentic palliative care, and the movement is in danger of becoming symptomatologists.[4,16,17]

The importance of the concepts of palliative care being integrated at an earlier point in the illness trajectory and in settings other than hospices and palliative care units is currently being explored in the MediCaring project,[18] extending the hospice concept to a larger population with a wider array of services over a longer time. The model will be tested in patients with congestive heart failure and chronic obstructive pulmonary disease with an estimated life expectancy of 1–2 years. The emphasis is on symptom management, maintenance of function, comfort, and family counseling. The model requires simultaneous efforts to secure a longer life and to make the patient and family ready for dying.[18]

The care of the dying is essentially a nursing and not a medical problem.[19] Good palliative care enables nurses to return to the root of our ability to care fully for people in a holistic manner. As patients shift from a sick to a dying role, it is the nurse that assumes the dominant role. As economics drives health care out of the hospital and toward community care, the supportive care required by patients and their carers will largely be the responsibility of the nurse.[20]

Nurses involved in palliative care are operating in a variety of settings—in well-integrated multidisciplinary teams, in solo practice and as advanced practice nurses, in hospices, oncology settings, AIDS clinics, chronic care settings, and in the community working to improve end-of-life care. The goal of good palliative care will be to preserve the core philosophy and principles of traditional end-of-life hospice care by incorporating it throughout the continuum of care. Such care is best provided by a multiprofessional team—a group of specialists who work together under appropriate leadership.

THE STRESSORS IN PALLIATIVE CARE

Palliative care work can be rewarding, but it can also be stressful. Using a broad perspective on palliative care, this section will review the literature on stressors associated with occupational role, the work environment, and interactions with patients and families. The review of the literature will focus primarily on studies conducted in the last fifteen years, with the emphasis on the decade of the 1990s. Elsewhere, the author has reviewed most of the literature from the 1970s to the mid-1990s.[21]

Occupational Role Stressors

Role overload has been identified as a major issue for oncology nurses in the 1990s.[22] In a study involving a random sample of hospice nurses throughout the United States, job pressure involving on-call duty, the need to travel to patients, and repeated crises were some of the least appealing aspects of hospice nursing.[23] The pressures of practice and work overload were associated with stress and burnout.[24]

Hospice initially prided itself on having the time to take to spend with patients and their families; however, as financial constraints have grown increasingly tight, hospice nurses are finding themselves more and more stretched to provide the type of care they want to provide. Further role overload could result if the potential for palliative care were ever to be realized. In one section of the United Kingdom it was predicted that an increase of around 65% of inpatient provision would be needed to accommodate all patients with chronic, progressive disease in that area.[25]

Oncology nurses experience difficulty with excessive demands, negative expectations from patients/families, unexpected crises, poor staffing, overwork, inadequate time, patient deaths, and balancing work and personal life.[26] In a Swedish study, hospital nurses' heavy workloads kept them from being able to attend continuing education courses to learn how to deal with the problems they were experiencing.[27] In another study, the more patients for whom the oncology nurse was responsible, the greater was her burnout score.[28] Heavy workload was the only job stressor associated with burnout, with emotional exhaustion being a particular stressor, in a study of Greek oncology nurses.[29]

Role conflict can result from inter-role or role-role conflict[30] when a person holds two or more roles and the demands of one role conflict with the demands of the other. Such conflict was found between hospice work and family obligations in several studies.[21]

Role conflict in palliative care can evolve from a variety of sources when one's role as a team member is in conflict with what one thinks might be in the best interest of patients. Such issues include: conflict about end-of-life care between nurses and physicians;[31] conflict with patients who may not yet be ready to accept the reality of impending death, when the nurse feels it is time for them to stop aggressive treatment;[31] "allowing" patients to maintain control, while feeling disappointed in not being able to fully discuss patients' expressed wishes to die; taking actions to help patients or families maintain a sense of control, while questioning the wisdom and morality of their decisions; dealing with the sometimes hazy distinction between patient autonomy and a professional ethic of care;[32] and the decision to transfer patients from active treatment settings to hospice and/or palliative care programs, primarily for economic reasons.[4] Inexperienced nurses caring for very symptomatic palliative care patients in the community may feel role conflict between the patient's right to good symptom control and the nurse's fear of hastening the patient's death.[33]

There may also be conflict between the "new nursing" and the "new consumerism."[34] Patients may not see themselves as active, collaborating partners in their care, may not see themselves as experts in their own health, or may fail to see the psychosocial aspect of care as one in which nurses have a right to intrude. Such patients may be classified as noncompliant and maladaptive. The role of nurse advocate may also be problematic. Johnstone[35] argues that if advocacy "is a reliable mechanism for protecting the patient's interest, then it should be a shared responsibility with family members and other health professions, not just the nurse or nurses in general" (as quoted in ref. 32 p. 256).

Role conflict is also associated with poor interpersonal relationships. Those who experience high role conflict are more apt to report that they have less trust in members of their role set, respect them less, like them less, and communicate with them less.[24]

Lack of control. Nurses have long struggled with issues related to power and control.[36–40] Protection and enhancement of the self are considered basic to human functioning. Mastery, the sense of being in control, and self-esteem, the assessment of one's worth, are resources that contribute strongly to the maintenance of one's identity.[41,42] Self-esteem and a sense of mastery have been shown to be effective in sustaining staff against the emotional distress associated with hospice work.[43,44] Situations that threaten or interfere with nurses' perceived ability to practice quality nursing care[45] and a lack of participation in planning and decision making have been associated with depression and increased stress.[32,46,47]

In Britain, the struggle around power and a lack of control and decision making are reflected in the fact that hospice medical directors rated their relationships with the matron as being most problematic.[48] "Encountering difficulties in relationships with nurses" was the only aspect of work in which palliative care physicians reported more stress than their colleagues in other specialties. This was hypothesized to derive in part from the lack of role clarity in the roles of consultants and senior nurses in palliative care, since historically some charitably funded hospices were run by matrons.[49] Recently, Hart and colleagues[32] used critical incidents from the practice of palliative care nurses to improve skills in psychosocial care. They found that in the practice incidents nurses identified, they repeatedly related roles in which they were mediating in a conflict situation in order to restore harmony and control. "The conflict was experienced within themselves and with others; the sense of control related to themselves, their clients and involved family and friends. Despite the magnitude of the issues they faced and perceived organizational constraints, most of the nurses related a sense of personal responsibility to mediate a successful outcome to the situation. When they were not able to 'fix' a situation, they expressed feelings of professional inadequacy" (p. 253). The incidents related by the nurses reflected how organizational policies and practices limited the flexibility of nurses to implement effective care. In order to support patient autonomy nurses need to experience professional autonomy within the work environment. Where they do not have this professional autonomy, they need to work toward achieving it, or recognize the limitations of the system in which they work and not assume personal blame and responsibility when this is inappropriate.

The personality characteristic of *hardiness*[50,51] has been found to be associated with decreased burnout in Greek oncology nurses.[29] *Hardiness* consists of three characteristics—commitment, control, and challenge. The sense of control over things that happen in life and in the work environment was found to protect nurses from emotional exhaustion, depersonalization, and a lack of personal accomplishment. Nurses who experienced higher degrees of burnout reported a lack of a sense of control over external events.

In a study of 1925 white- and blue-collar university employees in Australia,[52] *cognitive hardiness*, which assesses involvement, challenge, and control,[53] was found to be the best predictor of the ability to manage job stress, anxiety, daily hassles, and to maintain a healthy lifestyle.

Closely aligned with the concept of *hardiness* is the *sense of coherence*.[54,55] The sense of coherence is "a global orientation that expresses the extent to which one has a pervasive, enduring though dynamic feeling of confidence that one's internal and external environments are predictable and that there is a high probability that things will work out as well as can reasonably be expected."[54] With a sense of coherence the location of power is seen as being where it legitimately should be. That may involve the individual being in a position of power or it may involve power being vested in someone else, but the sense is that power is where it belongs.

A sense of coherence is partly personality-related and partly developed through life experience. It refers in particular to personal resourcefulness. Those with a broad repertoire and good flexibility are better able to adjust to most life challenges than those with poor repertoires.[56] "(T)he sense of coherence (SOC) construct is a generalized orientation toward the world which perceives it, on a continuum, as comprehensible, manageable, and meaningful."[55] The strength of one's SOC is a significant factor in facilitating the movement toward health.

Antonovsky[54] distinguishes between a sense of coherence and a sense of control, which implies that "I am in control." He states that a sense of coherence does not imply that one is in control, but rather that one is a participant in shaping one's destiny as well as one's daily experience.[24] In the case of palliative care nurses, the sense of coherence implies that nurses will have some ability to influence the care their clients receive—for some their influence may be great, and for others it may be more minor because of circumstances beyond their control, but they will be able to make a difference.

The sense of coherence is closely related to concepts such as optimism, will to live, self-efficacy, learned resourcefulness, and hardiness. Unlike concepts such as internal locus of control, mastery, empowerment, problem solving, and coping, the concept of self-coherence is not a culture-bound construct.[55] "The strength of one's SOC is shaped by three kinds of life experiences: consistency, underload-overload balance, and participation in socially valued decision making. The extent of such experiences is molded by one's position in the social structure and by one's culture—above all, I am persuaded, by the kind of work (including housework) one does and by one's family structure, with input from many other factors, ranging from gender and ethnicity to chance and genetics" (p. 15).[55]

Organizations exert a strong collective influence on the values, beliefs, and behavior of individuals.[57] If nurses, as individuals, do not have a strong sense of coherence, if they are working in a setting in which they consistently find themselves having a lack of control, and if they do not have the sense that those in positions of authority know what they are doing and understand the reality of the world of the palliative care nurse, the stage is set for feelings of powerlessness.

A study of 1,891 nurses,[58] most of whom were bedside nurses (80%), and the majority of whom worked full-time (58%), from six acute care hospitals in Quebec found that, *responsibility without power*, a combination of high psychological demands and low decision latitude, was associated with psychological distress and emotional exhaustion, one of the three dimensions of burnout. Current research suggests that restructuring high-demand, low-control jobs may enhance productivity and reduce disability costs.[59]

Schneider[60] reviewed the literature on decision making in situations in which ethical issues are involved and concluded that the evidence indicated that the nurse's role in such situations seems to be to participate in the sharing of information with other team members, but not to take part in actual decision making when an ethical dilemma existed. "If nurses perceive themselves as being less powerful than doctors, for example, in decision making, the nurses' own autonomy is compromised and their capacity to support patient autonomy effectively is limited" (p. 183). The author quotes a study by Erlen and Frost[61] involving how 25 nurses responded to ethical situations. Eighty-four percent of the participants reported feelings of powerlessness leading to anger, frustration, and exhaustion because of their inability to change the situation. "Reasons cited by the informants for their perceived powerlessness were a lack of knowledge about possible alternatives; a lack of recognition of their clinical knowledge and expertise and physicians resisting the nurses' attempts to advocate for the patient and intervene in ethical decision making."[60]

Recent practices, led by fiscal constraints, have raised increasing concern. Nurses are sometimes expected to perform procedures in the community for which they have not been prepared and for which no supervision is provided. When people are expected to assume responsibility with inadequate training, they have difficulty functioning.[27,62–66] In addition, there is sometimes the need to delegate tasks to unlicensed assistive personnel (UAP) while maintaining legal accountability. While nurses are told that legally it is inappropriate for an employer to require them to delegate when, in the nurse's professional judgment, this is not safe and not in the patient's best interest,[67] real-life situations may cause nurses to have to do just this.

Nurses report being in situations both in the hospital and in the community where they feel responsible for alleviating the pain of a palliative care patient yet do not have a physician willing to order the medication they feel will be sufficient to control pain. In addition, with the earlier discharge of sicker patients, nurses with limited experience may be expected to care for seriously ill palliative care patients in their home, without access to physicians skilled in effective palliative care and symptom management.

Power can come from external sources, such as a person's position and influence, or internal sources, such as knowledge, strength of personality, or state of mind. Both are needed.[66] Home care nurses who have the necessary knowledge and experience to adjust medications or route of administration to control difficult symptoms, but who do not have the necessary authority and power to make appropriate changes, are placed in untenable positions of knowing how to relieve the distress of the patient but not having the necessary power to do so.[33]

A sense of professional inadequacy and powerlessness marked many of the incidents identified by palliative care nurses in an Australian study.[32] The nurses had high expectations of their own performance and did not always take into account the organizational and professional constraints on their practice. Nurses tried to forge therapeutic relationships with patients, rather than coordinating a shared responsibility for care with family members, friends, and colleagues. They sought "individual" solutions to "organizational" and "family" problems. Much energy was expended to maintain harmony within family groups and the organization, and conflict was "viewed negatively and avoided rather than welcomed as a creative force for personal growth and organizational change" (p. 256).

Kanter[67] theorized that "to achieve work effectiveness, the individuals within an organization must have access to power and opportunity. Work effectiveness is measured by employee commitment to the organization and their perception of empowerment. Power is seen as access to support, information and resources as well as the individual's ability to use these resources to work toward the organization's mission and goals."[68] Powerlessness, or a lack of control over one's destiny, promotes a susceptibility to ill health for people who live in high demand or chronically marginalized situations and who lack adequate resources, supports, or abilities to exert control in their lives.[69,70] Such was the case in a number of studies of hospice nurses referred to above.[32,45–47] People with enough resources in their lives, such as decision making power, finances, or system access, can adequately cope with the psychological and actual demands in their lives.[71]

Role strain, or having difficulty performing various aspects of one's professional role, involves difficulty with constant exposure to needing to deal with the needs of dying persons and their families.[24] In a small study of palliative care nurses, staff reported difficulty in fulfilling their own performance expectations and felt pressured into a continuous commitment of time and energy to care for the dying because of the belief that the time to care is brief and the process happening now is the only meaningful measure of having cared well for this patient.[72] They reported struggling to narrow the gap between "real" and "ideal" as well as straddling the caring-vs.-curing dilemma, the stress flowing from the diffuse demands of home care and the challenge of being both a professional and a friend.[73]

Staff in a children's hospice were studied in the early years of the program[74] as well as more recently.[75] Whereas initially staff felt a sense of impotence when they were unable to relieve the perceived needs or distress of patients, they now have concerns about the increasing use of life-support equipment for the children, and about the balance between quality of life and technical support.

Role strain also involved feelings of isolation reported by matrons[46] and the burden of working with volunteers who were seen as extra people, creating extra strain.[76] Feeling inadequately prepared to deal with the emotional needs of patients and families and feeling that the nursing care offered was purposeless was associated with high stress scores.[77] Role strain has also been reported by nurses whose work makes them feel physically unsafe. This exposure included making visits to deserted country homes in the middle of snowstorms without access to cell phones or other ways of communicating if the nurse was in trouble; visiting in unsafe areas of the community, where the nurses do not feel safe during the day, and particularly at night; and visiting in homes where the family dynamics are such that nurses do not feel physically safe. When there are no organizational policies about how to handle these situations, nurses can feel quite stressed.

Nurses working with inner-city women dealing with AIDS found themselves becoming emotionally exhausted dealing with the physical abuse many of these women were suffering at the hands of their male partners and the women's apparent inability to leave their partners despite severe abuse. Gradually some of the most caring nurses became burned out and did not even bother to speak with the women about obvious signs of physical abuse. Gradually staff who had been employed in the center from its earliest stages began to leave, feeling they could not longer work with the changing population of patients.

Work Environment Stressors. Tension with others in the system was identified as a significant stressor early in the hospice movement.[24,78] This stressor involved difficulty with members of other specialties, who were seen as either not appreciating those in palliative care or not appropriately referring patients to the hospice.[21]

The problem continues with difficulty with timely referral.[10] Given the documented deficiencies in end-of life care,[79] it is to be hoped that the philosophy of palliative care could be incorporated into end-of-life care for increasing numbers of people. However, Byock[4] writes of the tensions between the "loyalists," who have generally been associated with the hospice movement, and the "progressives," who "tend to be caring, committed clinicians and administrators, often based in hospitals, nursing homes, or home health, who have awakened to the need to improve care for the dying in their own systems and are earnestly trying to do just that" (pp. 155–156).

Rivalries are encountered as programs try to determine with which agencies, if any, they will have preferred partner arrangements. The aggressive marketing techniques of some hospice programs have resulted in conflicts among the programs existing in and/or developing within some communities.[80] Other settings have developed palliative care programs in an apparent move to avoid referral to hospices, and to gain access to funding that might be made available for dying persons.

Hospice has also been limited in those it serves. One hospice administrator referred to "The Gates of Heaven" model, reflecting a narrow and inflexibly defined mission. "Patients must be just right, families in place, the disease one that the program is comfortable with, etc., etc. Such programs do not grow and over time they find themselves threatened by other providers whom they identify as somehow taking unfair advantage."[81]

Team communication problems were reported in numerous studies and continue to be an ongoing problem.[24,27,43–45,47–49,64,73–75,82] A lack of support from one's team members was implicated in high levels of depression.[83] Team communication problems involved dealing with a lack of team stability, intergroup conflict, and intragroup conflict.[24] Colleagues were found to be both a major source of stress as well as a major stress reducer.[24,45] Organizational factors, such as personality issues and team conflict, were more commonly reported stressors than were problems in dealing with patients and families and issues related to death and dying.[24,73] This finding has recently been replicated in a group of oncology nurses.[84] Organizational factors and coworker stress was rated as the most frequent and most intense stress cluster. However, stress clusters related to high patient contact (physician-related stress, death and dying, observing patient and family suffering, and ethical concerns) were also highly rated for frequency and intensity. The nurses believed they had the least control over the stress clusters related to dealings with others—that is: organizational factors, physician-related stress, and observing patients and family suffering. A lack of knowledge of team members[64] was noted to both lead to and reflect team communication problems. In addition, teams had difficulty if other team members were seen as having excessive emotional needs.[21,24,64] Staff in a children's hospice were surveyed ten years apart.[74–75] In both surveys, there were conflicts within the staff group. Most recently, the conflicts involved communication problems, reflecting the fact that many of the staff were working part time.

Palliative care requires the recognition that one cannot do this type of work alone or in isolation. Those attracted to the field often feel pressured to solve as many problems as possible within the shortest possible time. This type of pressure can lead to the conscious or unconscious belief that "I am the only person able to do what needs to be done." Such thinking does not respect the role of others on the team.[82]

Hospice team members need to learn to communicate with one another, to learn from one another, and in particular to deal effectively with conflict. Many palliative care teams have difficulty dealing directly with anger and may utilize a variety of obstructive behaviors. These may include *careerism* and *negative rivalry*—by concentrating on personal achievement and advancement, some team members' competitive instincts and energies may be channeled into rivalry among colleagues for career advancement and promotions, rather than on teamwork and effective patient care. Illusions of grandeur and interpersonal tugs-of-war occur on some teams where actual collaboration is low and mutual suspicion and antagonism is high. "Many team members engage in tugs-of-war, have territorial disputes, play one-upmanship, sabotage one another's programs, cut one another's throats, while all the time proclaiming what a great team they are."[85] *Lack of cooperation and discipline* occurs when teams have coordination without cooperation; they will go only so far. If team members are ordered about without consultation or participation, they will not give their best effort and will fail.[82]

Teams must recognize that buried conflicts will surface in other ways and will be detrimental to patient care. "Suppressed or disguised conflict is usually more harmful to teams than the possible discomfort and turbulence involved in confronting the conflict" (p. 19).[85]

The change to *managed health care* has threatened hospices. Administrative barriers may exist in which, in contrast to the philosophy and volunteer roots of hospice, health insurance coverage and financial concern dictate the hospice services provided[86] and palliative care providers often struggle to position their programs within the changing health care environment. The Medicare Hospice benefit has existing limitations. Tension results from the impact of the lack of reimbursement for physician involvement, per diem reimbursement, and an aggregate cap on reimbursement.[87]

In clinical care, the goal of actualizing patient choices, including the right to accept or reject treatment, is supported and protected through the informed consent process.[88] Yet patients are sometimes transferred to hospice or palliative care programs primarily because of economic considerations. Serving these "ambivalent clients" can be a considerable challenge.[89]

Palliative care in part seeks to avoid the regulations of the Hospice Medicare Benefit, enabling high-tech interventions to be reimbursed through routine Medicare and Medicaid. However, to the extent that the total costs of palliative care are actually less than those of hospice, there is concern that the fiscal advantage to the system may derive from providing fewer services or services of lesser quality to patients and their families.[4] As attempts are made to explore new models of care and to save money, there is the risk of developing "hospice lite" programs. Many of the new palliative care programs are not composed of interdisciplinary teams. Nor do most new palliative care programs genuinely incorporate goals that extend beyond relief of physical suffering and, perhaps, assistance with medical decision making.[4]

Patient and Family Stressors

Although it is logical to assume that caring for dying patients is the major stressor in palliative care, work environment and role stressors have generally been found to be bigger sources of stress.[21,24] Nursing a dying person can, however, still be a significant stressor. In addition, there is always the possibility that the stress nurses experience caring for dying patients gets displaced onto other aspects of their work.

Dealing with dying patients and inadequate preparation to deal with the emotional needs of patients and families were associated with higher stress scores in hospice nurses[77] and the final relationship and death trajectory were related to higher depression scores.[47] In a study comparing ICU, hospice, and medical-surgical nurses, hospice and ICU nurses perceived significantly more stress related to death and dying.[90] When hospice nurses were compared with medical-surgical nurses, hospice nurses were significantly higher on the death and dying dimension of the Nursing Stress Scale. For medical-surgical but not hospice nurses, death anxiety was significantly correlated with death and dying as a source of stress.[83]

The stress of decision making for nurses regarding the termination of treatment and the switch to a palliative approach was studied in intensive care units in the United Kingdom with nurses working with infants and adults.[60] The nurses were asked to identify the best and worst aspects of the situations. The themes of the worst incidents involved feelings of loss and helplessness, as the nurses often had a close relationship with the patient and/or family and empathized with the feelings of the family and had difficulty witnessing the pain and suffering of the family. The nurses often experienced feelings of failure after days of intensive treatment. If the patient seemed at all distressed, then the nurse was apt to feel helpless, because there is the expectation that with the current availability of drugs to handle pain or distress there should be no problem. Nurses had trouble with the unexpected turn of events when patients who were expected to get well suddenly took a turn for the worse. They found it difficult not to be able to organize and control events related to withdrawing active support and moving to comfort measures. They wanted to be able to give the family time to come to terms with the change of plans, but at the same time, they did not want to unnecessarily prolong the suffering. They had trouble when they could not predict the timing of the death, particularly if family members left and the patient died.

Patients coming to terms with dying was the main death-related concern of nurses working in acute care, hospice, and community settings[62] and in palliative care.[63] There can also be difficulties when patients do not want to die in the way nurses feel they "should" die.[32] Acute care oncology nurses may be susceptible to the more chronic situational stressors associated with the nature of their responsibilities and patient/family needs associated with deteriorating illness.[27,91] In a study comparing nurses and physicians in 54 different hospitals and clinics, working in oncology, cardiology, intensive care, and surgical units, those in oncology were found to suffer more from feelings of emotional involvement and self-doubt. The investigator hypothesized that the stress accompanying the care of people with cancer is no greater than that which accompanies the care of other medically ill people, but it is of a different quality. For oncology staff, institutional stressors move to the background when compared with the personal involvement of working with patients.[92]

One of the most significant areas of stress for oncology nurses can be watching people they have cared for over many years deteriorate. Staff may be torn when patients are then transferred from their care to be treated by palliative care or hospice programs. At times staff would prefer to care for patients as they die, while at other times staff would just as soon not have to witness the deaths of their patients who have struggled so long to live.

The difficulties associated with the care of dying persons may be due in part to the close connections palliative care nurses often develop with their patients. Whereas traditionally nurses and other professionals have been taught to maintain a boundary between themselves and their clients, in palliative care and oncology very close relationships can and do develop.[93] This closeness and exposure to repeated difficult illness experiences and deaths can lead to the experience of "secondary traumatic stress"

(STS), or compassion stress. Secondary traumatic stress is defined as "the natural consequent behaviors and emotions resulting from knowing about a traumatizing event experienced by a significant other—the stress resulting from helping or wanting to help a traumatized or suffering person."[94] Secondary traumatic stress disorder (STSD) is a more severe manifestation of STS and "is a syndrome of symptoms nearly identical to PTSD (post-traumatic stress disorder), except that exposure to knowledge about a traumatizing event experienced by a significant other is associated with the set of STSD symptoms, and PTSD symptoms are directly connected to the sufferer, the person experiencing the primary traumatic stress."[94] Compassion fatigue, which will be discussed below, is identical to STSD and is the equivalent of PTSD.[94] Unless nurses are helped to deal with their feelings when the people with whom they have close relationships die, compassion fatigue or other psychological symptoms can ensue.

Patient/family communication problems may occur when patients and family members come from a different social or cultural group than that of the caregiver or when the value systems of patients and families are different from those of the caregiver.[24] Communication problems also occurred when patients and families were ambivalent about continuing to use hospice care once it had been initiated. Sometimes there were areas of tension between patients, families, and staff regarding the proposed place of death, particularly if the family member wanted death to occur in a hospital and the staff felt an obligation to try to have a large proportion of their program's death occur at home.[89]

Australian nurses reported difficulty with patients who chose not to communicate their feelings about death and dying with either staff or their families and those who chose not to take medications in order that death might come more quickly. Patients' actions to take "personal control" of their situation and to refuse palliative care threatened the nurses' feelings about their role and function as palliative care nurses and made them feel they had not been good enough advocates for palliative care.[32]

Patients and families who were identified as having *coping or personality problems*, or else to be responding to their illness in a way that differed from the norm, presented problems to nurses. This group included patients or families who became extremely depressed, angry, withdrawn or psychotic; those who completely denied what was happening; those who acted out by drinking or taking drugs; and those who engaged in avoidance behavior.[24] Being concerned with patients selling their narcotic drugs to get money for food and dealing with family members and friends who steal the patient's narcotics can be very stressful for nurses. In general, staff found dealing with psychiatric symptoms more difficult than dealing with physical symptoms.[24,45,63] Nurses in the Hart and colleagues study[32] identified problems with clients who were difficult to manage, whose behavior had always been tolerated by their family members but was posing difficulty for nurses and dealing with aggressive clients.

In a study comparing hospital and hospice nurses with hospital matrons, both nursing groups reported greater levels of stress related to dealing with relatives and patients than did nurse managers.[47] Dealing with negative responses in family members was regarded as being more problematic than work with patients for staff in a children's hospice[74] as well as for medical directors and hospice.[48] The study of staff stress in the children's hospice was repeated in 1998 and the stressors were found to have changed.[75] Family issues involved staff feeling unable to meet a perceived need in siblings and fathers and coping with a difficult mix of families at any one time.

THE CAREGIVER'S RESPONSE TO LOSS AND GRIEF

Constant exposure to death and loss may leave nurses with grief overload and considerable distress. However, participating in the death of some patients may result in nurses' having intense positive responses that promote professional development.[95] Constant confrontation with the deaths of others causes caregivers to repeatedly reevaluate their own mortality and to reexamine the meaning of their life and living.[96]

Nurses have difficulty with grief if they hadn't been able to help the patient die a good death for whatever reason.[95] When the symptoms of dying patients are not controlled, the nurses feel responsible and "wanting," and if training and experience are lacking, this may well be the case.[33] Staff members often experience difficulty dealing with their feelings of grief and loss at the time of death because of other responsibilities that must be attended to immediately. There is often a strong covert institutional message as well as peer pressure not to dwell on the loss.[97]

Chronic compounded grief, defined as cumulative responses to losses over a period of time, has been found to be a powerful factor that contributes to resignations and turnover among oncology nurses and the ability of individual nurses to care for patients effectively. Feldstein and Gemma[97] suggest that what others refer to as burnout is really chronic, compounded grief. In a study of response to death in a Canadian continuing care and rehabilitation hospital, 42% of the staff felt themselves to have been "moderately" to "extremely" affected by patient deaths or they had lost time at work due to patient death, had low morale, experienced strain in personal relationships, had a loss of efficiency at work, or had health problems they attributed to patient deaths.[98]

Mount[96] has reflected on the *multiple losses* associated with working in oncology and notes that these losses become an integrated part of one's professional life. "Moreover, our losses do not occur in a vacuum. They interact with, modify, and often augment the other stressors in our personal and professional lives. Our reaction to loss may be repressed, only to surface later, associated perhaps with some other unrelated event" (p. 1127). He warns that the weight of these losses may lead to a burden that is increasingly intolerable and frequently difficult to define.

Particularly since the AIDS epidemic, the concept of multiple loss has been increasingly recognized. The concept of multiple loss in AIDS caregivers reflected in part the reality that many caregivers were caring for dying patients, while partners, friends, and members of their social network were dying at the same time.

Caregivers in palliative care may be caring for many patients who die within a short time of one another. Staff sometimes feel they do not have time to grieve for one person before another one has died. This grief can accumulate over the years, leading to significant depression. One pediatric oncology nurse said that she sometimes felt that she was carrying a "gunnysack" of dead children over her shoulder. As she met each new child she wondered if that child would someday go into her sack.

Multiple losses may result in chronic grief because there is no time to finish grieving for one loss before another one occurs. *Chronic bereavement* is distinguished from chronic grief in that chronic bereavement involves not only chronic grief but also anticipatory grief and unresolved grief, and most important, the experience of several losses *simultaneously*.[99] These losses may extend beyond the deaths of patients. Papadatou[100] has defined the losses as:

- loss of a close relationship with a particular patient;
- loss due to the professional's identification with the pain of family members;
- loss of one's unmet goals and expectations;
- losses related to one's personal system of beliefs and assumptions about life;
- past unresolved losses or anticipated future losses; and
- the death of self.

AIDS care has been described as being a never-ending cycle of perpetual grieving. Chronic bereavement includes *multiple loss syndrome*. "This syndrome includes the effects of chronic, anticipatory, and unresolved grief, as well as the compounding effects of experiencing several episodes of grief concurrently."[99]

Garfield[101] writes of the *compassion fatigue* that exists among AIDS/HIV caregivers. He suggests that the syndrome shares some characteristics with burnout: depression, anxiety, hypochondria, combativeness, the sensation of being on fast forward, and an inability to concentrate. However, with compassion fatigue caregivers can still be involved and care. In contrast to caregivers heading for burnout who unconsciously begin to wall off more and more strong feelings associated with their work, those with compassion fatigue are able to monitor their decrease in empathy and feeling and remain emotionally accessible. However, they have greater and greater difficulty in processing their emotions, are anxiety-ridden or distressed, have images that intrude on their days and nights, and have painful memories that flood their world outside the caregiving arena.

GIVING A VOICE TO THE NURSE

When caregivers were asked to identify what enabled them to cope with the stressors of dealing with the critically ill and dying, a sense of competence, control, and pleasure in one's work was a major coping mechanism.[24] This is closely related to both Kobasa's hardy personality[50–51] and to Antonovsky's sense of coherence.[54–56]

Some of the satisfactions received from palliative care work include:

- valuing each individual, experiencing the reciprocity of giving and receiving in relationships, a sense of interconnectedness and of mutual nurturing, being close to patients and sharing a part of one's self; the chance to make a difference in people's lives;[102]
- helping patients achieve optimum health by enabling them to do all they are capable of doing; being able to give patients options, recognizing that patients are the directors of their own decision making; being able to personalize the hospital environment so patients can feel more at home;[102]
- assisting patients and families to learn to cope with and adjust to caring for a dying relative at home, death at home, learning from patients and families;[103]
- experiencing positive feedback from patients and families, effective relating with and communicating with patients and families;[60,104]
- witnessing the smooth termination of life, initiating innovative, effective intervention for the patients, the right decision at the right time, peace for the patient;[60,104]
- being able to provide families with good memories in the midst of difficult times;[60]
- helping patients to find meaning in suffering;[17]
- an opportunity to learn skills and to develop as a person; the ability to constantly learn;[102]
- finding the challenge of working with cancer patients to be a reward that counterbalances the stressful aspects of the work;[29]
- relationships and support from colleagues;[60]

Perry[105] has used *nursing narratives* to explore exemplary nursing practice in palliative care and oncology nursing. She uses the themes of the dialogue of silence, mutual touch, and sharing the lighter side of life to illustrate aspects of exemplary nursing practice and identifies joint transcendence as the essence of exemplary nursing practice. "When both care providers and care receiver are co-participants in caring, the release can potentiate self-healing and harmony in both. The release can allow the one who is cared for to be the one who cares, through the reflection of the human condition that in turn nourishes the humanness of the care provider. In such connectedness they are both capable of transcending self, time, and space. Neither stands above the other.[105,106]

Case Study: Pattie Sun, a Breast Cancer Patient

Pattie Sun was a 48-year-old artist manager, piano player, amateur soprano, and dancer. She asked to see me because she wanted to explore meditation and visualization to deal with her relentlessly progressive breast cancer, which involved considerable bony metastases. Over the months we tried a few meditation sessions in which she was to go into a peaceful place and receive some insights from "helpers" who would appear. These sessions generally resulted in her going into fairly inhospitable settings. In a visualization a few weeks before her death, however, she envisioned herself lying in her bed at home, looking out the window at a beautiful garden. She was encouraged to imagine herself going out through the window and into the garden, but she chose to stay comfortably in her bed, knowing the garden was there when she was ready to visit it.

I suggested that she use a Prayer Wheel recently developed by a colleague, Dr. John Rossiter Thornton.[107] Using the Prayer Wheel, one focuses on several aspects of prayer, asks for what one needs for oneself and others, and listens with a pen in one's hand for whatever comes. As her disease progressed, Pattie used the Prayer Wheel most days.

A few months after we first met, I was away at a meeting. When I returned she had been readmitted to the hospital with pneumonia and had lost much of her voice. I went to visit her. She said that despite her progressive disease she was feeling a new sense of calm and joy. She said that she no longer feared death, although she was in no hurry to go there. She had a radiance about her that I had never seen. She said that she knew whatever happened to her would be okay. She acknowledged feeling that the spiritual transformation she had gone through was making it easier for her family and friends to face the possibility of her death, but she wondered what her role might be if she were to live for a longer time. We talked about her role in teaching those who surrounded her—family, friends, and staff—something about death by sharing with them the peace and joy she was experiencing.

The conversation felt very special to me. I reached out to hold her hand as I was about to leave. As I touched her, I felt a sudden surge of energy start in my toes and rush up through my body. As has happened only one other time, I found myself praying out loud for her and for the two of us that we would both be led to do whatever it was that we were meant to be doing. We had both been diagnosed with cancer. We had both been spiritually transformed by the experience. We were both using the Prayer Wheel for inspiration and direction, and both of our lives were changing in ways we could not have guessed. There was joy and laughter with that encounter quite unlike anything else I have ever experienced.

As Pattie lay dying three weeks later, this anecdote was read to her by her husband Jimmy and she smiled her permission to use it. In the brochure describing her life it was said that "Pattie passed away on October 26, 1999, peacefully and glowingly. At the end she felt she was 'close to God and close to her husband . . ."

Hart and colleagues[32] suggest that the sharing of practice experiences through narrative helps to tease out the assumptions underlying nursing actions. This reconstruction of nursing intervention through narrative gives meaning to the lived experience and creates opportunities for challenge and affirmation. The sharing of narratives can also help nurses to have a more reflective approach to their practice and their lives, to make their values more concrete, and to reaffirm the meaningfulness of their work. The sharing of narratives can also contribute to a collective culture of nursing care, and can lead to an opportunity to examine assumptions and collectively acknowledge the limitations of and constraints to practice. In this way nurses can generate creative solutions and mobilize collective action for organizational change.

As nurses begin to explore ways to change their practice situations to make them better for patients and more satisfying for the nurses, they will develop a sense of *empowerment* that "is the participation of individuals and communities in a social action process that targets both individual and community change outcomes."[71] Empowerment implies a group affiliation, community bonding, and collective action; it is not just an individual measurement such as self-esteem. Empowerment is not a fixed outcome of objectively changed conditions, but an ability to judge situations and determine whether the conditions are appropriate to demand change.[71] Palliative care nurses might work together in their own settings to determine which are the issues that are most in need of change. For example, nurses working in a hospice in South Africa were uncomfortable going into some settings, particularly at night. As a group they explored with administration the option of refusing to go into some areas, and it was agreed that this was a possibility. The hospice also provided them with cell phones. Brainstorming together, the nurses suggested the possibility of working with the police to develop a system whereby the police would be alerted when they were going to be in a potentially dangerous situation, and the nurses would consider asking the police to accompany them if they were really uncomfortable visiting certain areas but felt they should visit for the sake of the patient.

According to Antonovsky,[55] "People are, within limits, proactive and have some choice in life . . . and social institutions in all but the most chaotic historical situations can be modified to some degree" (p. 15). Participating in trying to change difficult situations can prevent damage to an individual's sense of coherence, can sometimes add some strength and in some cases, creates an opening for the beginning of a major change in life circumstances.[55] Hospice arose out of the attempt to change the care of the dying in institutional settings. Palliative care provides the opportunity to further expand these concepts to those at an earlier point in their illness trajectory.

When individuals participate in changing conditions and in the process of changing societal conditions become transformed, there is an improvement in their sense of self-efficacy and self-esteem. Work on empowerment has shown a change in group dynamics, an improved ability to communicate, a demonstrated change in levels of respect, and an improved ability to analyze situations and to act collectively when groups work together to effect a change.[71]

Given the need for role models for hospice and palliative care, the greater use of *advanced practice nurses* should be considered. The concept of the advanced practice nurse is more common in the United Kingdom than in North America.[13] "Attempts to devise systems for assessing the whole person with the disease and introducing programs aimed at addressing the physical, psychological, social and spiritual effects on the patient and family are more commonly found to have been introduced by nurses, usually those working in a specialist capacity. . . . These programs have been found to be effective in improving patients' quality (rather than quantity) of life and facilitating a greater degree of independence and control.[108]

Palliative care advanced practice nurses, skilled in combining the science of an active palliative treatment of pain-relieving care with the art and philosophy of holistic hospice healing,[13] could provide or oversee the provision of quality palliative care to patients and coordinate their care between home, hospital, clinic, or nursing home and do so in a cost-effective way, as has been demonstrated in a variety of settings.[13] Such nurses could provide in-depth knowledge of this specific patient population, decision making skills, leadership and the ability to negotiate a complex, integrated health care network.[13]

Advanced practice palliative care nurses can also act as advisers, enabling hospital staff nurses to improve the care they give to the dying, thus raising the general standard of care[109] and increasing patient satisfaction. In the community, advanced practice nurses can serve an important function for nurses in both community agencies and in some hospice programs wherein nurses are being asked to assume increasing responsibility without the proper preparation to do so.[33] The availability of 24-hour-a-day contact with a palliative care nurse practitioner with the knowledge, authority, and medical backup to make rapid changes in pharmacotherapy has proven to be very useful in such settings.[33]

Derry[108] notes that the key to significantly improving the future management of the large group of patients who could benefit from palliative care lies in the use of specialist nurse practitioners from a variety of clinical areas—including cardiology, Parkinson's disease, motor neurone disease, and respiratory disease—who have extensive knowledge and experience as well as proven communication skills. "Liaison between all disciplines and agencies, including providers of specialist palliative care, would be an integral part of this role. In this situation, education would be a two-way process, the specialist nurses gaining palliative care skills and knowledge, while the palliative care specialists learn more about the specific management of the particular condition" (pp. 81–82).

Social support has been found to be an essential variable for coping with many of life's stressors, including occupational stress.[21] "Although social support has many facets, a core dimension of it involves participating in a network of caring and reciprocal relationships with others and creating a sense of belonging and a reason for living that transcends one's individual self."[110]

Support from colleagues has been found to be very important for hospice nurses.[24,47] The overall mental health of hospice nurses was in part predicted by staff support,[47] and an association has been found between low burnout scores and social support in hospice nurses.[28]

When Greek nurses working with dying children in oncology and critical care were compared,[111] it was found that when the nurses were first hired they turned to family members and/or friends to discuss their work experiences and share their feelings, but they learned quickly that their friends and relatives found it difficult to listen to these accounts. The same finding was reported earlier.[24] Papadatou and colleagues found that overtime relationships with colleagues became progressively more important, and for some nurses this was their only source of emotional support. There was an intimacy that evolved involving friendships and quasi–family relationships outside of work and even marriage.

The support in that group of nurses was sought at four levels: informational, clinical/practical, emotional, and meaning making. The first two levels of support primarily benefited the patient; the latter two levels of support helped the nurses cope with the dying process and the death of children. There were similarities and differences in the levels of support used by both groups. Both groups valued *informational support*, although in different ways. Critical care nurses preferred information addressing clinical issues, while oncology nurses valued information exchange about the progress and treatment of individual patients and about acquiring new scientific knowledge. Both groups were dissatisfied with the level of *clinical/practical support*, primarily because of difficulty in cooperation among team members. In oncology this involved difficulties with role blurring between physicians and nurses; in the ICU it involved rivalry and closed subgroups due to educational differences.

The two groups were also different in the receipt of *emotional support*. In the ICU the ongoing presence of several colleagues provided emotional and clinical support, while the pediatric oncology nurses were more apt to be without a colleague or physician at night. The oncology nurses were more apt to share emotions and experiences openly when a child died, whereas the ICU nurses shared primarily in small groups or with "friends." They tended to try to avoid focusing on issues of death and to focus their energy on saving other children.

Both groups found *meaning* in their work, but this also differed. The ICU nurses tended to feel "we lost this one, but others also need our care and help." Oncology nurses tended to invest their work with meaning by dealing with issues that would lead to a good and peaceful death. The meaning of their work aimed at comfort and dignity instead of cure.

The development of supportive, collaborative work relationships may be fundamental to enhancement of self-efficacy and self-esteem. It is important that organizations create the opportunity for ongoing support, and that nurses have the time to attend support sessions, especially for those working alone in the community. This may consist of support through team meetings, easy access to consultants, a buddy or mentor system for ongoing support, and the opportunity to debrief after critical incidents.

The role of family and friends in supporting caregivers has been found to be important but to have limits.[24] When caregivers working in HIV and oncology were compared, it was found that one-third of staff without long-term emotional relationships felt that their work kept them from being involved in such relationships. Most subjects reported spending a considerable amount of time discussing their work with partners. Thirty-nine percent reported that their partners complained regularly about their commitment to work, and one-quarter reported that their relationship had suffered as a result of their work in oncology or HIV. While friends and family of HIV staff were more supportive of their working in the field, friends and family of oncology staff were more supportive of their actual work.[112]

A personal philosophy of illness, life, and death is an important *personal coping mechanism* in palliative care.[24] Inherent in a philosophy of practice is the right, and indeed obligation, to mourn for those who have died. Although not all patients will touch caregivers equally—indeed, if caregivers mourned for each patient they would never get beyond acute grief—in many situations patient deaths and the ensuing staff grief deserve recognition. Acknowledging the deaths of individual patients can enable practitioners to avoid the accumulation of grief that comes from repeated, unresolved losses.[96] However, at times multiple losses can lead to a sense of grief overload that may need to be dealt with in a variety of ways, including memorial services, journaling, staff "wakes," attending a funeral, sharing with the family of a client the joys the person brought into one's life, or the lessons that one will always remember from this person. At times it may be helpful to attend the funeral of one patient but to use it as an opportunity to reflect on the deaths of more than one person.

Interviews with caregivers in oncology revealed that many had memorabilia of patients who had died readily available in their offices. They pointed to pictures on the walls, small objects on their bookshelves, or reached into a file of letters in their desks thanking them for the work they had done with particular patients. This behavior was particular to caregivers in oncology. This is one of the ways in which professionals often maintain *continuing bonds*[113] with clients who have died. They carry the lessons learned from those who have died forward into the care of those they have yet to meet. This approach is helpful in avoiding "survivor guilt" or the feeling one can sometimes get with multiple losses that "all of one's energy is buried in the ground."[24]

Data from the AIDS field suggests that the flooding of emotion involved in multiple loss and grief may lead to incapacitation rather than healing. To defend against this flooding, some people might become emotionally numb.[114] Numbing and flooding have become very important skills for those in the HIV/AIDS field in order to deal with the intense emotion and "unbearable loss" caregivers experience. Numbing refers to the ability to turn off emotions, to avoid painful thoughts and images, to deny the full impact of grief. Numbing may feel like depression, but it allows caregivers to process the pain in small doses, to reduce anxiety while gradually coming to terms with the reality of losing so many loved ones so quickly. However, feeling numb is very far from feeling good. In fact, it can lead to hopelessness, fatigue, and suicidal feelings. Caregivers need to develop control in moving between the states of numbness and flooding. By moving between these states they can process the trauma over time and find some hope, peace, and inner strength again.[115]

Papadatou[111] describes dealing with the grief of multiple losses as being both an individual and social interactive process that may be understood in terms of an ongoing fluctuation between experiencing grief reactions by focusing on the loss experience, and containing or avoiding grief reactions by moving away from grief. This fluctuation allows professionals to attribute meaning to the dying and death of individual patients, and to transcend these losses by investing in life and living. She describes the losses as consisting of:

- the loss of a close relationship with a particular patient with whom one has shared a part of a significant journey;
- loss due to professional's identification with the pain of family members;
- loss due to one's unmet goals and expectations and one's professional self-image and role;
- losses related to one's personal system of beliefs and assumptions about life ;
- past unresolved losses or anticipated future losses; and
- the death of self (see also ref. 24 for earlier conceptualizations on the subject).

When caregivers focus on the loss, they experience a wide range of grief reactions on a cognitive, emotional, behavioral, and/or physical level and mobilize various emotion-focused and problem-focused coping strategies. Caregivers experience the emotions of grief and reflect on the lost person. They may withdraw into themselves for short periods, but this withdrawal may alternate with active searching for support, usually among colleagues. They may attend the funeral to bring closure to the relationship. They may feel a sense of relief over the person's death and have a sense of satisfaction at the care provided. Moving away from feelings of loss may vary from containing one's grief expressions to systematically denying them. Caregivers may shut out feelings of grief, avoid contact with the patient or the family, retreat to practical tasks, or dehumanize the dying person. Papadatou notes that difficulties occur in the grieving process when there is no fluctuation between experiencing and containing one's grief. In these situations, caregivers may be either totally overwhelmed by the experience or may systematically repress it.

While caregiving in the context of palliative care and multiple loss is difficult, there are also many rewards, including the ways in which one's deepest wounds can become one's greatest sources of strength. A number of authors have written of the *"wounded healer."*[101,116–118] This concept derives from ancient universal shamanic stories of Paleolithic times. These stories are of tribal priests, "the original wounded healers, whose ability to heal others was seen as being directly linked to their having journeyed in depth into their own wounded selves."[117]

Successful caregivers are often "wounded healers," with wounds sustained either in childhood, adulthood, or both. "In many cases, in trying to heal their respective wounds, these caregivers were drawn, consciously or not, to healing others."[101] Sulmasy,[118] a physician, philosopher, and Franciscan friar, contends that "all health care professionals are wounded healers. They cannot escape suffering themselves. Moments of pain, loneliness, fatigue, and sacrifice are intrinsic to the human condition. The physician or nurse's own bleeding can become the source of the compassion in the healer's art. From the physician or nurse's own suffering can come the wine of fervent zeal and the oil of compassion. . . . The physician's or nurse's wounds can become resources for healing . . ." (p. 48). Sulmasy warns, however, that wounded healers must not become so overwhelmed with the suffering of others that they are unable to offer effective care. "Competence remains the first act of compassion. Wounded healers do not ask their patients for help, but recognize the unity between their own neediness and the needs of their patients. Wounded healers issue an invitation to patients to enter into the space of the healing relationship" (p. 48). In this sense, the clinician offers hospitality.

Henri Nouwen[116] wrote of the minister as a wounded caregiver. His perspective provides interesting reflections for caregivers in palliative care. Nouwen quotes the Talmud as asking the question of how one might know the Messiah. "He is sitting among the poor covered with wounds. The others unbind all their wounds at the same time and then bind them up again. But he unbinds one at a time and binds it up again, saying to himself, 'Perhaps I shall be needed: if so I must always be ready so as not to delay for a moment' (taken from the tractate Sanhedrin)" (p. 82).

From Nouwen's perspective, the caregiver must bind her own wounds carefully in anticipation of the time when she will be needed. The wounded healer must look after her own wounds, but at the same time be prepared to heal the wounds of others. The signs that characterize the healing of those aware of their own woundedness are hospitality, concentration, compassion, and perspective.

Hospitality is the ability to pay attention to the "guest"—the client or patient with whom we work. Hospitality as a healing power "requires first of all that the host feel at home in his own house, and secondly that he creates a free and fearless place for the unexpected visitor. Therefore, hospitality embraces two concepts: concentration and community."[116] Feeling at home in one's own house implies both being comfortable in one's self as well as being comfortable in the work environment. Nouwen notes that hospitality is very difficult "since we are preoccupied with our own needs, worries, and tensions, which prevent us from taking distance from ourselves in order to pay attention to others" (p. 89). Concentration implies paying attention to the other person as an individual, not as someone on whom we should be imposing our own agenda. Too often caregivers in palliative care are so convinced of the rightness of their activity and desire the "best" for the person that they may impose their values onto those with whom they work. Concentration implies creating the "room and space where someone else can enter freely without feeling himself an unlawful intruder" (p.90). This implies a withdrawing into ourselves in order to create the space for another to be himself. Such an ability to withdraw into the self can come through meditation—an ability to enter into one's own center. "When we are not afraid to enter into our own center and to concentrate on the stirrings of our own soul, we come to know that being alive means being loved. . . . When we have found the anchor places for our lives in our own center, we can be free to let others enter into the space created for them and allow them to dance their own dance, sing their own song and speak their own language without fear. Then our presence is no longer threatening and demanding but inviting and liberating" (pp. 91–92). Through sharing pain with our patients "we become aware that we do not have to escape our pains, but that if we can mobilize them into a common search for life, those very pains are transformed from expressions of despair into signs of hope. Through this common search, hospitality becomes community" (p. 93).

The compassionate person stands in the midst of "people but does not get caught in the conformist forces of the peer group, because through his compassion he is able to avoid the distance of pity as well as the exclusiveness of sympathy. Compassion is born when we discover in the center of our own existence not only that God is God and man is man, but also that our neighbor is really our fellow man. . . . For a compassionate (person) nothing human is alien: no joy and no sorrow, no way of living and no way of dying" (p. 41). Compassion means, at the very least "feeling with" the patient. "To suffer is bad enough. To suffer alone is a far worse fate."[118] "The perspective required is to see the wounds of patients as true signs of God and as portals of hope."[118]

Michael Kearney,[117] a hospice physician, says that while there is an abusive and useless dimension to illness, pain, and suffering that needs to be removed if at all possible, there is also potential in such experiences. "It is as though the dragon (that is, the patient's distress) also guards a treasure—something essential for that particular individual's healing at that moment in time (p. 41). In *Mortally Wounded*[117] he speaks of "soul pain," which he defines as "the experience of an individual who has become disconnected and alienated from the deepest and most fundamental aspects of himself (p. 63). Palliative care patients experiencing severe and difficult-to-control symptoms are sometimes experiencing such pain. Our role is to help them by dealing with the symptoms—physical, emotional, and social—using the skills of a good multidisciplinary palliative care team. But Kearney warns this is only "surface work." "Depth work" is required. This is any approach or intervention that brings the individual to the experience of soul. The palliative care nurse who understands her own soul pain and has been through her own "depth" work of coming to understand her own "wounded healer" is in the position to be of considerable assistance to such patients. Personal work with meditation and exploring one's own spirituality can bring nurses into a position in which they are able to provide deeper healing for those we are called to serve and to help to heal as they come to terms with their personal death.

Christine Longaker[119] has written of caring for her young husband who died of leukemia. The experience led her to a search to find better answers in the care of the dying and a recognition of the spiritual aspects of dying. Her book contains meditation exercises that can be helpful for caregivers wanting to get in touch with their deeper selves as a way of maintaining their own psychic and spiritual health and of then being able to reach out to others.

Religion has been found to be a helpful coping mechanism for nurses.[120] In addition, for many caregivers a *spiritual or religious philosophy*, centered around a commitment to serve others, may be both helpful and key to deriving a sense of meaning in difficult times.[24] Nurses attracted to hospice work have been found to be more religious than others.[21,24,121] Compared with oncology nurses, hospice nurses reported a greater sense of personal spirituality, more frequent spiritual caregiving, and more positive perspectives regarding spiritual caregiving. Hospice nurses were also older and more experienced in nursing than oncology nurses. Hospices may attract nurses who have an existing sensitivity to personal spirituality, or the nature of the work might increase the nurse's spiritual sensitivity. It is also possible that more seasoned nurses may have both personal and professional factors that have led to more spiritual caregiving. Hospice nurses also reported receiving stronger employer support for spiritual caregiving than did those in oncology.[122]

A sense of spirituality can be helpful to caregivers as they struggle to find meaning in the work they are doing. It has been said that burnout has very little to do with work or overwork, but occurs because of the caregiver's having lost the ability to manage pain well and to keep balance in one's life. Being truly spiritual involved having a real balance in one's life.[123]

Many years ago the author heard Dr. Richard Lazarus, one of the world's greatest coping experts, speak about a variety of coping mechanisms. At the end of the lecture, an audience member asked Dr. Lazarus what was the single best coping mechanism. He replied with the "Serenity Prayer":

> God grant me the serenity to accept the things I cannot change,
> The courage to change the things I can,
> And the wisdom to know the difference.

The "Serenity Prayer" incorporates the *hardy personality*—commitment, control, and challenge; *empowerment* to be able to decide what is appropriate to do and to do it, and the *sense of coherence*—things will work out as well as can be expected, given the circumstances, and power is appropriately vested in someone who is capable of handling whatever might arise. At times when caregivers struggle to find meaning in the suffering of patients and families, or when they feel that the limitations of the health care system are keeping them from being able to provide the care they want to provide, a sense of spirituality and of something beyond the suffering of the moment can help us to carry on and may even provide inspiration for how to change what needs to be changed.

CONCLUSIONS

The world of the palliative care nurse is one of transition. As we are working with patients who are in process of their own transition, so too are we working to facilitate transition in the health care system. Transition could lead to transformation and transcendence in the care we are able to provide. Hospice attempted to change the way care was provided to the dying. At its best, hospice has provided excellent care, but not all hospices are equal and not all dying persons are, or can be, served by hospice. Bringing the best of hospice care to patients and families at an earlier point in the illness continuum through the use of integrated multidisciplinary palliative care teams will result in better care for all concerned.

But the road will not be easy. Nurses will need to continue to identify and deal with the stressors involved in their occupational roles, in their work environments, and with the patients and families with whom we work. Being well-integrated human beings with hardy personalities and a strong sense of coherence, and having a sense of empowerment to tackle the challenges ahead, will help us to succeed in doing the work that needs to be done. Working in environments that recognize the need for support and education for staff, the importance of mentors and advanced practice nurses will improve the quality of care for patients and families and the quality of work life for caregivers. Learning to deal with our own loss and grief, coming in touch with our wounded healers and spiritual selves, will help us to continue to survive and thrive.

REFERENCES

1. Cancer Pain Relief and Palliative Care. Technical Report Series 804, Geneva: World Health Organization, 1990.
2. Doyle D, Hanks G, MacDonald N. (1998). Introduction. In: Doyle D, Hanks GWC, MacDonald N, eds. Oxford Textbook of Palliative Medicine, 2nd ed. Oxford: Oxford University Press, 1998:3–8.
3. Last Acts Task Force. Precepts of Palliative Care. Princeton, N.J.: Robert Wood Johnson Foundation, 1997.
4. Byock I. Hospice and palliative care: a parting of the ways or a path to the future? Journal of Palliative Medicine 1998;1:165–176.
5. Hospice Fact Sheet. National Hospice Organization. July, 1999.
6. Newsline. National Hospice Organization. May 1999.
7. Christakis NA, Escarce JE. Survival of Medicare patients after enrollment in hospice programs. New England Journal of Medicine 1996; 335:172–178.
8. Nichols M. Coping with pain. Macleans August 16, 1999:52–55.
9. Connor SR. New initiatives transforming hospice care. Hospice Journal 1999;3:4:193–204.
10. Boling A, Lynn J. Hospice: current practice, future possibilities. Hospice Journal 1998;13:(1/2):29–32.
11. Vigano A, Dorgan M, Bruera E, Suarez-Almazor ME. The relative accuracy of the clinical estimation of the duration of life for patients with end of life cancer. Cancer 1999;86:172–176.
12. Magno J. The hospice concept of care: Facing the 90's. Death Studies 1990;14:109–119.

13. Weggel JM. Palliative care: new challenges for advanced practice nursing. Hospice Journal 1997;12:43–56.

14. DeVito R. Hospice and managed care: The new frontier. The American Journal of Hospice and Palliative Care 1995;12:2.

15. Doyle D. Special issues in palliative care. Henry Ford Hospital Medical Journal 1991;39:92–95.

16. Doyle D. Have we looked beyond the physical and psychosocial? Journal of Pain and Symptom Management 1992;7:302–311.

17. Kearney M. Palliative medicine—just another specialty? Palliative Medicine 1992;6:41.

18. Lynn J, Wilkinson AM. Quality end of life care: the case for a MediCaring demonstration. Hospice Journal 1998;13:151–163.

19. Benoliel JQ. Nursing research on death, dying and terminal illness: development, present state and prospects. Annual Review of Nursing Research 1983;1:101–130.

20. Jodrell N. Nurse education. In: Doyle D, Hanks GWC, MacDonald N, eds., Oxford Textbook of Palliative Medicine, 2nd ed. Oxford: Oxford University Press, 1998:1201–1208.

21. Vachon MLS. Staff stress in hospice/palliative care: a review. Palliative Medicine 1995;9:91–122.

22. Wilkinson SM. The changing pressures for oncology nurses, 1986–93. European Journal of Cancer 1995;4(2):69–74.

23. Amenta M. Study reveals hospice nurses have a high degree of role satisfaction. Fanfare 1995;IX:18.

24. Vachon MLS. Occupational Stress in the Care of the Critically Ill, the Dying and the Bereaved. New York: Hemisphere, 1987.

25. Wilson IM, Bunting JS, Curnow RN, Knock J. The need for inpatient palliative care facilities for non cancer patients in the Thames valley. Palliative Medicine 1995;9:13–18.

26. Bean CA, Holcombe JK. Personality types of oncology nurses. Cancer Nursing 1993;16:479–485.

27. Beck-Friis B, Strang P, Sjöden PO. Caring for severely ill cancer patients: a comparison of working conditions in hospital-based home care and in hospital. Supportive Care in Cancer 1993;1:145–151.

28. Bram PJ, Katz LF. Study of burnout in nurses working in hospice and hospital oncology settings. Oncology Nursing Forum 1989;16:555–560.

29. Papadatou D, Anagnostopoulos F, Monos D. Factors contributing to the development of burnout in oncology nursing. British Journal of Medical Psychology 1994;67:187–199.

30. Schmalenberg C, Kramer M. Coping with Reality Shock: The Voices of Experience. Wakefield, MA: Nursing Resources, 1979.

31. Kuuppelomäki M, Lauri S. Ethical dilemmas in the care of patients with incurable cancer. Nursing Ethics 1998;5:283–293.

32. Hart G, Yates P, Clinton M, Windsor C. Mediating conflict and control: practice challenges for nurses working in palliative care. International Journal of Nursing Studies 1998;35:252–258.

33. Coyle N. Focus on the nurse: ethical dilemmas with highly symptomatic patients dying at home. Hospice Journal 1997;12(2):33–41.

34. May C. Patient autonomy and the politics of professional relationships. Journal of Advanced Nursing 1995;21:83–87.

35. Johnstone M. Bio-ethics: A nursing Perspective. Sydney: Harcourt Brace Jovanovich, 1989.

36. Quint JC. The Nurse and the Dying Patient. New York: Macmillan, 1973.

37. Stein LI. The doctor-nurse game. Archives of General Psychiatry 1973;16:739–723.

38. Ehrenreich B, English D. Witches, Midwives and Nurses: A History of Women Healers. Old Westbury, N.Y: The Feminist Press, 1973.

39. Coburn J. I see and am silent. In: Acton J, Goldsmith P, Shepard B, eds. Women at Work 1850–1930 Toronto: Canadian Women's Educational Press, 1974:127–163.

40. Vachon MLS. The nurse in thanatology: what she can learn from the women's liberation movement. In: Earle A, Argondizo MT, Kutscher AH, eds. The Nurse as Caregiver for the Dying Patient and His Family New York: Columbia University Press, 1976:175–194.

41. Pearlin LI, Schooler C. The structure of coping. Journal of Health and Social Behavior 1978;19:2–21.

42. Pearlin LI, Lieberman MA, Menaghan EG, Mullan JT. The stress process. Journal of Health and Social Behavior 1981;22:337–356.

43. Yancik R. Sources of work stress for hospice staff. Journal of Psychosocial Oncology 1984;2(1):21–31.

44. Yancik R. Coping with hospice work stress. Journal of Psychosocial Oncology 1984;2(2):19–35.

45. Barstow J. Stress variance in hospice nursing. Nursing Outlook 1980;28:751–754.

46. Alexander DA, MacLeod M. Stress among palliative care matrons: a major problem for a minority group. Palliative Medicine 1992;6:111–124.

47. Cooper CL, Mitchell S. Nursing the critically ill and dying. Human Relations 1990;43:297–311.

48. Finlay IG. Sources of stress in hospice medical directors and matrons. Palliative Medicine 1990;4:5–9.

49. Graham J, Ramirez AJ, Cull A, Gregory WM, Finlay I, Hoy A, Richards MA. Job stress and satisfaction among palliative physicians: a CRC/CRF Study. Palliative Medicine 1996;10:185–194.

50. Kobasa SC. Stressful life events, personality and health: an inquiry into hardiness. Journal of Personality and Social Psychology 1979;37:1–11.

51. Kobasa SC, Maddi SR, Kahn S. Hardiness and health: a prospective study. Journal of Personality and Social Psychology 1982;42:172–177.

52. Sharpley CF, Dua JK, Reynolds R, Acosta A. The direct and relative efficacy of Cognitive Hardiness, Type A Behaviour Pattern, Coping Behaviour and Social Support as predictors of stress and ill-health. Scandinavian Journal of Behaviour Therapy 1995;24:15–29.

53. Nowack KM. Initial development of an inventory to assess stress and health risk. American Journal of Health Promotion 1990;4:173–180.

54. Antonovsky A. Health, Stress and Coping. San Francisco: Jossey-Bass, 1979.

55. Antonovsky A. The salutogenic model as a theory to guide health promotion. Health Promotion International 1996;11:11–18.

56. Antonovsky A. Unraveling the Mystery of Health: How People Manage Stress and Stay Well. San Francisco: Jossey-Bass, 1987.

57. Snyder M. Critical thinking: a foundation for consumer-focused care. Journal of Continuing Education in Nursing 1993;24:206–210.

58. Bourbonnais R, Comeau M, Vzina M, Dion G. Job strain, psychological distress, and burnout in nurses. American Journal of Industrial Medicine 1998;34:20–28.

59. Yandrick RM. High demand low control. Behavioral Healthcare Tomorrow 1997;6(3):41–44.

60. Schneider R. The effects on nurses of treatment-withdrawal decisions made in ICUs and SCBUs. Nursing in Critical Care 1997;2:174–185.

61. Erlen JA, Frost B. Nurses perceptions of powerlessness in influencing ethical decisions. Western Journal of Nursing Reseach 1991;13:397–407.

62. Copp G, Dunn V. Frequent and difficult problems perceived by nurses caring for the dying in community, hospice and acute care settings. Palliative Medicine 1993;7:19–25.

63. Alexander DA, Ritchie E. "Stressors" and difficulties in dealing with the terminal patient. Journal of Palliative Care 1990;6(3):28–33.

64. Paradis LF, Usui WM. Hospice staff and volunteers: Issues for management. Journal of Psychosocial Oncology 1989;7:121–139.

65. Delegation: an increasing part of nursing care. Clinical Journal of Oncology Nursing 1997;1:107–113; reprinted from Massachusetts Nursing Board News Summer, 1997;3:2.

66. Redfern L. Power and authority: Is there a difference? Nursing Times 1996;92(37):36–37.

67. Kanter R.M. Men and Women of the Corporation. New York: Basic Books, 1977.

68. Prince SB. Shared governance: sharing power and opportunity. Journal of Nursing Administration 1997;27(3):28–35.

69. Syme S. Social epidemiology and the work environment. International Journal of Health Services 1988;18:635–645.

70. Kaplan G, Haan M, Syme S, Minkler M, Miszcynski M. Socioeconomic status and health: Closing the gap. In: Amler R, Dull H, eds. Closing the Gap: The Burden of Unnecessary Illness. New York: Oxford University Press, 1987:125–129.

71. Wallerstein N. Powerlessness, empowerment, and health: implications for health promotion programs. American Journal of Health Promotion 1992;6:197–205.

72. McWilliam CL, Burdock J, Wamsley J. The challenging experience of palliative care

support-team nursing. Oncology Nursing Forum 1993;20:770–785.

73. Munley A. Sources of hospice staff stress and how to cope with it. Nursing Clinics of North America 1985;20:343–355.

74. Woolley H, Stein A, Forrest GC, Baum JD. Staff stress and job satisfaction at a children's hospice. Archives of Diseases of Children 1989;64: 114–118.

75. Forrest G, Woolley H. 15 Years of staff support in a children's hospice. 1999. (Unpublished data).

76. Robbins RA. Death anxiety, death competency and self-actualization in hospice volunteers. Hospice Journal 1991;7(4):29–35.

77. Power KG, Sharp GR. A comparison of sources of nursing stress and job satisfaction among mental handicap and hospice nursing staff. Journal of Advanced Nursing 1988;13:726–732.

78. Vachon MLS. Battle fatigue in hospice/ palliative care. In: A Safer Death Gilmore A, Gilmore S, eds.) pp. 149–160. New York, 1988: 149–160.

79. Field M, Cassel CK. Approaching Death: Improving Care at the End of Life. Washington, DC: Institute of Medicine, National Academy Press, Washington, 1997.

80. Vachon MLS. The stress of the professional caregivers. In: Doyle D, Hanks GWC, MacDonald N, eds. Oxford Textbook of Palliative Medicine, 2nd edition Oxford: Oxford University Press, 1998:919–920.

81. Mount BM. Keeping the mission. American Journal of Hospice and Palliative Care 1992; 9(5):32–37.

82. Vachon MLS. What makes a team? Palliative Care Today 1996;5:3:34–35.

83. Bené B, Foxall MJ. Death anxiety and job stress in hospice and medical-surgical nurses. Hospice Journal 1991;7(3):25–41.

84. Florio GA, Donnelly JP, Zevon MA. The structure of work-related stress and coping among oncology nurses in high-stress medical settings: A transactional analysis. Journal of Occupational Health Psychology 1998;3:227–242.

85. Heming D. The Titanic triumvirate: teams, teamwork and teambuilding. Canadian Journal of Occupational Therapy 1988;55(1):15–20.

86. Reese DJ, Brown DR. Psychosocial and spiritual care in hospice: Differences between nurses, social work and clergy. Hospice Journal 1997;12:29–41.

87. Walsh D. Palliative care: management of the patient with advanced cancer. Seminars in Oncology 1994;21(4 Suppl. 7):100–106.

88. Scanlon C. Unraveling ethical issues in palliative care. Seminars in Oncology Nursing 1998;14:137–144.

89. Hamilton CL, Neubauer BJ. Hospice nursing: serving ambivalent clients. Nursing and Health Care 1989;10:321–322.

90. Foxall MJ, Zimmerman L, Standley R, Bené B. A comparison of frequency and sources of nursing job stress perceived by intensive care, hospice and medical-surgical nurses. Journal of Advanced Nursing 1990;15:577–584.

91. Hansell PS. Stress on nurses in oncology. In: Holland JC, Rowland JH, eds. Handbook of Psychooncology. New York: Oxford University Press, 1989:658–663.

92. Herschbach P. Work-related stress specific to physicians and nurses working with cancer patients. Journal of Psychosocial Oncology 1992; 10:79–99.

93. Trygstad L. Professional friends: The inclusion of the personal into the professional Cancer Nursing 1986;9:326–332.

94. Figley CR. Compassion Fatigue As a Secondary Traumatic Stress Disorder: An Overview. In: Figley CR, ed. Compassion Fatigue New York: Brunner/Mazel, 1995:1–20.

95. Saunders JM, Valente SM. Nurses' grief. Cancer Nursing 1994;17:318–325.

96. Mount BM. Dealing with our losses. Journal of Clinical Oncology 1986;4:1127–1134.

97. Feldstein MA, Gemma PB. Oncology nurses and chronic compounded grief. Cancer Nursing 1995;18:228–236.

98. O'Hara PA, Harper D, Chartrand LD, Johnston SF. Patient death in a long-term care hospital. Journal of Gerontological Nursing 1996; 22(8):27–35.

99. Cho C, Cassidy DF. Parallel processes for workers and their clients in chronic bereavement resulting from HIV. Death Studies 1994;8: 273–292.

100. Papadatou D. A proposed model of health professional's grieving process. Omega 1999. (In press).

101. Garfield C, Spring C, Ober D. Sometimes My Heart Goes Numb: Love and Caring in a Time of AIDS. San Francisco: Jossey-Bass, 1995.

102. Perry B. Moments In Time: Images of Exemplary Nursing Care. Ottawa: Canadian Nurses Association, 1998.

103. Gotay CC, Crockett S, West C. Palliative home care nursing: Nurses' perceptions of roles and stress. Canada's Mental Health 1985; 33:6–9.

104. Krikorian DA, Moser DH. Satisfactions and stresses experienced by professional nurses in hospice programs. American Journal of Hospice Care 1985;2(1):25–33.

105. Perry B. Beliefs of eight exemplary oncology nurses related to Watson's nursing theory. Canadian Oncology Nursing Journal 1998;8:97–101.

106. Watson J. Human caring and suffering: A subjective model for health services. In: Watson J, Taylor R, eds. They Shall Not Hurt: Human Suffering and Human Caring. Boulder CO: Colorado Associated University, 1989.

107. Rossiter-Thornton SF. Prayer in psychotherapy. Ther Health Med 2000;6(1):125–128.

108. Derry S. Dying for palliative care. European Journal of Palliative Care 1997;4(3):80–82.

109. Bircumshaw D. Palliative care in the acute hospital setting. Journal of Advanced Nursing 1993;18:1665–1666.

110. Larson DG. The Helper's Journey. Champaign, Ill: Research Press, 1993.

111. Papadatou D, Papazoglou I, Petraki D, Bellali T. Mutual support among nurses who provide care to dying children. Illness, Crisis and Loss 1999;7:37–48.

112. Miller D, Gillies P. Is there life after work? Experiences of HIV and oncology health staff. AIDS Care 1996;8:167–182.

113. Klass D, Silverman PR, Nickman SL, eds. Continuing Bonds. Washington, DC: Taylor & Francis, 1996.

114. Grothe T, McKusick L. Coping with multiple loss. Focus 1992;7(7):5–6.

115. Bigelow G, Hollinger J. Grief and AIDS: surviving catastrophic multiple loss. Hospice Journal 1996;11(4):83–96.

116. Nouwen H. The Wounded Healer. Garden City, NY: Doubleday, 1972.

117. Kearney M. Mortally Wounded. New York: Scribner, 1996.

118. Sulmasy DP. The Healer's Calling. New York: Paulist Press, 1997.

119. Longaker C. Facing Death and Finding Hope. New York: Doubleday, 1997.

120. Heim E. Job stressors and coping in health professionals. Psychotherapy and Psychosomatics 1991;55:90–99.

121. Amenta MM. Traits of hospice nurses compared with those who work in traditional settings. Journal of Clinical Oncology 1984;40:414–419.

122. Taylor EJ, Highfield MF, Amenta M. Predictors of oncology and hospice nurses' spiritual care perspectives and practices. Applied Nursing Research 1999;12(1):30–37.

123. D'Shano J. Spiritual issues for patients and caregivers. Paper presented at Management of Terminal Illness: An Update, International Hospice Institute, Ann Arbor, MI, July 17–21, 1996.

47 Ethical Considerations

KAREN J. STANLEY and
LAURIE ZOLOTH-DORFMAN

I knew I could count on you to listen to my fears, and I often ran them by you to see if they were tolerable. . . . I always knew I could tell my wife anything, but I worried about her anguish over my suffering. You never stopped fighting for my comfort, and you never forgot that my pain was her pain. Thank you for that.

—A husband writing to his late wife's caregiver

Technologic advances in the diagnosis and treatment of chronic disease have resulted in longer life spans and in many cases an extended dying period. This ability to prolong life has been easily and almost seamlessly integrated into the medical profession's philosophical approach to treating disease as an adversary that can and must be conquered. The value of existence for its own sake, a false sense of security about technology's ability to rescue, and the human need to maintain hope and delay the end of life have obscured and postponed the inevitable need to confront critical issues.

Solomon and colleagues[1] demonstrated that physicians frequently recognized that they were overtreating patients at the end of life but did not know how to stop. It has become increasingly clear that the ability to prolong life has outpaced medical, philosophical, bioethical, and societal efforts to reach a value-based consensus on the goals of and criteria for care across the illness continuum. Ethical dilemmas on macro- and microlevels emerge daily as the debate on extending life versus postponing death continues. Nowhere is this more clear than in the palliative care arena, where decisions about life-supporting and life-ending interventions are made on a daily basis.

In the midst of this "white noise," palliative care as a viable and worthwhile choice for those at the end of life is often obscured by the focus on technology. From a societal perspective, demographic trends separate the generations, and cultural norms may no longer validate caring for one's aging family members in the home setting. Consequently, many individuals and families have not lived with or cared for a dying person. A generation that has no practical or emotional experience with the act of dying is bound to be uncomfortable with decisions that must be made and insecure about delivering care at home. Thus, patients and families continue to choose interventions that can only be delivered in the acute care setting versus a death at home under the care of a family member or significant other.[2]

Decisions regarding truth-telling and informed consent, withholding and/or withdrawing treatment, the definition of ordinary versus extraordinary medical intervention, and the right to assistance in ending one's life because of an unacceptable health condition are becoming further removed from those individuals most effected by the decisions. The argument is persuasive that these issues must be addressed through conversations, debates, and discussion groups in order to clarify individual and societal rights regarding end-of-life care. The inability to agree upon a health care decision making paradigm that allows the expression of diverse values endangers the individual's right to make personal choices about health care.

The rising costs of medical care have introduced another dilemma central to the whole spectrum of debate. The allocation of health care resources described as finite suggests that there can be a limit to medical intervention. The demand that society bear the cost of every possible medical intervention returns the debate to the most basic of issues. Are there circumstances such that existence is no longer intrinsically valuable? Whose values should drive the goals of care? How should these decisions be made, and by whom?[3]

These debates largely began with first cases in which patients demanded, first to their doctors, and then to the courts, to be rescued from the technological imperative. Karen Ann Quinlan's family contested her life on a ventilator, asking that this "artificial" but life-sustaining intervention be removed.[4] Nancy Cruzan's family requested that a feeding tube delivering enteral nutrition be discontinued.[5] These kinds of cases, in which the patient's wishes were not known or documented and/or in which patients and families' wishes were not honored without resorting to the courts, were common in the 1970s and 1980s. The ongoing public dialogue and legal activity sensitized the lay public to the concept of autonomy, and they began to insist upon greater control of health care decision making. The courts redefined what constituted extraordinary treatment and countenanced the wishes of patients and their families if patients were unable to speak for themselves, even to the extent that life-sustaining treatment could be withdrawn.[4–5]

Our abilities to understand current legal statutes, comprehend ethical discourse, and clarify our personal philosophies can be strengthened by a review of ethical methods and terminology. Nursing cannot be isolated from bioethical conflicts, and, in fact, has significant responsibility in understanding and articulating an ethical rationale for decision making and consequent actions.

TRADITIONAL METHODS OF ETHICS

Ethics asks these questions: What is the right act, the good human moral gesture, and what makes it so? What is the meaning of a good life and how is it made? How is justice best achieved among competing moral appeals? Who ought people to be, and how ought they to treat others, and what are the criteria for knowing such things? Ethics seeks to logically justify choices for right behavior, rules, and activities, particularly in situations that challenge established norms of behavior, or require new paradigms for judging behavior. It is this understanding of ethics as a methodology that distinguishes it from morality, rules of proper conduct, or descriptions of cultural norms.[6] In its normative capacity, ethics is an applied theory for the practice of medicine (bioethics), and the conduct of research, business, and political actions.

Ethical inquiry, in its interpretation of any act—for example, "that is the right thing to do"—traditionally has evaluated (*1*) the moral agent and their character; (2) the motive for the act itself; or (3) the effect of the action on others, with the assumption that humans are rational beings with the ability to justify their actions. While historically relying on sociability, accountability, conscience, and rationality, certain assumptions are currently being challenged. Can there be a single standard for rightness of action in a world so profoundly diverse? Can there be, if not agreement on the definitions of a good action, agreement on a common language of ethics?

The various ethical methods[7] have emerged at specific historic periods and are shaped by the culture, class, and gender of the theorists. At best, each is useful as a starting place in defining our approach to ethical dilemmas.

Virtue theory, the study of character attributes necessary for the achievement of a good life, was developed in the Greek philosophic tradition. The virtues described as good include courage, loyalty, and civic friendship and are developed through training and/or role modeling a virtuous person's behavior. The theory was expanded to include compassion, merging the Greek ideal with Christian philosophy. The arena of palliative care and its emphasis on caring, kindness, and respect for another person (virtuous attributes) is well suited to this methodological approach.

Deontological ethics focuses on rules and motives for behavior. It argues that certain qualities innate to a human being or a social order require specific obligations or duties. These obligations can be based in God's law, as in rabbinic text, with its emphasis on a life of commands and obligations to those commands, or in essential unconditional imperatives whose moral worth is to be found in the rule itself—for example, Kant's[8] imperative never to lie. This approach would incorporate the bioethical requisites to "do no harm" (the principle of nonmaleficence) or to "do that which is good" (the principle of beneficence).

Consequentialism is based in the nineteenth-century utilitarian philosophic tradition. The virtue of a behavior bears a direct relationship to its outcome. In contrast to deontological theories, which are rooted in commitments, essential obligations, or promises, consequentialist thinkers argue that assessment of a right action should be based on the possible outcomes of that action. In this theory, individual rights are more questionable, and individual freedoms depend on the outcome for the general good, the good for the greatest number,[9] or the avoidance of harm to the most.[10] This approach would argue that a dying individual's right to autonomous choice about assisted death is superseded by concern for society as a whole and the fear of imposing assisted death on those who do not wish for that outcome.

ETHICS AND PALLIATIVE CARE

An examination of ethical issues in palliative care requires an articulation of the standard to which all practice is compared. Ethical dilemmas surface as those comparisons draw attention to the inadequacies of current practice. Multiple perspectives on the essentials of palliative care are available, and each addresses important issues. However, in order for an ethical standard to be meaningful, it must reflect a comprehensive approach that simultaneously allows for each individual's particular needs. The incredible spectrum of requisites from the most basic of physical care concerns to the broad issues of existential distress is reflective of the daunting ethical responsibilities integral to palliative care.

Cassell[11] succinctly describes health care's ethical obligations as accountability for diagnosis and treatment plans made in terms of the patient rather than the disease, balancing quality versus quantity of life, and minimizing suffering for the patient and family. Ferrell's[12] quality-of-life model identifying the essential components of physical, psychological, social, and spiritual well-being is comprehensively reflected in a "paradigm of compassionate care" authored by the Supportive Care of the Dying Coalition. The Coalition, founded in 1995 by the Catholic Health Association and five Catholic health care systems across the country, has summarized their recommendations in a listing of the rights of the terminally ill.[13] This paradigm translates our larger obligations into specific accountabilities and can serve as a "checklist" for any health care professional caring for persons at the end of life. See Table 47–1.

The need for improving care at the end of life remains a constant in the midst of any ethically focused discussion. The results of the landmark SUPPORT study,[14] which examined how people died, were discouraging. The majority of people died in the hospital, often alone and uncomfortable, while receiving medical intervention they did not want. The current inadequacy of formal professional training[15–18] and the subsequent lack of a cadre of health care profession-

Table 47–1. Rights of the Terminal Patient

The Dying Person Can Expect to
1. Be treated with respect and dignity
2. Be given all necessary information in an honest manner
3. Be the primary decision maker (or choose a surrogate) concerning care, without fear of judgement from others
4. Be cared for by a compassionate, knowledgeable, and interdisciplinary team that provides excellent comfort care for the patient and family
5. Receive holistic, compassionate, skillful care through the trajectory of illness as goals transition from aggressive to terminal care
6. Be able to express emotional and religious or spiritual needs in the context of cultural values
7. Receive optimal and effective pain and symptom management
8. Have help from and for his or her family, friends, caregivers, and significant others in accepting death
9. Die with peace and dignity in the presence of those who have been faithful to them

Source: see Franey, 1996, reference 13.

als with palliative care expertise[19–22] impede excellence in end-of-life care. The professional's ethical obligation to provide excellent physical and psychosocial care is compromised by this lack of knowledge.

These variables have contributed to a decline in the public's historic belief in the integrity of the medical care system and in the confidence that the physician "knows best." The health care team is increasingly being held accountable for the delivery of skilled palliative care. Patients and their families are asking for the information necessary to make informed decisions and the right to be involved in the decision making process.[23]

Ironically, as this higher standard of accountability for quality care has emerged, end-of-life care is shifting from the inpatient to the home setting. Patients in the acute-care setting, including those who are no longer candidates for active medical intervention, are now being discharged home requiring more complex care. As a result, patients and their families are assuming responsibility for care that was previously delivered by health care professionals.

Demographic mobility, separation and divorce, and decreasing accountability for the care of elderly parents have changed the definition of family and the availability of support systems. Adequate caregivers for dying patients may not be readily available when spouses have predeceased them; adult children are geographically distant and dependent on dual incomes; and/or the primary caregiver also has health problems. Palliative medicine practitioners are ethically challenged to provide safe care in the ambulatory setting via education, support, and close supervision of the patient and caregivers.

The realities of the current health care delivery system have placed significant responsibility on nursing. Home health, hospice, and extended care facilities rely heavily on nursing assessment, intervention, and presence to ensure a high standard of comfort care. The profoundly existential issues that are the essence of palliative care can be double-edged swords. While presenting valuable caring opportunities, they may simultaneously generate ethical conflict. For nurses, those conflicts reflect differences in perspective from those of the patient, family, and/or other members of the health care team and occur, ironically, in the context of both providing care that may preserve and/or lengthen life or, conversely, hasten and/or end life.

Case Study: George, a Man Who Felt "His Whole Life Was Before Him"

George, a man in his mid-forties, was diagnosed with multiple myeloma, and the treatment regimen had not slowed the progress of the disease. As he began to deteriorate, he demanded that chemotherapy continue despite the healthcare team's strongly held opinion that it would not serve him well. The Clinical Nurse Specialist (CNS) caring for him understood his desire to be cured and grieved that it was not possible. She had been the nurse administering the chemotherapy and believed she was harming him. One night very late, George was open to conversation. The CNS and George had a frank discussion about the dilemma at hand. She spoke of quality of life, time at home with his family, and finishing up personal business as valuable goals. He spoke of the future that could not be. The two of them made a list of possible opportunities for George. He was discharged home the following day after talking at length with his physician. The CNS continued to see him at home and supported him as he made his way through the list of "opportunities." He died, knowing that he had accomplished his goals.

Ethical dilemmas emerge across the spectrum of care as nurses endeavor to provide the best possible symptom management, communicate appropriately and honestly with the patient and family, encounter cultural practices that demand a different approach, assist in making decisions to withhold or withdraw treatment, and/or respond to requests for interventions that may conflict with their personal value structures. As each patient and significant other confronts the realities of mortality and fragility, and as each nurse intervenes in the crisis, meaning and shape emerge from those choices made at the bedside. How we decide to act in any particular case is really the measure of how far we are willing to explore alternative diagnoses and treatments and of what we consider appropriate at the end of life.

CHANGING ROLE OF THE NURSE

As the health care delivery system has changed, historic role expectations have been adapted to meet the needs of patients and families, professional staff, and the health care delivery system itself. The multidisciplinary approach common in the palliative care arena requires that each team member contribute to overall excellence in patient care. While historically the traditional nursing role has been to carry out the physician's orders, that expectation has been expanded. The varied sites of palliative care, the nurse's primary role in case management, and the changing parameters of the health care delivery system require that nurses be expert practitioners. Assessment, intervention, evaluation, and reevaluation of symptoms are accepted nursing roles. It is not unusual for nurses to practice autonomously in providing expert symptom management under established standards of care. Nowhere is this clearer than in the hospice setting. It is not unusual for expert nurses to adjust medications and dosages, make multidisciplinary referrals, and engage patients at the most existential of levels as part of a normal day's work.

The enlarged arena of nursing responsibility translates into greater ethical obligations as well. The Task Force on End of Life Care[24] believes that nurses should play a primary role in facilitating self-determination about health care choices, and, in fact, it is not unusual for nurses to be involved in discussing advance directives, prognoses, do-not-resuscitate decisions, and a myriad of other palliative care issues.[25] Distinguishing quality versus quantity of life, providing objective feedback about the patient's current status, articulating outcomes of health care decisions, and offering to be present as health care choices are clarified demonstrates nursing's ability to assume these greater responsibilities.

Case Study: Nursing's Enlarged Role

Mike was an 84-year-old man in blast crisis. He became very ill during a weekend when his oncologist was out of town. The covering physician was prepared to begin the chemotherapy his colleague had ordered although he had hesitations. As he didn't know the patient, he felt uncomfortable in changing what had been agreed upon. The CNS was very concerned that Mike might not understand the whole picture. The high-dose chemotherapy was risky at best and not likely to provide any benefit. She went to his room, introduced herself, and spoke of the realities of the current circumstances. Her anguish at the information essential for informed consent was evident in her face and in the tears in her eyes. Mike and his wife and the nurse held hands as the three of them shed tears of grief. He elected to go home as soon as was possible so that he might spend time with his friends, play a few games of checkers, be with his family.

The opportunity to immerse one's self along with the patient in physical, psychological, social, and spiritual realms is rarely offered as frequently in any other nursing discipline. Establishing a trusting relationship in the midst of a frightening and anxiety-laden time requires effort and a significant investment of one's self but facilitates the transition from that of "kind stranger" to trusted clinician and confidante. This kind of relationship authenticates a partnered experience for addressing ethical issues.

As nurses assume increasing responsibility for the patient's care and well-being, it is important that they continue to hold themselves and each member of the multidisciplinary health care team accountable for the highest standards of ethical behavior. Open and thorough discussions regarding the rationale for care provide an opportunity for all team members to articulate personal values. This can be an opportunity for nurses to role model moral courage. By continuing to articulate concerns about circumstantial realities versus medical intentions and encouraging an ongoing dialogue with the patient/family, the nurse may facilitate the health care team's acknowledgment of its impotence and allow patients greater opportunities for a peaceful and dignified death.

SELECT ETHICAL ISSUES IN PALLIATIVE CARE

Ethical issues in palliative care involve and affect patients and their significant others, health care providers, the health care delivery system, and society as a whole. Issues central to discussion and debate center on concerns about individual autonomy versus societal norms and/or the state's interest; disparity between the patient's goals of care and those of family, friends, and the health care team; inadequacy of communication essential for informed decision making; inconsistency of care across the illness continuum; and the allocation of health care resources across the wellness/illness continuum. These broader issues reveal themselves in disputes regarding the appropriate timing of transition from curative to palliative care; withholding and withdrawing treatment; an individual's right to use personal value-based parameters—for example, quality of life, religious beliefs, or cultural norms—as the ultimate arbitrator of the value of existence; and the right to assisted death.

Death does not seem to visit us "gently." For many patients and families in the palliative care phase on the illness continuum, the simplest of decisions carries significant and often grave consequences. As nurses struggle along with patients and their significant others to make realistic yet comforting decisions, ethical issues are a constant. Nursing's obligations to those facing the end of life cover a wide spectrum of behaviors. Navigating the health care delivery system with its myriad professionals and sites of care can be daunting. Patients and families often lose sight of appropriate goals of therapy as they are cared for by one clinician after another. Some of the most critical nursing interventions are discussions about personal choices, about the type of medical intervention desired, or about ensuring informed consent.

Meaningful conversations cannot occur in the midst of unrelieved symptoms. Nursing must advocate for and contribute to effective pain and symptom management. They must become expert practitioners, hold others accountable for that same standard of excellence, and continue to advocate for the patient until symptoms are satisfactorily managed.

O'Connor[26] asked oncology nurses to identify situations indicative of personal moral and ethical dilemmas. Their responses reflected the normative bioethical principles of autonomy, beneficence, nonmaleficence, fidelity, and truth telling. However, as she reviewed nursing descriptions of moral conflicts in the care of the terminally ill, she categorized certain dilemmas as those of "suffering." Clinical scenarios describing terminal patients who were not allowed to die with dignity, critically ill patients who were resuscitated without a clear understanding of their circumstances; and terminal patients who were kept on life support until they died were identified by nurses as sources of great moral conflict. While the specifics of patient/family wishes regarding care were not identified, what is clear is that nurses experienced moral angst about the rightness of their actions.

Nurses must be involved in discussions regarding (*1*) withholding and withdrawing treatment; (*2*) providing care demanded by patients but deemed inappropriate by the healthcare team; (*3*) patient requests to stop eating or drinking; (*4*) appropriate criteria for sedation to relieve intractable distress; and (*5*) patient requests for assisted death. As central providers in palliative care, nurses must participate in these dialogues if they wish to remain valued members of the health care team and fulfill a primary responsibility of patient advocacy.

Pain and Symptom Management

Optimal pain and symptom management continues to be a priority and one of the most important of ethical issues in palliative care. Patients worry that pain and/or other symptoms will not be well managed[24] and articulate that the physical symptoms are far more stressful than the cancer diagnosis itself.[12] Pain, dyspnea, fatigue, nausea, sedation, and confusion are troublesome.[27] These unmanaged symptoms can strip patients of their dignity, impose tremendous professional and ethical burdens on nurses, and can destroy the quality of life of both the patient and family.[28]

While all symptoms are deserving of the same meticulous attention, pain continues to be the most prevalent of physical symptoms at the end of life. Overwhelming and unrelieved pain can cause anxiety, irritation, restlessness, sleeplessness, depression, fatigue, emotional withdrawal, and existential distress for both patients and caregivers. Its continued presence can provoke patients to request life-ending measures. Unrelieved pain is both an emergency and an ethical dilemma and demands the full attention of the palliative care team until resolved. This dilemma can be even more pronounced in the home care setting where nurses work independently with patients.[29] The standard to which all health care team members must be held is pain relief as defined by the patient. Nursing must assure that barriers to this standard are identified and overcome.

Case Study: Ethical Dimensions of Symptom Management

David had rapidly progressing mesothelioma. He was admitted to the hospital for intensive care secondary to obstipation. The Pain Management Nurse saw him on consultation and found a man in extreme pain with orders on the chart for NSAIDs and for "no narcotics." She determined that he had been previously discharged on an oral opioid without an accompanying bowel regimen. Three weeks of opioid therapy without any kind of laxative had, of course, caused the problem. His physician was reluctant to use opioids for fear of causing the same dilemma. The nurse discussed the use of opioids in tandem with an aggressive bowel regimen and recommended intravenous opioids immediately, titrating to effect, and concurrently titrating an effective bowel regimen.

She spoke to David, who was frantic for any kind of pain relief, of the plan. As she administered the initial dose of intravenous opioid, tears came into his eyes as he relaxed and allowed the medication to relieve the pain. Over the next few days, the opioid was titrated upward, and a bowel regimen that turned out to vary from the norm was instituted. As she prepared David for discharge, he gave her a napkin on which he had drawn a picture of an angel. "That's how I see you," he said. "Thank you for saving me from hell."

While aggressive pain management in terminal patients rarely causes death, the fear that it will do so continues to be a significant ethical barrier to adequate relief. Many nurses are reluctant to administer the analgesic doses necessary to adequately control pain for fear of causing respiratory depression. The Task Force on the Nurse's Role in End-of-Life Decisions[30] position paper regarding pain relief for dying patients states that nurses should not hesitate to use effective doses of analgesics for the proper management of pain in the dying patient, and that upward titration of an opioid to achieve adequate relief, even if life is compromised secondarily, is ethically justified. The Supreme Court in their 1997 ruling that disallowed an individual's right to physician-assisted suicide cogently argued, however, that palliative care may and should be aggressive even if the provision of such care should hasten death.

An ethical responsibility of advocacy emerges as the nurse anticipates and plans for expected sequelae to both the illness and any side effects of prescribed analgesics. Discussing expected symptoms and the plan for managing those symptoms should they occur relieves patients and caregivers and provides an opportunity to articulate concerns, be assured they're known and being addressed, and take comfort in that knowledge. Further advocacy responsibilities include suggesting pharmacologic and nonpharmacologic interventions to other members of the health care team, consulting with the physician for assistance in managing difficult symptoms or side effects, and continuing to attend to those issues until they are satisfactorily resolved.

In O'Connor's[26] study of the ethical/moral experiences of oncology nurses, the themes of suffering, secrets, and struggle emerged. The theme of struggle appeared in 73% of the responses and most often occurred when the physician had less experience in symptom management than did the nurse. A genuine collaborative approach to palliative care requires the acknowledgment that no one team member has exclusive domain over specific areas of knowledge. In the absence of a communal collaborative milieu, nurses must continue to advocate for the very best in pain and symptom management, role-model appropriate analgesic decision making, and should never apologize for what they know.

While less frequent in today's health care system, the use of placebos for the management of cancer pain does still occur. The Oncology Nursing Society has issued a position paper on this issue[31] stating that placebos should not be used to assess or manage cancer pain. Their use is deceitful, harmful to both patients and health care professionals who use them in a dishonest way, and can damage or destroy the nurse–patient relationship. Nurses, as moral agents, have an ethical responsibility to avoid the use of placebos and to assist in establishing institutional policies to prevent their use in pain management.

Issues of Truth-Telling

Effective and ethical communication is central to the highest standards of palliative care. Issues relative to every domain of quality of life—that is, physical, psychological, social, and spiritual—require communication such that goals and expectations can be articulated and those cared for know the comfort that a shared experience provides. Ethical principles, then, are reflected not only in behavior but in language.[32]

Delivering bad news is a reality in the palliative care arena, and truth-telling, while viewed as ethically appropriate behavior, can be troublesome in a multitude of situations. There is little disagreement in western European cultures that autonomous patients have the right to the complete facts about their illness, potential interventions (including risks and benefits), and prognoses in order to make informed decisions. However, the ability to function as an "existential messenger"[32] is far more complex than the verbalization of correct information. Issues such as presenting truthful information without destroying hope to both asked and unasked questions; providing information that has been purposefully "filtered" because of the patient's wishes or cultural background; and confronting other members of the health team who obscure information because of their own fears are not uncommon.

Truth-telling should occur in the context of the patient's wishes and emotional status. The nurse can confirm that the patient is ready to hear difficult news while concurrently giving permission to defer the conversation until greater emotional resources are available and/or family support is present. When difficult questions are asked, one of the authors responds in this manner: "I need to be sure that when you ask what must be very hard questions you want a truthful answer. I am an honest person and would feel I was honoring you by doing so. However, I want to hear from you how you believe these discussions would best be handled."

A reasonable ethical standard requires that patients receive answers to frightening questions as quickly as possible. While conveying distressing news has historically been the physician's domain, the multidisciplinary structure of palliative care allows a modification of these role expectations in deference to the patient's best interests. Patients often question nurses regarding test results that could confirm a life-threatening illness or progression of that illness. It has been common practice for the nurse to refer the patient to the physician at such times. But is it appropriate to ask the patient to wait and, of course, worry until the physician arrives? Is it unfair or unkind to postpone for what seems an interminable period of time answers to questions that carry such grave import? These circumstances offer nursing a unique opportunity. The best possible scenario under such circumstances would be a rapid resolution of the matter. Table 47–2 summarizes recommendations for a collaborative approach to truth-telling. Appropriate follow-up would include offering to be present when the patient discusses the information with others as well as leaving the door open to revisit any of the issues raised.

If the physician cannot be reached or a physician unknown to the patient is on call, and the nurse can answer the questions correctly and appropriately, they should be answered. If the nurse has established a close relationship with the patient, it can be argued that it is reasonable to hear difficult news from someone who is known and trusted. Remaining attentive to the primary goal of allowing the patient access to information as quickly and humanely as possible removes the focus from role issues to that of patient interests. However, nurses should not provide information that has not been verified or feel compelled to answer questions that they are not able to competently address. It is often necessary to provide compassionate understanding of the patient's anxiety regarding undisclosed information, yet defer to the physician to provide the actual information.

Table 47–2. A Collaborative Approach to Truth-Telling

Answering Questions Regarding Diagnostic Results

1. Report the patient's concerns to the physician, emphasizing the urgency of the matter.
2. Determine physician's availability.
3. If unavailable for a significant period, offer to discuss the test results with the patient. If available, plan to be present for follow-up questions and support.
4. Plan with the physician how best to respond regarding the meaning of the diagnostic results and the continued plan of care.
5. Explain to the patient that the physician is not available and is concerned that the information be provided in a timely manner.
6. Ask the patient's permission to discuss the questions asked. If positive, confirm those individuals the patient would like present and ensure they are there.
7. Use language the patient understands, answering all of the questions.
8. Stay present, both emotionally and physically, until the patient feels the conversation has ended.
9. Provide assurances that the physician will be available for further discussion.
10. Provide a detailed description of the discussion in the medical record and speak personally with the physician about the intellectual and emotional responses to the information.

The patient's wishes regarding access to information about the illness, prognosis, progression of the illness, and plans for care trump everyone else's wishes. However, it is not uncommon for members of the health care team to present an inaccurate, obscure, or overly hopeful description of the current physiologic circumstances; ask colleagues on the team to remain positive about outcomes regardless of current realities; or ask that the patient not be told of the current realities. Physicians may write a do-not-resuscitate (DNR) order for a patient without having a previous discussion with the patient and family because they are uncomfortable with the topic or believe that the patient and or family may refuse such a request. DNR orders, which have been upheld by the courts, disallow heroic measures should a patient suffer a cardiopulmonary arrest. They can serve patients well by preventing unwanted and unnecessary interventions, but they may also be improperly and unethically used to unilaterally prevent life-sustaining interventions. In each of the above circumstances it is the perceived physician/nurse power differential that may provoke a sense of impotence in nursing.

The tactic of using technical or purposely obscure language when breaking bad news to a patient is unethical. Patients are confused and unsure and may be reluctant to ask further questions. Family members, in describing communication techniques that are ambiguous, evasive, and elusive, identify these behaviors as contributing markedly to their own uncertainty.[33] If this behavior is indicative of the professional's own anxiety and sense of unease, it should be openly discussed. Nurses can act as both witness to and translator of the clinical conversation by articulating the inherent lack of understanding that occurs when clinical jargon is used to frame and distance an event.

If other members of the health care team request that the patient not be told, the nurse should ask for the rationale prompting the request. If self-protection or discomfort is evident, it is appropriate to speak to the ethic of truth-telling and offer to assist with the task. This predicament can be particularly difficult for nursing and requires a strong and sure knowledge of informed consent, advocacy skills, and a genuine sense of the moral weight of truth.

Family or friends may ask that the patient be "protected" from distressing news. A promise to keep silent would interfere with the nurse's truth-telling ethic and potentially compromise the relationship with the patient. However, the request should prompt a frank discussion with concerned family members in a quiet and protected environment. Family concerns and the adverse consequences of well-meaning attempts to protect the patient can be addressed. Potential solutions would include "checking in" with the patient about the amount of information wanted in the presence of a family member and offering the services of any member of the health care team to assist the family in difficult discussions with the patient.

Case Study: The Dilemma of Protecting the Patient

Fran was 64 when she was diagnosed with widespread ovarian carcinoma. Her family asked the health care team to avoid the term "cancer," as they argued that it would most certainly destroy all hope. Despite repeated conversations with the family that morning, they were adamant that this would be what she wanted. Fran had not been part of any conversation about her wishes, and the team was uncomfortable about the family's demands. Her family left to get breakfast, and the physician was writing treatment orders, still deliberating how he might best honor Fran and her family. The nurse was starting an intravenous line and assisting her in getting comfortable. Fran grabbed the nurse's hand and said, "I know there's something terribly wrong. I see those fake smiles and hear those words that don't make sense. Surely you can tell me what's wrong with me. I want to know, and I want to know now." Her grip was tight on the nurse's hand. The nurse looked into her eyes and replied "You have cancer of the ovary. Your doctor is planning treatment for you right now. I'll go and get him so that he can give you the details and you can ask as many questions as you want." Oddly enough, she visibly relaxed and said, "I just wanted the truth. It's frightening to be alone in a lie."

An equally complex dilemma arises when the patient's cultural norms are such that it is inappropriate to discuss diagnosis and prognosis. The Oncology Nursing Society[34] lists "access to culturally competent care provided by culturally competent caregivers" (p. 1) as a primary right of cancer patients. Clinicians, accustomed to the western model of informed consent, feel unsettled when patients abrogate autonomy to family members. However, asking individuals from culturally diverse groups to express their wishes may seem not only bewildering but also unnecessary, distasteful, or even immoral.[35] Cultural values may dictate that the family receive the frightening information and filter it for the patient. While it is ethically important to honor cultural dictates, it is equally important to query the patient regarding the information desired. Health care team members can wrongly assume that a patient's heritage reflects stereotypical behaviors and beliefs. In fact, individual variation is the norm.

HONORING PATIENTS' WISHES

The SUPPORT Study,[14] which examined how and where people died and if their deaths indicated previously expressed wishes, reflected the gaps in meeting the dictates of the Patient Self-Determination Act (PSDA).[36] The PSDA mandated that health care professionals educate patients about advance directives at the time of hospital admission and document their existence in the medical record. As previously mentioned, advance directives were not common, but most important, physicians routinely did not discuss end-of-life issues nor did they know patients' preferences for resuscitative measures.

Informed consent in end-of-life care is imperative for reasons beyond the fact that it is a basic legal requirement. Patients and families considering refusal of further treatment should be told of the consequences of their choice, just as they are informed of the benefits and risks of other interventions. Patients and families encountering the withdrawal of treatment may not have been fully informed of the risks and benefits of the therapy at the time it began, nor were they told of the possibility that treatment could be discontinued if no longer helpful.

When burdens of continued treatment are known, patients with decision making capacity may refuse or stop unwanted medical treatment even if such refusal may result in their deaths.[37–38] Those who lack capacity have the same rights, but those rights may be exercised through an authorized surrogate decision-maker.[39–40] This right may be ethically burdensome for nurses when they believe further intervention would markedly benefit the patient. In these circumstances, nurses are obligated to (*1*) reaffirm informed consent, (*2*) support the patient in the right to make personal choices, and (*3*) ensure that the patient is not abandoned, emotionally or otherwise.

The medical, legal, bioethical, and consumer advocacy communities are in agreement that support for and encouragement of individual preparation of written directives for health care would serve patients well and prevent needless tragedies. The articulation of health care preferences and identification of a surrogate agent to advocate for those preferences can reduce questions and conflict about what a patient would want, provide direction to the health care team, and relieve the burden of difficult decision making from family members.

However, a low completion rate of written (advance) directives as well as their inability to direct care in actual clinical situations[41–44] continues to be the norm. Individuals may choose to defer to the health care team for appropriate decision making, be reluctant to contemplate the issues at all, argue that they will complete a written directive when "it is really needed," or refuse to commit themselves to a specific course of action. When actually available in a time of crisis, the language may be too obscure to direct the course of care, or the choices challenged by the patient's family or members of the health care team.

It is not surprising, then, that a patient's values and wishes can be compromised in a multitude of ways, both intentional and unintentional. The inability to affirm a patient's care preferences can include, but is not limited to, (*1*) providing care that one believes the patient would want based on knowledge of that individual's value structure; (*2*) changing to a pattern of care that one considers appropriate but that does not reflect the patient's wishes when family members have left the clinical setting; (*3*) allowing family members to speak for a timid patient who has privately expressed health care choices that are at odds with the family; and (*4*) ignoring known preferences and/or honoring the preferences of assertive family members when the patient can no longer articulate personal wishes. In each of these instances, nurses have an ethical obligation to speak to the truths that exist and to hold all health care providers accountable to those truths. If necessary, the nurse may refer the case to the institution's bioethics committee.

Abandonment

Meaningful relationships require continued presence. The ability to remain available in the midst of considerable anguish, fear, sorrow, or profound grief requires tremendous courage. Nurses must be willing to set aside personal biographies, convictions about truth, and professional privilege. If nurses allow professional attitudes to provide distance from the intimacy of the experience, their role is diminished and the relationships lose meaning. They must be able to function in a partnership with patients, recognizing and acknowledging that one of the most meaningful parts of nursing's response to the dying experience is continued presence.[32]

Patients fear abandonment in response to decisions that conflict with those of the health care team. The idea of losing those whom one has known and trusted at a time of crisis can be overwhelmingly fearful. Abandonment can be very subtle. When a patient or their advocate chooses a course of care that is discomforting or unacceptable—that is, refusing treatment, stopping active treatment, demanding treatment deemed useless by the health care team, or asking for removal of life-prolonging interventions—health care professionals may withdraw in a multitude of ways. Time spent with the patient may become less frequent and direct verbal engagement limited. Each of these behaviors may be viewed by the patient and family as emotional withdrawal at the very least and abandonment at the very worst.

The ethical dilemma is evident: How can one balance one's own moral dictates with the patient's right to autonomous behavior and remain present in the process? Nurses are particularly vulnerable. They may feel "caught in the middle" when they are expected to provide care in circumstances that clash with their personal values. While wanting to remain loyal to the patient, they may be conflicted by (*1*) providing care they deem futile or inappropriate—for example, continuing artificial life support in the spite of a diagnosis of brain death; (*2*) following orders to provide care that is morally unacceptable—for examle, discontinuing hydration or nutrition or removing a patient from a ventilator; and/or (*3*) knowing how to respond to patients who make requests that they cannot honor—for example, a request for assisted death.

According to the Code for Nurses,[45] nurses may morally refuse to participate in care, but only on the grounds of patient advocacy or moral objection to a specific type of intervention. While it is ethically imperative to assure the patient/family unit that their decisions will be respected and they will not be abandoned if their goals differ from that of the health care team, nurses may remove themselves from the patient's direct care while simultaneously continuing to be available to the patient. These behaviors reflect a continuous partnership and acknowledge the importance of an ongoing personal commitment to caring and problem solving.[46]

Case Study: A Conflict in Care

Christine and her nurse became very close over the weeks while she was being treated for acute myelogenous leukemia. She was hopeful to receive a bone marrow transplant (BMT), which she believed would cure her. As she was 55, the health care team had reservations about her ability to withstand the rigors of a BMT but did not discuss those reservations with her. The task at hand was to get her into remission and ready for the transplant. A week after discharge from the hospital and successful completion of the induction therapy, she returned to the hospital with recurrent disease. When her nurse walked into the room, Christine looked at her face and said, "I'm going to die, aren't I? How will it be?" The nurse told her that another course of chemotherapy would be given, that the odds for cure had decreased markedly with this rapid recurrence, and that she might very well die either before or during the bone marrow transplant. She described complications that would occur if the cancer did not respond to treatment and how those symptoms would be managed. The leukemia did not respond to reinduction chemotherapy, and one night when it was quiet on the unit, Christine asked the nurse to sit with her. She seemed so fragile and frightened. The nurse sat beside her on the bed and held her. Christine said, "I can't do this anymore. I'm so tired. Please give me a shot to put me to sleep forever." The nurse was anguished at the request, for she had promised Christine she would never let her suffer. She felt cowardly and dishonorable in her refusal to provide the medication. The nurse's dilemma centered on her inability to honor her promise, the current state law that did not permit assisted death, and her mixed feelings about what would be appropriate in those circumstances. She promised Christine she would stay with her and make sure she was comfortable. The nurse asked if she should call someone else to be there with Christine, but she declined and died that night, never having spoken another word to the nurse.

This case brings attention to multiple issues that might have led to a better outcome for the patient, family, and health care team. Earlier and frank discussions with the patient and family about the course of the illness, the prognosis, and treatment expectations and realities might have allowed both the patient and family the opportunity to plan for death in a more comprehensive and meaningful way. These discussions might have presented opportunities for understanding the patient's perspective on assisted death and the circumstances that might trigger such a request. Finally, It would have allowed the health care team an opportunity to be clear about the kind of support they could offer.

Futility/Withdrawal of Treatment

Decisions in the clinical world are increasingly made under a new kind of pressure. With nearly every health care delivery institution facing financial constraints, health care providers are experiencing the tensions of "limits" imposed on comfortably established, professional standards of care. A powerful new vocabulary, that of "medical futility," has entered the discourse.

Health care professionals often find patient expectations and desires to be unreasonable, sometimes impossible, and on occasion, limitless. Nurses may find themselves searching for unilateral solutions to complex problems when historically they have acted in tandem with the patient and family. They, too, may feel that a patient's continued treatment serves no purpose, that increasingly scarce resources are being "wasted." They question what good comes from their actions and ask if these interventions may be refused. Influenced by outcome-based practice standards, reimbursement formulas, and a growing disenchantment with "hi-tech" interventions, these dilemmas evolve into questions of whether to withhold or withdraw treatment.

But it is precisely at this moment that patients and families insist on continuation of aggressive treatment and question the health care system's motives, wondering if the declaration of futility is a cover for cost containment or racial and/or other prejudice as they feel increasingly alienated and even abandoned. The dilemma is becoming increasingly common: Is it ever ethical to withdraw care deemed futile by the staff in the face of an intense patient or family desire to continue? A description of the nurse's role in such circumstances can only follow a clearer definition of futility, and an understanding of the legal and ethical dictates supporting the clinician's right to withdraw treatment.

Many definitions of medical futility have been proposed. Some have defined a futile treatment as one that does not serve a valid goal of medical practice (a standard of medical judgment),[47] and that it is the normative professional responsibility of the medical team to decide if desired treatment courses are realistic. Some have argued for a more precise definition, suggesting that a treatment is futile when it is unsuccessful more than 99% of the time (a standard of efficacy). Still others have indicated that treatment outside accepted community standards could be understood as futile (a standard of communal evaluation).

Rubin[48] suggests that futility exists when the treatment does not achieve the patient's intended goal. As Younger[49] noted early in the debate, futility is a concept that makes no sense when standing alone but is rather an evaluative judgment made on the basis of the worth of possible goals. The value of a treatment would depend on the meaning of the goals and who was empowered to select them, and that same treatment would be futile only if the goals could not be met. With that understanding, the contemporary futility debate could be understood in terms of power: the power to define the acceptable use of medical interventions, to determine whether and under what conditions limits can be appropriately set, and to negotiate the terms of the provider–patient relationship.

The demands of the current health care system ask us to assess a treatment's relative futility even though we have not agreed upon its definitions or determined criteria against which it can be measured. Further, we are asked to develop practice standards and institutional policies even though we do not have not a vision of how to set appropriate limits. Worst of all, we are offered the illusory hope that complex ethical dilemmas can be resolved merely by identifying treatments as futile and concluding that they need not be provided or paid for. Reframing the futility discussion in the language of goals is one of the most effective ways of addressing the moral appeals at stake in conflicts between patients and their providers, and it is the most significant intervention we think clinicians and ethicists can make when the new language of futility emerges as a way of talking about a case.

In the majority of situations in which death is imminent, consensus is reached and life-sustaining interventions are not provided. Conflicts in which questions of relative value arise do not represent straightforward issues of futility. Examples might include life-sustaining interventions for patients in a persistent vegetative state, resuscitation efforts in life-threatening illness, use of chemotherapy in patients with extensive, metastatic cancer, and the use of antibiotics or artificial hydration/nutrition for patients who are in advanced stages of an illness.

The concept of medical futility is more commonly invoked when values conflict. Those arguing from the provider's perspective feel that the health care team should neither offer nor provide therapy that is unlikely to work, or will only diminish quality of life. To do otherwise, they believe, would be to violate professional integrity, offer false hope to patients and families, and inflict harm on patients without the possibility of benefit. Others would disagree, wondering why the provider's values should override patient and family values, especially when those values are religiously based. Thus, the disagreements that arise are fundamentally moral and not medical in nature.

When a claim of medical futility arises, the investigation should first identify the goals and intentions of treatment and determine whose goals seem to be taking precedence. This offers a more productive method for discussion of concerns and the mutual exploration of goals and their meaning. Finally, it encourages the health care team to consider their ability and commitment to meet goals that differ from their own. If lack of communication is part of the problem, assessing and responding to misunderstandings by clarifying diagnosis and prognosis, eliminating medical jargon, discussing what "do everything" actually means, and checking for mistaken notions of legal requirements can be extremely helpful. Interpersonal issues such as distrust, grief, guilt, intrafamily issues, secondary gains, differences in values, and religious beliefs may contribute to the conflict and should be explored. The nurse, who is more likely to have developed a close relationship with the patient and family, should certainly be involved at every stage of the futility discussion. Opportune moments may arise when other members of the health care team are not available, and that particular nurse–patient conversation may help to resolve the conflict.

The withdrawal or withholding of life-sustaining treatment is very often at the heart of medical futility conflicts. Withholding or withdrawing life-sustaining medical interventions is considered neither homicide[50] nor suicide.[37] Courts have drawn a distinction between purposefully causing a patient's death and allowing a patient to die when life-sustaining measures are withdrawn. Courts have upheld the validity of do-not-resuscitate and other treatment limitation orders,[51] and there are no limits on the type of treatment that may be withheld or withdrawn. Ventilator withdrawal[4,37] and the withholding or withdrawing of parenteral nutrition and hydration[5] may occur under the same conditions as any other form of medical treatment.

The moment of nursing that perhaps demands the most elegant level of practice is the moment when patients and families decide to forgo aggressive care and elect a palliative approach. Patients and their families may need support for such difficult decisions and often require repetitive feedback about medical data, review of past therapies, reconsideration of any potential interventions, and, in some instances, retrospective permission to make that particular choice. Nurses have witnessed the dilemma of physician withdrawal when the medical team painfully confronts its inability to cure. The turn to palliation is not a defeat for the nurse, but rather an intensification and revaluing of the skills of nursing. The gifts of deferring to the patient's story, continued presence in the face of fear and anguish, and emotional intimacy involve interaction on multiple intellectual and emotional levels and enrich the lives of both the patient and the nurse.[32] In this context nothing is futile—no touch, no glance, no offer of assistance, and no silence held in common. The worth of the interaction is always based on nurturing and caring as an end goal. It is a stance that will require fierce protection and defense.

Despite legal support for withholding or withdrawal of life-sustaining treatment at the patient/proxy's request, the health care team can find itself at odds with patients and families who become suspicious, fearful, and often unmoving in their opposition when the subject is broached. Ethical differences exist in any pluralistic society, especially one in which resources are increasingly scarce. The desire to struggle aggressively with death is one of the most deeply rooted moral choices an individual can make, and there is little consensus about those choices, as evidenced by the right-to-life and assisted death debates.

While there are circumstances in which life-sustaining treatment can be stopped over the objections of patients and families—for example, when a patient meets the defined criteria for brain death—consensual standards should be developed after the fullest possible public discussion. As there is no authoritative legal definition of medical futility or clear resolution in the courts as to its meaning or jurisdiction,[48] the critical voices of physicians, nurses, and patients must be heard. The claims of medical futility cannot be made in order to transfer unwilling patients gratuitously into hospice settings as a cost-saving scheme.

The discussion cannot occur in a piecemeal fashion, at the bedsides of the most vulnerable or in the closed board-

Table 47–3. A Due-Process Approach to Futility Situations

A Paradigm for Preventing and Resolving Conflicts

1. Attempt to negotiate an understanding between patient, surrogate, and healthcare team as to what constitutes futile care in advance of the actual conflict.
2. Establish joint decision-making as the goal. Use the assistance of consultants as appropriate.
3. If disagreement persists, suggest use of other consultants, colleagues and the institution's ethics committee. This provides the maximum possible place for patient autonomy.
4. If institutional review supports the patient's position and the physician is uncomfortable with the decision made, transfer of care may be arranged.
5. If review supports the healthcare team's position and the patient/surrogate disagrees with the decision, transfer to another institution/provider can be arranged if both parties agree and if possible.
6. If no receiving institution can be found, the problem remains unsolved and further discussion must continue.

Source: American Medical Association (1999). Education for Physicians on End-of-Life Care.

rooms of individual institutions. Opening a communal debate rather than closing it with simplistic unilateral solutions is the only defensible decision making process, and the only way out of the futility challenge. Bioethics committees allow for such discourse, and their approach could become the template for (*1*) discussion of difficult cases, (*2*) justly evaluating new outcome data, (*3*) allowing for cultural differences in the selection of goals, and (*4*) facilitating end-of-life decision making. This would allow for a forum of careful debate before the inevitable crisis emerges, and for an appeals process that would permit a more detailed account of the decision making process. Whenever possible, joint decision making should occur. If resolution is not forthcoming after careful and deliberate discussion, a step-by-step process of communication and problem solving has been suggested by the American Medical Association.[52] See Table 47–3 for a "due process to futility situations" paradigm.

Case Study: Ethical Dilemmas When the Goals of Treatment Are Not Fully Explored

Mark was 42 when a virulent form of lymphoma recurred. He was admitted to the intensive care unit. He insisted he wanted everything done and was adamant that he meant everything. His wife Sue supported him in that decision, but as the hours passed and he became increasingly ill, she started to question their decision. Sue spoke at length with the nurse about their personal history. This was her second marriage, her first husband having died of cancer. Mark had promised Sue that he would never leave her, that he would not die before she did. The nurse gently suggested that Sue might want to consider giving Mark permission to die. Sue agonized for hours about that action but ultimately decided she must tell him. Sue could see he was going to die despite the high-tech interventions, and she wanted him to have a peaceful death. She did ultimately talk with Mark, and most of the interventions were discontinued after that conversation. The next day, as Sue held him, he died.

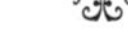

Assisted Death

The profound existential issues innate to end-of-life care are no more evident than in discussions regarding assisted death. The adult patient's right to control health care interventions has historically allowed individuals to refuse to seek medical care, refuse recommended care, stop hydration and nutrition and other prescribed recommendations, and/or forgo or discontinue life support. These historic methods of ending life sooner have become commonplace. They are legally and also morally acceptable to the majority of practitioners and, in fact, have become a standard of practice for patients and the health care team alike.[53–54]

The ability to exercise autonomy in health care decision making as reflected in these circumstances has engendered questions in both the medical and lay communities as to the "rightness" of extending autonomous behavior to other practices that have been described as humane interventions that would stop and/or prevent intractable suffering or unacceptably diminished quality of life. Certainly the courts have supported the individual's right to refuse or withdraw from life-sustaining treatment.[4,37,50–51]

It has been argued that withholding/withdrawing and/or refusing treatment are no different, from a consequential perspective—from physician-assisted suicide (PAS), voluntary active euthanasia, or sedation for intractable distress in the dying.[55–59] Others have argued that there is a distinct moral difference.[60–61] While a small part of the process of improving care for all dying patients and their families, the current and intense focus on the quality and scope of end-of-life care has added fuel to the debate about physician-assisted suicide. Scholars, lawyers, ethicists, health care personnel, religious organizations, and consumer organizations have taken varied stances as reflected in Table 47–4.[61–68]

Medical organizations such as the American Medical Association and American Society of Clinical Oncology have published position statements opposing PAS, as has the multidisciplinary American Pain Society. The American Nurses Association has based its position statement on assisted suicide from the philosophical stance of respect for patients that is extensively explicated in the Code for Nurses with Interpretive Statements.[45] Their position statement[69] maintains that nursing may not deliberately act to terminate the life of any person, that it has a social contract with society that is based on trust. It further states that while the nursing profession and its individual practitioners are committed to the patient's right to self-determination, nurses are not obligated to comply with all requests:

AMERICAN NURSE'S ASSOCIATION
POSITION ON PHYSICIAN-ASSISTED SUICIDE

The American Nurses Association (ANA) believes that the nurse should not participate in assisted suicide. Such an act is in violation of the *Code for Nurses with Interpretive*

Table 47–4. The Debate Concerning Assisted Death

Argument	Pro	Con
Liberty Interest vs. State's Interest	There is equal protection under the law that allows the right to refuse or withdraw treatment and to commit suicide.	There is constitutional power to override certain rights in order to protect citizens from irrevocable acts
Autonomy	Every competent person has the right to make momentous decisions based on personal convictions	Human beings are the stewards but not the absolute masters of the gift of life
Quality of Care	Removing legal bans would enhance the opportunity for excellent end-of-life care for all patients secondary to statutory requirements that the very best in palliative care has been provided.	The aim of medicine should be to facilitate a death that is pain free but also a human experience. A good natural death contributes value to the community.
Nonmaleficence	From the patient's perspective, there is no difference between ending life by providing a lethal prescription and by stopping treatment that prolongs life.	The role of the nurse has been to promote, preserve, and protect human life. Assisted death violates the oath to "do no harm" and destroys trust between the patient and nurse.
Beneficence	More patients could benefit from relief available illegally to many people who have strong relationships with physicians willing to risk assisting them to die.	A misdiagnosis of the illness, inadequate assessment of competence, and/or pressure from family or the physician might place patients in jeopardy.
Slippery Slope	The states could adopt regulations to insure informed, competent, and freely made decisions.	While assisted death might initially be restricted to competent, terminal patients, in time many other kinds of patients might be assisted to die in more aggressive ways.

Source: Adapted from Angell M, 1997; Annas GJ, 1997; Brock DW, 1992; Brody HR, 1992; Dworkin et al., 1997; Ethics Advisory Council, 1995; Pelligrino ED, 1992; Weir RF, 1992.

Statements (Code for Nurses) and the ethical traditions of the profession. Nurses, individually and collectively, have an obligation to provide comprehensive and compassionate end-of-life care which includes the promotion of comfort and the relief of pain, and at times, foregoing life-sustaining treatments.

Oregon voters approved PAS in 1994, and the appeal process ultimately sent the question to the United States Supreme Court. In June of 1997, the Supreme Court ruled that an individual does not have a Constitutional right to assistance with dying, nor does a physician have an obligation to provide that assistance.[70] Subsequent to the Supreme Court decision, in the fall of 1997 the citizens of Oregon again voted and legalized PAS with a 60%/40% majority.[71]

Terminally ill residents of Oregon are able to receive prescriptions from their physicians for lethal medications that may then be self-administered.[71] Criteria to protect citizens from coerced or involuntary action include (*1*) adults able to make and communicate decisions; (*2*) terminal illness expected to lead to death within six months; (*3*) one written and two oral requests separated by a two-week period; (*4*) confirmation of the terminal diagnosis, prognosis, and capability by both the patient's primary physician and a consultant; and (*5*) referral to counseling if either believes that the patient's judgment is impaired by depression or some other psychiatric disorder. The primary physician is also responsible for discussing all feasible alternatives with the patient—that is, comfort care, hospice care, and pain-control options.

Many reasons have been postulated as to what might instigate a request for physician-assisted suicide. The inadequacy of pain relief,[72–74] inadequate recognition and management of depression,[75–77] or inadequate management of other symptoms such as dyspnea, intractable nausea, and vomiting or diarrhea[59,78] are believed to be primary etiologies. In Oregon,[79] patient requests were more likely attributed to loss of autonomy and/or loss of control of bodily functions. In the first year's experience with PAS in Oregon, only one patient expressed concern about pain. This may reflect advances in pain management in Oregon, which ranks among the top five states in per capita use of morphine for medical purposes.[80]

Patients who have requested assisted suicide cite intolerance of physical disintegration, dependence, being a burden, extreme fatigue, and lack of meaning.[72] Those with access to a lethal dose of medication report that it provides them the freedom and reassurance to continue living knowing that they can escape if and when they choose.[81–82] In the midst of the ongoing deliberation, health care providers daily face ethical dilemmas as to the most appropriate response to patients who ask for such assistance. The spectrum of responses serves only to highlight the intensity of the dilemma. The moral weight of the decision despite legal countenance was evident in Oregon's first year of legalized PAS. Six patients had been refused by one or more physicians before finding someone who would assist them. The 14 physicians who did assist patients to die expressed diverse feelings about the emotional toll that was taken, feelings of isolation, and frustration that they were unable to share the experiences with colleagues for fear of being ostracized.

Suarez-Almazor, Belzile, and Bruera[83] surveyed the attitudes of the Canadian general public and physicians about euthanasia and physician-assisted suicide. They found that a slight majority of the public and terminally ill patients (50%–60%) agreed with their legalization while most physicians (60%–80%) opposed it. Interestingly, attitudes were markedly polarized, with sentiments strongly held at each end of the spectrum. Wolfe et al.,[84] in examining the stability of attitudes regarding PAS and euthanasia among oncology patients, physicians, and the general public, found a growing disparity between the public and the medical profession. As laypersons are becoming more comfortable with the concept, physicians are growing less supportive. This trend cannot help but engender further ethical conflict in end-of-life care.

Nurses have been and will continue to be asked to assist patients to die. Matzo and Emanuel,[85] in their survey of oncology nurses, reported that 30% of the respondents, 131 nurses, had been asked to assist with a patient's suicide. Nursing surveys continue to reflect the professional individual's ambiguity about this issue.[85–89] Nurses cannot help but be confronted by and struggle with the complicated moral and professional dilemmas regarding assisted suicide.[90] They see compelling cases wherein patients are devastated physically and emotionally by illness, and they are confronted with the torment and exhaustion of their families. Personal and professional tension and ambiguity about what is right are bound to occur.[91] At times it may be difficult to balance the facilitation of a dignified death with that of preservation of life,[78] and the willingness to consider participation in assisted suicide may be motivated by mercy, compassion, promotion of autonomy, and quality-of-life considerations.[91]

One of the most important ethical issues is the way in which the health care professional responds. Muskin[92] believes that the real violation of the patient's rights occurs when the motivation is not thoroughly explored. Dr. Ira Byock, who has publicly spoken out in opposition to physician-assisted suicide, suggests that our responsibilities, if PAS were legalized, would be to stand by the patient and family, whatever their decision, and continue to provide care. Byock also asserts that although patient choices may differ from the provider's preference, there is an obligation to respect that choice and struggle along with them.[93]

Nurses who are asked about or asked to assist with a patient's suicide are ethically bound to (*1*) respond nonjudgmentally to requests; (2) provide all relevant information about the state's legal restrictions as well as alternative treatments and options; (3) participate with the multidisciplinary team in a thorough evaluation of the patient's rationale for the request; (*4*) assist in the clarification of goals; and (5) ensure that all symptoms, including depression, are assessed and managed at a level acceptable to the patient and family. Ongoing emotional support and caring for the patient and family can be offered without regard for statutory law.

The Oregon Nurses Association (ONA) has published a white paper[94] on the Oregon Death with Dignity Act[71] that supports the ethical stances of nurses who choose to care for or discontinue involvement in the care of individuals who request physician-assisted suicide. The ONA supports both the patient's right to self-determination and the nurse's right to a professional practice congruent with personal moral values. Oregon nurses who choose to continue caring for the patient requesting assisted suicide may (*1*) explain the law as it currently exists; (2) discuss and explore options with the patient and make referrals when appropriate; (3) explore reasons for the patient's request, ensuring that depression is thoroughly evaluated and treated if found to be present; (4) maintain patient and family confidentiality; (5) provide care and comfort throughout the dying process; (6) remain present during the patient's self-administration of the medication and subsequent death to console and counsel the family; (7) continue to provide ongoing emotional support; and (8) be involved in policy development within the health care facility and/or the community. In addition to issues of confidentiality and judgmental behaviors toward patients and families, nurses may not inject or administer the medication that will lead to the end of the patient's life or make unwarranted judgmental comments to other members of the health care team who care for patients who have chosen assisted suicide.

Ethical imperatives for those Oregon nurses who choose not to be involved can offer some guidance for nurses whose legal jurisdiction does not legitimize assisted suicide and who want to respond appropriately and compassionately to the patients they serve. The nurse who feels ethically compromised in caring for a patient who has chosen assisted suicide is (*1*) obliged to provide for the patient's comfort and safety, (2) withdraw only when assured that alternative sources of end-of-life care are available to the patient, and (3) continue to provide ongoing care if unable to transfer that care to another provider. They may not breach confidentiality, subject patients or their peers to judgmental remarks about PAS, or abandon or refuse to provide comfort and safety measures to the patient.

Muskin's imperative[92] to explore the rationale for patient's requests needs to be translated into health care policies. Most health care systems do not provide written guidelines for their staff. The Hospice of Boulder County in Boulder, Colorado, has developed guidelines for caring for the patient who expresses interest in hastening death.[95] Modeled after the Oregon Nurses' Association white paper, it provides a thoughtful and caring structure for a multidisciplinary response to a distressed patient. Table 47–5 represents a paradigm of their policy.

Table 47–5. Identifying Vulnerability Factors and Responding to Those Patients Who Express Interest in Hastening Death

I Assessment

A. Patient Interview
1. What is happening now that makes you consider this action?
2. If we could relieve that problem, would you still be interested in dying now?
3. Have you thought about a method?
4. What do you know about the consequences of this method for your family?
5. Is this an idea that is yours alone or has someone suggested that you consider this?
6. Have you discussed this with family members, your doctor, or others who are caring for you?

B. Evaluation
1. Satisfaction with pain and symptom management?
2. Depression? Anxiety?
3. Fears? Anger? Family pressures?
4. Personal and spiritual philosophy?
5. History of depression or mental illness?
6. Weapons on the premises?

II Intervention

A. Team Meeting
1. Physician notification
2. Possible request for ethics committee consultation

B. Response to Unmet Needs
1. Aggressive efforts made to alleviate any unmet physical, emotional, or spiritual needs
2. Anxiety or depression? Offer pharmacologic treatment and/or psychotherapy

C. Response to Request
1. Description of current state law, its requisites, and the provider's rights/responsibilities
2. Information and counseling regarding the patient's request
3. Encouragement to discuss with family and others involved in care
4. Removal of weapons from the premises if they present a threat to staff or family
5. Notification of appropriate authorities if violent death (e.g. shooting) occurs

D. Staffing
1. Staff assignments made in terms of comfort/discomfort with patient request
2. Support offered to those who have cared for the patient but choose not to continue after a wish for hastened death has occurred
3. Review of case by involved staff and volunteers

E. Documentation
1. Assessment
2. Interventions

Source: Adapted from Hospice of Boulder County, Boulder, Colorado, Ethics Committee, 1997 and Oregon Nurses Association Guidelines.

Case Study: When the Patient Seeks to Hasten Death

Gertrude was a strong woman, who had barely lived through the Second World War, and emigrated to the United States as a child. When diagnosed with metastatic breast cancer, she stoically began treatment. As she and her nurse developed a relationship over time, she mentioned her fears of dependency, of losing her ability to think and communicate clearly, of losing her ability to control her bodily functions. She was absolutely clear that she did not want to die, having lost control of her physical and/or mental abilities. One day she asked her nurse if she would be able to "put her to sleep" when the time seemed appropriate. As her nurse explained why this was not possible from a legal perspective, Gertrude interrupted her and said, "They treat dogs better than they do human beings." The topic came up frequently over a few months, and each time the nurse would reiterate the difficulties while continuing to remind Gertrude that she would be supported with the very best in palliative care in order to ensure a death that was peaceful. Gertrude never stopped asking for assisted death. She ultimately became very confused in her final days. The nurse was with her when she died, and her last words, jumbled though they were, included the word "dog."

Gertrude's experience exposes the conflicts that nurses encounter every day. Many patients express fears as they near the end of life-losing control, fear of acting in a way that they regard as undignified, and/or fear of living beyond the time they consider acceptable. These fears may be at the most existential and intimate of levels and cannot be dismissed with easy answers. And so patients often ask for assisted death. The dilemma for the nurse and other members of the multidisciplinary team is how best to resolve the patient's deeply felt fears, how best to identify interventions that have meaning, and how to personally resolve the tensions generated by the inability to respond to another's plea for help. Gertrude might have benefited from more detailed discussions of how she could be helped at the end of life and more assistance from the hospice team's social worker in exploring her fears.

Voluntarily stopping eating and drinking (VSED) has been suggested as an acceptable moral alternative to PAS.[96] However, this choice requires considerable patient resolve, may last for weeks, and can initially increase suffering because the patient may experience hunger and thirst. While legally permissible, some patients, family, and members of the health care team may consider this method "dehydrating" or "starving" a patient and subsequently morally offensive. Should a patient choose this course of action, the nurse should continue meticulous comfort care and may need to implement sedative orders for the management of delirium. The choice to use VSED is based on the patient's values, and it would be egregious if the physician or nurse condemned the patient for this choice. Those health care professionals who believe it morally impermissible may excuse themselves from care after ensuring a suitable substitute caregiver.

Even with state-of-the-art care, a small number of dying patients will experience suffering that cannot be satisfactorily relieved—for example, pain, shortness of breath, intractable nausea/vomiting, delirium. Terminal sedation as a solution to these unmanageable kinds of suffering is a phrase that has appeared in the palliative care literature in the last few years. The Supreme Court[70] made terminal sedation legally acceptable in the same opinion that ruled PAS was neither a patient right nor a medical obligation.

However, consensus had not been reached as to a clear definition. Chater et al.[56] have suggested the following: "The intention of deliberately inducing and maintaining deep sleep, but not deliberately causing death in specific circumstances, i.e. for the relief of one or more intractable symptoms when all other possible interventions have failed and the patient is perceived to be close to death and/or for the relief of profound anguish (possibly spiritual) that is not amenable to spiritual, psychological or other intervention and the patient is perceived to be close to death" (p. 257). They have also suggested a less pejorative nomenclature to be "sedation for intractable distress in the dying."

Regardless of the terminology, there continues to be much debate in the bioethical and medical communities about the moral repercussions of sedation for intractable distress.[57–59,78] Some have argued that death with sedation for intractable distress is "foreseen" but not "intended," thereby invoking the principle of double effect—that is, the sedation itself is not causing death but is intended to relieve suffering, an accepted aim of medicine.[59] Those who take the middle ground allow the possibility that in some cases it may be morally acceptable when symptoms cannot be managed otherwise.[56] Finally, others see sedation for intractable distress as tantamount to euthanasia because the sedated patient may die from the combination of two intentional acts—the induction of stupor or unconsciousness and the withholding of food and water.[57] The American Nursing Association[69] has stated that the risk of hastening death through treatments aimed at alleviating suffering and/or controlling symptoms is ethically acceptable.

If sedation for intractable distress is evaluated to be necessary in light of current patient circumstances, the health care team must ensure that the patient's decision is informed and voluntary before initiating the intervention. If the patient lacks decision making capacity and appears to be suffering intolerably, it would be essential to discuss with family members or the health care proxy the exhaustion of all other palliative care interventions and the goals.

Case Study: Sedation for Intractable Pain

George was an older gentleman with widely metastatic colon cancer. Pain became the formidable adversary of the hospice team. Every possible analgesic intervention had been tried, all atypical analgesics, all anesthetic procedures, as well as intraspinal analgesia. He continued to experience severe pain and begged to have his life ended. After an emotional but carefully thought out discussion, the family supported the decision to begin intravenous sedating therapy in order to ensure his comfort. Many of the nurses who had been caring for him felt this was equivalent to euthanasia and asked to be excused from caring for him. They were forbidden to voice their concerns to George and his family but were allowed to offer comforting words and expressions of their feelings for George. Those nurses who were morally comfortable with the decision took responsibility for his care.

Ultimately, safeguards must be in place when considering any intervention, not just sedation to relieve intractable distress in the dying, that might end the patient's life sooner than would be otherwise true. They include: (*1*) informed and voluntary consent after detailed discussion; (*2*) diagnostic and prognostic clarity; (*3*) an independent second opinion from a consultant with expertise in palliative care; (*4*) a brief waiting period and reevaluation of the issues with the patient and family; and (*5*) documentation and review to ensure accountability.

When the goal of care is to manage a symptom, not hasten death, documentation of the whole process should be meticulous. The goals of care and discussion with the patient and family—that is, informed consent—should be clearly outlined in the progress notes. Careful documentation is not limited to sedation to relieve intractable distress in the dying. Withholding or withdrawing treatment and/or increasing doses of medication for symptom relief that may secondarily shorten life—for example, opioids for pain relief—must receive the same careful attention to documentation details.

THE ROLE OF THE NURSE IN A BIOETHICAL COMMUNITY

The struggles that surround the level and intensity of treatment are not the only ethical conflicts that emerge in the practice of palliative care. Choices about confidentiality, consent, research dilemmas, and family authority create a series of moral crossroads for the staff. When faced with a conflict of deeply held moral values, the nurse must first consider her or his own role in the clinical setting. Then a thoughtful conversation must begin within the "community" that includes the patient, the family (if the patient so desires), and the entire interdisciplinary health care team. It is at this point that institutions have turned to bioethics committees for the "moral architecture" of the clinical conversation.

As an integral part of the interdisciplinary team, nurses must sit at this table in order to provide descriptive, specific, and personal perspectives on moral issues; advocate for the patient and family; and emerge themselves in the milieu of accountability. A substantive discussion cannot occur without the clear and courageous voice of the bedside caregiver. Nurses must consider what is at stake in the nurse–patient relationship and the obligations of the role. They must evaluate how their own acts will shape both their characters and future practice. Finally, they must be vigilant for moral breaches in care and refer patients and their circumstances to the bioethics committee when a moral conflict cannot be resolved.

The nurse who is committed to palliative care will need to become comfortable addressing the bioethics committee with his or her concerns and involving the ethicist and committee in troublesome cases. Courage to speak of difficult issues, involving patients and family in the discussions, and developing both the patience and the perspective necessary to genuinely hear all voices will be required.

If there is not yet a committee at the institution (hospital, hospice, or home care agency), nursing should (*1*) be part of the endeavor to create a committee; (*2*) identify and recommend other health care providers and consumer and public members for membership; (*3*) advocate for training in bioethics provided by a qualified ethicist; (*4*) participate in the training and education; (*5*) assist in establishing a methodology for consistent, ongoing development and education for committee members, other health care providers, and the institution's lay members; (*6*) assist in formulating policies regarding treatment issues—for example, consent for treatment, treatment refusal, withholding and withdrawing of care, withholding nutrition and hydration, requests for assisted death; and (*7*) assist in formulating policies for education, case consultation, and documentation of the committee's work.[98] Nursing can assist in teaching the health care community about ethical norms and controversies, particularly drawing attention to end-of-life dilemmas.

When conflicts emerge and the patient/family/health care provider triad cannot reach consensus, the bioethics committee first assesses the patient's medical condition and wishes regarding medical intervention. They explore who the patient was prior to the illness and who the patient currently is, their circumstances, and their situation. This "photograph" of the patient allows for a discussion based on the realities of personhood as well as medical facts and allows the nurse an opportunity to provide details that might not be known by other members of the health care team. The nurse must also consider the duties of the nursing profession, including resistance to immoral actions or rules, and assess how the decisions made impact a patient's rights and responsibilities.

Next, the consequences of possible choices are considered. Can harms and wrongs be minimized and happiness maximized? After all the information has been gathered from every possible source, the committee makes a recommendation about the dilemma. See Figure 47–1.

As a contributing member of the bioethical community, the nurse will increasingly need to balance autonomy

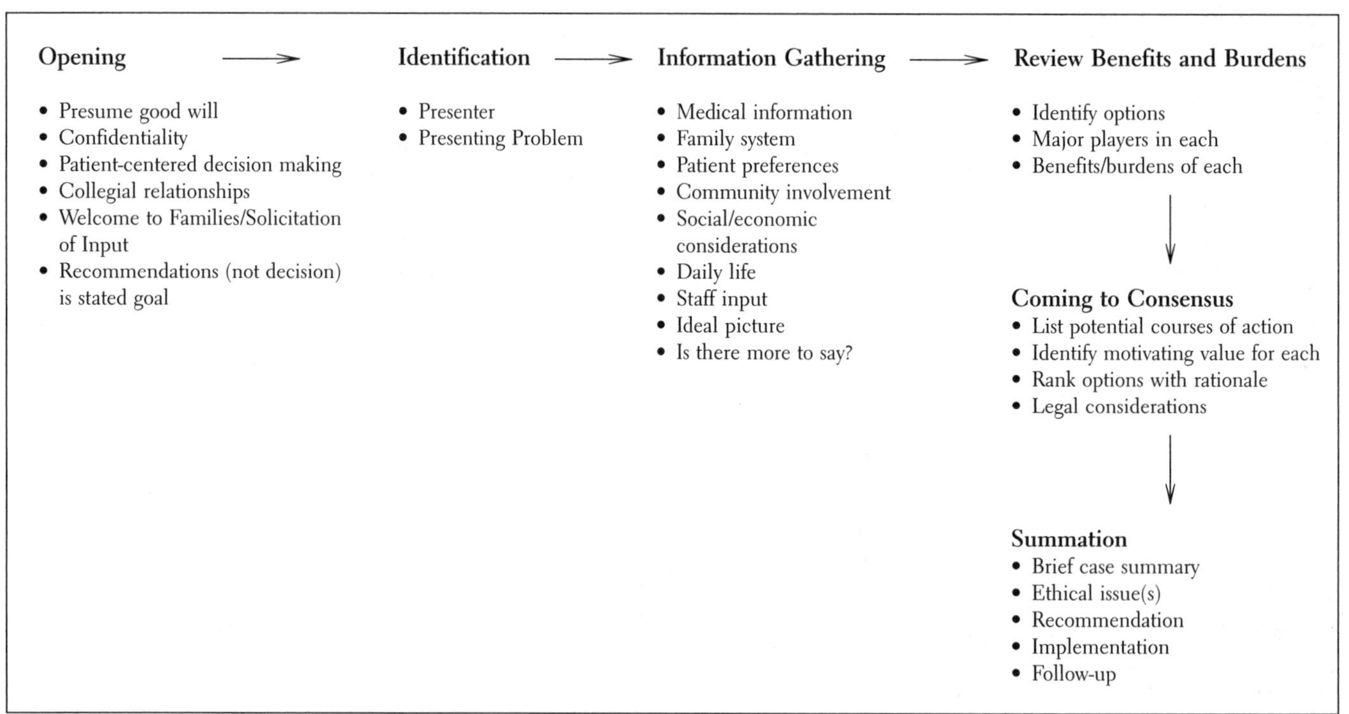

Figure 47–1. An Ethics Decision-Making Model. (From *Forming A Moral Community: A Resource for Healthcare Ethics Committees.* Bioethics Consultation Group, Berkeley, California 1992.)

with the issue of justice in the clinical setting, and that will be a challenge. Patients who might reasonably be considered candidates for palliative care may insist on active, aggressive medical intervention. Patients enrolled in hospice programs may demand interventions that would better serve the acute care population. The clinical setting must be a place not only of healing but of fairness, a fact that nurses understand and can articulate. Nurses must be vigilant in assuring that the patient who is poor, socially disadvantaged, or marginalized by race, ethnicity, language, or geography receives the same quality of care.

INHERENT TENSIONS IN MEANING, POWER, AND MORAL AGENCY

Our attention to ethical and spiritual issues as well as issues of justice, allocation, and marketplace realpolitic will shape the framing of our cultural responses to the dying process. In a world focused on productivity, illness and death are viewed as distractions and profoundly personal problems. Limits on our obligations to the dying are formulated within a milieu of legal and fiscal considerations in which health care and illness are viewed as "business." As Congress debates current legislation about how to adjudicate treatment constraints, small battles are being waged at the bedside of the dying every day.

A case in point is the use of EMLA Cream, a topically applied local anesthetic used to reduce pain and distress during the insertion of intravenous lines in children. This intervention is no longer covered by insurers for some patients. Nurses, aware that this simple treatment can significantly reduce discomfort, share the precious tube of medication, which costs all of $10. They do so because the process of an intravenous insertion for a terminally ill child can be an agonizing process or can be made pain free—a decision they feel must lie outside the business of profits and losses for insurance companies.

As mentioned previously in the chapter, nurses find themselves all too often "in the middle" when there are conflicts between providers, patients, and families about the most appropriate kind of care that should be delivered. Inherent in these tensions are *actual* ethical dilemmas that nurses encounter daily—that is, those circumstances wherein two competing moral appeals are in conflict. A classic example might be that of struggling to ensure informed consent when patients and/or families do not want to understand current realities and believe that information sharing will destroy the patient's hope and cause that individual to "give up" (veracity vs. maleficence).

However, *individual* ethical dilemmas occur when the practitioner's personal values are compromised. As each individual filters circumstantial realities through their own "mesh" of values, conflicts arise that may be particular to that person. Clinical issues of withdrawing treatment or providing sedation to relieve intractable distress in the dying can be morally impermissible to some while morally permissible to others. These dilemmas are distinct from legal constraints, fiscal considerations, and cultural implications. Practitioners will continue to struggle as they balance the demands of professional obligation and personal meaning and wonder if their roles as moral agents will be defended or defeated.

CONSIDERATIONS REGARDING NURSING'S FUTURE ROLE IN END-OF-LIFE CARE

The responsibilities of the nurse will include not only advocacy for patients but advocacy for the staff and team that support the patient. The discussion of the advance directive, to be effective, will need to begin much earlier and be a comprehensive part of the provider relationship—an admittedly difficult task in a changing health care environment. None of what any ethicist can suggest is revolutionary but rather focuses attention on oft-repeated truths. Advance conversations (not just "directives") about dying and the use of the hospice model merit particular attention.

First, in thinking about advance conversations and end-of-life planning, the professional must incorporate the constellation of friends and colleagues who support the patient. The notion that one is not alone, that one has comradeship and friendship, is embedded in advance conversations. Second, social support for this stage of life must be secured from health care systems that have the ability to provide real options for the dying patient. Nurses must speak strongly and courageously about the need for and value of palliative care to both policy makers and the public. Third, the meaning of the well self versus illness, autonomy versus limits, the importance of control versus the impotence of treatment interventions, the meaning of risk versus the potential for harm, and the place of faith will need to be understood by providers before a rigorous discussion with the patient can occur. Nurses, because of their ongoing contact with patients at the end of life, are well positioned to understand the nature of these discussions and insist upon these conversational "gold standards."

The second critical issue will be support for hospice and palliative care. Pioneering efforts by a multitude of practitioners and support from multiple segments of the public and private sectors are allowing a robust consideration of a variety of ways to create innovations in the care of the dying. The hospice and palliative care movement frames ethical reflections on the dying process. Hospice interrupts death as an unrelenting, fast-moving tragedy and slows the process with friendship, the claims of even the stranger, and a responsive community.

Hospice care resonates with the name itself—way stations for ones who wandered in war, far from family, moving into a wider and unknown world. Modernity necessitates the same passages. It will be the privilege of the nurse to hear the stories that travelers bring, and to recognize the importance of each, even the abandoned, as we collectively work to expand the hospice model. Taking on the care of the dying is an extraordinary responsibility, and calls on the development of a vision of a life of virtue, of serious personal consideration of what obligations the nurse will take on, and of a turn from the objective to the subjective. For such work, we will need to resist strong pressures to rescue and fix what cannot be repaired. We will need to learn to turn from the role of hero to the role of witness.

All of this will require a new sort of language, a language of a country that is fearful of death they find difficult to master. The speech is ordinary and very plain. It is tempting to pretend otherwise and discuss problems not in terms of befallenness, need, and loss, but in technological detail, the mother tongue of medicine. It will be not only patients and families but also nurses who will need to create internal communities of meaning and conversation. Such moral communities are the place for ethical reflection, conflict debate, closer examination of deep moral discord, and, finally for the development of new ethical visions that enrich the lives off all who participate in the experience.

REFERENCES

1. Solomon MZ, O'Donnell L, Jennings B, Guilfoy V, et al. Doctors near the end of life: Professional views on life-sustaining treatments. American Journal of Public Health 1993;83:14–27.

2. Schroeder SA. The president's message. On dying in America. 1998. Available at http://www.rwjf.org/library/annual/presint1.htm. Accessed April 8, 1998.

3. Stanley KJ. End-of-life care: Where are we headed? What do we want? Who will decide? Innovations in Breast Cancer Care 1998;4(1):3–8.

4. In re Quinlan, 70 NJ 10, 355 A2d 647, cert denied 429 US 922, 97 SCt 319, 50 Led 2d 289 (1976).

5. Cruzan v. Director of Missouri Department of Health 109 SCt 3240 (1990).

6. Robb CS, Casebolt CJ, eds. Covenant for a New Creation: Ethics, Religion, and a New Public Policy. New York: Orbis Books, 1991.

7. Jonsen AR. The Birth of Bioethics. Oxford, England: Oxford University Press, 1988.

8. Kant I. Fundamental principles of the metaphysics of morals. In Kant's Critique of Practical Reason and Other Works on the Theory of Ethics. London: Longmans, Green, 1898.

9. Mill JS. Utilitarianism. London: Longmans, Green, 1897.

10. Jonsen AR, Toulmin SE. The Abuse of Casuistry. A History of Moral Reasoning. Berkeley: University of California Press, 1990.

11. Cassel EL. The nature of suffering and the goals of medicine. The New England Journal of Medicine 1982;306:639–645.

12. Ferrell BR. The quality of lives: 1,525 voices of cancer. Oncology Nursing Forum 1996; 23:907–916.

13. Franey SG. Three factors critical for end-of-life care. Health Progress 1996;September–October:30–32.

14. SUPPORT Principal Investigators. A controlled trial to improve care for seriously ill hospitalized patients. The study to understand prognoses and preferences for outcomes and risks of treatment. Journal of the American Medical Association 1995;274(20):1591–1598.

15. American Board of Internal Medicine End-of-Life Patient Care Project. Caring For the Dying: Identification and Promotion of Physician Competence. Philadelphia: American Board of Internal Medicine, 1996.

16. Billings JA. Medical education for hospice care: A selected bibliography with brief annotations. Hospital Journal 1993;9:69–83.

17. Billings JA, Block S. Palliative care in undergraduate education: Status report and future directions. Journal of the American Medical Association 1997;278:733–738.

18. Ferrell B, Virani R, Grant M. Analysis of end-of-life content in nursing textbooks. Oncology Nursing Forum 1999;26:869–876.

19. Charlton R, Ford E. Medical education in palliative care. Academic Medicine 1995;70: 258–259.

20. Field MJ, Cassel CK, eds. Approaching Death: Improving Care at the End of Life (Report of the Institute of Medicine Task Force). Washington, DC: American Academy Press, 1997.

21. Lowden B. Introducing palliative care: Health professionals' perceptions. International Journal of Palliative Nursing 1998;4:135–142.

22. McCaffery M, Ferrell B. Nurses' knowledge of pain asessment and management: How much progress have we made? Journal of Pain and Symptom Management 1997;10:356–357.

23. Singer PA, Martin DA, Kelner M. Quality end-of-life care. Patient's perspectives. Journal of the American Medical Association 1999;281(2): 163–168.

24. Task Force on the Nurse's Role in End-of-Life Decisions, American Nursing Association. Position statements. Nursing and the Patient Self-Determination Act, 1991. www.nursingworld.org/readroom/position/ethics/etsdet.htm.

25. Haisfield-Wolfe ME. End-of-life care: Evolution of the nurse's role. Oncology Nursing Forum 1996;23:931–935.

26. O'Connor KF. Ethical/moral experiences of oncology nurses. Oncology Nursing Forum 1996;23:787–794.

27. Bruera E. Research into symptoms other than pain. In: Doyle D, Hanks GWC, MacDonald N, eds. Oxford Text of Palliative Medicine, 2nd ed. New York: Oxford University Press, 1998: 179–185.

28. Brant JM. The art of palliative care. Living with hope, dying with dignity. Oncology Nursing Forum 1998;25:995–1004.

29. Ferrell BE, Dean GE. Ethical issues in pain management at home. Journal of Palliative Care 1994;10:67–72.

30. Task Force on the Nurse's Role in End-of Life Decisions, American Nursing Association. Position statements. Promotion of Comfort and Relief of Pain in Dying Patients, 1991. www.nursingworld.org/readroom/position/ethics/etpain.htm.

31. Oncology Nursing Society. The use of placebos for pain management in patients with cancer. 1997. www.ons.org/ons/cross/position/placebos.htm.

32. Stanley KJ. Silence is not golden: Conversations with the dying. Clinical Journal of Oncology Nursing 2000;4:34–40.

33. Yates P, Stetz KM. Families' awareness of and response to dying. Oncology Nursing Forum 1999;26:113–120.

34. Oncology Nursing Society. Patient's bill of rights for quality cancer care. 1998. www.ons.org/ons/main/journals/bill.htm.

35. Ersek M, Kagawa-Singer M, Barnes D, Blackhall L, Koenig BA. Multicultural considerations in the use of advance directives. Oncology Nursing Forum 1998;25:1683–1690.

36. The Patient Self Determination Act of 1990 (PSDA) (Sections 4206 and 4571 of the Omnibus Budget Reconciliation Act of 1990, PL 101-508). Effective December 1, 1991.

37. Bartling v. Superior Court, 163 CalApp3d 186, 209 Cal Rptr 220 (1984).

38. Bouvia v. Superior Court, 179 CalApp3d 1127, 225 Cal Rptr 297 (1986).

39. Wis Sup Ct Case No 89-1197 4/1/92.

40. In re Jobes, 108 NJ 394 529 A2d 434 (1987).

41. Lynn J, Teno JM. After the Patient Self-Determination Act: The need for empirical research on formal advance directives. Hastings Center Report 1993;23(1):20–24.

42. Miles SH, Koepp R, Weber EP. Advance end-of-life treatment planning. Archives in Internal Medicine 1996;156:1062–1068.

43. Teno JM, Licks S, Lynn J, Wenger N, Connors AF, Phillips RS, O'Connor MA, Murphy DP, Fulkerson WJ, Desbiens N, Knaus WA. Do advance directives provide instructions that direct care? Journal of the American Geriatrics Society 1997;45:508–512.

44. Nolan MT, Bruder MT. Patients' attitudes towards advance directives and end-of-life treatment decisions. Nursing Outlook 1997;45: 204–208.

45. American Nurses Association. Code for Nurses with Interpretive Statements. Kansas City, MO, American Nurses Association, 1985.

46. Quill TE, Cassell CK. Nonabandonment: A central obligation for physicians. Annals of Internal Medicine 1995;122(5):368–373.

47. Teno JM, Murphy D, Lynn J, et al. Prognosis-based futility guidelines: does anyone win? Journal of the American Geriatric Society 1994; 42:1202–1207.

48. Rubin S. When Doctors Say "No". Bloomington: Indiana University Press, 1998.

49. Younger S. Futility: Saying no is not enough. Journal of the American Geriatric Society 1994;42:887–889.

50. Barber v. Superior Court 147 CalApp3d 1006, 195 Cal Rptr 484. (CalCt.App, 2nd Dist 1983).

51. In re Dinnerstein, 6MassAppCt 466, 380 NE2d 134 (1978).

52. American Medical Association. Education for Physicians on End of Life Care. 1999.

53. Jonsen AR. Physician-assisted suicide. Seattle University Law Review 1995;18:459–472.

54. Task Force on the Nurse's Role in End-of-Life Decisions, Center for Ethics and Human Rights, American Nursing Association. Position statements. Active euthanasia. 1994. www.nursingworld.org/readroom/position/ethics/eteuth.htm Accessed 9/4/99.

55. Quill TE, Lo B, Brock DW. Palliative options of last resort. A comparison of voluntarily stopping eating and drinking, terminal sedation, physician-assisted suicide, and voluntary active euthanasia. Journal of the American Medical Association 1997;278(23):2099–2104.

56. Chater S, Viola R, Patterson J, Jarvis V. Sedation for intractable distress in the dying-a survey of experts. Palliative Medicine 1998;12:255–269.

57. Orentlicher D. The Supreme Court and physician-assisted suicide. Rejecting assisted suicide but embracing euthanasia. The New England Journal of Medicine 1997;337(17):1236–1239.

58. Lynn J. Terminal sedation. The New England Journal of Medicine 1998;338(17):1230.

59. Rosseau P. Terminal sedation in the care of dying patients. Archives of Internal Medicine 1996;156:1785–1786.

60. Pellegrino ED. Doctors must not kill. Journal of Clinical Ethics 1992;3:95–102.

61. Pellegrino ED. Compassion needs reason too. Journal of the American Medical Association 1993;270:874–875.

62. Angell M. The Supreme Court and physician-assisted suicide—The ultimate right. New England Journal of Medicine 1997;336: 50–53.

63. Annas GJ. The bell tolls for a constitutional right to physician-assisted suicide. New England Journal of Medicine 1997;327:1098–1103.

64. Brock DW. Voluntary active euthanasia. Hastings Center Report March–April, 1992:10–22.

65. Brody HR. Assisted death—A compassionate response to a medical failure. New England Journal of Medicine 1992;19:118–124.

66. Dworkin R, Nagel T, Nozick R, et al. Assisted suicide: The philosopher's brief. The New York Review, March 27, 1997:41–47.

67. Ethics Advisory Council. Oncology Nursing Society's Endorsement of the American Nurses Association Position Statements on Active Euthanasia and Assisted Suicide. Pittsburgh: Oncology Nursing Society, 1997.

68. Weir RF. The morality of physician-assisted suicide. Law, Medicine, & Health Care 1992;20:116–126.

69. American Nurses Association. Position statement on assisted suicide. 1994. 600 Maryland Avenue, SW, Suite 100 West. Washington, DC 20024

70. Vacco v. Quill, 117 SCt 2293 (1997).

71. Oregon Death with Dignity Act (1997). Oregon Revised Statute 127800-127:897.

72. van der Maas PJ, von Dedden JJ, Pijnerberg L. Euthanasia and Other Medical Decisions Concerning the End of Life. An Investigation. New York: Elsevier, 1992.

73. Beck AL, Wallace JJ, Starks ME, Pearlman RA. Physician assisted suicide and euthanasia in Washington state. Patient requests and physician responses. Journal of the American Medical Association 1996;275:819–825.

74. Cummings NB, Eggers PW. Decision to forgo ESRD treatment. In: Nephrology and Urology in the Aged Patient. Orcopoulos DG, Michelis, MF, S. Mershorn, eds, Boston: Klower, 1993.

75. Breitbart W, Rosenfeld BD, Passik SD. Interest in physician-assisted suicide among ambulatory HIV-infected patients. American Journal of Psychiatry 1996;153:238–242.

76. Chochinov HM, Wilson KG, Enns M, et al. Desire for death in the terminally ill. American Journal of Psychiatry 1995;152:1185–1191.

77. Emanuel EJ, Fairclough DL, Daniels ER, Clarridge BR. Euthanasia and physician-assisted suicide: attitudes and experiences among oncology patients, oncologists, and the general public. Lancet 1996;347:1805–1810.

78. Quill TE, Meler DE, Block SD, Billings JA. The debate over physician-assisted suicide: Empirical data and convergent views. Annals of Internal Medicine 1998;128(7):552–558.

79. Chin AE, Hedberg K, Higginson GK, Fleming DW. Legalized physician-assisted suicide in Oregon—The first year's experience. New England Journal of Medicine 1999;340(7):577–583.

80. Drug Operations Section, Drug Enforcement Agency (1998). ARCOS 2 quarterly report. Report 4. Washington, D.C.: Department of Justice, 43–44.

81. Quill TE. Death and dignity. New England Journal of Medicine 1991;324:691–694.

82. Rollins B. Last Wish. New York: Warner Books, 1985.

83. Suarez-Almazor ME, Belzile M, Bruera E. Euthanasia and physician-assisted suicide: A comparative survey of physicians, terminally ill cancer patients, and the general population. Journal of Clinical Oncology 1997;15:418–427.

84. Wolfe J, Fairclough DL, Clarridge BR, Emanuel EJ. Stability of attitudes regarding physician assisted suicide and euthanasia among oncology patients, physicians, and the general public. Journal of Clinical Oncology 1999;17:1274.

85. Matzo ML, Emanual EJ. Oncology nurses' practices of assisted suicide and patient-requested euthanasia. Oncology Nursing Forum 1997;24:1725–1732.

86. Asch DA. The role of critical care nurses in euthanasia and assisted suicide. New England Journal of Medicine 1996;334:1374–1378.

87. Davis AJ, Phillips L, Drought TS, Sellin S, Ronsman K, Hershberger AK. Nurses attitudes toward active euthanasia. Nursing Outlook 1995; 43:174–179.

88. Leiser RJ, Mitchell TF, Hahn JA, Abrams DI. The role of critical care nurses in euthanasia and assisted suicide. New England Journal of Medicine 1996;335:972–973.

89. Young A, Volker D, Rieger PT, Thorpe DM. Oncology nurses' attitudes regarding voluntary physician-assisted dying for competent, terminally ill patients. Oncology Nursing Forum 1993;20:445–451.

90. Scanlon C, Rushton CH. Assisted suicide: Clinical realities and ethical challenges. American Journal of Critical Care 1996;5(6):397–405.

91. Curtin LH. Nurses take a stand on assisted suicide. Nursing Management 1995;26:71–76.

92. Muskin PR. The request to die: Role for a psychodynamic perspective on physician-assisted suicide. Journal of the American Medical Association 1998;279:323–328.

93. Hospice News Service. Box 31516. San Francisco, CA 94131. 1995.

94. Oregon Nurses Association. ONA provides guidelines on nurses' dilemma. 1995. www.oregonrn.org/services-whitepapers-0001.html Accessed 12/12/99.

95. Hospice of Boulder County Ethics Committee. Guidelines for caring for the patient who expresses interest in hastening death. Hospice of Boulder County, 2825 Marine Street, Boulder, CO. 1999.

96. Holden C. Caring for the patient who has a plan for hastened death. Fanfare 1998;12:5–6.

98. Fletcher J. Clinical Ethics Consultation. University Publishing Group, 1997.

48 Public Policy and End-of-Life Care: The Nurse's Role

COLLEEN SCANLON

Public policy options—whether legislative, regulatory, or administrative—have the potential to positively impact the quality and availability of palliative services and the care rendered to patients, families, and communities. The political and public demand for improved end-of-life care has moved to a prominent place on national and state agendas. Policy initiatives create a unique opportunity for nurses to influence present and future directions in end-of-life care.

The convergence of significant trends in clinical, research, social, legal, professional, economic, and political realities has dramatically influenced the evolution of palliative care within the last several decades.[1] It has become clear that end-of-life care is not just the concern of health care professionals, patients, and families. It is also a concern for the public at large and governmental entities. There has been increasing interest and activity within the public policy arena at the state and federal levels of government. Institutions and individuals also have a responsibility to inform and influence pertinent public policy initiatives.

THE EVOLUTOIN OF PALLIATIVE CARE

The enormous strides in research, prevention, detection, and treatment of disease have been incredibly promising. Scientific and medical progress has created significant options and desired choices for those facing life-threatening illness, yet these possibilities have also created poignant questions and dilemmas for those facing life's end, their families, and health care providers. This reality has drawn the attention and activism of health care professionals, the public, and policy makers.

While significant changes in health care, including end-of-life care, have occurred, and though these have been mostly positive, it is recognized that there is still a dramatic need for additional improvements. Intersecting trends have propelled palliative care to the forefront of American culture.

Changing Nature of Death and Dying

Significant scientific and technologic advances have created the possibility of extending life and delaying death. At times, the desire to preserve life has overshadowed the obligation to provide appropriate, compassionate, and dignified care.[1] With the expansion of technology there has been growing attention to the acceptability of limiting treatment interventions and focusing on the comprehensive, ignoring holistic needs of the person with life-threatening illness. Recent decades have witnessed the affirmation of the decisional authority of the individual, the dominance of self-determination, the acceptability of do-not-resuscitate decisions, the use of advance directives, and the acceptance of the withdrawal of life-sustaining therapies.

Judicial Decisions

End-of-life care has also been on the nation's judicial agendas. Judicial history is filled with cases, court decisions, and opinions that have influenced directly and indirectly the course of end-of-life care. From the middle of the 1970s, starting with the Karen Ann Quinlan[2] case through the 1997 United States Supreme Court decision,[3] the judicial system has dealt with complex issues in end-of-life care, including decisional authority, refusal of therapy, and physician-assisted suicide. While each of these decisions dealt with discrete legal questions, these and other judicial cases drew notable attention to the broader questions and concerns in end-of-life care.

Research Data

The acquisition of quantitative and qualitative research data has influenced care at life's end and has the potential to shape public policy. Multiple clinical, attitudinal, experiential, and health professional studies have been generated in the last several decades. In addition, public opinion polls and surveys have drawn attention to the challenges in providing quality end-of-life care. While these projects may generate important information, the ongoing challenge is to ensure that relevant data and knowledge garnered from ongoing research is integrated into care improvements that benefit individuals and communities.

The recent findings of the Study to Understand Prognoses and Preferences for Outcomes and Risks of Treatment (SUPPORT) and the Robert Wood Johnson Foundation national survey give a clear indication of some of the challenges and deficiencies present in end-of-life care.[4,5] SUPPORT was a 10-year project divided into two phases: the first focused on the assessment of the experience of patients at the end of life, including decision making and clinical outcomes, and the second phase involved testing an intervention designed to improve communication and decision making among patients, families, and physicians. Despite attempts to positively affect clinical outcomes, the conclusions of the study found the interventions to be ineffective in (*1*) ensuring that patient preferences were known and honored; (*2*) impacting the incidence and timing of do-not-resuscitate orders; (*3*) decreasing days in the intensive-care unit or on a ventilator before death; (*4*) improving pain management; and (*5*) controlling the utilization of hospital resources.[4]

In a recent national survey, Americans gave the medical system mixed reviews when it comes to how well it treats the dying.[5] About half the respondents believed that the current medical system does "only a fair/poor" job of helping patients remain pain free, helping them maintain dignity or including patients and families in decisions about care. Concern about the financial burden placed upon families was of greatest worry to the respondents. Additionally, by almost a three-to-one margin, respondents want attention directed to improving care at life's end and pain relief rather than legalizing physician-assisted suicide. It seems clear the public wants to see improvements in end-of-life care.

Legislation

Legislative initiatives have significantly influenced end-of-life care. From an historical perspective, one of the most significant pieces of legislation is the Patient Self-Determination Act (PSDA), which provides protection for the decisional authority of individuals.[6] The PSDA was the first federal act requiring all Medicare and Medicaid provider organizations to recognize the legal rights of the recipients of care to make decisions about their health care. This monumental legislation provided the impetus for legislative activity at the state level and the widespread acceptance of advance directives.

Simultaneous with legislative proposals related to protecting decision making authority has been the initiation of legislation regarding do-not-resuscitate orders, financing mechanisms, pain management, surrogate decision making, and physician-assisted suicide. These will be explored further.

Table 48–1. Institute of Medicine Recommendations for Improving End-of-Life Care

- Create and facilitate patient and family expectations for reliable, skillful, and supportive care
- Ask health care professionals to commit themselves to improving care for dying patients and to using existing knowledge effectively to prevent and relieve pain and other symptoms
- Address deficiencies in the health care system through improved methods for measuring quality, tools for accountability by providers, revised financing systems to encourage better coordination of care, and reformed drug-prescribing laws
- Develop medical education to ensure that practitioners have the relevant attitudes, knowledge, and skills to provide excellent care for dying patients
- Make palliative care a defined area of expertise, education, and research
- Pursue public discussion about the modern experience of dying patients and families and community obligations to those nearing death

Source: Field and Cassel, 1997, ref. 7.

FRAMEWORK FOR THE DEVELOPMENT OF PUBLIC POLICY

An initial step in the process of developing public policy proposals is to determine and clarify the particular issue or problem that needs to be addressed and to ascertain the perspectives of various stakeholders on the issue. Patients, providers, payers, and governmental entities may have very different goals and ends that they are seeking. The agendas and concerns of the multiple interested parties need to be considered, negotiated, and balanced.

A two-year comprehensive study conducted by the Institute of Medicine concluded that there were serious problems in end-of-life care and delineated steps to address this reality and lead to improvements in care.[7] One of the committee's tasks was to propose steps that state and federal policy makers and others could take to improve the organization, delivery, financing, and quality of care for persons with terminal illness. An outcome of the study was seven recommendations that could lead to significant improvements and provide a framework for public policy options (Table 48–1).

Also in the late 1990s, the Robert Wood Johnson Foundation, through the *Last Acts* project, promulgated a set of guiding principles, the "Precepts of Palliative Care," in an effort to explicate the non-negotiables of palliative care for the professional community and the public.[8] The precepts have been endorsed by numerous national and local organizations and disseminated widely to the public. One precept states that "palliative care relies on the formulation of responsible policies and regulation by institutions and by state and federal governments."[8] The precepts also provide a starting point for needed reform in end-of-life care (Table 48–2).

SPECTRUM OF ISSUES ADDRESSED IN PALLIATIVE CARE PUBLIC POLICY PROPOSALS AT THE STATE LEVEL

In nearly every state public interest in improving end-of-life care and the momentum for legislative initiatives at the state level has been growing.[9,10] There are town meetings, state commissions, community projects, grant allocations, seminars, active coalitions, and proposed legislation. State governors, attorney generals, and the medical community have all begun to initiate activities related to end-of-life care. While these interested parties may share a common

Table 48–2. Precepts of Palliative Care

Respecting Patient Goals, Preferences and Choices

Palliative Care
- Is an approach to care that is foremost patient-centered and addresses patient needs within the context of family and community.
- Recognizes that the family constellation is defined by the patient and encourages family involvement in planning and providing care to the extent the patient desires.
- Identifies and honors the preferences of the patient and family through careful attention to their values, goals, and priorities, as well as to their cultural and spiritual perspectives.
- Assists patients in establishing goals of care by facilitating their understanding of their diagnosis and prognosis, clarifying priorities, promoting informed choices, and providing an opportunity for negotiating a care plan with providers.
- Strives to meet patients' preferences about care settings, living situations, and services, recognizing the uniqueness of these preferences and the barriers to accomplishing them.
- Encourages advance care planning, including advance directives, through ongoing dialogue among providers, patient, and family.
- Recognizes the potential for conflicts among patient, family, providers, and payors, and develops processes to work toward resolution.

Comprehensive Caring

Palliative Care
- Appreciates that dying, while a normal process, is a critical period in the life of the patient and family, and responds aggressively to the associated human suffering while acknowledging the potential for personal growth.
- Places a high priority on physical comfort and functional capacity, including, but not limited to: expert management of pain and other symptoms, diagnosis and treatment of psychological distress, and assistance in remaining as independent as possible or desired.
- Provides physical, psychological, social, and spiritual support to help the patient and family adapt to the anticipated decline associated with advanced, progressive, incurable disease.
- Alleviates isolation through a commitment to nonabandonment, ongoing communication, and sustaining relationships.
- Assists with issues of life review, life completion, and life closure.
- Extends support beyond the life span of the patient to assist the family in their development.

Utilizing the Strengths of Interdisciplinary Resources

Palliative Care
- Requires an interdisciplinary approach drawing on the expertise of, among others, physicians, nurses, psychologists, pharmacists, pastoral caregivers, social workers, ancillary staff, volunteers, and family members to address the multidimensional aspects of care.
- Includes a clearly identified, accessible, and accountable individual or team responsible for coordinating care to assure that changing needs and goals are met and to facilitate communication and continuity of care.
- Incorporates the full array of interinstitutional and community resources (hospitals, home care, hospice, long-term care, adult day services) and promotes a seamless transition between institutions/settings and services.
- Requires knowledgeable, skilled, and experienced clinicians who are provided the opportunity for ongoing education, professional support, and development.

Acknowledging and Addressing Caregiver Concerns

Palliative Care
- Appreciates the substantial physical, emotional, and economic demands placed on families caring for someone at home, as they attempt to fulfill caregiving responsibilities and meet their own personal needs.
- Provides concrete supportive services to caregivers, such as respite, around-the-clock availability of expert advice, and support by telephone, grief counseling, personal care assistance, and referral to community resources.
- Anticipates that some family caregivers may be at high risk for fatigue, physical illness, and emotional distress, and considers the special needs of these caregivers in planning and delivering services.
- Recognizes and addresses the economic costs of caregiving, including loss of income and nonreimbursable expenses.

Building Systems and Mechanisms of Support

Palliative Care
- Requires an environment that supports innovation, research, education, and dissemination of best practices and models of care.
- Needs an infrastructure that promotes the philosophy and practice of palliative care.
- Relies on the formulation of responsible policies and regulations by institutions and by state and federal governments.
- Promotes equitable and timely access to the full array of interdisciplinary services necessary to meet the multidimensional needs of patients and caregivers.
- Demands ongoing evaluation, including the development of research-based standards, guidelines, and outcome measures.
- Assures that mechanisms are in place at all levels (e.g., systems, direct care services) to guarantee accountability in provision of care.
- Requires appropriate financing, including the development of new methods of reimbursement within the context of a changing health care financing system.

Source: Last Acts, Robert Wood Johnson Foundation, December, 1997, ref. 8.

goal, the focus can significantly vary from research, public dialogue, and grant projects to legislation.

Some of the impetus for public and professional interest in state policy initiatives may be the presence of controversial issues such as physician-assisted suicide or just a growing awareness of the present deficiencies in end-of-life care. Many, if not most, Americans have directly experienced or heard of the plight of someone facing death.

The overwhelming majority of states have some legislative initiatives proposed within the domain of palliative care. The following are examples of issues that are being addressed at the state level with specific public policy initiatives.

Advance Care Planning

Though all states have some type of advance directive legislation (e.g., living will, durable power of attorney for health care), there continues to be ongoing attention to the area of individual and surrogate decision making through proposed acts or amendments to existing legislation. Legislative proposals include simplification of form and process, combining approaches into one document, removing preconditions, and creating new approaches such as an open-ended, situation-specific response forms. In addition, separate advance directives have also been developed for mental health treatment.

A growing trend within the states has been the establishment of some form of surrogate consent provision in legislative codes. Given the paucity of individuals who complete advance directives, this protection of appropriate decisional authority becomes increasingly important.[11] While families have historically been considered the most natural decision makers and their involvement in clinical decisions is generally normative in practice, in many states it is not always legally sanctioned. States have begun to rectify the problems created by this reality with specific legislation.

Pain and Symptom Management

Statutory approaches are another avenue to address concerns about appropriate pain management. A state statute can affirm justifiable and legitimate pain-management practices, address appropriate disciplinary or prosecutorial actions, and provide guidance to professionals and to the courts.[12]

Several states have proposed intractable pain statutes or amendments to deal with the issue of pain management. The general goal of these state statutes and regulations is to mitigate barriers and improve pain and symptom management by creating a legal affirmation of the physician's appropriate role in prescribing controlled substances to relieve pain.[13] While the specifics of these statutes vary from state to state, they generally provide some level of protection for clinicians from disciplinary action for prescribing controlled substances for intractable pain. These statutes clearly have benefits in recognizing the legitimacy of appropriate pain management with opioids, yet there are some risks related to interpretation and application in varied situations.

States are also addressing legal, regulatory and other policy barriers that may interfere with the effective management of pain, such as restrictive prescriptive monitoring laws (e.g., the requirement to use triplicate forms), dosage limitations, and patient reporting.[14] In addition, state proposals have offered resolutions dealing with medical school education, the use of palliative care experts, and medical marijuana referendums.[15,16]

Do Not Resuscitate

Periodically there are initiatives to expand and/or strengthen standard do-not-resuscitate (DNR) laws (e.g., definition of a terminal condition) that are utilized within inpatient settings, but the more significant activity is around DNR orders in other settings such as home. Since the early 1990s states have begun to address the needs of the seriously ill and dying in the community. An area of particular attention has been the appropriateness of resuscitative interventions by emergency medical service (EMS) teams in the home. Generally, EMS is required to automatically institute cardiopulmonary resuscitation and other advanced lifesaving techniques in a crisis situation for the homebound. Many states have instituted nonhospital do-not-resuscitate orders to protect the wishes of individuals at home and avoid interventions that are unwanted.[9]

Reimbursement

Financing and reimbursement options are also included in state legislative initiatives. These include expansion of hospice and home health benefits, changes in eligibility requirements, reimbursement rates, Medicaid waivers, long-term care and nursing home reform, and attention to the care of seriously ill children.[10] The different types of payment sources for palliative care services can include Medicare, Medicaid, private insurance, out-of-pocket, and charity care, and can vary according to setting, which makes it difficult to understand the actual financing realities.[17,9]

Physician-Assisted Suicide

Throughout recent years there has been increasing attention to legislation on physician-assisted suicide. State legislative initiatives started with initial proposals in California and Washington, and those initiatives paved the way for an extensive "right-to-die" campaign.[18] The Oregon bill "Death with Dignity," the first state legislative initiative to legalize physician-assisted suicide, passed in 1994 and was reaffirmed by public vote again in 1997.[19] Since the emergence of this issue at the state level, a wide spectrum of proposals and perspectives has been offered.[20,16] States have proposals to criminalize or to legalize physician-assisted suicide, and some have both pending simultaneously. The expansion of several states' criminal laws include harsher penalties, including civil actions and the revocation of medical licenses.

FEDERAL LEGISLATIVE PROPOSALS

As is occurring at the state level, the federal government has been directing attention to issues of end-of-life care. Routinely, the attention occurs through a budgeting and appropriations process when funds are allocated through reimbursement mechanisms such as Medicare and Medicaid (e.g., hospice benefit) for health care services. Additionally, governmental entities have begun to address concerns about pain control, advance care planning, and physician-assisted suicide. Examples of current federal legislative proposals follow.

Advance Planning and Compassionate Care Act of 1999

This legislation, originally proposed in 1997, focuses primarily on the modification of the Patient Self-Determination Act (PSDA) and the expansion of advance directives. The legislation calls for the inclusion of the contents of the advance directive in the health care record if available and the use of "appropriately trained professionals" to offer the opportunity for discussion with individuals about advance directives, and provides for portability among states.[21] Under the provisions of the existing PSDA statute it is necessary only to document the existence of an advance directive and provide written information; there is no portability provision.[6] Portability allows an advance directive validly executed in one state to be honored in the state in which it is presented for enactment as long as the directive is consistent with the laws of that state. The implementation of the new amendments offered in this legislation is to be studied after 18 months of enactment.

In addition, this legislation calls for the development of outcome standards and measures to evaluate the performance of health care programs and projects that provide end-of-life care; a study of matters related to the creation of a national uniform policy on advance directives; creation of a toll-free hotline to provide consumer information about advance directives; an evaluation of existing innovative health programs that provide end-of-life care; conduction of demonstration projects; an annual report to Congress on the quality of end-of-life care and suggestions for legislation; and coverage for self-administered drugs prescribed for the relief of pain.

While this legislation offers some very constructive opportunities to improve advance care planning and responds to real concerns, it is not without differing assessments from various interested parties. There are concerns about the definition of "appropriately trained professional," risks of misapplication associated with portability, and the availability of funding necessary to enact this legislation.

Conquering Pain Act of 1999

Recognizing the significant concerns related to the appropriate and effective management of pain (e.g., untreatment and undertreatment of older adults, African-Americans, and children), this legislation was drafted and proposed. This legislation was developed with the input of multiple stakeholders, including organizations that represent health care professionals, consumer groups, religious organizations, providers, and end-of-life groups.

This comprehensive bill includes: the development of a website with pain-treatment guidelines; providing of informational materials on pain and symptom management; funding education programs; the inclusion of pain measurements in federal health plans; a report from the surgeon general on the state of pain management; grant awards for model programs and demonstration projects, particularly family/caregiver support networks and health care personnel education; research on barriers to pain and symptom management and palliative care services, including controlled-substances regulation; a survey of insurance providers to determine reimbursement policies; and the creation of a National Advisory Committee to assist in establishing a federal pain agenda.[22]

The comprehensive nature of this legislation responds to the complexities and challenges of creating an environment for pain improvement; however, the breadth of the bill makes it financially costly and possibly too difficult to garner the necessary support for enactment. The primary focus on pain improvement is very compelling and may override the challenges associated with the bill.

Pain Relief Promotion Act of 1999

This bill was introduced in the House of Representatives and Senate in June 1999. This legislation replaces the Lethal Drug Abuse Prevention Act of the previous year, which was aimed at blocking the use of Oregon's physician-assisted suicide law.[23] The new legislation is viewed as a significant improvement over the original legislation.

The Lethal Drug Abuse Prevention Act created a great deal of controversy within the health care provider community. Even organizations that have traditionally opposed physician-assisted suicide, such as the American Medical Association and National Hospice Organization, did not support this legislation because the harm potentially created by the legislation appeared greater than the benefit, that being to halt physician-assisted suicide. While it might have curbed physician-assisted suicide practices in Oregon, it was also predicted that it could have a chilling effect on appropriate pain-relief practices throughout the country. Basically, the legislation expanded the authority of the Drug Enforcement Agency (DEA), authorizing what appeared to be a new level of scrutiny over physician practices related to pain management. The legislation raised serious concerns and stimulated many differing viewpoints on issues of federalism, the potential negative impact on pain management, and the authority of law enforcement as it relates to medical practice.[24] Many thought that the positive outcome of limiting physician-assisted suicide was outweighed by the negative impact on end-of-life care in general. Ultimately this legislation failed.

The newly crafted Pain Relief Promotion Act has two main thrusts—to promote palliative care and pain management and to limit physician-assisted suicide.[25] It affirms the use of controlled substances in a medically appropriate manner to relieve pain and other symptoms. The bill recognizes that controlled substances can be legitimately used even if there is an increased risk of death. The underlying goal is to prevent federally controlled substances from being used to assist suicides in a state like Oregon that has legalized the practice.[19]

The legislation creates no new law, bureaucracy, or expanded authority for the DEA. It acknowledges that it is already against federal law to use controlled substances for assisted suicide in all states that have not acted to authorize the practice (i.e., 49 states). At present the Controlled Substances Act prevents the use of federally regulated drugs for the purpose of physician-assisted suicide.[26] A state may not exempt itself from this fact by passing a state law allowing physician-assisted suicide such as Oregon has done. Some concerns over unintentionally or negatively impacting appropriate pain management are diminished in the way this new legislation is crafted. In addition, the proposed legislation includes provisions addressing education, training, research, and funding of pain-management initiatives.

PUBLIC POLICY AND PHYSICIAN-ASSISTED SUICIDE

At both the federal and state level, attention to the legalization of physician-assisted suicide has escalated throughout the last decade. Since the early 1990s, the majority of states in this country have grappled with this issue. The highest court, the Supreme Court of the United States, addressed the issue of an individual's right to physician-assisted suicide. The fact that this issue found its way to the nation's highest court is symbolic of the growing acceptability of physician-assisted suicide as a tenable choice.

The United States Supreme Court reversed the holdings of two lower courts[27,28] and found that there is no constitutionally protected right to physician-assisted suicide on behalf of terminally ill patients.[3] The ruling of the Supreme Court does not prohibit individual states from legalizing such practices in the future. Probably one of the most significant aspects of the Court's decision was the attention directed at the urgent need to improve the quality of end-of-life care.[29] The Court demonstrated enormous sensitivity to the plight of the dying in the present health care system and emphasized the importance of effective pain relief for the dying.[29]

The nursing community became actively engaged in the debate and activities surrounding the physician-assisted-suicide issue. Major professional and specialty nursing organizations struggled with the complex moral and professional issues surrounding physician-assisted suicide. Undoubtedly nurses have invaluable experience and insight into care at the end of life, which informs the assisted suicide debate and guides the profession's response. The development of position statements (Table 48–3) and educational resources, involvement in professional collaborations and end-of-life coalitions, provision of testimony to congressional leadership and submission of an amicus curiae brief with other health-professional organizations to the Supreme Court of the United States were some of the important activities supported by and engaged in by the nursing profession.[30,31]

Table 48–3. Position Statements on the Nurse's Role in End-of-Life Decisions

Active Euthanasia

Summary: The American Nurses Association (ANA) believes that the nurse should not participate in active euthanasia because such an act is in direct violation of the *Code for Nurses with Interpretive Statements (Code for Nurses)*, the ethical traditions and goals of the profession, and its covenant with society. Nurses have an obligation to provide timely, humane, comprehensive and compassionate end-of-life care.

Assisted Suicide

Summary: The American Nurses Association (ANA) believes that the nurse should not participate in assisted suicide. Such an act is in violation of the *Code for Nurses with Interpretive Statements (Code for Nurses)* and the ethical traditions of the profession. Nurses, individually and collectively, have an obligation to provide comprehensive and compassionate end-of-life care, which includes the promotion of comfort and the relief of pain, and at times forgoing life-sustaining treatments.

Nursing Care and Do-Not-Resuscitate Decisions

Summary: The American Nurses Association (ANA) believes that nurses bear a large responsibility at the time a patient experiences cardiac arrest for either initiating resuscitation or ensuring that unwanted attempts to resuscitate to not occur. Nurses face ethical dilemmas concerning confusing or conflicting do-not-resuscitate (DNR) orders, and this statement includes specific recommendations for the resolution of some of these dilemmas.

Forgoing Medically Provided Nutrition and Hydration

Summary: The American Nurses Association (ANA) believes that the decision to withhold medically provided nutrition and hydration should be made by the patient or surrogate with the health care team. The nurse continues to provide expert and compassionate care to patients who are no longer receiving medically provided nutrition and hydration.

Nursing and the Patient Self-Determination Act

Summary: The American Nurses Association (ANA) believes that nurses should play a primary role in implementation of the Patient Self-Determination Act, passed as part of the Omnibus Budget Reconciliation Act of 1990.[6] It is the responsibility of nurses to facilitate informed decision-making for patients making choices, particularly at the end of life. The nurse's role in education, research, patient care, and advocacy is critical to the ongoing implementation of the Patient Self-Determination Act within all health care settings.

Promotion of Comfort and Relief of Pain in Dying Patients

Summary: The American Nurses Association (ANA) believes that the promotion of comfort and aggressive efforts to relieve pain and other symptoms in dying patients are obligations of the nurse. Nurses should not hesitate to use full and effective doses of pain medication for the proper management of pain and the dying patient. The increasing titration of medication to achieve adequate symptom control, even at the expense of life, thus hastening death secondarily, is ethically justified.

Source: American Nurses Association, 1996, ref. 37.

THE ROLE OF NURSES IN PALLIATIVE CARE PUBLIC POLICY

Advocacy is generally considered a prominent component of professional nursing practice. Advocacy is most frequently understood by nurses in their clinical, patient-centered experiences; however, a broader perspective of advocacy is called for. Professional commitment must also express concern for the wider community, for society, and particularly for those who are most vulnerable. The skills that nurses utilize in their clinical, research, education, and administrative roles can be extremely valuable and transferable in legislative and political arenas.[32]

Undoubtedly, public policy initiatives will continue to emerge at the state and federal level and nurses can assume an important role. Nurses need to remain in the forefront as advocates for improved end-of-life care and see public policy advocacy as yet another growing opportunity to demonstrate this commitment.

Nurses have most frequently been the professionals who have attempted to provide appropriate, competent, and compassionate care to individuals and families who confront the brevity of life. As the largest group of health professionals and those most connected to the comprehensive needs of the terminally ill and their families, nurses are obligated to provide leadership that advances improvements in end-of-life care.

Nurses, individually and collectively, must be interested in and become involved in the assessment of proposed end-of-life legislation and regulation. A proactive, responsible stance on the part of nurses can influence the creation and evaluation of needed end-of-life initiatives. Nurses bring an understanding of the present state of end-of-life care that helps in the analysis of appropriate public policy options and can craft future initiatives.

The *Code for Nurses with Interpretive Statements*, the profession's code of ethics, directs nurses to collaborate with other health professionals and citizens in efforts to meet the health needs of the public.[33] Ethical values that undergird professional responsibilities such as respect for autonomy, justice, professional integrity, beneficience and advocacy, interface with the goals of improving end-of-life care and provide a context for assessment of policy proposals.

While nurses may individually engage in public policy initiatives, it is most often through their involvement in entities such as professional associations or coalitions that advocacy efforts are effectively advanced. Depending on the importance of a particular issue, the nursing community will assume different roles and levels of activism. At times, the nursing community may act as the leader, advancing a particular public policy concern; at other times, it may choose to provide endorsement or support of an issue.

Nurses can and should become actively involved in the legislative and regulatory processes by gathering necessary information, providing the perspectives of not only professionals but also the recipients of care, evaluating policy proposals communicating with policy leaders, and lobbying on specific bills.[34,35] The more knowledgeable individuals are of the legislative process, the more

Table 48–4. Dimensions of Advocacy Activities for Nurses

Agenda Setting

- Identify palliative care issues/legislation of greatest importance to the profession and the public (often these are not evident to policy makers)
- Define and prioritize those issues and decide where time and resources will be concentrated
- Collect relevant data/information to validate the importance of particular health policy issues to the public, health care providers, and legislative leaders
- Evaluate policy proposals in light of professional goals and values
- Develop consensus positions and form recommendations on issues of highest priority
- Formulate new public policy proposals when needed

Coalition Building

- Identify other groups (e.g., health professionals, special-interest groups) with similar agendas where collaborative and coordinated efforts can be initiated
- Seek opportunities for combining, allocating, and sharing advocacy work
- Build grassroots networks within the profession through associations such as the American Nurses Association, the Hospice and Palliative Nurses Association, and the Oncology Nursing Society
- Recognize that in coalition building, broad policy positions are more successful and compromise may be necessary to advance a proposal
- Consider involving stakeholders that may not be typical partners in advocacy efforts, such as community members and employees
- Educate others to the importance of particular palliative care policy proposals

Political Activism

- Become involved with associations and groups that influence palliative care policy
- Develop strategic plans for advancing particular policy initiatives
- Establish and maintain reliable relationships with key legislators and regulatory leaders
- Mobilize and involve interested individuals in advocacy campaigns, including communicating with (e.g., letters, faxes, e-mails, phone calls) and visiting key contacts
- Invite policy makers and community leaders to care environments where they can learn more about the experience of patients and families receiving palliative care services and the needs of providers
- Engage the media in efforts through editorials, articles, and press conferences
- Testify before public policy makers to put a human face on the issue
- Monitor results of proposed public policy initiatives and communicate them with involved stakeholders
- Follow up with policy makers, either expressing satisfaction and gratitude or disappointment with public policy outcomes

effectively they can participate and influence outcomes.[36] Involvement by nurses in public policy and the political advocacy through various activities is yet another way to demonstrate professionalism and promote improvements in end-of-life care (Table 48–4). Nurses can provide a critical and valuable voice in professional, public, and governmental discourse about end-of-life care.

CONCLUSIONS

Public policy initiatives at state and federal levels of government can provide another avenue to advance improvements in end-of-life care. Nurses can inform and influence the process of developing, evaluating, and enacting palliative care public policy that benefits individual, family, and community end-of-life care. Involvement in public policy advocacy provides nurses an opportunity to assume their professional citizenship responsibilities and positively impact the quality of end-of-life care provided throughout the United States.

REFERENCES

1. Scanlon C. Unraveling ethical issues in palliative care. Seminars in Oncology Nursing 1998;14:137–144.
2. In re Quinlan, 70 N. J. 10, 355 A.2d 647, 1976.
3. US Supreme Court. (1997, June). No. 96-110, Washington, et al., Petitioners v. Glucksberg, et al and No. 95-1858, Vacco et al. v. Quill et al.
4. SUPPORT Principal Investigators. A controlled trial to improve care for seriously ill hospitalized patients. Journal of the Medical Association 1995;274:1591–1598.
5. Lake, Snell, Perry & Associates. Results from triads on end of life care. Princeton, NJ: Robert Wood Johnson Foundation, 1999.
6. Omnibus Reconciliation Act of 1990. Publ. No. 101-508, Sect 4206, 4751.
7. Field MJ, Cassel CK, eds. Approaching Death: Improving Care at the End of Life. (Report of the Institute of Medicine Committee on Care at the End of Life). Washington, DC: National Academy Press, 1997.
8. Last Acts. Precepts of palliative care. Electronic Newsletter of the Last Acts Campaign. Princeton, NJ: Robert Wood Johnson Foundation, 1997.
9. Merritt D, Fox-Grage W, Rothouse M, et al. State Initiatives in End-of-Life Care: Policy Guide for State Legislators. Washington, DC: National Conference of State Legislatures, 1998.
10. Tobler L, Gonzalez R, Flanders G. Health Care Legislation 1998. National Conference of State Legislatures, Washington, DC, 1999.
11. Nolan MT, Bruder M. Patient attitudes toward advance directives and end-of-life treatment decisions. Nursing Outlook 1997;45:204–208.
12. Johnson S. Disciplinary actions and pain relief: Analysis of the pain relief act. Journal of Law, Medicine and Ethics 1996;24:319–327.
13. Joransen DE, Gilson AM. State intractable pain policy: Current status. American Pain Society Bulletin 1997;7:7–9.
14. Joransen DE, Gilson AM. Regulatory barriers to pain management. Seminars in Oncology Nursing 1998;14:158–163.
15. Sabatino CP. State legislatures address legal issues. Last Acts: Care and Caring at the End of Life 1999;6:4.
16. Choice in Dying. Legislative update. Right-to-Die Law Digest New York: Choice in Dying, March 1999.
17. Stelzer L, ed. Major Health Care Policies: Fifty States Profiles, 1998. Washington, DC: Health Policy Tracking Service, 1999.
18. Hoefler J, Kamole B. Deathright: Culture, Medicine, Politics and the Right to Die. Boulder, CO: Westview Press, 1994.
19. Oregon Death with Dignity Act:. Ballot Measure 16. November 8, 1994, general election.
20. The New York State Task Force on Life and the Law. When Death is Sought: Assisted Suicide and Euthanasia in the Medical Context. New York: The New York State Task Force on Life and the Law, 1994.
21. Advance Planning and Compassionate Care Act of 1999. 106th Cong., 1st sess., S. 628, H.R. 1149.
22. Conquering Pain Act of 1999. 106th Cong., 1st sess., S. 941.
23. Lethal Drug Abuse Prevention Act of 1998. 105th Cong., 2nd sess., S. 2151, H.R. 4006.
24. Tuohey JF. Opposing moral error in society. Health Progress 1999;80:52–57.
25. Pain Relief Promotion Act of 1999. 106th Cong., 1st sess., S. 1272, H.R. 2260.
26. Controlled Substances Act of 1970. (1970). Publ. L. No. 91-513, 84 Stat 1242.
27. Quill v. Vacco, F3d, 996 US App (2d Cir), 1996.
28. Compassion in Dying v. Washington, F3d, 1996 (9th Cir), 1996.
29. Scanlon C, Rushton C. Assisted suicide: Clinical realities and ethical challenges. American Journal of Critical Care 1996;6:397–403.
30. Scanlon C. Assisted suicide: The contemporary controversy. Nursing Trends & Issues 1996;4:1–9.
31. Amicus Curiae Brief of the American Medical Association, the American Nurses Association, and the American Psychiatric Association as Amici Curiae in Support of Petitioners (1996, November). Vacco et al. v. Quill et al., United States Supreme Court, No. 95–1858.
32. deVries CM, Vanderbilt MW. The Grassroots Lobbying Handbook: Empowering Nurses through Legislative and Political Action. Washington, DC: American Nurses Association, 1992.
33. American Nurses Association. Code for Nurses with Interpretive Statements. Kansas City, MO: American Nurses Association, 1985.
34. Aiken TD, Catalano JT. Legal, Ethical and Political Issues in Nursing. Philadelphia, PA: FA Davis, 1994.
35. Davis A, Aroskar M, Liaschenko J, Drought T. Ethical Dilemmas in Nursing Practice, 4th ed. Stamford, CT: Appleton & Lange, 1997.
36. Neal T. Lawmaking and the Legislative Process: Committees, Connections and Compromises. Phoenix, AZ: Oryx Press, 1996.
37. American Nurses Association. Position Statements on the Nurses Role in End-of-Life Decisions. Washington, DC: American Nurses Association, 1996.

49 Nursing Education

DENICE SHEEHAN and BETTY R. FERRELL

One of the earliest responsibilities of the professional nurse was care of the dying. Florence Nightingale and other nurses provided care to soldiers dying on battlefields as well as to civilians dying as a result of epidemics. A major shift in patterns of disease and treatment began in the twentieth century as more effective treatment modalities became available. Today, student nurses are exposed primarily to curative-oriented care and are less likely to encounter comfort oriented care. Although many health care providers work with people at the end of their lives, nurses spend the most time with the dying and their families. Most nurses will provide palliative care to patients and their families no matter where they practice. Therefore, education in palliative care should begin in the nursing schools and extend through clinical inservices and continuing education courses.

THE NEED FOR IMPROVED PALLIATIVE CARE NURSING EDUCATION

It is imperative that nurses learn through both didactic and clinical experiences. Working with a palliative care or hospice team provides the best experience for learning about the interdisciplinary approach to patient care as the team members model excellence in care for the student. Many studies of end-of-life knowledge, attitudes, and skills of nurses provide evidence of the need to improve the education of nursing students, practicing nurses, and nursing faculty.[1–7] This chapter will focus on the role of nursing education in palliative care. An overview of the need to improve palliative care nursing education will include a brief history of nursing care of the dying, knowledge deficits, and the current focus on these deficits. Issues and challenges in palliative care education will be discussed. Several models of nursing education programs will be presented.

Many people, especially nurses and physicians, have been instrumental in developing a framework for the care of the dying and their families. Dame Cicely Saunders is credited as the founder of the modern hospice movement. She was educated first as a nurse and later as a physician in London. Her interest in pain management led her to the care of the dying. With support from the community and national government, she founded St. Christopher's Hospice in Sydenham on the outskirts of London in 1967.[8] About the same time, Dr. Elizabeth Kubler-Ross, a psychiatrist, began interviewing dying patients in hospitals. She found it difficult to find these patients because doctors and nurses repeatedly told her that there were no dying patients in their hospitals. She later proposed a theoretical framework that described the five stages of dying.[9]

Jeanne Quint's landmark study in 1967 revealed little emphasis throughout the nursing curriculum on teaching nursing students to care for dying patients.[10] Teaching and support were particularly lacking in the clinical setting. Nursing instructors were inadequately prepared to teach or support the students in care of the dying and were not comfortable with nursing problems associated with the dying patient. She recommended that faculty standardize death education curricula so they could be offered consistently throughout schools of nursing and continuing education, and through service programs.

RECOGNIZING DEFICITS IN PAIN EDUCATION IN THE 1980S AND 1990S

Many research studies have documented the lack of knowledge about pain management among student nurses, practicing nurses, and nursing faculty.[11–14] Studies have documented serious misconceptions in the assessment and treatment of pain and knowledge deficits in basic areas such as opioid pharmacology, use of adjuvant medications, and treatment of side effects. These studies have been instrumental in encouraging greater emphasis in nursing education programs and the significant need to provide pain education to practicing nurses.

The awareness of educational deficits in the specific area of pain education extended in the late 1990s to the broader area of end-of-life content in nursing education. Many studies have documented the inadequate preparation of nurses to care for people and their families at the end of life.[1,2,15–20] Several research studies have described important nursing behaviors in the care of the dying.[21–22] Inadequate professional education is often cited as a major barrier to appropriate end-of-life care. In Webster's 1981 study,[23] over 30% of the student nurses reported that they were not always told which of their patients were expected to die. Additionally, 60% were not told whether or not the patients knew they were dying. Care of the dying patient was not routinely incorporated into their curriculum. The type and amount of knowledge and support was dependent on the instructor. Although the students may have learned these skills by working with more experienced nurses, observations revealed that 25% of the students worked alone with the dying. The remaining 75% had only intermittent supervision.

Rittman and colleagues[24] identified five themes that were common among expert oncology staff nurses. They include knowing the patient and the stage of the disease, preserving hope, easing the struggle, providing for privacy, and responding to the spiritual aspects of living and dying. The nurses were able to maintain a high standard of practice by incorporating these themes into their clinical practice to provide for a peaceful death for their patients. They found that nurses who are able to deal with their own mortality become more comfortable with death.

Ferrell and colleagues[25] recently completed an analysis of nine areas of end-of-life content in nursing textbooks. Their review of fifty nursing textbooks revealed that only 2% of overall content was related to end-of-life care and much of the information was inaccurate (Table 49–1). Deficiencies were found in all areas. Palliative care was usually discussed in terms of the hospice model of care rather than the broader concept of palliative care. There was little information on quality of life, which was surprising in view of the recent explosion of research in this area. Pain was often included in the textbooks, but usually in the context of acute rather than chronic pain. Pain management during the end of life was virtually absent. Major gaps were found in symptom assessment and management. Information about communicating with patients and families at the end of life was also lacking. There was little information about the roles/needs of family caregivers as well as issues of policy, ethics, and law. A paucity of information was found about death awareness, anxiety, imminent death, or preparing families for the death. The stages and process of grief were described, but there was little information about nursing interventions or the nurse's personal grief.[25]

Another component of this project is the collaboration with the National Council of State Boards of Nursing (NCSBN), Inc., with the goal of improving end-of-life content in the national nursing licensure examination, the NCLEX. Presently, the Job Analysis Study activity statements are being reviewed for end-of-life care applications in conjunction with preparing test examination questions for end-of-life content. It is believed that end-of-life content in the NCLEX would be a significant force in increasing end-of-life content in nursing curriculum.

Each of the above studies has consistently echoed the strong message that improved patient care is contingent upon adequate preparation of nurses. The deficits cited in these studies provide direction for needed areas of education.

THE ISSUES AND CHALLENGES IN PALLIATIVE CARE EDUCATION

The World Health Organization has recognized the need for the development

Table 49–1. Analysis of End of Life (EOL) Content in Nursing Textbooks

Category of Nursing Text	No. of Texts Reviewed	% of Texts	No. of Pages	No. of EOL Related Pages	No. of Chapters	No. of Chapters Devoted to EOL Content
AIDS/HIV	1	2	526	20	16	0
Assessment/Diagnosis	3	6	1783	15.3	80	0
Communication	2	4	767	38	35	0
Community/Home Health	4	8	3108	21.3	116	0
Critical Care	4	8	4116	80.8	181	2
Emergency	4	8	1006	14.5	69	1
Ethics/Legal Issues	5	10	2018	143	88	4
Fundamentals	3	6	4353	114.9	140	3
Gerontology	3	6	2515	84.8	72	2
Medical-Surgical	5	10	9969	146.3	298	2
Oncology	2	4	3264	107.5	149	7
Patient Education	2	4	636	8.0	26	0
Pediatrics	3	6	2599	33.5	70.0	2
Pharmacology	4	8	3476	22.0	236	0
Psychiatric	3	6	2886	35.3	127	1
Nursing Review	4	8	2661	17.0	47	0
Total	**50**	**100**	**45,683**	**901.9 (2%)**	**1,750**	**24 (1.4%)**

Source: Ferrell, B.R., Virani, R., & Grant, M. (1999). Analysis of end of life content in nursing textbooks. *Oncology Nursing Forum,* 26(5), 869–876.[24]

of national policies and programs for palliative care and has issued several recommendations regarding the education and training of health care professionals. In addition, WHO has suggested that palliative care programs be incorporated into the existing health care system.[26] Another key document, the Institute of Medicine's (IOM) 1997 report on improving end-of-life care,[3] made several recommendations specific to improving professional knowledge. Three of these relate specifically to education:

Recommendation 2: Physicians, nurses, social workers, and other health care professionals must commit themselves to improving care for dying patients and to use existing knowledge effectively to prevent and relieve pain and other symptoms.

Recommendation 4: Educators and other health professionals should initiate changes in undergraduate, graduate, and continuing education to ensure that practitioners have relevant attitudes, knowledge, and skills to care well for dying patients.

Recommendation 5: Palliative care should become, if not a medical specialty, at least a defined area of expertise, education, and research. Palliative care experts should provide expert consultation, serve as role models for colleagues and students, supply leadership for undergraduate, graduate and continuing education, organize and conduct research.

The IOM report cites major deficiencies in professional education for end-of-life care. These include the relative absence of death in the curriculum, lack of educational materials pertaining to the end stages of most diseases and neglect of palliative strategies, and the lack of clinical experiences with dying patients and those close to them. The report suggests that educators can improve care by:

1. Conferring a basic level of competence in the care of the dying patient for all practitioners;
2. Developing an expected level of palliative and humanistic skills considerably beyond this basic level; and
3. Establishing a cadre of superlative professionals to develop and provide exemplary care for those approaching death, to guide others in the delivery of such care, and to generate new knowledge to improve care of the dying.[3]

Educational programs for nurses in palliative care vary widely throughout the world. There are established courses and programs in palliative care at universities as well as seminars, workshops, and conferences in the Americas, Australia, the United Kingdom, and elsewhere in northern Europe. In other parts of the world, education in palliative care is woven into other courses. Palliative care concepts are taught within oncology courses in Japan and Thailand. Since 1990, the Nairobi Hospice in Kenya has provided palliative care courses for health care professionals and have extended this program to nursing schools throughout Kenya. They are working to incorporate palliative care into the nursing curricula. An increase in the availability of charitable sources has resulted in support for the development of palliative care in Russia and the Czech republic.[27] Many additional examples are cited in the chapters of Part VIII, "International Perspectives" in this text.

There are many challenges in improving palliative care education. All educators stuggle with how best to integrate more content in an already packed curriculum. There also is tremendous need to increase the knowledge of faculty in palliative care so that they can lead the change in curriculum. Faculty also require current teaching guides such as audiovisual materials, case studies, and other resources to present this challenging content.

Teaching palliative care content is also not only a matter of didactic content. Preparing nurses to care for the terminally ill necessitates attention to the student's values, beliefs, personal experiences, and culture. It is also essential that palliative care education incorporate not only knowledge and skills, but also strive to identify methods to best enhance compassion, empathy, and the existential or "art" of palliative nursing.[28–35]

THE NURSING PROFESSION'S RESPONSE TO THE NEED FOR CHANGE

In recent years, several major professional nursing organizations have recognized the importance of nursing response to the mandate for improved end-of-life care. In 1997, the International Council of Nurses mandated that nurses have a unique and primary responsibility for ensuring that individuals at the end of life experience a peaceful death.[36] In the same year, the American Association of Colleges of Nursing convened a roundtable of expert nurses and other health care professionals to address this topic. The report from that meeting was titled "Peaceful Death."[37] This document outlines fifteen competencies necessary for nurses to provide high-quality care to patients and families during the transition at the end of life. These competencies should be attained prior to graduation from undergraduate programs of nursing. The group also made recommendations concerning the curriculum content areas where these competencies could be addressed (Table 49–2).

About the same time, the Nurses Section of the National Hospice Organization, under the direction of Cindy Yocum and Nancy English, developed the "Guidelines for Curriculum Development on End of Life and Palliative Care in Nursing Education."[38] Separate guidelines were prepared for undergraduate and graduate nursing programs. They include the biological, psychosocial, and spiritual responses to dying. Theory, assessment, interventions, and clinical placement are addressed within this conceptual framework (Table 49–3).

Another nursing project, the Nursing Leadership Consortium on End of Life Care, funded by the Open Society Institute, Project on Death in America, convened a meeting in 1999 to design an agenda for the nursing profession on end-of-life care.[39] This group, organized by the American Association of Critical Care Nurses, was developed to advance the nursing profession's commitment and efforts to improve end of life. Twenty-three nursing specialty groups participated in this meeting to mobilize nursing organizations in a shared agenda for better care of the dying.

Another related project, funded by

Table 49–2. Competencies Necessary for Nurses to Provide High-Quality Care to Patients and Families During the Transition at the End of Life

1. Recognize dynamic changes in population demographics, health care economics, and service delivery that necessitate improved professional preparation for end-of-life care.
2. Promote the provision of comfort care to the dying as an active, desirable, and important skill, and an integral component of nursing care.
3. Communicate effectively and compassionately with the patient, family, and health care team members about end-of-life issues.
4. Recognize one's own attitudes, feelings, values, and expectations about death and the individual, cultural, and spiritual diversity existing in these beliefs and customs.
5. Demonstrate respect for the patient's views and wishes during end-of-life care.
6. Collaborate with interdisciplinary team members while implementing the nursing role in end-of-life care.
7. Use scientifically based standardized tools to assess symptoms (e.g., pain, dyspnea [breathlessness], constipation, anxiety, fatigue, nausea/vomiting, and altered cognition) experienced by patients at the end of life.
8. Use data from symptom assessment to plan and intervene in symptom management using state-of-the-art traditional and complementary approaches.
9. Evaluate the impact of traditional, complementary, and technological therapies on patient-centered outcomes.
10. Assess and treat multiple dimensions, including physical, psychological, social and spiritual needs, to improve quality at the end of life.
11. Assist the patient, family, colleagues, and one's self to cope with suffering, grief, loss, and bereavement in end-of-life care.
12. Apply legal and ethical principles in the analysis of complex issues in end-of-life care, recognizing the influence of personal values, professional codes, and patient preferences.
13. Identify barriers and facilitators to patients' and caregivers' effective use of resources.
14. Demonstrate skill at implementing a plan for improved end-of-life care within a dynamic and complex health care delivery system.
15. Apply knowledge gained from palliative care research to end-of-life education and care.

Source: American Association of Colleges of Nursing. (1997, November). A peaceful death. Report from the Robert Wood Johnson End-of-Life Care Roundtable, Washington, DC.[37]

Robert Wood Johnson Foundation, is reviewing certification exams administered by nursing specialty organizations to encourage end-of-life content. This project, coordinated by the Oncology Nursing Certification Corporation, will promote changes in nursing practice by introducing changes in continuing education materials focused on prepared candidates for the certification examinations and by promoting increasing content on end-of-life care in the examinations.

Involvement of the certification corporations is a vital force in promoting palliative nursing care. In addition to integration of end of life content across multiple specialty organizations, the Hospice and Palliative Nurses Association (HPNA) also has provided leadership to this evolving discipline. HPNA is the leading nursing organization supporting the development of palliative nursing. This organization provides numerous educational programs, publishes extensive educational materials, and also has a certification arm that administers the specialty certification in Hospice and Palliative Nursing.

MODEL NURSING PROGRAMS

Undergraduate and Graduate Education

The coauthor of this chapter (Sheehan) has identified many important strategies in teaching palliative care to nursing students. It is important to include both didactic and clinical components in both the undergraduate and graduate curriculums. An example of an undergraduate model includes content on loss, grief, and bereavement and pharmacologic interventions for symptom management at the sophomore level. Content on the physiology of dying, psychosocial and spiritual issues, and the hospice model of care are presented at the junior level with a minimum of 12 hours with nursing faculty at an inpatient hospice facility. Students tend to learn best during teachable moments. These include real events with real people. For student nurses this usually means the clinical setting. During the clinical expeience, the students work with an experienced hospice nurse. The students attend the morning report and choose one or two patients with the guidance of the hospice nurse. The nursing instructor asks questions of the student and hospice nurse to facilitate learning. She also meets with the students as a group early in the day to clarify the assignments for the day and check on how the students are feeling in this environment.

The instructor brings the students together as specific learning opportunities arise, such as the death of a patient, unusual dressing changes, or pharmacologic interventions. The use of reflection is a powerful tool to assist students and faculty to learn about themselves and about their practice from situations they encounter in the clinical setting and integrating personal and professional learning experiences. For this reason, the students write a reflection on practice for each hospice clinical day. Students are prepared for the hospice experience through a group meeting with the nursing instructor early in the day. An example of instructions for clinical assignments is listed below.

- **Undergraduate Clinical Preparation**
  1. You may feel exhausted by the end of the day even if you have done very little physical work. You may be emotionally drained.
  2. Take time to discuss your fears and experiences with death with your clinical instructor, the hospice nurse, or your peers.
  3. You may leave the unit (or classroom) at any time. Please let your instructor know how you are feeling.
  4. You will be given the option to see someone who has just died to discuss physical changes in the body and the feeling in the room. You may decline this opportunity.
  5. Take time to reflect on your practice.

Table 49–3. The Human Response to Dying (Approaching Death)

Level I (entry-level nursing students): Theory and Clinical practice to be integrated within the two years of a generic nursing education curriculum.

Biological Response	Psychosocial Response	Spiritual Response
Theory		
• Physiology of dying (physical decline) • Adaptive responses to approaching death • Palliative nursing care	• Family dynamics in crisis • Loss-grief continuum • Exploration of attitudes regarding death and dying: Society/physicians/nurses Self • Legal issues: Advance directives Proxy decision maker • Ethics—Dying • Community health nursing aging caregivers • Belief systems and cultural customs (Rural/urban, minority, etc)	• Death as a final stage of growth • Meaning of death from a philosophical view • Meaning of the human spirit • Meaning of suffering • Fears surrounding dying Loneliness and abandonment • Role of hospice interdisciplinary team
Nursing Theory		
		• Carative model of nursing practice • Role of hospice-caring and comfort • The carative role of the nurse • Palliative nursing
Assessment/Nursing Diagnosis		
• Nutritional needs • Fluid volume needs and processes • Elimination needs • Skin and tissue integrity • Delirium • Pain: Acute-Chronic-Terminal • Confusion • Cycles sleep-rest • Cardiovascular processes • Respiratory processes Agitation Anoxia	• Coping strategies in response to loss Anticipatory grieving Powerlessness • Age-related responses to loss	• Patient/Family assessment of needs • Assess the process Spiritual distress Fear Anxiety Ineffective coping individual/family
Interventions		
• Palliative care (symptom management to provide comfort and alleviate suffering) • Emphasis on comfort measures • Complementary therapies • Pain-management guidelines	• Communication Therapeutic vs. nontherapeutic use of reflection storytelling Empathetic listening	
Complementary therapies as a focus of interventions		
		• Touch with intent • Therapeutic touch • Massage • Music therapy • Prayer • Imagery
Clinical placement		
• Nursing care centers (nursing homes) • Assisted-living centers • Inpatient hospice centers • Senior-level optional community health nursing • Hospice in the home	• Same as those listed under biological responses • Psychosocial competencies identified	• Same as those listed under biological responses

(continued)

Table 49–3. The Human Response to Life-Threatening Illness (Palliative Care) (*Continued*)

Level II (Registered Nurses with 6 months to 1 year of experience in clinical nursing). Time required to complete Level II: three semesters (or four quarters) in a university setting; including at least 12 weeks in a palliative care hospice setting.

Biological Response	Psychosocial Response	Spiritual Response
Theory		
• Palliative care History and present day Application in health care • Pathophysiology (end-stage disease processes) Malignancies Immune deficiency disease Dementia Chronic illness • Neurophysiological mechanisms of acute/chronic/terminal pain • Principle of pain management • Physiology of symptoms Anoxia Dyspnea Fluid volume changes Changes in ADH and kidney function Nutritional changes A. Nausea B. Constipation Restlessness • Agitation • Delirium	• Palliative nursing care role • Nursing role in hospice In-home vs. residential care Teaching: families, caregivers, and nursing assistants Liaison with community health organizations/resources Health-enhancing work habits • Recognition of personal needs and attitudes regarding death/pain/loss • Interdisciplinary team • Family dynamics—pathological families Abuse and neglect Closed systems Addictive/manipulation Enmeshed • Cultural differences Rituals Customs Values Funeral preparations Religious influence • Symbolic communication • Communication/interaction Interviewing techniques Reflection Empathetic listening Silence	• Philosophical and historical role of healers • The spiritual process and spiritual distress Religiosity vs. spirituality • Meaning of suffering • Consciousness and dying • Transpersonal meaning of existence • Theories of Jung-Cassel • Nursing theory • Carative model • Addressing the intuitive process within the nurse Centering Journaling
Assessment/nursing/diagnosis		
• Emphasis on physical assessment/ symptoms/behaviors in end-stage processes • Pain assessment—types and analogies of measurement • Pain behaviors in: Infants Children Preadolescents Adolescents Middle adulthood Aging	• Human response to loss of individual/family • Coping strategies Denial/anger/bargaining/ depression/acceptance Grief and grieving Anticipatory grief • Bereavement meaning and importance in hospice High-risk families • Social isolation	• Suffering • Spiritual distress • Hopelessness • Powerlessness • Anxiety • Fear
Interventions		
• Palliative nursing role • Advanced practice role • Common approach to symptom management Pharmacological Nonpharmcaological • Complementary therapies • Pain management as established for: Cancer pain Acute pain Chronic pain • Terminal pain	• Therapeutic communication Patient/family Hospice team • Crisis intervention • Teaching Patient/family Staff Community • Conflict resolution Patient/family Staff Hospice team • Complicated bereavement	• Establishing criteria for the efficacy of complementary therapies • Scientific and historical evidence in support of: Therapeutic touch Massage Acupressure Aroma therapy Music therapy Guided imagery Visualization Prayer Relaxation techniques Breathing Homeopathy

(*continued*)

Table 49–3. The Human Response to Life-Threatening Illness (Palliative Care) (*Continued*)

Biological Response	Psychosocial Response	Spiritual Response
Clinical experience		
• Inpatient hospice • Assisted living • In-home hospice or residential setting • Correctional institutional (hospice center)		
Management Role of the Nurse		
• Strategies for reimbursement • Health maintenance organizations • Medicare/Medicaid • Regulatory agencies Federal State • Standards/Accreditation JCAHO CHAP NHO Standards • Liaison with specialized agencies • Quality assurance standards	• Supportive intervention for staff • Facilitate communication with team members • For profit vs. nonprofit hospice • Regulations interval Policy Procedural guidelines • Education/training Inservice/staff Community Management/leadership training • Support and interface with community	

Source: See ref. 38.

6. Be open to learning from a variety of people, including patients, families, interdisciplinary team members, peers, and yourself.

- **Undergraduate Clinical Assignments**
  1. Listen to full report on your unit.
  2. Review Patient/Family Guidelines for Signs and Symptoms of Approaching Death.
  3. Make rounds with the hospice nurse to see all of his/her patients.
  4. Choose one or two patients with guidance from the hospice nurse.
  5. Review patient/family information with the hospice nurse.
  6. Assess one specific physical symptom which is most important to the patient. Use the literature to link the diagnosis with the pathophysiology. List the appropriate nursing interventions and expected outcomes. This information will be presented during the clinical conference.
  7. Listen to the patient's story throughout the day.
  8. Reflection on practice: What happened today that made a difference in the way you will practice nursing?

At the senior level, content on the dying child is covered in the Developing Families rotation.

Madonna University in Livonia, Michigan, was the first institution in the United States to offer interdisciplinary hospice education programs. The programs of study at Madonna University are available at the undergraduate and graduate levels under the direction of Sister Mary Ceclilia Eagan. A certificate of achievement in hospice is also offered.

The Breen School of Nursing at Ursuline College in Pepper Pike, Ohio, was the first graduate program in the United States to prepare advanced practice nurses in palliative care. The Master of Science in Nursing program officially began in August 1998, under the direction of Denice Sheehan, although Palliative Care I was first offered during the 1998 spring semester. The program builds on the college's mission to provide an education based on values. Contemplation and reflection on practice are hallmarks of this program. The core curriculum of the master's program concentrates on theory, informatics, research, critical thinking, and leadership. The advanced practice courses include pathophysiology, pharmacology, and health assessment. Students in the palliative care program also take three specialized palliative care courses and 500 hours in the palliative care practicum. Table 49–4 lists the required courses. A post-master's certificate is offered to nurses with a Master of Science in Nursing degree.

Table 49–5 summarizes the topical outlines for the palliative care courses in the graduate program. Palliative Care I is an introductory course that provides an overview of palliative care with re-

Table 49–4. Ursuline College's Master's Degree Program and Post-Master's Certificate

Master's Degree Program

I. **Nursing Core: 15 Credits**
Nursing Informatics
Concepts and Theories
Advanced Statistics
Applied Nursing Research
Health Policies, Roles and Issues

II. **Advanced Practice Core: 9 credits**
Advanced Physiology and Pathology
Advanced Pharmacology
Advanced Health Assessment

III. **Area of Concentration: 12 credits**
Palliative Care I
Palliative Care II
Palliative Care III
Palliative Care Practicum

Post-Master's Certificate

Nursing Informatics
Advanced Physiology, Pathology
Advanced Pharmacology
Advanced Health Assessment
Palliative Care I
Palliative Care II
Palliative Care III
Palliative Care Practicum

Table 49–5. The Breen School of Nursing

Topical Outlines for Palliative Care Graduate Courses
Palliative Care I
• Introduction to Palliative Care • Personal and Societal Perspectives on Dying • The History and Philosophy of Palliative Care and Hospice • The Interdisciplinary Team • The Importance of the Narrative • Physiology of Dying • Spirituality, Religiosity, and Culture • Ethical Issues • Legal Issues • Loss, Grief, and Bereavement • Reimbursement Issues • Culminating Seminar
This course also includes fifteen hours of clinical time to learn about the role of the palliative care or hospice nurse.
Palliative Care II
• Personal Perspectives on Dying • An American Profile on Death and Dying • Setting Professional Boundaries • Nursing Standards and Competencies • Communication and Counseling • Pediatric Issues • Nursing Care of the Patient with Selected Symptoms • Clinical Emergencies • Ethical Issues—end-of-life decision making • Loss, Grief, and Bereavement
Palliative Care III
• Advanced Practice Nurse Role Development in Palliative Care • Quality Process Measurement • Continuous Quality Improvement and Analysis • Impact of Economic and Political Factors on the Delivery of Palliative Care • Resource Management • Enhanced Communication Skills Used in Collaborative Practice • Influencing Legislation Related to Palliative Care and Hospice • Cultural Issues Related to Loss, Grief, and Bereavement • International Perspectives in Palliative Care

spect to history, philosophy, the interdisciplinary team model, and reimbursement mechanisms. Students have opportunities to explore personal beliefs, attitudes, and reactions to progressive illness, dying, and death. They discuss ways in which these attitudes can influence the care of terminally ill people and their families. Students also explore the professional health care provider's role in legal and ethical issues. Spirituality is explored within a framework of individual values and beliefs. The essence of the self is analyzed as the physical being deteriorates at the end of life. Religious and cultural beliefs, traditions, and rituals are discussed as they pertain to end-of-life issues. Research, case studies, and personal and professional experiences are used to emphasize key concepts. Classical literature is woven throughout this course in the form of case studies. Students begin a personal clinical resource book to use in the care of patients and families. They add to this book as they progress through the program. They also begin a personal reflective journal to record thoughts and feelings throughout the program.

In Palliative Care II students have an opportunity to analyze personal attitudes toward progressive illness, dying, and death and compare their current analysis to that developed in Palliative Care I. They also continue the discussion about how these attitudes can influence the care of terminally ill people and their families. Professional boundaries and personal wellness are emphasized. Students are encouraged to think and write about their own personal wellness, including their personal stress-reducing techniques. Ethical issues are explored in relation to treatment decisions and quality of life. This course integrates pathophysiology, pharmacology, psychosocial issues, and spirituality in the assessment and management of symptoms in the person with a terminal illness. Loss, grief, and bereavement are also explored as they relate to the terminally ill person and the family. Communication and counseling techniques are woven throughout this course. Current research in palliative care is analyzed and applied in the clinical setting. The practicum may be taken concurrently or after Palliative Care II.

Students in Palliative Care III explore leadership roles for the advanced practice palliative care nurse in administration, education, consultation, and clinical practice. Quality process and measurement is presented within the framework of continuous quality improvement. The impact of economic and political factors on the delivery of palliative care in a variety of settings is analyzed. Issues related to loss, grief, and bereavement are analyzed from a variety of different cultural perspectives. International perspectives in palliative care are presented by guest speakers who have spent time in countries outside the United States.

During the Palliative Care Practicum students have opportunities in the clinical area for direct contact with expert palliative care practitioners. This includes direct patient–family contact during home visits, team conferences, and clinical forums with the clinical group and the instructor. The students work with the dying and their families in the home, hospice and palliative care inpatient facilities, hospitals, and extended-care facilities. Students meet with an assigned faculty member to tailor the practicums to meet the learning needs of the student. The students work with patients and their families through the dying process and participate in grief support groups. The students keep a clinical journal, including learning objectives, personal/professional strengths identified during the practicum, and reflections on their thoughts and feelings during the clinical experience. They will also participate in team meetings, research and educational presentations to staff, patients and their families, and the community. The student's individualized research project progresses throughout the course.

Another model nursing program is located at New York University (NYU) in New York City. NYU was the first in the United States to offer a Palliative Care Nurse Practitioner program. Under the direction of Dr. Deborah Sherman, the palliative care program builds on the core curriculum of the master's program, focusing on theory, research, critical thinking, human development, community, and leadership. In addition to advanced science courses in pathophysiology, pharmacotherapeutics, and advanced health assessment, students take five specialized palliative care courses, a role development course, and 640 hours of palliative care practicums. A post-master's certificate is an option for those individuals who already have a master's in nursing. A summary of the curriculum is included in Table 49–6.

Continuing Education

While palliative care education in undergraduate and graduate programs will provide an important foundation for the nursing profession, continuing education is also needed to reach nurses already in practice. Continuing education will be needed to reach nurses in all settings involved in end-of-life care. A wide range of methods, from conferences, self-study courses, computer- and Web-based approaches, simulated clinical experiences, and other education approaches, are needed.

An example of a continuing education program initiated to improve end-of-life care in home care was developed by nurse researchers at the City of Hope National Medical Center in Duarte, California. This project is titled HOPE: *H*ome Care *O*utreach for *P*alliative Care *E*ducation.[40] Table 49–7 summarizes the major content of the HOPE curriculum across five modules.

The focus of Module 1 of the HOPE curriculum was a general overview of end of life issues. The participants were provided a perspective on national activities related to improved end-of-life care, such as the Supreme Court's consideration of the right to die, and recent studies that have confirmed the need for improved care. This session also discusses the differences in home care versus hospice care and the need for home care agencies to gain additional expertise in palliative care. This introductory session also provides an opportunity to introduce the importance of cultural issues in end-of-life care.

Module 2 emphasizes pain management at the end of life. The content focuses on the importance of pain assessment in determining the etiology of pain and specific causes of pain occurring at the end of life. The content includes the impact of pain on both the patient and family caregivers as well as common barriers to effective pain management. Basic content is provided on pharmacologic management of pain and nonpharmacologic interventions with an additional emphasis on special concerns at the end of life.

Module 3 presents symptom management. The content introduces the importance of distinguishing various symptoms for optimum comfort. A review of the literature is presented to illustrate the many symptoms commonly present in terminal illness. Priority symptoms are identified by the investigators in order to provide more detailed content on the symptoms of dyspnea, fatigue/weakness/immobility, hydration/nutrition, and delirium/agitation/terminal restlessness.

Table 49–6. New York University Master's Degree Program in Palliative Nursing

I. Nursing Core: 18 credits
Nursing Science and Unitary Human Beings
Patterns of Inquiry in Nursing
Research in Nursing
Nursing Issues and Trends within the Health Care Delivery System
Group Behavior: Development of Collaborative Skills
Basic Statistics II
II. Advanced Practice Core: 12–15 credits
Palliative Care I: The Care of Individuals and Families Experiencing Loss, Grief, Death, and Bereavement
Advanced Comprehensive Health and Physical Assessment: Pract. I
Clinical Practice: Advanced Practice Roles
Advanced Pathophysiology
Clinical Pharmacotherapeutics
III. Electives: 3 credits
Nursing or Free Elective or Independent Study
IV. Area of Concentration: 12 credits
Palliative Care II: Enhancement of Quality of Life Through the Management of Pain and Suffering
Palliative Care Practicum II: Comprehensive, Holistic End-of-Life Care
Palliative Care III: Enhancement of Quality of Life Through Symptom Management
Palliative Care Practicum III: Advancing Nursing Practice and Leadership in Palliative Care

Table 49–7. Key Content of the Home Care Outreach for Palliative Care Education (HOPE) Curriculum

Module 1: General Overview of End-of-Life Issues
- Current status and issues of end-of-life care
- Need for improved end-of-life care in home care
- Home care versus hospice care
- Cultural consideration in end-of-life care

Module 2: Pain Management at the End of Life
- Pain assessment
- Impact of pain on quality of life and family caregivers at the end of life
- Barriers to pain management
- Pharmacologic management of pain
- Nonpharmacologic management of pain

Module 3: Symptom Management at the End-of-Life
- Signs versus symptoms
- Priority symptoms in end-of-life care
  - Dyspnea
  - Fatigue/Weakness/Immobility
  - Hydration/Nutrition
  - Delirium/Agitation/Terminal Restlessness
- Characteristics of symptoms
- Symptom distress and duration
- The meaning of symptoms
- The impact of symptoms on quality of life

Module 4: Communication with Patients and Family Members at the End of Life
- Definition and goal of communication
- Importance of communication at the end of life
- Concerns/factors of patient and family members at the end of life
- How to communicate with patients/families at the end of life
- Strategies to help patients and family members at the end of life

Module 5: The Death Event
- Importance and goal of improving care at the time of death
- Signs and symptoms of approaching death
- Fears of the patient and family members at the end of life
- Signs and symptoms of death
- Care following death
- Nurse's role in the death event

Source: See reference 40.

The final two modules address important psychosocial considerations in end-of-life care. Module 4 focuses on the communication with patients and family members at the end of life, reviewing basic communication patterns and the importance of verbal and nonverbal communication at the end of life. Common concerns and barriers between health care providers, patients, and family members at the end of life are explored. Strategies for more effective communication are also provided.

Module 5 focuses on the actual death event. Based on input from a needs assessment survey, many home care agencies voiced feeling that while they are comfortable in care of the terminally ill patient at home, there still remains great discomfort in managing the actual death at home. This module stresses the importance of the actual death event and the need to anticipate and address barriers to provide the best death at home. Participants are provided information regarding signs and symptoms of approaching death for use in patient and family education. Content includes discussion of the common fears of patients and family members at the end of life as well as care provided following the death event in the home.

Future Directions

Clearly there is much work to be done to advance nursing education in palliative care. Improving the care of patients will be accomplished only when nursing education within undergraduate, graduate, and continuing education is improved.

In February 2000 a major initiative to contribute to this demand for enhanced nursing education in palliative care was begun. The project, End of Life Nursing Education Consortium (ELNEC), is cosponsored by the American Association of Colleges of Nursing (AACN) and nurse investigators at the City of Hope National Medical Center. The project is funded by the Robert Wood Johnson Foundation and includes development and implementation of a

Table 49–8. End-of-Life Nursing Education (ELNEC) Consortium

Module	Description of Content
1	*Nursing Care at the End of Life*—Goals of care, cost issues in palliative care, use of aggressive interventions, personal death awareness, broad review of end-of-life care to encompass all age groups and across various disease trajectories or acute illness.
2	*Pain Management*—Assessment, pharmacological, and nonpharmacological/complementary therapies.
3	*Symptom Management*—Assessment, pharmacological, and nonpharmacological/complementary therapies.
4	*Cultural Considerations in EOL Care*—Cultural assessment, beliefs regarding death and dying, afterlife and bereavement.
5	*Ethical/Legal Issues*—Assisted suicide, euthanasia, advance directives, decision making, advance care planning.
6	*Communication*—Breaking bad news, communicating with other disciplines, interdisciplinary collaboration.
7	*Grief, Loss, Bereavement*—Assessment, interventions, nurses' experiences with cumulative loss and grief.
8	*Preparation and Care for the Time of Death*—Nursing care at the time of death, including physical care, support of family members, saying good-bye.
9	*Achieving Quality of Life at the End of Life*—Including physical, psychological, social, and spiritual well-being and discussion of needs of special populations.

comprehensive palliative care curriculum for nurses. The components of the ELNEC program are listed in Table 49–8.

Progress over the next decade will require collaboration internationally and a close commitment by both nursing education and practice. Collectively, these efforts can advance the profession of palliative nursing and dramatically improve care at the end of life.

Evaluation of Palliative Care Education

Evaluation of education is a challenge in any program and for any content but is of special challenge in palliative care education. As the core content of this education evolves, so will the methods of evaluation. There is a need for standard knowledge assessment measures as well as means for evaluating clinical skills, decision making, and a broad range of physical, psychosocial, and spiritual care skills necessary in palliative care.[41–43] New technologies, such as Web-based teaching and evaluation tools, will be important resources for educators.

REFERENCES

1. Copp G. Palliative care nursing education: A review of research findings. Journal of Advanced Nursing 1994;19(3):552–557.

2. Farrell MJ. National palliative care education and training needs analysis. Contemporary Nurse 1998;7(2):60–67.

3. Field MJ, Cassel CK, eds. Approaching Death: Improving Care at the End of Life. Report of the Institute of Medicine Task Force on End of Life Care. National Academy of Sciences, Washington, DC, 1997.

4. James CR, MacLeod RD. The problematic nature of education in palliative care. Journal of Palliative Care 1993;9(4):5–10.

5. Ferrell BR, Grant M, Ritchey K, et al. The pain resource nurse training program: A unique approach to pain management. Journal of Pain and Symptom Management 1993;8:549–556.

6. Kristjanson L, Balneaves L. Directions for palliative care nursing in Canada: Report of a national survey. Journal of Palliative Care 1995; 11:5–8.

7. Manias E, Kristjanson L, Bush T. Palliative care nursing education: Australian and Canadian challenges. Contemporary Nurse 1997;6(3–4): 96–97.

8. Bennauhum, DA. The historical development of hospice and palliative care. In: Sheehan DC, Forman WB, eds. Hospice and Palliative Care Boston: Jones and Bartlett, 1996:3–5.

9. Kubler-Ross E. On Death and Dying. New York: Macmillan, 1969.

10. Quint JC. The Nurse and the Dying Patient. New York: Macmillan, 1967.

11. Sheehan DK, Webb A, Bower D, et al. Level of cancer pain knowledge among baccalaureate student nurses. Journal of Pain and Symptom Management 1992;7:478–484.

12. Grant MM, Rivera LM. Pain education for nurses, patients, and families. In: McGuire DB, Yarbro CH, Ferrell BR, eds. Cancer Pain Management Boston: Jones and Bartlett, 1995:289–319.

13. International Association for the Study of Pain. Pain curriculum for basic nursing education. IASP Newsletter September/October 1993:4–6.

14. Coolican M, Stark J, Doka K, Corr C. Education about death, dying, and bereavement in nursing practice. Nursing Educator 1994; 16:35–40.

15. Field D, Kitson C. Formal teaching about death and dying in UK nursing schools. Nurse Education Today 1986;6:270–276.

16. Pickett M, Cooley ME, Gordon DB. Palliative care: Past, present, and future perspectives. Seminars in Oncology Nursing 1998;14(2):86–94.

17. Samaroo B. Assessing palliative care educational needs of physicians and nurses: Results of a survey. Greater Victoria Hospital Society Palliative Care Committee. Journal of Palliative Care 12(2):20–22.

18. Sellick SM, Charles K, Dagsvik J, Kelley ML. Palliative care providers' perspectives on service and education needs. Journal of Palliative Care 1996;12(2):34–38.

19. Webber J. New directions in palliative care education. Support Care Cancer 1994;2(1): 16–20.

20. Degner LF, Gow CM, Thompson LA. Critical nursing behaviors in care of the dying. Cancer Nursing 1991;(14)5:246–253.

21. McClement SE, Degner LF. Expert nursing behaviors in care of the dying adult in the intensive care unit. Heart and Lung 1995;24: 408–419.

22. Webster NE. Communicating with dying patients. Nursing Times, June 4, 1981:999–1002.

23. Rittman M, Rivera J, Godown I. Phenomenological study of nurses caring for dying patients. Cancer Nursing 1997;(20)2:115–119.

24. Ferrell BR, Virani R, Grant M. Analysis of end of life content in nursing textbooks. Oncology Nursing Forum 1999;26(5):869–876.

25. World Health Organization. Cancer Pain Relief and Palliative Care. WHO Technical Report Series 804. Geneva: World Health Organization, 1990.

26. Jodrell N. Nurse education. In: Doyle D, Hanks G, MacDonald N, eds. Oxford Textbook of Palliative Medicine, 2nd ed. Oxford: Oxford University Press, 1998:1202–1208.

27. Davies B, Oberle K. Dimensions of the supportive role of the nurse in palliative care. Oncology Nursing Forum 1990;17:87–94.

28. Hanson EJ, Cullihall, K. Images of palliative nursing care. Journal of Palliative Care 1995;11(3):35–39.

29. Nishimoto P. Venturing into the unknown, cultural beliefs about death and dying. Oncology Nursing Forum 1996;23:889–894.

30. Rooda LA, Clements R, Jordan ML. Nurses' attitudes toward death and caring for dying patients. Oncology Nursing Forum 1999; 26(10):1683–1687.

31. Scanlon C. Unraveling ethical issues in palliative care. Seminars in Oncology Nursing 1998;14(2):137–144.

32. Redman S, White K, Ryan E, Hennrikus D. Professional needs of palliative care nurses in New South Wales. Palliative Medicine 1995;9(1): 36–44.

33. Sheldon F, Smith P. The life so short, the craft so hard to learn: A model for post-basic education in palliative care. Palliative Medicine 1996; 10(2):99–104.

34. Vachon ML. Caring for the caregiver in oncology and palliative care. Seminars in Oncology Nursing 1998;14(2):152–157.

35. Yates P, Hart G, Clinton M, McGrath P, Gartry D. Exploring empathy as a variable in the evaluation of professional development programs for palliative care nurses. Cancer Nursing 1998; 21(6):402–410.

36. International Council of Nurses. Basic Principles of Nursing Care. Washington, DC: American Nurses Publishing, 1997.

37. American Association of Colleges of Nursing. (1997, November). A peaceful death. Report from the Robert Wood Johnson End-of-Life Care Roundtable, Washington, DC, November 1997.

38. National Council of Hospice Professionals. Guidelines for Curriculum Development on End-of-Life and Palliative Care in Nursing Education. Arlington, VA: National Hospice Organization, 1997.

39. Sheldon F. Will the doors open? Multicultural issues in palliative care. Palliative Medicine 1995;9:89–90.

40. American Association of Critical-Care Nurses. Designing an agenda for the nursing profession on end of life care: Report of the Nursing Leadership Consortium on end of life care. Washington, DC, Author. 1999.

41. MacLeod RD. Education in palliative medicine: A review. Journal of Cancer Education 1993;8(4):309–312.

42. Sowell R, Seals G, Wilson B, Robinson C. Evaluation of an HIV/AIDS continuing education program. Journal of Continuing Education Nursing 1998;29(2):85–93.

43. The SUPPORT Principal Investigators. A controlled trial to improve care for seriously ill hospitalized patients: The study to understand prognoses and preferences for outcomes and risks of treatments (SUPPORT). Journal of the American Medical Association 1995;274:1591–1598.

50 Nursing Research

BETTY R. FERRELL and MARCIA GRANT

From the cellular to the social level, much remains to be learned about how people die and how reliably excellent and compassionate care can be achieved. Important, unanswered questions exist about the fundamental physiological mechanism of the symptoms that cause so much suffering among dying patients and about the kinds of interventions that will relieve these symptoms. Basic epidemiological information on how people die is limited, and the influence of attitudes and beliefs on people's experience of dying and on caregiving practices is little charted. In addition, a better understanding of the reasons for the inadequate application of existing knowledge would help in identifying organizational, economic, and other incentives for the provision of accessible, effective, and affordable care at the end of life.[1]

—Field and Cassell, Institute of Medicine, 1997

The words from the Institute of Medicine's 1997 report on improving care at the end of life capture the breadth of palliative care research. Uniform agreement across disciplines and among authors confirms the paucity of palliative care research and resultant absence of a scientific foundation for practice, thus impacting care of patients at the end of life.[2–7] Better patient care is dependent on both the quantity and quality of palliative care research.

A major component of palliative care research is nursing research. The patient experience of dying is an ideal health care concern appropriate for nursing inquiry.[8–9] As nurses are concerned with patient responses to illness, the physical, psychological, social, and spiritual responses of the terminally ill and their families are prime areas for nursing research.

The ultimate goal of nursing research, and thus nursing knowledge, is to improve patient care. Palliative care offers a rich opportunity for research to directly influence patient care in areas such as symptom management, psychological responses to a terminal illness, and the family caregiver experience of terminal illness.[10–14]

Some of the earliest contributions to palliative care research were made by nurses. Pioneering work by Jeanne Quint Benoliel and others raised our awareness of deficiencies in care of the dying.[15–16] Early descriptive studies documented the influence of nursing attitudes and beliefs about death on the care provided to patients.

From the earliest studies in the 1960s to the "awakening" of attention to palliative care in the late 1990s, research in palliative care has been limited. Nurse investigators have addressed aspects of end-of-life care such as pain management, bereavement, settings of care, and special populations such as AIDs care. However, there has been a lack of cohesive commitment to palliative care nursing research.

In 1997, the National Institute of Nursing Research (NINR) led an initiative regarding end-of-life care research across several National Institutes of Health (NIH) institutes. Specific recommendations of an NINR-sponsored conference on end-of-life care are described later in this chapter.[17] It is appropriate and commendable that the NINR is providing leadership at the NIH in this research agenda.

As has been true in other areas of health care, the research agenda has lagged behind the demands of clinical practice and education. Hospice programs and palliative care settings face increased demands for improved end-of-life care with little scientific knowledge to guide clinical decisions. Nursing schools have begun to develop undergraduate and graduate courses in palliative care, and some have launched degree or certificate programs in palliative care, again with limited research as a scientific foundation of their programs. Obviously, developing a solid research agenda and supporting nursing science in palliative care are overdue.

GOALS OF PALLIATIVE CARE RESEARCH

The goals of palliative care nursing research are similar to goals of other areas of nursing inquiry. Nursing research serves multiple functions such as quantification of information, discovery, description of phenomenon, quality improvement, and problem solving.[9] *Quantification* is accomplished through descriptive studies or through epidemiologic approaches. For example, there is a need to quantify the symptoms present in terminal illness, their severity and impact. The field of palliative nursing care is relatively unexplored, and thus there is great opportunity for discovery. What are the greatest needs of terminally ill patients and their family caregivers? What is the unique role of nursing within the interdisciplinary team?

The subjective nature of terminal illness and the existential experience of dying will require research methods that *describe phenomena*. Death, as a subject that has been avoided in society, is still a relatively unknown aspect of life. On a more specific level, palliative care is also a field that would benefit tremendously from research linked to *quality improvement*. Numerous reports have identified serious deficits in end-of-life care and efforts to improve the quality of end-of-life care will undoubtedly benefit from research. And finally, a major goal of palliative care research should be basic *problem solving*. What drugs are most beneficial for dyspnea or agitation? What is the best treatment for pressure ulcers in a dying patient? What education best prepares family caregivers for signs and symptoms of approaching death?

ETHICAL/METHODOLOGICAL CONSIDERATIONS IN PALLIATIVE CARE RESEARCH

There are many unique aspects of research in palliative care. The multidimensional nature of care at the end of life and the vulnerability of the population are but two examples of factors that pose special challenges to this area of research.

The challenges of nursing research in palliative care should be prefaced by a discussion of the benefits. While even the mention of conducting research with dying patients and their burdened families immediately creates concerns, there are in fact many benefits to participants. Participating in research, even at this most vulnerable and sensitive time of life, provides opportunity for research subjects to contribute to others. Research participation often provides an opportunity to derive meaning from illness and to feel that one's suffering will provide benefit to others.[8,18]

In our research at the City of Hope over numerous studies in sensitive areas such as pain, quality of life, and fatigue, we have consistently received positive feedback from research subjects. Patients and family caregivers often have thanked the researchers for studying these topics perceived to be of great importance. Subjects have also frequently related that completing written instruments or participating in interviews provided a mechanism for communicating needs that had not previously been voiced.

However, research in palliative care is very challenging and includes many obstacles. Nurses are often conflicted in balancing roles of clinician versus researcher. For example, in conducting research related to pain in terminally ill cancer patients, we have often had to carefully balance our roles as both clinicians and researchers. Identifying a patient with severe pain has often meant we must end the patient's participation in a study in order to seek treatment for their pain. Research must always respect the more important ethical consideration of protecting the patient's well-being.

Seeking informed consent in rapidly declining, weak patients is a challenge, as is the need to constantly protect patient and family autonomy. Subjects in palliative care research may feel obligated to participate in research, particularly if they have been the recipients of good care. While all patients in palliative care are considered vulnerable, we know that certain subgroups such as the cognitively impaired poor or elderly are of special concern.[19–23]

The sensitive nature of palliative care research provides inherent challenge. The areas of concern at the end of life are highly emotional and may invoke heightened distress. Exploring areas such as grief, fears, spiritual concerns, family conflict, and other common dimensions of terminal illness is highly challenging. Participation in research can bring to the forefront previously undisclosed problems. In our research experience, we have found that palliative care research necessitates highly skilled research staff. Collecting data from palliative care subjects is very different from research in healthy or chronically ill subjects. Research nurses in palliative care studies must be clinically competent, highly skilled nurses equipped to balance the rigor of research with extreme sensitivity.

Palliative care research, perhaps more than any other field of inquiry, must carefully weigh subject burden. The time required of research subjects in palliative care, a precious commodity amidst terminal disease, must be carefully protected. Special consideration

Table 50–1. Barriers to Nursing Research in Palliative Care

- Overall limitations in funding for nursing research and in the limited number of nurse researchers.
- Research establishment and associated funding has been focused on rehabilitation or cure.
- Lack of political or consumer advocates to promote research agenda in end-of-life care.
- Limited focus on palliative care in graduate nursing education to promote end-of-life research within master's or doctoral nursing education.
- Few established relationships between nurse researchers and clinical settings of palliative care.
- Ethical considerations of conducting research with vulnerable populations, including issues related to ability to provide consent.
- Rapidly declining status limits subject accrual and opportunity for longitudinal measures.
- Lack of conceptual frameworks appropriate for palliative care research.
- Participation in research interferes with demands of patient care.
- Late referrals to hospice or palliative care programs severely restricts opportunities for accrual to studies.
- Lack of research instruments and methods appropriate for this population.
- Challenge of conducting research in a sensitive area.
- Balancing demands of rigorous research, such as the need for randomization with awareness of patient needs.

Source: Adapted from refs. 1 and 29.

Table 50–2. Funding Sources for Pilot Studies

1. Hospital Continuous Quality Improvement Programs
2. Oncology Nursing Foundation
3. Sigma Theta Tau
4. American Nursing Foundation
5. American Society of Pain Management Nurses
6. Local Community Foundations
7. Pharmaceutical Companies

must be given to selection of research instruments and procedures to minimize subject burden.

A useful resource for nurses researchers in palliative care is a "Tool Kit" project, supported by a grant from the RWJ Foundation to researchers at the University of Rhode Island. This project has reviewed and compiled a list of research instruments recommended for use in palliative care. The tool kit is available on the Web at www.chcr.brown.edu/web-pubs.htm#top.

Subject attrition is another common problem area in palliative care research. Accounting for higher attrition has serious implications when determining sample sizes and also has budget implications. This problem area becomes an even greater concern when attempting longitudinal studies, a definite need in palliative care.[19–23] New approaches to handling data are needed to improve data analysis.

Palliative care research also necessitates diversity in research methods. Our experience has been that a combination of qualitative and quantitative approaches is needed.[24] Qualitative approaches are especially important in descriptive studies. Quantitative approaches are essential when studying symptoms, their frequency, nature, and response to treatment.

We also have found that nursing research in palliative care is greatly enhanced by interdisciplinary collaboration. The problems studied are multidimensional and are best defined from the viewpoints of various members of the health team. Participation from our colleagues in psychology, theology, social work, and other disciplines has enhanced our work considerably.

A final special consideration in palliative care research is the importance of including family caregivers. Terminal illness is a shared experience, and including family caregivers as subjects enriches the benefits to be derived from the research.[10,12,13]

Table 50–1 summarizes some of the key challenges of conducting palliative care research. Advancement of the nursing profession in palliative care will require attention to overcome these obstacles.

A RESEARCH AGENDA IN PALLIATIVE NURSING

The IOM report identified priority areas for end-of-life care research, including pain, cachexia-anorexia-asthenia, dyspnea, cognitive, and emotional symptoms. Also addressed was the need for social, behavioral, and health services research. Nursing as a profession has much to contribute to each of these identified priorities.[8,9]

There is a tremendous need to bring together nurse researchers and nurse clinicians in palliative care. Historically,

Table 50–3. Research Proposal Evaluation Criteria

Abstract
- Accurately reflects the proposal
- Includes problem statement and purpose
- Summarizes key variables, sample, and methods

Study Aims, Hypotheses, or Study Questions
- Clearly stated
- Hypotheses or study questions are consistent with the study aim
- Encompasses all proposed study procedures and data to be collected

Significance of the Study
- Contributes to the science of palliative nursing care
- Has the potential to lead to further investigation
- The research offers a unique contribution to the literature
- The research is clinically relevant to end-of-life care

Literature Review
- Relevant and current literature is reviewed
- Literature primarily includes research rather than opinion
- Literature is critiqued, synthesized, and analyzed

Conceptual/Theoretical Framework
- Framework identified is appropriate to the study and consistent with study questions and methods
- Framework is consistent with the philosophy of palliative care

Procedures
- The procedures are feasible
- Includes methods for training and supervision of personnel
- Procedures provide sufficient description of precisely what will be required of subjects

Data Analysis
- Identifies specific statistical procedures. Analysis is appropriate for the type of data and study design and answers the study questions.
- Describes computer facilities and consultation
- Investigator has sought consultation if necessary in preparing the proposal

Human Subjects Considerations
- IRB approval is given or documentation of pending review is given
- The investigator is clearly aware of the impact of participation in the study on the subject
- Addresses concerns regarding the length, intrusiveness, and energy expenditure required
- Researcher has acknowledged special considerations of terminal illness

Investigators and Research Team
- Consultation is available for the less experienced researcher
- Establishes the role of co-investigators or consultants

Overall
- Strictly adheres to format restrictions and page limitations

Source: Adapted from the Oncology Nursing Foundation, 1999.

Table 50–4. General Tips for Preparing Research Proposals

1. Grant writing is not a solo activity—seek consultation and collaboration from others. Seek opportunities to involve clinical palliative care settings, such as hospices in nursing research.
2. Have your proposal reviewed by peers before submitting it for funding. A proposal submitted for funding is generally the product of numerous revisions.
3. Follow the directions in detail, including margins, page limits, and the use of references and appendices. Communicate directly with the funding source to clarify any directions you are unsure of.
4. State ideas clearly and succinctly. Word economy is essential to a fine-tuned proposal.
5. Use high-quality printing and use a good-quality copier. Give attention to spelling and grammar.
6. Plan ahead and develop a time frame for completing your grant. Avoid the last-minute rush that will compromise the quality of your proposal. It is better to target a future deadline for submission than to compromise your score due to a lack of time for preparation.
7. Use appendices to include study instruments, procedures, or other supporting materials. Adhere to funding agency criteria, but maximize the opportunity for a complete proposal.
8. Include support letters from individuals who are important to the success of your study. This includes medical staff, nursing administration, consultants, and co-investigators.
9. Do not hesitate to contact experts in your subject area to seek their input. They are often able to review your work and direct you toward related instruments or literature.
10. Start small. Successful completion of a pilot project is the best foundation for a larger study. Efficient use of small grant funding is influential when seeking larger-scale funding for major proposals.
11. Be realistic. Design research projects that can be realistically accomplished within the scope of your other responsibilities and the limitations of your work setting.
12. Keep focused on the patient. Design and implement research that is relevant to patient care and improves quality of life at the end of life for patients and families.

Source: See ref. 30.

few nurse researchers have focused on palliative care, and likewise, few expert clinicians in palliative care have had opportunities or expertise in research.

While an exhaustive review of research methods or grant writing is not possible in this chapter, a few comments are worthy of attention. Palliative care clinicians are encouraged to seek collaboration with nurse researchers in order to initiate clinically relevant and scientifically sound studies. Another key issue of advice is to begin small. Conducting small pilot studies is an essential foundation to launching larger-scale studies. Potential sources for funding are found in Table 50–2.

Table 50–3 includes an example of criteria used in evaluating small-scale research projects. These criteria, adapted from the Oncology Nursing Foundation, depict the essential elements of a research proposal. Many professional organizations provide small grant support to novice investigators. Table 50–4 includes some general tips for preparing a research proposal.

Another useful guide for nurses initiating research proposals is included in Table 50–5. This includes the review considerations used by grant reviewers at the

Table 50–5. Review Considerations in NIH-Sponsored Research

1. Significance

Does this study address an important problem? If the aims of the application are achieved, how will scientific knowledge be advanced? What will be the effect of these studies on the concepts or methods that drive this field?

2. Approach

Are the conceptual framework, design, methods, and analyses adequately developed, well integrated, and appropriate to the aims of the project? Does the applicant acknowledge potential problem areas and consider alternative tactics?

3. Innovation

Does the project employ novel concepts, approaches, or methods? Are the aims original and innovative? Does the project challenge existing paradigms or develop new methodologies or technologies?

4. Investigator

Is the investigator appropriately trained and well suited to carry out this work? Is the work proposed appropriate to the experience level of the principal investigator and other researchers (if any)?

5. Environment

Does the scientific environment in which the work will be done contribute to the probability of success? Do the proposed experiments take advantage of unique features of the scientific environment or employ useful collaborative arrangements? Is there evidence of institutional support?

In addition, the adequacy of plans to include both genders and minorities and their subgroups as appropriate for the scientific goals of the research are reviewed. Plans for the recruitment and retention of subjects is also evaluated.

Table 50–6. Potential Areas for Research in End-of-Life (EOL) Care

Critical Areas of End-of-Life Care	Examples of Area Content	Examples of Potential Areas of Inquiry
1. The Concept of Palliative Care	A. Importance of palliative care for nurses B. Definitions of palliative care C. Important goals/characteristics of palliative care: 1. Dignity/Respect 2. Relief of symptoms 3. Peaceful death 4. Ethical issues 5. Patient control/choices D. Importance of interdisciplinary collaboration E. Recognition of nurses' own discomfort/anxiety	1. Refinement of definitions/criteria for palliative care 2. Descriptive studies of interdisciplinary involvement and related outcomes 3. Evaluation of methods to provide staff support in palliative care
2. Quality of Life (QOL) at the EOL	Recognition of Multiple Dimensions of QOL @ EOL A. Physical well-being B. Psychological well-being C. Social well-being D. Spiritual well-being	1. Development/testing of QOL instruments for use in palliative care 2. Refinement of research methods to decrease patient burden in QOL assessment 3. Development/testing of QOL instruments for family caregivers
3. Pain Management at EOL	A. Definition of pain B. Assessment of pain C. Assessment of meaning of pain D. Pharmacologic management of pain at EOL E. Use of invasive techniques F. Principles of addiction, tolerance, and dependence G. Nonpharmacologic management of pain H. Physical pain vs. suffering I. Side effects of opioids J. Barriers to pain management K. Fear of opioids hastening death L. Equianalgesic dosing M. Recognition of nurses' own burden in pain management at EOL	1. Methods of assessing pain in the nonverbal or confused patient 2. Refine methods for pain assessment to decreasepatient burden 3. Development of pain measures that incorporate all dimensions of pain at EOL, i.e., spiritual pain 4. Intervention studies to treat common pain syndromes at EOL 5. Testing of protocols to treat pain at EOL, including changing routes of analgesia 6. Development/evaluation of teaching programs for patients/families to decrease fears regarding pain management 7. Development/evaluation of programs to educate/support nurses in managing pain
4. Other Symptom Management at EOL	A. Assessment and management of common EOL symptoms 1. Dyspnea/cough 2. Nausea/vomiting 3. Dehydration/nutrition 4. Altered mental status/delirium/ terminal restlessness 5. Anxiety/depression 6. Weakness/fatigue 7. Dysphagia 8. Incontinence 9. Skin integrity 10. Constipation/bowel obstruction 11. Agitation/myoclonus	1. Descriptive studies to better understand symptom prevalence and patterns at EOL 2. Evaluation of pharmacologic treatments for each symptom 3. Development of patient/family caregiver education for symptom management, including pharmacologic and nonpharmacologic treatments 4. Evaluation of protocols/algorithms to enhance nurse's effectiveness in symptom assessment and management

(*continued*)

Table 50–6. Potential Areas for Research in End-of-Life (EOL) Care (*Continued*)

Critical Areas of End-of-Life Care	Examples of Area Content	Examples of Potential Areas of Inquiry
5. Communication with Dying Patients and Families	A. Definition/goals of communication B. Importance of listening C. Barriers to communication D. Delivering bad news/truth-telling E. Recognizing family dynamics in communication F. Sensitivity to culture, ethnicity, values, and religion G. Discussion of options/decisions with patients/family H. Communication among interdisciplinary team members/collaboration I. Responding to requests for assisted suicide	1. Descriptive studies to better determine common areas of concern regarding communication at EOL 2. Studies that describe the role of nursing in communication 3. Evaluation of protocols for delivering/reinforcing bad news 4. Studies that explore cultural issues influencing communication 5. Evaluation of methods that support communication (i.e., written materials, family conferences) 6. Exploration of decision making by patients and family caregivers 7. Exploration of causes of requests for assisted suicide and preparation of nurses to respond to requests
6. Role/Needs of Family Caregivers in EOL Care	A. The importance of recognizing family and caregivers needs at EOL B. Assessment of family needs C. Family dynamics D. Recognizing ethical/cultural influences E. Coping strategies and support systems	1. Descriptive studies to enhance our understanding of the family caregiver perspective of terminal illness 2. Studies that explore family dynamics and the family as a unit rather than focus only on single caregivers 3. Exploratory studies to enhance understanding of cultural influences
7. Care at the Time of Death	A. The nurse's personal death awareness B. Death as natural process C. Recognizing signs/symptoms of impending death D. Patient/family's fears associated with death E. Preparing for the death event 1. Health care providers 2. Patient 3. Family Caregivers F. Physical care at the time of death G. Spiritual care at the time of death	1. Evaluation of educational/support approaches to enhance personal death awareness 2. Evaluation of teaching approaches to prepare families for impending death 3. Development and evaluation of protocols for care at the time of death—i.e., physical and spiritual care
8. Issues of Policy, Ethics, and Law	A. Patient preferences/advance directives B. Assisted suicide C. Euthanasia D. Withdrawing food/fluids E. Discontinuing life support F. Legal issues @ EOL G. Need for changes in health policy H. Confidentiality	1. Evaluation of approaches to enhance use of advance directives 2. Testing of educational methods to enhance nurse's ability to respond to requests for assisted suicide/euthanasia 3. Development and evaluation of protocols that promote patient comfort while discontinuing food/fluids and life support 4. Identification of legal and regulatory barriers to optimum EOL care
9. Bereavement	A. Stages/process of grief B. Assessment of grief C. Interventions/resources D. Recognition of staff grief	1. Descriptive studies of grief by patients, families, and staff with attention to cultural considerations 2. Refinement of efficient methods of grief assessment 3. Testing of approaches to facilitate staff grieving

NIH. The five criteria of significance, approach, innovation, investigator, and environment can serve as a useful guide in designing research proposals.[17]

Several initiatives have begun to establish an agenda for palliative care research. Topics frequently identified as priority topics for palliative care research include pain, symptom management, epidemiologic studies of terminal illness, family caregiver needs, bereavement, cultural considerations, spiritual needs and health systems considerations such as costs of care.[4,25–27]

At the City of Hope, we have developed a framework of nine areas of palliative nursing care that is used in our nursing education efforts as described in Chapter 49, on nursing education. Table 50–6 includes a summary of these nine topic areas, with examples of potential research that is needed.[28]

Another excellent resource for identifying future areas of palliative care research comes from the conference convened by the NINR as described previously.[17] An excerpt of the Executive Summary from this NIH research workshop, which focused on symptom management in terminal illness is included as Appendix A, together with the specific recommendations from that conference, which identified research needs in the symptoms of pain, dyspnea, cognitive disturbances, and cachexia.[17]

SUMMARY

Advances in the care of patients and families facing terminal illness is contingent on advances in palliative nursing research. Control of symptoms, comfort for families, and attention to psychosocial and spiritual needs will improve when nurse clinicians have a stronger scientific foundation for practice. Research will require collaboration with other disciplines and unity of nurse clinicians and researchers.

REFERENCES

1. Field M, Cassel C. Approaching death: Improving care at the end of life. Committee on Care at the End of Life, Institute of Medicine. National Academy Press, 1997.

2. Cohen SR, Bultz BD, Clarke JY, et al. Well-being at the end of life: Part 1. A research agenda for psychological and spiritual aspects of care from the patient's perspective. Cancer Prevention Control 1997;1(5):334–342.

3. Cohen SR, MacNeil C, Mount BM. Well-being at the end of life: Part 2. Research for the delivery of care from the patient's perspective. Cancer Prevention Control 1997;1(5):343–351.

4. Corner J. Is there a research paradigm for palliative care? Palliative Medicine 1996;10(3): 201–208.

5. Hearn J, Higginson IJ. Outcome measures in palliative care for advanced cancer patients: A review. Journal of Public Health Medicine 1997; 19(2):193–199.

6. Pickett M, Cooley ME, Gordon DB. Palliative care: Past, present, and future perspectives. Seminars in Oncology Nursing 1998;14(2):86–94.

7. Richards MA, Corner J, Clark D. Developing a research culture for palliative care. Palliative Medicine 1998;12:399–403.

8. Barnett JW, Richardson A. Nursing research. In: Doyle D, Hanks GWC, MacDonald N, eds. Oxford Textbook of Palliative Medicine, 2nd ed. Oxford: Oxford University Press, 1998: 193–200.

9. Ferrell BR, Funk B. Hospice Research. In: Sheehan DC, Forman WB, eds. Hospice and Palliative Care. Sudbury, MA: Jones and Bartlett, 1996;167–174.

10. Change E, Daly J. Priority areas for clinical research in palliative care nursing. International Journal of Nursing Practice 1998;4(4):247–253.

11. King CR, Haberman M, Berry D, et al. Quality of life and the cancer experience: The state of the knowledge. Oncology Nursing Forum 1997;24:27–41.

12. Kristjanson LJ. Quality of terminal care: Salient indicators identified by families. Journal of Palliative Care 1989;5:21–28.

13. Leis AM, Kristjanson L, Koop PM, Laizner A. Family health and the palliative care trajectory: A cancer research agenda. Cancer Prevention and Control 1997;1(5):352–360.

14. Yates P, et al. Families' awareness of and response to dying. Oncology Nursing Forum 1999; 26(1):113–120.

15. Benoliel JQ. Death influence in clinical practice: A course for graduate students. In: Benoliel JC, ed. Death Education for the Health Professional. Washington, DC: Hemisphere Publishing, 1982;31–50.

16. Benoliel JQ. Health care providers and dying patients: Critical issues in terminal care. Omega 1987;18:341–363.

17. National Institutes of Health website http://www.nih.gov/ninr/end-of-life.htm. Symptoms in Terminal Illness: A Research Workshop. September 22–23, 1997.

18. Bruera E. Ethical issues in palliative care research. Journal of Palliative Care 1994;10(3): 7–9.

19. Cohen SR, Mount BM. Quality of life in terminal illness: Defining and measuring subjective well being in the dying. Journal of Palliative Care 1992;8:40–45.

20. American Geriatric Society Panel on Chronic Pain in Older Persons. (1998). The management of chronic pain in older persons. JAGS 1998;46:635–651.

21. DeRaeve L. Ethical issues in palliative care research. Palliative Medicine 1994;8:298–305.

22. Rinck GC, van den Bos GA, Kleijnan J, et al. Methodological issues in effectiveness research on palliative cancer care: A systematic review. Journal of Clinical Oncology 1997;15(4): 1697–1707.

23. Van Eys J. The ethics of palliative care. Journal of Palliative Care 1991;7:27–32.

24. Clark D. What is qualitative research and what can it contribute to palliative care? Palliative Medicine 1997;11:159–166.

25. Dudgeon DJ, Raubertas RF, Doerner K, et al. When does palliative care begin? A needs assessment of cancer patients with recurrent disease. Journal of Palliative Care 1995;11:5–9.

26. Emanual EJ. Cost savings at the end of life. What do the data show? Journal of the American Medical Association 1996;26;275(24):1907–1914.

27. Aaronson NK, Meyerowitz BE, Bard M, et al. Quality of life research in oncology: Past achievements and future priorities. Cancer 1991; 67:839–843.

28. Ferrell BR, Virani R, Grant M. Analysis of end of life content in nursing textbooks. Oncology Nursing Forum, 1999;26(5):869–876.

29. Doyle D, Hanks GWC, MacDonald N, eds. Oxford Textbook of Palliative Medicine, 2nd ed. Oxford: Oxford University Press, 1993.

30. Ferrell BR, Nail LM, Mooney K, et al. (1989). Applying for Oncology Nursing Society and Oncology Nursing Foundation Grants. Oncology Nursing Forum 1989;16(5):728–730.

APPENDIX A: NIH RESEARCH WORKSHOP ON SYMPTOMS IN TERMINAL ILLNESS—EXECUTIVE SUMMARY

Patients at the end of life experience many of the same symptoms and syndromes, regardless of their underlying medical condition. Pain is the most obvious example, but others are difficult breathing (dyspnea), transient episodes of confusion and loss of concentration (cognitive disturbances and delirium), loss of appetite and muscle wasting (cachexia), as well as nausea, fatigue, and depression. Taken together, these and other symptoms add significantly to the suffering of patients and their families, and to the costs and burden of their medical care. Yet in many cases the symptoms could be treated or prevented.

Pain, for example, is a multibillion-dollar public health problem in the United States. Over half of all cancer patients experience pain related to their disease or its treatment. Similarly, half of all cancer patients and 70 percent of all hospice patients experience shortness of breath in the last weeks of life. Yet dyspnea remains under-diagnosed and under-treated. Forty percent of all patients experience cognitive disturbances during the final days of life, and high numbers of terminally ill patients experience cachexia regardless of their primary disease. Significantly, these symptoms occur not in isolation but in clusters, with most patients experiencing combinations of symptoms that vary greatly in their prevalence and severity, as well as in the suffering they cause.

Basic research has improved our understanding of the underlying mechanisms of symptoms that are commonly experienced at the end of life, particularly with respect to pain. Clinical research has in some cases translated this knowledge into new drugs and other interventions that can effectively relieve or prevent these symptoms, even where the underlying disease cannot be cured. At present, however, there remain a number of important gaps in knowledge.

Clinical care would benefit from an integrative, multidisciplinary research initiative that brings basic and clinical researchers together to address the constellation of symptoms at the end of life. The following areas should receive priority:

- Epidemiology—There is a need for better data on the incidence and combinations of symptoms that are experienced at the end of life in specific populations. Epidemiological data will demonstrate the magnitude and costs of the problem, as well as suggest specific topics for basic and clinical research.
- Basic research—Additional research is needed on the mechanisms and interactions of these symptoms, including biochemical, neuronal, endocrine, and immune approaches. The possibility of common factors, mechanisms, and pathways across different symptoms should be examined There is also a need for research on the mechanism of action of successful therapies, with particular attention to the role of opioid receptors. This research could lead to therapies that are better targeted, more selective in their action, and thus produce fewer side effects.
- Clinical research—Because these symptoms have multiple determinants, and occur in clusters, successful interventions will also be multifactorial, including behavioral as well as pharmacological approaches. Combination therapies and off-label drugs should be explored. Researchers should be alert to differences in outcome based on age, gender, and underlying disease. Interventions to mobilize psychosocial and spiritual resources may be of help mediating the perception and interpretation of symptoms. The goal of research should be to test a wide range of interventions that could be successfully implemented in the home or hospice, as well as in the hospital.
- Methodology—Researchers will need better tests for diagnosing and assessing the level of severity of these symptoms, as well as for monitoring the effectiveness of interventions. Standardized terminology and definitions of symptoms should be established. Particular attention should be paid to validating subjective and nonverbal measures. Better data and tools are also needed for evaluating outcomes, in order to determine costs and strengthen accountability for the quality of care at the end of life. It is important to develop and use measures which reflect the subjective experience of the effects of symptoms on quality of life.

Research is also needed on the ethical issues that may be barriers to research at the end of life, including the needs and protection of vulnerable populations, especially the role of privacy during this important phase of life. Attention must be paid to community and individual preferences about the relative value of symptom management at different points in the dying trajectory, and to the development of comprehensive strategies for the early detection and treatment of the full range of symptoms at the end of life—an approach that will reduce costs as well as burdens, while preserving the patient's dignity and quality of life.

Recommendations for Research on Specific Symptoms

The following preamble for the recommendations reflected the consensus of the entire workshop:

To adequately address symptom control in the terminally ill, an important first step is to invest resources in the development of new methodologies for assessing symptoms and evaluating treatments. These tools will allow us to elucidate the extent of the problem and to set national priorities to improve quality of life for those facing life-limiting illness.

Pain

1. Epidemiology—There is still a great need for epidemiological data on the incidence and types of pain at the end of life. Research in this area will provide direction for researchers regarding what specific topics should be tackled next.
2. Treatment—There is a clear need to discover new drugs for the treatment of pain, including analgesic combinations. Neuropathic pain, because of its incidence and burden, should be a particular priority. There should also be studies of the relationship between disease, pain, and suffering at the end of life, which would also include psychosocial mediators. Clinical Trials Groups should be developed to study promising interventions.
3. Measurement—Methods should be developed for collecting valid data on pain in the home, in nursing homes, etc., possibly using telephones or computer technology. Measurement of other outcomes of subjective experience, such as the suffering caused by pain, should also be developed and utilized.

Dyspnea

1. Epidemiology—What are the incidence and impact of dyspnea in different populations? There is some information about dyspnea in cancer and COPD patients, but almost none in cardiac disease, and other terminal conditions.
2. Mechanisms—Relatively little is known about the various determinants of dyspnea, including respiratory muscle strength, exercise capacity, respiratory controller, gas exchange, and psychosocial factors. Neurobiological models, like those developed for pain, will be useful, but the overall approach must be integrative. The determinants are almost certainly multifactorial, necessitating multidisciplinary strategies.

3. Measurement—Research is needed to refine available instruments and develop new ones for measuring both the causes of symptoms and the effects of treatment. There is at present no standardized approach for assessing the degree of dyspnea in a given disease (e.g., chronic vs. acute, COPD vs. cancer). The goal would be to formulate guidelines for optimal assessment, which would point to optimal treatment.
4. Treatment—A number of potential treatments are available, but there is little information on their relative effectiveness. Particular attention should be given to the choice and timing of anxiolytics, phenothiazines, oxygen, opiates, and exercise. Attention should also be given to the timing and management of terminal weaning (removal of ventilation), including the role of families.

The collaborative and integrative nature of this research is well suited to sponsorship and funding by NIH. It would be useful, for example, for the various NIH Institutes to sponsor a series of joint workshops that would characterize clinical experience and impact of therapies on dyspnea in diseases other than lung cancer.

Cognitive Disturbances. There is a considerable amount of epidemiological data on delirium already, and while it might be useful to gather additional information on specific patient populations, this symptom is known to be under-recognized and under-treated. Consequently, the research priorities in this symptom area are as follows:

1. Measurement—Research is needed to enhance the recognition of delirium in different treatment settings (homes, hospices, hospitals), including common diagnostic criteria and terminology. Also needed are better instruments to describe and rate the severity and course of episodes of delirium. This research will lead to a better understanding of the phenomenology of delirium—its signs, patterns, and subtypes—which in turn should produce benefits in terms of newer, more sensitive, and more effective treatments.
2. Treatment—Two aspects of treatment research deserve simultaneous attention. First, there should be randomized, placebo-controlled trials to systematically assess the efficacy of currently available therapies, as well as emerging approaches, including both pharmacological and nonpharmacological strategies. Second, there should be research on the relation between the mechanism of action of these therapies and the underlying pathophysiology of delirium. In both cases, studies should include both random populations and populations with delirium of homogeneous etiology.
3. Epidemiology—Finally, there is a need for additional research on the interactions of delirium between delirium and other symptoms at the end of life.

A concurrent policy issue that must also receive priority attention is the need for guidelines for research in patients who are incapable of giving informed consent because of serious medical illness.

Cachexia

1. Epidemiology—High priority should go to epidemiological studies of anorexia-cachexia, in order to establish the magnitude of the problem, its impact on the patient and family, and its costs to society. However, it is important that cachexia not be studied in isolation from other symptoms. If the ultimate goal of cachexia research is prevention and early intervention, then it would be useful to conduct studies that examine the epidemiology of several related symptoms—e.g., pain, dyspnea, delirium—at an earlier stage in their development.
2. Mechanisms—Basic and clinical research on cachexia should be done in parallel. Basic research should emphasize the interactions among multiple underlying pathophysiological mechanisms, both central and peripheral, including biochemical, neuronal, metabolic, endocrine, and immunological. Research is also needed on the varying clinical manifestations of these mechanisms, both neuropsychiatric and gastrointestinal. This calls for a multidisciplinary approach.
3. Treatment—Similarly, since it is unlikely that any single therapeutic intervention will be successful, clinical research should emphasize multiple combination therapies that include nutritional, pharmacological, and nonpharmacological components. Combination therapies should be evaluated for their effects on other symptoms such as pain, dyspnea, and delirium. Particular attention should also be paid to differences in outcome based on age, gender, and underlying disease. In considering drug trials, NIH should concentrate on studies that would not otherwise be funded by drug companies.

Given the wide range of mechanisms and therapeutic strategies in cachexia, it would be useful to convene a preliminary, integrative workshop that would include both basic and clinical researchers

Cross-Cutting Recommendations. Methods issues that need to be addressed in all four symptom areas include the following:

1. Statistical handling of missing data.
2. Proxy reporting for subjective symptoms.
3. Outcome measures that indicate quality care.
4. Ethics issues are also important. What are the barriers to research at the end of life, including the needs and expectations of vulnerable populations? What are community and individual preferences with respect to symptom management of dying persons?
5. Economics questions include the direct and indirect costs and burdens of symptoms.

Part VIII

International Perspectives

51 South Africa

HOSPICE ASSOCIATION OF SOUTH AFRICA WORKING GROUP and KATHLEEN M. DEFILIPPI, PAMELA E. FOWLER, PAULINE A. HANNA, KAREN C. HINTON, JOAN A. MARSTON, and NKOSAZANA NGIDI

The vision and message of hospice was brought to South Africa in 1979 by Dame Cecily Saunders, who had been invited by the University of Cape Town, Medical Campus. She subsequently did a tour of lectures and introduced the hospice movement to South Africa. A few years prior to this, a seed was planted in Port Elizabeth when a network of people, working in conjunction with the Cancer Association, St. Johns Ambulance, and the Radiotherapy Department of the local Provincial Hospital, became aware of the lack of support for terminally ill patients. The lack of support and counseling for their families was also taken into consideration, and the group set about creating a home based care service founded on the British hospice model.

During 1980, other groups formed in Cape Town, Durban, and Johannesburg leading to the development of hospice programs in these cities and subsequently in other areas. Between 1982 and 1988, the first inpatient units were opened in these cities providing around-the-clock care. The emphasis was and still is on home care.

In South Africa, hospice nurses work closely with the patient's family, general practitioner (if there is one), or traditional healers to ensure best-quality care in view of the limited community resources. Patients with medical insurance can afford private hospital care and medical attention. However, the majority of the South African population do not have this and are therefore totally reliant on government-funded medical services. It is estimated that at least 75% of the total number of patients cared for by South African hospice programs have no medical insurance whatsoever; hence the need for a free-of-charge hospice service. During the early stages of development, medical involvement was minimal. Fortunately, there were some medical practitioners interested in this field of medicine and they provided free medical service to patients and support to the nurses.

During 1984, Professor Eric Wilkes from St. Lukes Hospice in Sheffield, England, came to South Africa, and his visit played an important role in influencing doctors to become more aware of the necessity for palliative care. Four years later, a visit by Dr. Robert Twycross further enhanced knowledge of palliative care. Today in South Africa, there are two doctors with diplomas in palliative medicine and more medical practitioners are attending hospice-initiated training courses and conferences.

Nurses have played a pivotal role in initiating the majority of hospice programmes in the country. In the early pioneering days, few had formal training in palliative care. Experience was gained by traveling overseas, usually to England, working in a hospice, or otherwise from books, videos, and audiotapes, which were the only resources available apart from workshops and conferences.

In view of the fact that all South African hospices are autonomous nongovernmental organizations, financial constraints have limited the number of inpatient units to 12 out of the current total of 47 hospices.

The first provincial organization was formed in KwaZulu Natal in 1982. There are now four other provincial organizations: Hospice Association of Western Cape, Eastern Cape, Gauteng and Free State/Northern Province (see Fig. 51–2). The Hospice Association of South Africa (HASA) was formed in 1988, evolving from a need to have a national body to support the development of the hospice network and to fundraise. Today, in addition to a small administrative office, there are three active HASA development committees, which deal with (*1*) patient care, education, and training; (2) hospice organization and development; and (3) fund-raising and public relations.

Education and training has always been considered a priority. A short course in palliative nursing care for professional nurses was developed by HASA in 1989 and accredited by the South African Nursing Council. This course has served professional nurses working within hospice as well as increasing numbers from hospitals and primary health care settings. During 1999, a HASA short course in palliative care for enrolled nursing auxiliaries was piloted and was successful.

ADAPTATION OF THE BRITISH HOSPICE MODEL

The social conditions and geographical layout of South Africa made it imperative for hospice programs to adapt the British model. As far back as 1984, the South Coast Hospice (Port Shepstone—see Fig. 51–2) introduced their rural outreach program, which empowered state-employed primary health care nurses to render palliative care in areas inaccessible to the mainstream hospice program.

The implementation of a district health care system, which coincides with the unprecedented demand for palliative care because of the rampant HIV/AIDS epidemic, has provided South African Hospices with both a unique opportunity and a unique challenge. It is imperative that hospice recognize and respond to this situation to ensure its long-term survival. The opportunity of taking the first meaningful steps to integrate into the National Health System has, in fact, been recognized and acted upon by HASA. HASA is currently piloting the Integrated Community Home Care–based (ICHC) model via a research tender awarded by the HIV/AIDS Directorate of the National Department of Health (Fig. 51–1). The challenge of ensuring the incorporation of the concepts of both "wellness" and "caring," which are central to both the primary health care and palliative care approach, has been addressed.[1] HASA has also developed a curriculum for training community caregivers, guidelines for palliative care, and an audit tool for measuring the standard of care given to the vast numbers of patients and families affected by HIV/AIDS.

The ICHC (see Fig. 51–1) is in accordance with the view that, in South Africa, limited health care resources and the economic demands of transformation make *collaboration* at every level necessary. In order for hospice care to survive and thrive in this millennium, it will need to share and empower health care professionals in both the public and private sector with palliative care, knowledge, and skills.

Formal health care in South Africa is currently engaged in a process of transformation toward a system known as United National Health System, which is based on the primary health care approach and committed to the development of a district health system. Notably, this is in accordance with the health objectives of the Reconstruction and Development Programme (RDP). The RDP was formulated in 1994 as the vehicle for socioeconomic upliftment as poverty, and its resultant environmental hazards have a profound effect on nutrition, immune status, general health, and access to health care.[2]

The health district model subdivides the entire country into manageably sized, geographically coherent, and continuous districts. District Health Authorities, supported and guided by the Provincial and National Health Departments, are responsible for managing comprehensive health care services for the population in the district.[3] The system promotes cooperative governance with appropriately defined roles, coordination of policy-making and services, and joint participation in monitoring and evaluation for each sphere of government—national, provincial, and local.[4] There is a considerable decentralization of powers and functions to local government level where community participation by non-governmental organisations (NGOs) is actively encouraged.[2]

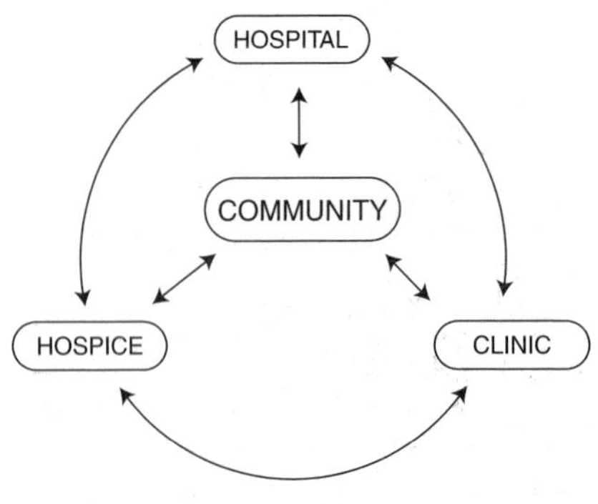

Figure 51–1. Diagram of ICHC Model.

CULTURAL ISSUES INFLUENCING COMMUNICATION, PATIENT AUTONOMY, DECISION MAKING, AND DEATH RITUALS

The Republic of South Africa is a multicultural, multilingual country enjoying its sixth year as a new democracy. It is divided into nine provinces, each administered autonomously but ultimately under the control of central government (see Fig. 51–2).

Traditionally, the population of South Africa fell into four main categories legislated through parliament. Today, the ethnic grouping remains, but only as a self-perception. The African (black) population is by far the largest group, numbered at 31.5 million, followed by the Caucasion (white) group at 4.05 million, the colored* group at 3.05 million, and, finally, the Asiatics (Indians) at 1.05 million.

Under South Africa's new constitution, everybody, regardless of origin, language or color, is considered equal. The net result is that cultural divides are closing and South Africans are beginning to find each other (Table 51–1).

There are eleven official languages in South Africa, and there are others that have not been given this status. It is not at all unusual for a South African to be proficient in three, four, or even more languages. Despite this, most of our main newspapers are in English or Afrikaans (see Fig. 51–3).

In keeping with the new constitution, all religious faiths are now recognized and religious affiliation is protected by law (see Fig. 51–4).

Palliative care has to fit into many economic milieu—from the sumptuous to the desperately poor—and into many cultural settings in South Africa. According to the last census, done in 1996, approximately 52% of the population of South Africa live in rural areas—often without clean water, electricity, and water-borne sanitation (see Fig. 51–5).

Cross-cultural communication presents varied problems in any society. Difficulties arise over language ability, understanding of various religions, and traditional customs. If a health care worker of any category cannot understand his patient's language and vice versa, an interpreter needs to be found. In the translating of one language to another, nuances of meaning can be lost, which can sometimes be misleading,

*It is important to clarify the term "colored." In the South African context, it is a word used to describe a person of mixed ethnic origins.

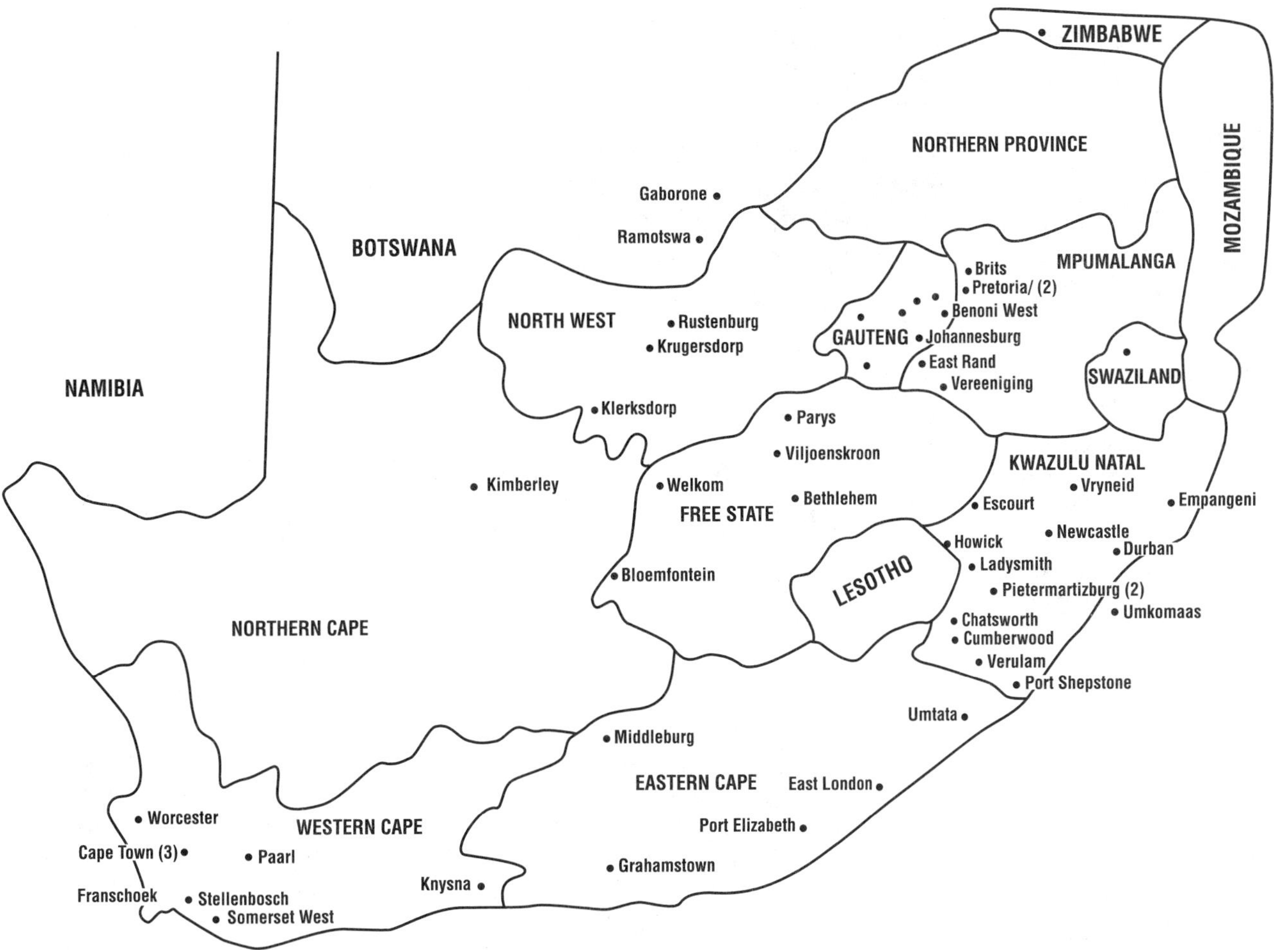

Figure 51–2. Geographical location of Member Hospices in South Africa, Botswana, and Zimbabwe. It is of interest that the single hospice in Zimbabwe now has 17 branches.

particularly when talking of abstract concepts like emotions.

When a palliative care nurse has to rely on an interpreter in order to communicate with his or her patient, problems can arise. How can the nurse develop a good, trusting relationship with the patient?

Teaching basic communication skills to the students of palliative care can sometimes present problems. The concept of reflective empathy is foreign and difficult to learn.

Table 51–1. Population Groupings in South Africa, According to the 1996 South African Census[6]

Africans	31,127,631
Colored	3,600,446
Asian	1,045,596
White	4,434,697
Unspecified	375,240
Total	40,583,573

Gender and age can also be a barrier to communication. For example, an elderly African male patient would be unaccustomed to a young female addressing him. In their normal cultural environment, she would wait to be spoken to first. Palliative care nurses need to be culturally aware in order not to misinterpret body language—for example, not having direct eye contact is a sign of respect.

To many black South Africans, the words "death" and "dying" are not culturally accepted. The words "very sick" instead of "dying" and "passed away" instead of "died" are more common terms. The deceased is more often than not referred to as "late"—for example, "my father is late." The words "death" and "dead" are more applicable to the demise of animals.

Within many black South African family systems, there is a strongly entrenched hierarchical tradition. When illness, misfortune, or death occurs within the family, the senior chronological member assumes leadership and responsibility. In the case of a family member dying, the elders will take control and actually bar the younger ones from seeing and knowing as a form of protection in case the misfortune should spread. In a palliative care setting, it is important to know this because the senior family members are to be informed first about the patient care program, especially in the inpatient unit. This is rather contrary to the Western tradition.

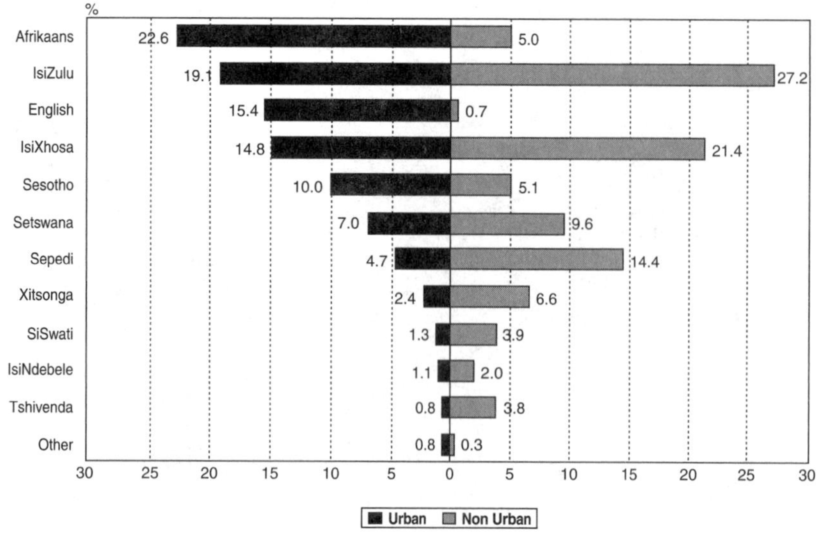

Figure 51–3. Language distribution of South Africa.

Myths abound in some communities. The nondisclosure of HIV status may lead to the assumption of bewitchment and the family may want to take revenge. Revenge in some communities takes the form of raping young girls. In the African community, traditional healers play an important role that has resulted in more hospices liaising with them.

Death Rituals

In a multicultural country like South Africa, there are many rituals surrounding death and dying. Most of these are also encountered in the United Kingdom.

Many people of the African culture attach great importance to dying at home among their own people. The reasoning behind this is that the person's spirit is thought to be also *at home,* wherever that may be. With urbanization, however, the notion of dying at home poses a dilemma for families renting rooms, as it is traditionally required to cleanse the whole building to avoid misfortune. If the death occurs elsewhere, it can cause great concern and the family are obliged to go to the place where the death occurred to fetch the spirit and take it home. If this is not done, the funeral rituals are not completed satisfactorily. Many a family has come back to a hospice inpatient unit asking to "fetch the spirit," which can be a somewhat disconcerting request.

Funeral rites and rituals are symbolically rich and are attended to with meticulous care. In both an urban and rural setting, the night before the internment takes place, the deceased is returned home by the undertakers for a vigil. The family should not be visited by an outsider between the death and the funeral. The coffin or casket is open so that everybody can see the person, candles are placed around the coffin, and the family sit with the body all night singing hymns or praying.

In the morning the undertakers return and the body is then taken to the church and the funeral service takes place, which is followed by the committal. The family sit on a special matting next to the grave. Once the coffin has been lowered into the grave, the males who are present fill the grave to the top, a mound is fashioned, and flowers (often artificial) are placed on top. Thereafter, the whole company goes to the home of the deceased and a meal is provided. Before the meal is served, the mourners have to wash their hands, which is a ritual cleansing of any bad influences that may be lingering.

There are striking similarities between the Jewish customs and the African ones, notably hand washing, care of the immediate family, and unveiling of the tombstone. There are various meaningful rituals that occur during the mourning process, such as "ukugeza amapiki" (washing of the picks). Various implements are used by the mourners to dig the grave. After the burial, these implements are washed by the deceased's family and returned to their rightful owners (see Fig. 51–6).

Babies and toddlers who have not been weaned are not allowed to attend the funeral service. The older children have to inhale incense in order to protect them from evil spirits.

It is common for many people to combine Christian and traditional practices.

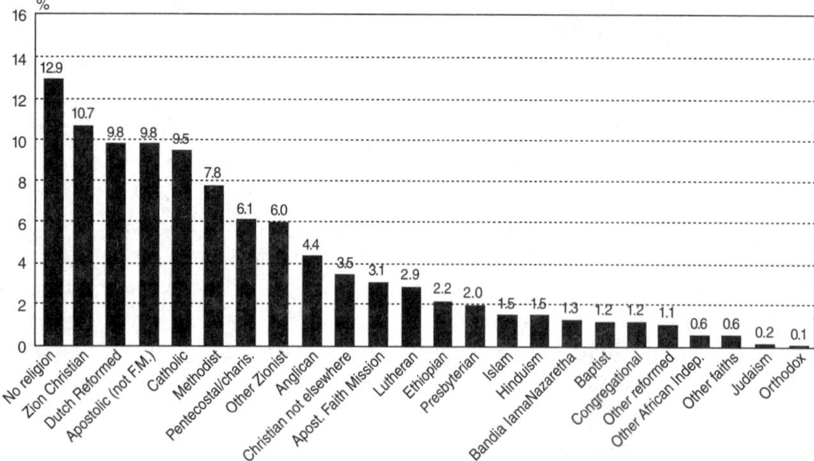

Figure 51–4. Religious affiliation in South Africa.

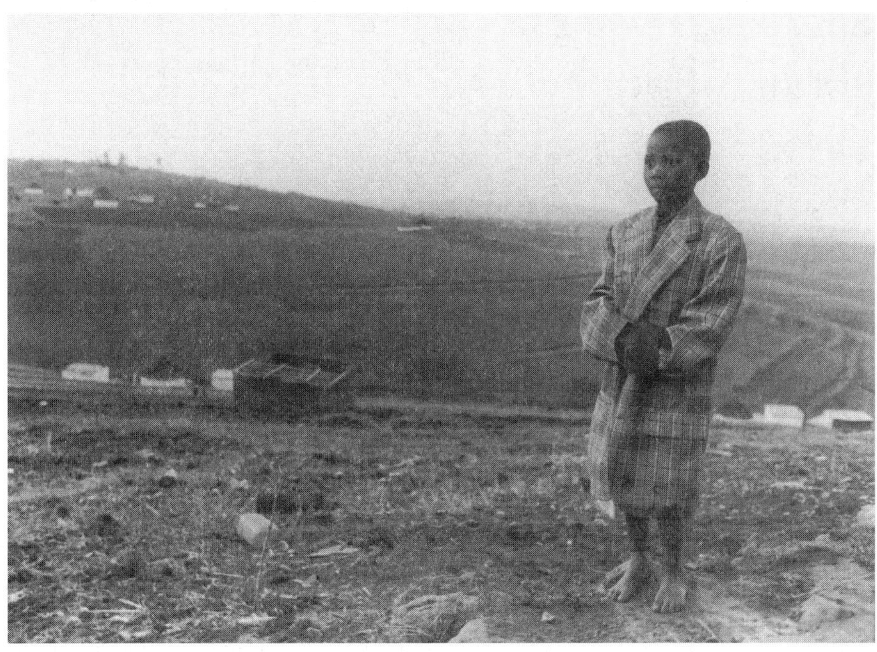

Figure 51–5. Photograph depicting the rural areas in South Africa.

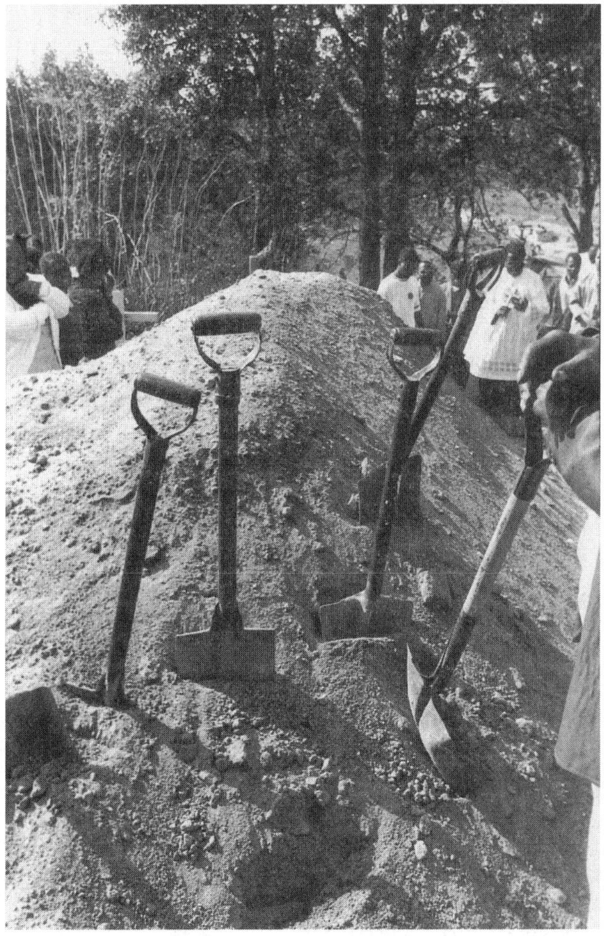

Figure 51–6. Photograph depicting "Ukugeza Amapiki."

Patient Autonomy and Decision Making

In South Africa's multicultural environment, despite women's rights being entrenched in the constitution, signs of patriarchy are still very evident, and all too often male family members will make decisions on behalf of the patient. Patient autonomy is only starting to emerge in South Africa, and it is occurring across the ethnic spectrum.

Despite adequate availability of opioids on the essential drug list, they are occasionally unavailable.

CONCLUSION

In South Africa, hospice care has played an important role in building bridges across racial divides. From the outset, hospices have been nonracial organizations caring for people from all cultures and faiths and has survived the apartheid years of isolation from the international palliative care community.

The palliative nurse in this country needs to continue to play a pivotal role in advocating for palliative care and for the standards of best practice to be integrated into the health care service while maintaining the ethos and identity of hospice.

REFERENCES

1. Defilippi K. The Palliative Primary Health Care Interface. In: The European Journal of Palliative Care 1997;4(3):86–89. Oxon, England: Hayward Medical Communication.
2. South African Department of Health. (1997). Towards a National Health System. In: South African Government Gazette, vol. 382. Pretoria: Government Publishers, 1997.
3. Owen CP. A Policy for the Development of a District Health System for South Africa: South African Department of Health Pretoria: Government Publishers, 1995:3,18.
4. Magwaza N. Report on Co-operative Government in Health Workshops in the National Progressive Primary Health Care Network, 1999.
5. Hospice Association of South Africa. Publication Depicting the Geographical Location of Member Hospices, 1999.
6. South African Government. The South African National Census. Pretoria: Government Printers, 1996.

52 Zimbabwe

AUXILIA CHIDEME MUNODAWAFA

Zimbabwe is a southern African landlocked country, classified as low-income based on a per capita GNP of U.S. $610 in 1996.[1] The population is estimated to be 11 million, of which 70% reside in rural areas. According to the census of 1992, national report, the average intercensual (in between census period) population growth is 3.13%. The economic growth was reported as 1.9% per annum.[2] Life expectancy at birth is 62 years for females and 60 years for males.

Between independence in 1980 and 1984, Zimbabwe went through different phases of socioeconomic developments. In the early 1980s, the new government's commitment to equity and development resulted in remarkable progress in health care, correcting some of the serious inequalities that the government had inherited from the British rule (National Health Strategy[21]).

PROVIDERS OF HEALTH CARE

The majority of health services in Zimbabwe, especially in the rural areas where 70% of the population reside, are provided for by the Ministry of Health and Child Welfare (MOH&CW), mission facilities, and rural District Councils. The municipalities of cities and larger towns provide primary services, and some have a thriving private sector.

HEALTH CARE FINANCE

The government provides the bulk of the finance for rural health service provision. Government financial allocations are made available to districts on an annual basis, but the funds are not transferred to a district fund. All revenues from central payment of services and resources are made at the central treasury payment office in the capital city.[3] The cost of providing health services has risen tremendously over the past few years. This is especially the case at the quaternary and tertiary levels of the health system, which require more specialists and more expensive equipment.

Following the introduction of the Economic Structural Adjustment Programme (ESAP), the government sought to protect the social sectors through establishment of the Social Dimension Fund as a basic safety net for the vulnerable. However, this fund is continuously affected by the health budget, which continues to decline. Public resources are currently stretched thin, largely due to the provision of a limited health package free of charge to the majority.

HEALTH CARE POLICY

Primary Health Care

At Independence, in 1980, the government of Zimbabwe adopted the Primary Health Care (PHC) concept as the strategy of health care delivery system to provide affordable, accessible, and culturally acceptable health care, so as to achieve "health for all by the year 2000." The strategy was in harmony with the national goal of "equity in health," which the government embarked on at independence. Policies were then developed by the Ministry of Health and Child Welfare (MOH & CW), which defined processes designed to reallocate resources from mainly central hospitals and urban areas, to the districts and health centers in rural areas. The overall government policy focused on resources for rural development. The health for all action plan reemphasised the principles of the Primary Health Care (PHC) approach, focusing on critical elements in addressing the most urgent health needs of the rural disadvantaged, including:

- education concerning the diagnosis, prevention and control of locally prevalent problems;
- food supply and security (nutrition);
- drinking water and sanitation;
- maternal and Child Health Care, including family planning;
- immunization against major infectious diseases;
- appropriate treatment of common diseases and injury.

The elements were to be implemented within the following principles:

- community participation;
- accessibility;
- affordability;
- culturally acceptable; and
- use of appropriate, scientifically proven technology.

HEALTH CARE REFORM

Decentralization

A policy decision was made by the government to fully decentralize the management of health care services to rural district councils. The government's policy toward decentralization is to implement new mechanisms for providing health services in ways that further national health objectives such as access, equity, efficiency, patient satisfaction, and improved outcomes.

Decentralization helps in minimizing bureaucracy, by reducing levels of decision making and thereby achieving greater efficiency of operations. It is intended that implementation of the reformed structures of health will give district authorities control over the financing and operation of their health services, thereby promoting and strengthening democracy and responsibility as citizens to participate in their governance. Decentralization is under way in some countries of the sub-Sahara Region, and has been completed in countries such as Zambia.

Providers of Care. Health services are provided for at four central and several specialized hospitals (the quaternary level): provincial hospitals (tertiary level); district hospitals (secondary level); and rural hospitals, health centers, and clinics (primary level). Health care services are provided at various levels in the country: the quaternary level, made up of the ministry of health, responsible for planning, policy making, and regulating the health care system; the tertiary level consisting of four central, multidisciplinary training hospitals; the secondary level, made up of ten provincial hospitals, which are also training hospitals; and the primary level, with fifty-two district hospitals and several rural health hospitals and clinics. Before independence, hospitals and polyclinics provided mainly curative services, while the rural populations relied on mission hospitals, rural hospitals, and a few district hospitals. Preventive and promotive services were run from the center through the provincial medical officer of health. The health care services have since been redirected away from a curative bias to integration of promotive and preventive services at all levels.

A referral system does exist, which is based on the four levels of health care provision, with each level providing specified forms of care in keeping with resources and mission statement at that level. In theory, patients are required to present at the primary level first, and then to be progressively referred to the secondary up to quaternary level, depending on the complexity of illness. The structure of the health care services is also linked with local government structures at all four levels, to ensure consistency and integration of activities or programs (Figs. 52–1 and 52–2).

In this dynamic environment of the shifting epidemiological and economic foundations of health care, the Ministry of Health, after extensive description and analysis of the past and present situation in Zimbabwe from time to time, provides a broad descriptive outline of the future priorities.

The Current Priority Diseases and conditions in the country are:

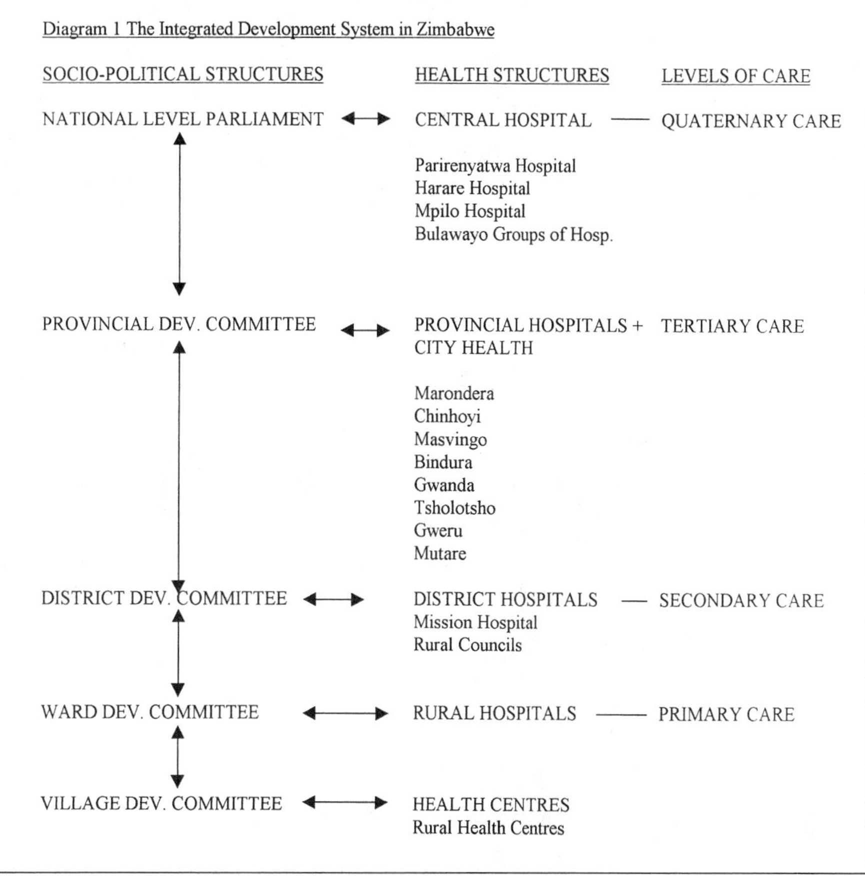

Fig. 52–1. The integrated development system in Zimbabwe.

- human immunovirus/acquired immunodeficiency syndrome (HIV/AIDS), sexually transmitted diseases (STI), and tuberculosis;
- malaria;
- integrated management of childhood illness, including family planning conditions;
- cardiovascular conditions (e.g., hypertension);
- diarrhea diseases;
- nutritional conditions (e.g., PEM, micronutrients);
- injuries, accidents, suicides; and
- mental disorders.

(Strategic Plan 1997–2007[21]).

The Nursing Fraternity

The nursing fraternity forms the backbone of PHC and the largest portion of the workforce. Presently, it is estimated that 17,000 to 18,000 nurses, including both registered general nurses (SRNs) and state-certified nurses (SCNs) form part of this workforce.[4] Government employs about half of this number; they are in hospitals and in preventive services in all the ten provinces of the country. Nurses constitute 60%–70% of health human resources within the national service. Nurse education in Zimbabwe is still, to a large extent, hospital-based diploma programs. The post–basic degree in nursing was established in 1987 and the master's degree in nursing science in 1995. The generic degree, a four-year BSc NS, started in 1998. All these programs produce a small number of nurses compared to the number required—hence the perpetual shortage of nurses. Meanwhile, there is a total of 1,697 physicians in the country, 7857 midwives, 830 environmental health technicians, 538 pharmacists, 212 radiographers, and dietitians with the least number of 11 people. Due to increased

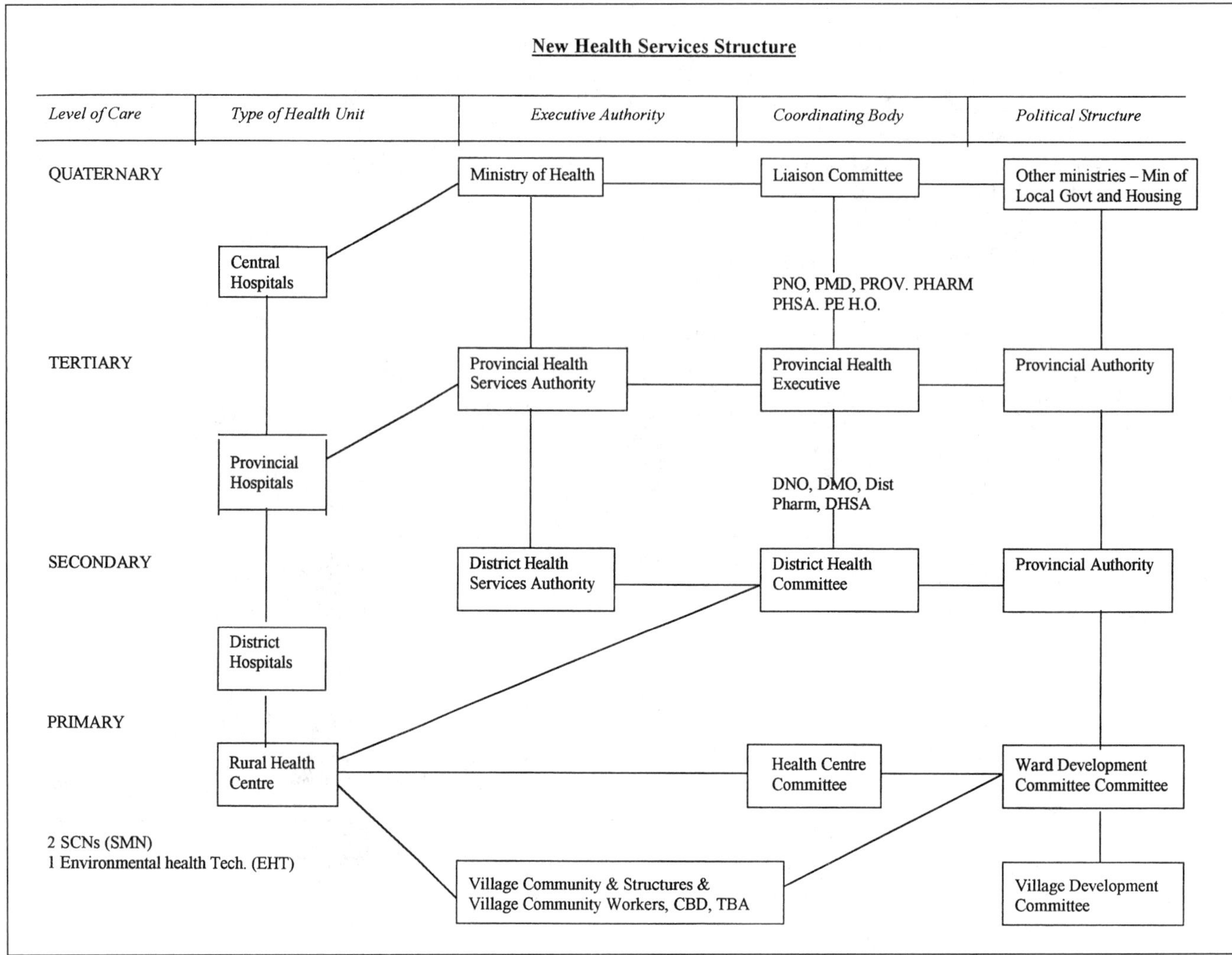

Fig. 52–2. New Health Services Structure: Patient referral ladder. Patient referral is according to need for further higher level management. From Rural Health Clinic which is at Primary Level to Secondary, Tertiary and up to Quaternary Level where the highest specialist patient services are available.

disease burden, the patient/nurse ratio has gone up to 2951 (of state-registered and state-certified nurses). The doctor/patient ratio stands at 10 to 100,000 population in the 1993–1997 health master plan. The Economic Structural Adjustment Programme (ESAP) has seen a reduction in the buying power of civil servants. This has led to reduced staff morale and exodus of health workers to neighboring countries and abroad.

A HISTORICAL PERSPECTIVE OF PALLIATIVE CARE IN ZIMBABWE

The history of palliative care in Africa probably dates to before the nineteenth century, when modern medicine was introduced to the continent. Palliative care has traditionally concentrated on the last days of life, a time when pain and other symptoms, such as psychosocial and spiritual distress, are often prominent and difficult to control. WHO extended the scope of palliative care by stating that many aspects of palliative care are also applicable earlier in the course of illness, especially when used in conjunction with anticancer treatment.[5]

Within the Zimbabwean setting, palliation was in most cases what the herbalist or traditional healers could offer. The herbs offered relief to untreatable conditions, and to various symptoms like headaches, stomachache, and other discomforts. The nursing care was offered mostly by women in the form of hygiene, good nutrition, and psychosocial and spiritual support. The gatekeepers of care were the spirit mediums or traditional healers (personal conversation in June 1983 with a 103-year-old man).

An individual who was chronically or terminally ill would be moved to the outskirts of the village to a "musasa," a temporal home. An individual would be allocated to cater for the total patient needs. The traditional healer or herbalist usually directed the care. The carer, who in most cases was an old lady, would see to the nutrition and comfort of this individual. The patient would be nursed to recovery before rejoining the rest of the clan or till death. It is quite apparent that palliative care was being practiced without the modern term attached to it. The practice was similar even after delivery of a child, where the newly delivered mother would be given time to recuperate and would have a female aide cook for her, bathe the baby, and do all the other chores. During this period, the women would receive nutritious food and herbs for pain, to strengthen her and the baby, and to prepare her to be sexually ready for her husband. This practice is still applicable in some areas.

Modern nursing was introduced to Zimbabwe in 1890 by two Roman Catholic nuns, Mother Patrick and Mother Jacob, who set off on April 13, 1890, from King William's Town, South Africa, in the company of Father Hatman and Dr. Rand as the medical doctor.[6] Their leadership saw the opening of several health structures in the country, which later established nurse training. Only acute care was offered at these institutions. Palliative care, as it is known today worldwide, was not part of the health care delivery system at that time.

Introduction of Palliative Care

Palliative care was introduced to Africa by the formation of hospice organizations, particularly in southern Africa. Island Hospice of Zimbabwe, which operates as a registered welfare organization, was formed in 1979, as the first of its kind not only in Zimbabwe but in Africa.[7] Island Hospice currently operates with 17 branches in various urban centers of Zimbabwe. In Kenya, hospice services were introduced seven years ago; Sirengo's presentation at a biennial conference for nurses in cancer care stated that the organization, which was the first of its kind in the whole of the East African Region, would provide and promote the highest quality of holistic care possible for people with advanced cancer, and provide counseling and support services for their families and other individuals important to their care.[8] The team would combine consultative and hands-on-care, as well as education and training of health care professionals in palliative care. At the same conference, Katjine of Namibia highlighted the lack of patient preparation for discharge, the omission of family involvement in planning care, and the lack of follow-up and support systems as being the reasons of failure to achieve an effective palliative care system in Namibia.[9]

Island Hospice

Island Hospice of Zimbabwe offers its services to people with life-limiting illnesses, their families and bereaved people. The guiding principles embraced by palliative care offered by Island Hospice include the following:

- control of pain, of other symptoms, and of psychological, social, and spiritual problems;
- provision of the best possible quality of life for patients and their families;
- reinforcement of life, while regarding dying as a normal process;
- recognition that hospice neither hastens nor postpones death;
- belief that hospice is not only applicable immediately prior to death, but many aspects of palliative care can be instituted early in the course of illness in conjunction with anticancer treatment;
- radiotherapy, chemotherapy, and surgery have a place in palliative care, provided the symptomatic benefits of such treatment clearly outweigh its disadvantages;
- offering of support systems to help the patients live as actively as possible until death, and a support system to family members to help them cope during the patient's illness and in their bereavement;
- requirement of an interdisciplinary approach;
- emphasis on advanced planning, rather than crisis intervention.

The Palliative Care Team

The team consists of the referring doctor, who continues to direct and monitor patient care, the registered nurses or practical nurses, the social worker, the rehabilitation officer, volunteers, spiritual or religious leaders, or any other relevant team members. The number of people or team members will vary according to availability of resources and, as already indicated, the needs of the patient.

PALLIATIVE CARE ACTIVITIES

Home Care Visits

Teams consisting of professional nurses, social workers, or volunteers visit patients and their families. These teams will assess the patient's condition, review and adjust pain-control drugs, or carry out other nursing care procedures required for the total comfort of the patient. The team will arrange transport for patients for hospital visits where possible, refill prescription drugs for them, or just provide company or an ear to listen when needed.

The hospice centers also offer lending facilities for items such as mattresses, wheelchairs, commodes, and walkers. The team members are available on 24-hour-telephone-contact services to patients or clients.

Bereavement Services

The services are offered to those who experience any loss or death of a loved one, within the existing family or social structures as support systems. Services are also available to families of patients in hospice care, as well as to those who come for assistance without patient involvement. In particular, the team offers special services for bereaved parents, and offers both individual and group therapy to them. Similar children's groups are also conducted, and the same team is responsible for production of newsletters for bereaved parents and other bereaved people.

Training Department

The training department is responsible for teaching all aspects of palliative care at the center. The team will give presentations and lectures to nursing, medical, or any other health care students, and to professionals such as doctors, nurses, and physiotherapists. In-service training programs for various groups are organized and groups like service clubs and other interested members of the public. Occasionally, the team is involved in outreach training program of caregivers in various communities. Currently, the training department is coordinating an educational program in palliative care programs, which the Ministry of Health & Child Welfare, Nursing Directorate, is running for various provincial teams.

Fund-Raising Committee

As a registered charitable organization, Island Hospice runs on donation and fund-raising monies, so this team is concerned with gaining financial support from the community and donors. The group organizes fund-raising activities to meet its annual budget, as well as appeal to and invite organizations to be patrons of hospice or donate in cash and kind. There are shops at various centers that sell donated items such as books, clothing, and miscellaneous gifts. The shops are manned by volunteers who greatly assist in all fund-raising activities.

The Cancer Association

The association serves as a resource center for information on cancer and educates the public on the prevention, control, and treatment of cancer. Prevention is promoted by offering talks to schools and clubs, and by disseminating information via the newspapers and radio. Psychosocial support and counseling is offered to cancer patients and their families. The cancer association also helps to raise funds for equipment for departments like the radiotherapy centers. The National Cancer Association owns and administers two 40-bed hostels in the country. These hostels provide a home free of charge for cancer patients from the rural areas, while they undergo chemotherapy and radiotherapy treatment.

Ministry of Health's Role in Palliative Care

Palliative care has not been fully funded by governments in most countries in Africa, probably because of poor economies, the devaluation of currencies, and the diminishing resources from the high demands of care caused by chronic conditions like the HIV/AIDS pandemic, as well as increasing cancer cases. Zimbabwe is currently among the hard-hit countries in the sub-Saharan region by the HIV/AIDS infection. Seven hundred people have been estimated as dying of HIV/AIDS every week.[10] The number of cancer patients increased consistently between 1990 and 1994.[11] At present, cancer deaths in the country account for approximately 10% of all deaths registered annually. Based on incidence, probably 15,000 new cases of cancer occur in Zimbabwe per year, and this figure is expected to double in the next two decades.[12] This has increased tremendously the number of chronically and terminally ill patients in the country who require palliative care.

Although hospice services have existed in the country for as long as 20 years, the services have mostly been available only to a few urban families. The existing 17 branches of Island Hospice serve a total of about 1,000 families at any one given time in the country. This is a drop in the ocean compared to a population of 11 million people and the escalating numbers of chronically or terminally ill patients.

Prevention and Control of Cancer Committee of Zimbabwe

Oncology nursing is not a specialty area in Zimbabwe, yet information on how symptoms associated with cancer or its treatment, both in hospital and in the primary health care setting, must be given to health care workers. To address this knowledge gap and reduce cancer-related morbidity and mortality, the Ministry of Health and Child Welfare (MOH & CW) established (*1*) a National Cancer Control Program, and (2) a Prevention and Control of Cancer Committee of Zimbabwe (PCCZ). This is a multidisciplinary group that was formed to map out and prioritize prevention and control of cancer activities in Zimbabwe. It consists of the epidemiology department within the MOH & CW, who chair the committee, and oncologists, hematologists and radiologists, who are either faculty members of the University of Zimbabwe or are working within the MOH & CW. The committee also has the Nursing Directorate representation, pharmacists at MOH & CW level who are responsible for acquisition and distribution of pain-control drugs in the country, the Department of Nursing Science, University of Zimbabwe, Island Hospice, Cancer Registry, as well as the Cancer Association of Zimbabwe, where the bimonthly meetings are held. Traditional healers from the Zimbabwe National Association of Traditional Healers, ZINATHA, are also included.

The committee operates under several other subcommittees, including:

- the Cancer Registry Committee;
- Oncology Committee/Palliative Care Committee;
- Cancer of the Cervix/Breast Committees; and
- prevention, early detection, and screening in cancer care, counseling, and any other services are offered within these committees.

The Oncology Committee

The Oncology Committee has since produced a practical guide for management of patients with cancer, designed especially for doctors. Acknowledging that nurses, who are at the primary health care level, have a crucial role to play in early diagnosis, referral, and management of cancer, the committee produced a second cancer guideline, the cancer module. This module aims at helping health care workers to have cancer in mind at all times when making a diagnosis. It includes guidelines for the type of management possible at a referral center, aims to provide a better understanding of cancer, and the various related signs and symptoms, and will enable the health worker to inform and prepare a patient whom they are going to refer about cancer.

Many patients in Zimbabwe seek help only after having tried other alternative treatment, such as traditional healers, herbs, and others. They present to hospital when their cancer is too advanced for cure. These patients can, however, still be helped in many ways within the palliative care framework. Surgery, radiotherapy, or drugs can reduce the cancer to some extent, and symptoms (in particular pain), can be relieved and patients may live good-quality lives for months or years. In all cancers, whether or not a cure can be achieved, all efforts must be made to maintain a good quality of life for the patient.[13]

The Cancer Registry Committee

The Cancer Registry is responsible for compilation of all cancer data and production of annual registers. The committee has also produced a cancer module. This module assists primary health workers in the rural areas with knowledge in early detection of cancer, diagnosis, management of pain, and the appropriate referral of patients.

Cancer of the Cervix

Educational efforts to alert the public about risk factors for cervical cancer, such as sexual activities at an early age, multiple sexual partners, and sexually transmitted diseases (STI), are carried out in an effort to curb HIV transmission. Research studies in screening methods are also carried out.

Breast Cancer Activities

The breast cancer group develops educational material for the public. The group also organizes annual activities in observance of October as breast cancer awareness month. Pink ribbons are worn during this month, and all mass media channels are used to educate the public on breast cancer early detection, screening, management, and support for those affected.

Cancer Treatment

Treatment of cancer in Africa is very expensive, as cancer drugs are imported from outside the country. Treatment is also highly specialized; in Zimbabwe, chemotherapy and radiotherapy are available only at two of the central hospitals in the country. The rest of the other central, provincial, and district hospitals can perform surgery only in the form of diagnostic biopsies, which are then sent to the two centers for confirmation of absence or presence of cancer. Patients in Africa generally present at a late stage of the disease, when no meaningful treatment except palliation is possible. This only confirms further the need for and importance of palliative care knowledge and education in Africa.

Shortage of Resources

Besides oncology education, there is the issue of scarce resources. More than half of the world's cancer patients live in developing countries, but less than 10% of the world resources committed to cancer are available to them. Of this 10%, most of the resources are devoted to curative treatment at a relatively high cost, but with limited effect.[14] Many people with terminal illness suffer unnecessarily because they do not receive effective systematic management. Symptom management requires an understanding of underlying causes. Symptoms in the terminal illness are caused by the disease itself, either directly or by the treatments given, or by coexistent disorders that are unrelated to the main disease. In sub-Sahara Africa, excluding South Africa, there are less than 1,000 cancer experts for a population of 300 million.[14]

Palliative Care Training

The nursing directorate, in conjunction with Island Hospice training department and the PCCZ, have mounted an in-service training program in palliative care. Nurse educators and clinicians from all over the country representing the ten provinces have been trained as educators in palliative care. The idea is to produce hospital teams at each institution, who will then coordinate the discharge planning, implement the home-based-care policy, while delivering palliative care to ensure fluent delivery health care services. The nursing directorate has since facilitated the development of the discharge plan guidelines, and a home-based-care policy has also been developed so as to enable planning and budgeting for home care nursing, which includes palliative care.

Apart from the palliative care in-service training program by the Ministry of Health and Child Welfare, a palliative care program has been developed at a post–basic degree level under the Open University of Zimbabwe by Distance Education. This will enable nurses, for the first time ever in Zimbabwe, to engage in formal palliative care education. The course consists of similar topics covered under the in-service training program, which are:

1. elements of palliative care;
2. nurse's role;
3. palliative care as a cancer-control strategy;
4. barriers to delivering palliative care;
5. pain management;
6. management of other symptoms;
7. communication in palliative care;
8. approaches to specific problems;
9. loss and grief;
10. spiritual issues;
11. legal and ethical issues.

The course's aim is to produce a nurse who can easily integrate as a team member in the treatment and service of all cancer patients or life-threatening illness, and to provide the best possible quality of life for the patients and their family.

Other curricula, within both the University of Zimbabwe and the hospital-based training diploma schools, are being reviewed to include oncology care, including palliative care. Palliative care should be in corperated into health care delivery systems in Africa. All health professionals require training in palliative care so as to effectively render services to terminally ill patients. The development of home-based-care policies is long overdue.

Palliative care adds life into days where days cannot be added into life, and should be accorded as a human right to every terminally ill patient. To prepare clients well, nurses need to have a good understanding of normal cell function, so as to be able to interpret the etiology and pathology of various cancers. Knowledge of pathology will also enable the nurse to critique research in cancer, and to develop assessment techniques that can aid in early detection of the disease. Hence the need for oncology education for health professionals, as either in-service training or continuing education programs.

SETTINGS OF CARE AND WHERE PEOPLE DIE

Acute Care Settings

Acute care settings remain the traditional places where people die. The 1996 Permanent Secretary for Health Report shows an increasing trend in hospital mortality from 2.3% in 1987 to 4.3% in 1996. The increase in the number of chronically ill and terminally ill inpatients continues to create a heavy demand on nursing manpower in the midst of the acute shortage and exodus of nursing staff. Pulmonary tuberculosis and malaria contributed to a large number of inpatient admissions.[21]

Home Care Settings

As the number of chronically and terminally ill patients continues to rise and resources dwindle, hospitalization increasingly is being reserved for acute short-term patients. In the face of the HIV/AIDS epidemic in sub-Saharan Africa—and Zimbabwe in particular, where 20% of the population is said to be positive and 2000 new infections occur every week—the future perspective on health care delivery is that care has to move out of hospitals into homes.[15] Community-based care is becoming the core of the biggest practice areas for health care professionals. More and more people now prefer to die at home among their loved ones. Apart from freeing hospitals for more acute conditions, this health care delivery approach gives the patient time to put their affairs into order and bid their good-byes to loved ones. While being attended to at home, patients are nursed in familiar surroundings and can, to a certain extent, continue with some of their roles.

In community-based Care, a health care provider has to be able and willing to carry out different roles, such as counseling, patient confidant, teacher, and family's observer. The health care provider has to be knowledgeable about the resources within the community in a setting where sometimes other health care workers are not available to validate findings. Careful evaluation is the essential basis for symptom management. The evaluation should include not only physical problems but also psychological help to build a picture of the disease itself, of the patient as a whole, and, in particular, of the effects of the illness on the patient's quality of life.

Quality of life is an abstract and complex term representing individual response to the physical, mental, and social factors that contribute to normal daily living.[16]

CULTURAL ISSUES INFLUENCING COMMUNICATION, PATIENT AUTONOMY, DECISION MAKING, AND DEATH RITUALS

In the African culture, many people believe that illness has either a normal or an abnormal cause. When a headache or a stomach ache persists over a long time, it ceases to be a normal illness and may be believed to have been sent by the ancestral spirits.[17] The kin group feels the illness of one of its members to be a crisis for them all, and whenever possible, the group participates in decisions about treatment. The decision of whether or not a patient seeks hospital treatment does not always lie with the patient. The patient relies on and is dependent on this group for psychological, mental, and physical support.

Most chronic incapacitating illnesses, such as cancer, arthritis, and HIV/AIDS, are referred to the traditional healers. The belief in witchcraft, for example, is not only a causative principle, but it also interlocks with the moral code and the social structure. Many Shona and Ndebele people in Zimbabwe take some of their illnesses to scientific medical practitioners in hospitals and clinics. Yet others still go to traditional healers. In some families, both systems are used simultaneously. Traditional healers can be diviners (an individual with ancestral powers to cast off evil spirits), diviner-therapeutists, and therapeutists (otherwise known as herbalists).[18]

Thus, if a man should consult a diviner about his child's illness, he may be told that the disease was sent by the spirit of his mother's brother, who is annoyed because the father of the child has left some part of his marriage payment unpaid. The action here is for the father of the child to right the wrong and to make a sacrifice to the spirit in the hope of appeasing his wrath.[17] The Mashona tribe, who occupy most of the country except the southern part, occupied by the Ndebele tribe in Zimbabwe, believe that there are four spiritual causes of disease. They are: the spirit of their ancestors—"Vadzimu"; the alien and patronal spirits—"mashave"; the aggrieved spirit—"ngozi"; and the evil spirit of the witch—"muroyi."[6]

Quite a lot of Africans who are educated or have become Christians consult both church and the "nganga," the traditional healer, when they are in trouble or face abnormal illnesses. They do not see any contradiction in accepting Christianity and believing in the power of the spirit elders. Thus, an African often feels that he can be a Christian and still, as a last resort, if ill fortune or sickness persists, consult a nganga and make a suitable sacrifice to his guardian spirit. If a man is dying, close relations, such as a nephew and brother, sit with him. A married man will die in his first wife's hut, and she should be with him at the time.[18]

AVAILABILITY OF OPIOIDS IN THE COUNTRY

Zimbabwe has adopted the WHO three-step ladder for cancer pain relief (see Figure 52–3). The first step is when nonopioids and adjuvant drugs are given to control pain. The second step is given if pain persists or is increasing. Weak opioids, nonopioids, and adjuvant drugs are given in this category. The third step is given if pain persists or increases. Strong opioids, morphine, nonopioids, and ad-

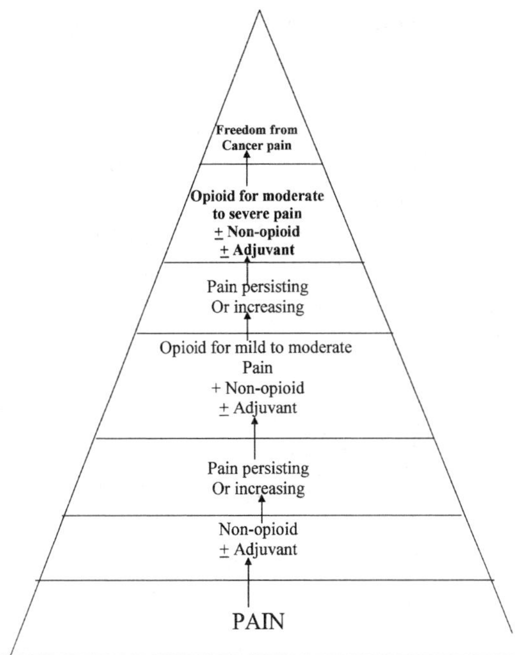

Fig. 52–3. The World Health Organization's three-step ladder for cancer pain relief.

juvant drugs are used for this highest level. The modern approach to pain is to control and then prevent pain, not to wait until pain is severe and then try to relieve it. Therefore, strong opioids like morphine are administered "by the clock"—that is, every 4 to 6 hours—rather than "on demand." It must also be remembered that morphine does not cause addiction in cancer patients and does not hasten death.

Morphine is given orally, by subcutaneous injection or rectally. The usual starting dose for oral route is 5–10 mg every 4 hours. If pain persists after 24 hours, the dose is increased by 50% each day until pain is controlled. Usual dose range is 5–60 mg every 4 hours, but occasionally, higher doses are required (e.g., 200 mg every 4 hours). Side effects such as constipation, nausea, confusion, and intolerance are to be watched for and appropriate interventions implemented.

Other Symptoms

Symptoms often arise out of the treatment that has been administered for the cancer. But other symptoms could be from concurrent conditions. All symptoms are potentially distressing, but symptoms such as anorexia and weakness, nausea and vomiting, dry or painful mouth, hypercalcemia, constipation, intestinal obstruction, anxiety, and depression are of paramount importance to note and manage.

Morphine Distribution in the Country

In 1993, morphine manufacturing was taken over by a local drug company in Zimbabwe. A problem arises when the company runs out of raw material or powder to manufacture the drug. The tablet form, which is said to be popular, especially with the rural population because of easy storage, is sometimes unavailable. Due to the stigma attached to morphine as a cause of respiratory distress and the suspicion of its use in passive euthanasia, many doctors, patients, and relatives are very reluctant to use it despite its capacity to control pain. This leads to under-utilization of morphine and under-treatment of pain.

The third issue is that of morphine's cumbersome forms. Morphine in Zimbabwe is bound by the dangerous-drug act, and therefore only doctors can prescribe it. According to Zimbabwe's levels of care, doctors are available only up to district levels of care. This means patients seen at rural health centers can only have weaker opioids and nonopiods for pain. Morphine cannot be stored at rural health centers.

The last issue is that of price; 100 mg/5ml of morphine costs $72 Zimbabwean dollars (ZD) and tablets $463 each (U.S. $1 = $38 ZD). It becomes an ordeal for the rural population to find their way to central levels when they require pain-control drugs unless they are covered by the Social Dimension Fund (SDF). The Zimbabwe government's health expenditure as a proportion of the growth domestic product (GDP) grew from 2.2% in the early 1980s to over 3% by 1990. Since 1996, the MOH & CW total health expenditure has declined from the 3% to 2.1% of the GDP, depicting a declining expenditure on health.

As a way of monitoring morphine availability, the chief pharmacist in the MOH & CW, who is a member of the PCCZ, publishes an account of morphine consumption in the country every month. This record highlights the name of the institution, the description of opioid used—either powder, tablets, or injections—amount used, stock in hand expiration date, number of prescribing doctors, and number of patients on morphine every month. These records are then presented to the PCCZ, problem areas are identified, and solutions are sought as a multidisciplinary group.

CONCLUSIONS

Palliative care in Zimbabwe, and in Africa as a whole, will be most effective when it is integrated into the country's comprehensive health plan. This will allow coordinated action on common risk factors for several diseases. The major focus of the government of Zimbabwe, through the Ministry of Health, has been the establishment of the Cancer Registry and a cytotoxic (anticancer) drug list, and the development of supportive palliative care therapy. The Ministry of Health and Child Welfare needs to provide leadership in collaboration with nongovernmental organizations interested in cancer control and palliative care activities. Comprehensive cancer control requires a multisectoral approach—one that includes the Ministries of Finance and Economic Affairs, Education, Information, Industry, and Agriculture—because factors that contribute to the causes of cancer have a broad base in society. There is a need for explicit commitment by governments in Africa and provision of resources and policy measures to effectively implement cancer control and palliative care programs. There is also a need for continuing education of the medical and nursing fraternity, and other workers in the health service, especially regarding prevention of cancer, early signs and symptoms, diagnosis, referral, and symptom control in palliative care.

REFERENCES

1. World Population Data Sheet, 1998.

2. Census Report, Harare: Government Printer, 1992.

3. Health Sector reform. Ministry of Health and Child Welfare, Government Printers, Harare (Government Document), 1997.

4. Ndlovu R, Bakasa RV, Munodawafa A, Mahlangu N, Nduna. Situation analysis of Nurses and Nursing in Zimbabwe. (Produced as a Zimbabwe Government Planning Document by the Government Printers, Ministry of Health, Harare), 1998.

5. Doyle D, Hanks GWC, McDonald N. Palliative Medicine. Oxford: Oxford Medical Publishers, 1997.

6. Gelfand M. Witch Doctor. London: Harvill Press, 1964.

7. Hospice Fact Sheet. Harare (Non-Governmental Policy Document), 1997.

8. Sirengo. Hospice Care in Kenya (unpublished). Presented at the 10th International Conference on Cancer Nursing, Jerusalem, Israel, 1998.

9. Katjine (unpublished). Presented at the 10th International Conference on Cancer Nursing, Jerusalem, Israel, 1998.

10. National AIDS Co-ordination Programme. Ministry of Health, Harare (Government Report), 1998.

11. Chogunongwa E, Borok Z, Levy L, et al. Annual Cancer Registry Report. Harare: Government Printers, 1997.

12. Prevention and Control of Cancer Committee of Zimbabwe 10-Year Strategic Plan, 1994–2003, (Government document, Guidelines for Cancer Management).

13. Levy L, Chitsike I, Banderson C, et al. Cancer Module, Zimbabwe Essential Drug Control Programme, Ministry of Health, Harare.

14. WHO Report, 1997.

15. Sunday Mail. The Herald, Harare (newspaper article), 1998.

16. Fisher RA, MacDaid P. London: Pub Hodder Headline Group, 1996.

17. Chavunduka GL. The Traditional Healers and the Shona Patient, Gweru: Mambo Press, 1976.

18. Gelfand, M. Medicine and Magic of the Mashona. Cape Town: Juta and Company Limited, 1956.

21. Ten-Year Strategic Plan 1997–2007. Government printers, Harare, Zimbabwe.

53 People's Republic of China

WANG YING and JUDITH A. PAICE

Palliative care is a very new and emerging field in the People's Republic of China. The development of the first palliative care unit in China began in 1987 when two nurses from the Tianjin Cancer Institute and Hospital were sent to the Royal Marsden Hospital in London for specialized training in oncology nursing. After a one-year training program, they returned to their hospital and began to work with hospital administrators to develop a "continuing care" or palliative care unit. The goal of this unit is to care for patients with terminal illness, to improve pain and symptom control, and to allow patients to die peacefully. This five-bed unit was first established in 1989 within the Department of Traditional Chinese Medicine. Owing to its success, the unit has since expanded to 27 beds.

There is a new and increasing awareness among medical professionals and the government of China about the need for enhancing quality of life in persons with advanced disease. To that end, the National Hospice Society within China was established in 1992. The overall goal of this society is to advance the care of the dying patient. Additional goals of this organization include: (*1*) to conduct academic exchange and improve the level of hospice care in China; (2) to enhance awareness of hospice care; (3) to train professionals in hospice care; and (4) to exchange information with hospice organizations outside of China. The National Hospice Society is located in the Tianjin Medical College, Qixiangtai Road, Tianjin 300070, People's Republic of China.

Although attitudes toward death and dying are more naturalistic in China, illustrated by such comments as "let nature take its course," several cultural variables impact the development of palliative care.[1] Many Chinese believe that the discussion of death should be avoided and fear that revealing a terminal diagnosis might cause the patient to wish to die sooner, or even commit suicide. This makes frank discussion between the patient and the health care professional difficult and serves as a barrier to the advancement of palliative care.

The eldest son is expected to provide physical and emotional support to the parent, a reflection of filial piety that is highly regarded in Chinese culture. However, the advent of one-child families instituted by the government to control population growth may place undue stress on children who lack siblings or other extended family. Furthermore, direct requests for assistance from family members may mean "losing face." Food and other offerings may be symbols of this support, rather than direct discussion of the issues surrounding end of life.[1]

Government and health care professionals have only recently addressed one aspect of palliative care—cancer pain management. Previous historical events assist in explaining the delayed attention to palliative care and pain relief. Understanding these events allows health care professionals to view the barriers to good palliative care and pain relief in their own countries with a different perspective and renewed awareness. This new outlook can lead to the development of effective strategies for improved palliative care and pain control, both internationally and in our own settings of care.

CANCER IN CHINA

Cancer is widely recognized as one of the most formidable of human afflictions. The number of new diagnoses of cancer in China is approximately 1.8 million per year, and the number of deaths due to cancer is about 1.4 million a year. The most common malignancies include lung cancer, stomach cancer, and hepatic carcinoma in men. In women the most common diagnoses include lung, breast, and colon cancer. The widespread popularity of smoking in part accounts for the high prevalence of lung cancer.[2,3,4,5] In a prospective study of 9351 adults in Shanghai aged 35–64, the percentage of males who smoked was estimated to be 61%, while only 7.0% of the female population smoked.[6] After 16 years, 12% of the study population had died. The majority of these deaths were due to cancer (40%), primarily lung, stomach, liver, esophageal, and intestinal cancer. Smokers had a relative risk of 1.8, suggesting that one-third of all male cancer deaths were due to tobacco. Air and water pollution, associated with the increase in industrialization, probably contributes to this high rate of lung and other cancers.[7,8]

Hepatic carcinoma, also highly prevalent, is believed to be associated with pervasive hepatitis infection.[9] In fact, cancer-prevention activities include immunization programs to reduce the rate of hepatitis infection. Other factors contributing to the high prevalence of hepatocellular carcinoma include exposure to aflatoxins in food and alcohol intake.[10] Increasing rates of colon cancer and breast cancers (in women), are believed to be associated with many factors, including the introduction of Western foods and lifestyles.

Previously, the majority of cancer patients were diagnosed with advanced disease. This is evidenced in part by the fact that the number of new diagnoses is approximately equal to number of deaths due to cancer. Late diagnosis is largely due to lack of availability of health care resources, particularly in more rural areas. Additionally, surveys of individuals in China revealed lack of knowledge regarding cancer risk factors and early warning signs.[11] Furthermore, past health care emphasized the treatment of acute illnesses, such as infections, which were treatable and were associated with significant mortality. As acute illnesses are more successfully treated, greater emphasis is being placed on early detection and treatment of cancer. As these efforts become more widely available, people with cancer are diagnosed earlier and the course of the disease is longer. Thus, cancer in China is becoming a chronic syndrome.

CURRENT STATE OF CANCER PAIN

Prevalence of Pain

Cancer pain is one of the most common symptoms associated with cancer. It is estimated that 30%–45% of patients with cancer in China have moderate to severe pain. Thus, in China, there are 2 million people suffering from cancer, and about 1 million suffering from cancer pain. In 1997, the Ministry of Public Health began a study of the prevalence of cancer pain in China.[12] The total number of patients with cancer in this investigation was 1555 cases. According to this study, which employed patient self-report, 958 cases (61%) experienced cancer pain. Physicians also were asked to estimate the number of these patients experiencing cancer pain. They reported that 967 of these patients experienced cancer pain (62.2%). This difference is not statistically significant

Barriers to Cancer Pain Relief in China

The barriers to cancer pain relief in China are similar to those of other nations, although unique historical factors greatly influence these obstacles. The Agency for Health Care Policy and Research (AHCPR) *Cancer Pain Management* clinical practice guidelines categorized the barriers to cancer pain relief as those related to the health care professional, the health care system, and the patient.[13] Of these barriers, fears related to opioid use are most pronounced in China. Much of this fear has evolved from historical factors in which opium played an important role.

Historical Factors: Fear of Addiction. Beginning in the 1700s, opium was imported into China by the British, Dutch, and Americans. Although importation was illegal, unscrupulous Western and Chinese merchants became willing partners. By 1838, more than 5.25 million pounds of opium was imported annually, representing the extract of 4.8 trillion opium poppies.[14] An estimated 1%, or 4 million, Chinese were addicted, primarily men between the ages of 20 and 55.[15] Social decline resulted, with the establishment of opium dens and the increasing cultivation of poppies rather than grains and vegetables. The Chinese rulers realized the devastating effects that opium produced within their country and asked England to cease import. Because the opium trade was extremely lucrative, England refused and several battles ensued. As a consequence of China's losing these battles, Hong Kong was ceded to Britain. Although Hong Kong returned to Chinese rule in 1997, this loss continues as a potent reminder to modern-day Chinese of the cost of opium.

The result of this history, and subsequent fears, is limited availability of opioids for health care, both in variety and quantity. In 1993, the per capita morphine consumption in China was 0.01 mg, compared to 20.80 mg in the United States.[16] Pethidine (Dolantin), also called Demerol (meperidine,) remains the most commonly available opioid. Morphine is available in select centers, and long-acting formulations have only recently been introduced. Other opioids include codeine, tramadol, dihydroetorphine, and buprenorphine. Supply is severely restricted as hospitals receive quarterly shipments of these drugs. Outpatient use of opioids remains uncommon.

Inadequate Assessment. Another barrier to good analgesia is the lack of systematic assessment. To improve pain assessment, the Brief Pain Inventory was translated into Chinese (BPI-C) and validated in a large group of cancer patients at three cancer treatment hospitals in Beijing.[17] In comparing the pain interference data derived from this population with similar patients in France and the United States, the Beijing patients had greater interference (6.55 vs. 4.64 and 4.72, respectively). The Pain Management Index (PMI), an estimate of adherence to the World Health Organization guidelines, revealed that 67% of these patients had inadequate treatment.

Lack of Knowledge. Information related to the treatment of cancer was not widely available to many health care professionals in China. To answer this need, the Bureau of Drug Administration and Policy translated the abbreviated form of the AHCPR *Cancer Pain Management* clinical practice guideline into Chinese and disseminated the document to health care professionals. More recently, the Pain Research Group headed by Dr. Charles Cleeland from M.D. Anderson Hospital in Houston, Texas, published the translated version of the complete text. This translation occurred in cooperation with colleagues from the Tianjin Medical University and other experts from China.

The Cultural Revolution, which occurred from 1966 to 1976, presented another obstacle to adequate medical and palliative care. Universities were closed during this period and converted to factories.[18] Nursing schools were also closed, so that for over 30 years China had no baccalaureate nursing program.[19] Many health care professionals and college professors were forced to relocate to rural settings and were not allowed to practice or teach. In effect, they were cut off from the rest of the world. Although the Cultural Revolution ended in 1976, there remains a shortage of health care professionals.

Table 53–1. Nonopioids Available in the People's Republic of China

Drug	Dosage, Frequency	Route
Paracetamol (acetaminophen)	500–1000 mg, q 4–6 hours	Oral
Aspirin	250–1000 mg, q 4–6 hours	Oral
Brufen (ibuprofen)	200–400 mg, q 4–6 hours	Oral
Indomethacin	25–50mg, q 4–6 hours	Oral

Other Barriers. In a survey of 89 health care professionals attending a pain conference in 1993, lack of education about cancer pain management was cited as the chief barrier. Other barriers included lack of education for the public, low priority given to pain management and palliative care, lack of education and training opportunities for health care professionals, and an insufficient number of health care professionals who know how to manage cancer pain.[20]

Treatments for Cancer Pain in China

The three-step analgesic ladder advocated by the World Health Organization is an effective model for pain management in many countries in the world, as well as in China.[21] Approximately 90% of patients can obtain adequate cancer pain relief when this method is applied appropriately. For the patients who need anticancer therapy, radiation therapy, chemotherapy, and surgery also may be included in the treatment regimen.

Available Analgesics. At present, the main kinds of analgesics available and in use in China are nonopioids (nonsteroidal anti-inflammatory drugs [NSAIDs] and paracetamol [acetaminophen]), opioids, and adjuvant agents. Nonopioid drugs are primarily nonprescription. Table 53–1 shows the nonopioids typically available in China.

At present, the main stronger opioids used in China are morphine, pethidine (meperidine), and fentanyl injection. Other opioids include codeine with aspirin or paracetamol, hydrocodone, tramadol, qiang tong ding (AP-237), buprenorphine, and dextropropoxyphene, although these are prescribed less frequently. In addition, there are several complexes of opium drugs, such as Galake, lufendaiyin No. 1, and lufendaiyin No. 2. If the patient is not able to take drugs orally, patient-controlled analgesic (PCA) may be chosen. Table 53–2 shows the opioid consumption in Tianjin Tumor Hospital during the period 1991–1997. Tianjin Tumor Hospital is a large cancer hospital that has hosted several intensive cancer pain training seminars.

Adjuvant drugs include antidepressants (the most common in China is amitriptyline), anticonvulsants (commonly carbamazepine), and corticosteroids (usually dexamethasone or prednisone). For very severe pain that is localized, nerve block therapy may be chosen.

Traditional Chinese Medicine in Cancer Pain Management. Traditional Chinese Medicine (TCM) has been practiced in China for more than 2,000 years. This medicine plays an important role in the supportive therapy of cancer patients. Their main effects are to enhance blood circulation and resolve blood stasis, to nourish *qi* (the life source) and blood, and enhance immune function. Some Chinese herbal medicines are believed to enhance the action of analgesics. Other herbal medicines cause sedation to improve sleep or relieve constipation (e.g., senna leaves). A recent review of complementary and alternative therapies details the known positive and adverse effects of these treatments.[22]

EFFORTS TO RELIEVE CANCER PAIN IN CHINA

In the early 1990s, physicians and other health care professionals within China identified the need for improved cancer pain relief.[23] In 1990 Dr. Jan Stjernsward of the WHO introduced the concept of the three-step analgesic ladder at a conference in Guangzhou (formerly called Canton).[24] In 1991 the People's Republic of China established a national policy for cancer pain relief and disseminated this proclamation to hospitals and public health organizations throughout the country. This "red-headed" document and subsequent documents supported the need for cancer pain control. The term "red-headed" is used when documents and policy statements are of special importance. In June 1992 the International Workshop on Cancer Pain Relief and Research was

Table 53–2. Consumption of Opioids (mg) in Tianjin Cancer Institute and Hospital, 1991–1997

Drug	1991	1992	1993	1994	1995	1996	1997
Codeine	650,430	450,390	951,240	1,148,160	1,831,500	1,410,330	1,418,820
Morphine injection	0	3000	39,400	28,220	60,000	116,580	189,080
Morphine tablets	0	26,060	130,365	512,790	693,860	1,448,810	1,847,750
Dolantin*	151,000	1,679,100	2,327,000	3,106,800	4,428,100	1,808,000	1,908,600
Fentanyl injection	113	123	131	266	223	300	350

The reduction in consumption of Dolantin (also called pethidine or meperidine [Demerol]) is in contrast to the increases seen in the other opioids. These changes, increases in opioids and a reduction in Dolantin, are believed to be due to extensive educational efforts and enhanced availability of appropriate opioids.

presented in Beijing. This conference was held in collaboration with the Ministry of Public Health, the Pain Research Group, the Beijing Cancer Institute and Hospital, the Chinese Academy of Medical Sciences, the WHO Collaborating Center/Saitama Cancer Center (Japan), the Beijing Jushuitan Hospital, and the Beijing International Medical Exchange Center. Presentations were given by Chinese and foreign experts, including Charles Cleeland, Ph.D., David Joranson, M.S.S.W., David Borsook, M.D., Ph.D., Karen Syrjala, Ph.D., and Judith Paice, Ph.D., R.N. Topics included the barriers to cancer pain relief in China, physiology of pain, pharmacological management, and nonpharmacological approaches.

The Ministry of Public Health then sought guidance from Dr. Charles Cleeland (currently at M.D. Anderson Cancer Center) and David Joranson of the Pain Research Group at the University of Wisconsin to develop a comprehensive plan to improve cancer pain relief. The three-year plan included a broad program of education, training, research, and evaluation.[25]

One of the primary components of this plan included education. National training seminars were held in geographically diverse sites throughout the country: Beijing, Shanghai, Chengdu, Guangzhou, Xian, and Wuhan. Content included pain assessment, pharmacological therapy, the use of the WHO three-step ladder, and regulatory issues. More than 500 physicians, nurses, pharmacists, and administrators attended these sessions. Not only were foreign advisers involved in teaching, but also Chinese experts were vital to the success of these seminars. This core group of leaders includes Professor Li Tong Du, a surgeon from Bengbu Hospital in Anhui province; Professor Cai Zhi-ji, director of the National Institute on Drug Dependence; and Professor Hao Xi-shan, the director of Tianjin Tumor Hospital. Their efforts have been supported by the leadership of Gu Wei-ping and her colleagues at the Bureaus of Drug Administration and Policy, Ministry of Public Health. These individuals and others continue to tirelessly provide educational offerings throughout this vast country.

In addition to these seminars, an extended training program was conducted at the Tianjin Tumor Hospital. This three-week course incorporated morning lectures and afternoon rounds, followed by case conferences in the hospital. The educators included experts from the United States as well as China. The attendees represented professional triads (nurse, physician, and pharmacist) from hospitals throughout China. The goal was to train those individuals so that they would return to their respective settings to educate their colleagues. They were given monographs, slides, videotapes, and other materials to assist them in this process.

Regulatory Issues

Along with educational efforts has been the change in laws intended to reduce diversion of opioids. These include allowing increased manufacturing of analgesics and dispensing needed doses to hospitals around the country. In part as a result of these efforts, the consumption of morphine has increased from less than 10 kilograms per year to more than 140 kilogram per year in 1998.

SUMMARY

Palliative care is in the midst of a revolution in the People's Republic of China. Through the efforts of a committed group of individuals, knowledge is being disseminated and laws are being modified in this vast and populous country. These efforts, not unlike those taking place in other countries around the world, will result in improved quality of care at the end of life.

REFERENCES

1. Chan KS, Lam ZCL, Chun RPK, Dai DLK, Leung ACT. Chinese patients with terminal cancer. In: Oxford Textbook of Palliative Medicine, 2nd ed. (D.Doyle, GWC Hanks, and N MacDonald, eds.), pp. 793–795. Oxford University Press, Oxford.

2. Liu BQ, Peto R, Chen ZM, Boreham J, Wu YP, Li JY, Campbell TC, Chen JS. Emerging tobacco hazards in China: 1. Retrospective proportional mortality study of one million deaths. British Medical Journal 1998;317:1411–1422.

3. Niu SR, Yang GH, Chen ZM, Wang JL, Wang GH, He XZ, Schoepff H, Boreham J, Pan HC, Peto R. Emerging tobacco hazards in China: 2. Early mortality results from a prospective study. British Medical Journal 1998;317:1423–1424.

4. Yuan JM, Ross RK, Wang XL, Gao YT, Henderson BE, Yu MC. Morbidity and mortality in relation to cigarette smoking: A prospective male cohort study in Shanghai, China. Journal of the American Medical Association 1996;275: 1636–1650.

5. Yu JJ, Mattson ME, Boyd GM, et al. A comparison of smoking patterns in the People's Republic of China with the United States: An impending health catastrophe in the Middle Kingdom. Journal of the American Medical Association 1990;264:1575–1579.

6. Chen Z-M, Xu Z, Collins R, Li W-X, Peto R. Early health effects of the emerging tobacco epidemic in China: A 16-year prospective study. Journal of the American Medical Association 1997;278:1500–1504.

7. Xu ZY, Blot WJ, Xiao HP, et al. Smoking, air pollution, and the high rates of lung cancer in Shenyang, China. Journal of the National Cancer Institute 1989;81:1800–1806.

8. Lynge E, Anttila A, Hemminki K. Organic solvents and cancer. Cancer Causes & Control 1997;8:406–419.

9. Yu MC, Henderson BE. A case-control study of hepatocellular carcinoma and the hepatitis B virus, cigarette smoking and alcohol consumption. Cancer Research 1987;47:654–655.

10. Riegler JL. Preneoplastic conditions of the liver. Seminars in Gastrointestinal Disease 1996;7:74–87.

11. Myhre SL, Li VC, Guan JH, Wang ZJ. Cancer knowledge and perceptions among Chinese factory workers: Implications for cancer control and prevention. Cancer Detection & Prevention 1996;20:223–233.

12. Liu Z-M, Zhou W-H, Lian Z, Mu Y, Cao J-Q, Cai Z-J. Survey of cancer pain in China. Proceedings of the Workshop on Cancer Pain Relief and Palliative Care. Beijing, China (Chinese). 1998:22–40.

13. Jacox A, Carr DB, Payne R, et al. Management of Cancer Pain. Clinical practice guideline No. 9. AHCPR Publication No. 94-0592. Rockville, MD. Agency for Health Care Policy and Research, U.S. Department of Health and Human Services, Public Health Service, March 1994.

14. Wilson SM. Coffee, tea, or opium? Natural History 1993;102:74–79.

15. Booth M. Opium. New York: St. Martin's Press, 1996.

16. United Nations International Narcotics

Control Board: Narcotic Drugs; Estimated World Requirements—Statistics for 1993.

17. Wang XS, Mendoza TR, Gao SZ, Cleeland CS. The Chinese version of the Brief Pain Inventory (BPI-C): Its development and use in a study of cancer pain. Pain 1996;67:407–416.

18. Huang J. Medical education and medical education research and development activities in modern China. Medical Education 1992;26:333–339.

19. Davis AJ, Gan LJ, Lin JY, Olesen VL. The young pioneers: First baccalaureate nursing students in the People's Republic of China. Journal of Advanced Nursing 1992;17:1166–1170.

20. Joranson DE, Cai Z, Gilson A. Barriers to opioid availability in China. Chinese Bulletin of Drug Dependence 1995;4:88–91.

21. World Health Organization. Cancer Pain Relief and Palliative Care: Report of a WHO Expert Committee. Geneva: WHO, 1990.

22. Cassileth BR. Evaluating complementary and alternative therapies for cancer patients. CA-A Cancer Journal for Clinicians 1999;49:362–375.

23. Sun Y. Status of cancer pain and palliative care. Journal of Pain and Symptom Management 1993;8:399–403.

24. Joranson DE. Availability of opioids for cancer pain: recent trends, assessment of system barriers, new WHO guidelines, and the risk of diversion. Journal of Pain and Symptom Management 1993;8:353–360.

25. Hong Z, Gu W, Joranson DE, Cleeland C. People's Republic of China: Status of cancer pain and palliative care. Journal of Pain and Symptom Management 1996;12(2):124–126.

54 India

GILLY BURN and GEOFFREY BOWRING

Each country needs to work out the best way of looking after dying people in accordance with its culture and resources.

—Jan Stjernswärd

The diversity and color of the terrain—from the mountains of Ladakh and Kashmir to the golden beaches of Kerala and Goa, and the deserts of Rajasthan to the deltas of the Ganges—are some of the natural wonders of this vast subcontinent. There are as many religions and races as there are spices in an authentic Indian meal. Hinduism is the majority religion, but there are more Muslims in India than in any country apart from Indonesia. There are also Buddhists, Christians, Jews, and Jains; animism survives among tribal peoples (adivasis). This richness and range is reflected in the multitude of languages, cultures, and peoples in India: there are 19 official languages (including English), but more than 1,600 dialects. The literacy rate is nationally about two-thirds for men and one-third for women. This varies from only 30%–40% in some of the northern states to over 90% for both sexes in the southern state of Kerala. Life expectancy in India is 63 for both men and women. India is still predominantly a rural economy, and the vast majority of the billion population live in villages. A nuclear power, India is also the world's largest producer of tea, has huge mineral reserves, and creates high-quality textiles and handicrafts for export, as well as being the largest producer of opium.[1]

BACKGROUND

India has more poor people per capita among its one billion population than any other country in the world. Three quarters of India's population lives in rural areas with minimal health care facilities.[2] Although there is a well-planned community health network, most of this is related to disease-prevention programs, child and maternal welfare, family planning, inoculation programs, and public health. Cancer-detection camps are offered in the community, but they do not encompass palliative care. Unfortunately, these camps are not always able to offer effective therapy even when a curable cancer is detected, and patients may be put on a long waiting list for treatment. Even then they may not be able afford the treatment offered.

District Government Hospitals offer general medical and surgical facilities, and more than 150 of these hospitals offer some surgery or radiotherapy service to treat cancer patients. In addition, there are eleven Regional Cancer Centres in Allahabad, Ahmadabad, Bangalore, Calcutta, Chennai, Cuttack, Delhi, Gouhati, Gwalior, Mumbai, and Trivandrum. These Centres provide comprehensive surgical, radiotherapy and medical oncology services. Some, but not all, currently offer a degree of palliative care service. There are many private and charitable hospitals, some with a religious foundation, that offer a wide range of acute and chronic services. In all of the above, the majority of patients are expected to make at least some contribution, if not a total contribution, for their treatment. As will be discussed later, there is a paucity of doctors and nurses per head of population. In India, palliative care is not a specialty, although it forms an integral part of the National Cancer Control Programme.

The health care budget for India is less than 1% of the gross national product. Illiteracy, lack of awareness, fear of serious disease and of subsequent treatment, and long distances from medical centers make treatment for many sick and terminally ill people inaccessible. This is compounded by the fact that the majority of people cannot afford what is offered, even where treatment is available.

Lack of resources, broken equipment, and lack of drugs such as oral morphine (and the fears surrounding its use) are serious barriers in themselves. Add to these the low ratio of health personnel to patients and their lack of education about palliative care, and even simple, indigenous, cheap and effective pain relief is not a certainty for hundreds of thousands of patients.

In 1986, the Indian National Cancer Control Programme (which included palliative care) was set up with the assistance of the Cancer and Palliative Care Unit of the WHO. There is nothing complicated about palliative care. The straightforward approach recommended by the WHO holds that governments should:

- establish national programmes for cancer pain relief and palliative care;
- ensure that palliative care programmes are incorporated into their existing health care systems;
- ensure that health care workers are adequately trained in cancer pain relief and palliative care;
- review national health policies to ensure that equitable support is provided for programs of palliative care in the home;

Table 54–1. WHO Proposals for a National Cancer Care Program

Evaluation Category	Palliative Care Measures
Foundation	Pain relief policy adopted Education of health professionals Legislation passed to ensure availability of oral morphine
Implementation	>80% cancer hospitals adopt WHO guidelines >50% general hospitals adopt WHO guidelines
Short-term outcome (up to 5 years)	>50% cancer patients in pain receive oral morphine
Medium-term outcome (within 10 years)	>30% abolition of peak cancer pain
Long-term outcome (within 20 years)	>80% abolition of peak cancer pain

- ensure that hospitals are able to provide appropriate backup and support for home care;
- ensure the availability of both opioid and nonopioid analgesics, particularly morphine for oral administration.[3]

The WHO "triangle" of education, drug availability, and legislation should be the keystone of the success of palliative care in India. It shows the interdependency of state and federal legislation, the availability of oral morphine for pain relief (along with other drugs), and education and training of health care professionals.[3]

Table 54–1 lists additional WHO proposals for the evaluation of the palliative care component of a national cancer control program.

ACCESSING HEALTH CARE

There is no social security system anywhere in India. No work equals no money for the household, and therefore no means of obtaining treatment or providing food and essentials for the family. Often, the main wage-earner will carry on working despite disease symptoms, as he or she cannot take time off to visit the doctor and has no money to pay treatment fees.[4] In many cases, severe pain or other symptoms prevent the wage earner from working, and finally force him or her to seek medical attention. Local remedies, which are easier to access, may be inappropriate, and may also drain the financial resources of the family.

The fact that most centers offering cancer treatment are in major cities compounds the problems of poverty. Villagers may have to travel hundreds of miles, in extreme heat, in overcrowded buses or trains. The roads may be crumbling where the monsoon rains have caused craters, and even major thoroughfares can be reduced to dirt tracks. The experience of traveling in such conditions with, for example, multiple bone metastases or severe pain are beyond the imagination of those in the affluent West. A far higher cost of living and strange surroundings may confront the patient and family upon their arrival from their village. They may also be vulnerable to exploitation owing to a lack of familiarity with the harsh realities of urban life and loss of their social network. Whole families may be seen camping outside hospitals, perhaps with a primus stove, as they await admission; even then, patients are not guaranteed a bed, and some sleep on the floor in overcrowded wards.[5]

The world of cancer strikes terror in the hearts and minds of those who suspect they may have it, and their families. Fear of the unknown—and a lack of awareness that if detected and treated early, many cancers are curable—means that many people, even the highly educated, delay seeking treatment in case their worst fears are confirmed. The social stigma associated with the diagnosis of cancer means that in India, some people with the disease become social outcasts. This may be because other family members are sometimes not able to endure the patient's symptoms and suffering. The problem is now being compounded by the increased number of people diagnosed with HIV/AIDS, which is associated with other, perhaps even more virulent forms of stigma and oppression.

PIONEERING INDIGENOUS PALLIATIVE CARE SERVICES IN INDIA

Dr. L. J. de Souza, a surgeon from a major cancer center, built the first hospice in India. Opened in 1986, Shanti Avedna Ashram in Mumbai is closely modeled on the design of St. Christopher's Hospice in London.[6] Since then two other Shanti Avedna Ashrams have been opened, in Goa and in Delhi. The hospice in Delhi opened in 1994 and is staffed by dedicated and caring missionary sisters. When the hospice was visited by the author 16 months after it opened, there was a low bed-occupancy rate, despite major public and professional publicity, although the Ashram is built within a mile of a Regional Cancer Centre and within half a mile of another general hospital with cancer facilities. Patients from both these hospitals could benefit greatly from admission for symptom control and psychosocial support at some time during their illness. At that time, the policy was that patients receiving "active" treatment could not be admitted, even if they needed symptom control as well. One needs to consider the reasons for low occupancy: Is it because doctors are not informing their patients of available facilities? Is it due to lack of awareness or inability to collaborate with colleagues? Is it because of ignorance of the potential of palliative care? Does referral for palliative care represent "defeat" on the part of the referring physician or surgeon? Or is it the stigma and fear sometimes associated with this type of institution in India by an uninformed public? As palliative care develops, we hypothesize that this situation will gradually change through exposure to examples of good practice.

Other hospices are developing in other parts of India. A community-based team in Bangalore now has inpatient facilities for 55 patients, and an education facility has attracted major funding from the Rotary International because of the educational emphasis of the service. There is considerable patient demand at another hospice, Jeevodaya, in Chennai, opened in 1995. Because of lack of funds, this hospice has been able to function to its full capacity only since early 1999. Good preparatory work in terms of working relationships has been undertaken with both professionals and the public to generate support. Cooperation with medical colleagues has ensured supplies of oral morphine. In the words of their newsletter, "the bottom line . . . is quality of life and freedom from pain."[27] The hospice also offers a limited community outreach service. Community palliative care is vital if coverage is to be achieved, especially as potential service-users are rural-based. The overriding principle must be to develop appropriate models of care.

EXTERNAL INITIATIVES

In 1988, at the International Cancer Nursing Conference in London, attended by more than 2,000 nurses from around the world, the author heard an inspired address by Dr. Jan Stjernswärd, then Chief of the Cancer and Palliative Care Unit of the World Health Organization (WHO). Moved into action, the author took four weeks' annual leave in 1989 to visit and teach in various centers in India. What became obvious was the fundamental need for education of health care professionals. As a result, a registered charity "Cancer Relief India" (CRI) was set up in 1990 in the United Kingdom, with two aims—education of doctors and nurses in palliative care and practical provision of pain and symptom relief for cancer patients.[4,7] Doctors and nurses were invited to come to the United Kingdom for training in palliative care under the aegis of CRI.

The first senior nursing position—associate professor in palliative care—was set up in Kerala in 1992 and was funded by CRI. Appropriate clinical placements in palliative care settings were organized and educational materials to take back to India provided. The first doctor in India to undertake and successfully complete the Diploma in Palliative Medicine in the United Kingdom in 1993 was supported by CRI. CRI has since supported three other doctors to complete the Diploma in Palliative Medicine, qualifying in 1996, 1997, and 1998. In 1998–99, a staff nurse (B.Sc. qualified in nursing) from the Regional Cancer Centre (RCC) in Trivandrum, Kerala, studied at Oxford Brookes University, supported by CRI. She became the first nurse from India to obtain the Diploma in Palliative Nursing. Upon her return to Trivandrum in October 1999 she was appointed as nursing officer in charge of developing palliative care nursing services at the RCC.[8]

The director of CRI has led a variety of initiatives for health care professionals, from multidisciplinary workshops to conference lectures, from hands-on clinical teaching to teaching on ward rounds, where her role as both the patient's and nurse's advocate was put to the test. Heightened public awareness of palliative care through the media—newspaper interviews and articles, radio and television interviews, and public lectures—was also sought. This often resulted in inquiries from the public by telephone or visits to local centers that might offer palliative care.[8]

From 1993 to 1995, Cancer Relief Macmillan Fund (CRMF), in collaboration with the Cancer and Palliative Care Unit of the WHO, built on these earlier endeavors. The director of CRI became project director/palliative care consultant (nurse educator) and was involved in peripatetic teaching in India and organizing the course in the United Kingdom for Indian nurses and doctors. During this time, 20 doctors and eight nurses were selected for a specially created course in palliative care. Disciplines within medicine included radiotherapy, surgical oncology, anesthesiology, medical oncology, general surgery, and head and neck surgery, and ranged in status from lecturer to professor and head of department. The nurses were managers, staff nurses, educators, and a superintendent. None of the doctors or nurses had received any previous formal training. The course involved the theoretical components of palliative care and relevant clinical placements, with a module that included presentation and teaching skills, communication skills, and the management of change.[5]

WORKING CONDITIONS

Working conditions are difficult for health care professionals in India. Hospital wards are overcrowded and understaffed, with often 40 to 60 patients per nurse. Nurses are outnumbered by doctors 3:1. In 1993, there was approximately one doctor per 2,500 people. Clinics are often attended by 70 to 100 patients per day. There is little time to accurately examine and assess a patient's needs.[8] Promotion in medicine and nursing is frequently age-related and not necessarily based on interest or experience. The hierarchical structure makes it difficult to advance palliative care, especially if the person is seen as "young." Entrenched attitudes may crush enthusiasm. Hence there is a need for networking locally and nationally with like-minded spirits and ongoing external support until there is a critical mass and palliative care is recognized as an integral part of the continuum of cancer care. At least 450,00 out of nearly a million registered doctors in India have a recognized qualification in a traditional form of medicine such as ayurveda, unani, or siddha.[9] The status of the nurse is relatively low, and therefore it is not a profession that many people enthusiastically pursue. Unlike in the West, there is minimal patient advocacy by nursing staff, and because of the shortage of nurses there is less nurse–patient contact. In addition, interprofessional communication is not on an equal level with that of the West. This means that to achieve coverage it is essential to use the great strength of the Indian extended family structure, to support and empower them to deliver the care. It is therefore vital to teach nurses to teach others—that is, the patient and family.[8]

To this end, a Palliative Care Centre with specific objectives related to family teaching and support was built in Pune in the state of Maharastra, approximately 180 miles from Mumbai. This center is described later in this chapter.

TEAMWORK

In many hospitals, the concept of teamwork is not evident. Professionals work more as individuals within a group, each with their own tasks and objectives. Doctors may fear losing their patients, as they would also lose the patient's fees, and therefore there is an element of understandable competition with colleagues. Conversely, the atmosphere among nurses is more passive. The doctors' competition and the nurses' passivity appear to block interprofessional communication, which in turn can affect patient care. There is also a lack of awareness regarding what other team members (e.g., occupational or physiotherapists, dietitians, and chaplains) can offer to palliative care. Despite lack of financial resources, patients and their families frequently seek several opinions regarding treatment. This is often due to a lack of information regarding treatment options.

HOSPITAL-BASED PALLIATIVE CARE—CALICUT SHOWS THE WAY

Recall the face of the poorest and the most helpless man whom you may have seen, and ask yourself if the step you contemplate is going to be of any use to them.

—Mahatma Gandhi

Several regional centers are endeavoring to develop palliative care alongside curative therapy. The most exciting development has been the hospital-based pain and palliative care clinic set up by the professor of anaesthetics at Kozhikode (Calicut), Dr. M. R. Rajagopal. It has been singled out by the WHO for its pioneering work, and it is unique for a variety of reasons.

Dr. Rajagopal attended a CRI workshop using an interactive videodisc teaching program in Trivandrum in 1992. His awareness raised, he showed a keen interest in the subject and was therefore selected for a ten-week training course in the United Kingdom in 1993. Upon returning to India, he converted an old anaesthetic storeroom at the teaching hospital into a clinic for pain and palliative care advice. With his excellent team-building skills, Dr. Rajagopal created a dedicated multidisciplinary team, made up mostly of untrained volunteers and medical students. At the beginning there was one full-time paid doctor (CRI funded), who took more than a 50% drop in the salary he had earned in the private sector to bring him in line with government salaries. Since the first clinic opened in 1994, when 387 patients presented, the numbers rose to more than 1800 new patients in 1998.

The team works on a referral basis, giving advice, not taking other consultants' patients. Team members visit the wards daily and teach by role modeling. Potential professional and public communication barriers are prevented by skillful interaction among team members. Colleagues, patients, and families alike are empowered to deliver care. The team includes more than 40 volunteers actively involved in patient contact—something that is virtually unheard of elsewhere in India. The Chief of the Cancer and Palliative Care Unit of the WHO declared this innovative and farsighted unit a demonstration model for developing countries during a visit there in 1995. Individuals thinking of setting up palliative care services in India are encouraged to visit this center, which has introduced a culturally sensitive model of palliation.[8,10,11]

When the unit at Calicut was opened, it was planned that there should be a realistic delivery system of palliative care, in line with the WHO policy of "coverage."[12,13] It would be aimed at reaching as many of the needy as possible, the patient's needs taking priority.[11] In line with the WHO, the caregivers would establish a partnership in care with the patient: doctors would not force decisions on patients. At Calicut, volunteers—by design—became the backbone of the palliative care facility from its inception. The founders acknowledged the essential direction that would be needed for this group of volunteers in saying, This strong work force only needs to be organized and channeled properly. Religious or social convictions of the carers should never be imposed on patients, even subtly. This is particularly important in India, with its diverse religious and social beliefs." The volunteers are valued and are acknowledged publicly.[18]

Referrals are mainly by doctors, but about 12% of patients approach the clinic directly. The new patients are "clerked" first by volunteers, who have been trained to fill in a chart, including a list of symptoms, a body chart and a scale for pain, a family tree, any social and emotional problems, and the patient's insight about the illness recorded in his or her own words. (This is similar to the British situation, where a patient will talk openly to a cleaner or porter, but stay silent to a staff nurse or doctor!). The doctor then cross-checks the data, performs a physical examination, and listens to the patient. Enough time is spent with the patient to bring out emotional problems. The team have recognized that formal education and intelligence are not synonymous and that illiteracy is no excuse for insufficient communication with the patient. As observed in other parts of India,[14] the average villager is capable of decisions regarding treatment options. Patients are aware of the implications for family finances in such discussions.

The delivery of care is geared to giving service to the poorest of the poor. Expensive equipment or drugs such as sustained-release formulations are considered justifiable only if their use does not detract from the service available to the very poor. Patients are encouraged to give their feedback anonymously by filling out a questionnaire and by adding their comments.

A home care project, covering a radius of 20 kilometers from the parent clinic, was funded by the Overseas Development Agency of the British High Commission. It aims to see patients who cannot be transported to the clinic because they are too sick or too poor. By 2000, 20 satellite clinics had been established in the area around Calicut, as well as the home care program.

One of the major strengths of the medical personnel are their excellent listening skills and their ability to really hear what the patient's needs are. A man in his late thirties with four children had his leg amputated for a osteogenic carcinoma. As a result, he was unable to work, lost his job, and therefore had no money to feed his four children. As a consequence, his children had to be cared for by a charitable agency. Although the patient suffered considerable physical pain, his doctor was also able to elicit his social, emotional, and spiritual distress. Dr. Rajagopal approached a local foundation and asked it to buy a coffee vending machine. This provided a service for patients and visitors in the hospital and enabled the man to be employed. The minimal profit that he made from working on the vending machine and selling the beverages enabled his four children to return home within two months.

Four years on, the patient was still alive, working the machine every day, as well as working voluntarily in the clinic. He donated 25% of his earnings (of his own volition) back to the Palliative Care Society, which had restored his family unit. This is just one example where attention to all components of "total pain," plus lateral thinking and commitment to the patient, has resulted in truly compassionate and holistic care. A self-help group has also been created.[15]

Several alternative systems of medicine, particularly ayurvedic medicine, are practiced in India and are widely used by patients. The Calicut Centre employs an ayurvedic doctor who is carrying out research, comparing ayurvedic and allopathic treatments. One study currently being undertaken is looking at the role of allopathic and ayurvedic laxatives and comparing their efficacy.

The Calicut team have demonstrated their indices for evaluation of their work:[11] Monthly consumption of oral morphine rose in three years, from 0.018 kg in January 1994 to 0.737 kg in December 1996. Patient attendance at the clinic increased from 4.92 patients seen per day in January 1994 to 53.72 in December 1996. In terms of cost-effectiveness, the Calicut unit saw 2,205 new patients and 55 patients each day, six days a week, in 1999. They calculate the cost to be about the cost of running a ten-bed British hospice for one week. These are impressive achievements in any country, and in one where there are so many impediments to palliative care, they are unique. Overall, the Calicut centre demonstrates the symbiosis that can be achieved through working together by the local community, government, the Pain and Palliative Care Society, and other agencies.

COMMUNICATION CHALLENGES

With its hundreds of dialects and several official languages, not all people speak the national language of Hindi. The educated language and the "jargon" of the medical profession may be totally incomprehensible to a patient, who may be not only unable to read or write but may not understand what the doctor or nurse is trying to convey. This makes the whole issue of informed consent, for example, particularly fraught with problems, and in most instances it is not achieved.[16]

The social status of most patients in relation to doctors makes it difficult to communicate fears, needs, and queries, and thereby almost impossible to understand the implications of the treatment. In most instances there are no simple explanatory leaflets—useless anyway for those who are illiterate—and no nurse acting in an advocacy role. Direct and honest communication between patient and doctor is rare. Constraints on the doctor's time make meaningful explanations difficult. In addition, the relatives may see the doctor first and tell the doctor not to tell the patient about diagnosis and prognosis. A "conspiracy of silence" isolates the patient early on, denying the opportunity of attending to "unfinished business" and imprisoning him or her in a lonely world of silence and secrecy in which all treatment choices are denied. Even if it proves possible to overcome the obstacles of communication in terms of travel and information, the person may be confronted with the news that there is no treatment available, as either the relevant equipment has broken down or the drugs are not available or are unaffordable.

The concept of the strong family support network in India is currently under threat. It still exists, but the culture is changing—more women go out to work as opposed to working at home, and more families are becoming "nuclear." The move away from the village to the cities continues apace as people search for work. There are even reports of patients with advanced cancer being abandoned by their families. Several questions come to mind here: Is it because financial resources are so drained that the family has gone in search of work in the cities? Or is it because family members cannot cope with their own terrible suffering and feeling of impotence at the sight of someone they love in uncontrollable pain or with the smell of suppurating lesions? Supportive palliative care could have enabled those families to cope and share together their burden of suffering.

TECHNOLOGY AND TRUTH-TELLING

One of the problems confronting doctors is the high expectations of both professionals and the public regarding the preservation of life at all costs. Unaware of what palliative care encompasses, some doctors are prescribing a "living death" for their patients in the mistaken belief that it is the best option.[11] Western death-denying attitudes have undoubtedly reached countries like India. Of course, advanced technology has its place, and just because a country is financially poor does not mean it should be denied the latest machinery and professional updating in latest techniques. In the context of acute life-threatening crises, with appropriate treatment there is a good chance of a positive outcome.

At present, however, health care technology is used indiscriminately and patients with advanced cancer are often dying alone in intensive-care units, wired up to every possible machine and with no nurse in attendance. Outside the hospital, the patient's family, denied access to the bedside, wait for the inevitable. Both family and patient therefore suffer the final stage in separation, alone, at a time when they most need to be united. The relatives are left with the recurring nightmare of a loved one's traumatic, solitary death, with none of them able to complete their "unfinished business."

Compounding the emotional, social, and spiritual suffering, the financial burden to the family can often be hundreds of dollars per day. Inappropriate use of technology, often camouflaged as "hope," has left families bankrupt. Cows, land, jewelery, tractors, even houses are sold, or money is borrowed because patients have been denied a true appraisal of the situation. The ethics of informed consent are as relevant in India as anywhere else in the world.[14] Feelings such as love, guilt, or desperation to stop the suffering on the part of the family, and the fear of abandonment for the patient, make all of them vulnerable to grasping at any treatment, irrespective of whether or not it is medically or ethically sound. One patient, seen by a British doctor, had a large neck tumor. He had had surgery, the wound was breaking down, and he was unable to turn his head in any direction, as it was solid with tumor. He was staying in a hospital more than 100 miles from his home and his family had spent literally thousands of dollars, having been told that the man had at least five to eight years to live. They were completely bankrupted, and in addition the patient and his family were separated at a time when they most needed to be together. He was also suffering from the side effects of the chemotherapy and had an oral stomatitis. The patient and family were advised that further attempts at cure would be counterproductive. His pain and other symptoms had not been addressed. After exploration and explanation they all came to the conclusion that the patient should go home with his family.

The concept of multidisciplinary teamwork is poorly developed in most centers, and the nurse tends to have a low status. What has been encouraging to observe is that after doctors and nurses have been exposed to multidisciplinary teaching sessions, the communication between the two groups and the understanding of the role of the other is enhanced.

Specialization within nursing in India is not common practice, and it would be interesting to undertake a survey to find out how many nurses would prefer to follow a specific career path of their own choosing. Often, trained nurses are moved at random, not only to other wards but to other hospitals, within the same state, but perhaps three or four hundred miles from their home. They may well need to live away from the family and return home for a day on weekends.

Of those nurses who attended the CRMF courses in the United Kingdom between 1993 and 1995, one has written a booklet in Hindi about palliative care aimed at general nurses and teaching programs. A nursing superintendent from south India has fought to raise the status of nurses in her RCC, and has concentrated her practical efforts on lymphoedema care and massage. Two nurses from Pune—with minimal exposure to palliative care—returned to India with experience and knowledge to set up a comprehensive palliative care nursing program within their unit and for nurses from surrounding hospitals. Having observed them speaking at conferences, all of them have benefited from the work in presentation and teaching skills.

It is easy for experts in palliative care from the Western world to tell Indian doctors about the correct use of oral morphine, but in a country where the use of morphine is not legal in several states, the issue is more complex and needs persistent unraveling. Teaching needs to motivate students into continuing to strive to obtain morphine. Alternative drugs, such as buprenorphine, may or may not be available, but often the cost of such drugs is prohibitive to the majority who could benefit. If morphine *is* legal, bureaucratic hurdles have to be jumped, from transport and import permits (from one state to another), to licenses to prescribe, hold, and dispense morphine.[17] It is not available in the community—that is, it cannot be prescribed by a community physician, only a hospital doctor. Some hospitals stipulate that only inpatients can have morphine—and that means the chance of dying pain-free in a hospital but separated from family and home, or at home in pain. Patients and carers often choose the former in an attempt to avoid intolerable suffering and potential abandonment by both health care professionals and family/informal carers. Witnessing the effectiveness of morphine in the clinical setting is more convincing than any number of formal lectures.

LEGISLATION AND MORPHINE

Extensive legislation and the numerous bureaucratic hoops through which the medical profession has to jump in order to acquire drugs makes the use of morphine more problematic than less efficacious analgesics.[19] Many of the laws date back to British rule and are aimed at preventing drug addiction rather than preventing pain. In India each state has its own laws regarding morphine, including transport, export, import, prescribing, and the licenses needed before the drug can be used.[13] In one instance it took four years of bureaucratic battling for a professor of radiotherapy to obtain oral morphine. Even then, he was told that the hospital had a license to dispense only oral morphine solution, not tablets. In some states, licenses have to be renewed annually. Not all doctors can prescribe morphine, and often only one doctor per hospital has this burden/privilege. This means that even within a hospital that *has* morphine, a patient in pain may not get pain relief if the physician does not have permission to prescribe, or is not able to refer the patient to another doctor who can.

The WHO has made several proposals to ensure that morphine is made available.[12,3] However, even where it is available, there is a further impediment: government officials, doctors, and the public are afraid of addiction in the patient, or that it might spread to widespread abuse of the drug because of theft from pharmacies stocking the drug or from patients. There is a concern that the relatives may abuse the drugs. Respiratory depression and tolerance leading to ever-escalating doses are also feared. Both health care professionals and the general public see morphine as synonymous with death. The problem of constipation as a side effect is rarely addressed, but it is the symptom that often causes patients the greatest distress.[18,10] Action and side effects of morphine must be stressed in both clinical and theoretical teaching: It is not enough merely to state drug doses and timings. In a drug such as morphine, which is surrounded by a plethora of myths and misconceptions, its safe and effective use needs to be seen, to be believed and understood. Therefore, visiting lecturers need to work alongside colleagues at the bedside or in the clinic, and to facilitate and support practitioners in their prescribing. This must also include a continuing evaluation of the effectiveness of the drug prescribed. There needs to be competence and confidence in prescribing morphine—just as someone learning to drive can learn the theory (competence) but must also practice on the road (confidence) to become a good driver.

The state of Kerala in south India, with a population of only 30 million, has seen major key developments in palliative care in the last ten years. At the time of writing, Kerala is poised to become the first state to simplify the regulations regarding the use of morphine. The role of the World Health Organisation and in particular of the Pain and Policy Unit from Wisconsin has been crucial in this development. They have worked closely with the policy makers and health care professionals within Kerala. The Pain and Palliative Care Society, the Indian Association of Palliative Care, and David Joranson of the WHO Collaborating Center for Policy and Communications in Madison, Wisconsin, have worked together on opioid availability. As of June 2000, five Indian states have now amended and simplified the narcotic regulations.

Education of health care professionals is a key step in getting palliative care to the needy. This is vital because palliative care is not yet part of the medical or nursing curriculum.

Palliative care is slowly becoming recognized in India. The impetus for this came with the formation of the Indian Association of Palliative Care in 1994.[20] The inaugural meeting was held in Banaras (Varanasi), considered to be the most holy city in India. The river Ganges flows through Varanasi, and this is the place most Hindus would choose to die if it were possible. When it is not possible, water from the Ganges River is given to the dying person. One of the exciting features of that first meeting was that it was not uniprofessional—in fact, it was attended by nurses, occupational therapists, physiotherapists, nursing aides, religious leaders, volunteers, and—within the medical community—surgeons, physicians, anesthetists, neurosurgeons, and radiotherapists. At that time, there was only one trained palliative care physician in India, the radiotherapist who had undertaken the Diploma in Palliative Medicine from the University of Wales in 1992. At the Sixth Annual Meeting in 1999, held in Calicut, 300 delegates attended from all over India.

PUNE PALLIATIVE CARE CENTRE

In 1992, the author was approached by trustees of the Cipla Cancer and AIDS Foundation in Mumbai. They had plans to build an AIDS hospice on a site outside Pune, Maharasthra. The original plans were amended and the concept of a "living" palliative care center, influenced by ideas put forward by CRI, were wholeheartedly endorsed.[21] When Pune Palliative Care Centre was built, it was very much on the outskirts of the town. However, in the two years since it opened, the town has expanded its boundaries, and local buses now service the area. The Centre has 50 beds, in four wards, which form a quadrangle that has an eight-foot veranda and a children's playground in the middle.[22] This is an unusual feature for a palliative care facility, and patients and relatives enjoy the area, particularly in the evenings. By mid-2000, a wide-ranging program of social activities meeting the needs of not only the patients but also their carers was in place. The Centre endeavors to be as self-sufficient as possible and uses solar-heated water and grows its own vegetables. The essence of the Centre is education—education of health care professionals, training programs for 16-year-olds (pre-nursing), and education and training of patients' relatives. Total admissions in the year 1999–2000 were 604—369 new admissions and 265 readmissions. As of June 2000, the Centre had, since its opening, over 800 new admissions. Survival rates after discharge from the Centre were as follows: 64, 6 months or over; 12, 10–15 months; 13, 15–20 months; and 2 over 2 years.

The principles underpinning the Pune Centre are[23] the following:

In keeping with the family structure and Indian traditions, a relative is required to stay at the Centre when the patient is admitted. The relative is involved in the training program during this period. The training given is as follows:

- importance of cleanliness and hygiene at the personal and family level;
- wound care and dressing;
- ryles tube: How to keep it clean. How to feed the patient?
- palliative care—general;
- death or discharge of the patient: the relative's responsibility in this matter
- pain chart;
- patient's medication: How relatives learn about the patient's medicines and the patient's timetable at home. How to keep the patient occupied.
- morphine—all aspects related to the proper and careful use of morphine.
- wound dressing—from readmission patient's relatives;
- coping mechanism—for patient and their relatives.[23]

The medical staff at Pune are acutely aware of the palliative care needs of patients with a noncancer diagnosis,[23] something that will surely become more center-stage in the near future.

USING AVAILABLE KNOWLEDGE

"Compassion not combined with wisdom is inefficient in relieving suffering."[13] As in many Western countries, palliative care has not yet been included in the undergraduate curriculum of either nursing or medicine in India. Continuing education of staff in palliative care is still uncommon, and there is even a lack of awareness of what palliative care is. Often confused with "pain control," the concept of "total pain," relevant in any care setting, is rarely appreciated. In spite of the vast body of research that already exists regarding cheap and effective oral analgesia, the professional attitudes of many Indians regarding the use of opiate medication prevents millions of cancer patients from having their pain adequately controlled. Stjernswärd has summed up this state of affairs: "There is—even in many resource-rich countries—an inadequate application of available knowledge."[13]

It is important to understand the different levels of nurse training that exist in India. The diploma nurse (three-year training) remains at the bedside but tends to be regarded by the public and professional peers as a "second-class citizen." Reasons for nurses not liking their job include the poor status afforded to their role. At first, to be sure, many diploma nurses are enthusiastic. Our experience is that they welcome interactive teaching, as opposed to traditional didactic sessions in large classes, and their ideals are high. It is not helpful that they are frequently taught by graduate and postgraduate nurses who do not always want to be in nursing, have not had training in teaching methods, or do not have access to teaching resources such as up-to-date books or journals. The hierarchical nature of both nursing and medicine means that many young people do not have a chance to develop their creativity for the benefit of their patients, and enthusiasm upon entering the profession may soon be dissipated, turning to disillusionment at qualification. Despite this, there are of course nurses and doctors who do retain their professional enthusiasm and ideals in the face of overwhelming challenges.[8]

It is vital to teach in the practical, realistic situation. Very often people are keen to impose Western values and methods, which may be demoralizing, and irrelevant, and wholly inappropriate—if not impossible to achieve. In the West we have much to learn from our counterparts in countries less developed economically than ours—technically or in terms of financial resources. We from the West have become a "waste-disposal" society—in terms of both human and practical resources. The resource-fulness of Indians in all aspects of their daily lives, both at home and at work, means that whereas we wait for a brochure describing the latest high-tech invention, Indians are already inventing an indigenous solution. Perhaps Western medicine needs to reassess its basic human values and realize that, for instance, having family members involved in basic care during the illness trajectory is valuable.[24] We can learn from India by looking at their strong family and community values and their wonderful sense of practicality.

It is important to adapt what is relevant from an advanced health care system. Thankam looked at the symptom distress scale of McCorkle and Young and translated it into malayanam and asked 100 patients with advanced cancer to indicate the severity of their symptoms. She demonstrated that pain is what drives patients to seek treatment, but even when they do present they do not get their symptoms assessed correctly. Very often there is no comprehensive symptom assessment methodology—and even more sadly, all attention may be focused on trying to cure a tumor that, because of its late stage of presentation, is probably incurable. Owing to cultural factors, patients will not divulge their symptoms, or even severe pain, unless asked. The shortage of staff and the enormous patient overload means that nonverbal expressions of pain are either not noticed or ignored. Symptoms related to appearance, particularly in head and neck tumors, were the most distressing, followed by bowel problems, pain and appetite.[26]

Even professors may not get subscriptions to their specialist journals. CRI has endeavored to get around this problem by compiling a digest of relevant articles on palliative care and distributing it free of charge to health care professionals all over India. The feedback received from the first two digests showed that a gap had been identified and filled. The ideal now is the establishment of a journal in print and online, giving multidisciplinary papers on palliative care in India.

Education should also consist of learning through real-life stories—"our patients are our best teachers"—and certainly this has been the case in India. In 1990 when the availability of morphine in India was very low, many were scared of its potential for addiction, respiratory depression, and potential theft by patients. Someone who has posthumously helped in teaching and dispelling those myths was a bright young man of 20 with osteosarcoma of his leg and metastases, who had severe pain. It was found that the disease had progressed. He was offered an amputation but refused surgery, as he wanted to die with two legs, but he did request that something be done for the intractable pain. When seen in the clinic by the author, he was taking 70 mg of oral morphine every 4 hours for his pain. He was bright, alert, pain free, had no respiratory depression, was not addicted to the drug, had continued working in the shop, and was leading a full life. He continued to live pain free for another nine months.[25] I told his story during teaching sessions in India, and showed his picture—looking alert and pain free. It has been interesting to note how many people remember this example of morphine use even years later.

From the beginning of these activities, multidisciplinary/interdisciplinary workshops in India have been encouraged and palliative care is one of the first disciplines in medicine/nursing to be taught in such a collaborative fashion. Nurses have a voice at last in medical meetings, and they are beginning to be recognized for what they can offer and are not see as just handmaidens to doctors.

The philosophy of education practiced, the teaching methods used, and the relationship between facilitator and students should mirror the care as practiced in the clinical setting between clinician and patient. It should be one of partnership. It requires knowledge, skills, and attitudes that foster trust and create a supportive environment that enables both partners to grow and learn from the experience. Another innovation in India started by CRI in the early 1990s is the use of interactive teaching sessions rather than the traditional didactic methods common in unidisciplinary nursing and medical teaching.

Nurses can and must make a difference in whatever ways are available to them. After hearing the author speak at an oncology conference in Mumbai in 1989 during which a British nurse spoke out for the need for palliative care, Dr. C. D. Joseph was the first doctor to get oral morphine in Kerala. Several doctors were horrified that a nurse should even be attending a medical meeting, let alone speaking. Many thought the nurse was a doctor and gave her 30 minutes as a guest speaker. Upon finding out she was a nurse, her speaking time was halved! Undeterred by the bell that rang after 15 minutes as an indication to stop, she continued to talk about the need for pain relief and providing relevant treatment, including oral morphine, for patients. One doctor listened, and set about to get oral morphine. Nine months and many bureaucratic hurdles later, Dr. Joseph succeeded and became the first doctor in Kerala (the third in India) to get oral morphine. Subsequently, he set up a pain clinic in the cancer hospital with funds from Cancer Relief India.

CONCLUSION

There cannot be one ideal future for the developed nations and another future for the developing nations. It is either one joint future or none.[13]

There are some brilliant individuals in India who have the vision to promote palliative care as a relevant treatment. Bringing people to the United Kingdom for training can be useful in some instances, but it is not always an ideal solution. The way forward is to develop usable and dynamic educational initiatives within India from model palliative care teaching centers attached to inpatient or community units, thereby making a close and relevant partnership between theory and practice. Such centers for palliative care teaching, offering high-quality education that is culturally sensitive and relevant to the Indian situation, have already been developed. They need to be sensitive to the challenges that face health care professionals who are trying to promote palliative care in a developing country.[8]

Suresh Kumar, of the Calicut Pain and Palliative Care Society, has written: "My exposure to the UK system [of palliative care] helped me to see for myself the possibilities of palliative care. It was a different atmosphere, where as a palliative care man I didn't have to worry much about the available resources or the poverty of the patients, but it showed me the actual potential of the care. It also threw up the irresistible challenge of adapting the model to an entirely different socio-political and cultural situation in India. Palliative care in the U.K. was the springboard from which I could jump into the Indian situation."

By comparing initiatives around India, we can discern factors that enable effective delivery of palliative care: inspired leadership, teamwork, empowerment of colleagues, patients and families, humility, recognition of the importance of communication skills, constant review of progress, and acknowledgment of the dynamic and diverse nature of palliative care. Contrary to commonly held beliefs, buildings per se, big budgets, and high technology are low on the list of priorities. Stjernswärd rightly observed that "institutions, organisations and countries have no excellence in themselves . . . and therefore individuals and their initiatives remain essential" and this is clearly apparent in the context of palliative care.[13]

Of course, the future belongs to our children and grandchildren. Children in the West, from youngsters to medical students, need to think responsibly about cancer, palliative care, death, and health care. They may learn certain from their Indian counterparts-courage, bravery, and independence. Will young people around the world be committed to the philosophy and best practice of palliative care? Indian people tend to be more outward looking than people in West. Children in India will have encountered death, and are expected to contribute and be actively involved in the home. A 17-year-old English boy, Benjamin Ford, who raised money for CRI, reported following a visit to India in September 1999:

"I appreciated the openness of Calicut and was particularly impressed with the spiritual care. I felt a wonderful addition was the ayurvedic doctor. I am not religious, but we need to see to see the person as spiritual—the body is not only mind and body but has a spiritual essence. Patients were given the opportunity to express their spirituality, made to feel at ease. In the U.K. more medical students and doctors need to see patients in their entirety, their physical, emotional, and spiritual needs; cancer is not just a physical disease. There is not so much spiritual care in the U.K. I noticed how well old people look 'spiritually at ease'—they could be thin bony men but their heads were held high. Old men in the U.K. seem to be alone in the world. The most important thing is education so that people would be self-sufficient."

This boy and the author are motivating others at his school to think not only about health issues but about ethics, philosophy, and ecological issues.

The development of palliative care in India during the last ten years has relied heavily upon input and models taken from the West, particularly England. The authors predict that in years to come the West will have much to learn from the authentic approaches that are being developed in several parts of the subcontinent.

Calicut Palliative Care Centre was developed in answer to the question "How can we achieve coverage and meet the needs of as many of those requiring palliative care in our area?"—patients first. Pune Palliative Care Centre was developed in answer to the question "How can we achieve coverage and enable the families and carers to be fully involved in patient care?"—families first. With the increasing pressure on health care resources in the West, these examples of dynamic responses to the challenges of achieving coverage in palliative care must serve as beacons. Their attention to the concerns for education and drug availability can serve to enlighten others, not only in under-resourced countries like India, but also in countries with ample economic and health care resources.

REFERENCES

1. The Huthinson Almanac 1999. Oxford: Helicon Publishing, 1998.
2. Tulley M. No Full Stops in India. Penguin: New Delhi, 1992.
3. National Cancer Control Programmes. Policies and Managerial Guidelines. Geneva: WHO, 1995.
4. Burn GL. A personal initiative to improve palliative care in India. Palliative Medicine 1990; 4:257–259.
5. Burn GL. An educational initiative to promote palliative care in a developing country. European Journal of Palliative Care 1996;3(3): 113–117.
6. De Souza LJ. India's First Study Centre for Palliative Care. Hospice Bulletin (Hospice Information Service) No 21; 12.93.
7. Webb PA. Cancer relief in India. European Journal of Cancer Care; 1993;2:2.
8. Burn GL. Progress in palliative care in India. Progress in Palliative Care 1996;4:161–162.
9. Mudhur G. Panel defends India's traditional doctors. BMJ 1997;314:1573 (1.5.97)
10. Suresh Kumar K, Rajagopal MR. Palliative Care in Kerala: Problems at presentation in 440 patients with advanced cancer in a south Indian state. Palliative Medicine 1996;10:293–298.
11. Rajagopal MR, Kumar, S. A model for delivery of palliative care in India—the Calicut experiment. Journal of Palliative Care 1999;5(1): 44–49.
12. Stjernswärd J, Koroltchoul V, Teoh, N. National policies for cancer pain relief and palliative care. Palliative Medicine 1992;6:273–276.
13. Stjernswärd J. Palliative medicine—a global perspective. In: Doyle D, Hanks GWC, MacDonald N, eds., Oxford Textbook of Palliative Medicine. Oxford: Oxford University Press 1993.
14. Sanwal A, Kumar S, et al. Informed consent in Indian patients. Journal of the Royal Society of Medicine 1996;89:196–198.
15. Suresh Kumar K. Occasional Letter, Calicut Pain and Palliative Care Society. Calicut, August 1995.
16. Burn GL. From paper to practice. Quality of life in a developing country: challenges that face us. Annals of the New York Academy of Sciences. Communication with the Cancer Patient: Information and Truth. New York, 1997.
17. Sharma DL. Hindu attitude toward suffering, dying and death. Palliative Medicine 1990; 4:235–238.
18. Sebastian P, et al. Evaluation of symptomatology in planning palliative care. Palliative Medicine 1993;7:27–34.
19. Kaye P. A letter from India. Hospice Bulletin (Hospice Information Service). 1995;2(2).
20. Proceedings of the First International Conference of the Indian Association of Palliative Care, Varanasi, January 27–29, 1994.
21. First Annual Report, May 1997–April 1998. Cipla Cancer Palliative Care Centre. Warje Pune.
22. Second Annual Report, May 1998–April 1999. Cipla Cancer Palliative Care Centre. Warje Pune
23. Paranjape SY. Personal Communication. 1999.
24. Hope J. Our Third World wards, a startling request to relatives—NURSE YOUR OWN PATIENTS (front-page headline). London, Daily Mail, January 8, 1999.
25. Removing the pain out of cancer's sting in Indian Express (Bangalore) 25.12.93.
26. Thankam K. Symptom distress—Are you really measuring it? Presentation at Oxford Brookes University for Diploma in Palliative Nursing.
27. Jeevodaya Newsletter. Chennai, October 1999.
28. Ford B. Personal communication. October 1999.

55 Japan

YASUKO ISHIGAKI, MEGUMI TESHIMA, and KEIKO HAMAGUCHI

From 1981 until the present, the leading cause of death in Japan has been cancer. In 1998, this accounted for 30.3% of total deaths in Japan (n = 283,827). The Regional Cancer Registration research group, under the Ministry of Welfare, estimated that 592,500 new cancer diagnoses would occur in the year 2000, and that half of these cancers would occur in individuals aged 70 years or older. The research group also noted that cancers with low cure rates, such as cancer of the lung, liver, or pancreatic cancer, would become problematic. Japan has an aging population, with those aged 65 or older exceeding 16% of the general population. Life expectancy for males is 77.19 years and for females 83.82 years (1997 figures). End-of-life care for the elderly, therefore, is of great concern to Japanese society. The study of *Tenju-gann*, a popular "ideal" means of cancer therapy for those of an advanced aged, has increased rapidly. In Japanese, *ten* means "heaven" and *ju* means celebrated long life. The definition of *Tenju-gann* is "cancer in people of advanced age that leads to a peaceful death with minimal suffering." This field has gained attention as an important area for study in end-of-life care.[1]

THE HOSPICE MOVEMENT IN JAPAN AND THE INCREASE IN HOSPICE/PALLIATIVE CARE UNITS

In 1977 the number of people who died at a hospital in Japan (50.6%) exceeded the number of people who died at home (49.4%). In response to these figures and to better understand the needs of the dying, the Japanese Association for Clinical Research on Death and Dying was formed.[2] In 1981, the first hospice unit in Japan, the Hospice of Seireimikatagahara, was opened in Shizuoka prefecture. The Ministry of Welfare strongly supported the hospice movement and endorsed the need for standards and funding for end-of-life care in Japan. Standards were set, and in 1990 a fixed amount of medical insurance remuneration for hospice/palliative care units (PCU) that met those standards was established. As of 1999 (18 years after the first hospice program in Japan began), 68 such facilities exist, with a total of 1230 beds approved by individual prefectural administrators in Japan. In 1991, the Japanese Association of Hospice and Palliative Care Units was established. The aim was to improve medical care of the dying and to better understand and provide for their overall needs. The Association predicts that the number of hospices/PCUs in Japan will exceed 100 within the next few years. The Association has also identified the need for ongoing study of the system and specialty of hospice/palliative care as practiced in Japan.[2]

PROFESSIONAL NURSING ASSOCIATION AND RESEARCH GROUPS AND EVIDENCE OF CITIZEN CONCERN ABOUT END-OF-LIFE CARE

In 1986, the Japanese Society of Cancer Nursing was formed. Annual conferences and seminars are held, with a focus on assessment and control of pain. In 1987, the Institute of Hospice Care was established. The Institute holds training seminars with a format of case studies, lectures, and consultation among patients and their families. In addition, support is given to medical professionals, including nurses, who engage in palliative care and hospice care. Since 1994, the Institute has conducted a nationwide support project for cancer patients and their families, based on the "I Can Cope" program developed in the United States. Overall, a paradigm shift has occurred in Japan, and quality of life is now regarded as an important part of cancer therapy. Recognition of the importance of expert end-of-life care is part of this paradigm shift. With this as a background, in 1996 the Japanese Society for Palliative Medicine was inaugurated. The society aims to develop palliative medicine as a specialized scientific discipline.[2]

Various other types of associations with a focus on end-of-life issues are being formed all over Japan. In many cases, nonmedical citizens in collaboration with some medical professionals lead activities, including lectures on end of life; care of the families of the deceased; and consultations and support for hospice care. An example is the Japan Association for Death Education and Grief Counseling. Based in Tokyo, the Association was established 20 years ago. There are 16 branches nationwide, and the number continues to grow. The Sapporo-based association established for "the development of hospice care with people" is another example. This association was established through the efforts of some medical professionals specializing in palliative care, hand-in-hand with nonmedical people. More than 10,000 citizens have participated in a series of 70 lectures and seminars to date. The seminar themes cover such topics as "truth-telling," "death in dignity," "euthanasia," and "cancer pain control." Nonmedical volunteer members of the association have expanded their activity to include issuing regular newsletters, holding study classes, organizing the association's support for patients and families, telephone consultations on hospice care, and organizing the grassroots movement to increase the number of institutionally based hospice programs. On a national level, more than 100 end-of-life–related associations have been organized and managed by nonmedical people. This national grassroots phenomenon can be seen as the Japanese people's attempt to sincerely face the question of "how to live and how to die" in an aging society.[3]

DEATH AND DYING IN JAPANESE CULTURE

The words heard from a person approaching death are usually a calling for "Mom." Stories that friends or family already deceased have "come to fetch" the dying person, or that when dying one "goes to see" those who have died before, are not uncommon. However, historically it has been taboo for Japanese to talk about death. This avoidance of death talk can be seen in everyday life throughout society. For example, the Japanese word for "death" and the word for "four" are pronounced identically; therefore, the words "four" and number "four" are often avoided.

Religion has an important role in the meaning of life and death and how life or morals should be. However, religions in Japan focus on ceremonies such as marriage and funerals. Few Japanese judge things in their daily living based on the standards of a religion. The majority of Japanese believe in Buddhism. In this religion, it is told that the deceased crosses the river Styx. Therefore, after the deceased's body is purified at a hospital or institution, it is dressed with the white attire of the dead in preparation for the journey across the river to the other world. Then the body is laid in a coffin with some objects needed for the journey, things that the deceased liked and treasured. For 24 hours after death, the family wake and sit by the body all through the day and night. This is called *O-tsuya*. Cremation is carried out 100% of the time in Japan, the body is cremated within two to three days after death. After the death, memorial services are held every seventh day from the first seventh day, *Sho-nanoka*, till the 49th day, *Shiju-ku-nichi*. Then the urn is placed in the cemetery. At these rites, where family and relatives of the deceased gather, the Buddhist priest chants sutras.

It is believed that spirits of the deceased come back on *O-bon*, in the middle of August. Accordingly, the family and friends gather and have memorial services on *O-bon* of the first, third, seventh, thirteenth, and so on up to the fiftieth year after death, this being an opportunity to remember the deceased. This system of remembrance and ceremony characteristic of Japanese culture supports the bereavement process.

Confucianism influences Japanese culture greatly and has become the standard of order in the social life for Japanese who were born before World War II. In Confucianism, mutual harmony is most important, and the whole harmony is prioritized to individuals. It is uppermost in the mind not to make other persons feel bad due to any emotional expression. The Confucianism characteristics of value influence the clinical issues at the end of life. For example, it is reported that many physicians do not tell their patients about prognosis and diagnosis because they consider it as being merciful to their patients not to do so.[4,5]

In Japan, individual autonomy or individualism has been denied.[6] *Omakase* (entrustment) is the idea symbolizing Japanese non-autonomy. This word means not only their trusting in authorities, but also their belief in the responsibility of authorities to take care of them.[7] In Confucianism, strict adherence to authority is expected, and individuals respond to health care providers' authoritative directives with a high level of conformity.[8] Recently, individuals have shown more positive attitudes toward "truth-telling"; however, 58% of families still do not want the patient to be told bad news about their illness.[9] Because of this attitude, even though a physician may wish to tell the diagnosis to a patient, the family may want to "protect" the patient from such information. In most cases, the families are informed as patient substitutes and provide consent for needed treatment to avoid "disturbing the patient emotionally."[5]

Among the Japanese, the capacity to endure difficult situations is a virtue. The ability to suppress complaints, conceal discomfort, and demonstrate a tolerance for adverse circumstance is seen as an opportunity to display courage, resourcefulness, and personal stamina.[6] This may lead to difficulty in pain and symptom control among the traditional Japanese. A study of 59 advanced cancer patients found that they tended to deny expressing their needs and to be patient in their situation.[10]

CHANGING VALUES AND FACING ISSUES

Especially after World War II, Western culture has made a strong impact on Japan. Since that time, education has emphasized more individualism. In addition, the nuclear family has become popular as a Japanese family style. However, although cultural values may be changing in the generation born after World War II, the majority of the population who currently receive hospice care still have traditional values.

Due to their cultural uniqueness, the Japanese are facing two major issues in providing care at the end of life. One is pain control, although knowledge and strategies for pain control in Japan are becoming advanced, and the other is telling the truth to the patient. The World Health Organization's (WHO) pain treatment approach was introduced into Japan in 1987. This method of cancer pain control treatment, mainly with use of morphine, has become popular. It is reported, however, that pain management remains a problem in some cancer hospitals.[11]

Issues surrounding informed consent continue to need attention. The nurse, as a patient advocate, is an ideal person to participate in a clinical ethics review on this topic. However, only a few hospitals in Japan have a clinical ethics team. The report of a survey regarding clinical ethical issues indicated those of informed consent and goals of care were problematic. For example,

"The hospitalization period is prolonged by the patient's or family's intention, while the medical goal remains undefined" or "Due to family's opposition, the truth cannot be told to the patient." These were listed as problems in daily clinical practice.[12] Palliative care teams need to obtain a greater cultural understanding of these issues in order to address them in a culturally sensitive manner.

THE NURSE'S ROLE IN PALLIATIVE CARE

The nurse's role in palliative care in Japan is essential. The Japanese Nurses' Association, recognizing this importance, developed a system of certification and training for nurses working in the fields of palliative care and oncology. One such system, initiated in 1994, is for a clinical nurse specialist in oncology nursing, Such a nurse must have a total of five years' clinical experience (including three years in oncology nursing), be master's prepared, and have passed an examination. A second system, initiated in 1998, involves certification of qualified nurses in hospice care. After a six-month training period, and following successful completion of an examination, the nurse obtains certification. These nurses are expected to assume leadership roles in providing end-of-life care in Japan.

END-OF-LIFE CARE IN GENERAL HOSPITALS

Although over 280,000 persons die of cancer annually in Japan, there are currently only 1230 hospice/PCU beds. Consequently, most patients die in hospitals that do not specialize in palliative care. In palliative care, the control of pain and other symptoms has the highest priority. The amount of morphine administered is frequently used as an index for adequacy of pain management in individual countries. The use of morphine in Japan continues to increase annually and reached 757 kg in 1998. However, the amount is far less that of other developed countries—for example, about one-tenth of that consumed in the United Kingdom.[13]

General hospitals are struggling to address the concerns of citizens regarding end-of-life care. Provision of end-of-life care to a patient in a general hospital, however, can be problematic in that the physician in charge of the patient has primary influence. The frequency of use of a specialized end-of-life team varies, and is dependant on recognition by the physician in charge of the patient of the need for input from such a team. The specialized team also strives to conduct education and research and to improve the quality of end-of-life care throughout the facility. Recently, palliative care specialists in general hospitals have developed a network and organized research groups in palliative care in many regions in Japan. Participation of local nurses and physicians in such groups has increased. Originally, the intent was for patients to be able to receive appropriate end-of-life care at any facilities. It is recognized that to foster interest in end-of-life care by physicians and nurses in general hospitals, education is important. There is an urgent need to introduce end-of-life curriculum into the basic education for physicians and nurses. Concomitantly, there is a need for continuous education for many physicians and nurses who are currently engaged in cancer care, and to disseminate recent research findings and updated clinical practice through specialized journals such as *Japanese Journal of Palliative Medicine* and *Japanese Journal of Hospice and Palliative Care.*

PALLIATIVE HOME CARE

In Japan, there is a movement in the twenty-first century for cancer care to expand from facility-type care to outpatient/home care. Although home care for cancer patients' is facing a turning point, at present medical care in hospitals overwhelmingly predominates. In a 1997 survey on where people die in Japan (n = 913,402), 76.2% died in hospitals and 16.1% died at home. When cancer deaths alone were looked at (n = 275,413), 89.9% were in hospitals and 6.9% were at home. It was estimated that about two-thirds of the patients who wanted to die at home actually died in the hospital, so the desire of the patient was not always realized. The reasons for hospital deaths included the following: the diagnosis and pathologic condition were not always told to the patient; the system of home hospice care is in the developmental stage; and medical expenses paid directly by the patient are less for hospital care than for care at home.

A system of home care programs, called the "visit nurse station," started in 1992. By 1998, 2756 sites for home care programs had been established all over Japan. A 24-hour on-call system has been instituted in 44.9% of these programs.[14] Unfortunately, if the emergency department is called at night, the plan for the patient's end-of-life care, which had been agreed upon by the patient and medical workers, does not bear weight, and lifesaving emergency treatments may be initiated. Individuals over 70 years of age account for over 80% of patients who are followed by home care programs, while patients with cancer account for only 4.5% of those who participate in the program[15] (Figure 55–1).

THE TRANSITION FROM HOSPITAL CARE TO HOME HOSPICE CARE FOR PATIENTS IN JAPAN

In 1996, the Japanese Foundation for Multidisciplinary Treatment of Cancer, initiated a collaborative research initiative on home cancer care, to evaluate the effectiveness of home care for cancer patients.[16] The subjects were 208 patients receiving home cancer care—namely, nursing visits, at 26 institutions all over Japan. The patients were assessed every two weeks, commencing on transfer to home and continuing until the home care was completed. The key findings from this research are as follows:

1. *Understanding of diagnosis.* In Japan, as previously stated, diagnosis and conditions are not always explained to the patient, especially for younger age groups where treatment is aimed at healing and prolongation of life. However,

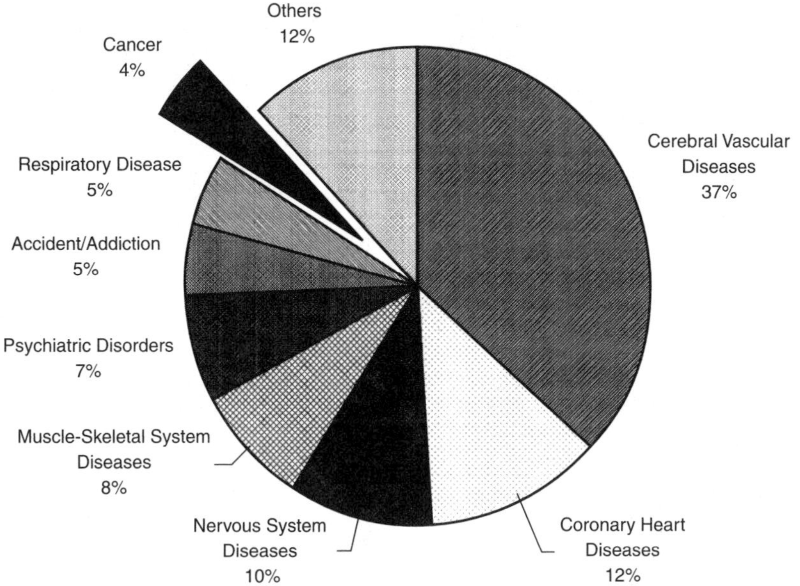

Fig. 55–1. Users' diagnosis of Visiting Nurse Station in 1997.[15] Population 1997 [On-line]. Available: mhw.go.jp/toukei/rkango98_8/sec02.html 16.

to choose home care in Japan, it is necessary for patients to know their diagnosis and condition. When patients were asked questions about having knowledge of their disease state, 60% of individuals answered "I was informed of my disease" and 24% answered "I have not been informed of my disease." The notification of the disease was made more often in younger age groups[16] (Table 55–1). The number of patients who died at home was 82 of 208 (39.4%). The frequency of death at home showed significant correlation among four factors: "Patients knew their cancer diagnosis"; "Patients and their family had requested home care originally"; "Patients desired to stay at home until their death"; and "Families desired patient to stay at home until death." Death at home was not related to age. These findings indicate that sufficient informed consent and a patient's understanding of the disease condition are important elements to continue care at home until death.[16]

2. *Patient's satisfaction with care and influential factors.* The patient's satisfaction with care was marked on an 11-point scale from 0 to 10, where 0 indicated very unsatisfied and 10 showed very satisfied. The patients with satisfaction of 8 or higher accounted for 50% and increased slightly with the passage of time. Factors influencing patient's satisfaction included family's satisfaction, patient's psychological factors such as anxiety, depressive feeling, and sleeplessness, or fatigue. From these findings, care of the family, alleviation of symptoms, and psychosocial care are shown to be important factors to enhance patient's satisfaction.

3. *Patient's anxiety.* Variation in patient anxiety eight weeks after the care was changed from hospital to home care was evaluated. The age group of less than 70 years included some patients who had strong anxiety from the beginning of home care, and showed slightly increased anxiety as a whole. In the age group 70 years or older, the patients who had no anxiety at the beginning of home care accounted for about 50%, and the anxiety then increased only slightly. A significant difference was seen between the age groups. Feelings of depression showed similar trends. These findings indicate that attention to anxiety and depression should be continued from the beginning of home care, especially for the younger age group. The findings suggest that specialists such as psychiatrists and social workers should be included in the home medical team.

Table 55–1. Relationship Between the Age and Disclosure of Cancer Diagnosis

	Age $p < 0.001$					
	*49	50–59	60–69	70–79	*80	Total
Patient knew	21 (84%)	16 (62%)	41 (73%)	38 (56%)	8 (24%)	124 (60%)
Patient guessed	1 (4%)	1 (4%)	6 (11%)	7 (10%)	1 (3%)	16 (8%)
Patient didn't know	3 (12%)	8 (31%)	6 (11%)	12 (18%)	21 (64%)	50 (24%)
Other	0 (0%)	1 (3%)	3 (5%)	11 (16%)	3 (9%)	18 (8%)
Total	25 (100%)	26 (100%)	56 (100%)	68 (100%)	33 (100%)	208 (100%)

*Japanese Foundation for Multidisciplinary Treatment of Cancer (1998). Specific research 22–A survey for developing home care systems for cancer patients.

FACING FUTURE EOL ISSUES IN JAPAN

Twenty years have passed since the end-of-life movement began in Japan. Future needs include facilitating research on end-of-life care. At present, in the Japanese Society for Palliative Medicine, many specialists, including nurses, are developing cancer pain management guidelines based on evidence from use of medicine. In addition, studies on the development of a rational system of care for cancer patients at home and the study of clinical and ethical practice systems are being conducted, mainly by nurses. Ongoing research in other aspects of end-of-life care in Japan continues.

Modeling of End-of-Life Care

End-of-life care is medical care for the whole human being, including mental/psychological, sociological, philosophical/

ethical aspects, as well as biological aspects of the whole person. A medical model based on Japanese cultural values is needed. Because of the rapid increase of the elderly population, Japan is urged to reform various social systems as well as the means of medical treatment and welfare activities. In such a period, end-of-life care, the model of care for the whole human being, should be applied to wider medical fields. It is especially desired as a mode of care for the aged and handicapped, and for people with chronic diseases. Numbers in these groups of individuals are anticipated to increase in Japan.

Education

It is very important to combine the curriculum of end-of-life care into the basic education for physicians and nurses. At present there are few classes on end-of-life care at medical schools, and many subjects of this field remain to be taught to medical students. In 1999, there were 76 undergraduate nursing programs, 30 graduate programs, and 9 doctoral programs in nursing in Japan. However, there are few systematic, independent courses on end-of-life care taught. For end-of-life care to acquire a field in nursing and medicine and to be settled in the future, it is necessary to develop a curriculum on end-of-life care that is firmly established in the basic education of medical professionals. In addition, to develop end-of-life care in the future, it is most important for professionals engaged in end-of-life care to cooperate with medical professions engaged in the traditional biological field and to support them in attempts to improve the quality of hospice and palliative care.

Cost-Effectiveness of End-of-Life Care

Analysis of cost-effectiveness of end-of-life care is important. As stated previously, the hospice/PCU which meets a certain standard is paid 38,000 yen for medical treatments, medications, and daily care expenses by the medical insurance. It is necessary to analyze how the cost actually contributes to the patient and family outcomes. When research demonstrates that care by hospice/PCU specialists truly contributes to patients and family outcomes, end-of-life care will be reflected in education for medical professions and in construction of the social system.

SUMMARY: END-OF-LIFE CARE AS SOCIAL MOVEMENT

End-of-life care is a social movement that influences people's awareness and ideas. Progress in the medical field in Japan in the 50 years following World War II has been remarkable. However, a sociological approach is needed for medical care as it is applied to human beings. For the society in the twenty-first century to respect human rights, it will be necessary for medical professions to network with various people such as public officers, economists, and sociologists, and to strive to spread end-of-life care as a social movement. Education and enlightenment of general citizens, as well as education of professionals, is essential to improve end-of-life care for all. In the past, Japanese lived naturally with four sufferings called, in Buddhism, *sei* (life), *byo* (disease), *rou* (aging), and *shi* (death). However, due to current scientific advance, these "natural events" have become "special events" occurring in special places. The Japanese, with the longest life expectancy of any country in the world, continue to search for a longer life. There is a beginning realization, however, that extension of life may result in very unnatural living. It needs to be recognized that to learn about death and dying is to learn about life and living. It makes sense, therefore, to combine education about preparation for death with health education.

REFERENCES

1. Kitagawa T, Hara M, Sano T, Sugimura T. The concept of Tenju-gann, or "natural-end cancer." Cancer 1998;83:1061–1065.

2. Ishitani K. The development for the Japanese Society for Palliative Medicine. Support Cancer Care 1999;7:62–63.

3. Japanese Association of Hospice and Palliative Care Units. Terminal care network. Japanese Journal of Hospice and Palliative Care 1999; 9:292–295 (Japanese).

4. Paton L, Wicks M. The growth of the hospice movement in Japan. American Journal of Hospice & Palliative Care 1996;14(3):26–31.

5. Tanida N. Japanese attitudes towards truth disclosure in cancer. Scandinavian Journal of Medicine 1994;22(1):50–57.

6. Johnson FA. Dependency and Japanese socialization. New York: New York University Press, 1993.

7. Suzuki S, Kirschling JM, Inoue I. Hospice care in Japan. American Journal of Hospice & Palliative Care 1993;10(4):35–40.

8. Sagara M, Pickett M. Sociocultural influences and care of dying children in Japan and the United States. Cancer Nursing 1998;21:274–281.

9. Public opinion about cancer. (1994, July 19). Yomiuri Shinbun. p.12 (Japanese).

10. Teshima M, Kojima M, Tamura M, Watanabe M, Tanaka K, Hamaguchi K, Suzuki K. Advanced cancer patients' needs. Proceedings of second international research conference, Kobe, Japan, 1995;188–189. The Japan Academy of Nursing Science.

11. Hiraga K. Honpou ni okeru ganseitoutsuukanri no genjou to kongo no tenbou [Pain control for cancer patients: Now and future vision in Japan]. Pain Clinic 1999;20:479–484 (Japanese).

12. Hamaguchi K. A survey for a clinical ethics committee and issues of clinical ethics. 1999 (Japanese).

13. The Ministry of Health and Welfare in Japan. (1999, Sept.) Dynamic statistic report of the morphine consumption in Japan. [Online]. Available: mhw.go.jp/search/docj/houdou/1101/h0111-2_15.html (Japanese)

14. The Ministry of Health and Welfare in Japan. (1999, Sept.). Activity report of visiting nurse station in 1998. [Online]. Available: mhw.go.jp/toukei/rkango98_8/sec03.html (Japanese)

15. The Ministry of Health and Welfare in Japan. (1999, Sept.). Users' diagnosis of visiting nurse station in 1997. [Online]. Available: mhw.go.jp/toukei/rkango98_8/sec02.html (Japanese)

16. Japanese Foundation for Multidisciplinary Treatment of Cancer (1998). Specific research 22–A survey for developing home care systems for cancer patients (Japanese).

56 Taiwan

SIEW TZUH TANG

Palliative/hospice care is a new development in Taiwan in reaction to the insufficient and inhumane treatment of dying patients by conventional medical care. Although death is feared and remains a taboo subject for the majority of people in Taiwan, a wealth of thought about death in terms of ancient philosophy, social customs, and morals can be found in Chinese literature dating back thousands of years. In this chapter, attitudes toward death and dying in Chinese culture will be explored, followed by a discussion of the evolution of the hospice movement in Taiwan. The current practice of palliative nursing care, exploring the following issues, will be presented: (*1*) sociodemographic data and common symptoms of hospice patients, (2) truth-telling and disclosure of diagnosis and prognosis, (3) pain management, (*4*) traditional Chinese medicine and alternative treatment, and (5) place of death. Additionally, challenges and future directions of palliative nursing care will be discussed.

ATTITUDES TOWARD DEATH AND DYING IN CHINESE CULTURE

Death remains a taboo subject for the majority of people in Taiwan. From an ancient age, Confucius taught his disciple Zilu that " not yet understanding life, how could you understand death?"[1] Traditional beliefs maintain that the deceased become invisible spirits who remain with the living. Such spirits may exercise their power to benefit or haunt the family, depending on how well they are treated. If proper attention is not paid to the details of the ritual, the dead person's spirit or ghost may return to plague the living family.[2] Therefore, Confucius advocated respect for ghosts and spirits while keeping them at a distance.[1] In *The Analects of Confucius*, the Master had nothing to say about strange happenings, the use of force, disorder, or spirits. In folk stories, however, it is suggested that talking about death will speed it up or even bring it about. In fact, many people believe that talking about death will bring bad luck. Consequently, a common strategy to cope with the fear of death is to escape or avoid that topic. The avoidance of death can be manifested in different ways in everyday examples throughout the society. For example, the pronunciation of the Chinese word for death and the word for "four" sound very similar; the Taiwanese word for "crying" and the word for "nine" also sound alike. The words "four" and "nine" are therefore often purposely avoided. When people must mention death, they often use expressions such as "passed away" or "went back to meet his Maker."

In addition to the profound negative traditional beliefs and thoughts about death and dying, thinking about death may arouse amorphous and unspecified anxieties about the many unknowns connected with death. This particular reaction is related to the difficulty of comprehending fully the existence of the world in the absence of consciousness. It is this anxiety, of "not being," that makes thinking about death unsettling and incomprehensible. Dying and death represent the ultimate loss, the loss of the self and those with whom we relate. Whatever is gained in life must be given up in its entirety. Therefore, it is difficult to examine one's own dying and death. A common idiom in Chinese is that throughout history dying and death is the most difficult human experience. Chinese people believe that "a living ass is better than a dead lion," which means that to live a rotten life is better than to have a good death.

However, a wealth of thought about death in terms of ancient philosophy, social customs, and morals can be found in Chinese literature dating back thousands of years. Ju-Chia, Taoism, Mohism, Legalism, and Buddhism have had tremendous impacts on Chinese culture and philosophy. Each elucidates many positive attitudes toward death in their doctrines. In *The Analects of Confucius*, Confucius taught that life and death are a matter of one's lot; if at dawn you learn of and tread the Way (Tao), you can face death at dusk; for the resolute scholar-apprentice and the authoritative person, while they would not compromise their authoritative conduct to save their lives, they might well give up their lives in order to achieve it.[1] In *Xunzi*, Confucius recognized that life in this world is full of obligation and suffering and that death will bring a release to a better afterlife and an eternal rest. In *Mencius*, Mencius said: "I want fish, and I also want bear paws. If I can't have both, I'll give up fish and take bear paws. I want life, and I also want Duty. If I can't have both, I'll give up life and take Duty.[3]

Taoism's philosophy recognizes that the principal characteristic of the Tao is the cyclic nature of its ceaseless motion and change. All developments in nature, those in the physical world as well as those of human situations, show cyclic patterns of coming and going.[4] Taoism's philosophy envisages the cosmos/universe and man as one; humans are expected finally to be absorbed in the ultimate energy that is the reality. Death means a return to nature.

Mohism and Legalism endorse the belief that the national interests outweigh an individual's life. Mohism advocates that, to pursue the benefits for their own country, people should proceed without hesitation. That means even to sacrifice their life, they will take it for granted. "Taking the vicissitudes of nation as an individual's first responsibility and leaving personal life and death out of consideration" is a typical example of Legalism's philosophy about life and death.[5]

Buddhism contends that there is a cycle of reincarnation. Death leads to a change of living state via numerous reincarnations on earth, until ultimately merging with energy, reality, atma. The Buddhist declares that what people reap, they have already sown. One's eternal destiny is decided in part by the kind of life one has led. The cumulative "weight" of an individual's deeds are of central importance to one's destiny. However, one's actions and state of mind during the process of dying can decide the final destiny of his next reincarnation. Buddhism therefore encourages dying patients to retain tranquility and understanding at the time of death.[6]

MEDICAL TREATMENT FOR TERMINALLY ILL CANCER PATIENTS IN TAIWAN

Since 1982, malignant neoplasms have been the leading cause of death in Taiwan. In 1997, more than 29,000 people died of cancer, accounting for 24.3% of the total deaths.[7] The immense technological advances in health care in recent years have improved the potential for cures in many previously fatal malignant diseases. Current health care systems continue to value life above living productively and meaningfully, with their overemphasis on life-prolonging treatment for the terminally ill. Thinking of options for management in terms of disease reversal has led to an overestimate of medical successes and has even misrepresented the benefits of therapy. Small but statistically significant improvements in survival have been enthusiastically heralded, whereas the effects of therapy on patients' symptoms and quality of life have been ignored. When some patients face the terminal disease, every effort is made to encourage the patient to keep on fighting; it has even declared a patriotic duty to do so. Family wishes are honored by physicians. It is commonly agreed that "rescue work for dying patients should be done according to the requests of the relatives in order to avoid or prevent unnecessary disputes." Therefore, aggressive treatment is frequently kept up right to the moment of death. In a survey of more than 1,000 physicians, results showed that over 40% of hospitals didn't have a do-not-resuscitate (DNR) order in place for terminally ill patients.[8] Recently, Yang and Ying[9] found that 80% of terminal cancer patients continued to receive active treatment during their hospitalization.

However, there is a growing recognition of and dissatisfaction with the futility and indignity of continuing expensive and intrusive medical treatments for terminally ill cancer patients. Standard or even extraordinary medical treatment is largely ineffective in the terminal illness and does not adequately relieve physical and emotional symptoms or family distress.

The hospice movement was a reaction against the inhumane treatment of the dying by conventional medical care. By introducing and incorporating hospice care into the medical care systems, the spirit of revolutionary humanitarianism and the glorious moral faith of the human being, which has long been embodied in traditional Chinese culture, can be reclaimed. The hospice approach, including its emphasis on quality of life, can fit with traditional Chinese virtues (compassion, piety, propriety, righteousness, wisdom) and the more recent "revolutionary humanitarianism." The essence of hospice care is that it gives highly personalized attention to a dying person and the family. The goals of hospice care are to help terminally ill patients and their families accept the impending death, receive mutual emotional care and support, mitigate the dying person's discomfort and isolation, and complete all "unfinished business." The ultimate aim is for the patient to die peacefully and with dignity (Shan-Zhong), and for the bereaved families to live without regrets.

THE HOSPICE MOVEMENT IN TAIWAN

In Taiwan, the introduction of the concept and philosophy of hospice and palliative care started in 1983 after several oncologists visited hospices in the United States. Under the promotion of the organizing hospice committee, which was set up in 1987 at Mackay Memorial Hospital, the first inpatient hospice started to operate in February 1990. At the end of 1990, the Hospice Foundation of the Republic of China was organized to promote education, publicity, and medical subsidies for terminal cancer patients.[10] In April 1991, the first oncology home care program in Taiwan was established at Sun Yat-Sen Cancer Center under the support of a grant from the Department of Health, the Executive Yuan, R.O.C. Approximately 80% of patients who received this home care service were terminally ill. Afterward, the hospice movement grew like "green bamboo shoots after a spring rain." According to statistics from the Department of Health, at the end of 1999 there were 20 inpatient units, which provided a capacity of 249 beds, and 26 hospice home care programs, with an average of 153 cases per month.[11]

In the National Cancer Control Programs, the government of Taiwan has offered a strong recognition of the need for hospice care and has taken a proactive role in the development of hospice care programs. The Department of Health has been involved in the hospice movement since 1995. First of all, the term "hospice and palliative care" was officially recognized in Chinese by the Department of Health. There is no equivalent term in Chinese for the English word "hospice." When government officers, scholars, and practitioners of palliative care decided on the appropriate translation of "hospice care," they not only considered the same basic meanings as the English term, but also incorporated the moral value of caring for dying patients in traditional Chinese culture and the essence of active care of the terminally ill. "Hospice care" or "palliative care" is finally translated as "An-Lin-Liau-Hu." The policy of reimbursement of hospice home care was initiated in 1996. Continuing education programs for all professionals in hospice care have been funded since 1996. In order to assure the quality of hospice care, standards of inpatient and home care hospice were formulated in 1995. Afterward, guidelines for cancer pain management and other care procedures were established and systems of monitoring and measuring quality of hospice care are currently under development. Also, grants for palliative research are funded each year. In May 2000, the Do-Not-Resuscitate had finally been enacted to legitimate the right of self-determination for terminally ill patients to decide the way they prefer to die. Starting from July 2000, inpatient hospice care will be included in the national health insurance system. It is estimated that by the year 2001 there will be more than 30,000 people who will die of cancer each year. The Department of Health has made the policy to revise the national health insurance system to appropriately reimburse inpatient and home care hospices toward the goals of at least one inpatient and one home care hospice program in each county in Taiwan.[11]

Hospice has gained high recognition and acceptance among the people in Taiwan. From a survey of Chao and colleagues,[12] over 90% of health care providers (including physicians, nurses, and social workers) and 77% of the general public have heard about hospice care. Chao and colleagues,[12] as well as Sheu and Duo,[13] both demonstrated that 80% of the general public and approximately 85% of terminal cancer patients and their families, respectively, were willing to receive hospice care.

THE CURRENT PRACTICE OF HOSPICE/PALLIATIVE CARE IN TAIWAN

Social-Demographic Data and Common Symptoms of Hospice Patients

From the most recent and largest-scale studies,[14–16] slightly more than 50% of hospice patients were male, with an average age of around 60 years old (Table 56–1). Lung cancer, hepatoma, colon-rectal cancer, head and neck cancer, and cervical cancer were the most common diagnoses. For inpatient hospice, the average length of stay was 17.4 days. The average length of service for hospice home care patients was around 40 days. The most prevalent terminal symptoms were pain, fatigue, constipation, and edema (Table 56–2).

Truth-Telling and Disclosure of Diagnosis and Prognosis

As the family is often more highly valued than the individual in Chinese culture, frequently, the degree of truth-telling has to be adjusted in the family's wishes. Results from the study of Chen[17] showed that 59% of families proclaimed that patients should not know about their cancer diagnosis. Traditionally in Taiwan, a terminal diagnosis is fully disclosed to the patient's family but not to the patient. According to a study conducted to investigate the attitudes of general medical and surgical physicians toward caring of terminally ill cancer patients, approximately one-third of physicians will respect family's opinions not to disclose the terminal diagnosis and prognosis to patients.[8] Under such a condition, a commonly observed phenomenon is that terminal cancer patients may not know about their own life-threatening diagnosis. Ger and Ho[18] found that only 37.2% of cancer patients knew about their own diagnosis. Yang and Ying[9] indicated that one-third of terminal cancer patients in their study did not know about their prognosis.

At the surface level, it appeared that patients and family were attempting to spare each other the anxieties aroused by the acknowledgment of death. It was considered cruel and tactless to speak directly of death, especially to people who were anticipating or had experienced a loss. Many Chinese believe that disclosure of a fatal diagnosis "will make the illness more serious" or "take away all hope." Some health professionals indicated that to tell the patient the diagnosis is to "encourage him or her to give up." Nevertheless, it was obvious that the considerate people who were avoiding

Table 56–1. Social-Demographic Data of Hospice Patients

	Studies			
	Chen[14]	Lai and Luh[15]		Tang[16]
	Care Setting			
Characteristics	Inpatient	Inpatient	Home Care	Home Care
Total number of patients	452	357	217	354
Sex				
Male	50.2%	50.4%	50.2%	51%
Female	49.8%	49.6%	49.8%	49%
Age				
Average ± SD	54.7	61.4 ± 15.6	63.4 ± 15.5	61.1 ± 14.4
Most Common Diagnosis				
Lung cancer	17.3%	16.5%	19.4%	17%
Hepatoma	17.3%	16.0%	16.1%	7%
Colon-rectal cancer	10.6%	15.4%	12.4%	16%
Head/neck cancer	5.1%	7.6%	7.3%	8%
Cervical cancer	4.4%	6.4%	6.9%	10%
Gastric cancer	8.6%	5.3%	6.0%	8%
Breast cancer	5.1%	4.8%	4.1%	12%
Pancreatic cancer	8.4%	3.6%	2.3%	6%
Prostate cancer	2.2%	2.0%	1.8%	5%
Length of Stay				
Average ± SD	17.5	17.3 ± 25.9	39.9 ± 68.1	45.1 ± 55.2

Table 56–2. Common Symptoms of Hospice Patients

	Studies				
	Chiu[27]	Lai and Luh[15]		Tang[16]	
	Care Settings				
Symptom	Inpatient	Inpatient	Home care	Home Care	Average
Pain	85.5%	81%	82.5%	70%	79.8%
Fatigue	89.7%	59.7%	68.2%	57.3%	68.7%
Constipation	67.8%	39.5%	52.1%	20.1%	44.9%
Edema	50.0%	—	—	30.6%	40.3%
Dyspnea	56.5%	38.7%	35.5%	18.2%	37.2%
Nausea/Vomiting	44.0%	32.4%	31.8%	26.6%	33.7%
Dysphagia	30.4%	21.0%	33.2%	—	28.2%
Insomnia	48.1%	22.4%	20.7%	8.1%	24.8%
Lymphedema	—	20.4%	28.1%	—	24.3%
Ascites	32.2%	16.8%	14.7%	16.3%	20%
Bleeding	34.1%	—	—	5.4%	19.8%
Malignant ulcer	22.5%	7.0%	8.8%	—	12.8%

the subject of death were also attempting to control their own anxieties. Since many patients and their families have difficulties in talking about their life-threatening situations, hospice nurses often have a major role in facilitating understanding and communication between patient and family. With the support of hospice nurses, the patient and the family are encouraged to communicate openly, offer mutual support, and settle unfinished business before the patient dies. In situations where the family is unwilling to communicate openly with the patient, hospice nurses who are willing to listen and support can minimize the feelings of isolation and loneliness.

Hospice care has initiated a change from the long-established practice of not telling patients their prognosis, to one that respects the patients' right to know and facilitates open communication. This new approach has produced positive results among Taiwanese patients. Dying patients in Taiwan do talk about their impending death if given permission. Chiu[19] demonstrated that 97.4% of interviewed subjects indicated that, if they got a cancer disease, they preferred to be informed of diagnosis. In a retrospective review of the first 497 patients served in the first inpatient hospice in Taiwan, Lai[20] found that awareness of dying was evident in 86% of patients. Similar findings were reported from the study of Wang.[21] The proportion of terminal cancer patients who have an insight into their own diagnosis was 87%, and 53.4% of those patients understand that their disease is incurable and their life span may be limited. Cheng and colleagues[22] demonstrated the significant effect of hospice care on improving awareness of impending death for terminal cancer patients, from 54.2% at admission to 72.9% before death.

Cancer Pain Management

There is a widespread impression among people in Taiwan that cancer patients eventually will die, with intolerable pain and suffering.[23] However, prevalence of cancer pain in Taiwan has not been extensively studied. Results from the only existing two studies[24–25] demonstrated that the prevalence of moderate to severe pain at all stages of cancer ranges from 31% to 38%. It is estimated that 36,000 cancer patients in Taiwan suffer from pain each day.[26] Among those who have advanced cancer, 70%–85.5% suffer from moderate to severe pain.[15–16,27–29]

There are major insufficiencies in cancer pain management in Taiwan. The majority of cancer patients with pain receive inadequate pain management, if they are treated at all. According to the research findings from Ho and colleagues,[25] 69% of cancer patients with pain were undermedicated and 44% of cancer patients with moderate to severe pain were not treated with opioids. Cherng[30] and Lin and Ward[31] also reported that 47% and 61.6%, respectively, of cancer patients in the study group were categorized as using a less-than-optimal potency analgesic as measured by the Pain Management Index. A survey from more than 600 nurses about their experience, attitudes, and knowledge of cancer pain management revealed disappointing results. Approximately 50% of respondents reported that from their experience cancer pain has been relieved in less than 50% of cases, and only 1.4% of nurses indicated that cancer pain can be completely relieved.[32] Eighty-one percent of nurses rated pain management in their own practice as fair, poor, or very poor.

The reasons for such inadequacies in cancer pain management in Taiwan may include attitudes of health care providers and the general public toward cancer pain management, specifically toward use of morphine, and the lack of knowledge of physicians and nurses for appropriate cancer pain control.

Physician-Related Barriers. Cherng[30] suggested that physician-related barriers were the most important factors for optimal pain management in Taiwan. Huang, Liao, and Yeo[28] showed that 51% of interviewed physicians failed to acknowledge the content of the WHO three-ladder cancer pain control method. Sun and colleagues[33] demonstrated that 50% of physicians believed that prolonged opioid medications may potentially induce addiction. Even with the well-established evidence that chronic pethidine (Demerol) usage might induce neurological toxicity, intramuscular pethidine was the drug of choice for cancer pain relief for 46.9%,[27] 83%,[25] and 98% of the physicians[28] surveyed in three separate studies. This opioid was reported as prescribed in an "as needed" fashion by 63.9%–83% of physicians.[26–27]

Nurse-Related Barriers. From the survey of Tang,[32] approximately 60% of nurses believed that more than 50% of cancer patients overemphasize their pain. Only one-third of nurses believed that cancer pain can be relieved for over 80% of patients. Fifty-eight percent of nurses believed the incidence of opioid addiction is less than 1%, and over one-fifth of nurses believed that the incidence of addiction is equal to or greater than 25%. Fear of side effects of morphine was the primary reason for prohibiting them from using opioids for cancer pain management. Specific side effects recognized by nurses as prohibitive factors are as following: respiratory depression (90.4%), conscious disturbance (57.4%), drowsiness (52.9%), nausea and vomiting (42.5%), addiction (42.1%), urinary retention (33.1%), and constipation (30.1%). Factors identified by nurses that may influence effective and appropriate cancer pain management include: attitudes of patients toward cancer pain management (72.7%), barriers from physicians (60.3%), family resistance to using opioids (55.8%), lack of personal experience and knowledge of cancer pain relief and management of side effects of opioid treatment (37.4%), and restrictions on narcotic utilization (27.7%).

Patient-Related Barriers. From the study of Lin and Ward,[31] 62% of the patients reported that they had hesitated to report pain to their health care providers in the past month, and 59% of the study participants indicated that they had hesitated to use pain medication in the past month. Concerns about tolerance, disease progression, time interval, and addiction were the most frequently mentioned barriers for these cancer patients to requesting opioids to relieve their pain.

Sun and colleagues[33] also confirmed that attitudes of cancer patients and their families toward morphine affect the acceptance of use of morphine for pain relief and influence the number of requests for discontinuation of morphine prematurely. They prospectively investigated the cancer pain management for 627 patients who were referred to a special pain clinic at a national teaching hospital. Fourteen percent of the referred patients refused to enter the study mainly because they or their families objected to use of morphine for pain relief. Forty-nine percent of the patients under morphine treatment asked for discontinuation of the medication. However, only one-fifth of this group of patients could be successfully managed by tapering the dosages of morphine. The majority of these patients were treated with various antineoplastic treatment for curative or palliative purposes. The other 79.7% of patients who requested termination of morphine suffered predominantly from an exaggeration of preexisting pain on premature discontinuation of morphine. This result indicated that the fear of addiction is highly prevalent among cancer patients who suffered from severe pain in Taiwan and sometimes took precedence over the desire for pain relief.

Achievement of Cancer Pain Management among Hospice Patients. Introducing hospice care for terminal cancer patients remarkably improves the status of cancer pain management in Taiwan. First, there is increasing knowledge of the use of morphine by oral route as the first choice for severe cancer pain management. By 1995, the national consumption of morphine in Taiwan had increased 11-fold over that of 1988.[26] The average increment of morphine consumption has been 35% per year. The rise in consumption of oral formulation (1,260% increase) has exceeded the rise in injection formulation use (585% increase). Opioid availability has been improved to allow clinicians to have more flexibility to manage cancer pain. In addition to morphine and pethidine, propoxyphene, codeine, tramadol, and fentanyl are available in Taiwan to treat cancer pain. To improve the quality of life for terminal cancer patients, slow-release formula (such as MS Contin), transdermal patch, and patient-controlled analgesia are frequently used in appropriate patients. Recently, the National Narcotics Bureau had revised the regulations of opioids to allow terminal cancer patients, when they are under appropriate supervision, to use opioids at home.

Chen and colleagues[29] reported that satisfactory pain relief was achieved in two-thirds of hospice patients. Successful pain management also has positive impacts on sleep and appetite for those patients, thereby increasing their quality of life. Specifically, Tang[16] demonstrated statistically significant decreases of average pain intensity (on a scale of 0 = no pain to 10 = worst pain) from 4.23 at the initiation of pain control to 2.43 at the end of care for hospice home care patients ($p < 0.000$). At the end of home care service, 27.9% of terminal cancer patients with pain were at a pain-free status. Forty-nine percent of patients didn't require any increment of morphine dosage, and 38% of patients increased their morphine dosage with an average of 59 mg oral dosage increment per day. Decreases of morphine dosage occurred in 13% of patients, with an average of 33 mg oral dosage decrement per day.

Traditional Medicine and Alternative Treatment

Traditional Chinese medicine is frequently used in the treatment of cancer either as the principal approach or complementary to Western medicine. These treatments are based on the theory of balancing ying and yang, qi, and five elements—namely, metal, wood, water, fire, and earth. The effectiveness of traditional medicine for cancer pain and other terminal symptom management is uncertain due to few scientific data.

Hsin and colleagues[34] conducted a study to investigate the proportion of inpatient hospice cancer patients who had ever used alternative therapies. Results showed that 81.9% of patients have used at least one alternative therapy. The most common alternative therapy was herbs prescribed by Chinese medicine doctors (51.4%). The other popular alternative therapies in order of use were herbs not prescribed by Chinese medicine doctors (50%), special diets (34.8%), the therapies of gods (18.1%), breathing therapy (10.9%), and acupuncture (5.1%). Most users hoped the alternative therapies could cure their disease or impede the progression of disease. However, the majority (67.3%) of users indicated no obvious effects of those treatments, and only 23.7% of users had experienced relief of symptoms from those alternative therapies. Similar findings were reported by Chang.[35] In this multicenter study, 46.9% of cancer patients had ever tried alternative treatments. Among those who had used alternative therapies, 91.6% of them finally abandoned those treatments due to ineffectiveness.

One phenomenon of clinical importance is that many cancer patients in Taiwan hide the fact that they are currently using alternative therapies from their health care providers. Results from the studies of Hsin and colleagues[34] as well as Chang[35] showed that 56.3% and 71.3%, respectively, didn't tell or discuss with their doctors that they used herbal drugs. Notably, Hsin and colleagues[34] found that 12.3% of study participants had abandoned standard Western medical treatments so as not to conflict with Chinese herb drugs. Hospice nurses need to understand and accept the practice of alternative therapies among terminal patients and try to act in accord with the value system of patients and their families. Only when terminal patients and their families can perceive the nonjudgmental, supportive attitudes from hospice nurses can they openly discuss their utilization of alternative therapies with them. Then hospice nurses may incorporate the alternative therapies into palliative nursing care in order to achieve the maximal benefits for dying patients.

Place of Death of Hospice Patients

To maintain dignity, terminal patients must be able to do things in their own way, to make their own decisions and to preside over their own dying. Among the tasks considered essential for terminal cancer patients is the decision of where to die. Hospice care strives to do this. The actual place of death can provide a measure of whether this particular outcome is being achieved, and it has been recognized as an indicator of quality of care of hospice care.[36]

Approximately two-thirds of cancer patients, when asked about their preferred place of death, wished to die in their own homes.[37–45] Terminal cancer patients who die at home may find physical and emotional comfort there. Home is a place where people may feel safety and a sense of belonging. Terminal cancer patients who die at home also may have a greater chance to control their environment, more autonomy and privacy, and a greater sense of normality. Furthermore, for Chinese people, dying at home has a special cultural meaning to dying patients and their families. Chinese refer to dying in the main hall of one's own house as "dying peacefully in one's bed." Dying there is the most glorious and fortunate way to die.[46–49] When death occurs at home, the spirit of the dead can reunite with the forebears, and thus, "the fallen leaves can return to their roots." When one dies at home, the spirit of the dead have a place to rest and the dead will not be a koo'un' ia' kui (literally, spirit wanderer), a solitary soul with no one to depend on.

Dying at home not only benefits the dying person but is also believed to be crucial to the well-being of living descendants. The Chinese believe that if departed ancestors can exercise the necessary influence upon the supernatural world, the dead family member will be able to intercede with a supernatural power on behalf of the descendants for special blessings. However, if an individual has died outside the home, the person lacks the domain through which to shelter his descendants.[47–48,50–55] In addition, the Chinese also believe that when a person dies, he takes the misfortune of earthly life and leaves good fortune to the family. Owing to these traditional Chinese customs and beliefs, dying at home is especially important for the people of Taiwan.

Although there are many advantages to dying at home and the majority of terminal cancer patients prefer to do so, the reality is that few of them see their wish come true. According to the vital statistics from the Department of Health in 1995,[56] 83% of all deaths in Taiwan occurred in hospitals and 17% at home. From the study of Tang,[44] terminal cancer patients identified obstacles of receiving terminal care and dying at home as the following: lack of home care services, inability of family to provide care at home, insufficiency of pain management, lack of opioids at home, and deficiencies in insurance reimbursement for providing care at home. Provision of hospice home care can overcome the aforementioned obstacles of dying at home and can achieve the goal of helping terminal cancer patients remain at home with their family and therefore realize their preference of place of terminal care and death. Statistics from hospice home care programs[15–16,45] demonstrated that 66.7%–72.5% of patients under the home care services could die at home (Table 56–3) and

Table 56–3. Place of Death for Terminal Cancer Patients

	Studies				
	Lai and Luh[15]		Tang		
	Care Settings				
Place of Death	Inpatient	Home care	Home care[16]	Inpatient[45]	Home care[45]
Home	28.5%	72.7%	69.5%	20.7%	66.7 %
Inpatient hospice	45.8%	10.9%			
General hospital	21.1%	13.6%	30.5%	79.3%	33.3 %
Others	4.4%	2.7%			

24.5%–33.3% of patients under such care died in the institutions (including general and cancer wards and inpatient hospices). The availability and accessibility of comprehensive and coordinated home care services are pivotal in making death at home a realistic option.

Mor and Hiris[57] demonstrated that patients served by a hospice that had its own beds or was affiliated with a hospital were three times more likely to die in a medical setting than were patients served by hospices without beds or direct access to them. Results from the studies of Lai and Luh[15] and Tang[45] were similar. Lai and Luh[15] found that 45.8% of terminal cancer patients served by inpatient hospices died there and another 21.1% of patients died in general hospitals (for a total of 66.9% institutionalized death). Results from the study of Tang,[45] which was conducted to compare the quality of terminal care received by patients at a cancer center or at home, showed that 79.3% of hospitalized patients died in the hospital.

CHALLENGES AND FUTURE DIRECTIONS OF PALLIATIVE CARE IN TAIWAN

Nurses are currently able to take on leadership roles in the development of palliative care in Taiwan. Their success depends not only on a solid base of knowledge and skills in the delivery of palliative care, but also on a high level of political awareness and political activity to influence policymaking in the field of palliative care. For the further development of palliative nursing in Taiwan, nurses need to be aware of challenges and potential opportunities inherent in the progress of palliative care in the future.

Expansion of Coverage and Scope of Palliative Care

Although, as mentioned earlier in this chapter, a high percentage of people have heard of hospice care, only a small proportion of them have personal experience with hospice care. From a survey of Chao and colleagues,[12] less than 30% of health care providers (24.5%, 14.6%, and 27.7% for physicians, nurses, and social workers, respectively) and only 5.9% of the general public have a personal experience with hospice care. This phenomenon may be related to two causes: (*1*) there still is misunderstanding or lack of acceptance of the concept and philosophy of hospice care; and (2) inadequate coverage of hospice care. In the survey of Chao and colleagues,[12] more than 20% of physicians, nurses, and the general public misrecognized hospice as nursing home or long-term-care facilities, and 11% and 14.5% of physicians and general public, respectively, identified hospice as euthanasia. Yao and colleagues[58] demonstrated that only 53% of the patients who searched for palliative care consultation finally accepted the options of inpatient hospice admission. The primary reasons for the decision to not receive hospice care from families were unacceptance of the philosophy of palliative care and insistence on continuing life-sustaining treatments. At the same time, in the survey of Chao and colleagues,[12] the majority of participants identified psychosocial, spiritual, and physical care as the essential components of hospice care; fewer subjects, especially the general public, recognized pain management (32.7%) and symptom control (35.5%) as the primary functions of hospice care. However, findings from the studies of Sheu and Duo[13] as well as Yao and colleagues[58] showed that terminal cancer patients and their families identified pain and terminal symptom control as the first priority of care needs. Therefore, the general public may not actually understand or recognize that hospice care can meet the needs of the terminally ill. Palliative nurses can play an active role in clarifying these misconceptions and demonstrate the effectiveness of hospice care in relieving the physical suffering of dying patients.

By the year 2001, it is estimated that more than 30,000 people will die of cancer per year in Taiwan. However, currently the capacity of hospice care in Taiwan is 249 beds and 26 hospice home care programs, with an average of 153 cases per month. There is obviously inadequate coverage of hospice care in Taiwan. One of the major goals of hospice care is to allow terminal cancer patients to remain at home as long as possible, using in-hospital days only when absolutely necessary.[59–60] In addition, under cost-containment pressure in today's health care systems, hospice home care may be more feasible and cost-effective for the large number of terminal cancer patients who die every year in Taiwan.

Stjernswärd and Pampallona[61] suggested that a broader approach to palliative care is needed from the outset and that institutionalization should be avoided. Home care is the dominant form of service across all geographic regions globally.[62] As Wilson and Kastenbaum[63] suggested, the dominance of home care services is an economic necessity that service providers tend to make a virtue. An alternative view is that the development of outpatient or home care services reflects an important attempt to improve access across the population.[62] Empowerment of family members as effective caregivers in palliative care is the most realistic approach to achieving meaningful coverage.[61]

In addition, future development of hospice care in Taiwan should integrate the palliative care approach into the everyday practice of medical care and into the management of all patients with incurable diseases from diagnosis to death. The knowledge achieved in cancer palliative care should be applied to as many of the terminally ill as possible, including the elderly, individuals with chronic diseases, and AIDS patients.

If the trend toward home care continues, there will be an urgent need to address the educational needs of the nurses who will provide the primary care for terminal patients and who will be required to function more independently than their counterparts in hospitals. Palliative nurses should be prepared to function in diverse care settings for a wide range of disease populations.

Quality Assurance and Research in Palliative Care

If hospice programs are to continue to grow as the health care system changes, their services will have to be at a consistently high level of quality. Hospice programs still vary considerably in the quantity and quality of services they deliver. It is necessary to prove that value for money and improved quality of life can be achieved in the treatment of the terminally ill. Quality measurement could be used for external audit, for internal improvement in the care process, and for giving patients and families choices in facilities and programs. Studies that evaluate the outcomes of palliative nursing care are urgently needed.

MacDonald[64] suggested that progress in a particular field depends on its research base. "Evidence-based medicine" will increasingly influence the decisions of policy makers responsible for setting priorities and supporting health care programs. Palliative care will be unfairly hampered if research in the field is not supported and the lack of research is then used as a reason not to support palliative care initiatives. Quantification of the efficacy of varied interventions for care of the terminally ill is difficult and requires several measures, including indicators of quality of care such as quality of life, quality of symptom management, amount of hospital use, containment of costs, place of death, family distress, and patient and family satisfaction. A national database is needed that can show how caregiving can be measured across all settings. The sum of measuring quality in various settings is more than the sum of measurements of individual settings. Appropriate application of pertinent methodology in this area is essential. Assessment tools for quality of care should be reliable, sensitive, specific, have predictive value, and reflect indigenous characteristics of Chinese and Taiwanese culture.

Studies of a patient-driven or family-driven nature are needed to gain the perspectives of patients and families in relation to the needs of terminal care, definition of quality of life, evaluation of effectiveness of symptom management and psychosocial support, satisfaction with the care given, outcomes achieved, the extent to which opportunities were provided to complete life in a meaningful way, and the reasons for end-of-life decisions. Listening to the voices of patients and families, a central tenet embedded in the philosophy of palliative care, may extend our understanding of their unique needs and help to clarify our directions for the future.

With the emphasis in palliative care on home care and shortened hospital stays, there is an increased demand for family assistance in the management of health problems for terminal patients. While many caregivers value their caregiving role, it is not without emotional and physical sacrifice and profound economic consequences. Family care burden, including financial and emotional effects, is another area that needs to be investigated. Interventions that empower family caregivers and make them more effective also need to be identified and evaluated.

Improvement of Palliative Nursing Education

Benoliel[65] stated that care of the dying is essentially a nursing, and not a medical, problem. However, caring for and dealing with dying patients can be extremely stressful for caregivers, as it forces each of us to confront our mortality and arouses our preconceptions about dying. Nurses are asked to understand and respond to the dying person. Yet to understand another person's life requires that we understand the same conflicts, the same feelings, and the same situations located within ourselves. Such self-understanding may provoke recognition of our own mortality and the potential for the loss of our own self. The death of a patient may also threaten the professional curative goals of health care. Death in this sense is seen as a failure.

The interpersonal relationships between terminally ill patients and nurses can be intense and intimate. When a patient dies, a part of the nurse may die with him or her. Death induces a loss of relationship, which many nurses value very much. Therefore, caring for dying patients causes great emotional strains on nurses in Taiwan. Findings from the study of Duo[66] showed that nurses experience considerable anxiety when caring for dying patients. The most common feelings brought on by taking care of dying patients are powerlessness and depression. The majority of nurses (83.4%) who participated in the study wished patients would not die on their shift, and only 37.3% of them had the motivation to work on units with high mortality rates.

Jodrell[67] suggested that it is only through education that we are likely to dispel the concept that death is a failure of nursing care and instill in those caring for patients in a palliative care setting the belief that delivery of palliative care is active care and should be scientifically, clinically, and educationally sound. Compassion that is not combined with wisdom is inefficient in relieving suffering.

There is a need for a more systematic approach to nurse education on death and dying in Taiwan. Duo[66] found that only 21.7% of nurses who participated in her study had gained palliative nursing care knowledge from their undergraduate education, and only 57.1% of them attended in-service education focused on palliative nursing care. Undoubtedly, there are profound and serious deficiencies of knowledge in pathophysiological changes in the dying process, signs and symptoms of impending death, pain management, emotional and psychosocial care of dying patients, and bereavement care for the family.

The goal of palliative nursing education is to provide nurses with the appropriate knowledge, skills, and attitudes for taking care of dying patients and their families, together with a commitment to ongoing personal and professional development. In addition to basic concepts and philosophy of palliative nursing care, more endeavors should be emphasized that teach practical knowledge and skills for the management of common terminal symptoms,[15–16,27] and that offer clinical demonstrations of effectively communicating with dying patients, providing psychosocial support, dealing with ethical dilemmas, and giving hope and spiritual care. Palliative nursing education also needs to address family care, especially given the trend toward home care of dying patients and the tremendous burdens and stress they might experience in providing care to dying patients. Until now, bereavement care has not been regularly provided to bereaved families. Nurses need to cooperate with social workers and other team members to extend palliative care to families after the death of a patient.

CONCLUSION

In reaction to the insufficient and inhumane medical care of dying patients, palliative/hospice care has been actively developed since 1983 in Taiwan. The philosophy of palliative care matches the essence of nursing—humane caring. Palliative nursing care has accomplished much in helping terminally ill patients and their families accept impending death, relieve dying persons' discomfort and suffering, let patients die peacefully and with dignity, and permit bereaved families to live without regrets. Even so, palliative nurses in Taiwan need to be aware of the coming challenges and to be prepared to take an active role in the further development of palliative care. With the unique input from palliative nursing, dying patients in Taiwan may be helped to experience the final stage of life with traditional Chinese wisdom of death and dying.

The author thanks Tzay Jinn Chen, M.D., M.P.H. Director-General, and Dan Rony Chang, P.R.N. Senior Technical Officer of Bureau of Promotion and Protection, Department of Health, The Executive Yuan, R.O.C., for supplying information and input for this chapter.

REFERENCES

1. Ames RT, Rosemont H. The Analects of Confucius: A Philosophical Translation. New York: Ballantine, 1998.

2. Gudmundsdottir M, Martinson PV, Martinson IM. Funeral rituals following the death of a child in Taiwan. Journal of Palliative Care, 1996; 12(1):31–37.

3. Hinton D. Mencius. Washington, DC: Counterpoint, 1998.

4. Capra F. The Tao of Physics, 3rd ed. Boston: Shambhala Publications, 1991:101–120.

5. Jeng SJ. The contemporary values of traditional Chinese wisdom of death. Journal of Philosophy and Culture 1993;20(8):795–802. (In Chinese.)

6. Hamel RP, Lysaught MT. Choosing palliative care: Do religious beliefs make a difference? Journal of Palliative Care 1994;10(3):61–66.

7. Department of Health. Public Health in Taiwan, Republic of China. Department of Health, The Executive Yuan, R.O.C, Taipei, 1998: 42.

8. Chao CS, Wang MS, Chen MJ, Jiang AB. Attitudes of Physicians Concerning Care of Terminally Ill Cancer Patients. Final report of project supported by grant DOH86-TD-061, DOH. Kang-Tay Medical Educational Foundation, Taipei, 1997. (In Chinese.)

9. Yang KP, Ying TC. Health-related quality of life for terminal cancer patients. Nursing Research of Taiwan 1999;7(2):129–143. (In Chinese.)

10. Lai YL, Su WH. Palliative medicine and the hospice movement in Taiwan. Supportive Care in Cancer 1997;5:348–350.

11. Chen TJ. Reports on Overseas Assignments. by officals of Executive Yuan, R.O.C. Taipei, Taiwan, 1999. (In Chinese.)

12. Chao CS, Chen MJ, Lai YL, Chou SL, Lee ZH. Recognition and Acceptance of Physicians, Nurses, Social Workers and General Public Toward Hospice/Palliative Care. Final report of project supported by grant DOH87-TD-1060, DOH. Kang-Tay Medical Educational Foundation, Taipei, 1998. (In Chinese.)

13. Sheu DT, Duo IT. An investigation of the cognition and its related factors of cancer patients and their families forward the terminal care needs. Journal of Veteran Nursing 1997;14(1):11–22. (In Chinese.)

14. Chen CY. Principle of palliative care. Formosan Journal of Medicine 1997;1(2):186–192. (In Chinese.)

15. Lai YL, Luh YC. Establishment of Indicators for Monitoring Quality of Care of Hospice. Final report of project supported by grant DOH87-HP-5H04, DOH. Mackay Memorial Hospital, Taipei, 1998. (In Chinese.)

16. Tang ST. Outcomes of Home Care for Cancer Patients at Sun Yat-Sen Cancer Center in Taiwan, 1998. (Unpublished Study.) (In Chinese.)

17. Chen CH. Attitude of family toward telling the truth to the cancer patient. Journal of Nursing 1982;29(3):29–38. (In Chinese.)

18. Ger LP, Ho ST. Awareness of diagnosis among cancer patients. Newsletter of Narcotics 1997; 1. (In Chinese.)

19. Chiu TY. The Attitudes Toward Terminal Care in Rural Communities in Taiwan and Japan: A Comparative Study. (Thesis), pp. 1–31. University of Tokyo, 1995.

20. Lai YL. Continuing hospice care of cancer—A three year experience. Journal of the Formosa Medical Association 1994;93:98–102. (In Chinese.)

21. Wang MS. The Factors Influencing End-Phase Cancer Patients and Their Families to Accept Hospice Services. Final report of project supported by grant DOH87-TD-1071, DOH. National Yang-Ming University, Taipei, 1998. (In Chinese.)

22. Cheng SY, Chiu TY, Hu WY, Guo FR, Wang Y, Chou LL, et al. A pilot study of good death in terminal cancer patients. Chinese Journal of Family Medicine 1996;6:83–92. (In Chinese.)

23. Dodd MJ, Chen GG, Lindsey AM, Piper BF. Attitudes of patients living in Taiwan about cancer and its treatment. Cancer Nursing 1985; 8(4):214–220.

24. Cherng CH, Ho ST, Kao SJ, Ger LP. The study of cancer pain and its correlates. Journal of Anesthesiology Taiwan 1991;29:653–657. (In Chinese.)

25. Ho ST, Ger LP, Cherng CH. Epidemiology of cancer pain in Taiwan. In: Sun WZ, Cancer Pain Management. Taiwan Cancer Foundation Publisher, Taipei, 1996:30–36. (In Chinese.)

26. Sun WZ, Hou WY, Li JH. Republic of China: Status of cancer pain and palliative care. Journal of Pain and Symptom Management 1996; 12(2):127–129.

27. Chiu TY. Pain control in terminal cancer patients. Formosan Journal of Medicine 1997; 1(2):198–208. (In Chinese.)

28. Huang MC, Liao JH, Yeo CY. Study on the applicability of narcotics self medication for terminal cancer patients. Chinese Journal of Pain 1993;3:S515. (In Chinese.)

29. Chen MH, Chiu TY, Hu WY, Chen CY. Pain management for terminal cancer patients. Chinese Journal of Family Medicine 1997;7:24–32. (In Chinese.)

30. Cherng CH. Patient-Related Barriers to Management of Cancer Pain. Final report of project supported by grant DOH86-TD-081, DOH. Tri-Service General Hospital, Taipei. (In Chinese.)

31. Lin CC, Ward SE. Patient-related barriers to cancer pain management in Taiwan. Cancer Nursing 1995;18(1):16–22.

32. Tang ST. Experience, Attitudes, and Knowledge of Nurses of Cancer Pain Management, 1997 (Unpublished study.) (In Chinese.)

33. Sun WZ, Chen TL, Fan SZ, Peng WL, Wang MS, Huang FY. Can cancer pain attenuate the physical dependence on chronic morphine treatment? Journal of Formosan Medical Association 1992;91:513–520. (In Chinese.)

34. Hsin LS, Chiu TY, Hu WY, Cheng SY, Chen CY. The behavior of alternative therapies among terminal cancer patients. Chinese Journal of Family Medicine 1996;6:127–137. (In Chinese.)

35. Chang LY. "Patient, physician and hospital: An exploration of the illness experience of the cancer patients." A manuscription for the project entitled The Organization-Entered Studies of

Modern Social Structure. Academia Sinica, Taipei, Taiwan, 1999.

36. Toscani F. Classification and staging of terminal cancer patients: Rationale and objectives of a multicentre cohort prospective study and methods used. Support Care Cancer 1996;4:56–60.

37. Toscani F, Cantoni L, Di Mola G, Mori M, Santosuosso A, Tamburini M. Death and dying: perceptions and attitudes in Italy. Palliative Medicine 1991;5:334–343.

38. Dunlop RJ, Davies R, Hockley JM. Preferred versus actual place of death: a hospital palliative care support team experience. Palliative Medicine 1989;3:197–201.

39. Townsend J, Frank AO, Fermont D, Dyer S, Karran O, Walgrove A, Piper M. Terminal cancer care and patients' preference for place of death: a prospective study. British Medical Journal 1990; 301:415–417.

40. McWhinney IR, Bass MJ, Orr V. Factors associated with location of death (home or hospital) of patients referred to a palliative care team. Canadian Medical Association Journal 1995; 152(3):361–367.

41. South Australian Parliamentary Select Committee on the Law and Practice relating to death and dying. Interim Report of the Select Committee of the House of Assembly on the Law and Practice Relating to Death and Dying.

42. Gilbar O, Steiner M. When death comes: Where should patients die? Hospice Journal 1996; 11(1):31–48.

43. Kai I, Ohi G, Yano E, Kobayashi Y, Miyama T, Niino N, Naka KI. Communication between patients and physicians about terminal care: a survey in Japan. Social Science and Medicine 1993;36:1151–1159.

44. Tang ST. Preferred and perceived actual site of death for Chinese cancer patients in Taiwan. [Thesis]. North Carolina: Duke University, 1990.

45. Tang ST. Comparison of quality of care for home and hospital terminal cancer patients. Journal of Pain Symptom Management 1998; 15(Suppl 4):S32.

46. Gau SC, Ferng TM. Chinese custom, folklore, and belief. Taipei: Chung Wen, 1981: 223–288 (In Chinese.)

47. Parish WL. Village and Family in contemporary China. Chicago: University of Chicago Press, 1978:248–399.

48. Thompson LG. Chinese Religion: An Introduction, 3rd ed. Belmont: Wadsworth, 1979: 34–56.

49. Wu YT. Chinese Folklore. Taipei: Chung Wen, 1987:145–162. (In Chinese.)

50. Addison JT. Chinese Ancestor Worship. Taiwan: Chung Hen Sheng Kung Hui, 1925.

51. Baker HR. Chinese Family and Kinship. New York: Columbia University Press, 1979:26–106.

52. Chao P. Chinese Kinship. London: Kegan Paul International, 1983.

53. Eisenbrach M. Cross-cultural variations in the development of bereavement practices. Cultural, Medicine, and Psychiatry 1984;8:315–347.

54. Hsu FLK. Americans and Chinese: Passage to Differences, 3rd ed. Honolulu: The University Press of Hawaii, 1900:238–269.

55. Jochim C. Chinese Religions: A Cultural Perspective. Englewood Cliffs: New Jersey: Prentice-Hall, 1986:157–181.

56. Department of Health. Statistics of Public Health in Republic of China. Part II—Vital statistics. Taipei: Department of Health, The Executive Yuan, Republic of China, Taipei, 1995.

57. Mor V, Hiris J. Determinants of site of death among hospice cancer patients. Journal of Health and Social Behavior 1983;24(4):375–384.

58. Yao CA, Chiu TY, Hu WY, Chong RB, Cheng SY, Lee LT, et al. A study of initial assessment of palliative care: The viewpoints of caregivers. Chinese Journal of Family Medicine 1998; 7:174–181. (In Chinese.)

59. Doyle D. Domiciliary palliative care. In: Doyle D, Hanks GWC, MacDonald N, eds., Oxford Textbook of Palliative Medicine, 2nd ed. Oxford: Oxford University Press, 1998:957–976.

60. Vinciguerra V, Degnan TJ, Sciortino A, O'Connell M, Moore T, Brody R, Budman Eng M, Carlton D. A comparative assessment of home versus hospital comprehensive treatment for advanced cancer patients. Journal of Clinical Oncology 1986;4 (October):1521–1528.

61. Stjernswärd J, Pampallona S. Palliative medicine—a global perspective. In: Doyle D, Hanks GWC, MacDonald N, eds., Oxford Textbook of Palliative Medicine, 2nd ed. Oxford: Oxford University Press, 1998:1227–1245.

62. Aranda S. Global perspectives on palliative care. Cancer Nursing 1999;22(1):33–39.

63. Wilson M, Kastenbaum R. Worldwide developments in hospice care: Survey results. In: Saunders C, Kastenbaum R, eds., Hospice Care on the International Scene. New York: Springer, 1997:21–38.

64. MacDonald CM. Palliative care—an essential component of cancer control. Canadian Medical Association Journal 1998;158(13):1709–1716.

65. Benoliel JQ. Nursing research on death, dying and terminal illness: development, present state and prospects. Annual Review of Nursing Research 1983;1:101–130.

66. Duo IT. The knowledge, attitude and its related factors toward caring dying patients by nurses in central Taiwan. Journal of Veteran Nursing 1997;14(1):1–10. (In Chinese.)

67. Jodrell N. Nurse education. In: Doyle D, Hanks GWC, MacDonald N, eds., Oxford Textbook of Palliative Medicine, 2nd ed. Oxford: Oxford University Press, 1998:1201–1208.

57 Australia and New Zealand

SANCHIA ARANDA

Palliative care nursing in Australia and New Zealand shares many features of the specialization as practiced elsewhere in the world. Nurses working in the area believe that care of the dying and their families epitomizes the essence of nursing, with an emphasis on excellence in what is commonly understood as "good nursing care." This supports Bradshaw's[1] argument that palliative care captures the "quintessential" spirit of nursing.

As the field has developed increased specialist status, one challenge facing nurses in palliative care is the articulation of how their work differs from nursing practice in other areas. If palliative nursing is fundamentally about the essence of nursing, is the concept of specialization a tautology? Palliative care is also increasingly being integrated into mainstream health care, accompanied by significant changes in service delivery and major imperatives to improve population access to services. The role of specialist palliative care nurses in providing direct "hands on" care to the dying is perceived to be under threat in Australia and New Zealand as a result of government imperatives that emphasize the role of all health practitioners in providing appropriately for the needs of people dying in their care.

At the same time, palliative nursing is also subject to changes in nursing more broadly, particularly development of advanced and expanded practice roles. Advanced practice roles challenge existing power structures in health care. Many of the changes to the role of specialist nurses in palliative care taking place as a result of mainstreaming can be understood as moves toward advanced practice—for example, less direct care provision and increased consultancy to generalist nurses. However, few nurses in the field of palliative care are adequately prepared for the requirements of advanced practice.

This chapter seeks to explore contemporary issues facing nurses in the delivery of palliative care in Australia and New Zealand. Given the limited number of publications available to support the perspectives of Australian and New Zealand palliative care nurses, this chapter was developed following consultation with palliative nurses in both countries. The consultation aimed to support the author's broad knowledge of Australian palliative care and limited knowledge of the New Zealand perspective despite being a New Zealander by birth. The head nurses of all palliative care services in New Zealand ($n = 39$) were consulted about the following six questions related to palliative care nursing in that country. In addition, a small group of Australian palliative care nurses were also consulted. The six questions asked were:

1. To what extent is palliative care included in undergraduate curricula in your country?
2. What opportunities exist for education of specialist palliative care nurses in your setting/country?
3. What is the scope of practice of nurses working in palliative care in your context? What roles exist? What care do nurses deliver? What constraints are there on practice?
4. What are the current issues facing nurses in the delivery of palliative care in your setting?
5. What impact are the changing directions in nursing likely to have on palliative nursing in the near future?
6. What are the future directions in palliative care that will have an impact on nursing in palliative care?

Acknowledgment of participating nurses is included at the end of the chapter. The perspectives on palliative nursing gained from them have been invaluable in development of the chapter. The chapter begins with an overview of the Australian and New Zealand care context and current status of palliative care within each country, including an exploration of issues in the delivery of palliative care for indigenous and migrant populations. Palliative nursing is then considered in terms of its scope of practice and factors influencing the education and preparation of nurses for palliative care. Important issues identified by survey respondents were similar for both countries and relate to mainstreaming of palliative care and advanced practice developments in nursing. Each of these factors has the potential to result in significant change to the scope and practice of palliative nursing.

SOME ESSENTIAL DIFFERENCES BETWEEN AUSTRALIA AND NEW ZEALAND

Australia and New Zealand are often considered together—consistently labeled as "down under" and far away in world consciousness. Despite being close geographically and sharing a predominantly British heritage, these countries have significantly different personalities that are important to understand before exploring palliative care developments within them.

New Zealand is a small country consisting of two large islands and one smaller, sparsely populated island. The total population is 3.6 million, according to the 1996 census.[2] The population is unevenly spread between the two main islands, with almost 75% living in the North Island. European/Pakeha (white) make up almost 80% of the population; 14.5% are Maori and 5.6% are Pacific Islanders. Industry is predominantly agricultural, located in a mix of rural and urban areas. Specialist health services are likely to be confined to large cities in each of the two main islands, but most general health services are available locally. However, New Zealand's population density, 12.6 people per km^2 compared to 234.5 per km^2 in Britain, has some effect on access to health services.[3]

In contrast, Australia is a large island continent of five states and two territories plus Tasmania, a small, island state to the south of the main island. The population is 18.5 million, of which only 2.1% are indigenous or Australian Aboriginal people. Australia has undergone significantly more migration than New Zealand, with 23% of the population born overseas. Overseas-born Australians are predominantly from the United Kingdom and Ireland (28.6%), although this percentage is falling. Significant migration occurs from New Zealand to Australia, with 7.4% of the population born there. This means that more than 1 million Australians were born in New Zealand, or just over 1 quarter of the total New Zealand population. Italy (6%), Greece (3%), and Germany (3%) contribute the three next-largest groups of Australians. Twenty-two percent of overseas-born Australians come from Asian countries and make up 5% of the total population.[4]

Australia ranges from dense urban cities such as Sydney, with approximately 4 million people, through rural communities surrounding large towns, to isolated remote areas where the nearest neighbor may be a day's drive away. Despite the Aboriginal population constituting only 2.1% of the population, they make up 30% of the population of central Australia, and in some communities they are the main clients of health services.[5]

It is clear, then, that Australia and New Zealand have similarities and differences. Both countries feature a predominance of people from Anglo-Celtic origins and were populated by these settlers at a similar time, although under different circumstances—Australia was established as a penal colony and New Zealand with free settlers. Both were colonialist settlements featuring disinfranchishement of the existing population—in Australia the native Aboriginal people, and in New Zealand the Maori. Since that time, New Zealand has remained largely bicultural despite limited migration from other parts of the world, while Australia is considered a multicultural society. Despite many languages being spoken in Australia, English is the only official language. In contrast, both English and Maori are recognized national languages in New Zealand, and significant effort has been made to maintain Maori cultural identity and influence at a national level. Resurgence in Maori nationalism over recent years has been more effective in influencing national policy than has similar Aboriginal nationalism in Australia.

AUSTRALIAN AND NEW ZEALAND MODELS OF HEALTH AND PALLIATIVE CARE

Both countries have a long history of universal health insurance or "welfare state" systems that provide a basic level of care to all people. This universal health care approach is supported by a limited system of private health care, perhaps more developed in the Australian context. There is a consistent valuing of universal access to adequate health care within the two populations despite increasing trends toward user payment for some services. User payments are more common in New Zealand, where services such as visits to the local doctor are user pay, while they remain predominantly government-funded in Australia.

The countries have a similar trend toward privatisation of public facilities that affects health care services to a limited but growing extent, perhaps most noticeably in the aged care sector. Privatization of nursing home facilities has resulted in an increased need to profit from care of the elderly, with considerable potential impact on access to palliative care services in the shift toward user payments. Health care is of a high standard, with access to a range of generalist and specialist services at a level consistent with that of the United States and Europe. In rural communities most generalist services are available, but specialist services such as radiotherapy are likely to require travel to a large city. In remote areas of Australia, access to health care may be limited to a regular monthly clinic by the Royal Flying Doctor Service and limited access to outreach telephone services.

Cultural Issues

A key feature of New Zealand health care is responsiveness to Maori nationalism, which calls for greater control over their own health and services compatible to cultural beliefs. Cultural safety is a feature of Maori demands for appropriate health service development, and is a concept that moves beyond cultural sensitivity featuring both acknowledgment and respect for difference, toward implementation of strategies to promote and nurture the cultural identity of the person who is ill.[6,7] Some New Zealand hospices embrace these concepts and have established relationships with local Maori communities (personal visit, North Haven Hospice, 1998).

In contrast, the Australian Aboriginal people remain a marginalized group with a health status significantly below that of other Australians. A long history of neglect and suffering as a result of ethnocentric government policy has left a legacy of difficulties for this ancient race. The provision of sensitive care to dying Aboriginal people is beginning to feature in national consciousness, and some research in this area is emerging.[6,7] However, outside of Central Australia and Northern Australia and some areas of Western Australia, South Australia, and Queensland, it is rare for palliative care services to encounter Aboriginal clients. Current models of palliative care delivery with an emphasis on terminal illness are unsuitable for Aboriginal Australians whose concept of life-death-life is at odds with Western notions of death.[6,8]

Palliative nursing literature is beginning to feature the needs of Aboriginal Australians,[9] and attempts to develop culturally safe models of service delivery are beginning with projects such as the "Many Ways of Caring" art project in Central Australia.[5] The use of Aboriginal art depicting looking after people who were 'finishing up' in this project became an important medium for communication about palliative care to local Aboriginal communities. Importantly, the paintings identified that these Aboriginal depictions of "finishing up" feature similarities with Western concepts such as providing care in the place of choice and the role of family in providing care. However, unlike the individualism dominant in Western health care, these Aboriginal depictions feature the primacy of family decision making, a mix of Aboriginal and Western health care practices, and the need for a cross-cultural health care team. These are important issues if services are to deliver appropriate care to indigenous Australians. The large number of migrant Australians also places different demands on palliative care services. The provision of palliative care for these groups is beginning to be featured in national research and service delivery efforts,[10,11,12,13,14] with nurses often leading the call for improved service provision to people of non-English-speaking backgrounds.[15] Importantly, Kanitsaki's research has challenged a dominant palliative nursing belief in open discussion about death and dying. Participants in her studies of Italian, Chinese, and Greek Australians often perceived nurses "who attempted to discuss with them death and dying and were negative, insensitive and transmitted to them a sense of hopelessness" (p. 39). In addition, nurses who were accepting of death and told them they were dying were interpreted as giving up on them, producing fears that they would stop caring.

Two Australian states have recently launched palliative care information brochures in five non-English languages, with 20 more languages to follow,[16] but attempts to improve information access are just a beginning. Systematic attention to cultural safety should move beyond access to interpreters, multilingual information, and liaison with ethnic community organizations and religious groups,[6] a point that appeared to be missed in the recommendations of the one major Australian study in this area.[14]

Structure and Delivery of Palliative Care

Hospice and palliative care developments in Australia and New Zealand are well advanced, with services required to meet established standards of service delivery and care[17,18] and increasing emphasis on education and nursing standards.[19,20] Models of palliative care delivery in these countries feature inpatient, home care, and hospital support teams, with New Zealand evidencing more use of palliative day care than Australia. Urban cities tend to feature all service elements, with home care provision showing the most variation. In rural areas, small specialist services are offered in some larger centers providing support and consultancy services to generalist nurses and local doctors. Palliative care developments in both countries are notable for their lack of homogeneity, with models of care dependent on historical factors, financial support, population density, and the makeup of the local community.

The first hospice service in New Zealand opened in 1979,[3] and by 1997 the Hospice New Zealand directory listed 40 services. Thirty-two of these services responded to a recent study aimed at determining benchmarks for staffing ratios and skill mix.[21] Of the 32 responding hospices, 18 were eligible for full analysis. The distribution of service type of these 18 services was as follows:

- 6 provided inpatient and direct care in the community;
- 4 provided inpatient beds and community consultancy services;
- 2 provided inpatient beds;
- 5 provided community direct care; and
- 1 provided community consultancy services.

Nurses were predominantly registered nurses with a ratio of 5 RNs to 1 enrolled nurse and 15 enrolled nurses to 1 nursing assistant or personal care attendant. (In the Australian and New Zealand context an enrolled nurse undergoes 1–2 years of training and provides most direct patient care provided by a registered nurse, usually excluding care associated with medications.) All services provided 24-hour nursing, and inpatient units provided a mean of 7.75 hours of nursing care per patient per day. Thirty percent of the registered nurses in these services were undertaking or had completed postgraduate training in palliative care.[21]

By contrast, Australian palliative care developments since the advent of the modern hospice movement have mainly occurred in the community. The first Australian hospices predate the opening of St. Christopher's in London (1969) by 79 years—the establishment by the Sisters of Charity of Hospices in Sydney (1890) and Melbourne (1938). Redpath[22] argues that modern hospice developments were largely separate from these institutions, which were perceived to be out of step with modern developments. Therefore, Australian palliative care is predominantly made up of a vast network of small community hospice services, a few small hospices in the St. Christopher's style, and several large Catholic hospices. However, significant change is taking place in service delivery, with increased emphasis in both state and federal government health policy to improve access to palliative care by equitable service distribution across the community. Beds in large city hospices are being redistributed across the community. For example, Caritas Christi Hospice (CCH) in Melbourne has begun to be changed from a single 70+ bed facility to a multi-part institution split across two, and in the future three, sites of care. The model envisioned by the Victorian state government is 15 bed units linked to public hospitals and, where possible, located with them. Twenty-six of the CCH beds are now located at St. Vincent's Hospital Melbourne, a large teaching hospital linked to Melbourne University. The hospice beds are located on one floor of the hospital and are colocated with a palliative home care service, an acute pain service, and the nursing branch of an academic research and teaching program linked to Melbourne University. In the first year of operation these changes have allowed for improved relationships with acute care services (particularly oncology), the development of collaborative research projects, a planned nursing education program, and a range of joint appointments for nurses to work across inpatient and community settings. A key emphasis in both countries is to support the patient's decision to die at home whenever possible. Australian state government policy directions clearly support the care of people in their own homes.[23,24] While the majority of people die in hospital,[25,26] most people are cared for at home until a short period before death. This is supported by falling average length of inpatient hospice stay (now 18 days at CCH, falling from 25 days in 2 years).

Funding

Initial distribution of government funding for palliative care was uneven for Australia and New Zealand, with recent increases seeking to provide funding in areas previously under-resourced.[26,27,28] In 1997–98 New Zealand spent 12.4 million on palliative care;[27] however, individual services received Government support ranging from 20% to 100%, while three services were totally charity funded.[3] New Zealand's 40 hospice and palliative care services are supported by active volunteer fund-raising and contributions to service delivery. Seventeen of the hospices surveyed by Macready[21] received a combined total of 84,600 hours of volunteer service per year, frequently filling roles, such as provision of meals, that in Australia would be undertaken by paid employees.

However, maintaining public interest in financial support of hospices is difficult in an environment of competition for charity dollars.[29] Indeed New Zealand services are asking questions about "how far you can sell death" in a competitive environment of 30,000 other organizations seeking the same charitable dollar.[30] In contrast, palliative care services in Australia receive most of their funding through government sources and lead the world in this area.[31] Government policy recognizes the role of palliative care in improving care of the dying, and this support is apparent in the major expansion of palliative care funding and service development that has taken place over the past 20 years. Government policy at state and federal levels places palliative care as a vital part of mainstream health care services—an issue considered by many to be of both advantage and danger to palliative care. Services see attraction of charity funding as important, as it provides them with some independence from government. This independence allows delivery of services that go beyond the other minimalist support possible under total government funding.

Palliative care services in Australia and New Zealand are accessed in the main by people with cancer. In New Zealand, most services are also available to people with HIV/AIDs, while in Australia this group is more likely to access specialist HIV/AIDS palliative care units and community services, particularly in large cities. People with other terminal illness, such as motor neurone disease and respiratory failure, can access services, but a major difficulty surrounds determination of prognosis in this group. Increasingly, access to palliative care is being defined on the basis of need rather than diagnosis or prognosis, which increases the potential for access by people with illnesses other than cancer. Only one children's hospice was identified, the "Very Special Kids House" in Melbourne. This hospice cares for children with terminal and debilitating illnesses such as muscular dystrophy and has a significant role in the provision of family respite in long-term-care situations.

Rural and Remote Communities

Nurses working in rural areas believe there is significant work to be done to assist them to provide for the palliative needs of the community.[32] Rural and remote communities are not homogeneous; they offer various challenges to health delivery based on demographics, local culture, physical environment, and distance from health services. Rural nurses providing palliative care as one aspect of a broader health role in the community suffer significant professional isolation. In some settings, particularly in remote areas, the nurse may be the sole health practitioner in a community, receiving telephone support from a doctor located some distance away. The challenge is to find sustainable models of palliative care provision in many of these communities.

The provision of palliative care to people in rural areas is a major component of government attempts to improve access to palliative care. In many rural communities, a specialist palliative nurse consultant has been employed to work with a local team of interested people to provide palliative care support to local health services. Many rural local doctors have taken up the challenge to improve their palliative care skills and work in partnership with the nurse. There is now evidence that these approaches are working.

Sach[33] undertook a major study to explore the provision of rural palliative care in Australia. This study found the role of palliative nurse consultants to be vital in the provision of quality palliative care in rural areas. The rural palliative care nurse was identified as maintaining a contemporary knowledge of treatments and drugs that was vital for their support of local doctors. The consultative nursing role was appreciated as being in the background supporting the family and community nurses to provide care. Despite the fact that rural palliative care services were likely to visit less often than city services, there was a greater use of telephone support, use of community members, and innovative use of nursing support through access to specific funds available for rural health. Overall, the study found rural communities to not be disadvantaged in the quality of palliative care provided. Major issues surrounded nursing travel time and the need to improve access to training through linkage programs with city specialist services and technological advances.

SCOPE OF NURSING PRACTICE IN PALLIATIVE CARE

In both New Zealand and Australia, nurses are key to providing specialist palliative care services. The role of the nursing profession is considered essential in the continuance of hospice values and philosophy at a time of increasing medicalization[34] and funding limitations that challenge the ability of many services to employ the full range of disciplines necessary for multidisciplinary palliative care. Nonmedical and nursing staff are often part-time and depend on expert nursing assessment and referral for their services to be mobilized for those clients with specific need for pastoral care, physical therapy, and psychological support. Yet relationships between nursing and other disciplines in palliative care are often difficult, with major issues over role delineation and perceptions that nurses gatekeep access to the client and family[35]. Specialist palliative nursing is delivered across hospital, hospice, and community settings. Nurses employed as palliative specialists are engaged in a range of roles, including provision of direct care, consultant support to nonpalliative care services (including nursing homes), education, and management—all varying according to the setting of care and care delivery model.

Two models of community palliative nursing exist in both countries. The first model links specialist community teams providing consultant support and education to generalist nursing services who provide most of the direct care to clients and families. In this model the specialist nurse provides minimal direct care. In the second model specialist nurses are employed by community palliative care teams and provide direct care to a caseload of patients in addition to providing consultant support to other services.

Where direct care is a component of the specialist nursing role, this is mainly confined to a maximum of one or two short visits a day, making the need for a family carer important to the success of palliative home care, particularly in the last few weeks of life. In some New Zealand settings, nurses are also involved in providing full shifts of home nursing where significant care relief or respite is required. Funding restrictions limit this element of the service to a maximum of eight shifts of care for the period of illness. Volunteers can be used in a similar capacity where nursing care is not required. In Australia such care relief services would be available only to those families able to purchase them. However, new models of funding may give more flexibility in this area. For example, the Victorian government recently established a new category of funding, titled the "unassigned bed fund." This gives community hospice services access to a pool of money equivalent to an inpatient bed that can be used at home to support clients who would otherwise require inpatient care. For example, the funding could be used to provide an overnight nurse when the person was close to death and in need of significant intervention to manage problematic symptoms.

Recent changes in palliative care delivery, aimed at improving access to palliative care, have required specialist services to work more closely with generalist community nurses, and as a result the direct care role of specialist nurses is likely to decrease. It is likely that over the next decade of palliative care developments in Australia and New Zealand, as mainstreaming of palliative care increases, the model of specialist nurses providing direct care in the community will be replaced by one of nurses in a predominantly consultant role to generalist services.

Inpatient palliative nursing roles in both countries are similar. While registered nurses are predominant in community settings with some use of care attendants, inpatient facilities are more likely to utilize the services of enrolled nurses and care attendants. Enrolled nurses are similar in both countries, undertaking approximately 12–18 months of training and able to perform most nursing activities with the exception of medications and intravenous management. In some settings additional training is offered to enrolled nurses to allow delivery of some medications under the supervision of a registered nurse. Care attendants or nursing assistants predominantly work in supporting patients in activities of daily living under the instruction of a registered nurse. These personnel do not have formal health care qualifications but undertake either in-service or short-course preparation for their roles.

In both countries and in all care settings, registered nurses working in palliative care assume key roles in the following areas:

- patient and family assessment;
- provision of direct care such as hygiene, wound dressings, and other treatments;
- management of distressing symptoms, including adjustment of complex drug regimens and use of drug delivery technology;
- liaison with related services, particularly local doctors;
- referral and coordination of multidisciplinary team input, including volunteers;
- provision of patient, family, professional, and community education; and
- provision of bereavement support, although this is increasingly an area of role friction in the multidisciplinary team.

Patients requiring inpatient care tend to be elderly, frail, and dependent, or suffer from complex symptoms. Inpatient beds are also used for family respite at times, a necessary service given the elderly carers of patients, many of whom have their own health issues. These patient characteristics mean that inpatient palliative nursing is heavy and physical care demands are high. A recent study of admissions and discharges from CCH shows that a significant proportion of the clients admitted to the hospice subsequently require transfer to an aged care facility.[36] This may be because the clients have received inadequate symptom management prior to admission, and after attention to these issues and good nursing interventions they improve and are no longer considered close to death. The significant overlap between these people and clients of aged care facilities demand the formation of closer relationships between them. One survey found that up to 10% of nursing home residents may require palliative care at any one time.[37] The directors of nursing at these facilities see palliative care as part of their normal work but identify barriers such as resources and inadequate education and training in palliative nursing as limiting what they can achieve. This overlap between aged care and palliative care makes visible the essential tension between generalist and specialist models of palliative nursing.[38]

Generalist and Specialist Models of Nursing Delivery in Palliative Care

As stated in the introduction to this chapter, palliative nursing can be considered to capture the essence of nursing.[1] It is, in fact, difficult to argue how specialist palliative nursing differs from nursing in general. Alistair Campbell[39] argued that "an ethic for hospice means a commitment to become redundant, to be replaced by a better and more universally available social system for caring for the dying." Such an ethic would see the philosophy of palliative care enshrined in the practice of all health professionals, in this case nurses, and in theory make specialist palliative nursing unnecessary.

Payne[3] identified three service models in New Zealand on the basis of whether they supplanted, supplemented, or supported existing health services. Services that supplant other services add another layer of care to those already existing, with the danger of service overlap. Supplemental services are likely to be offered as a means of filling gaps in care, the main emphasis for the establishment of the hospice movement. Supporting services work alongside existing health care organizations to support their care of people requiring palliative care. Given that people requiring palliative care and those who are dying can be found in all settings of health care delivery, it seems obvious that the supportive model of palliative nursing is most sustainable. Moves toward mainstreaming in both Australia and New Zealand[26,27] indicate the replacement of direct care provision by specialist palliative care nurses and increased provision of consultative support in the delivery of palliative care by generalist nurses. At least one difficulty lies in the fact that status in nursing is frequently identified by demarcation of care roles and is in tension with imperatives to transfer palliative nursing knowledge and skills to all nurses.[38] Further difficulties lie in the current absence of palliative care content outside of specialist education programs and the limited preparation of specialist nurses for consultative roles.

Palliative Care in the Undergraduate Nursing Curriculum

Despite the belief that palliative nursing embodies the "quintessential" spirit of nursing, there is little evidence to suggest that this is reflected in undergraduate nursing curricula. In both Australia and New Zealand, nursing education occurs in the higher-education sector, although in New Zealand the qualification has until recently been a diploma, while in Australia all nurses exit their educational programs with a bachelor's degree. There has not been a formal attempt to explore the inclusion of palliative care content in undergraduate nursing programs in either country; however, there is general recognition that inclusion is patchy. Nurses consulted for this chapter confirm the lack of consistent inclusion of palliative care in undergraduate curricula across the two countries. Where respondents identified a discrete module of palliative care, this was predominantly in the form of an elective offered to a small subgroup of students. In only one Australian state, New South Wales, is there a developing process to include palliative care content in all undergraduate programs, despite research into this area having been identified as a national priority in a recent Delphi study of palliative care experts (Hanson 1999, personal communication). This initiative serves as a good model for other parts of Australia and New Zealand.

Topics such as pain management are the most commonly included palliative care content in undergraduate programs, but survey respondents believe more content is required. Hospice and palliative care staff in surveyed agencies were commonly involved in the provision of education to undergraduate students, at their personal initiative. Services also offered clinical placements for students undertaking palliative care elective courses. However, the small size of most agencies and the large numbers of undergraduate students necessarily limit the number who can access such placements.

Graduating nurses are unlikely to choose palliative care as an area of practice early in their career, with most preferring to work in large hospitals to gain acute care skills, yet all will come in contact with dying people sooner or later. Since transfer of nursing to the tertiary sector, it is now more likely that a newly graduating nurse has never been in contact with a dying person or more specifically cared for someone at the time of death. If this first experience comes following graduation, it is likely that few supports exist to assist the nurse to process this experience. Despite the inconsistency of palliative care content in undergraduate programs, the need for preparation in working with dying patients is not featured as an area of preparation in programs offered to newly graduated nurses. For example, in Victoria a survey of coordinators conducting graduate nursing programs failed to identify palliative care as an area of importance or content in most programs.[40] All nurses are likely to encounter dying people and their families in practice, yet their preparation for doing so appears inconsistent and under-recognized. Support of generalist nurses in the acute setting is an identified important role of palliative nurses working in hospital support teams,[41] and there was some evidence in the Hordern and Cockayne study[40] that this support was being utilized, although inconsistently. Indeed, a perceived lack of preparation in palliative care was a potential source of stress identified by community nurses in New South Wales.[42]

Opportunities for Specialist Education

In both countries access to postgraduate education generally and palliative care education specifically is often a product of geography, with more educational opportunities in large urban centers than elsewhere. There is a recognized need to research different models of education delivery in palliative care in order to find appropriate models to support education of nurses from different practice settings and geographical locations, and with varied levels of experience and education.[43] There is an increasing emphasis on the provision of specialist courses via distance education, in some cases supported by information technology such as teleconferencing and Internet delivery, in order to overcome some of these access issues.

Postgraduate education is more developed in Australia than in New Zealand. Australian nursing has a long history of certificate courses offered in the health industry to prepare nurses in a range of specialist practice areas. Since the transfer of nursing education to the higher-education sector, many of these certificate courses have also transferred to universities and redeveloped as graduate diplomas. In the Australasian context a graduate diploma consists of 50% of a two-year master's by coursework program, and many articulate to master's degrees. However, participation in such courses is quite small, with little recognition of the master's degree as an essential requirement for clinical nurse specialist status (see below). Graduate diploma courses in palliative nursing or multidisciplinary palliative care are available in at least eight Australian universities, and another two offer cancer nursing courses that include cancer-related palliative care. In addition, other universities offer palliative care elective subjects in broad nursing graduate diplomas. The need for cross-over of subject areas at the graduate level is suggested by the finding of Wilkes et al.[42] that generalist community nurses feel unprepared to deliver palliative care after completion of child and family nursing courses. In New Zealand, specialist education is predominantly offered within bachelor of nursing (postregistration) and generalist master's programs undertaken by registered nurses.[44] A pediatric palliative care course commenced in 1998 at the Auckland Institute of Technology, the first of its kind in Australasia.

Specialist palliative nursing education is also offered through professional bodies such as the Royal College of Nursing and Hospice New Zealand. The Royal College of Nursing Australia provides an introductory palliative nursing course via distance education. This course is significant in its ability to bring palliative care education to generalist nurses working in all parts of Australia, including remote regions, and the course is recognized for credit by some universities. Four palliative care modules are offered via a number of hospices linked to Hospice New Zealand. As yet these are not recognized for credit points within university-based courses, although there are moves toward accreditation. Service providers, such as the Royal District Nursing Service (RDNS) in Victoria, also offer formal courses of study in palliative nursing that may be accredited at the graduate diploma level. Indeed, RDNS Victoria could be considered to set a benchmark for education at the entry to practice level in palliative nursing. All nurses identified as palliative care nurses complete the in-house course as a minimum requirement.

Issues related to the identification of nurses who are specialists in palliative care link to current changing directions in nursing more broadly. Despite identification of fairly consistent areas of practice focus for palliative nurses across all settings of care, the skill and education of nurses self-defining as specialists in palliative care varies widely. The increasing emphasis on a consultative role for palliative nurses, particularly those working in the community and in hospital support teams, means that these nurses are likely to be affected by moves toward advanced practice role recognition and credentialing.

CHANGING DIRECTIONS IN NURSING

The most important changing direction in nursing for both Australian and New Zealand palliative nurses is the development of advanced practice roles. The nurses consulted for this chapter consistently identified issues to do with the movement toward specialist recognition, credentialing, role change in terms of both erosion and expansion, the development of advanced practice, and nurse prescribing. These issues are all linked in some way to the development of advanced practice nurses.

New Zealand developments in this area are well established in midwifery and are extending to other areas of practice. The report of the Ministerial Taskforce on Nursing[45] identified a key role for advanced practice nurses in the context of the breakdown of the welfare state. The report recommended the recognition of nurse practitioner and clinical nurse specialist roles as central to improvements in client services. The report supported recent moves toward nurse prescribing and saw this as logically linked to rights for nurses to order diagnostic tests and make referrals to specialists. A call to no longer exclude nurses from reimbursement and to recognize nursing autonomy and accountability within their present and expanding scope of practice were major steps forward for nurses in this part of the world. However, the task force correctly identified the absence of enforceable competencies in the area of advanced practice as an immediate barrier to the profession's ability to make a greater contribution to health care.

In Australia, considerable debate has taken place with discussion documents produced by key nursing organisations.[46,47] New South Wales undertook demonstration of advanced practice nurse projects,[48] with one of the outcomes in that state being a move toward nurse prescribing. Similar projects are taking place in Victoria in 1999, with one of the ten projects occurring in palliative care and in South Australia. The South Australian project evaluated the role of palliative nurse practitioners in aged care.[49] While this project found that the nurse practitioner contributed to pain and symptom management and provided more than 200 hours of education for staff, significant barriers existed to role development, including the low level of funding to aged care facilities. Despite this, during the 6 months of the project it was estimated that the nurse practitioner enabled 17 residents to die in their aged care facility who would otherwise have been transferred to an acute hospital.

The debate is at a critical point. Australian and New Zealand nursing draws on nursing developments in both the North American and British settings, creating an interesting cultural mix. Any exploration of nursing in these countries demonstrates evidence of these influences but an ultimate creation of local approaches to the issues. While Australia and New Zealand followed the lead of the United States in the transfer of nursing education away from hospital schools of nursing and into the higher-education sector, advanced practice developments vary in terms of academic preparation. Similar to the debate in the United Kingdom,[50] there has been a less strong endorsement of a master's qualification as mandatory for advanced practice roles. This key difference is evidenced by differences in the title of clinical specialist between Australia and New Zealand and other countries, particularly the United States.

The title of clinical nurse specialist is frequently used by palliative nurses in both community and inpatient settings and denotes their dedicated involvement in care of the dying rather than specific educational qualifications or demonstrated competence. Some change in this area is expected following the recent release of generalist competencies for advanced practice nurses.[51] The expectation is that these competency standards will now be applied to the development of specific competencies for specialist advanced practice, including palliative care. However, neither Australia nor New Zealand has a process or established body for the credentialing of nurses who meet advanced practice requirements. The New Zealand Taskforce[45] identified credentialing as a role for the New Zealand Nursing Council. In Australia, the debate about the merits of credentialing continues, with calls by the RCNA to undertake this role despite its limited membership and influence.

SOME THOUGHTS ABOUT THE FUTURE

Palliative nursing in Australia and New Zealand is undergoing significant change. This is particularly related to a need to move away from what have been identified as ideological perceptions of hospice care,[52] to consideration of contemporary and sustainable models of palliative care delivery as part of the mainstream of health care. Palliative nurses, like nurses everywhere, are being asked to demonstrate their contribution to the health and outcomes of palliative clients. There has been limited research in this area owing to considerable belief that the provision of palliative care is inherently of benefit. Recent projects being undertaken by me in Victoria and colleagues in Western Australia[53] attempt to provide nurses with a framework for documenting the outcomes of their interventions around a range of symptoms. However, the relative ease of measuring outcomes in areas such as pain means that there is a danger that other aspects of the nurse's work in palliative care go unexplored. Australian and New Zealand nurses are also attempting to articulate the more aesthetic aspects of the nurse's role in palliative care. A consistent area of importance identified in the delivery of palliative nursing is the nurse–patient relationship.[54,55] This work attempts to move beyond the glowing testimonials of clients and families about nursing work and suggestions that palliative nursing is just good nursing care, toward a more rigorous investigation of the nursing practices involved in establishing therapeutic relationships with clients.[56] This beginning research to articulate the knowledge, skills, and practices involved in palliative nursing offers a significant contribution to global efforts in this area.

The author would like to thank Linda Devilee for secretarial assistance in preparing this manuscript and Donna Milne for editorial comment. In addition, this chapter would not have been possible without the input of the following people:

New Zealand

Ester Sweet, Te Omanga Hospice, Lower Hutt; Sue Wood, Coast Health Care, Greymouth; Suzanne Brocx, Hospice Bay of Island, Kerikeri; Roberta Vaughan, South Canterbury Hospice, Timaru; Yvonne Boyes, Whakatane Hospital; Faye Gillon, Community Hospice, Whakatane; Yvonne Bray, Hospices of Auckland; June Connor, Arohanui Hospice Service Trust, Palmerston Nth; Jan Nichols, St. Joseph's Hospice, Auckland; W Alward, Hospice Wanganui; Helen Blaxland, Walter Naserek & Jo Loney, North Haven Hospice, Tikipunga; Sharon Dickel, Otago Community Hospice, Dunedin.

Australia

Peter Hudson, Formerly of Bethleham Community Palliative Care Service, PhD student, Victoria; Caroline Short, Cessnock Community Health, Palliative Care Team, New South Wales; Di Krutli, Royal District Nursing Service, South Australia; Catherine Duck, Melbourne Citymission Palliative Care, Victoria; Denyse Haseman, Mt. Olivet Community Service, Queensland; Jacqui Burch, Blue Nursing Service, Brisbane, Queensland; Tara Worby-Beck, Territory Palliative Care, Northern Territory.

REFERENCES

1. Bradshaw A. The spiritual dimension of hospice: the secularisation of an ideal. Social Science and Medicine 1996;43:409–420.

2. New Zealand Population Census. 1996. Online: www.stats.gov.nz/statsweb.nsf

3. Payne S. To supplant, supplement or support? Organisational issues for hospices. Social Science and Medicine 1998;46:1495–1504.

4. National Multicultural Advisory Committee. Australian Multiculturalism for a New Century, Commonwealth of Australia, 1999. Online: www.immi.gov.au.

5. Fried O. Many ways of caring: reaching out to Aboriginal palliative care clients in Central Australia. Progress in Palliative Care 1999;7:116–119.

6. Prior D. Palliative care in marginalised communities. Progress in Palliative Care 1999a;7: 109–115.

7. Ramsden I. After Kia ora—what next? Paper presented at the Hospice New Zealand Conference, Wellington, June 24–26, 1998.

8. Prior D. Life-Death-Life: Aboriginal Culture and Palliative Care. Unpublished Thesis for Master of Science. Flinders University, South Australia, 1997.

9. Prior D. (1999b). Culturally appropriate palliative care for indigenous Australian people. In: Aanda S, O'Connor M, eds, Palliative Care Nursing: A Guide to Practice. Melbourne: Ausmed Publications, 1999b:103–116.

10. Roddy Y. Cultural Sensitivity in Palliative Care. Paper presented at the National Hospice and Palliative Care Conference, Melbourne, October 27–29, 1993.

11. Sforcina J. (1993). Education in diverse cultural attitudes—stereotyping or increasing cultural sensitivity. Paper presented at the National Hospice and Palliative Care Conference, Melbourne, October 27–29, 1993.

12. Cotterill D. The hospice in a multicultural society. Paper presented at the National Hospice and Palliative Care Conference, Melbourne, October 27–29, 1993.

13. Balmain V. Attitudes to death: differences between Anglo-Australian and Darwin Chinese people. Paper presented at the National Hospice and Palliative Care Conference, Melbourne, October 27–29, 1993.

14. Campbell S, Small G, Moore G. Improving palliative care in a multicultural environment. Hope Healthcare Limited and Northern Sydney Area Health Service, Sydney, 1997.

15. Kanitsaki O. Palliative care and cultural diversity. In: Parker J, Aranda S, eds. Palliative Care: Explorations and Challenges pp. Sydney: MacLennan and Petty, 1998;32–45.

16. Palliative Care Victoria. Relief, Comfort Support. Palliative Care Information Brochures. Author, Melbourne, 1999.

17. Hospice New Zealand. Standards for the Provision of Hospice/Palliative Care. Author, Wellington, 1994.

18. Palliative Care Australia. Standards for palliative care provisions, 2nd Edition. Author, Yarralumla, 1998.

19. Hospice New Zealand. Education Standards. Author, Wellington, 1997.

20. Hospice New Zealand. Professional Standards for Hospice/Palliative Care Nurses. Author, Wellington, 1997.

21. Macready J. Staffing Ratios and Skill Levels in New Zealand Hospice/Palliative Care Provision. Paper presented at the Hospice New Zealand Conference, Wellington, June 27–29, 1998.

22. Redpath R. (1998). Palliative care in Australia. In: Ramage J, ed. Australian Nursing Practice and Palliative Care: Its Origins, Evolution and Future Royal College of Nursing, Canberra, 1998: 1–16.

23. Queensland Health. Guidelines: Palliative Care Program. Queensland Department of Health, Brisbane, 1995.

24. Department of Human Services. Palliative Care in Victoria: The Way Forward. Victorian Government Publishers, 1996.

25. Prior D, Poulton V. Palliative care nursing in a curative environment: An Australian perspective. International Journal of Palliative Nursing 1996;2:84–90.

26. Nichols J. Is home death rate a good quality indicator for a community palliative care service? Paper presented at the Hospice New Zealand Conference, Wellington, June 24–26, 1998.

27. English W. Address by the Honorable Bill English Minister of Health. Paper presented at the Hospice New Zealand Conference, Wellington, June 24–26, 1998. Online: www.executive.govt.nz/minister/english/s980624.htm

28. Clark R. Palliative care—a right or a privilege? Kai Tiaki: Nursing New Zealand 1997–98; Dec./Jan.:13–15.

29. Joblin M. Hawke's Bay: A New Zealand Approach to Hospice Care. In: Saunders C, Kastenbaum R, eds., Hospice on the International Scene New York: Springer, 1997:117–122.

30. Brown D, Ross A. Ethics: Broadening the dimensions of care. Paper presented at the Hospice New Zealand Conference, Wellington, June 24–26, 1998.

31. Wilson M, Kastenbaum R. Worldwide Developments in Hospice Care: Survey Results. In: Saunders C, Kastenbaum R, eds. Hospice on the International Scene. New York: Springer, 1997:21–38.

32. McCarthy A, Hegney D. Rural nursing in the Australian context. In: Aranda S, O'Connor M, eds, Palliative Care Nursing: A Guide to Practice. Melbourne: Ausmed Publications, 1999:83–101.

33. Sach J. Issues for palliative care in rural Australia. Collegian 1997;4(3):22–27.

34. Rumbold B. Implications of mainstreaming hospice into palliative care services. In: Parker J, Aranda S, eds. Palliative Care: Explorations and Challenges Sydney: MacLennan and Petty, 1998:3–20.

35. Aranda S, Kelso J. The nurse as coach in care of the dying. Contemporary Nurse 1997; 6:117–122.

36. Aranda S, O'Connor M, Milne D. Inpatient Palliative Care: Admission and discharge review project report. Caritas Christi Hospice, Fitzroy, 1999.

37. DeBellis A, Parker D. Providing palliative care in Australian nursing homes: issues and challenges. Geriaction 1998;16(3):17–23.

38. Aranda SK. The role of the specialist nurse in palliative care. Palliative Care Today 1997; November (Issue 12).

39. Campbell AV. An ethic for hospice. Paper presented at the First Australian Hospice and Palliative Care Conference, Adelaide, 1990.

40. Hordern A, Cockayne M. A review of palliative care related education within graduate nurse year programs. Paper presented at the Palliative Care Australia Conference, Canberra, September 16–19, 1997.

41. White K. The role of the nurse consultant in the Acute Hospital Setting. In: Parker J, Aranda S, eds. Palliative Care: Explorations and Challenges. Sydney: MacLennan and Petty, 1998;218–228.

42. Wilkes L, Beale B, Hall E, Rees E, Watts B, Denne C. Community nurses' descriptions of stress when caring in the home. International Journal of Palliative Nursing 1998;4(1):14–20.

43. Yates P, Clinton M, Hart G. Design of a professional development programme for palliative care nurses (Part 2). International Journal of Palliative Nursing 1997;3:70–75.

44. Robertson G. Guest Editorial—Palliative Nursing in New Zealand. International Journal of Palliative Nursing 1997;3:244.

45. Ministerial Taskforce on Nursing. Report of the Ministerial Taskforce on Nursing: Releasing the potential of nursing. Ministry of Health, Wellington, 1998. Online: www.moh.govt.nz

46. Royal College of Nursing Australia. Discussion paper No. 4 1996. Credentialling Advanced Nursing Practice and Accreditation of Continuing Education Programs: An Exploration of Issues and Perspectives. Author, Australia, 1996.

47. Australian Nursing Federation. Specialisation and credentialling in nursing, Author, Melbourne, undated.

48. Nurse Practitioner Project (Stage 3). Final Report of the Steering Committee. New South Wales Department of Health, Sydney, 1996.

49. Maddocks I, Parker D, McLeod A, Jenkin P. Palliative Care Nurse Practitioners in Aged Care Facilities. Report to the Department of Human Services. International Institute of Hospice Studies, Adelaide, 1999.

50. United Kingdom Central Council (UKCC) for Nursing, Midwifery and Health Visiting. "A higher level of practice." Author, London, 1998. Online: www.ukcc.org.uk

51. Australian Nursing Federation. Competency Standards for the Advanced Nurse, Author, Melbourne, 1997.

52. Aranda S. Palliative care principles: masking the complexity of practice. In: Parker J, Aranda S, eds. Palliative Care: Explorations and Challenges Sydney: MacLennan and Petty, 1998a:21–31.

53. Kristjanson L. Development and testing of a symptom assessment tool. Paper presented at the 20th Annual Scientific Meeting, Australian Pain Society, Fremantle, April 1999.

54. Taylor B, Glass N, McFarlane J, Stirling C. Palliative nurses' perceptions of the nature and effects of their work. International Journal of Palliative Nursing, 1997;3:253–258.

55. Aranda S. A critical praxis study of nurse-patient friendship, Unpublished Ph.D. thesis. La Trobe University, Melbourne, 1998b.

56. Aranda S, Street A. Being authentic and being a chameleon: Nurse-patient interaction revisited. Nursing Inquiry 1999;6:75–82.

58 Great Britain

ANDREW KNIGHT

It is now 32 years since St. Christopher's Hospice in Sydenham, a suburb of South East London, opened its doors to patients. St. Christopher's had been long in gestation. Cicely Saunders had been thinking about, praying for, traveling, in effect what we would now call "networking," and generally organizing her hospice for the previous 20 years. The amount of organizational effort meant that it could not fail, although Saunders and her supporters were never sure it would wholly succeed. The building itself, a large concrete and glass structure, architecturally very much of its time, proclaims a bold statement that few could ignore. Here was something new, something that would not go away.

Yet Cicely Saunders and those early pioneers did not imagine that the concept of hospice—a philosophy of care that would encompass all needs of the terminal patient and their family—would lead to a movement replicated across the world in hundreds of settings and cultures, and a new form of medicine that would change forever how systems of care are delivered: palliative care.

Students of the origins of hospice are indebted to the ongoing careful work of Professor David Clark. He makes the important point "that to claim an arbitrary starting point for such a complex and far-reaching movement is unsatisfactory. Indeed it may be preferable to see the opening of St. Christopher's in 1967 as a crucial outcome of ideas and strategies . . . in which can be located the essential characteristics of the subsequent hospice movement".[1] Many of the principles of hospice care are as sound and applicable now as they were then. Furthermore, they neatly embrace the postmodern concept of holistic care and new ageism.[2]

Cicely Saunders's sense of a calling to undertake this work and the idea of a religious community operating outside the mainstream of the health service is prevalent throughout the decade prior to the opening of St. Christopher's.[3] It is now interesting to speculate what would have happened had she not decided, in a pragmatic way, to embrace the need to practically work within the world of modern medicine and social services. Would the movement have had so much influence? Certainly in the 1960s there was a greater openness to question the norm, to challenge tradition; and the public was beginning to become interested in alternative therapies such as Eastern and homeopathic medicine.[4] But would politicians, administrators, and planners of health care have been so influenced by an evangelical religious community? This is not known. However, it is clear that the originators of St. Christopher's and those that followed in its wake were religiously motivated; they carried with them a religious zeal to change the way that society and, in particular, the medical establishment cared for the dying.

Would St. Christopher's have been established if it were to be proposed now, at the end of the millennium? Many of the advisers to Cicely Saunders were religious and established figures in the church. The church in secular Great Britain has much less influence and power than it did in the 1950s and early 1960s. The concept of hospice care remains popular with the public; its ideas are easily understood and thought to be necessary. Many public figures sit on hospice boards of trustees, giving voluntarily of their time. But it is not at all clear in a world where health budgets are being cut and stretched to deal with pressing needs that another seat at the table labeled "palliative care" would be at all welcomed.

INFLUENCE ON NURSING

From the beginning, the need to publish and spread the new principles of the care of the dying were recognized. Cicely Saunders had an article on euthanasia published in Britain's most widely read nursing journal, *Nursing Times*, in October 1959. This was the first of a seminal series of six articles on care of the dying whose influence has been immeasurable. They contain advice on "should a patient know"; pain control; mental distress in the dying; and principles of and the nursing care of the dying. It is not surprising that they can still be purchased in reprint form today, as they contain many of the founding principles of palliative care.[5] Many nurses, like the author, came to know about hospice through a reading of these articles (in my case in 1977).

The Joint Board of Nursing Studies, later to be divided into national boards, formed to oversee the burgeoning number of postgraduate courses for nurses in the United Kingdom, recognized the need to formulate a course in the "Care of the Dying Patient and their Family" in 1974, the first course appropriately being run at St. Christopher's. Despite the diminishing number of colleges of nursing that run this certificated course, it remains as popular as ever, containing as it does a synthesis of the subject.[6]

The impact that this had on nursing throughout British hospital nursing care was matched only by the care being given in intensive-care units. The rise of a movement in the United Kingdom and the growth of hospice facilities was fired by inspired nurses wanting to practice this form of care and frustrated by the lack of resources in the National Health Service. It was mirrored by a growing sense of professionalism in nursing and need to formulate philosophies of care. Virginia Henderson's model[7] seemed to many to come closest to an ideal model of care and was readily taken up by the influential Royal Marsden Hospital. However, it was not until the 1980s that a full model of care, embracing palliative and cancer care, came into being, the Royal Marsden Hospital adding palliative care to it's curriculum in 1986.

The Acquired Immune Deficiency Syndrome (AIDS) pandemic in the mid-1980s took many by surprise. Wells[8] and others felt, rightly, that those who were equipped and trained to deliver palliative and cancer care were best equipped to deliver the care of this largely dying population.

However, the providers of mainstream hospice care were, with some notable exceptions, seen to be indifferent, fearing the difficulties of an unpredictable human immunodeficiency virus (HIV) trajectory and the effects on a largely voluntary income. Criticisms of homophobia were not unjustified. Two hospices specifically for the care of the HIV patient were formed: the London Lighthouse in North West London, an area that had and still has the largest group of HIV patients in the United Kingdom, and the resurrected Mildmay Mission Hospital in East London. Those who practiced the care of the HIV patient have much to learn from the palliative care nurse, while she had much to learn about from them, not least the proper practice of confidentiality and patient rights. The self-determination and questioning spirit of the HIV patient is a good foil to an apparently unquestioning elderly cancer patient. Proponents of the two systems of care coexist side by side, and while the HIV population is now relatively healthy, enjoying the effect of combination drug therapies, there is felt to be little reason to cross-reference each other's work. It remains a matter of concern that two nursing specializations continue to work in parallel but not with each other.

HEALTH CARE SYSTEMS

The National Health Service (NHS), promising free health care for all, was nineteen years young in 1967 and still considered successful. Its modes of operation were well established and took up much of the resources and time. There was largely indifference to care of the dying. Systems of nursing, based on the traditional work-based apprentice model, were designed so that each block of extensive work practice was preceded by a (hopefully) appropriate block of classroom teaching. The Committee on Senior Nursing Staff Structure,[9] known universally as the Salmon Report, refashioning nursing management and crucially introducing a tier of nursing officers that were to stay in nursing for thirty years, had yet to bite. Matrons and assistant matrons still ruled in a world where little audit of care or questioning of practice took place. The first degree program in nursing, at Manchester University, would not appear until 1969. From the outset there had been a need for the NHS to control costs, and the sense of actually running a free service was not matched by the reality of dental, ophthalmic, and prescription charges.[10]

The first hospices emerged into this system. Independent in nature, they relied on charitable giving and voluntary labor, raising funds to provide for capital building and staffing. At the same time, they looked to the health service, in the form of hospital boards and regional health authorities, for contractual arrangements for patients. Some, like St. Christopher's, also received grants from the Ministry of Health for research into pain.[11]

The emotional appeal of terminal care was strong. Its zealous founders were convincing in their moral arguments that society address the need to care for the dying, languishing without adequate pain control in hospitals. It easily caught the public imagination, as all families would experience death; in particular, the way that the dying were cared for, good and bad, had special meaning. Taking health care planners unawares, the spread of hospice facilities was rapid and ad hoc. Indeed, the need for hospice care and the question about the use of resources allocated to it was not carefully examined until the advent of the so-called purchaser-provider split as part of the conservative government health reforms of the 1980s.[12] To question the motivation of benefactors providing for worthy services was thought incorrect, to say the least. Although clearly the hospice movement could not exist outside, with its charitable foundations it was difficult for it to survive unchecked inside the NHS. Perhaps reluctantly, they were mutually dependent, and for hospices to survive some regulation on their growth and some organizational sense had to be brought to bear. This was gradually taken up by regional, area, and local health authorities. A sense of need for hospice facilities was sought.

In 1980, the Working Group on Terminal Care produced the first report on the provision on hospice serves. Believing that a lack of specialist staff and financial resources would limit the growth of independent hospice facilities, it recommended a concentration on home care (care of the terminally ill in their own home) and day care. Fundamentally, its members held the view that the dying should not be "hidden away" from the provision of wider, hospital and community-based services.[13] However, their prediction that the number of stand-alone services would be self-limiting was found to be false: the number of such units trebled in the next decade.[11] This also ran contrary to the recommendation of a survey by Lunt and Hillier,[14] who, in the following year, recommended that inpatient services be limited and that community services be coordinated to ensure equity of access across regions.

In 1987, 20 years after the first "modern" hospice started treating patients, the Department of Health set out its stall. In the first official circular on the subject, it firmly recommended that district health authorities gauge the need for and control the provision of hospice services.[11] It underscored the need to control hospice finances to ensure that facilities were financially secure to meet all contingencies, such as nurse salaries.

In 1990, in what was quickly to become a controversial departmental press release, the government seemed to be prepared to commit "a pound for a pound" of charitable giving. This announcement was indeed followed by a large injection of some £8 million and an unequal and divisive scramble among hospices and NHS providers of palliative care for funds. It seemed to say that monies for this health sector were limitless and, in turn, led to much ill feeling among other, apparently equally deserving, providers of health care. Deeply unpopular except among hospice providers, the scheme was dropped in 1995 and the age of earmarked monies for palliative care was over.

The 1980s had seen the beginning of health care reforms that continue to this day. Believing that the NHS was bureaucratically badly managed by ill equipped managers who could not compete with the vested self interests of its professionals, the conservative government finally introduced a system of general management in 1983. Writing in the report that was to carry his name, Sir Roy Griffiths, the head of a supermarket chain, famously declared that "if Florence Nightingale were carrying her lamp through the corridors of the NHS today, she would almost certainly be searching for the people in charge."[15] It was felt by commentators that with the introduction of "general management" and its business ethos, professional and clinical staff had lost out. Certainly a paradigm shift in power had taken place.

Fundamentally for the provision of hospice care, these management reforms ensured that there was now a clear demarcation between the purchasers of care, the district health authorities and the newly formed General Practitioner fund holders, and its providers, independent hospices and charitable providers of funds, notably Macmillan Cancer Relief. Crucially, purchasers brought to bear four key components to the planning of palliative care services: an overall strategy; a service specification (of assessed need); the contracting process to allocate funds; and need for clinical audit and quality assurance.[16]

The multidisciplinary Standing Medical Advisory and Standard Nursing Advisory and Midwifery Committees (SNAC/SNMAC), reporting in 1992, again recommended that palliative care should not be concentrated in hospice units, and that need should be assessed demographically and care delivered as an integral part of the local health service. This report served as a blueprint for purchasers and providers alike, and by 1995, 97% of hospices had entered into a contracting relationship with health authorities.[17]

"The idea that health care services should be predicated upon a rational assessment of need rather than upon emotional pleading, political lobbying, or the vested interests of particular providers is one with which it is difficult to disagree."[11] The palliative care community were enthused at the opportunity to state the needs of their population group and lobby for a properly financed commitment based on that need. However, it became clear that the needs of the cancer patient are many and include needs previously not considered by cash-strapped health authorities: psychosocial, social, and emotional. The strategy developed to one of prioritizing need and hoping that the limited resources would be shared equitably.[18]

The remaining years of the conservative governments saw the conclusion of their health care reforms. The number of general practitioner (GP) fund-holders expanded, and from 1994 were enabled to purchase palliative care services.[19]

Fund-holding was abandoned with a change of government in May 1997. It has been replaced by Primary Care Groups (PCGs), who essentially have a not dissimilar role to assess, plan, and commission a local health strategy. At the time of writing, there is ongoing controversy over the need for a strong nursing voice on PCGs.[20]

In 1995, the Expert Advisory Group on Cancer published its findings on the provision of cancer services in the United Kingdom. Known universally as the "Calman-Hine Report," it found a significant inequality of services—an absence in some areas, a plenitude in others. It recommended a three-tier system of primary care provision, for prevention and initial consultation; cancer units at district level for the treatment of common cancers; and cancer centers to deal with rarer cancers, covering larger populations.[21] It highlighted that palliative care should be a seamless service across all three tiers, effectively underlining the need for palliative care. To enable this, teams of palliative care nurses and consultants should work in cancer units and centers.

The Calman-Hine Report did much to raise the profile of cancer within the NHS, but as Richards found, the provision of palliative care services was patchy at best, with the most success at the cancer unit level where physicians had built on previously good relationships.[22]

The providers of palliative care have had to learn how to promote their services; they have had to learn a business culture. "At the dawn of the Conservative reforms of the 1990s the position was crystallised completely: join the contract culture or be condemned to obscurity. The independent hospices, after the briefest of vacillations, climbed on board and rarely looked back."[11] To enable them to do this, many hospices have appointed their own chief executives, often from outside a health service background. The current U.K. Hospice Directory lists 60 chief executives in post.[23]

Hospices have had to evolve to survive, and this has been a logical step in the process. However, the appointment of chief executives as business managers meant that the tripartite management system of matron/director of nursing, medical director, and administrator is now effectively a dying model. There have been casualties, as those holding professional values in powerful positions have met managers empowered to promote business- and market-based value systems.[24] These sources of conflict have been accentuated by the formation and rise of the specialty of palliative medicine,[25] the perception that nursing is not held in sufficient regard, and a power split on gender lines.[26]

The National Council for Hospice and Specialist Palliative Care Services (NCHSPCS)

Formed in 1991 as a representative and coordinating body for the hospice movement in England, Wales, and Scotland, the NCHSPCS has done much to ensure that hospices have been faithfully represented at every level. Its membership comes from national cancer charities, professional organizations, and regional representatives. Through its working parties and guidelines it has been instrumental in affecting the practice of palliative care. Examples of this work include guidelines on artificial hydration and cardiopulmonary resuscitation, care in the general hospital, and the management of the last days of life.[27] Its work with purchasers of palliative care, ensuring that a high profile is maintained, include guidelines on contracting; needs assessment and research in palliative care; and a statement of definitions of palliative care.[28]

SETTINGS OF CARE

An important piece of work undertaken by the NCHSPCS has been the gathering of information about the activities of specialist palliative care services, the Minimum Data Sets Project (MDS). In conjunction with and building on the excellent work undertaken by the Hospice Information Service, based at St. Christopher's Hospice, the MDS provides valuable information on numbers of inpatient and home care services, hospital support service, and day care, as well as how these services are used (Table 58–1).

Marie Curie Centres are administered by a national charity, Marie Curie Cancer Care. In addition to the 10 centers, there are some 6,000 part-time nurses who nurse patients in their own homes.

Sue Ryder Homes are administered by a national charity, the Sue Ryder Foundation, providing palliative care for patients with cancer in their Homes. Several homes have visiting nurses who visit patients prior to and after admission.

The growth of hospices in recent years has been considerable. In the early 1970s, Macmillan Cancer Relief began a program of capital funding to provide units within NHS hospitals, or on their grounds, with hospital authorities ensuring the responsibility for their running costs. Hospices catering to the terminally ill child and family are currently being established at the rate of 3 per year, with many at the planning stage.

The number of adult inpatient hospice services can be said to have reached a saturation point. Very few patients are more than 60 miles from an inpatient unit in England, and most are within 30 miles of some form of specialist palliative care provision. The original model of care, much is owed to these inpatient institutions. They broke new ground with their nonhierarchical teams of professionals and volunteers, incorporating patients' needs and wishes into the care that they gave. Hospice involves "a personal non institutional approach, promoting psychological care and physical well being through good symptom control."[29] Important, too, has been the research and, lately, the audit that continues and that has been linked to the delivery of this care.[30]

But inpatient units are costly. A recent analysis of nine London hospices showed that an average day of inpatient care cost £250, compared to £6.89p for an average day of patient care at home.

Table 58–1. Inpatient Services in Great Britain and N. Ireland as of January 2000

Service	Units	Beds
Independent or voluntary hospices*	143	2448
Marie Curie Centres	10	270
Sue Ryder Homes	7	145
NHS-managed units	56	600
Total	216	3323

*This figure includes 21 hospices for children, with a total of 159 beds, and three hospices for the HIV patient, with 72 beds (HIS).[23]

An average occupancy of available beds in these units was (only) 79%, an average length of stay 15.7 days.[31]

Sixty-fve percent of patients admitted to hospices in 1994–95 were over the age of 65, hardly surprising given that cancer is a disease of the elderly. Approximately 17.5% of people who died from cancer in the United Kingdom in 1994–95 were cared for in a hospice. The largest percentage of admissions come from home.[32]

A survey conducted by the Hospice Information Service at St. Christopher's has shown that there are approximately 40,000 new patients admitted to an inpatient hospice in the UK each year. There are 56,000 admissions and 29,000 deaths per year, which means that about half the admissions result in discharge.[23]

SOME ISSUES FACING INPATIENT HOSPICES

Criteria for Admission

Criteria for admission to what is, in effect, a valuable and limited resource, has always been an important issue for hospices.[33] Admission is likely to be because the patient has symptoms that the hospice can play an active part in treating, or because the patient is dying and the patient and/or their family believe that admission is appropriate.

A review of requests for admission are usually decided each working day by a small representative team of senior staff. They take into account the patient's physical, psychosocial, and other needs; whether they live alone and who is at home to care for them; and what packages are already in place. A visit by a member of the hospice's medical staff may be necessary, but often there is little time to accomplish this. Many hospices have a businesslike understanding with their referring community or hospital-based teams, trusting their estimation of the patient's prognosis, present condition, and needs.

A study of a random sample of people who had died in 1990 investigated which terminally ill cancer patients received inpatient care in hospices and other specialist palliative inpatient units.

This study interviewed families and others who knew about the last year of life. Interviews were obtained for 2,074 cancer deaths. Of these, 342 had been admitted to 31 different hospices. Five factors were found to independently predict hospice inpatient care: having pain in the last year of life, having constipation, being dependent on others for activities of daily living for between one and six months before death, having breast cancer, and being under the age of 85 years. A third of patients with all five factors were admitted, compared with no patients with none of these factors. It was found that symptom severity, age, dependency level, and site of cancer played a role in determining hospice admission but had limited predictive value. The study's salutary conclusion was that "admission seems to be governed more by chance than by need."[34]

It is generally unlikely that a hospice will agree to the admission of a patient with a prognosis of longer than three months. In the United Kingdom, the complex social services banding procedures for estimating residential and nursing home care mean that few hospices willingly admit patients who may require referral for this care on discharge.

Patient Dependency

So that the resources of the hospice's clinical staff can be maximized and the care of the inpatient population is not put in jeopardy by the admission of another patient, many hospices have adopted dependency scales.[35] When successfully implemented, they can provide an impartial view of the patient, family, and bereavement needs on the hospice ward.

Range of Services

The range of services offered by hospices is now considerable, the days long past when hospices cared only for the terminal patient. Johnson and colleagues reported that "our findings suggest that their [patients] management is likely to include a range of investigations and procedures that are usually associated with acute hospital care."[36] St. Christopher's and other hospices now routinely admits patients who are still having chemotherapy and radiotherapy for their cancer. Logistical problems are inevitably encountered when patients require daily transfer to acute centers and hospices, with limited drug budgets causing fear of incurring extra expenditure for chemotherapy.

Blood transfusions and injections of biphosphanates either as a day case or overnight inpatient admission are performed. Proponents of this rather more accommodating and enabling position have felt it important that patients come to see hospices as places where they can be successfully treated and discharged. Critics believe that we lose much if we forget the original binding ethos and principal aim: the holistic care of the dying in the rush to diversify and to be seen as therapeutic, a process universally known as the "routinization and medicalization of hospice."

"Routinization"

Cicely Saunders, as we have seen, chose to work in a way to influence the care of the NHS. St. Christopher's was never meant to be an isolated project. "To suggest that such care could only be based in a separate building, still more only one with some form of religious foundation, would have been to close doors when the commitment from the beginning was to open them and spread such care as widely as possible."[37] That hospice principles have been accepted and adopted by practitioners in the health service is therefore welcome.

However, James and Field, in the oft-quoted paper on routinization, adopt a Weberian thesis. Examining the charismatic personality and style of leadership of Cicely Saunders, they note that the movement depended upon "a singleness of vision, an intensity of purpose and a narrowness of focus."[38] They note the chord that this "vision" struck and the impact on the public, the subsequent demand for education, research, and pressure to disseminate the ideas and ideals of hospice care to noncancer patients, and the bureaucracy that has grown to meet this demand and the blurring of the vision, "a displacement of focus and practice back toward the more traditional medical conceptions of disease and it's treatment, to the possible detriment of other 'softer' aspects of care."[38]

Medicalization

The emergence of the new specialty of palliative care in 1987 was thought to be further evidence that the hospice movement was changing from a unique specialty to one dominated by mainstream medical thinking and practice. Hospice was in effect losing its special holistic edge.[25,38] Field[39] noted a number of concerns: a lack of clarity regarding the role of palliative medicine, a tendency to use technology, a threat to the autonomy of other professionals, and a lack of emphasis on dying.

The arguments put forward by Field are in part based on work by Johnson and colleagues,[36] which showed a higher tendency toward technological interventions when a full time medical consultant is employed. Recent work by Meystre et al. show that the routinization and medicalization debate is far from clear-cut, "given the proliferation of palliative care in many different settings of care and the movement of patients with palliative care needs from one setting to another."[40]

Clive Seale, in his comparative study of hospice and "conventional" care, concludes: "What the study reveals beyond question is that the process of hospice care, in both inpatient and home care settings, was rather different from conventional care and that hospice care was in many respects seen as valuable."[41] For the time being, palliative care continues to occupy a middle ground between the mainstream, the so-called conventional, and the holistic world of complementary medicine, bringing together an often loose but fundamentally family-centred collection of ideas. For the time being.

Respite Admissions

The majority of hospices are able to admit for a period of one to two weeks to enable the family or carers to have a rest. The concept of providing this form of care is not new. Families who "battle their way through" the journey from diagnosis to death and beyond require considerable information from the palliative care team and attention to their emotional and health needs.[42] They need empowering to undertake their role. Early identification of family members who may not cope well in the bereavement period is also important so that resources can be mobilized in a preventive manner. The admission of a patient for respite care easily affords this.

The problems associated with respite admission have been well identified. Raeside and Ellershaw, in their retrospective analysis of 34 respite admissions to St. Christopher's, found that patients admitted were enabled to receive a range of services, including anaesthetic referral. However, 24 (71%) died during the admission in the hospice or during a subsequent admission.[43]

A retrospective study of the first 20 patients admitted to St. Christopher's for respite care in 1995 showed that 13 (76%) died during the admission.[44] This study noted that eight (23.5%) were admitted from hospital, which "challenges the definition of respite care as being temporary care . . . to permit family caregivers to relinquish their duties, stress and responsibilities."[45] As a consequence of this study, respite admissions were defined in a hospice policy this way: "Short admissions will be considered for patients whose disease is advanced in order to give carers respite. The date of discharge will be determined before admission. It is expected that the family will resume care at the conclusion of the admission."[46]

This has met with limited success, and in effect the problem remains. The results of a retrospective audit of the first 45 patients admitted for respite this year revealed that 27 (60%) died while an inpatient, 11 (24%) were discharged, and 30, (66.6%) were admitted for "symptom control" as well as respite. Despite evidence that those patients who were admitted purely for a time-defined respite admission were more likely to be in the discharge group, there remains a need to properly quantify respite admissions to ensure that optimal interdisciplinary care is made available during the patient's brief stay and that appropriate goals are set for patient and family.

Admission for Rehabilitation

Despite the assertion by the World Health Organization that "the goal of palliative care can be summed by the word 'rehabilitation,'"[47] hospices in the United Kingdom struggle to provide rehabilitation uniformly. A report into the provision of services for rehabilitation at the Royal Marsden Hospital described "an un-programmed approach . . . due to a lack of understanding of the concept of rehabilitation by members of the caring team, and lack of communication and cohesiveness among those responsible for rehabilitation."[48] This could serve as a summary of the position of rehabilitation in U.K. hospices today. Hockley warns that hospices, in their "cocooning" of patients, run the risk of failing to make the patient the center of care and giving them back a degree of choice, control, and independence.[49] Although most hospices have many of the health professionals necessary to promote a rehabilitative approach, there is a failure to capitalize on their collective potential. Rehabilitation can require space and specialized equipment, and it is unfortunate that the modern hospice practice of placing emphasis on symptom control has meant that the long-haul, time-consuming aspects of rehabilitation are all but forgotten.[50]

The Question of Segregation

Many hospices in the United Kingdom, following a model first promoted at St. Christopher's, place their patients in bays of four beds. After observation of (only) 11 patients Honeybun concluded that "all things being equal, retaining the dying patient in the room with other patients would appear to be in the best interests of these other patients."[51] Payne and colleagues in a larger, more comprehensive study, support the hypothesis that patients who have witnessed the death of a fellow patient are significantly less depressed than those who have not. This careful study points out the apparent contradictions in its findings and its methodological limitations.[52] At St. Christopher's there is considerable anecdotal evidence that placing short-term patients alongside those who are terminally ill is detrimental to their overall well-being. Many patients report being distressed and subsequently reluctant to be readmitted. Research into the effects of placing patients for short-term admission—for example, for respite or rehabilitation—alongside those that are dying is required.

Ethnic Minorities

The need to meet the needs of all cultural and ethnic groups residing within a hospice's catchment area is recognized by a movement anxious to help hospice shed its white, middle-class image. After all, a hospice not only serves, but also depends on, its local population.

The National Council for Hospice and Specialist Palliative Care Services report "Opening Doors"[53] attempted to:

- identify the extent and reasons for low uptake by hospice and specialist palliative care services;
- ensure that those purchasing and providing these services were aware of ways in which the service could be improved;
- develop guidelines to assist hospice services; and
- help purchasers measure uptake.

It found that:

- the ethnic minority population had a lower proportion of elderly people and
- the incidence of cancer in the black and Asian communities was lower than that of the indigenous white population.

However,

- there was a lack of data about the supposed low uptake of hospice and palliative care services, and
- there was little or no information available to ethnic minority patients and their carers about these services.

Its recommendations included:

- the need for cultural awareness for all grades of staff;
- that codes of conduct for staff include information on acceptable and nonacceptable behavior;
- that increased efforts be made to attract staff and volunteers from ethnic minorities;

- the provision of a translation, interpreting, and advocacy service in each locality; and
- that information in the community on hospice and palliative care services be translated into the relevant local services.

This strategy document, widely welcomed and adopted by hospices as a blueprint for the provision of care for ethnic minorities, has given attention to this important issue by which many hospices and indeed the movement in the United Kingdom is judged.

Dying from Other Diseases

The use of hospice and specialist palliative care services by patients without a cancer diagnosis is another important issue for and measure of a service that is openly diversifying and trying to shed its old image. For those with a noncancer diagnosis, palliative care is most likely to be delivered by a primary care team. Provision of specialist palliative care to this group is rare or even extremely rare. Few services advertise their willingness to extend their services to the noncancer patient, and as a consequence patients' symptoms that might be met remain inadequately treated and carers' needs remain unmet.[54]

An interview survey of 600 informal carers of patients who had died from heart disease found that they had experienced a wide range of often distressing symptoms that often lasted for longer than six months. Little or no symptom relief was reported for 35% of patients with pain, 31% with constipation, 24% with nausea and vomiting, and 24% with dyspnea.[55] A retrospective study of 170 patients with dementia concluded that many had symptoms and health care needs comparable with cancer patients.[56] These two pieces of research support much anecdotal evidence that an improvement in the palliation of other diseases is required. However, despite the knowledge that palliative care teams and units have the means to address these symptoms, the fear that services could be overwhelmed is very real.[57,58] Until the funding for the provision of the required extra resources, both financial and human, is secure the movement is likely to remain reticent.[59]

Sadly, it would be a generalization to say that nurses would welcome an extension of their nursing care to other disease groups, as, even where they are instrumental in dictating patterns of care, they have remained reluctant to widen their scope. Other factors preventing wider uptake by the noncancer group are an uncertainty and lack of hard data about the progression of chronic diseases.

Ultimately, as the process of purchasing palliative care continues, a questioning of the need for inpatient units will prevail, particularly as care in the community becomes more sophisticated.

However, at the present time, "in the UK, the emphasis has been on the collection and evaluation of evidence to improve care within units, rather than a critical analysis of the continued benefits of in-patient hospice provision."[11]

COMMUNITY PALLIATIVE CARE SERVICES

In January 2000 the results of a survey of the services provided for patients in the community were published (see Table 58–2).

A survey conducted by the Hospice Information Service at St. Christopher's has shown that in the UK over 120,000 patients per year (principally suffering from cancer) are seen at home by palliative care nurses. This is well over half of all patients dying from cancer.[23]

"Macmillan Nurses," long a feature of the provision of specialist palliative care, are named after Macmillan Cancer Relief, the funding charity that pump primes these posts in community and hospital settings. Their principal role remains one of personally assessing and delivering care to patients and families and giving advice to and empowering primary caregivers. However, this has evolved to one that promotes high standards of cancer and palliative care. This is achieved by acting as a catalyst and change agent; contributing to pre- and postregistration educational curricula, and promoting and participating in clinical research and audit.[60]

Table 58–2. Community Palliative Care Services in Great Britain and N. Ireland

Community palliative care services including Macmillan Nurse Services)	338
Extended nursing care at home	61
Day hospices/services	234
Hospital support nursing services	118
Hospital palliative care/ support teams	215

Source: See ref. 23.

Extended nursing care at home, a relatively new initiative, is a service that employs registered and auxiliary nurses in the patient's home, providing physical care and psychosocial support. Although the amount of time spent at home is small, it is thought that this type of service reinforces the patient's confidence to remain in their own surroundings and in their ability to stay there.

Day centers afford the chance for patients to express their creativity, be among others in a similar situation, and the opportunity to receive symptom control as required. An estimated 16,000 new patients attended day facilities in 1995–96, with an estimated total attendance of 7700 per week.[32]

Hospital support nursing services consist of one or two nurses based in hospitals, acting as a resource. Hospital support teams may have the support of a specialist doctor. Access to patients who require palliative care but who may be in a surgical or gynecological bed is vital, and a doctor facilitates this. In 1995–96 there were an estimated 50,000 to 60,000 new patients seen by these services.[32]

Writing of her work with 1,500 patients, McNulty (1978) noted the need to provide 24-hour care: "Once the surgery has closed and the telephone number has been referred to a central agency or to another doctor, the patient is cut off from the familiar source of help, comfort and reassurance upon which he has come to depend."[61] The community palliative care team now often provides that support; indeed they will lead the care in the patient's own home, directing and advising general practitioners and community nurses. However, although McNulty recommended 24-hour medical and nursing coverage as a basic essential of home care, a number of services, particularly those that are hospital based, do not provide this.

OTHER ISSUES

"Ethical Decision Making in Palliative Care" is the title of a series of short papers prepared by the National Council for Hospice and Palliative Care Services. Two of these papers, one on artificial hydration and one on cardiopulmonary resuscitation for people who are terminally ill, are most in demand.[62,63] Four ethical issues—the two named above, coping with the patient's spiritual needs, and euthanasia—can be said to be those that will always engage the palliative care nurse's interest.

As Dunlop et al., in a review of the literature, point out, there is no clear evidence to support the prescription of intravenous or subcutaneous fluids in the terminally ill. Increased nutritional support or fluid therapy does not appear to alter the comfort, mental status, or survival of patients who are dying. As long as the wishes of the patient are not contravened, they believe, a therapeutic trial of fluids may be warranted in the case of a sudden onset of dehydration and an uncertain diagnosis. Similarly, where families are not satisfied with a decision not to commence systemic fluids a small amount of fluid, one liter per 24 hours, is given subcutaneously. In the author's experience, this latter situation arises only two or three times per 1,000 admissions at St. Christopher's.[64]

The conflict of needs between the acutely ill and terminally ill patient,[65] and the pressure placed on medical and nursing staff in hospitals, makes this an emotive and tough ethical dilemma. Even in a controlled environment like a hospice, careful explanations to relatives and carers are required to help them understand that we are not abandoning the patient to their fate "but it is the appropriate treatment decision at this stage of their illness."[66]

Cardiopulmonary resuscitation in hospice is an equally difficult area if the patient is young and wishes to receive the care and expert symptom control of a hospice, continue with active treatment, and receive resuscitation. Hospices are not equipped to undertake resuscitation, the nursing staffs' training and experience of resuscitation may be out of date, and resuscitation may not fit with the central belief of a hospice to support but not to prolong life. The NCHSPCS Document attempts to allay fears that nurses may have about this essentially alien, but nonetheless occasionally encountered, area of practice.

The regulation of hospices and specialist palliative care services gives concern to nurse managers. At present registered under the Nursing Homes Act (1984), a convenient place to lodge a facility that did not fit in with the mainstream hospital sector, hospices find that they are both over-regulated and burdened by the regulations that apply to nursing homes, be they for six beds or 500. Sadly, the current arrangement does not reflect the comprehensive, multiprofessional work that hospices provide. The regulation and inspection teams are interested in inpatient facilities only, not in the important work in the community and how it impacts on these facilities. The present government has recently taken evidence and published its proposals for the provision and regulation of services in the independent sector. These suggest a separate regulatory body to set and inspect hospices against new, defined standards.[67] As yet it is too early to see if these will be specific enough for the complex work of inpatient units and community palliative care services, be they in the independent sector or NHS.

SPIRITUALITY AND PALLIATIVE NURSING

Few issues appear as difficult for the nurse new to palliative care as the need to address the patient's spiritual needs. Few issues underscore the difference between nursing in a hospice and elsewhere as does the constant exposure to death and dying. This subject matter is covered elsewhere in this book, but I would like to briefly look at spirituality as it affects palliative nursing.

Bradshaw, writing cogently of the secularization of hospice, brings a criticism to bear on the practice of nursing that, in its need to be professional, has lost something precious. Hospice is the "quintessential" place for fundamental nursing care.[68] She describes how, in our efforts to ensure a good death, we have become too concerned with the process and are in danger of losing our role as "spiritual anchor." "Real love" is replaced by the "self-conscious application of psychosocial skills and techniques." Certainly one can agree with Bradshaw that the delivery of holistic nursing care to the dying patient is fundamental to the art of nursing, even appreciate the sentiment that spiritual care of the dying patient is akin to "standing on holy ground."[69] However, her warnings are largely unheeded by an increasingly secular and professionally motivated nursing workforce.

Nurses relate to Saunders's concept of "total pain," the combination of social, psychological, and spiritual need. Indeed, "the professionalization of nursing has resulted in the enhancement and wholehearted pursuit of the holistic values associated with palliative care, making the experience of dying more bearable and meaningful for people in many settings of care."[11]

CONCLUSIONS

But nursing is struggling. Faced with a reduced number of newly qualified practitioners, and a dearth of experienced nurses coming through a "graying" profession,[70] palliative care services are beginning to experience a difficulty in the recruitment of suitably qualified nurses. This situation has not been helped by a switch to post-registration diploma, first and master's degree programs that, while comprehensive, are time-consuming and difficult to accomplish on top of a busy clinical workload. What is the most suitable course for palliative care nurses? That this question is still being asked may be unremarkable given the ongoing uncertainty of the content and length of our "P2000," preregistration nurse courses. The national nursing shortage, which has gained much tabloid newspaper interest throughout 1999, has had even the nursing profession asking itself if it needs to be baccalaureate based.

Nursing in the United Kingdom has to learn to be more adaptive to a changing environment. Privatized health care continues to make inroads into traditional NHS territory and, through more elaborate purchasing arrangements, will expect more from palliative care.

As Lipscomb states, "The post-war consensus on welfare is dead, and the beliefs and assumptions that once underpinned health and social welfare are no more. The unassailable 'right' of health care to be financed from general taxation, to be organised nationally and delivered by unaccountable professions, has disintegrated. Nursing would do well to recognise this fact."[71]

Sophisticated outcome measures to evaluate the effectiveness of palliative care are now in an advanced state of readiness,[72,73] yet are not universally understood, much less adopted. A system of organizational audit for specialist palliative care,[74] successfully tried by many hospice services in the United Kingdom, have been incorporated into the prestigious King's Fund Quality Service.

Despite this important stamp of approval, the movement remains reluctant to take them up and shies away from any system of accreditation. Nurses are the main deliverers of care and the main upholders of standards of care. They should also take the lead by demanding that hospices remain centers of clinical excellence and ensure that the hospice ideal is kept alive.

REFERENCES

1. Clark D. Originating a Movement: Cicely Saunders and the development of St. Christopher's Hospice, 1957–1967. Mortality 1998a;3(1):43–61.

2. Walters T. Developments in Spiritual Care of the Dying. Religion 1996;26:353–363.

3. Clark D. An annotated bibliography of the publications of Cicely Saunders—1:1958–1967. Palliative Medicine 1998b;12:181–193

4. Wald FS. Hospice's path to the future. In: Strack S, ed., Death and the Quest for Meaning New Jersey: Aronson Northvale, 1997.

5. Saunders C. Care of the Dying. Nursing Times reprint. London: Macmillan, 1976.

6. English National Board for Nursing, Midwifery and Health Visiting (ENB). Post Registration Studies Programmes. Circular 1999/03/RLV. London: ENB, 1999.

7. Henderson VA. The Nature of Nursing. Reflections after 25 Years. New York: National League for Nursing, 1991.

8. Wells R. AIDS and Its Impact on Cancer Nursing. Lampada, Royal College of Nursing 1987;10:8–11, 45–46.

9. Ministry of Health, Scottish Home and Health Department. Report of the Committee on Senior Nursing Staff Structure (Salmon). London: HMSO, 1996.

10. Timmins N. The Five Giants: A Biography of the Welfare State. London: Fontana, 1996.

11. Clark D, Seymour J. Reflections on Palliative Care. Buckingham: Open University Press, 1999.

12. Clark D. The Future for Palliative Care. Buckingham: Open University Press, 1993.

13. Working Party on Terminal Care [The Wilkes Report]. Report of the Working Party on Terminal Care. London: DHSS, 1980.

14. Lunt B, Hillier R. Terminal care: present services and future priorities. British Medical Journal 1981;283:595–598.

15. Department of Health and Social Security. NHS Management Enquiry [The Griffiths Report] DA (83)38. London: DHSS, 1983.

16. Clark D, Malson H, Small N, Mallett K, Neale P, Heather P. Half-full or half-empty? The impact of health reforms on palliative care services in the United Kingdom. In Clark D, Hockley J, and Ahmedzai S, eds., New Themes in Palliative Care. Buckingham: Open University Press, 1997.

17. Standard Medical Advisory Committee / Standing Nursing and Midwifery Advisory Committee. The Principles and Provision of Palliative Care. London: HMSO, 1992.

18. Clark D, Malson H. Key issues in palliative care needs assessment. Progress in Palliative Care 1995;3:53–55.

19. Department of Health. EL(94)14. Contracting for Specialist Palliative Care Services. London: Department of Health, 1994.

20. Wheatley M, Sweeting J. Nurses on board. Nursing Management 1999;5(10):7–8.

21. Expert Advisory Group on Cancer [The Calman-Hine Report]. A Policy Framework for Commissioning Cancer Services: A Report by the Expert Advisory Group on Cancer to the Chief Medical Officers of England and Wales. London: Dept. of Health and Welsh Office, 1995.

22. Richards M. Calman-Hine two years on (editorial). Palliative Medicine 1997;11:433–434.

23. Hospice Information Service (HIS) at St. Christopher's. Directory of Hospice and Palliative Care Services in the United Kingdom and Republic of Ireland. London: HIS, 2000.

24. Anning P. Have hospices lost their way? Nursing Management 1998;5(5):6–7.

25. Biswas B. Medicalization: a nurse's view. In Clark D, ed. The Future for Palliative Care. Buckingham: Open University Press, 1993.

26. Clay T. Nurses, Power and Politics. London: Heineman, 1987.

27. Gaffin J. Achievements and intentions—the work of the NCHSPCS. European Journal of Palliative Care 1996;3(3):100–104.

28. National Council for Hospice and Specialist Palliative Care Services. Specialist Palliative Care: A Statement of Definitions, Occasional Paper No. 8. London: NCHSPCS, 1995.

29. Salisbury C. What models of palliative care services have been proposed or developed in the UK, Europe, North America and Australia? In: Clark D, Seymour J, eds. Reflections on Palliative Care. Buckingham: Open University Press, 1999.

30. Higginson I. Palliative care: a review of past changes and future trends. Journal of Public Health Medicine 1993;15:3–8.

31. Clark C. Hospice Benchmarking Exercise. Unpublished. St. Christopher's Hospice, London, 1999.

32. Eve A. Hospice and Palliative Care in UK 1995/6. Report of First National Survey of the Minimum Data Sets Project The Hospice Information Service, St. Christopher's Hospice, London, 1997.

33. Hockley J. In: Clark D., ed. New Themes in Palliative Care. Buckingham: Open University Press, 1997:84–100.

34. Addington-Hall J, Altmann D, McCarthy M. Which terminally ill cancer patients receive hospice in-patient care? Social Science and Medicine 1998;46(8):1011–1016.

35. Williams A. Dependency scoring in palliative care. Nursing Standard 1995;10(5):27–30.

36. Johnson IS, Rogers C, Biswas B, Ahmedzai S. What do hospices do? A survey of hospices in the United Kingdom and Republic of Ireland. British Medical Journal 1990;300:791–793.

37. Saunders C. Some challenges that face us. Palliative Medicine 1993;7(suppl.1):77–83.

38. James N, Field D. The Routinization of Hospice: Charisma and Bureaucratisation. Social Science Medicine 1992;34(12):1363–1375

39. Field D. (1994) Palliative medicine and the medicalization of death. European Journal of Cancer Care 1994;3:58–62.

40. Meystre CJN, Burley NMJ, Ahmedzai S. What investigations and procedures do patients in hospices want? Interview based survey of patients and their nurses. British Medical Journal 1997; 315:1202–1203.

41. Seale C. A comparison of hospice and conventional care. Social Science and Medicine 1991;32:147–152.

42. Saunders C, Baines M. Living with Dying: The Management of Terminal Disease. Oxford: Oxford University Press, 1983.

43. Raeside D, Ellershaw J. What does respite care offer to cancer patients admitted to hospice? Palliative Medicine 1994;8(1):68.

44. Pridmore M, Armes J. Respite Audit Report, St. Christopher's Hospice, London, 1996. Unpublished.

45. Dewi Rees W. The mortality associated with respite care in a hospice. Palliative Medicine 1987;1(2):163–164.

46. Knight A. Admissions Policy, St. Christopher's Hospice, 1999. Unpublished.

47. World Health Organisation. Palliative Cancer Care. Policy Statement. Leeds, 1987.

48. Wells R. Rehabilitation: making the most of time. Oncology Nursing Forum 1990;17(4): 503–507.

49. Hockley J. Rehabilitation in palliative care—are we asking the impossible? Palliative Medicine 1993;7(suppl. 1):9–15.

50. Hunter M. Rehabilitation in cancer care: a patient focused approach. European Journal of Cancer Care 1998;7:85–87.

51. Honeybun J, Johnston M, Tookman A. The impact of a death on fellow hospice patients. British Journal of Medical Psychology 1992;65: 67–72.

52. Payne S, Hillier R, Langley-Evans A, Roberts T. Impact of Witnessing Death on Hospice Patients. Social Science and Medicine 1996; 43(12):1785–1794.

53. National Council for Hospice and Specialist Palliative Care Services. Opening Doors: Improving Access to Hospice and Specialist Palliative Care Services by Members of the Black and Ethnic Minority Communities, Occasional Paper No. 7, London: NCHSPCS, 1995a.

54. Addington-Hall J, McCarthy M. Dying from cancer: results of a national population based investigation. Palliative Medicine 1995;9:295–305.

55. McCarthy M, Lay M, Addington-Hall J. Dying from heart disease. Journal of the Royal College of Physicians of London 1996;30(4):325–328.

56. McCarthy M, Addington-Hall J, Altmann D. The experience of dying with dementia: a retrospective study. International Journal of Geriatric Psychiatry 1997;12(3):404–409.

57. National Council for Hospice and Specialist Palliative Care Services. Dilemmas and Directions: The Future of Specialist Palliative Care. Occasional Paper No. 11. London: NCHSPCS, 1997a.

58. Gibbs LME, Addington-Hall J, Gibbs JSR. Dying from heart failure: lessons from palliative care. British Medical Journal 1998;317:961.

59. Pettingell Y. Palliative care for all. Nursing Management 1999;6(4):8–9.

60. Webber J. The evolving role of the Macmillan Nurse. Nursing Times 1994;90(25).

61. McNulty BJ. Out Patient and Domiciliary Management from a Hospice. In: Saunders C, ed. The Management of Terminal Disease. London: Edward Arnold, 1978.

62. National Council for Hospice and Specialist Palliative Care Services. Ethical Decision Making in Palliative Care: Artificial Hydration for people who are terminally ill. London: NCHSPCS, 1997b.

63. National Council for Hospice and Specialist Palliative Care Services. Ethical Decision Making in Palliative Care: Cardiopulmonary Resuscitation(CPR) for people who are terminally ill. London: NCHSPCS, 1997c.

64. Dunlop R, Ellershaw J, Baines M, Sykes N, Saunders C. On withholding nutrition and hydration in the terminally ill: has palliative medicine gone too far? A reply. Journal of Medical Ethics 1995;21:141–143.

65. House N. The hydration question—hydration or dehydration of terminally ill patients. Professional Nurse 1992;8(1):44–48.

66. Malone N. Hydration in the terminally ill patient. Nursing Standard 1994;8(43):29–32.

67. Department of Health. Regulating Private and Voluntary Healthcare. London: Department of Health, 1999.

68. Bradshaw A. The spiritual dimension of hospice: the secularisation of an ideal. Social Science and Medicine 1996;43:409–420.

69. O'Brien ME. Spirituality in Nursing: Standing on Holy Ground. Sudbury, MA: Jones and Bartlett, 1999.

70. RCN. Carry on Nursing? Employment Brief 21/98 Royal College of Nursing Employment Information and Research Unit. London: Royal College of Nursing, 1998.

71. Lipscomb M. A dose of reality. Nursing Management 1999;6(3):5.

72. Hearn J, Higginson I. Outcome measures in palliative care for advanced cancer patients: a review. Journal of Public Health Medicine 1997; 19(2):193–197.

73. Hearn J, Higginson I. Validation of a core outcome measure for palliative care—The palliative care outcome scale (The POS). Journal of Public Health Medicine (in press).

74. CRMF. Cancer Relief Macmillan Fund, [Macmillan Cancer Relief] Organisational Audit for Specialist Palliative Care. London: CRMF, 1994.

59 Ireland

ANNE HAYES and MAURA MCDONNELL

Ireland has a long tradition in hospice care. In the late nineteenth century the Irish Sisters of Charity opened two hospices in Ireland: Our Lady's Hospice in Dublin, and Marymount in Cork, to meet the needs of the terminally ill. At that time patients with tuberculosis formed the majority of their admissions. The same sisters opened St. Joseph's Hospice in Hackney, London, at the turn of the century, where Cicely Saunders was later to do her pioneering work establishing the value of regularly administered morphine as the cornerstone of cancer pain control. In 1967 she opened St. Christopher's Hospice in South London, which heralded the start of a rapid period of development of this area of care known as the hospice movement. In the last 20 years, hospice care or as it is now widely known, palliative care, has gone through a time of renaissance in Ireland, stimulated by developments in the United Kingdom and growing public and professional interest.

Palliative care has been described as both a philosophy and a practice of care and is inextricably linked to quality of life. Its ethos provides for sensitivity to personal, cultural, and religious beliefs, and to values and practices. Stjernsward[1] stressed the fact that each country must develop the best approach to caring for dying people relative to its culture and resources. The metaphor of journey when applied to the patient with advanced disease can also be applied to the development of hospice and palliative care in Ireland. This chapter will provide an overview of these developments and of the central role played by nurses, highlighting the fact that nurses are the key to the delivery of palliative care services.[1]

HISTORICAL PERSPECTIVE

Larkin, reviewing the historical development of palliative care services, suggests that the Republic of Ireland owes a legacy to the Irish Sisters of Charity as well as other religious orders.[2] In caring for the poor as a vocation, religious sisters, many of whom were nurses, sought to alleviate the poverty of dying through their vision of helping the terminally ill on the road home.[3] The place of religion in the historical development of Irish palliative care reflects the legacy of the church-state relationship dating back to the late nineteenth century, when Our Lady's Hospice, Harold's Cross, was founded. The Church, supported by Catholic political movements, fought to regain control of health care and education from British administration.[4] Institutional developments such as hospitals and health care facilities helped to consolidate the Church and indeed the Irish identity at a time of British rule in Ireland.[5]

Inglis[6] clearly documents the spread of the Catholic Church's organization and influence from the foundation of the Free State in 1922 to the visionary speeches of Eamonn deValera in 1943,[7] in which Catholic nationalist orthodoxy was endorsed. The social context of religious change since that time, through a policy of modernization, is now well documented.[4,8] However, it is important to acknowledge the debt owed to Irish religious orders in the establishment of a caring and nursing service for the dying in Ireland.[2]

From this we can see that since the end of the nineteenth century the role of the state has evolved from the provision of essential services, funded locally to the poor, to playing a major role in the provision and funding of services, as well as the regulation and setting of standards for input to the health system and, in recent times, an increasing emphasis on setting targets and objectives. Today a combination of government, Department of Health and Children, advisory and executive agencies, and voluntary organizations all play a role in service delivery and development, though their degree of power and influence varies.

In Ireland, the home of hospice, the first dedicated palliative care unit for people with advanced cancer, was opened in Our Lady's Hospice in 1978, when a full-time medical director was appointed. Since that time, the nationwide demand for hospice services has increased dramatically. This demand has primarily been driven by both local communities and a concomitant heightening awareness by nurses for specialized knowledge in the whole area of palliative care. Out of this has evolved the growth in services that have developed through the predominantly joint efforts of local communities, national charitable agencies (i.e., the Irish Cancer Society), the Irish Hospice Foundation, regional health boards, and the Department of Health and Children. This arrangement, whereby different services have been funded by different agencies, has not been without its problems. To understand palliative service development and delivery, and the problems associated with it, one must first have an understanding of the structural and organizational arrangements of the present Irish health system.

THE IRISH HEALTH SYSTEM

The Irish health system is a mix of both public and private institutions and funders. Approximately 75% of health care is funded by the government, mainly through general taxation, and 25% is funded mainly through voluntary health insurance premiums. Public health expenditure makes up approximately 20% of government spending, and in 1997 was 6.8% of GNP (gross national product). Private health expenditure accounts for nearly 25% of health expenditure, and approximately 2% of GNP.[9] However, as Dwyer and Taaffe[10] note, Ireland is one of the few OECD (Organisation for Economic Co-operation and Development) countries that has reduced its share of GNP devoted to health. During the period 1980 to 1993, the fall in our share of GNP devoted to health was approximately 23%. This contrasted with an average 24% increase experienced in 13 other OECD countries over the same period.

Over 36% of the population are eligible for all health services free of charge, based on means testing of income. The remainder of the population are entitled to public beds in public hospitals/hospices, and if they wish they may avail themselves of voluntary health insurance to cover private accommodation in public and private hospitals. Over 40% of the population are enrolled in the two voluntary health insurance schemes.[9] It should be noted here that all specialist home care services are free at the point of delivery to the patient. This has largely been through the aegis of local hospice groups' commitment and fund-raising efforts, together with varying degrees of support from statutory bodies. Indeed, many of the new care programs that have been initiated in, for example, inpatient units have also been dependent on local fund-raising efforts.

In 1994 one of the most significant health policy and planning documents, "Shaping a Healthier Future,"[11] was launched by the Department of Health and Children. Its main focus was the reorientation and reshaping of the Irish health services so that improving people's health and quality of life became the primary and unifying focus of the health services. The Department of Health and Children also committed itself to the further development and promotion of palliative care services. Since the strategy was launched, there have been further policy documents produced that tie in with the implementation of programs to meet the targets and objectives of "Shaping a Healthier Future." One of these documents is a cancer strategy and a cancer action plan. In terms of defining palliative care development policy, this is a very important document, outlining a structure that recognizes the importance of providing a comprehensive patient-focused cancer service that includes palliative care. This is relevant because, among other things, cancer accounts for one-third of all deaths in Ireland among those aged under 65 years and Ireland has a higher mortality due to cancer than the EU (European Union) average. However, it should also be noted that many of the palliative care services have been extended to provide care for other patients—for example, people with Motor Neurone Disease and AIDS. Palliative care services in Ireland have in the past and will increasingly face the challenge of providing accessible high-quality care in an effective way. This is being achieved in the context of, among other things, increasing demands for service and budgetary controls. However, since the launch of the Cancer Strategy in 1996 a total of almost £4.3 million has been allocated to palliative services.

PALLIATIVE CARE SERVICES

Today specialist palliative care services are provided in a range of settings, including inpatient hospice units; home care programs; palliative care services within a general hospital; and day-care and outpatient centers that are attached to inpatient units. There are also a number of general and other local hospitals that provide either a palliative care unit or "backup beds." All of these care settings are not isolated entities, but together comprise a comprehensive and integrated service,[12] which is essential if the aims as outlined in the National Cancer Strategy[13] are to be achieved, namely that:

> patients should be enabled and encouraged to express their preference about where they wish to be cared for and where they wish to spend the last period of their life; services should be sufficiently flexible and integrated as to allow movement of patient from one care setting to another depending on their clinical situation and personal preferences; the ultimate aim should be for all patients to have access to specialist palliative care services where these are required.

Whereas in 1987 there were two Home Care Services in the Irish Republic, there are now 31, with more than 100 specialist nurses employed; every county is covered. It should be noted that the majority of these services are nurse-led and in partnership with the primary health care team. In 1989 the first hospital-based palliative care service was set up in St. Vincent's University Hospital, Dublin. Today, there are six such services in general hospitals, comprising ten palliative care nurses. In the coming years this is expected to be one of the main areas of growth in the field. The first day-care unit was set up in 1993, and there are now four such units attached to inpatient hospice units. At the close of 1999 there were six inpatient palliative care units. From this we can see that experienced nurses working in palliative care services are making a valued and substantial contribution to the care of patients and their families in every setting.

EDUCATION OF THE PALLIATIVE CARE NURSE

As the nationwide demand for palliative care has increased dramatically, so the demand for both practitioners with specialist knowledge and skills as well as those with a palliative approach to care has increased. However, until 1987, when the first courses were set up, there were no education programs available in Ireland to prepare nurses for their role. Many at that time had learned their skills "on the job." A very few had completed a Diploma in Oncological Nursing, and still fewer had attended a six-week course in the United Kingdom on "Care of the Dying Patient and the Family." Our Lady's Hospice in Dublin, recognizing this deficiency in training, set up the first education unit, developing programs for nurses and other health care professionals. These courses ranged from one-day to eight-week programs on different aspects of palliative care and culminated in 1997 with the commencement of a two-year part-time Higher Diploma in Nursing Studies (Palliative Care), now run in partnership with University College in Dublin.

This development needs to be placed within the context of changes that have and are taking place in nurse education in general in Ireland. Until 1994 nurses were trained in apprenticeship programs, entirely in hospitals, with no involvement in third-level institutions. In 1994 the first university-based preregistration education program in nursing was established. Since 1998 all preregistration education of nurses in Ireland has been college based. In 1993 An Bord Altranias, the Irish Nursing Board, produced a document on the Nature of Nurse Education and Training in Ireland. One of the recommendations was that postregistration continuing education should be structured in such a way as to ensure the development of nurses for clinical nursing roles in specialist areas. They also recommended that links with higher-education institutions be developed to accredit such courses for nurses and that all courses should be subjected to a joint professional (An Bord Altranais) and academic (Higher Education) validation and accreditation. In Ireland, though we call particular nurses specialists, this is more by convention than actual academic and career structure. However, this is changing. In 1997 a commission on nursing was established to examine and report on different aspects of the role of nurses. In its report the need for a coherent approach to the progression of nursing specialization, and the development of a clinical career pathway,[15,16] was identified. These objectives are already being pursued.

IRISH PALLIATIVE NURSING

Much has been written in previous chapters on the nature of palliative nursing and the knowledge and skills necessary to fulfill this specialized role as a member of a multidisciplinary team. Intrinsic to palliative nursing, as it has developed in Ireland, is a belief in and nuturance of the soul and spirit of the patient; a desire to serve and to help alleviate suffering of the patient; and a deep compassion and love for the patient, whether a patient or family member. Larkin,[2] in his seminal work on the lived experiences of Irish palliative care nurses, identified a number of themes that seem to encapsulate the unique expression of Irish palliative care nursing: closeness—the emotional and spiritual closeness of one person to another rather than just physical closeness; friendship—anam chara, or soul friend; loving—which encompasses the ideals of giving, sharing, reciprocity, and rapport; humor; caring about and caring for the person; and spirituality—"having positive concern for the spirit beyond religion." These themes suggest that the Irish perspective on caring for the dying encompasses a philosophy of being, "being there," which involves a presence at an existential level without the need to perform an action or duty,[2] although this may be important too. This speaks of the person who is the nurse—his or her own experiences, feelings, and intuition. The basic belief here is that who we are as persons underlies, informs, and complements all of the knowledge and skills necessary in our caring. Irish palliative nursing, therefore, is about tending and nurturing the flow of life in ways that facilitate growth in the direction of wholeness and healing.

At this time a transformational process is evident in Irish palliative care nursing that will continue well into the twenty-first century. In the late twentieth century, Irish palliative care nurses were concerned with, for the most part, service initiation, provision and development, and gaining recognition for both these services and their own positions. These nurses were pioneers in the true sense of the word, often exploring new ground, many times as the lone member of a team expressing the palliative nursing concepts of caring, compassion, love, intuition, and healing, in addition to exhibiting the knowledge and skill required for palliative nursing. In the twenty-first century, palliative nurses are likely to seek, in addition role and service enhancement; service innovations aimed at connecting with the healing of the patient; empowerment; recognition of their complementary rather than subsidiary relationship with medicine, and the opportunity to participate in shared governance[10] of their hospital/hospice and home care program.

CONCLUSION

If nursing is about caring, and we believe it is, and palliative care is about a specialized and a particular approach to care, then Irish palliative nurses, the largest occupational group in this specialty, must remain alert and responsive to their ongoing professional needs and development, as well as to those people who use the services. This presents many challenges and issues for the future. At a time when increasing demands are being made on resources for treatment programs, it is imperative that equal energy and enthusiasm be devoted to exploring and making known the unique contributions of Irish palliative care nurses and services. This is important not only because of the strong foundations Ireland has in the development of palliative care from the nineteenth century on.[2] It will also maintain the art of caring as central to this role and all that that implies. It is important to find ways to articulate and exemplify this and gain the necessary resources for "caring" from health service providers and funders. At heart, the philosophy of palliative care is about quality of life. It is about wholeness in the healing journey.

For a person living with a life-threatening illness, palliative nurses, through their specializing in, for example, complementary touch therapies, offer another dimension to whole-person care on both a surface and a deep level.[17] All of this is particularly pertinent at a time of increasingly strident debates over care versus cure; issues relating to matters of life and death; sustaining or withdrawal of treatment; easing death's pains or hastening its arrival, and resource allocation.

People always have ideas and expectations different from those of a generation earlier,[18] and this challenges us to adapt the original objectives of palliative care to the changing needs of the populations we serve. Worldwide, and Ireland is no different, there is a danger that a "professional/public" gulf could open up,[18] leading to the professionalisation of death and dying, as well as demands for further health care structures. It could be postulated that these structures will only meet the professional's needs. The danger if this happens is that the structure can become the ultimate objective. Ensuring ongoing equal partnership with local communities, professionals, and health service providers guards against this and helps us, the professionals, to remember the fundamental fact that palliative care is part of how communities care for their dying. It is easy to forget in the rush of modern life that the first hospice in Ireland was not a sudden spontaneous flowering but arose from the surrounding culture and community.[19] Above all, palliative care nursing must continue to create an environment that listens to the dying person, because only in listening can we know and learn.[20]

REFERENCES

1. Stjernswärd J. Nurses in the frontline of Palliative Care. International Journal of Palliative Nursing 1995;1(3):124–126.

2. Larkin PJ. A Hermeneutical Inquiry into the Lived Experiences of Irish Palliative Care Nurses. Unpublished Thesis. The University of Huddersfield, England, 1997.

3. Butler K. We Help Them Home. A History of Our Lady's Hospice, Harold's Cross. Dublin, Ireland: Caritas Press, 1980.

4. Breen R, Hannon D, Rottmann D, Whelan C. Understanding Contemporary Ireland: State Class and Development in the Republic of Ireland. London: Macmillan, 1990.

5. Kirby P. Is Irish Catholicism Saying? Dublin, Ireland: Mercier Press, 1984.

6. Inglis T. Moral Monopoly: The Catholic Church in Modern Irish Society. Dublin, Ireland: Gill and Macmillan, 1984.

7. Murphy JA. Ireland in the 20th Century. Gill and Macmillan, Dublin, Ireland, 1975.

8. Hornby Smith M, Whelan C. Religious and moral values. In: Whelan C., ed. Values and Social Change in Ireland, Chapter 2, 1994:7–45.

9. O'Hara T. Current structure of the Irish health care system: Setting the context. In: Leahy AL, Wiley MM, eds. The Irish Health Care System in the 21st Century. Bodmin, Cornwall: MPG Books, 1998:3–36.

10. Dwyer M, Taaffe P. Nursing in 21st century Ireland: Opportunities for transformation. In: Leahy AL, Wiley MM eds. The Irish Health Care System in the 21st Century. Bodmin, Cornwall: MPG Books, 1998:237–253.

11. Department of Health and Children. Shaping a Healthier Future. Dublin, Ireland: Department of Health and Children, 1994.

12. O'Brien T. Specialist palliative care services in Ireland. Palliative Care Today 1998; VIII(1):Issue 7.

13. Department of Health and Children. Cancer Services in Ireland: A National Strategy. Dublin, Ireland: Department of Health and Children, 1996.

14. An Bord Altranais. The Future of Nurse Training and Education in Ireland. Dublin, Ireland: An Bord Altranais, 1993.

15. Commission on Nursing. Report of the Commission on Nursing: a Blueprint for the Future. Dublin, Ireland: Government Publications Office, 1998.

16. An Bord Altranais. Review of Scope of Practice for Nursing and Midwifery. Interim Report. Dublin, Ireland: An Bord Altranais (Nursing Board), 1999.

17. Kearney M. Palliative medicine—just another speciality? Palliative Medicine 1992;6:39–46.

18. Clark D, Seymour J. Reflections on Palliative Care. Philadelphia: Open University Press, 1999.

19. Donnelly S. Folklore associated with dying in the west of Ireland. Palliative Medicine 1999;13:57–62.

20. McDonnell MM. Patients Perception of their Care at Our Lady's Hospice, Dublin. Palliative Medicine 1989;3:21–27.

60 Israel

SUSAN BRAJTMAN and RUTH GASSNER

During the Middle Ages, Christian hospices offered bed and board to the Christian pilgrims and crusaders who traveled to the Holy Land. The ill and the dying who managed to find their way to them were also taken in and cared for. During this same period, the Jewish Diaspora throughout Europe was in the process of developing the institution of the "hekdesh." The word "hekdesh" originally referred to property that had been designated for charitable purposes.[1] These institutions eventually evolved to become communal shelters and infirmaries for wayfarers, the destitute, and the ill. During this period most of the sick people were cared for at home; therefore, the "hekdesh" serviced mainly those who were without family or were passing through the community. Many years later, various forms of these institutions that cared for the sick arrived along with the Jewish immigrants who were the early founders of the future State of Israel.

THE MODERN HOSPICE MOVEMENT

The modern hospice movement in Israel began during the early 1980s. The medical, nursing, and social service professions began to indicate a growing awareness of the deficiencies that existed in regard to the care of patients with advanced disease. Pilot trips to both Germany and England (which included a visit with Dr. Cicely Saunders at St. Christopher's Hospice) enabled the early pioneers in the field of palliative care in Israel to obtain valuable knowledge concerning the needs and treatment of this patient population.

Israel's first hospice, the Tel-Hashomer Hospice, opened in Tel-Aviv in the year 1983. Based on the British model, palliative care was from the beginning provided by a multidisciplinary team. In 1984, the first hospice home care service was established by volunteers in Tivon, and in 1986 the Hadassah University Hospital at Mount Scopus, Jerusalem, established a 14-bed palliative care unit. Staffed by a multidisciplinary team, this hospice has the added distinction of being the only one in Israel that has had from its establishment a nurse serving as its director. In 1986 both of these hospices initiated a hospice home care service in an attempt to meet the needs of the terminally ill patients and their families who were being cared for in the home.

PALLIATIVE CARE SERVICES

In Israel today there are 13 hospice services located throughout the country, from the Lebanese border in the north to the Negev in the south. These services include three in-patient hospices; home care services; and one integrated medical oncology and palliative care service. There are 2.6 hospices per 1 million population, providing 1.1 inpatient hospice beds per 100,000 population.[2] Home care services are distributed throughout the areas of major population, with efforts under way to improve service to the more remote areas of the country. Inpatient hospice beds are concentrated in Jerusalem, Tel-Aviv, and Haifa, with the majority of the patient population being composed of cancer patients. Plans are under way for the development of two more inpatient palliative care departments, one in Beer-Sheva and one in Jerusalem.

In Israel, hospice is not the only framework in which palliative care is provided. Terminal care is also provided by nonspecialist services in general hospitals. In certain areas throughout Israel, the chronically ill patient with end stage disease is cared for in the home and receives care provided by nurses who are part of the continuing care units of the various Sick Funds. Oncology nurses who have received additional training in palliative care and who work either in the hospitals or in the community are a resource of information and support for these units.

Pain clinics exist in a number of the major hospitals throughout the country. They are actively involved in treating patients suffering from advanced disease and offer both treatment and consultation services. Palliative care consulting teams operate in a number of the larger hospitals in Israel and are available to any ward or clinic that may require their services.

Patients who suffer from cancer or other chronic terminal illnesses may be cared for in a number of different private or public frameworks that exist throughout the country. Both the municipal authorities and the Ministry of Health are involved in the funding and in the provision of long-term institutional care, for both the physically and the mentally incapacitated. Not all of these institutions have special facilities or resources developed specifically for the provision of palliative care. The various Sick Funds are responsible for the provision of short-term institutional care for patients requiring more complicated nursing care and/or rehabilitation services. The special units of continuing care belong to the Sick Funds and care for acutely ill patients in their home who require short-term intensive care in order to avoid hospitalization. They also provide care for the terminally ill patient who is able to remain in the home.

THE ISRAELI HEALTH CARE SYSTEM

In 1918, following the downfall of the Ottoman Turkish rule at the end of World War I and the granting of the mandate for Palestine by the League of Nations to Great Britain, health care in the Holy Land was in the hands of the charitable institutions. The first of these organizations to make its stamp on the development of health care services was the Medical Aid Group of American Zionists, which within a few years became the Hadassah Medical Organization. It was soon to become the most progressive medical institution in the country, establishing a network of clinics and hospitals that brought modern health care to the population.

With the founding of the modern State of Israel in 1948, the health care system of the country came under the auspices of the Ministry of Health. A comprehensive health care system was developed that provided equal rights to health care for all, irrespective of their economic status. The Sick Funds provided the framework for the delivery of these services.

The first Sick Fund in Israel began functioning in 1912 when a small group of immigrant workers joined together to form a mutual aid health care association. Today there are four Sick Funds operating in Israel. Since the implementation of the new National Health Law in January 1995, Israeli residents pay a tax in proportion to their income and everyone is entitled to the same quality and range of basic medical services. Voluntary supplementary health insurance plans are offered by the various funds. These plans provide access to services not covered by the law. The Sick Funds receive their share of the health tax collected from residents and employers by the National Insurance Institute (a governmental agency) on a capitation basis according to the number and age of their members.

Residents may belong to whatever health fund they choose. The various health funds provide comprehensive health insurance and medical care to the majority of the Israeli population through a countrywide network of community clinics, pharmacies, hospitals, laboratories, and X-ray and specialist centers. Housebound and bedridden patients in the home are cared for by multiprofessional home care teams.

The Law of Nursing Care was enacted in 1988. Its purpose is to ensure that the elderly population in the country receive benefits from the government according to their social and health care needs. This law is administered by the National Insurance Institute in cooperation with the Ministry of Labour and Welfare, the Ministry of Health, and the Sick Funds.

In 1995, based on the recommendations of a prominent State Commission of Inquiry into the Israeli Health System (the Netanyahu Commission), a new Health Insurance Law was enacted in Israel.[3] The impetus for the reorganization of the health care system was a result of changes in consumer needs and demands and an increase in the costs of providing comprehensive health care to a growing population. Some of the major reforms included ensuring that all citizens have obligatory health insurance and securing the right of the insured to a law-defined parcel of health care services.

Unfortunately, the care of the terminally ill cancer patient and other needs and services related to palliative care were not included in the parcel of obligatory health care services. Terminally ill patients were not accorded a specific status, in contrast to, for example, diabetic or geriatric patients. As a result, funds are not presently allocated toward the provision of specific palliative care services for this population. Not all of the hospice programs are funded as an integral part of the health services provided by the health insurance funds. Many of the hospice programmes are funded partly or fully by the Israel Cancer Association or other voluntary associations.

Major efforts continue by the organizations involved in palliative care to have these needs legally recognized. The Ministry of Health working committees today include experts in palliative care, and it is hoped that their presence will influence the inclusion of palliative medicine in the reorganization of the services.

THE MANAGEMENT OF CANCER PAIN

According to a report from the World Health Organization, between the years 1984 and 1992 Israel was in first place in relation to other countries regarding the increase in its per capita consumption in the use of opioids for medical purposes.[4] The use of opioids for medical purposes, according to the WHO, is a reflection of the level of pain treatment in the country.[4] There is excellent availability of opioids in Israel. Cancer patients are entitled to receive a prescription that provides opioid medication for one month without any dosage limitation. Prescriptions must be written by physicians in a specific format, according to the law.

Recently the Ministry of Health announced new regulations for the prescription of opioids for cancer patients. The major reforms included the lifting of ceiling doses for all opioids and authorization of the direction "as needed" for immediate release formulations.[5]

In Israel there are a wide range of opioid analgesics available and they appear in various doses and formats. These include codeine, oxycodone, methadone (oral only), hydromorphone HCl (oral only), propoxyphene, morphine (in a wide range of oral and parenteral formulations) and fentanyl (parenteral and transdermal). Special formulations, such as high-concentration or preservative-free morphine, are not easily available in all areas of the country. There is also a need to have available more soluble forms of parenteral opioids.

Surveys that assessed the knowledge and attitudes of medical practitioners, nurses, and pharmacists were conducted as part of a quality-improvement project in Israel in the management of cancer pain. The results of the surveys conducted with physicians and nurses indicate that the major barriers to the effective relief of pain include: inadequate assessment of pain and pain relief, inadequate knowledge of pain management, medical staff reluctance to prescribe opioids, and patient reluctance to take opioids.[6,7] Data collection of the survey conducted with the pharmacists is still in progress.

These results indicate the necessity for ongoing teaching of the principles of pain management, both at the academic level and at the clinical level. Remedial interventions to improve the standard of clinical practice are currently being implemented. These interventions include the following : publication and dissemination of guidelines in the management of cancer pain in the Hebrew language, the initiation of two postgraduate diploma programs for physicians in palliative care, the introduction of formal examination of pain and palliative knowledge in Oncology Board Certification exams, multiple brief hospital- and community-based education programs, the publication of a quarterly update on cancer pain and palliative care that is sent to all family practitioners, oncologists, and palliative care physicians, and the formation of a palliative care division within the Israel Medical Association.[7]

EDUCATION AND PALLIATIVE CARE

In recent years there have been significant developments in Israel in the realm of professional education and the field of palliative medicine. However, at present courses in palliative care are not included in the formal curricula of the medical schools. The Family Medicine Department of the Ben-Gurion University of the Negev provides its students with extra instruction in palliative care. Since 1996 this same department has offered a 120-hour basic course in palliative care for general physicians. In 1998, the School of Continuing Education in Medicine at the University of Tel-Aviv initiated a two-year certificate course for physicians in palliative care. In some of the general hospitals, trainees in internal medicine, family medicine, and geriatrics receive practical experience in palliative care during hospice rotations that are included in their specialty training.

Since 1996 the Ministry of Health in Israel has included palliative care as part of the curriculum that is taught to student nurses. Schools of nursing include a basic unit requirement of 24 hours in palliative care and provide elective courses in death and dying and in palliative care. The oncology advanced nursing courses include both academic instruction and clinical experience in palliative care as part of their program of instruction. There has been interest expressed for the development of an advanced nursing course in palliative care, but presently it is at the level of discussion. In the last four years, selected nurses from the fields of education, community health, and internal medicine were sent to England to participate in an intensive Macmillan program in palliative care.

The basic principles of palliative care are reflected in the professional ethics of the profession of social work.[8] In Israel the schools of social work are located in the universities. Courses are offered in the general area of health care, plus there are elective courses available that focus specifically on the needs of the terminally ill patient and the family. The Israel Cancer Association offers in-service education courses in palliative care to social workers working in the field of oncology and for those caring for HIV and AIDS patients and their families.

The Israel Cancer Association and Ministry of Health offer professional seminars on the subject of palliative care, and most hospitals and medical centers have followed suit. In 1997–1998, the Israel Association of Palliative Care and the Ministry of Health provided for the training and development of community professional and volunteer home care support teams for dying cancer patients and their families. This program was carried out in three different towns.

Israeli authors have published, both nationally and internationally, numerous articles plus books on the subject of palliative care. *The Handbook of Palliative Care in Cancer*, by Israeli physicians Waller and Caroline, has been recommended by the WHO as a basic textbook of palliative care.[9,10] In 1996, the Hematology Oncology Clinics of North America published *Pain and Palliative Care*.[11] One of the editors, Dr. Nathan Cherney, is Israeli, and Israelis were among the various authors who contributed to this book. The *Israel Journal of Symptom and Pain Control* published its first issue in 1999, and is the first journal published in Israel that specifically addresses the problems and issues involved in the field of palliative medicine. An Israeli nurse is a member of the editorial board of the *International Journal of Palliative Nursing*.

Research studies in the fields of palliative care and pain are ongoing, and the results of many of these studies have been presented at both national and international conferences. The increasing number of participants at these conferences is a reflection of the growing interest in palliative care among all of the caring professions in Israel.

NATIONAL AND INTERNATIONAL ORGANIZATIONS

A number of organizations in Israel are involved with the field of palliative care (see Table 60–1). The Israel Cancer Association is a voluntary organization that was founded in 1952. Since its inception it has been actively involved in the following areas related to cancer: prevention, early detection, treatment, and research. It also provides telephone information and telephone support services, contributes funding toward a number of hospice services that operate in the country, and organizes workshops and continuing education programs both for the professional sector and for the public.

The Israel Association of Palliative Care (IAPC) was established in 1993 as a voluntary association under the auspices of the Israel Cancer Association. It is involved in issues of education, development of services, and public policy. Its members are professionals and trained

Table 60–1. Israeli Organizations Associated with Palliative Care

Organization	Address	Telephone	Fax
The Israel Cancer Association	7 Revivim Givatayim, P.O.B. 437,Israel, 53103	972-3-5721616	972-3-5719578
The Israel Association of Palliative Care(Tmicha)	P.O.B. 157, Kiryiat Tivon, Israel 36101	972-3-5663222	972-3-5604914
The Israel AIDS Task Force	P.O.B. 56110,Tel Aviv Israel 61561	972-3-5253053	972-3-5253071
The Israel Oncology Nurses Society	P.O.B. 613, Givatayim, Israel 53106		
The Israel Palliative Medicine Society	Family Medicine Department, Ben Gurion University of the Negev, P.O.B. 653,Beer Sheva Israel 84105	972-7-6477436	
The Israel Pain Association	Ichilov Hospital 6 Weitzman, Tel-Aviv, Israel	972-3-6974716	972-3-6974583
The Israel Family Physicians Association	Ben Gurion University of the Negev P.O.B. 653, Beer Sheva Israel 84105	972-7-6477436	

volunteers from the many disciplines who tend and care for dying patients and support their families. There are among its members laypersons who support the principles of palliative care. IAPC members are active advocates of developing palliative care services within the Health Insurance Law.

In 1996, the Israel Association of Palliative Care became a collective member of the European Association of Palliative Care. With the collaboration of the EAPC, the Israel Association of Palliative Care organized an international conference on palliative care that was held in Jerusalem in March 2000. The subject was Palliative Care in Different Cultures. The conference focused on the diversity of approaches to palliative care and examined the unifying principles that cross cultures.

The Israel Palliative Medicine Society was established in 1997. The association holds annual conferences and is actively working toward the development and recognition in Israel of palliative care as a medical specialty.

The Israel Oncology Nurses Society is a growing organization in Israel. Topics related to palliative care, and specifically to palliative care nursing, are published in its periodicals and are presented at its annual national conference.

There are a number of other national organizations in Israel whose activities are related to the field of palliative care. Among these organizations are the Israel Pain Association and the Israel Family Physicians Association. Cooperation between these associations, combined with ongoing meetings and discussions between professionals from the various disciplines, the public institutions, and the government agencies is working toward meeting the needs of the terminally ill patient and the family.

AIDS SERVICES

In comparison to other countries, Israel has a small number of people who are either actively ill with AIDS virus or are HIV positive. According to the National TB & AIDS Unit of the Ministry of Health, at the end of the year 1998 there were 2,000 reported AIDS carriers in Israel.[12] Overall, there has been a reduction in the number of reported AIDS cases in Israel within the last several years. However, there has been an increase in the number of AIDS carriers within the population. Most of those infected with the AIDS virus have contracted the virus outside the country.[12]

Both testing centers and treatment centers for AIDS exist in a number of hospitals located throughout the country. Testing may be carried out anonymously. There is a five-bed AIDS hospice located at the Tel-Hashomer Hospital in Tel-Aviv. Since the introduction of the "cocktail" treatment, the number of terminally ill AIDS patients has decreased dramatically.[13] As a result, in order to meet the changing needs of this population the focus is now on the development of more day-care treatment facilities. Depending on their specific problem, AIDS patients who require hospitalization are treated on the appropriate ward of an acute care hospital.

The Israel AIDS Task Force is a voluntary association founded in 1985 whose purpose is to provide support and assistance for people living with HIV and AIDS. It also provides information to the public about the virus and the means of preventing its transmission. The Israel AIDS Task Force maintains contact and cooperation at both the national and international level with the government bodies and organizations that are involved with the prevention, identification, and treatment of AIDS. In addition, health instruction in the schools and in the army includes discussions surrounding the topic of AIDS.

PEDIATRICS AND PALLIATIVE CARE

In Israel, most terminally ill children are cared for in hospitals up until the time of their death, and these children are usually hospitalized on pediatric oncology wards. Recently the first pediatric hospice was opened at the Tel Hashomer Hospital in Tel Aviv. The unit has 4 beds and cares for infants, children, and young adults up to the age of 20. It also provides a pediatric home hospice service. Both the unit and the home hospice service are available on a round-the-clock basis to meet any needs that might arise.

BEREAVEMENT COUNSELING SERVICES

Within the framework of the National Insurance, bereavement counseling services are available for those who require them. When a spouse or family member applies for their benefits, these services are also offered. Depending on the individual's financial situation, a fee for these services may or may not be requested. Mental health clinics provide bereavement counseling but do not do active reaching out. Those who wish to do so may receive counseling within a private fee-for-services framework. Both the hospice in Jerusalem and the hospice in Tel-Aviv provide bereavement counseling for the family members of the patients who were cared for in their units. There are also a number of voluntary organizations and support groups throughout the country who offer these services.

CULTURAL ISSUES

Israel is a country that over a relatively short period of time has absorbed a large number of immigrants from a multitude of different countries. Differences in attitudes among the various cultures toward terminal illness, death, dying, and bereavement have not been widely studied. As a result, conclusions must be carefully qualified. The differences that tend to exist between the generations must also be acknowledged. The younger generation, while being influenced by the social and cultural context of their individual families, are also those who tend to be more quickly and easily absorbed into the mainstream of society. There is the need to avoid the danger of stereotypes and to recognize the fact that each person is simultaneously a citizen of Israel, a member of some particular cultural or religious group, and an individual in his or her own right.

New immigrants have been and continue to be absorbed into Israeli society at many levels: in the defense of the country, socially, politically, and economically. Nevertheless, Israel remains a country that hosts a population that is composed of individuals with a wide variety of languages and diverse cultural and religious backgrounds (Jews, Moslems, and Christians). In the following section, three of the many different sectors of the Israeli population will be discussed in order to highlight some of the unique aspects of each different group. It is imperative that palliative care be tailored to the individual needs and values of the patient and the family in order to provide a service that is both sensitive to and respectful of the unique spheres of people's lives within their cultural and religious context.

The Ethiopian Population

Until 1977, the Ethiopian Jewish community (Beta Israel) lived in Ethiopia mostly in the Gondar and Tigre regions. During the 1980s, about one-third of the community immigrated to Israel. In 1991, most of the Jews who had remained in Ethiopia were airlifted to Israel in "Operation Solomon" and Ethiopia no longer was an active living center for members of the Jewish Ethiopian community.[14] Today there are more than 40,000 Jewish Ethiopians living in Israel.[15]

Their family structure is strongly patriarchal and is centered around extended close-knit families. Traditionally, family members lived in close proximity to each other, sometimes even in the same dwelling. Their outlook regarding key concepts may be very different from modern Western-centered perspectives—for example, with respect to time or pain.[16] Serious diseases are usually not openly spoken about. Decisions pertaining to methods of treatment and/or disclosure and discussion of the patient's illness are usually made by the most prominent male member of the family. Mourning rituals involve a display of crying and wailing. During the seven days of mourning following the burial, all mourners are invited to a mourning booth erected at the home of the bereaved family.

The Russian Population

Since the breakup of the Soviet Union in the late 1980s, approximately 800,000 Russians have immigrated to Israel.[15] The concept of hospice and palliative care was unknown in Russia, and as a result may be initially received with fear and suspicion. Patients are usually aware of their diagnosis and are involved in the decisions surrounding their treatment. Within the family, end stage disease states are usually not discussed openly with the patient. The emphasis is on hope and curative treatment. Death and mourning rituals and practices are usually those of the general Israeli population.

The Arab Population

Approximately 20% of the population of Israel is Arab, the majority of them Moslems. Within the Arab community, the majority of terminally ill patients are cared for by their families within the home. The family has both a cultural and social obligation not only to physically care for the patient themselves but also to allow the patient to die at home. The patient is hospitalized toward the time of death only if there is no choice on the part of the family. A very small number of patients are cared for within the hospice framework.

It is usually not acceptable to discuss a serious illness with the patient. Major decisions concerning treatment and hospitalization are usually made by the most prominent male member of the family or by the older sons. Fear and suspicion exist surrounding the use of opioids, and there is concern expressed about the possibility of addiction.

Among Moslems it is customary to make every effort to bury the deceased on the very day of death, even late at night. Mourning booths are put up for the mourning period of 40 days.

In some of the Arab towns and villages located outside the major centers of the country, the medical teams are less aware of the availability and need for palliative care services. The family doctor of the town or village provides the medical support, but many of the physicians and nurses are not sufficiently knowledgeable in the principles of pain management and palliative care. There is a need for improvement of palliative care services in those parts of the country in the areas of support services, delivery of care, and professional and public education.

JEWISH RELIGIOUS LAWS AND VALUES

There are many religious, ethical, social, and legal dilemmas involved in the care of dying patients. According to the Jewish religious law (Halakha), the value of life is infinite and absolute, and there is an obligation to preserve life under any and all conditions.[17] One is commanded to preserve life even if one must break another commandment in order to do so. The Halakha takes certain conditions and situations into consideration and provides rulings and guidance that deal with pain, suffering, terminal illness, and the prolongation of life. There are many acceptable interpretations of the Halakha. Within the religious community itself there may be differences in the degree to which the religious leaders are involved in the decisions concerning the treatment of the terminally ill patient.

In the Jewish Halakha there is a definition for almost every concept. The patient is defined as a person who is in pain because of illness or from injury, whether the illness is general and serious or whether the injury is localized.[18] Even the patient's role is defined. The Halakha provides detailed guidelines concerning specific types of diseases and their treatments. For example, a tube-fed patient or one fed by gastrostomy does not say the blessing over food because he does not enjoy it, but it is good for him to hear the blessing over food from another person.

The Halakha deals with the subjects of decision making and informing the patient of his condition. Decision making in medical matters should be based upon the opinion of specialists most qualified to treat the patient. Final decisions concerning the prolongation of life should be taken by three persons: the doctor, the patient, and the rabbi.[19]

The decision to inform the patient of his condition should be based on moral, factual, and Halakhic considerations. It is necessary to decide who is authorized to tell the patient the truth and in what manner this should be done. There is a moral obligation to tell the patient the truth based on the person's basic right to know, mutual respect, and the right of free choice. The patient must also be accorded the opportunity to prepare for death by drawing up a testament, by confession, repentance, and prayer.[20] There are interpretations that say that if the patient's life or health would be endangered by hearing this information, it should be withheld.

Treatment by pain-relieving drugs is intended to relieve the pain and not to hasten the patient's death. However, pain and suffering are a state of disease and may be treated as any other disease despite the risk. The administration of opioids may be seen as prolonging life, in view of the fact that when the patient is relieved of pain he will feel better and may therefore be more capable of eating and drinking.[17] There are recent rabbinical rulings that have sanctioned the administration of powerful analgesics, including opioids, even if their cumulative effect may be to hasten death, as long as this is not the intended aim but the incidental by-product of the treatment.[21]

The Jewish Halakha defines the dying patient and therefore the treatments associated with the patient's care. There are laws pertaining to what is and what is not permitted in the treatment of the dying, who remains by the patient's bedside, and what prayers are to be said for the benefit of the person's soul. It is forbidden to hasten the soul's leaving the body, and therefore it is forbidden to carry out any act that will hasten a person's death.[17] Customs associated with the act of dying or the soul's leaving the body involve opening a window, lighting candles, and reciting the prayer of Sh'ma Israel.

Once death has occurred, the principles of respect for the dead and concern for the welfare of the living provide the basis for many of the laws and customs pertaining to death and mourning. The laws are clear and detailed in order to avoid confusion and provide guidance. Jewish law requires that burial take place within 24 hours unless there are extenuating circumstances. The initial period of mourning, called Shiv'a, lasts for seven days. In the home of the deceased or a close family member, the bereaved sit on the floor, prayers are recited at specific times during the day, and family and friends pay condolence visits to those who have suffered the loss.

According to Dr. Abraham Steinberg, a rabbi and physician, the Jewish position as formulated by leading Halakhic authorities can be summarized as follows:

> Any action that directly and deliberately hastens death is forbidden and is equated to murder. Hence, active euthanasia, physician-assisted suicide and withdrawal of life-sustaining measures are unacceptable. In patients who are terminal and who are suffering, it is permissible to withhold any treatment that is aimed at treating the terminal situation. Hence, it is permissible to withhold resuscitation and ventilation, chemotherapy, radiotherapy, dialysis, etc. However, any treatment that is required to sustain life which is unrelated to the terminal condition ought to be continued. Hence, food and fluid, oxygen, antibiotics, blood and the like should be administered. Pain and suffering should be treated adequately, including the use of narcotics.[22]

There does not appear to be any fundamental contradiction between the approach of palliative care and the approach of Halakha. Both approaches emphasize the holiness of life, the unacceptability of shortening a person's life, and the intensive care of the dying.[1] Recent medical knowledge about the effects of certain treatments on the well-being of the dying patient have resulted in new rabbinical rulings in this area.[21] For example, the decision to administer intravenous fluids to a terminally ill patient who is not capable of drinking is not made automatically. The decisions should be based on the results of a careful medical evaluation of the possible risks and benefits involved in order not to cause any harm to the patient.[17]

The rapid development of the modern hospice movement in Israel and the establishment of a solid base of palliative care services throughout the country is evidence of the successful integration of the philosophy of palliative care and the religious law of the Jewish people.

FUTURE TRENDS AND CHALLENGES

It may be said that a firm base has been developed in the country in the field of palliative care since the opening of the first hospice in Israel 15 years ago. This base is composed of a number of components, which include the delivery of care both in the hospital and in the community, professional education, the development of volunteer services, and the establishment of organizational structures.

However, there remain a number of significant challenges to be met. Academically, instruction in the principles and practice of palliative care needs to be included in the curriculum of all of the schools of medicine, nursing, psychology, social work, and physiotherapy. These courses should be offered both at the basic level and at an advanced level through continuing education programs. Palliative medicine needs to be recognized as a distinct discipline within the medical and nursing fields.

At the governmental level, palliative care services need to be included in the parcel of services to which every Israeli citizen is entitled under the National Insurance Law. In addition, physiotherapy, occupational therapy, and music therapy should be made available and included as part of a comprehensive treatment plan available to every terminally ill person requiring these services.

There is a need for the knowledge and services of palliative care to be made available to all chronically and terminally ill patients, not just those suffering from advanced-stage cancer. Within the framework of the hospitals, palliative care consulting services should exist in order to provide advice whenever and wherever needed.

Throughout Israel there is the need for further development of hospices, hospice home care programs, hospice day care centers and ambulatory services, information centers, and consultation services. The Israel Association of Palliative Care is currently involved in the development of policy papers that include information on palliative care and suggestions for the implementation of palliative care services in the community, in hospitals, and in institutions for the aged.[23]

There is a need to make both the public and the various health care personnel more aware of the existence of the available palliative care services and the potential that they have to help the terminally ill patients and their families.

Palliative medicine in Israel has expanded dramatically in the past number of years with the development of research and education, services, resources, public awareness, and drug availability.[24] The goal remains to continue this momentum and to strive toward the day when all patients will receive appropriate palliative and supportive care.

REFERENCES\

1. Waller A. Hospice and palliative care services in Israel. In: Hospice Care on the International Scene. New York: Springer, 1997:235–241.

2. Waller A, Bercowitz M, Aronski A. Palliative care: Past, present, future. Bamah, Journal for Health Professionals in the Field of Cancer, Israel Cancer Association 1998;10:4–9.

3. Chernichovsky D, Chinitz D. The political economy of health system reform in Israel. Health Economics 1995;4:127–141.

4. Pain Research Group /World Health Organization Collaborating Centre for Symptom Evaluation. From: International Narcotics Control Board data, 1994.

5. Cherney NI, Sapir R, eds. Update in Pain and Symptom Control, Jerusalem. The Cancer Pain and Palliative Care Service, Dept. of Oncology, Sha'are Zedek Hosp., Jerusalem, 1997;1:4.

6. Sapir R, Cherney NI, Livneh J. Pain management: Knowledge and attitudes of nurses in Israel. Cancer Pain and Palliative Medicine Services. Dept. of Medical Oncology, Sha'are Zedek Hosp., Israel. The Hospice, Israel Cancer Association, Sheba Medical Centre; 1998.

7. Sapir R, Catan R, Cherney NI. Cancer pain: Knowledge and attitudes of physicians in Israel. Journal of Pain and Symptom Management 1999;17(4):266–276.

8. Organization of Social Workers. The Ethical Code of Social Workers in Israel, May 1995.

9. Waller A, Caroline LN. Handbook of Palliative Care in Cancer. Newton, MA: Butterworth-Heinemann, 1996.

10. WHO Collaborating Centre for Palliative Cancer Care. Looking Forward to Cancer Pain Relief for All. CBC Oxford, 1997:23–61.

11. Cherney NI, Foley KM, eds. Hematology/Oncology Clinics of North America. Pain and Palliative Care. 1996;10(1).

12. State of Israel, Ministry of Health. The National TB & AIDS Unit. HIV/AIDS Quarterly Report, No. 4, 1998.

13. Yedioth Ahronoth, May 7, 1999. Interview with Prof. Z. Bentwich, Kaplan Hosp., Rehovoth, Israel.

14. JDC-Falk Institute. Preface. In: Barasch M, Lipsky D, eds. Cross-cultural Issues in Mental Health: Ethiopian Populations. 1995:5–7.

15. State of Israel, Ministry of Immigration, 1998.

16. Workneh F. Issues in the treatment of Ethiopian immigrants. In: Barasch M, Lipsky D, eds. Cross cultural issues in mental health: Ethiopian Populations. JDC-Falk Institute, 1995: 37–41.

17. Steinberg A, ed. Encyclopaedia of Jewish Medical Ethics. Jerusalem. 1994; Vol. IV.

18. Steinberg A, ed. Encyclopaedia of Jewish Medical Ethics. Jerusalem. 1991; Vol. II.

19. Steinberg A. Ethical issues involved in the care of dying patients: A problem-oriented approach. Israel Journal of Medical Sciences 1987; 23:305–311.

20. Steinberg A, ed. Encyclopaedia of Jewish Medical Ethics. Jerusalem. 1992; Vol. II.

21. Jakobovits I. Death and the dying: Treating the hopeless patient. Israel Journal of Medical Sciences 1996;32:600–601.

22. Steinberg A. The terminally ill: Ethical and Jewish perspectives. Israel Journal of Medical Sciences 1996;32:601–602.

23. Cibulski O. Israel Association of Palliative Care, Support, 1998;10:1–3.

24. Cherney NI. Israel: Status of cancer pain and palliative care. Journal of Pain and Symptom Management 1996;12(2):116–117.

61 Canada

CARLEEN BRENNEIS and
SANDY McKINNON

Canada is a country of great cultural, ethnic, and linguistic diversity. Four main cultural groupings include the Aboriginal Peoples, British and French "founders" of Canada, and a composite of cultural groups from all over the world who have immigrated since the early nineteenth century.[1] A declining birth rate (25% from 1980 to 1998) coupled with record-high immigration rates is increasing the heterogeneity of Canadian culture.[2] Our "Canadian Mosaic" has resulted in a rich variety of beliefs and a potential for very different perspectives about end-of-life issues. This chapter describes the status of palliative care in Canada and identifies factors that influence development of palliative care services, education, and research.

The modern era of palliative care in Canada began in 1974 with the establishment of palliative care units at the Royal Victoria Hospital in Montreal and the St. Boniface Hospital in Winnipeg. These specialized, publicly funded units were located within tertiary university hospitals (McGill University and the University of Manitoba, respectively), thus providing an academic connection that had previously been lacking in hospice and palliative care settings.[3–6] Modeled after the British system of palliative care, and influenced by the pioneering work of Dame Cicely Saunders, the units offered an interdisciplinary, comprehensive approach to care that included attention to symptom control as well as psychosocial and spiritual support. Palliative care programs soon followed in other large urban centers. Services generally evolved from hospital-based programs to include outpatient clinics and limited home-based care.[7,8] In the last several years, many other Canadian settings have also begun to develop palliative care programs, often with improved linkages between hospitals and the community.

In the 1970s and '80s, during the initial development of palliative care, health care was strongly institution based. While Canadians normally died at home in the first few decades of the twentieth century, there was a steady increase in hospitalized deaths and a decrease in the availability of home-based caregivers during the mid- to later decades.[9] In the mid-1990s, 77.3% (1994) to 72.8% (1996) of total Canadian deaths occurred in hospitals.[9] We are now beginning to see a reversal of the trend toward dying in hospital. Growing numbers of patients, families, care providers, and planners are now advocating for increased community care and more opportunities for home deaths.

Canada's vast territory has led to many regional subcultures with differences in resources, attitudes, and ways of thinking.[1] With ten provinces, and three Northern Territories, two official languages (English and French), a mix of urban and rural populations, and the rich composite of cultural groups, it is an ongoing challenge to define common goals and beliefs. For example, the definitions of hospice and palliative care will vary between care settings. The term "hospice" may indicate a philosophy of care, a freestanding building, a unit in a long-term-care facility, or a home-based program. Although there continues to be ongoing debate about definitions, the Board of Directors of the Canadian Palliative Care Association (CPCA) currently offers the following definition of palliative care: "Hospice palliative care is aimed at relief of suffering and improving the quality of life for persons who are living with or dying from advanced illness or are bereaved."[10]

RESPONSIBILITY FOR PALLIATIVE CARE

The Constitution Act of Canada (1982) defines health care as a provincial rather than federal responsibility. In practice, responsibility for health care is shared between the federal and provincial governments. The federal government can influence health care through legislation and control of financial resources. The federal government can also impact areas of health care through regulations and activities of its various departments. For example, Health & Welfare Canada published a document in 1981, updated in 1989, with guidelines for palliative care services that included such areas as philosophy, components, staffing, and space allocation.[11–12]

Health care in Canada is publicly funded and universally accessible. The Canada Health Act is federal legislation that facilitates reasonable access to health services without financial or other barriers through the five key principles of public administration, comprehensiveness, universality, portability, and accessibility.[13] However, the Act is generally viewed as a barrier to community-based palliative care.[14] The principle of "comprehensiveness" has been defined to include only health care provided in hospitals, or by medical practitioners in any setting. Each province decides which other services, if any, will be funded. The result is that home care coverage varies between provinces, and within regions of a province.

Resource allocation is a central issue in all aspects of health care planning in Canada. The Canadian health care system must remain affordable if we are to be able to maintain our current system of publicly funded, universally accessible care.[15] As a response to growing federal and provincial deficits, funding for health care has been decreased in the 1990s. The majority of provinces are combining individual hospital boards into larger regional boards, often including community care and public health. This process of regionalization has, in most areas, resulted in a decrease of acute care beds.

The move to community-based care is seen as appropriate and fitting for palliative care.[7,14,16] Most palliative patients do not need to be in acute care hospitals, and quality palliative care can be provided in a home or hospice setting. However, the issue of transferring the cost of care from hospitals to patients and families has not yet been adequately addressed in most settings. People cared for at home may assume responsibility for the costs of medications, supplies, additional home care services, and transportation.[14] Reimbursement for medications in the home is now being addressed by some provinces. For example, Alberta and Saskatchewan will now cover the cost of palliative medications such as opioids and laxatives for patients who are designated as palliative by their physicians.

CANADIAN PALLIATIVE CARE ASSOCIATION

The Canadian Palliative Care Association (CPCA) is the recognized national organization for leadership of palliative care in Canada. Founded in 1991, the mission of the CPCA is to promote palliative care awareness, education and research, advocating at a national level for policy development, resource allocation, and support for caregivers (Table 61–1).[8,17] Each province has a provincial palliative care association that is linked to the CPCA.

A priority of the CPCA has been to develop national standards for palliative care delivery. Canadians have generally supported organizations with a strong central focus, employing a consensual approach to decision making, combined with respect for groups and individuals.[2] The evolution of early programs and the proliferation of services in the 1980s highlighted the need to develop a Canadian consensus of palliative care standards. There was a clear need for linkages between various care settings and an urgency to begin to identify common goals and appropriate outcome measures.[8] Sensitive, reliable measurements to assess if palliative care services are making a difference for patients and families are needed to further clarify and integrate palliative care services into broader areas of health care.[18–24]

In 1993, the CPCA launched a national initiative that resulted in a working document titled "Palliative Care: Towards a Consensus in Standardized Principles of Practice." Included in the document were suggested definitions, statements of philosophy, principles, and suggested standards of practice.[8] A second document, completed in 1999, outlines the present status of national consensus around palliative care.[25] The work group has reached national consensus on over 70 of the 101 items identified in the document. As expected, complex areas that require further development include definitions and models of care. Statements of philosophy and principles of palliative care were considered to be more acceptable, requiring minor modifications. Consensus building will continue until at least 2001. Once completed, the standards of practice will provide a conceptual framework for the delivery of palliative care services in Canada, and could form a template for use in other countries.[25]

Table 61–1. Contact Information

Canadian Palliative Care Association 43 Bruyère Street, Suite 131C Ottawa, Ontario KlN 5C8 1-877-203-4636 (toll free)

PRESENT STATUS OF PALLIATIVE CARE

Access to Resources

The number of people able to access palliative care in Canada has not been clearly identified. In general, it is believed that only a small minority (5%) have access to palliative care services.[26,27] The population of Canada is more than 28,847,000 (1996 census). There is a significant rural population (22.1%), spread out over large areas, particularly in the north. Rural population ranges from 17% (Ontario) to 58% (North West Territories).[28] Although there are growing numbers of Canadian programs, usually in large urban centers, providing excellent clinical care, for those in rural areas factors such as geography, access to resources such as specialists, and knowledge of and relationship with consultants affect the pattern of referral of terminally ill patients to palliative care services.[29] A study of referral patterns to a central palliative care service in Halifax, Nova Scotia, found that people were more likely to be referred if they were younger, receiving radiation therapy, or lived closer to the center.[30]

Literature on existing types and numbers of Canadian programs, model designs, numbers of patients, and costs of palliative care is limited. The 1997 palliative care directory lists over 600 palliative care services, an increase from 432 in 1994.[17] The information in the directory should be viewed with caution, since it is based upon self-reporting.[22,26] There is no consistency within the directory on what delineates a program of care versus a site of care within a program. Some services listed are voluntary organizations, while others are components of broader programs. The development of common terminology and standards by the CPCA will assist in future reporting.

Provinces have begun to recognize palliative care as part of basic health care services. Some, such as Manitoba and British Columbia, acknowledge palliative care as a core health care service. Others, such as Saskatchewan, Nova Scotia and Alberta, have developed provincial guidelines for services.[31–33] Program structures and services provided are highly variable between provinces, and within regions of provinces. Bringing guidelines to life involves integration within several existing or changing health care services, since programs include multiple levels of care, such as home care, hospice, continuing care (long term care), and acute care. As health care restructuring and regionalization proceeds, program planners face the task of developing "seamless" systems that have the best interests of patients and families in mind.[34,35]

Models of Care

Recent reports have called for the development of coordinated, integrated palliative care services as a top priority.[6,7,14,26,35] In particular, the Expert Panel of Palliative Care, in their report to the Cancer 2000 Task Force (responsible for providing recommendations on priorities and coordination for cancer to national cancer agencies), strongly recommended support of development based on regional plans, containing essential components such as home-based care, acute care, chronic palliative care beds, consultation services, and a tertiary, regional unit that would act as a learning and research center.[6] The development of secondary and tertiary levels of care are necessary for the collaborative management of complex cases and for the much-needed education and research development in this field.

Other authors have echoed the need for regional approaches with primary, secondary, and tertiary levels of care based on the needs of patients and families.[6–8,35–37] A needs-based approach will recognize that the majority of care will be primary care and will, therefore, be provided by family physicians in conjunction with the community interdisciplinary teams. Canadian physicians have adequate access to a wide variety of analgesics for pain management and do not have to contend with the daunting regulatory impediments faced by care providers in many other countries.[38] In many regions, programs must advocate for adequate reimbursement for family physicians, as they provide home visits, spend the necessary time with patient and family, work with team members, and provide 24-hour coverage.[34,35,39] Only a handful of provinces have addressed palliative care codes for physician remuneration (Nova Scotia, New Brunswick, Ontario, and Alberta). Palliative care consultants in their secondary or tertiary roles must develop strong relationships with family practitioners and home care teams, as they provide the link between various providers of care.

Provinces generally report emerging models utilizing generic services, complemented by specialized services. Model development includes essential components such as pain and symptom management, interdisciplinary teams, medical consultation, psychosocial/counseling care, spiritual care, and volunteer and bereavement programs.[14] The impact of a comprehensive, regionalized palliative care program on patterns of care for terminal cancer patients has been studied in Edmonton.[40] A regional palliative care program was established in Edmonton in July 1995 with four levels of care: home, hospice (palliative continuing care units), acute care, and tertiary unit. Criteria for admission were established for every level of care, with patients at each level having access to palliative care consultation. In 1996–97, 35% of the region's family physicians referred patients for consultation. Access to consultation, which was defined as a referral to a palliative care consultant, increased from 22% in 1992 to 84% in 1996 ($p < 0.0001$) of a population of approximately 1300 cancer patients. Location of death shifted from acute care (86% in 1992–93 to 49% in 1996–97 ($p < 0.0001$)) to the palliative hospices and home (30% and 18%, respectively, in 1996–97). Patient days in acute care hospitals decreased by 16,523 in 1996–97 compared to 1992–93 as care was transferred to the community. The results suggest that a comprehensive regional palliative care program can lead to a significant increase in access to palliative care and a decrease in the number of cancer deaths in acute care facilities.[40] Although patients with a noncancer diagnosis were included in the program of care, 92% of the total number of patients had a cancer diagnosis (excluding home care patients), and the end points of the study used the more reliable data from provincial cancer statistics.

In most Canadian regions, palliative care models must address the rural and remote components as part of comprehensive care. In her recommendations about palliative care services to Health Canada (the federal department of health), Kristjanson describes a mixed model, structured as a continuum of care weighted toward care in the home.[7] The model includes two consultative services: a centralized service accessible by telephone or written consultation, and a mobile team to provide consultation to rural and remote communities.[7] For example, in Nova Scotia, the Palliative Care Unit, located in the Queen Elizabeth II Health Sciences Center, provides tertiary-level consultative support to regions throughout the province. Nurses and physicians from the unit provide phone consultation to front-line staff and to the regional consultants (personal communication J. Simpson Palliative Care Educator, Halifax, May 31, 1999). Although hospice and a specialized palliative care unit are part of the mixed model, Kristianson acknowledges that some individuals would continue to be cared for in settings where they have received the majority of their prepalliative care, such as renal dialysis, pediatric, or medical units. Canadian communities with large populations with special health needs, such as AIDS, may have specialized units.[7]

Pediatrics

The provision of pediatric palliative care is usually undertaken in children's hospitals, oncology centers, and some home care programs. Although there are palliative care programs in some areas, availability remains inconsistent.[41,42] Care is usually provided in a pediatric setting, where staff develop long-term relationships with patients and families. Children's hospitals in Canada tend to be tertiary referral centers covering large geographic areas. Therefore, rural pediatric issues will be similar to those faced by adults with palliative care needs. An early link between palliative care and the primary health care team would allow combined expertise and resources to be available for the child and her/

his caregivers. In the rural or semirural setting, this link may be by phone/teleconference.[7,41]

PALLIATIVE CARE WITHIN THE CANADIAN CULTURE: INFLUENCING FACTORS

Care providers, legislators, administrators, and the public have been involved in broad discussion and debate related to end-of-life issues. In part, these discussions are spurred by high-profile cases addressing euthanasia and assisted suicide.[43,44] Two recent national reports have enhanced the prominence and debate about the direction of palliative care. Both reports, the Canada 2000 Task Force Expert Panel on Palliative Care[6] and the Special Senate Committee on Euthanasia and Assisted Suicide,[26] offered strong support for the development of palliative care services in Canada. Influencing factors on these discussions are described as follows:

Lack of Understanding About Palliative Care

Canada shares with many other countries the challenge of delineating the exact nature of our palliative care patient population.[16] Although palliative care practitioners are working toward a common understanding, as a relatively new area of specialization, our practitioners have yet to reach full consensus on many issues.[25] Most members of the general public and many health care practitioners are unfamiliar with the field of palliative care. Definitions that are outdated, reflecting palliative care that is offered only when all else fails, remain active in the minds of many health professionals and the public. This limited understanding is a barrier to the integration of palliative care services within the health care system.[7] The single-sentence definition espoused by the CPCA in 1998, pared down from the 1995 seven-sentence definition, reflects the wish to simplify the meaning, understanding, and acceptance of palliative care in Canada.

Aging Population

The Canadian population is clearly growing larger and getting older. The "baby boomer" population (born 1947–1964), which comprises one-third of Canada's population, will soon begin to retire.[45] Although the increase in age-adjusted cancer mortality rates is beginning to slow down, the increase in the need for palliative care is evident.[27,46] In 1999 the expected number of cancer deaths in Canada was 63,400. By the year 2010, the number of cancer deaths is expected to be 95,000, a 50% increase from 1999.[47] MacDonald[4] describes a Canadian paradox, in which we are facing growing numbers of elderly and people with chronic life-threatening illnesses, during a period of continued downsizing in the health care system, while at the same time, societal expectations for access to excellent care are rising. Canadian society, with a culture oriented to youth and health, is challenged to refocus efforts to address the needs of people experiencing pain and suffering.[35]

Relationship of Palliative Care with Oncology

In most care settings, patients with advanced cancer comprise the majority of the palliative population and many palliative care providers have a strong background in oncology. However, the field of oncology has been slow to accept palliative care into cancer centers, academic journals, and education and research programs.[4] Care of the dying has not been regarded as topics of academic interest for cancer centers, and the Canadian Cancer Society slogan, "Cancer Can Be Beaten," identifies the strong focus on cure in the "battle" against cancer.[4,7]

Many authors argue strongly for better articulation between the disciplines of oncology and palliative care.[4,36,37,48,49] The structure of the Canadian health care system, which includes provincial cancer care networks, should permit the development of a fully integrated cancer care system if appropriate planning, priorities, and resources are identified.[4,48] The Expert Panel on Palliative Care, in its report to Cancer 2000 Task Force (1991), recommended reallocation of cancer resources to palliative care. To a large extent, this reallocation has not occurred.[4]

We continue to be challenged to address the end-of-life needs of the noncancer population. Many Canadian palliative care programs have intentionally avoided a formal connection with oncology in order to maintain accessibility for people with noncancer diagnoses. For these patients, there can be complicated issues, and the course of illness is often longer and less predictable compared to the cancer population. Furthermore, it may not be appropriate to apply knowledge regarding the physical, psychosocial, and emotional needs of people dying from cancer to those dying from a disease other than cancer. Fortunately, there is growing attention to the following questions: Who should have access to palliative care? and When should palliative care become involved with patients whose disease cannot be cured?.[4,8,49,50]

Movement to Community-Based Care: Impact on Caregivers

Quality care can be provided in the home, giving the patient further options for care and potentially increasing autonomy and quality of life. However, a shifting of care from hospital to home presupposes that care providers will be available in the home. The availability of professional care providers will depend on setting (i.e., rural vs. urban) and program. Most programs do not fund 24-hour care over a long term and there are regional differences in availability of home support.[51] Unless families are able to afford private funding of care providers, the burden of care will fall to family and friends.[27,52,53] Although many Canadian palliative programs advocate for care in the home setting, there are several potential concerns to be considered:[35,51]

- the average size of families has been decreasing since the Second World War, leaving fewer children to care for the wave of aging "baby boomers";

- children may live too far away to provide routine care;
- family caregivers, women in particular, often work outside the home;
- most terminal care is provided to elderly people by elderly spouses with chronic illness;
- people are being discharged home sooner, while more acutely ill, and this can increase the stress to care providers;
- there is a growing shortage of family physicians, nurses, and paraprofessional staff; and
- there are notable regional differences in availability of home support.

Other concerns that have not yet been adequately addressed by supporters of home-based care and home deaths, including the costs of lost wages for care providers, anxiety regarding the need to carry out unfamiliar tasks, possible exhaustion of care providers, and the decreasing prominence of church as a source of support in an increasingly secular society.[20,27,46] Another issue requiring clarity is whether the decision to plan for a home death (rather than planning for admission) changes over the illness trajectory for patients and families.[52–54]

The use of acute care beds for palliative care has been well entrenched in Canada since the turn of the century.[9] The movement toward more people choosing to die at home is requiring a shift in our expectations and socialization. It may require a review of a fundamental issue in Canadian health care previously described in this chapter: all expenses for care are covered by provincial plans as long as people remain in an acute care hospital bed.[46]

At present, there has been insufficient research into the issues and outcomes of caring for family members at home.[9,55,56] Since we are likely to see increasing demands for home-based care, in part because of economic pressures in the Canadian health care system, solid research investigating all aspects of such care is needed.

Ethical Issues: Communication, the Euthanasia Debate, and Advance Directives

Canada and the United States hold many ethical issues in common. Recent decades have seen increasing attention to self-determination and autonomy, especially in decisions surrounding the beginning and the end of life.[35] The challenge of addressing our North American attitudes to truth-telling within a multicultural society is experienced by both countries. Latimer describes "truth with tenderness" as the goal of communication, with the patient determining how much they wish to know and who should have access to their information.[43] Ideally, communication regarding the goals of care should include discussions about the use of hydration, antibiotics, and artificial feeding as well as the potential use of cardiopulmonary resuscitation (CPR). A Joint Statement on Resuscitative Interventions, endorsed by the Canadian Medical Association, the Canadian Hospital Association, and the Catholic Health Association of Canada, notes that while conversations about CPR are encouraged, physicians are not obligated to offer futile treatments to patients.[57] In practice, many treatment decisions, including no-CPR orders, are often made at a time when patients are no longer able to participate in decision making.[58] Advance directives, or living wills, are beginning to gain attention, and provinces such as Newfoundland, Alberta, and British Columbia have passed legislation to compel health care providers to follow the previously written wishes of patients in the event that they are unable to speak for themselves.

Euthanasia and physician-assisted suicide have been discussed extensively in both the professional literature and in the press.[9,43,44,59] In Canada, as in many other countries, there is little endorsement for euthanasia or assisted suicide within the palliative care community of professional care providers. A few very high-profile cases of requested euthanasia and physician-assisted suicide have led to increased public support for these practices. In 1995, the Canadian government convened a Special Senate Committee to study the issues of euthanasia and assisted suicide.[26] The Committee acknowledged in the final report that it had not anticipated a key finding that effective palliative care could be a viable alternative to euthanasia. Witnesses consistently spoke to the Committee of the need for improved access to palliative care throughout Canada for people dying of any disease, and of the need for adequate funding, increased educational opportunities, and more research into pain and symptom management. The committee expressed concern that the demand for palliative care remains greater than the available services, and urged "governments, at all levels, as well as health care planners, providers, and educators to make the development of a comprehensive system of palliative care in Canada a priority" (1995, p. 23).

Since most Canadians remain unfamiliar with palliative care, or unable to access a palliative care program, it remains ethically untenable to consider euthanasia in the absence of such care.[46,59] Ethical arguments aside, the practice remains illegal throughout Canada. The Senate Committee stated that voluntary euthanasia must remain a criminal offense. They also recommended that the Criminal Code be amended to allow for a less severe penalty in cases where compassion or mercy are appropriate.[26] A report updating the Senate Committee findings is expected in 2000.

EDUCATION

There are both shared and unique issues regarding palliative care education for all members of interdisciplinary care teams in Canada. Many team members would describe their basic education as inadequate for the demands of current practice.[60–62] Continuing education opportunities of various kinds have helped to fill in the gaps as the body of palliative care knowledge grows. For example, the International Congress on the Care of the Dying, held every two years in Montreal, with the national CPCA conference held in alternate years, and many provincial and regional conferences reflect an ongoing commitment to continuing professional education in palliative care.[63] The Ontario Ministry of Health has sponsored educational initiatives over the past several years for coordinating pain- and symptom-control teams, community nursing, support for volunteer hospices and community caregivers and long-term care, as well as for family physician education (personal communication Larry Librach, July 8, 1999).

With insufficient academic faculty able to teach palliative care to nurses and physicians, basic training in the care of the dying has been underdeveloped, and universities have generally been slow to recognize and correct this deficiency.[38,64] If nurses and physicians have difficulty finding adequate training, there appear to be even fewer opportunities for team members such as social workers, chaplains, and rehabilitation practitioners to obtain discipline-specific training in palliative care.[64] The current educational initiatives toward integrated or case-based learning, with an interdisciplinary approach, may actually be more appropriate for teaching palliative care at an undergraduate level.[63] Many Canadian programs welcome volunteers as part of the interdisciplinary team and will provide specialized training to prepare them for their work.

Nursing

Providing care for the dying has been a part of nursing practice throughout the history of the profession. Indeed, much of nursing care in the early half of the twentieth century was "palliative" in the sense that little could be done to cure most illness.[9] Despite the contact that nurses have had with dying patients, training programs have historically been deficient in directly addressing the need for education about death and dying, a concern that has continued to the present.[9,29,65] In our current practice of treating people very aggressively until the point of death, this aspect of care has become even more challenging to teach and learn.[66–68]

The Expert Panel on Palliative Care, in their report to the Cancer 2000 Task Force (1991),[6] included several recommendations for nursing education:

- Nursing schools from across Canada should develop a working group to establish national learning objectives in palliative care.
- Nursing schools should ensure that palliative care is a compulsory and evaluated subject in both clinical and nonclinical components of nursing curricula.
- Nursing schools should develop faculty members with specific training in palliative care and seek funding to create chairs in palliative care nursing, with the assistance of the Canadian Cancer Society.
- A one- and/or two-year postcertificate fellowship in palliative nursing should be developed in several sites across Canada.
- Specialized programs in Oncology, Geriatrics, and Pediatrics should include palliative care training.

Although these recommendations have not yet been fully addressed, they were the "driving force" behind a 1993 gathering of palliative care nurses from across Canada who met to address key issues.[69] Following the meeting, a survey was conducted to explore the attendees' perceptions of professional and practice issues. The top three issues identified were: development of standards of practice, educational needs of palliative care nurses, and clinical care issues. Most respondents supported the need for a palliative care nurses' organization, but were divided on the question of affiliation under the umbrella of the CPCA or CANO (Canadian Association of Nurses in Oncology). The authors note that the lack of consensus may originate in concerns about palliative care being identified too strongly with cancer care. Since 1994, the Nurses' Interest Group of the CPCA has continued to advocate for recognition of palliative care nursing as a specialty within the Canadian Nurses' Association (Pat Elliot-Miller, Chair of Nursing Interest Group for CPCA, personal communication, June 10, 1999).

In Canada, palliative patients and their families may receive care delivered by nursing personnel with educational preparation ranging from advance practice degrees to unlicensed attendants with limited formal nursing education. In response to diminishing financial resources as well as a growing shortage of nurses, many care settings have elected to employ unlicensed care providers instead of licensed or registered nurses.[46] Clearly, research is urgently needed to help care planners determine the best skill mix for appropriate care, and to guide educators in developing training programs to meet the needs of palliative care patients and families. The CPCA has produced a training manual for support workers designed for use in all care settings for the nonprofessional health caregiver.[70]

Many Canadian universities offer programs of advanced practice education for either nurse practitioners or clinical nurse specialists, some with an opportunity to focus on palliative care. Postgraduate nursing education focusing on palliative care is dependent on faculty members with adequate preparation and background. Employment options for advanced practice nurses continue to evolve and will depend on several factors, such as regional politics, resources, and needs.

Postdiploma certificate programs are offered at several community colleges and range from single courses to full university credit programs. Many include a "distance learning" and/or an Internet option to meet the needs of nurses and other team members in remote areas, since it is particularly difficult for practitioners to access education in rural or remote communities that have limited access to palliative care specialists.

Medical Education

Several authors report concerns about inadequate attention given to palliative care education in both undergraduate and postgraduate medical training.[4,7,71] A recent survey of Canadian physicians that explored their understanding of cancer pain management asked the physicians to rate their medical school education in pain management.[38] Only 5% gave a rating of excellent, and 67% rated their basic education in pain management as fair to poor. Canada now has three designated chairs in palliative medicine and seven recognized academic divisions out of a total of 16 schools of medicine. However, a recent survey of all 16 schools showed considerable variability in education programs and identified a need for consensus in undergraduate curriculum.[72] The authors make several suggestions for medical training, including the need for mandatory palliative care rotations, written examinations to assess knowledge and direct changes in curriculum, and an increase in faculty positions for palliative medicine.

The question of whether palliative care should be recognized as a legitimate medical specialty with a unique body of knowledge, skills, and attitudes has been debated in Canada since the mid-1980s.[71] Recently, the answer has come in the form of an agreement between the College of Family Physicians of Canada and the Royal College of Physicians and Surgeons of Canada to develop a conjoint Postgraduate Program in Palliative Medicine (personal communication, Robin Fainsinger, May 18, 1999). The accreditation process for certification of training programs has been determined, paving the way for recognizing palliative care as a medical specialty. Credible training programs are essential if we are to be able to address current deficiencies in practice, education, and research in palliative care.[35,69,71]

RESEARCH INITIATIVES

In spite of a significant increase in our understanding and ability to treat common symptoms in palliative care, there is still considerable disagreement in certain areas of practice, such as when and how to use antibiotics or hydration. Some aspects of care perceived to be invasive or "high tech" may be viewed with suspicion by some members of the health care community. There are ongoing discussions regarding depersonalization of care and futility of treatment near the end of life.[7,73] The controversy underscores the need for disseminating recent advances in palliative care research and education to care providers outside of the specialty of palliative care.

Through the last decade, owing to ongoing efforts of many researchers within Canada and elsewhere, we have begun to develop a body of knowledge upon which to base practice. It is becoming increasingly critical that evidence-based practice underpin all aspects of palliative care, from symptom management to program development, and patient, family, and staff support. Without research evidence to support policy and practice decisions, palliative care may remain unrecognized and undervalued when illness care priorities are determined.[46]

With Canada's great social and cultural diversity, many research findings cannot simply be transferred from another country without first determining applicability to the Canadian context.[74] While a number of individual Canadian researchers have contributed to the growing body of knowledge in palliative care, Canada has yet to develop a coordinated and systematic approach to end-of-life research. Research agendas and recommendations advanced throughout the 1990s by contributors to such forums as the National Cancer Institute of Canada (NCIC)–sponsored workshops, have been hampered by the small number of dedicated researchers and difficulties in securing ongoing operating grant funding.[74] The availability of financial support and the existence of role models and mentors are critical factors in attracting new researchers to the field of palliative care.[4]

In late 1998, the CPCA received a grant from Health Canada to develop an agenda for palliative care research in Canada. Within a few months, the CPCA had created the National Research Advisory Committee (NRAC), which included leading nursing and medical palliative care researchers in Canada and consumer representatives. Driving forces for the development of NRAC included an announcement by the federal government in February 1999 of plans to establish the Canadian Institutes for Health Research and the recent formation of the Palliative Care Foundation of Canada.

The Committee used three approaches to develop the research agenda: a literature review to identify gaps and priorities for Canadian research in palliative care/end-of-life issues, focus group interviews with family and professional caregivers regarding significant clinical and health service concerns, and a thorough analysis of the current status of available funding, including a national survey of key researchers.

NRAC identified several issues and priorities necessary for the Canadian Agenda for Research in Palliative Care. The following key issues were noted:[74]

- research questions and approaches in Canadian palliative care research are similar to those of other countries;
- the Canadian research infrastructure is underfunded and not currently able to ensure the timely production of useful knowledge;
- methodological and ethical challenges of palliative/end-of-life research must be addressed;
- an agenda of research priorities would be useful for the development of coherent, multicenter trials; and
- research efforts have not adequately reflected Canada's cultural and social diversity

As a first priority, NRAC acknowledged the need to stimulate capacity development through supporting senior investigators and training a new generation of researchers. Second, NRAC recommended that funding be made available in the form of operating grants and targeted requests for funding from major national granting agencies, New Idea Grants, and Centres of Excellence Grants.

The Committee provided recommendations for further research into areas including, but not limited to: symptoms, ethics, clinical decision making, communications, family and family caregiving issues, interdisciplinary team issues, health systems and services, existential and spiritual concerns.[74]

Regarding nursing research, there are many master's and doctoral students completing research in the area of palliative care. However, these researchers need to be encouraged to publish their work, as the body of nursing research in the area of palliative care is limited.

CONCLUSION

Palliative care is gaining recognition in Canada. The aging population, and the prominence of several high-profile cases of euthanasia, has brought to the forefront the need to ensure that access to palliative care is widely available to Canadians. Reports such as Cancer 2000 Task Force,[6] Senate Report on Euthanasia,[26] and Symposium on Palliative Care: Provincial and Territorial Trends and Issues in Community-Based Programming,[14] have advanced a clear rationale for universal access to competent, effective palliative care that is integrated with other health services as a priority for all levels of government and for health care educators and planners. The majority of provincial governments have recognized palliative care, through palliative care guidelines or through identifying palliative care as a core service. The certification of palliative care for physicians as a recognized specialty is an important step in increasing the availability of palliative care within the health care structure. Nursing has expressed interest in beginning the process of identifying palliative care as a nursing specialty. The Canadian Palliative Care Association has contacted the Canadian Nurses Association, which was supportive. However, the process however, has just begun (personal communication, Edna McHutchin, September 1, 1999).

The CPCA's work toward drafting national standards will provide the necessary common terminology and principle functions for palliative care programs. Health care has changed significantly in the 1990s as provinces have grappled with diminishing resources and begun to look for new ways to provide health care services. Palliative care is well positioned to succeed in a community-based model of care. The call for adequate resources in these programs of care must be heeded to ensure that palliative care is widely accessible.

The authors thank Catherine Neumann, Karen MacMillan, Joanne McKinnon, and Robin Fainsinger for their assistance in editing this chapter.

REFERENCES

1. The Canadian Encyclopedia, 2nd ed. Edmonton: Hurtig Publishers, 1988.

2. Purvis A. The changing tapestry. Time 1999;154(21):30–44.

3. Doyle D, Hanks G, MacDonald N. Introduction. In: Doyle D, Hanks G, MacDonald N, eds. Oxford Textbook of Palliative Medicine pp 3–8. New York: Oxford University Press, 1998:3–8.

4. MacDonald N. Palliative care—an essential component of cancer control. CMAJ 1998; 158(13):1709–1716.

5. Bruera E. Palliative care in Canada. Eur J Palliat Care 1998;5(4):134–135.

6. Report to Cancer 2000 Task Force. The Expert Panel on Palliative Care, 1991.

7. Kristjanson L. Generic versus specific palliative care services. Final report to Health Care and Issue Division Systems for Health Directorate. Health Canada, 1997.

8. Ferris FD, Cummings I, eds. Palliative care: towards a consensus in standardized principles of practice. First phase working document. Ottawa, Ontario: Canadian Palliative Care Association, 1995.

9. Wilson DM, Anderson MC, Fainsinger RL, et al. Social and health trends influencing palliative care and the location of death in twentieth-century Canada. Final Report to Health Canada. National Health and Research Development Program, 1998.

10. Canadian Palliative Care Association. Board of Directors. AVISO 1999; Spring 27:2.

11. Report of the working group on special services in hospitals. Palliative care services in hospitals, guidelines. Ottawa, Ontario: National Health and Welfare Canada, 1981.

12. Report of the subcommittee on institutional program guidelines. Guidelines for establishing standards. Palliative care services. Ottawa, Ontario: Health and Welfare Canada, 1989.

13. Canada Health Act, 1984, C.6, s.1, pp. 1–12.

14. LaPerriere B. Proceedings of the invitational symposium on palliative care: provincial and territorial trends and issues in community-based programming. Health Canada. Health System and Policy Division, 1997.

15. Dossetor J, MacDonald N. Ethics of palliative care in the context of limited resources: an essay on the need for attitudinal change. J Palliat Care 1994;10(3):39–42.

16. Doyle D. The provision of palliative care. In: Doyle D, Hanks G, MacDonald N, eds. Oxford Textbook of Palliative Medicine New York: Oxford University Press, 1998:3–8.

17. Canadian Palliative Care Association. The Canadian Directory of Services Palliative Care and HIV/AIDS. Canadian Palliative Care Association, 1997: Ottawa ISSN 1200–8699.

18. Broadfield L. Evaluation of palliative care: current status and future directions. J Palliat Care 1988;4(3):21–28.

19. Maltoni M, Travaglini C, Santi M. Evaluation of the cost of home care for terminally ill cancer patients. Suppl Care Cancer 1997;5: 396–401.

20. Scott JF. Palliative care 2000: What's stopping us? J Palliat Care 1992;8(1):5–8.

21. Munn B, Worobec F. Data collection as the first step in program development: The experience of a chronic care palliative unit. J Palliat Care 1997;13(2):39–42.

22. Cummings Ajemian I. Palliative care in Canada: 1990. J Palliat Care 1990;6(4):47–5.

23. Jarvis H, Burge FI, Scott CA. Evaluating a palliative care program: methodology and limitations. J Palliat Care 1996;12(2):23–33.

24. Degner LF, Henteleff PD, Ringer C. The relationship between theory and measurement in evaluations of palliative care services. J Palliat Care 1987;3(2):8–13.

25. Ferris FD, Adams D, Balfour HM, et al. How close are we to consensus? A report on the first cycle of the national consensus-building process to develop national standards of practice for palliative care in Canada. Ottawa, Ontario: Canadian Palliative Care Association and Frank Ferris, 1999.

26. Of Life and Death. Report of the Special Senate Committee on Euthanasia and Assisted Suicide. Ottawa: Senate of Canada, 1995.

27. Chochinov HM, Kristjanson L. Dying to pay: the cost of end-of-life care. J Palliat Care 1998; 14(4):5–15.

28. Statistics Canada. Catalogue No. 93-357-XPB. http://www.statcan.ca/english/consus96/table15.htm.

29. Langley GR, Minkin S, Till JE. Regional variation in nonmedical factors affecting family physicians' decisions about referral for consultation. CMAJ 1997;157(3):265–272.

30. Johnston GM, Gibbons L, Burge FI, Dewar RA, Cummings I, Levy IG. Identifying potential need for cancer palliation in Nova Scotia. CMAJ 1998;158(13):1691–1698.

31. Guidelines for the Establishment of Palliative Care Services. Nova Scotia Department of Health and Fitness, September, 1988.

32. Guidelines for Developing an Integrated Palliative Care Service. Saskatchewan Health, April 1994.

33. Palliative Care: A Policy Framework. Alberta Health, December 1993.

34. MacKenzie MR. The interface of palliative care, oncology and family practice: a view from a family practitioner. CMAJ 1998;158(13): 1705–1707.

35. Latimer EJ. Caring for the dying in Canada. Canadian Fam Phy 1995;4:362–365.

36. MacKenzie MR. Oncology and palliative care: bringing together the two solitudes. CMAJ 1998;158(13):1702–1704.

37. O'Donnell NM. A regional approach to palliative care services. J Palliat Care 1992;8(1): 43–46.

38. MacDonald N, Findlay HP, Bruera E, Dudgeon D, Kramer J. A Canadian survey of issues in cancer pain management. J Pain & Symptom Manage 1997;14(6):332–342.

39. Brenneis C, Bruera E. The interaction between family physicians and palliative care consultants in the delivery of palliative care: clinical and educational issues. J Palliat Care 1998; 14(3):58–61.

40. Bruera E, Neumann C, Gagnon B, et al. Edmonton Regional Palliative Care Program: impact on patterns of terminal cancer care. CMAJ 1999;161:290–293.

41. Davis B. The development of pediatric palliative care. 19.7.3 Development in Canada. In: Doyle D, Hanks G, MacDonald N, eds. Oxford Textbook of Palliative Medicine. Oxford: Oxford University Press, 1998:1100–1102.

42. Frager G. Pediatric palliative care: building the model, bridging the gap. J Palliat Care 1996;12(3):9–12.

43. Latimer EJ. Ethical care at the end of life. CMAJ 1998;158(13):1741–1747.

44. Robb N. The Morrison ruling: the case may be closed but the issues it raised are not. CMAJ 1998;158(8):1071–1072.

45. Purvis A. A new generation gap. Time 1999;154(21):7.

46. MacDonald N. A march of folly. CMAJ 1998;158(13):1699–1701.

47. Cancer Bureau. Laboratory Centre for Disease Control, Health Canada. Unpublished.

48. Scott JF. Palliative care 2000; mapping the interface with cancer control. J Palliat Care 1992;8(1):13–16.

49. Dudgeon DJ, Raubertas RF, Doerner K, et al. When does palliative care begin? A needs assessment of cancer patients with recurrent disease. J Palliat Care 1995;11(1):5–9.

50. O'Neill WM, O'Conner P, Latimer EJ. Hospital palliative care services: three models in three countries. J Pain Sympt Manage 1992; 7(7):406–413.

51. Grunfeld E, Glossop R, McDowell I, Danbrook C. Caring for elderly people at home: the consequences to caregivers. CMAJ 1997; 157(8):1101–1105.

52. Hinton J. Can home care maintain an acceptable quality of life for patients with terminal cancer and their relatives? Palliat Med 1994;8: 183–196.

53. McWhinney IR, Bass MJ, Orr V. Factors associated with location of death (home or hospital) of patients referred to a palliative care team. CMAJ 1995;152(3):361–367.

54. Dudgeon D, Kristjanson L. Home versus hospital death: assessment of preferences and clinical challenges. CMAJ 1995;152(3):337–340.

55. Vachon MLS. Psychosocial needs of patients and families. J Palliat Care 1998;14(3): 49–56.

56. Kristjanson LJ, Sloan JA, Dudgeon D, Adaskin E. Family members' perceptions of palliative cancer care: predictors of family functioning and family members' health. J Palliat Care 1996;12(4):10–12.

57. Canadian Hospital Association, CMA, Catholic Health Association of Canada, Canadian Bar Association. Joint Statement on Resuscitative Interventions 1994;151(8):1176A–1176C.

58. Wilson D. A report of an investigation of end-of-life care practices in health care facilities and the influences on those practices. J Palliat Care 1997;13(4):34–40.

59. Chochinov HM, Wilson KG. The euthanasia debate: Attitudes, practices and psychiatric considerations. Can J Psych 1995;40(10): 593–602.

60. Samaroo B. Assessing palliative care educational needs of physicians and nurses: results of a survey. J Palliat Care 1996;12(2):20–22.

61. Haines CS. Assessing needs for palliative care education of primary care physicians: results of a mail survey. J Palliat Care 1993;9(1):23–26.

62. Sellick SM, Charles K, Dagsvik J, Kelley ML. Palliative care providers' perspectives on service and education needs. J Palliat Care 1996; 12(2):34–38.

63. Scott JF. Palliative care education in Canada: attacking fear and promoting health. J Palliat Care 1992;8(1):47–53.

64. Kristjanson L, Dudgeon D, Nelson F, Henteleff P, Balneaves L. Evaluation of an interdisciplinary training program in palliative care: addressing the needs of rural and northern communities. J Palliat Care 1997;13(3):5–12.

65. Benoliel JQ. Nursing research on death, dying, and terminal illness: development, present state, and prospects. In: Annual Review of Nursing Research (Werley HH, Fitzpatrick JJ, eds.). New York: Springer, 1983;1:101–130.

66. Degner LF, Gow CM. Preparing nurses for care of the dying. A longitudinal study. Cancer Nurs 1988;11(3):160–169.

67. Degner LF, Gow CM. Evaluations of death education in nursing. A critical review. Cancer Nurs 1988;11(3):151–159.

68. McClement SE, Degner LF. Expert nursing behaviors in care of the dying adult in the intensive care unit. Heart Lung 1995;24(5):408–419.

69. Kristjanson LJ, Balneaves L. Directions for palliative care nursing in Canada: report of a national survey. J Palliat Care 1995;11(3):5–8.

70. Canadian Palliative Care Training Manual. Canadian Palliative Care Association, 1998.

71. Seely JF, Scott JF, Mount BM. The need for specialized training programs in palliative medicine. CMAJ 1997;157(10):1395–1397.

72. Oneschuk D, Bruera E. Access to palliative medicine training for Canadian family medicine residents. Palliat Med 1998;12:23–27.

73. Downing GM, Braithwaite DL, Wilde JM. Victoria BGY model—a new model for the 1990's. J Palliat Care 1993;3(5):287–292.

74. Report by the National Research Advisory Committee of the Canadian Palliative Care Association: Canadian agenda for research in palliative care. Unpublished. March 31, 1999.

62 South America: Argentina

CLARA MARIA CULLEN and MANUEL MARIO VERA

Argentina is a federally governed country with a total land area of 3,761,274 square kilometers and, according to the 1996 census, a population of 35,219,612. Large cities, distributed in its 23 provinces, are home to half of this population.[1] There are marked differences in health care development among regions: some regions have excellent medical facilities, while in others basic primary care is insufficient.

The health service is made up of three sectors, which are the Public Health Services, health plans, and the Medical Health System. Public Health Services comprise 81,000 hospital beds and 6880 facilities and are free of charge to the patient or involve a minimum payment. The Public Health Services exist under federal, provincial, or municipal jurisdiction. In contrast, health plans, which number approximately 300, are usually managed by trade unions. They are financially dependent on employers' and employees' dues. The Medical Health Systems comprise some 200 institutions, and affiliation is on a voluntary basis.[1] According to 1995 data, 62% of the population of Argentina has some type of health insurance through health plans or the Medical Health System.[1] The country's public health expenditure in 1995 was 1.75 % of the national gross income, or 388 $U.S. per inhabitant.[1]

The situation of health care workers in Argentina presents some particular features. For example, a graph of the numbers of medical doctors and paramedics looks like an inverted pyramid. There are approximately 150,000 medical doctors and approximately 85,000 paramedics.[2] In addition, there are more doctor specialists than general practitioners, and more doctors than nurses (0.3 professional nurses for each doctor). The life expectancy of Argentinians is 75.6 years and the mortality rate is 7.7 per 1000 inhabitants. The three most common causes of death are cardiovascular diseases, cancer, and cerebrovascular disease.[1] The incidence of HIV and AIDS in Argentina is growing every year. The first cases were reported in 1982. In 1998, 14,289 cases of AIDS were reported, but these numbers are thought to represent only 40% of existing cases.[3]

The health system in Argentina is complex and is presently undergoing major changes. The economic resources currently assigned to public health do not effectively solve the problems, and poor administration combined with bureaucracy at the professional and administrative levels aggravate the problem. As a consequence, a high percentage of the population has difficulty obtaining qualified and efficient medical care. This is most evident in patients belonging to lower socioeconomic classes.

NURSES' CONDITIONS IN ARGENTINA

It is estimated that Argentina has 8 nurses per 1000 inhabitants.[2] "Nursing staff" designates all those individuals who care directly for patients, whether or not they have the corresponding professional degree. According to this definition, there are four types of nurses practicing in Argentina, including those with a master's degree in nursing, those with a college or university degree, licensed nursing auxiliaries, and "Empiricals" (without diploma or qualifications). In 1994, there were 85,000 individuals working as "nurses"[2]: 1,000 (1.7%) had a master's degree in nursing; 25,000 (29.4%) had a college or university degree; 49,000 (57.7%) were licensed nursing auxiliaries; and 10,000 (11.7%) were Empiricals. This data indicates that there is an important lack of professional nurses—that is, those with college or university qualifications—in Argentina.

Wages are low, in most cases ranging from 500 to 700 U.S dollars/month, and many nurses must hold more than one job to make ends meet. This situation can adversely affect the lifestyle of the nurse and at times the quality of the patient care given. However, in recent years, and in spite of the unfavorable working conditions (low wages, multiple jobs, insufficient number of professionals per service to carry out the necessary tasks), nurses have shown a high level of participation and dedication to continuous training programs in different areas. At present there are 103 nursing schools in Argentina. Of these, 25 are attached to universities, eight of which award a master's degree in nursing, and 78 are nursing specialist schools (institutions of further/higher education that give training in more practical subjects than universities and award certification, but are not universities).

PALLIATIVE CARE DEVELOPMENT IN ARGENTINA

Since 1982, and due to the influence of the Hospice Movement and the World Health Organization's (WHO) Cancer Pain Program, the modern palliative care concepts began to spread in an organized manner across Argentina in both the Federal District and the Provinces simultaneously.[4–7] The development was unlike that found in Europe or the United States, because cultural and economic characteristics made it difficult to follow those models exactly. Essentially, the development of palliative care in Argentina followed three paths in consecutive and interrelated stages.

These paths are described as horizontal, ascendant, and descendent models.[8]

The Horizontal Model was the first model implemented and has had a sustained development. This model reflects the need for an increasing interest in palliative care in Argentina. It draws upon and expands "on a surface or grassroots level" motivation and dedication coming from within community and nongovernmental entities. In numerous cities, volunteers and professionals of different health disciplines assist patients in different ways: individually or in a team, single discipline or interdisciplinary teams, in institutions or at home, as paid or as nonpaid professionals.

The Ascendant Model is the result of promoting and achieving more awareness of the needs of patients with incurable illnesses and of the palliative care benefits in higher levels of organization in the community (i.e., municipalities and hospitals) by motivated professionals in diverse executive positions. The results obtained with the policy and organization of voluntary work in the private sector or nongovernmental organizations have attracted the attention of political and health authorities. The practical aspect of this model is that it provides hospitals and universities with the two most important team activities initiated and developed in the community: assistance and teaching.

The Descendent Model occurs at a planning and/or management level. Official institutions, such as health ministries or medical federations, propose palliative care programs to be implemented by and/or developed in different institutions, mainly concerned with teaching or providing clinical assistance. This model represents an attempt to share responsibilities and associated work with health authorities, professional organizations, and the community. Results for this model are mixed.

OBSTACLES TO THE IMPLEMENTATION OF PALLIATIVE CARE

Distribution of Resources

The lack of an equitable distribution of resources remains an obstacle to the provision of palliative care in Argentina. For example, palliative care as a medical specialty and medical practice is not recognized, and therefore payment for palliative care is not included in most health plans. A 1996 survey indicated that less than 10% of both medical health systems and health plan institutions would pay for palliative care services.[9] In addition, a 1998 poll revealed that only six out of 36 public hospitals in Buenos Aires have active palliative care teams.[10] As a general rule, most of the human and material resources in Argentina are dedicated to curative treatments and few or none to palliative care.

Availability of and Access to Opioid Analgesics

Since 1999, twelve different opioid analgesics have been available in Argentina (Table 62–1).[8] According to the International Narcotic Control Board, the annual consumption of morphine is increasing.[11] However, the high cost of opioid analgesics places a restriction on use.[8] Considering an average monthly income of $400 for most individuals, and the fact that some health systems only partially cover the cost of commercial preparations, these drugs remain very expensive for the average patient. Consequently, only some patients can afford pain management through the use of opioids. In addition, most of the public hospitals in Buenos Aires City do not have oral morphine or other strong opioids.[10] Because commercial products of opioids are expensive, the need for prescribing cheaper magistral medicines arises. A problem that has arisen, however, is that in some instances magistral medicines have actually become more expensive than the commercial ones.

CONTEMPORARY MODELS FOR PROVIDING PALLIATIVE CARE

Discussions about death and dying, and the different options and provisions for care at the end of life that are available, are infrequently held either in the professional teaching setting or in the media in Argentina. However, the great diversity of the health system resources in different regions has determined different ways to provide palliative care at this time.[12–15]

There are approximately 25 to 30 active palliative care teams throughout the country. Team structure varies depending on the characteristics of each institution as well as other factors. In general, teams have a predominance of doctors over nurses and psychosocial professionals. This also occurs in other specialized fields, as there are few general-practice doctors compared to the number of specialists, and fewer nurses compared to the overall number of doctors. Teams can include two or more disciplines, depending on the availability of professionals in each area; all have at least one doctor. Nurses, psychologists, social workers, pharmacists, volunteers, and chaplains are added to the team depending on their availability. Most teams consist of part-time dedicated palliative care professionals. Very few of these professionals are able to work full-time in palliative care, because they cannot afford to live on the low remuneration received. Some team members are paid; some work "ad honorem." Few health systems pay fees for palliative care services, and most of the remunerated teams have inadequate funding. In the public system teams, a high percentage of professionals work ad honorem.

Teams in the country are at different stages of development, with some in the

Table 62–1. Opioids Available in Argentina since 1999

Morphine	Codeine	Buprenorphine
Hydromorphone	Hydrocodone	Nalbuphine
Oxycodone	Dextropropoxyphene	
Methadone	Tramadol	
Fentanyl		
Pethidine		

beginning stages and others fully implemented. There is an increase in the number of teams in the development and implemented stages, and also an increase in the number of professionals interested in creating new palliative care teams. All teams teach within their institutions and frequently lend a hand in meeting teaching needs outside of their institutions. Research in palliative care is in the initial phases of development in Argentina, but there is a growing awareness among several palliative care teams of the importance and need to generate local data. In this way the palliative care needs of the local population can be better met. Some collaborative national and international research is also being done.

Most of the team's work is dedicated to cancer patients, but lately the scope has widened to include patients with AIDS and other chronic and/or degenerative diseases. In addition, there are a larger number of palliative care teams treating adult patients compared with those who treat pediatric patients. There are two pediatric teams in the city of Buenos Aires, and one pediatric team in each of the following cities: Rosario, Mendoza, and Neuquén. There are a few other pediatric palliative care teams in the preliminary stages of development. Generally, these teams care for patients with congenital/degenerative pathologies.

Outpatient consultation services are available in all palliative care programs. Admission to the hospital, however, requires admission to a different specialty ward. At present there are no specific pain and palliative care areas available for inpatients. Day hospital services are provided in a few institutions, but this concept is still in the development stages. Home care, although practically nonexistent in the public system—exceptions are the cities of Rosario and Buenos Aires—has been widely developed in the private sector and in social organizations. The scarcity of specific home care teams and the great distances to be traveled are obstacles for the small portion of the population that can have access to palliative care. In addition, the common belief that only health institutions are capable of providing all resources and services needed in the care of the dying is also a factor in the general preference for in-hospital palliative care treatments.

SOCIOCULTURAL ASPECTS INFLUENCING PALLIATIVE CARE CONDITIONS IN ARGENTINA

Argentina is a country with a strong Latin culture. Some of these sociocultural characteristics influence trends related to palliative care.[8]

Diagnosis and Prognosis Disclosure

Upholding the paternalistic doctrine, the majority of the health community considers that it is important to keep patients uninformed about cancer diagnosis. They argue that in this way they shield the patient from the anxiety and the suffering of a fatal diagnosis. Frequently, family members filter and influence information with the same intent. As a result of this behavior, many cancer patients are not aware of the gravity of their illness and undergo antineoplasic treatment while lacking all the information necessary for making informed therapeutic decisions. Nevertheless, a more open discussion of incurable diseases like cancer, AIDS and others appears to be taking place at the individual level—doctor-patient and family-patient—and in the media.[16]

Patients' lack of information or misinformation about their disease and prognosis varies with the type and location of the facility at which they receive care. In a group of 76 consecutive terminally ill cancer patients being cared for by a community volunteer palliative care group in San Nicolás, only 25% knew of their diagnosis at the first consultation with the team.[17] In another group of 100 cancer patients receiving both palliative care and active oncological treatment at a university hospital, 55% fully knew their diagnosis and 14% had a partial knowledge of their diagnosis at the first consultation with the palliative care team.[18] This data suggests that an early palliative care consultation model interfacing cure and palliation facilitates the disclosure of diagnosis and prognosis.

Nurses find themselves at times adopting a paternalistic attitude toward patients. This is due in part to their lack of training in how to talk with patients about their diagnosis and prognosis, and in part by fear of causing them pain. The team members join in a conspiracy of silence. Because nurses are frequently asked by patients about their diagnosis, prognosis, and treatment, it is important that they have good communication with the rest of the palliative care team and are aware of what information patients and their families have been given.

Misconceptions on the Use of Morphine and Other Strong Opioids

Morphine and its derivatives are strongly associated in the minds of many patients and families with drug addiction and imminent death.[19] One of the limiting factors in achieving pain control is patients' reluctance to increase the doses of opioids. In a study involving 40 cancer patients looking at barriers to adequate pain control, two distinct patterns were noted. At the time of initial consultation, the most prevalent limiting factors in pain control were those regarding incorrect prescriptions (drugs, doses, intervals). However, by the third week, patients' attitudes (reluctance to increment opioid dosage, nonutilization of rescue doses, or noncompliance with prescribed indications) were prevalent as limiting factors.[20] Barriers to the appropriate use of morphine to manage pain may be reinforced by inadequate knowledge on the part of nurses in the use of these drugs. Studies on nurses' knowledge of palliative care demonstrate that during their undergraduate training, education on opioid use is scant. Consequently, it is not unusual to hear nurses who have not been trained in the principles of palliative care make inaccurate statements on the use of morphine. There is even less knowledge about the use of alternative strong opioids such as oxycodone, methadone, or fentanyl.

End-of-Life Decision Making

Discussions around resuscitation or the benefit versus burden of admitting a patient to an intensive care unit if chances for improvement are small or nonexistent are held infrequently in Argentina. Most patients have difficulty addressing these subjects, and few palliative care teams broach them. In addition, the use of living wills and other advance directives are still uncommon and such documents do not carry much legal weight. Some palliative care teams, however, appear to be making inroads in addressing these issues. Discussions around diagnosis and prognosis, recognizing the ethical necessity of an informed consent from the patient regarding treatment and other important decisions, appear to be more frequent and to be approached with less discomfort. For the last five years, interest in ethical issues at the end of life has increased.

Notwithstanding this increasing interest in ethical concerns at the end of life, a recent survey of young doctors with less than 10 years of experience ($n = 407$), asking about practices related to care at the end of life, indicated a strong need for ongoing discussion and education on the subject.[21] The survey included questions about nontreatment, assisted suicide and active euthanasia without patient's consent; 70.5% ($n = 287$) agreed with the decision of nontreatment, 24% ($n = 97$) favored assisted suicide, and 61% ($n = 257$) agreed with active euthanasia without the patient's consent. In this last group, 63% ($n = 162$) (39.8% of the overall survey) had actually ended terminal patients' life without their explicit consent.[21] The need for ongoing discussion on ethical issues in end-of-life care and for continuing education in palliative care for physicians in training is evident. The same need for ongoing discussion and education on ethical dilemmas faced by nurses who provide end-of-life care is clear. Some nurses express feelings of guilt and unethical practice when asked by a doctor to sedate a patient; some feel that they are being asked to practice euthanasia by following medical orders.

SPECIFIC CHARACTERISTICS OF THE PALLIATIVE CARE NURSE'S ROLE IN ARGENTINA

In Argentina there are substantial differences between the role of palliative care nurses and those in other medical specialties. For example, the palliative care nurse, among other responsibilities, participates in multidisciplinary patient consultations; takes an active part in the assessment, diagnosis, treatment, and decision-making processes with the patient and the patient's family; and actively participates in the palliative care team meetings with the patient and family. In addition, the palliative care nurse monitors the therapeutic effect and side effects of the opioid analgesics, and informs, educates, and trains the patient and family on various aspects of symptom management prior to discharge. The palliative care nurse also supervises home care through visits or telephone support.

Nurses' Participation in Palliative Care Teams

In Argentina only a small number of professional nurses and licensed practical nurses are part of a specialized palliative care team. It is estimated that in the city of Buenos Aires there are no more than ten nurses working as members of a total of six palliative care teams. This is a very low percentage when compared to the total number of nurses in our country. These nurses are frequently designated to other hospital services, and their dedication to palliative care varies. They generally work part-time in palliative care teams. The situation for palliative care teams working in the provinces is even more variable, with fewer nurses specializing in palliative care. In October 1999, during the Medicine and Palliative Cares Argentine Association's national meeting, the first census of professionals and teams in Argentina was held.

PALLIATIVE CARE KNOWLEDGE IN NURSING

There is a growing interest on the part of students and nurses in end-of-life care and palliative care. This is evidenced by their large participation in scientific and educational activities related to the specialty. Although there are few nurses with a formal and systematic training in palliative care, their desire to assist patients following palliative care guidelines is evident. In actual clinical practice, a broader range of application of palliative care medical standards is observed on the part of nurses than in any other health discipline. It is usually the nurse who focuses on the goals of care and the appropriateness or inappropriateness of certain treatments for the patient. However, in Argentina, as in other countries, there is insufficient knowledge about pain treatment and palliative cares among nursing professionals.

Palliative Care Nursing Education in Argentina

In Argentina there is no systematic palliative care education in the medical or nursing schools. There are still few training opportunities for professionals in this field. Training is generally done by the professional, on his own initiative, and it is generally theoretical with few opportunities for clinical practice. At the moment a fundamental change is occurring in palliative care training opportunities. A variety of training systems have been implemented including university or non-university courses, single discipline or interdisciplinary courses, distance education systems, or with a marked emphasis on clinical activities. These diverse types of learning methods facilitate the professional's ability to acquire or complete their pain and palliative care education. In addition, topics on pain treatment, palliative care and mourning are being included at the undergraduate level in nursing schools and universities. At a postgraduate level activities are carried out at the main educational centers in Argentina, such as: Palium Teaching Center, the Palliative Care Unit of the Tornú Hospital and FEMEBA Foundation, the Roemmers Foundation, the Pain Foundation, the Argentine Chapter of the International Association for the Study of Pain, among others. The programs offered vary in their content and structure.

Palliative Care Nursing Research

The aim of research in nursing is to develop knowledge to sustain and guide nursing practices. However, health research in Argentina is mostly carried out by medical doctors, and nurses' participation in these projects is minimal. The overall number of nurses that are involved in research is very low. The reasons for this scant nursing participation in research include inadequate training at an undergraduate level on the principles of clinical research, the need to work two or three jobs because of low wages, and the limited number of grants available for nursing research. However, as a relatively new discipline, palliative care nursing has generated some innovative ideas—for example, the creation of a fellowship for nursing research by the FEMEBA Foundation in the Palliative Care Unit of the "Enrique Tornú" Hospital. The methodology of this fellowship includes participation in presenting work guidelines, explaining informed consent, gathering information personally or by phone, entering statistical data for future analysis, and presenting and discussing results. Some research areas generated by this fellowship include treatment of constipation by using brewer's yeast as a laxative; treatment of pain with methadone; monitoring opioids and usage patterns in Argentina; monitoring symptoms and cognitive failures in patients who attend the palliative care unit; and thalidomide treatment of cachexia in oncologic or chronically ill patients.

CONCLUSIONS

In Argentina, palliative care was introduced approximately 17 years ago. A high degree of interest on the part of nurses has been evident since that time. Active participation by nurses at every event or conference where a nurse can obtain knowledge regarding palliative care reflects this interest. This interest is probably due in part to nurses' recognition that illnesses are not always curable, but that nurses have an important role in supporting patients and families at the end of life so that a patient can die with dignity and surrounded by affection. This interest has also led schools and universities to progressively include palliative care topics in courses such as "Medical and Surgical Nursing." It is predicted that palliative care will become an important part of nursing in Argentina and will allow nurses to respond in an informed way to the unmet social and medical needs of an enormous group of people in this developing country.

REFERENCES

1. Argentina. In: La Salud en Las Américas. Eds Oficina Sanitaria Panamericana. Oficina Regional Organización Mundial de la Salud. Washington DC, EUA;1998; Vol II: 24–48.
2. Davini C, Heredia AM, Malvárez SM, Muñoz SE. "Desarrollo de Enfermería en Argentina 1985–1995. Análisis de situación y líneas de trabajo." Publicación científica No. 42. Organización Panamericana de la Salud. OPS/OMS, 1995.
3. Boletín sobre el SIDA en Argentina. Ministerio de Salud y Acción Social, VII, No. 16. Marzo 1999:9–20.
4. World Health Organization. Cancer Pain Relief and Palliative Care. Geneva: World Health Organization, 1990.
5. Stjernswärd J, Colleau S, Ventafridda VJ. The WHO Cancer Pain and Palliative Care Program. Past, present and future. J Pain Symptom Manage 1996;12(2):65–72.
6. Saunders C. Foreword. In: Doyle D, Hanks G, MacDonald N, eds. Oxford Textbook of Palliative Medicine. Oxford: Oxford University Press, 1993:v–viii.
7. Stjernswärd J, Koroltchouk V, Teoh N. National policies for cancer pain relief and palliative care. Palliat Med 1992;6:293–298.
8. Wenk R, Bertolino M. Models for delivery of palliative care in Argentina. In: E Bruera, R Portenoy, eds. Topics in Palliative Care. Volume 4. New York: Oxford University Press, 1999.
9. Wenk R, Marti G. Palliative care in Argentina: deep changes are necessary for its effective implementation. Palliat Med 1996;10:263–264.
10. Bertolino M, Laje E, Contissa D, Vugalter B, Ponczeck B, Wenk R. Disponibilidad de opioides en los hospitales públicos de la Ciudad de Buenos Aires. II Jornada de la Unidad de Cuidados Paliativos Hospital Tornú-Fundación FEMEBA. November 1998.
11. Joranson DE, Gilson AM, Nelson JM, Colleau SM. Disponibilidad de opioides para el alivio del dolor en cancer: puntos relevantes en America Latina (monografía). Division of Policy Studies; University of Wisconsin Pain Research Group/WHO Collaborating Center, Madison, Wisconsin. 1999.
12. Wenk R, Diaz C, Echeverría M, et al. Argentina's WHO Cancer Pain Relief Program: A patient care model. J Pain Symptom Manage 1991; 6:40–43.
13. Wenk R. Los Cuidados Paliativos en la República Argentina: la necesidad de centros de asistencia y entrenamiento. Rev Arg Anest 1993; 51(2):107–111.
14. Wenk R. Argentina: Status of cancer pain and palliative care. J Pain Symptom Manage 1993; 8:385–387.
15. Wenk R, Pussetto J. Resultados de la actividad de una hot-line de cuidados paliativos. Fifth Congress of the European Association for Palliative Care. Barcelona, 1995.
16. Bertolino M, Felippo R, Leone F, Aresca L, Mammana G, Curci C, Vera M, Wenk R. Condiciones del final de vida en pacientes con cáncer tratados por una Unidad de Cuidados Paliativos. VII Congreso Nacional de Medicina 1999;S-04-01:316.
17. Wenk R, Marti G. Palliative Care in Argentina: deep changes are necessary for its effective implementation. Palliat Med 1996;10:263–264.
18. Bertolino M, Wenk R, Aresca L, Bagnes C, Rogel M, Vicente H. Awareness of cancer diagnosis in patients at the first consultation with a palliative care team in Argentina. Fifth Congress of the European Association for Palliative Care 1996;P-133:S57.
19. El miedo a la adicción: Obstáculo al alivio del dolor de cáncer. Cancer Pain Release 1998;11(3):1–8.
20. Bertolino M, Lassauniere JM, Marchand H, Leone F, Wenk R, Zittoun R. Prognosis factors in the relief of cancer pain. A French-Argentinian Study. Fifth Congress of the European Association for Palliative Care 1996; P-003:S29.
21. Przygoda P, Saimovici J, Pollán J, Figar S, Cámera MI. Posición de los jóvenes médicos sobre las prácticas relacionadas con el fin de vida. Rev Arg Med 1999;1(3):135–139.

63 South America: Brasil, Chile, Paraguay, Peru, and Uruguay

MARTA H. JUNIN

Palliative care as a medical discipline began to grow throughout South America in the mid-1980s. Pioneer initiatives of multiprofessional health teams, which worked with an holistic approach, promoted the care of dying people. These first initiatives were supported by the enthusiasm of their leaders and were able to prosper with few available resources, both inside and outside of the hospital setting. At times institutional recognition was either partial or nonexistent. The teams were small and the job was hard. Many difficulties still remain, and the need to provide skilled and compassionate care for seriously ill and dying patients is now being recognized as a major challenge in most South American countries.

This chapter addresses, from a nursing perspective, the ways in which palliative care came about in South American countries, including Brasil, Chile, Paraguay, Perú, and Uruguay. Included is historic background of palliative care in all these countries; a description of the health care systems, settings of care, and places where people die; and cultural issues influencing communication, patient autonomy, and decision making. Nursing views on these topics, availability of opioids and other resources, barriers, and religious and spiritual issues influencing end of life care are also examined.

BRASIL

Brasil is the biggest country in South America, occupying a territorial area of 8.511.965 km^2 and populated by 140 million inhabitants distributed geographically in five great regions, each one with its own cultural characteristic.The initial population was indigenous, and was followed by the Portuguese colonization and African slaves. At the end of the nineteenth century to the middle of the twentieth, there was an increasing European migration to Brasil by Italians, Poles, Ukrainians, Germans, and Japanese Asians. The official language is Portuguese. Brasília is the capital city, and governmental system is presidencialism. The economy is based on capitalism. The country is considered "in development" by the World Health Organization (WHO), and the national health system, denominated SUS (Central System of Health), includes the whole population without distinctions of race, economic situation, and religion.[1]

The Brasilian historical context in palliative care is not very different from that of other South American countries. This movement began, as in other countries, with a concern for the care of terminally ill patients where there were no protocols with specific attention to those patients. The first palliative care service began its activities in 1983 in the State of Rio Grande do Sul;[2] today there are 17 teams registered by Brasilian Palliative Care Society (ABCP), founded in October of 1997. Prior to the formation of this organization dedicated to palliative care, teams could count only on the support of the Brasilian Association for the Study of Pain, Brasilian Society of Oncology, and on the previous experience of neighbor countries like Argentina and Chile.[3]

Brasilian teams have worked in palliative care in a way similar to the other teams throughout the world. They have developed modalities of ambulatory care, home care, and care in the hospital setting when necessary. Some teams haven't attended patients at home, but there is already a movement to provide such care. Palliative care teams have received only informal support from the national health system, because palliative care is not recognized as a specialty and because it is still considered unimportant. Some trends for development in the future include the improvement of a home care public system, but this would not be specific for palliative care. Some teams that provide private care already exist, and there is a health institution in Jaú (São Paulo) similar to a hospice.[4]

In spite of the large size of Brasil, there are palliative care teams working from one point to another in the country. There is an increasing interest by health professionals in improving knowledge of their respective area. However, Brasil continues to depend on the palliative care education and training support of more experienced countries, such as Argentina. As an example of this, the Erasto Gaertner Hospital in Curitiba (Parana), and its "GISTO" (Interdisciplinar Group of Oncologic Therapeutic Support), has contributed its own experience to the regional South American teaching program called PALLIUM Río de la Plata Study Center in Palliative care. Nurses from different regions of Brasil get their university postgraduate training through this program.[4]

Relatives are not usually caregivers of the great majority of terminally ill patients, because patients are frequently sent to hospitals far away from their homes. It also means that family doctors are not involved in this type of care; rather, the main responsibility for terminal care remains with the hospital doctors and nurses where the patient has been admitted. Even though these doctors and nurses are improving their knowledge and skills in palliative care, the challenge is still great because most

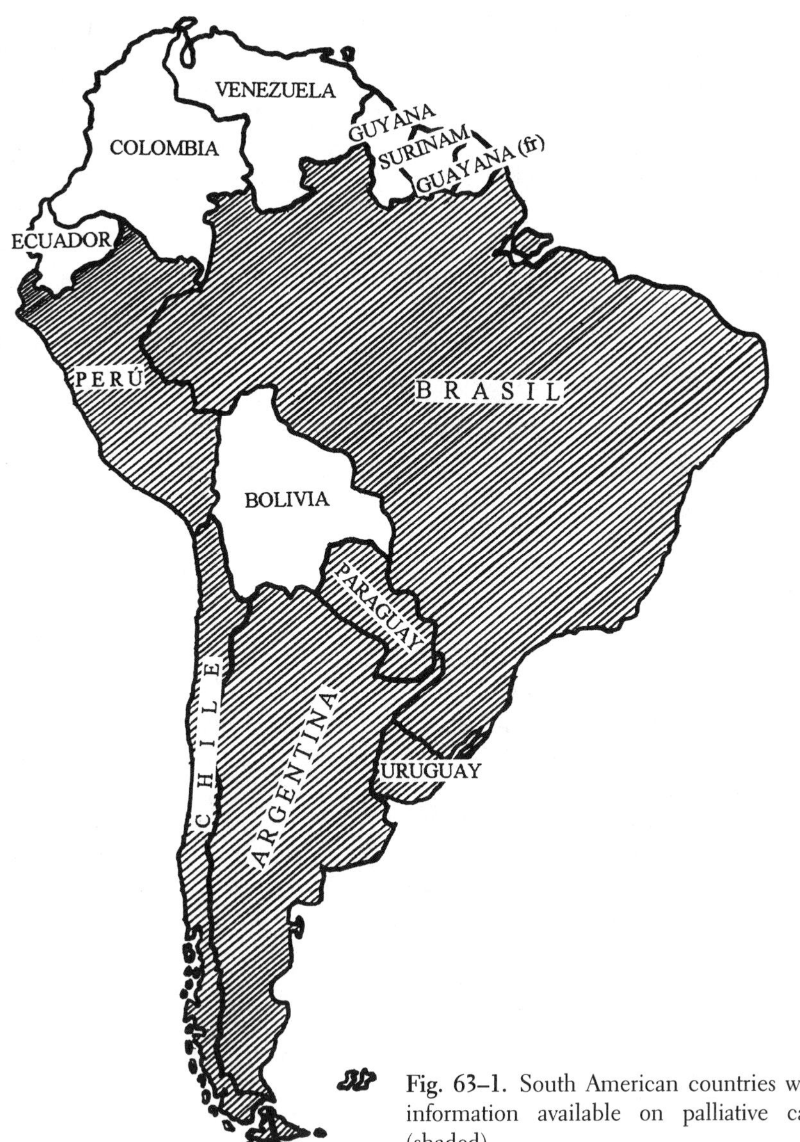

Fig. 63–1. South American countries with information available on palliative care (shaded).

patients and families do not participate in the decision-making process.

Brasil is predominantly a Catholic country, in spite of its cultural diversity. The presence of a spiritual assistant at the hour of the death is still very much needed. There is also a strong influence from African culture in the northeast of the country, with its own rituals that are mixed with Christian beliefs.

There are still some difficulties with the treatment of cancer pain in Brasil. The Health Police do not favor the importance of opioid analgesic. As a result, many cancer patients still die with their pain uncontrolled. Additionally, patients and their families have many taboos related to the use of these opioids, necessitating that the palliative care teams spend much time educating the family about the use of opioids such as morphine.

The number of interdisciplinary teams working in palliative care is being expanded in all regions of the country. The nursing interventions in outpatient, home care, and inpatient hospital settings is increasing day by day, and nurses have independent roles in this area. Nurses attend to the patient and the family, taking the responsibility of care for hygiene, comfort, administration of medicines, and other procedures. But the most important nursing task is family support and education, because without appropriate education, care of the terminally ill patient by the family at home becomes impossible.

CHILE

Chile is a narrow, long strip of land located at the southernmost part of South America. The Chilean population is 15 million people. It has a territorial area of 2.006.626 km^2. It includes a continental, insular, and Antarctic Chile, which is geographically divided for political and administrative reasons into 12 regions plus the metropolitan region (MR), where the country's capital, Santiago de Chile, is located. The population is mainly "crossbred"—descendants of Europeans and American Indians. The official language is Spanish; the Mapuche Indians also have their own language—"mapudungun." Ninety percent of the people are Catholic. The metropolitan region involves 40% of the total population (6 million habitants). However, the rural population has been decreasing.[5]

Despite a rapid growth in the country economy during the last several years, there has also been an increase in the inequality of incomes, which creates important differences in people's lives. In addition, the population is aging, with a life expectancy of 75 years. This indicates to the health sector the need to assure services such as disease prevention, recuperation, rehabilitation, and palliative care for older people. Deaths by cardiovascular diseases are the most frequent, followed by tumors, traumas, poison, and lung diseases. Cancer and AIDS, plus the causes of many traumas and cerebral vascular diseases, must be the most important concerns of the Chilean palliative care movement.

Palliative Care and Pain Relief National Program

The first initiative of palliative care in Chile goes back to 1990. Several interdisciplinary teams organized the "special local program" in their respective health centers. Later, each one of them was consolidated as "motor team"—the driving force of the future National Programme. Supported by the Chilean chapter of the International Association for the Study of Pain (IASP), this program developed an outreach experience, with national seminars and events on the subject of palliative care. The aim was to wake up awareness in the health sector, which had been indifferent until that time. These pioneer groups have organized together, reviewed the international literature, and revised all similar programs in other countries. A higher level of interest from the Health Ministry/Ministerio de Salud (MINSAL) regarding palliative care was sparked and a wider meeting was called for in 1994. At this time, a Ministry resolution resulted in the formation of a National Commission, with representatives from all sectors and regions of the country with the aim of addressing the problems of terminally ill people and describing the situation and the standards to be used as a guide to all health teams of both Public and Private Sectors.[6]

In 1995, the "Pain Relief and Palliative Care National Programme"/Programa Nacional de Alivio del Dolor y Cuidados Paliativos (PAD y CP) was officially recognized for cancer patients. The First National Meeting Programme resulted in a two-year study project to evaluate the use of morphine and codeine, neither of which is available in the public system in Chile.

In 1996, five existing Health Primary Services/Servicio de Salud (SS) were consolidated as Palliative Care Programmes. The Second National Meeting will analyze the development level of the palliative care programs in each one of the 28 SS. The clinical skills of nurses in the PAD y CP will be evaluated. Efforts have begun to elicit the support of local authorities and financial resources for the public SS to help increase the number of patients. The costs of coverage of the program have been estimated.

In 1997, standards for the program were introduced to the Juridical Accessory Departments of MINSAL for its reviews and approval. Simultaneously a study of the needs and resources of PAD y CP presented a proposal to the Health National Fund/Fondo Nacional de Salud (FONASA) for its financial support. Five SS were proposed to start this process. Also, an official Chilean Journal of Palliative Care on Terminal Cancer was begun as a way to maintain the constant communication between the services of public health in the country, given the large distances and geographic differences.

By 1998, five Health Primary Services had received the financial support of FONASA for 5,800 patients in Palliative Care. In the Third National Meeting, the programs were evaluated and strategies were designed for local and regional development with the presence of local authorities and MINSAL. Eleven other centers of PAD y CP were proposed to receive the support of FONASA. A Technical General standard, to be applied on the Public Health System as a guide for the Private Health System, was approved.[7]

By 1999, there were 16 accredited centers, with a national coverage of 50% of all terminally ill cancer patients and support for 14,880 patients in palliative care at an approximate cost in U.S. dollars of $46 patient/monthly. The global national coverage, including accredited centers, is 40% in all territories after three years of consolidation. The morphine consumption in the country is now about 38 kg. MINSAL has recognized PAD y CP as a program of high social and medical importance, with high quality, proven effectiveness, and satisfaction by users.

All of the SS have a palliative care team consisting of a doctor, a pharmacist, a nurse, and volunteers. The nurse plans the organization and continuing home care, self-care patient education, volunteer use, and training of colleagues. The volunteers are coordinated by the nurse, and they visit patients at home as a link between the primary center and a home. The pharmacist's role is to prepare the oral magistral opioid formula. The primary team receives annual training from the Palliative Care Education Programme, resulting in the higher level of dedication and skill that SS primary teams bring to terminally ill patients. There is different training for secondary- and tertiary-level teams who refer to this program.

For the year 2000, it is projected that 15 more centers will be accredited, creating a total of 31 accredited centers in the national territory. The financial support of these additional centers has been approved. This is a clear example of the constant development of palliative care in a Latin American country with support from the Health System administration.

PARAGUAY

Paraguay is a country with a territorial area of 406.752 km^2. The population is 3.1 million—most descendants of "Guaraní" Indians and Spanish conquerors. The capital city is Asunción and the official languages are Spanish and "Guaraní." The Paraguay River runs north to south and divides the country into two regions: the western and the eastern—the latter having a denser population.

Paraguay's first initiative in palliative care was born in the National Cancer Institute, situated in Capiatá, a city near Asunción. Some doctors saw the need to address the growing increase in the number of sick people in the terminal stage of disease, and the absence of attention to their needs by basic care services. These motivated doctors worked for the creation of a palliative care service. The management of the hospital trusted the psychologist of the institution to coordinate the operation of the service and arranged for the use of a physical space that comprised an office, a room for procedures, and six patient rooms with a total of 12 beds. After some time, this was modified to include only one bed per room so as to provide privacy and improve the relationship between patient and family.

In the beginning, none of the team members had proper training and skills in palliative care. In spite of the refusal of some doctors to use the service among many other problems, the service was inaugurated on May 12, 1995. It received the name "Palliative Care Unit," and now is known as the Department of Palliative Care and Medical Clinic. The initial staff was composed of a psychologist as the coordinator, a third-year resident doctor, and five auxiliary nurses, and had the support of doctors for interdisciplinary consultation (radiation oncologist, surgeon, clinicians, etc.). This group of professionals evaluates the patients to determine who can be considered terminally ill. This service is the only one in the country that deals with terminal care, and also it does not appear in any plan or program of the Ministry of Public Health and Social Welfare.[8]

From the beginning, interdisciplinary meetings were held twice a month to reinforce collaboration among staff. The clinical skills of the nursing staff was performed through workshops initiated by doctors, and members of the team were sent to train in palliative care centers in Argentina and Brasil, to carry out university postgraduate course run by PALLIUM Study Centre in Buenos Aires. The nurse in the palliative care service is trained in the administration of morphine and symptom management. She reports patient assessment data to other members of the team—for example, physical complaints, fears, or any personal or familiar conflict. The present staff comprises seven auxiliary nurses supervised by a registered nurse.

Although opioids can be easily found in the capital city, prescriptions for controlled substances require four copies. Ready availability of opioids is not true for the inner country; therefore, people in pain must come to the capital city to get opioid medications for pain relief. The most used opioid is morphine (ampoules and syrup), because of its effectiveness and cost. Morphine pills are very expensive. The ampoule is used via subcutaneous injection or through the use of a subcutaneous winged needle which is left in place for intermittent infusion for one or two weeks.

Because of cultural barriers, most doctors have difficulty in communicating with the patient regarding his or her cancer disease and terminal status. The doctor usually informs the family, but the relatives often desire to protect the patient from knowing the truth. The patient progressively loses his autonomy and the family makes the decisions without the patient's explicit consent. In an attempt to change this situation, the palliative care team now runs weekly workshops and support groups with the families and the patients, where they speak about subjects such as feelings, myths of morphine, doubts and fears about death, and any worries that the family or the patient have.

The predominant religion in Paraguay is Catholicism. Most people have a deep faith, so the spiritual aspect of care is very important to terminally ill patients. A person who realizes that he or she is terminally ill may lean a lot on religion, as does the family. As a result, most patients prefer to spend their last days at home, surrounded by relatives. In addition, confession to a Catholic priest may be very important at this time, since in Paraguayan culture many patients think that illness is a punishment of God and that only God can grant salvation, relief, and even healing.

With respect to the place where people die, the situation is changing. Because most of the patients who come to a palliative care service arrive from the rural areas of the country, they prefer to stay in the hospital, where they may feel safer because of the presence of staff. They have added spiritual support to the palliative care service, since these patients do not have a home care service to ensure that they will be cared for in their homes. In 1995, 23% of the patients who died did so at the hospital palliative care service and 77% died at home. In 1998, 35% of the patients who died did so inside the service and 65% died at their homes.[8] Some family doctors working outside the palliative care service try to convince patients to be admitted, believing patients will get better care than they would at home. This is a result of what they have been able to see when they visit the National Cancer Institute Palliative Care Department. However, this means a new challenge for the team: to convince others that home care is a good option to fulfil the philosophy of palliative care.

PERÚ

Perú is a country with a territorial area of 1.285.222 km^2 and 26 million inhabitants. The Incas were the most prevelant native population, with the Spanish conquerors and black Africans arriving later, resulting in a mixture of races. There are three geographical regions with distinctive characteristics: the coast, the mountain range, and the Amazonian. People from each of these regions are clearly different in terms of culture and beliefs. The capital city is Lima, and the government's system is a constitutional republic, with 24 political division departments and a province. The official languages are Spanish and Quechua/Aymara.[9] The National Health Service provides assistance for about half of the population with primary health centers in the community and general/specialist public hospitals. Five percent of working people have an Insurance Social System. The Private Health System assists a small percentage of the population.

The first initiative in the care of dying persons was developed in 1709 when camilians (Catholic priest congregations) built the "Good Death Chapel" for the care of native terminaly ill patients (Incas, Mulattos, and mongrel people) with the active help of volunteers. This was the genesis of Hospice/Palliative Care, a religious group with few resources but tasked with providing love and comfort to ill persons at the end of life.

In 1989, the first outpatient pain clinic was created, in the National Peruvian Police Hospital in Lima. Initially the clinic provided pain relief for victims of the country's internal subversive struggle; afterward they also provided for care of cancer patients. This was the beginning of the modern palliative care movement in Perú. It is now known as the Pain and Palliative Care Service, and it has ten years of professional work behind it. It is important to emphasize that this team included a home care program in 1998 that was run by volunteers. Science and compassion are growing jointly![10]

There are other initiatives that deserve mention. Since 1995, the "PADOMI" Programme/Programa de Atención Domiciliaria del Instituto Peruano de Seguridad Social has seen to the care of patients with pain, including domiciliary care, supported by the National Social Security. Since 1998, there has been a Quality of Life Committee in the Medical Oncology Department of the National Neoplasic Diseases Institute (INEN/Instituto Nacional de Enfermedades Neoplásicas), which is a multidisciplinary team with the aim of organizing a palliative care and pain service. The palliative care service began its work in June 1999 as a consulting team for inpatients and also for the ambulatory setting. There is also a project that includes a volunteer group committed to providing home care.

Even though most patients would prefer to die at home, there are many reasons to explain why the majority of patients nowadays die in hospitals in Perú. These reasons include low educational level, lack of socioeconomic resources, fears harbored by relatives (about the development of the disease and end of life), past bad experiences, lack of relatives, and difficulty in symptom control. An informal educational family program was established with the aim of helping the family become aware of their importance and role in the care of the patient at home. Palliative care teams keep in touch with relatives by phone to offer help in case of unexpected home events.

In Perú there is a strict and rigid legislation regarding the prescription of opioids. This has been a great barrier to good pain relief, and until now there has not been a national palliative care program. The Peruvian Association for the Study of Pain (Peruvian chapter of the IASP) organized their first meeting with National Health authorities and Drug Administration National Department in February 1999. Their goal was to promote the delivery of free palliative care and pain relief, given that average family daily expenses are five U.S. dollars and a daily morphine treatment has a similar cost.

The culture inherited from the Inca Empire follows a strong principle to adore and venerate the Father Sun and to live just like him—being mild, pious, stoic, benign, and gentle. This is the reason why most people in the mountain range have adopted a stoic behavior in the face of painful experiences. In villages far away from large cities there is also a strong influence of folk medicine and quackery.[11] All of these beliefs and practices hinder dying persons from accepting medical treatments such as pain and symptom control.

To change popular myths about opioids, the Peruvian Association for the Study of Pain (a multidisciplinary nongovernment organization devoted to the promotion of palliative care) offers professional health care education and training in all regions of the country. The educational role of nurses is crucial because they are especially sensitive and aware of the importance of care for the terminally ill at home.

Catholicism is also the predominant religion in Peru, and nurses have a hard humanistic role to carry out in accordance with Catholic principles. They are the first contact when the patient consults at a Health Institution, and they usually hear and are exposed to all the family problems, worries, anxieties, feelings, and grief. Nurses recognize the absence of undergraduate education in palliative care and the need to incorporate a specific palliative care subject in their university nursing curricula. Peruvian nurses express their committment for joining forces with all Latin American nurses, with the aim of promoting palliative care in their region.

URUGUAY

Uruguay is a small country in South America with 3 million inhabitants, half of whom live in Montevideo, the capital city. Almost all the population is descendended from foreigners, mostly Euoropeans; "pure" natives practically don't exist. Most Uruguayans are Roman Catholics. Life expectancy is 70 years in males and 76.7 years in females. Cancer mortality is very high, the highest in the South American countries, causing 22% of all deaths in the country, just surpassed by cardiovascular diseases. As in Western countries, the most common tumors are lung cancer in males and breast cancer in females.

Since cancer is a leading cause of death in Uruguay, there are many terminally ill patients. Nevertheless, there are no governmental training programs in palliative care. There are two reasons for this. First, palliative care is not a priority for health authorities, either because they are unaware that it is the most holistic treatment for both patients and their families, or because some of them still think that palliative care is "second-rate" medicine and they would prefer to invest their money in newer and more expensive technology. Second, people involved in palliative care have failed to demonstrate to the health authorities the cost-effectiveness of this work, and the need to plan for more palliative care services in the future. This point is very important, because the state funds health care for approximately 50% of the population.

In the private health care sector, two programs designed for the care of the terminally ill person are home care nursing and hospice: Asociación Española Primera de Socorros Mutuos (started during the 1980s) and Servicio Médico Integral (since 1997). However, less than 10% of the population has access to them. In general, people covered by private health care (40%) have easier access to medical assistance and drugs than do the poor.

For the 50% of the population dependent on the state for health care, it is sometimes difficult to get good care in the battle against a terminal disease. The Public Health Ministry provides no palliative care teams or palliative care units in any of its health centers, and only a few psychosocial support teams. However, in the Paysandú, Soriano, and Durazno departments of the country, a procedure exists to provide training for palliative care teams.

In public health, the only palliative care unit is in the Clinicas Hospital—the University Hospital—the largest in the country (500 beds) and part of the National Healthcare system and therefore a "poor" hospital in terms of financial support. It was created in 1993 as an outpatient clinic and a Palliative Care Team at the Oncology Service. When patients are discharged, they are provided treatment and support at home with a palliative care interdisciplinary team consisting of a social worker, a psychologist, four oncologists, a geriatrician, a nurse, and some volunteers, all of whom have many problems and difficulties in performing their work because of a lack of resources.[12] Uruguayans belong to a Latin culture, where family ties are still strong. The duty of health professionals is to support the family members. In almost all cases, the terminally ill who die at home do so under the care of only a general practitioner who usually has no palliative care training.

The University Hospital is the only medical school in the country, and therefore access to the palliative care approach is possible for all medical students. There are a few lectures each year in palliative care to all students in the last year of their training. This is surely an important way to improve patients' access to palliative care in the future. Members of the hospital Palliative Care team are part of a regional organization called PALLIUM Río de la Plata, concentrated on teaching palliative care, and also involves centers from Argentina and Brasil.

Morphine is available all over the country, and the law and regulations are good with respect to opioid use. Nevertheless, morphine consumption by terminally ill patients is still low in Uruguay, mainly because of insufficient medical prescription and morphine myths in the population and among health professionals. This suggests another area where pressure should be exerted on the government to support the teaching of palliative care in public education programs.

In summary, there are still many challenges and many things to do to improve palliative care in Uruguay. The current focus on palliative care in the educational system gives hope for real change in the future.

CONCLUSIONS

The WHO has promoted clear recommendations about the urgent need for the development of effective, skilled palliative care services that are readily accessible to all. In addition, public and private organizations have articulated different programs in response to the urgent need for more education and research in the areas of pain relief and the alleviation of suffering. This has been described as a "number one priority" for health care programs.

In South America there is evidence of growth in palliative care initiatives to improve availability of opioid analgesics for the treatment of cancer pain, as well as more educational opportunities for physicians, nurses, social workers, psychologists and, at the community level, volunteers. There are multidisciplinary nongovernment organizations devoted to the promotion of palliative care services, research, and education, including national palliative care associations in many countries.

There is still a great need to develop national health policies that promote and implement palliative care as an effective and efficient way of assisting people suffering from advanced and terminal disease. Such policies must address justice in the allocation of resources for the delivery of care, increased undergraduate and postgraduate education, and research on palliative care topics, including ethics. There is also a need for promotion of home care as a low-cost option (making it an important resource for developing countries and for evaluation systems to ensure that home care is of high quality. Active participation by the entire health care system, by members of community groups, and, most important, by patients and families is needed.

Today, the majority of people in South American cities die in hospitals, and provision must be made for their care in this setting. But it is also important not to forget the Latin American traditions that identify relatives as the main caregivers. This will mean active participation of families even in the hospitals.

The field of palliative care has been a prototype in developing a model of care based on the concept of an interdisciplinary, multiprofessional team: nurses, physicians, social workers, psychologists, pastoral care providers, pharmacists, physio/occupational therapists, and also volunteers. In South American countries palliative care strongly highlights nurses'

I acknowledge with gratitude the helpful reports about the real situation in each South American country of the following colleagues working in palliative care:

- Danielle Sellmer Ramos, R.N.—GISTO, Erasto Gaertner Hospital. Curitiba, Brasil.
- María Lea Derio Palacios, R.N.—Pain Relieve and Palliative Care National Programme, Health Ministry. Santiago, Chile.
- María de Lourdes Cardozo, R.N.—Department of Palliative Care and Medical Clinic, National Cancer Institute. Capiatá, Paraguay.
- Marlene Goyburu Molina, R.N.—Palliative Medicine and Pain Treatment Service, INEN. Lima, Perú.

I am grateful for assistance in preparing this chapter to:

- Gustavo De Simone, M.D.—Medical Director, PALLIUM Río de la Plata Study Center in Palliative Care. Buenos Aires, Argentina.
- Norma Raquel Molinas Pietrafesa, Ph.D.—Department of Palliative Care and Medical Clinic, National Cancer Institute. Capiatá, Paraguay.
- María Berenguel Cook, M.D.—Palliative Medicine and Pain Treatment Service, INEN. Lima, Perú.
- Eduardo García Yanneo, M.D.—Palliative Care Unit, Clinicas Hospital. Montevideo, Uruguay.

role, and nurses are beginning to be considered as important members of the team. We must also remember, however, that the doctor's role was traditionally hierarchical and physicians maintained a paternalistic relationship with other team members, a situation that is beginning to change.

South American nurses have been a driving force in their respective teams' fight against the difficulties in providing palliative care. There has been much personal effort by individual nurses to improve their own scientific knowledge and professional skills. However, there is still much to be done to allow dying people in our region to live with dignity until the end of their lives. We South American nurses have assumed the burden of this commitment.

REFERENCES

1. Brasil. Ministério da Saúde. Secretaria Nacional de Assistência à Saúde. Instituto Nacional do Câncer (1997)—INCA Coordenadoria de Programas de controle de Câncer Pro-Onco. O Alívio da Dor no Câncer, Pro-Onco, Rio de Janeiro, 1997.
2. Schulze CMN. Dimensões da Dor no Câncer. 1ªed Robe Editorial, São Paulo, 1997.
3. Figueiredo MTA. Lista de Equipes de Cuidados Paliativos no Brasil. São Paulo, 1999.
4. Bettega RTC. Cuidados Paliativos no Brasil. Subject not published. Curitiba, 1999.
5. National Chilean Statistic Institute. Santiago de Chile, 1998.
6. Florianapolis Declaration. Palliative Care Latin American Congress, Florianapolis, Brasil, 1994.
7. Concepción Declaration. Palliative Care Latin American Congress, Concepción, Chile, 1998.
8. Millot V. Palliative Care in Paraguay. Subject not published. Asunción, 1998.
9. Universal Calendar Navarrete. Lima, Fondo Editorial Navarrete, 1998.
10. Cordero Luján R. Anthropology of Pain. Subject not published. Lima, 1999.
11. Rostworowski M. Tahuantinsuyo History. Perú: IEP Ediciones, 1992.
12. García Yanneo E. World News. Newsletter European Association for Palliative Care 1999; 35 (March/April): N2–N3.

Part IX

"A Good Death"

64 Narratives of Dying Aimed at Understanding a "Good Death": A Spouse's Story

DAVID L. KAHN and RICHARD H. STEEVES

Thinking about a good death is not something most people do. For most people, thoughts and talk about death are avoided as much as possible, except when fictionalized and trivialized in the mass media or when it becomes unavoidable due to existential circumstances of life. Practitioners of palliative nursing care, however, confront this issue every day. It is the focus, aim, and goal of good, expert practice. The point of palliative nursing care is, after all, to try to the extent possible to create the environmental and therapeutic conditions in which a dying person can experience a good death. A good death is difficult to define, however, for a good death is as complex as the good life of which it is an extension. Thus, our goal in this chapter is not to offer a definition of a good death but to convey some of the rich and multilayered facets of human experience that should be considered when thinking about dying, and how those facets affect palliative care nursing.

The overall goal of a good death is the "forest," and practice is of necessity often focused on the "trees." To add another metaphor, when we were practitioners of palliative nursing care or hospice nurses, as we called ourselves then, we often characterized our daily work as "fighting fires." With each patient and each day, there was another fire to be addressed, attended to, and put out to the extent possible. There was pain, then fatigue, then constipation, then depression and/or anxiety, then nausea, then a dry mouth, and so on; the daily work of our care and practice embraced all the subjects of this book, covered in preceding chapters. These issues, while not present for each patient, and certainly never in the same order, were the crux of our clinical practice.

The metaphor of firefighting worked on another level as well. Each fire had to be fully attended to in the present moment—pain had to be relieved and other symptoms controlled as soon as possible. Often there was little time to step back and look at the situation from a longer temporal perspective. Our clinical practice with suffering and dying people took place in the immediate present. This is true for other practitioners of palliative nursing care. In this immediacy, practitioners work for comfort. The first aspect of the good death is to make sure that a person living while dying maintains a decent quality of life in multiple dimensions for as long as possible.

The second aspect of a good death occurs at the point when the focus of the person shifts from quality of life to dying well, a subtle shift since dying well can be seen as a matter of living well until the very last moment. As an 87-year-old man, dying of lung cancer, who was an informant in our ongoing study of cancer patients in hospice, stated: "I'm going downhill now, and I don't like it. It just gets harder to breathe. I can see that eventually I'll be far enough down that hill that it will be better to be at the bottom and dead then still sliding down." Usually the focus of practitioners and that of the family shifts in the same direction in recognition and understanding of the patient's experience.

In our research, we have the luxury of stepping back from fighting fires, so to speak, into a more distanced position of participant-observer. In this role, we watch the events of dying unfold, and we document the experiences of dying people and their caregivers in their own words. We then transform the transcripts of our interviews and the notes about our observations into narratives that aim to tell the story of a single death and can be read by anyone with interest. This method is in keeping with the "narrative turn" of recent social science, predicated on the belief that narratives of illness and other forms of suffering provide access to the private and cultural life-worlds of individuals, including the meaning they make of their experiences.[1–5] This turn or trend toward narrative has been put to good use in understanding the experience of death, dying, and bereavement.[6–10]

In these narratives, the complexity of what constitutes a good death is clear; the stories are multilayered and often fraught with ambiguity and tension. While the purpose of these stories is to allow insight into and advance understanding of the complex human experience of dying, they often raise more questions than can be answered given the current state of knowledge about death and dying. For those who practice palliative care or do research about it, the narratives are an opportunity to step back and view practice, theory, and scholarship from a perspective that is longer in time, broader in framework, and deeper in reflection. In this regard, we present the narrative below. This narrative is one of more than a hundred we have collected in our research on suffering and making meaning of suffering at the end of life, aimed at understanding what is a good death. This narrative, which takes the point of view of a husband caring for his dying wife, is typical in structure in that the themes, timing, and events of the story are familiar and recognizable to us both from practice and research. Like all narratives of suffering, however, the specific details of an individual's experience are unique as lived.[2]

*Case Study: Calvin and Lucille**

April 19

Calvin is caring for his wife, Lucille, who is dying of leukemia. She had been ill for months, had gone through chemotherapy, and now her doctor has finally said she is ready for hospice care at home. She continues to receive whole-blood transfusions and platelets as part of her palliative care. Calvin and Lucille never use the word *palliative*, but they expect the transfusions to continue as a normal part of her treatment.

Both Calvin and Lucille are in their early seventies, and they have been together for almost 50 years. Calvin met his wife soon after he came home from World War II, during which he served in the Navy and saw action in most of the major engagements of the Pacific Theater. He was only 18 or 19 then, and the war seemed a great adventure. He told me that sailing through a tropical typhoon was much more frightening than the Japanese bombers.

He showed me a photograph of Lucille and him in downtown Charlottesville, Virginia, sitting on the grass at the foot of Robert E. Lee's statue. She is blond and pretty, and he is dressed in a suit and fedora in a Humphry Bogart pose. A line under the photo says simply that Lucille will soon share Calvin's name.

After the war, Calvin went to work in a dry-cleaning plant and has been working there ever since. He says he works more now that he is 70, because the extra pay will not decrease his social security check. Lucille has been working as a school crossing guard for the last 15 years. Calvin and Lucille have two grown children and one grandchild. Calvin tells me that his son had mumps late in life and is sterile. Their daughter, Carolyn, has a seven-year-old daughter. Just this month Carolyn was diagnosed with Hodgkin's disease and began treatment.

Calvin has taken constant care of his wife since she became ill. But he and Lucille have always been caregivers. They cared for Lucille's mother for years. Calvin tells me: "Her mother was sick a long time. She had a stroke and she was down five years. We went every Friday evening. After our week's work, we took off and went to the country to give her sisters a chance to have a break. So we took care of her from Friday until Sunday night, and when we come back to work, her sisters of course would come back."

Lucille has asked Calvin to watch over her when she sleeps to make sure she does not die alone in the night. A couple of times she has stayed awake most of the night, telling him that she thinks her end is near and she is going to die before morning. Calvin sleeps very little. He never goes to bed until she is asleep, and he wakes before her.

Calvin tells me he cries nearly every day: "I get like that just about every day. I even have to get out, you know, and take a walk and cry. Just get it off me. I don't want her seeing me doing it. I try to be normal around her. Do you know what I mean? I just try to be that old normal Calvin. I just talk to make it sound like it's nothing wrong. I tell her, you gonna get all right now. But she knows better than that. She knows she's going to get no better. She said she knows her time is short. And she said, 'Why do they do what they have to do to keep me living?' She wishes the Lord would take her on."

Calvin says Lucille weighed 165 pounds before she became sick, and he thinks she is in the 90s now. But he does not believe she is in pain: "I can see her weaken. She lost a tremendous lot of weight. When I look at her and see the way she frowns, she looks like she's in pain, but it's just she's wrinkling and whatnot, and I think probably that makes me think she's in pain, but she's not, but she's just going down."

The bleeding bothers Calvin a lot: "She will get up in the night because she is swallowing that blood, you know, and it's making her sick, and she gets up and goes into the bathroom and swabs her gums and everything. These swabs, she just swabs all between her teeth. There are two of 'em that's bleeding; two at the top bleeds real bad. I don't know why they bleed. It will finally ooze, start to ooze on her bottom teeth, too, and seep around her gums."

June 7

Lucille is receiving platelets, and I talk with Calvin under the maple tree in the front yard: "It is very hard for the person who has to watch his wife go down. Almost as hard as it is on the sick person. Sometimes I watch her sit with her head in her hands, and I know that she is thinking: *How long have I got to live?* Sometimes she says, 'Why have I got to go on. I am ready to die if it's God's will.' But he don't take her."

Calvin has trouble continuing at work. Sometimes at work he goes into the bathroom and cries until he feels better. He cannot stop working, because he needs to continue to pay his medical insurance. He says he needs his "medi-gap" insurance even though hospice is taking care of all of Lucille's expenses. He is afraid he will become ill and not be able to care for himself or her. "I am paying four hundred dollars a month over and above my regular insurance. They take out about ninety dollars a month for Medicare, so it's forty-five dollars apiece."

Calvin and Lucille have bought plots in a local cemetery and paid in advance for a headstone with both of their names on it. All that needs to be filled in are the dates of death. He had paid $500 for a vault for Lucille several years ago, but recently a salesman talked him into paying $300 for a better one. He says he will buy the best vault so he can buy a plain pine casket. Lucille wants to be buried in a "plain pine box, just like President Eisenhower." Nobody has explained to Calvin that vaults are not necessary in this state and he could have buried her in a pine casket without a vault.

The oncologist at the University Hospital who sent them to hospice tells Calvin and Lucille that it is "plain determination" that is keeping Lucille alive. Calvin is proud of her for this. Calvin tells me about last night: "Her body was just like it was on fire. But yet I felt her forehead, and she didn't seem to have too much of a fever. It just seemed like her body was so hot. And she moaned and groaned all night long. Every time she goes to turn, and if I bump her the least little bit, she would just scream in pain. She couldn't stand it if she rolls over or something in the bed, hit a headboard or something. Honest to God, she's getting weaker and weaker all the time, and it's just, it's just so hard."

July 26

Lucille is in the hospice unit in the hospital now. She has come in to die. Calvin wanted her to die in the hospital. Lucille looks awful. She is cachectic. She has a large lesion on her lower lip that is oozing blood and multiple purpuric lesions on her arms, face, and neck. But she is talking and making sense. I am convinced her time is very short.

*Both names have been changed to ensure confidentiality. The use of first names reflects the relationship established with both people and their own wishes in how they wanted to be addressed and written about. The appropriate university committee for the protection of human subjects approved the procedures of the research study from which this narrative evolved.

I have a brief conversation with the hospice chaplain, who is worried that Calvin may be "losing it." Calvin has been very emotional and crying in the hall outside Lucille's room. When I find Calvin and talk with him, he is upset but very lucid. "I have gone through my whole life waking up in the morning and thinking that this day is going to be better than the last one. Now I wake up, and it ain't true anymore.

"Nobody should ever say in their life that they will never do this or never do that; you never know what you are going to face, and when the time comes, if it's your family member who is sick, you will end up doing things that you wouldn't expect yourself to do. I clean her and take care of the bedpan and everything. I spend every night here sleeping on this cot.

"I don't understand why she is suffering. Jesus suffered for all of us, but why have we got to continue to suffer anyway? It don't make sense to me. I probably ain't supposed to ask those kinds of questions; we just gotta accept things with faith. I have to believe that in the next world there won't be any suffering, and maybe what we are doing now is getting some suffering out of the way so that there won't be any suffering in the next world.

"I really want her to go out easy. I don't want her to be struggling for life at the end. And I don't want her to have no hemorrhage. But I think the doctors are working really hard to make sure that she don't hurt."

Calvin says sometimes Lucille sees things and hears things that nobody else does. He believes that she is in the "other world" during those times. Her soul has moved on and left her body here. But most of the time she is still in this world.

August 9

Lucille did not die in the hospital. She went home for several days and now has returned to the hospital again. When I go to see her, I have a brief conversation with the physician who is the medical director of the hospice unit. He explains that Calvin is the major reason Lucille is back in the hospital. She wants to die at home, and her sisters want to honor her wishes, but Calvin wants her in the hospital. When a hospice nurse asked how he was doing caring for her at home, he began to cry. That is when the nurse arranged for her to be admitted to the unit.

The medical director explains that his goal is to provide a death that is not too ugly. He talks a little about the aesthetics of death. He thinks exsanguination is not a good option for the family, and therefore, he plans to continue with the platelets. But he will not continue to administer the whole blood or packed cells. He is guessing that Lucille will die of heart failure, and he will give her enough morphine so that she probably will not have to experience the angina that will accompany that. When I ask, he says he is not sure how much the family understands that these considerations will be part of Lucille's treatment.

I find her room, and Lucille is pale and yellow and bleeding from her gums. She looks tiny and thin and crumpled up in the bed. But she is awake and alert and knows who I am. Calvin is there with her. He says: "I am gonna spend all my nights up here with her. Her sisters didn't like it much that she is here. But they come in, and they can all say, well, good night, Lucille, see you tomorrow. But I'm the one who has to be with her all the time, and I would be in the hospital myself if I didn't bring her in. It was just becoming too much for me. They can care for her much better here, give her the platelets and all that sort of thing.

"Everybody comes to visit at the same time when I had her at home. And her sister brings this dog. A little bitty lap dog that whines all the time. Once when Lucille was getting her platelets, this dog jumps up in her lap. It really scared her, and now Lucille sees this dog all the time, sees it when it's not there and all. She is not thinking clear. But at home there was too many visiting and nobody helping."

As I watch Calvin, he washes Lucille's face and straightens her covers. When I ask, he tells me he helps her with the bedpan and rolls her. He bathes her and makes certain she has clean, dry linen. He seems to be doing as much and in fact the same work in the hospital he did at home. But for him, there is an important difference, it seems.

August 16

Lucille is still alive. She was sent home from the hospital again a couple of days after I last saw her. But she has returned to the hospital now, and this is where I visit Calvin and her. Calvin appears to be right on the edge of being overwhelmed by emotion, teary-eyed, and flushed. "She is really sick, and she had a really bad day." Calvin has been given lorazepam by his doctor and usually takes it to sleep. But he is taking it during the day today.

Their daughter Carolyn is coming in from North Carolina. Lucille's oncologist has arranged to have Carolyn's chemotherapy for Hodgkin's disease given here so she will not miss a dose.

Lucille is not responsive anymore. She is stretching her arms in the air, reaching out and scratching, and then resting awhile. She is having Cheyne Stokes respirations and looks agonal to me.

Calvin tells me about a conversation he and Lucille had a few days ago: "We talked about whether she was right with God. I am completely satisfied that she is right with God, and Jesus is her Savior, and she is going to go to heaven. I been praying, too, and asking for forgiveness. I want to go to the same place she is going to go, and she would want to go to the same place that I am going to go. And I said to her, whoever gets there first will wait for the other. That's what I said to her, because who knows who's going to really die first? None of us came here to stay forever. We came to die. But it's very hard to think about it."

October 4

Lucille died the morning of August 17, the day after I last visited. I have been trying to visit with Calvin for weeks, but he has been putting me off. After the funeral, Calvin went into a cleaning and remodeling frenzy. He cleared out all of Lucille's clothes and her collection of knickknacks from the basement and had a yard sale. He sold almost everything she owned. Now he is repainting his house inside and out and refinishing the floors. He is working frantically, and says he feels better when he is busy. He now has a prescription for Prozac along with the lorazepam. Calvin says he has stopped losing weight. He lost weight as his wife lost weight and weighs little more than 125 pounds now. He tells me Lucille weighed 78 pounds when she died.

Calvin tells me some of the details of Lucille's last hospital stay, but I am not sure he has the facts about hospice and Medicare straight: "Last time I had to take my wife back up to the hospital, I got a thing from Medicare saying that they were going to pay it this time but wouldn't pay it again, because I took my wife back in the hospital without the authority from the doctors having told us to come back. Medicare says they will pay hospice for 100% if you're home, but they will only pay 80% if you go into the hospital. That don't make no sense to me. I got good insurance, too, and what is that for unless you are real sick and she was as sick as somebody could get."

"Her doctor even got me a little upset there when he was going to let her go home. I told him, naturally, she's gonna say she wants to go home, whether she is able to, or should go home or not. He said she wanted to spend all her last days with me at home, if there was any way possible she could stand it. But it got to the point where she couldn't stand anything that was happening, and I couldn't tend to her. I couldn't take care of it. It was just worrying me, worrying me to a pretzel. I couldn't. I was getting weaker all the time. I was growing as weak as she was."

"At the end she got really down. She said, 'Why have I gotta live? I just as soon go on.' And I would try to say don't talk like that. But I think she had given up."

The night before Lucille died, Calvin said he knew she was going: "They'd given her an increase of medication, because they said she was in a lot of pain. I didn't want them throwing any more drugs into her, but she was in a lot of pain. I didn't want to see her suffer no more. I just accepted the fact that she was gonna go, and I just didn't want to know when it was gonna be. I just wanted her to be eased on off. Like I told her doctor, you can ease her off easy as you possibly can. Let her go on off in her sleep.

"My daughter got there. She got there between eight and nine. She came in and walked over to the bed and said, 'Mom, you feeling bad?' She looked at Carolyn and her eyes got big and bright, and she tried to reach up, but she was just so weak. She couldn't reach up to hug her. And she knew who she was. She said, 'You know who this is?' and she nodded her head. She knew it was Carolyn. But she was in so much pain, and then they turned up the medication on her. But she went on through the night. I came on home; just a little after 11, I reckon, it was. My son said, 'I'm gonna stay, you go ahead on home, Daddy, and try to shut your eyes if you can for a couple hours.' I was just wore out. So I came on home, and I knew it would be a matter of hours because they done drugged her up so heavy with morphine.

"My son said she passed away 10 minutes after 6. He said, 'I woke up at 6 o'clock, and she was still breathing then, but she wasn't saying nothing. Then I fell off to sleep for about 15 minutes.' Then the nurse came in and woke him up and said, 'I think your mother's passed.'"

DISCUSSION

The use of stories to reflect on practice has long been a tradition in nursing.[11–12] What the narratives add to nurses' understanding of treating suffering at the end of life is an opportunity to see palliative care in all its complexity. Each narrative, like the one above, is complex not only thematically but also in its portrayal of the reality of human experience as often nonlinear, nonrational, and contradictory. Certainly the story of Calvin and Lucille can stand alone in portraying that complexity, but a few comments on the story might also be helpful. Calvin and Lucille can be seen as experiencing this death on a number of different levels, as a political/economic event, as a spiritual event, and as an aesthetic event.

Politics/Economics

Because of the nature of the research question in the study from which this story of Calvin and Lucille was taken, the events are seen from the point of view of Calvin. For Calvin, the politics of his situation are manifest at the most basic level and the highest level. At the basic level is the politics of family. From Calvin's point of view, Lucille's family visits but does not help. In fact, her sisters make caregiving harder than it needs to be; from the lap dog that seems to terrify Lucille, to the fact that her sisters want a say in her care while not providing any care themselves. It is interesting that Calvin never says he is due their help after spending so much of his time caring for their mother. He seems to have taken caregiving for granted, as something he must do. He does not consider relinquishing the job of caring for Lucille to anyone else. Even while insisting she be in the hospital, he continues to do the same for her there as he has been doing at home.

It is interesting that the emotional burden of caring for Lucille at the end is lessened for Calvin by hospitalization in the inpatient palliative care unit. An inpatient setting, however, is more expensive, and thus there is a bias in the present system toward having patients stay at home; in fact, many practitioners and families believe it is inherently better to die at home, surrounded by family, than anywhere else. Recent research has noted that the economic contribution of the caregiver is both invisible and considerable,[13] and that the burden of caregiving increases tremendously in the last stages of life.[14–15]

On a larger scale, the politics of aging in the United States as it affects national policies has a large effect on Calvin. Because he is over 70, he can work full-time again without fear of losing his Social Security Benefit. In effect, being older allows him to work harder, and he feels the need for the money since Lucille can no longer work. Calvin does not seem to understand fully the hospice Medicare benefit. It is not clear why he believes he needs expensive "medi-gap" insurance. He does not understand why his wife cannot be in the hospital all the time, since hospitals are for the sick and no one could be sicker than Lucille; she is dying, after all. The Medicare regulations are not clear to Calvin (but then, how long does it take a well-educated nurse to figure them out?). Also, it could be argued that a well-regulated funeral industry would not be allowed to market to vulnerable people expensive vaults that they do not need.

The lessons in this part of Calvin's story for palliative care nurses are ones we already know but need to keep ourselves reminded of. Health-care financing regulations are incredibly complex, and we must keep teaching families over and over so they can make the best choices. The second lesson is that there are none better than us, palliative care nurses, at knowing when and how the system does not work. We have an obligation to be politically active on behalf of the people whose lives are so deeply affected by this system of rules and regulations. Families suffering the imminent loss of a loved one, struggling to care for themselves and their family member, are perhaps more vulnerable than at any other time and need professionals advocating for them.

Spirituality

In the nursing literature in cancer and palliative care, there is recognition that dying is a spiritual event for most people and that part of providing for the good death means the availability of spiritual care.[16–20] In the above story, Calvin seems to balance on the edge of a spiritual crisis but manages on his own to come back from the brink. He wrestles with what is arguably the central question in all religions: Why must human beings suffer? He answers this question in terms of faith, a faith in the joyousness of an afterlife. But his basic optimism has been shaken. He says he can no longer wake in the morning, thinking that this day will be better than the last. He does not succumb to hopelessness, however, because in the end he invests his hope in heaven.

Palliative care nurses are not expected to be experts in spiritual care, but we need to have expertise in recognizing a spiritual crisis and make referrals. Our part in spiritual care is our own recognition that the basic questions of life are shared by all of us: Why is there something rather than nothing? Why do bad things happen to good people? Why do we so badly need to have life be meaningful? What seems to be common to all spiritual thought is that everyone shares these questions. No matter what answers we have found or have failed to find, we are all in this together. The shared questions make us a single family. Our patients and families need to hear that recognition from us.

Aesthetics

It may seem odd that the medical director of the hospice unit talked about the aesthetic of dying, but that approach appears to add to the understanding of what families go through at the end of life. Art is considered by some the highest form of human achievement. It is the conscious molding of the raw experiences of life into something that is important, meaningful, and has the potential of enlightening us in some way. Ceremonies such as weddings, graduations, baptisms and funerals can be seen as art forms. These ceremonies are culturally constructed to make them beautiful and give them all the meaning and portent that beauty implies. To some degree, births and deaths fall into this same category. Although what is under our control seems often to be very little in birth and death, the parts of the experiences over which we do have control can be judged—and, we would contend, are often judged—for their aesthetic qualities.

On its most basic level, the qualities used to make aesthetic judgment are boundaries, rhythm, and clarity (these are adapted from Aquinas).[21–22] In terms of boundaries, works of art are seen as creative narratives, and these narratives have beginnings, middles, and endings.[23] While it is true that some of the boundaries of Calvin's story are established by our telling of it, much of the actual experience fits well into a self-contained story that Calvin can understand. The story of Calvin and Lucille, their narrative of dying, started with the referral to hospice. The cast of characters was established, family and the hospice team, and the action began to move toward the inevitable.

In this narrative, Calvin at first is pleased that Lucille has determination or willpower that is keeping her alive. This implies a common metaphor used in Western culture to organize narratives: the metaphor of war or another kind of a contest. The cancer is the enemy, and one is heroic as long as he or she continues to fight. Near the end of Calvin's story, he believes she has given up. She has decided not to fight anymore. Then the enemy (death) will surely win soon. Yet by this point the metaphor begins to fail as Calvin also realizes that death is inevitable and an ally in that it means an end to Lucille's suffering. The failure of the war or battle metaphor marks in this story, and many others we have collected, the transition from living as well as possible while dying to dying well.

Calvin and Lucille also have strong ideas about the elements that should and should not be in the narrative. Lucille does not want to die alone in her sleep. From her point of view, this is not how the narrative should go. She should be home with Calvin, but she does not want to be surprised by death arriving stealthily in the night. Calvin does not want her to hemorrhage. He does not want her to struggle at the end of life, crying out in pain or gasping for breath. Finally, he wants to have the doctors "ease her on off," so that she will die in her sleep, taking a stance that is presumably the opposite of what she asks for earlier, not dying in her sleep, alone.

But this seeming contradiction leads to the second criterion for an aesthetic death, rhythm. What is true early in the narrative is not true later on. Dying peacefully in her sleep is desirable at the end of the story but would seem wrong at the beginning of the story. Dying needs to be played out, so to speak. The rhythm of Calvin's and Lucille's story is not all that it should be, however. Everyone appears frustrated that she goes into the hospital to die, then comes home again. She is admitted a second time to die, and once again she does not and is sent home. Finally, on the third try, the timing is correct and she goes to the hospital to die. This uncomfortable break in the expected rhythmicity of the story seems to be aggravating to everyone concerned and is an aesthetic flaw.

The third aesthetic criterion is clarity. By this we mean a sense that things generally happened in the way they were supposed to happen. Not that Lucille was supposed to die. Her death was tragic and sad. But there was a sense of the inevitable about it. Lucille did not die because of something done or left undone by others or herself. The medical staff did not make a mistake that killed her, nor did Calvin fail to seek treatment for her when she needed it. An aesthetically satisfying story does not leave one with anger or guilt. Instead, one is left with a sense of clarity. That is, the sadness is deep and profound, but the reasons are clear and not confused with regrets about what was done or left undone.

So much of palliative care is about helping a narrative about dying come as close as possible to having good aesthetic qualities. Deaths are to some degree orchestrated and directed (in the sense that one directs a play or movie) by palliative care nurses and physicians. Whether we want that responsibility or not, we often have it. We have to learn the rhythm of the narrative to know when enough analgesic to relieve the pain but leave the patient incapable of social interaction is appropriate and when it is not. The rules of aesthetics may dictate treatments such as platelets to prevent exsanguination, even though this treatment could be seen as prolonging death. Even issues of when to hospitalize have large aesthetic elements.

Certainly, what is aesthetically satisfying to one family may not be to another. Calvin seems to believe that the staff was using morphine to help Lucille die on that last night. Regardless of the truth of this belief from the staff's point of view, Calvin saw this as appropriate and to be desired. In another family, this might be anathema to beliefs about a "natural death." We are not suggesting that medical treatments such as the titration of morphine be dictated by the aesthetic sensibilities of the family only. We are arguing that nurses and physicians must realize that this sense of aesthetics should be a part of the considerations.

Ending

We have asserted that a good death, to the extent possible, is the aim of palliative care. We have also presented a narrative from our research, which is aimed at better understanding exactly what a good death means. We have carefully avoided defining a good death or predicting or prescribing how to achieve one. The complexity of the experience stands out in the narrative above, in other stories we have collected in our work, and in the everyday life of palliative nursing practice. Striving to provide for a good death for each unique patient is a useful goal. Trying to better understand elements of the complexity as a research question is also worthwhile. But abstraction to the point of prescription seems impossible, unrealistic, and counterproductive when attending to individuality, uniqueness, or the "suchness" of people's lives and deaths.

What we mean by this is that there are no general cases; there are no theoretical lives; living is never done in the abstract. This seems obvious, but it may sometimes be lost in the science of our practice. Usually we base our interventions on what works most of the time for most people. This is the essence of science-based nursing practice. We do things to help our patients based on a high probability that it will work, and that probability is based on an abstraction. It is based on looking at many cases and generalizing about what usually happened. Necessarily, the specifics of individuals must be lost in the process of making general statements. For example, in bowel regimens we depend on knowledge of what works for most people.

What works for most people in terms of parts of palliative care, such as a bowel program, are one thing; what works for most people in terms of the whole experience of a good death is another. A narrative approach to understanding palliative care can rescue the individual particularities of life from being lost in our practice. Listening to Calvin's story—his teenage sojourn in the South Pacific, posing jauntily with his fiancée under Robert E. Lee, his daughter receiving chemotherapy as his wife is dying—makes it impossible to see him as anything but a real man with a complex life that is uniquely his. Recognizing this suchness of his life cannot help but make us care for him in a different way.

The authors acknowledge the financial support of the National Institute of Nursing Research (R15 NR02482 and R01 NR04693) and the National Institute of Aging (R01 NR03517), National Institutes of Health.

REFERENCES

1. Brody H. Stories of Sickness. New Haven: Yale University Press, 1987.

2. Kahn DL, Steeves RH. The significance of suffering in cancer care. Seminars in Oncology Nursing 1995;11:9–16.

3. Kleinman A. The Illness Narratives: Suffering, Healing and the Human Condition. New York: Basic Books, 1988.

4. Polkinghorne DE. Narrative knowing and the human sciences. Albany: State University of New York Press, 1988.

5. Sandelowski M. Telling stories: Narrative approaches in qualitative research. Image 1991; 23:161–166.

6. Steeves RH, Kahn DL, Wise CT, Sepples SB, King MG. Loss and bereavement: A man's perspective. Quality of Life: A Nursing Challenge 1997;5(1):4–8.

7. Steeves RH. Grief, loss, and bereavement: the Flaharty Memorial Lecture. Oncology Nursing Forum 1996;23:897–903.

8. Steeves RH, Kahn DL. Family perspectives: The tasks of bereavement. Quality of Life—A Nursing Challenge 1995;3(3):48–53.

9. Steeves RH, Kahn DL, Wise CT, Baldwin A. The tasks of bereavement for burn center staffs. Journal of Burn Care and Rehabilitation 1993; 14:386–397.

10. Steeves RH. Patients who have undergone bone marrow transplantation: Their quest for meaning. Oncology Nursing Forum 1992;19:899–905.

11. Gadow S. Response to "Personal knowing: Evolving research and practice. Scholarly Inquiry in Nursing Practice 1990;4:167–170.

12. Maeve MK. The carrier bag theory of nursing practice. ANS 1994;16(4):9–22.

13. Sarna L, McCorkle R. Burden of care and lung cancer. Cancer Practice 1996;4:245–251.

14. Weitzner MA, Jacobsen PB, Wagner Jr, H, Friedland J, Cox C. The Caregiver Quality of Life Index-Cancer (CQOLC) Scale: Development and validation of an instrument to measure quality of life of the family caregivers of patients with cancer. Quality of Life Research 1999;8(1–2): 55–63.

15. Weitzner MA, McMillan SC. The Caregiver Quality of Life Index-Cancer (CQOLC) Scale: Revalidation in a home hospice setting. Journal of Palliative Care 1999;15(2):13–20.

16. Burton LA. The spiritual dimension of palliative care. Seminars in Oncology Nursing 1998;14:121–128.

17. Highfield MF. Spiritual health of oncology patients. Cancer Nursing 1992;15:1–8.

18. Highfield MF. Spiritual assessment across the cancer trajectory: Methods and reflections. Seminars in Oncology Nursing 1997;13: 237–241.

19. McGrath P. Putting spirituality on the agenda: Hospice research findings on the "ignored" dimension. Hospice Journal 1997;12(4): 1–14.

20. Millison MB. A review of the research on spiritual care and hospice. Hospice Journal 1995; 10(4):3–18.

21. Aquinas T. Selected Writings (R. McInerny, trans.). New York: Penguin Books, 1998.

22. Eco E. The Aesthetics of Thomas Aquinas (H. Brendin, trans.). Cambridge: Harvard University Press, 1988.

23. Aristotle. Poetics (K. McLeish, trans.). New York: The Theater Communication Group, 1999.

Appendix

Pain and Palliative Care Resource List

ROSE VIRANI

Contents

AUDIO RESOURCES

Pain lectures from recent national conferences are often available from professional organizations, including:

ONS: Oncology Nursing Society
501 Holiday Drive
Pittsburgh, PA 15220-2749
(412) 921-7373
(412) 921-6565 Fax
Website: http://www.ons.org

APS: American Pain Society
4700 W. Lake Avenue
Glenview, IL 60025
(847) 375-4715
Website: http://www.ampainsoc.org

IASP: International Association for the Study of Pain
IASP Secretariat
909 NE 43rd St., Suite 306
Seattle, WA 98105
(206) 547-6409
(206) 547-1703 Fax
Website: http://www.halcyon.com/iasp
E-mail: IASP@locke.hs.washington.edu

Patient Education Teaching Kit. The Cancer Pain Education Program provides a comprehensive approach to pain management in the home by helping patients learn how to assess their pain and actively participate in its management. The pain education kit includes a patient booklet, self-care log, information regarding non-drug interventions, and two audiocassette tapes. To receive order form, or send $45.00 (this includes sales tax, shipping, and handling) to:

- City of Hope National Medical Center
  Marketing Department
  1500 E. Duarte Road
  Duarte, CA 91010
  (626) 359-8111 X2356

Academy for Guided Imagery. Interactive guided imagery self-paced audio/video study course.

- P.O. Box 2070
  Mill Valley, CA 94942
  1-800-726-2070
  (415) 389-9324
  (415) 389-9342 FAX
  Website: http://www.interactiveimagery.com

Coping Skills for Bone Marrow Transplantation. Relaxation, imagery, distraction, and conversation with yourself (e.g., positive thoughts). These approaches to pain management are helpful with pain experiences other than bone marrow transplantation. To order booklet and accompanying audiotape for relaxation:

- Behavioral Sciences
  Fred Hutchinson Cancer Research Center
  1100 Fairview Avenue N., FM815
  Seattle, WA 98109-1024
  (206) 667-5022
  (206) 667-6356 Fax

Exceptional Cancer Patients. This is a healing center founded by Bernie Siegel, M.D., which sells self-help materials and audiotapes, including relaxation tapes.

- Touch Star Productions
  522 Jackson Park Drive
  Medville, PA 16335
  (800) 759-1294
  (814) 337-0699
  Website: http://www.touchstarpro.com
  E-mail: kcb@touchstarpro.com

Source. Has a catalog with a wide variety of relaxation and stress-management tapes based on specific techniques such as muscle tension release, breathing, visualization, and self-hypnosis. "Letting go of stress" is a good overall tape; however, other tapes on managing pain are available.

- Source
  P.O. Box 6028
  Auburn, CA 95604
  (800) 52-TAPES
  (800) 527-2737
  Website: http://www.docmiller.com

BOOKS AND MONOGRAPHS

American Medical Association's Institute of Ethics. (1999). *Education for Physicians on End-of-Life Care (EPEC): Trainer's Guide.* Chicago, IL: American Medical Association.

Berger A, Portenoy R, Weissman, D. (eds). (1998). *Principles and Practice of Supportive Oncology.* Philadelphia, PA: Lippincott-Raven.

Buckman R. (1992). *"I Don't Know What to Say . . .": How to Help and Support Someone Who Is Dying.* New York: Vintage Books.

Byock I. (1997). *Dying Well: The Prospect for Growth at the End of Life.* New York: Riverhead Books.

Callanan M, Kelley P. (1992). *Final Gifts: Understanding the Special Awareness, Needs, & Communications of the Dying.* New York: Bantam Books.

Davies B, Reimer J, Brown P, Martens N. (1995). *Fading Away: The Experience of Transition in Families with Terminal Illness.* Amityville, NY: Baywood Publishing Company.

De Hennezel M. (1997). *Intimate Death: How the Dying Teach Us How to Live.* New York: Alfred A. Knopf.

Dossey L. (1996). *Prayer Is Good Medicine.* New York: HarperCollins.

Doyle D. (1994). *Caring for a Dying Relative: A Guide for Families.* New York: Oxford University Press.

Doyle D, Hanks G, MacDonald N (eds). (1998). *Oxford Textbook of Palliative Medicine.* 2nd Edition. New York: Oxford University Press.

Dunlop R. (1998). *Cancer: Palliative Care.* London, UK: Springer-Verlag London.

Faulkner A, Maguire P. (1994). *Talking to Cancer Patients and Their Relatives.* New York: Oxford Medical Publications.

Ferrell BR. (1996) *Suffering.* Sudbury, MA: Jones and Bartlett.

Field MJ, Cassell CK. (1997). *Approaching Death: Improving Care at the End of Life.* Report of the Institute of Medicine Task Force. Washington DC: National Academy Press.

Fine PG. (1998). *Processes to Optimize Care During the Last Phase of Life.* Scottsdale, AZ: VistaCare.

Furman J, McNabb D. (1997). *The Dying Time: Practical Wisdom for the Dying and Their Caregivers.* New York: Bell Tower.

Groopman J. (1997). *The Measure of Our Days.* New York: Penguin Putnam.

Harrold J, Lynn J. (1998). *Good Dying: Shaping Health Care for the Last Months of Life.* Binghamton, NY: The Haworth Press.

Haylock PJ, Curtiss CP. (1997). *Cancer Doesn't Have to Hurt.* Alameda, CA: Hunter Press Publications.

Holland JC. (ed.) (1998). *Psycho-Oncology.* New York, Oxford University Press.

Hospice Nurses Association. (1996). *Hospice and Palliative Care Clinical Practice Protocol: Dyspnea.* Pittsburgh, PA: Hospice Nurses Association.

Hospice and Palliative Nurses Association. (1997). *Hospice and Palliative Care Clinical Practice Protocol: Terminal Restlessness.* Pittsburgh, PA: Hospice and Palliative Nurses Association.

Hospice and Palliative Nurses Association. (1999). *Hospice and Palliative Care Clinical Practice Protocol: Nausea and Vomiting.* Pittsburgh, PA: Hospice and Palliative Nurses Association.

Kemp C. (1999). *Terminal Illness: A Guide to Nursing Care.* 2nd Edition. Philadelphia, PA: J.B. Lippincott.

Lang SS, Pratt RB. (1994) *You Don't Have to Suffer.* New York: Oxford University Press.

Lattanzi-Licht M, Mahoney J, Miller G. (1998). *Hospice Choice: In Pursuit of a Peaceful Death.* New York, Fireside Publishers.

Lynn J, Harrold J. (1999) *Handbook for Mortals: Guidance for People Facing Serious Illness.* New York: Oxford University Press.

Lynn J, Schuster JL. (in press, 2000). *Improving Care for the End of Life: A Sourcebook for Health Care Managers and Clinicians.* New York: Oxford University Press.

MacDonald N. (1998). *Palliative Medicine: A*

Case-Based Manual. New York: Oxford University Press.

McCaffery M, Pasero C. (1999). *Pain: Clinical Manual.* 2nd Edition. St. Louis, MO: Mosby.

Mundy RR, Rohaly-Davis JA, Sivesind DM, Johnston Taylor E, Chamberlain Wilmoth, M. (1998). *Psychosocial Dimensions of Oncology Nursing Care.* Pittsburgh, PA: Oncology Nursing Press.

Nelson EC, Batalden PC, Ryer JC (eds). (1998). *Joint Commission Clinical Improvement Action Guide.* Oakbrook, IL: Joint Commission on Accreditation in Healthcare Organizations.

Portenoy RK, Bruera E (eds). (1998). *Topics in Palliative Care* (Vol. 3). New York: Oxford University Press.

Ray MC. (1996). *I'm Here to Help: A Hospice Worker's Guide to Communicating with Dying People and Their Loved Ones.* Mound, MN: McRay Company.

Remen RN. (1996). *Kitchen Table Wisdom: Stories That Heal.* New York: Riverhead Books.

Saunders C, Baines M, Dunlop R. (1995). *Living with Dying: A Guide to Palliative Care.* 3rd Edition. New York: Oxford University Press.

Sheehan DC, Forman WB. (1996). *Hospice and Palliative Care: Concepts and Practice.* Sudbury, MA: Jones and Bartlett.

Storey P, Knight CF. (1998). *UNIPAC One: The Hospice/Palliative Medicine Approach to End-of-Life Care.* Dubuque, IA: Kendall/Hunt.

Storey P, Knight CF. (1997). *UNIPAC Two: Alleviating Psychological and Spiritual Pain in the Terminally Ill.* Gainesville, FL: American Academy of Hospice and Palliative Medicine.

Storey P, Knight CF. (1996). *UNIPAC Three: Assessment and Treatment of Pain in the Terminally Ill.* Gainesville, FL: American Academy of Hospice and Palliative Medicine.

Storey P, Knight CF. (1996). *UNIPAC Four: Management of Selected Nonpain Symptoms in the Terminally Ill.* Gainesville, FL: American Academy of Hospice and Palliative Medicine.

Storey P, Knight CF. (1998). *UNIPAC Five: Caring for the Terminally Ill—Communication and the Physician's Role on the Interdisciplinary Team.* Dubuque, IA: Kendall/Hunt.

Storey P, Knight CF. (1996). *UNIPAC Six: Ethical and Legal Decision Making When Caring for the Terminally Ill.* Gainesville, FL: American Academy of Hospice and Palliative Medicine.

Tycross R. (1999). *Introducing Palliative Care.* 3rd Edition. Oxford, UK: Radcliffe Medical Press.

United Hospital Fund. (1998). *The Challenge of Caring for Patients Near the End of Life: Findings from the Hospital Palliative Care Initiative.* New York: Author.

Waller A, Caroline NL. (1996). *Handbook of Palliative Care in Cancer.* Newton, MA: Butterworth-Heinemann.

Webb M. (1997). *The Good Death: The New American Search to Reshape the End of Life.* New York: Bantam Books.

Young-Mason J. (1997). *The Patient's Voice: Experiences of Illness.* Philadelphia, PA: F.A. Davis.

CD-ROM RESOURCES

A Practical Guide to Communication Skills in Clinical Practice (CD-ROMs with pocket guide)

- Medical Audiovisual Communication Inc.
  Niagara Falls, NY, 1998
  (800) 757-4868
  E-mail: DWC@MABC.com

Easing Cancer Pain: Fireside Retreat. Interactive CD-ROM program designed to empower people with cancer who suffer from pain. Available from:

- The American Cancer Society
  Great Lakes Division Headquarters Office
  Attention: Cancer Control Department
  1205 E. Saginaw Street
  Lansing, MI 48906
  (800) 723-0360
  (517) 271-2605 Fax

Graceful Passages. Interfaith audio resource (CD) to assist caregivers, dying persons, and their families to help transition from denial to acceptance. To order:

- Companion Arts
  PO Box 2528
  Novato, CA 94948-2528
  (415) 209-9408
  (888) 242-6608
  E-mail: music@gracefulpassages.com
  Web: www.gracefulpassages.com

Pain Education That Feels Good, interactive multimedia on CD-ROM and the Internet; *Pain Management,* written by Susan Pendergrass, M.S.N., Med, R.N.C.S., F.N.P. 7 contact hours (ANCC) Multimedia courseware.

- Graphic Education Corporation
  903 Old Highway 63 North
  Columbia, MO 65201
  Website: http://www.graphiced.com/pain.html

EDUCATIONAL RESOURCES

About Caregiving
About Dying

- National Hospice and Palliative Care Organization Store
  200 State Road
  South Deerfield, MA 01373-0200
  (800) 646-6460
  (800) 499-6464 Fax
  Website: http://www.nhpco.org

Active Euthanasia and Assisted Suicide, Cancer Pain Management, and *ONS and Association of Oncology Social Work Joint Position on End-of-Life Care.* Oncology Nursing Society positions that may be downloaded and printed at no charge from ONS online at www.ons.org or contact:

- Oncology Nursing Society
  501 Holiday Drive
  Pittsburgh, PA 15220-2749
  (412) 921-7373
  (412) 921-6565
  Website: http://www.ons.org

Agency for Healthcare Research and Quality (AHRQ) Pain Guidelines [formerly AHCPR (Agency for Health Care Policy and Research)]:

- **Acute Pain Guidelines from AHRQ:**
  - *Acute Pain Management in Adults: Operative Procedures,* Quick Reference Guide for Clinicians No. 1a, AHCPR Pub No. 92-0019, February 1993.
  - *Acute Pain Management in Infants, Children, and Adolescents: Operative Procedures,* Quick Reference Guide for Clinicians No. 1b, AHCPR Pub No. 92-0020, February 1993.
  - *Pain Control After Surgery, A Patient's Guide,* Consumer Guideline Number 1, AHCPR Pub No. 92-0021, February 1993. Spanish version, AHCPR Pub No. 92-0068, September 1992.
  - *Acute Pain Management: Operative or Medical Procedures and Trauma,* Clinical Practice Guideline 1, AHCPR Pub No. 92-0032, February 1992.
- **Cancer Pain Guidelines from AHRQ:**
  - *Management of Cancer Pain,* Clinical Guideline Number 9, AHCPR Pub. No. 94-0592, March 1994.
  - *Management of Cancer Pain: Adults,* Quick Reference guide for Clinicians Number 9, AHCPR Pub. No. 94-0593.
  - *Managing Cancer Pain,* Consumer Guide Number 9, AHCPR Pub. No. 94-0595, March 1994. Spanish version, AHCPR Pub No. 94-0596, March 1994.

To order:

- AHRQ Publications Clearinghouse
  2101 East Jefferson Street
  Rockville, MD 20852
  (800) 358-9295
  Website: http://www.ahcpr.gov

Or:

- U.S. Government Printing Office
  GPO Order Desk
  (202) 512-1800

Building an Institutional Commitment to Pain Management: The Wisconsin Resource Manual for Improvement. (Gordon, DB, Dahl, JL, Stevenson, KK).
The Handbook of Cancer Pain Management, 5th Edition (Weissman, DE, Dahl, JL). A pocket-size handbook for health care professionals about diagnosis and management of cancer pain.
The Wisconsin Cancer Pain Initiative: Helping Health Professionals Help Cancer Patients in Pain.
To order:
- Wisconsin Cancer Pain Initiative
  1300 University Avenue, Room 4720
  Madison, Wisconsin 53706
  (608) 262-0978
  (608) 265-4014 Fax
  Website: http://www.wisc.edu/wcpi or http://www.Medsch.wisc.edu/
  E-mail: wcpi@facstaff.wisc.edu

Cancer Pain Management. This brochure discusses why cancer causes pain, how to describe different types of pain, and pain treatment options. Spanish version available.
Available from:
- Cancer Pain Information Center
  PO Box 37
  Norwood, MA 02062
  (800) 767-7246

The Cancer Pain Education Program: A Comprehensive Approach to Pain Management in the Home
City of Hope Patient Handbook for Cancer Pain Management (English)
Folleto Sobre Como Tratar con el Dolor del Cancer para los Pacientes de City of Hope (Spanish)
- City of Hope National Medical Center
  Marketing and Communications
  1500 East Duarte Road
  Duarte, CA 91010-0269
  (626) 359-8111, Ext. 2356
  Website: http://www.coh.org

Cancer Pain Relief and Palliative Care in Children (1998). World Health Organization (WHO) guidelines on the management of pain in children. Available in English, Spanish and French. To order:
- WHO Publication Center
  49 Sheridan Avenue
  Albany, NY 12210
  (518) 436-9686 x118
  E-mail: QCORP@compuserve.com

Children's Cancer Pain Can Be Relieved (for parents). A 12-page booklet in Q&A format. Preview copy free of charge, additional copies $0.50 plus postage.
Dispelling the Myths About Morphine. Patient brochure. Information for safe and effective use of morphine in managing moderate to severe pain. Spanish version also available.
Eight Facts Everyone Should Know About Cancer Pain. Facts about cancer pain. Order from:
- The Resource Center
  1300 University Avenue, Room 4720
  Madison, Wisconsin 53706
  (608) 262-0978
  (608) 265-4014 Fax
  Website: http://www.wisc.edu/wcpi/

Chronic and Recurrent Pain in Children and Adolescents: Progress in Pain Research and Management, Vol. 13 Authored by Patrick J. McGrath, Ph.D., and G. Allen Finley, M.D., F.R.C.P.C., provides in-depth reviews of important issues relating to chronic pain in children. To order:
- IASP Press
  909 NE 43rd Street
  Seattle, WA 98105-6020
  (206) 547-6409
  Website: http://www.halcyon.com/iasp
  E-mail: IASP@lock.hs.washington.edu

City of Hope Pain/Palliative Care Resource Center. Clearinghouse to disseminate information and resources on pain management and end of life care. Index of materials and order information available on web.
- City of Hope Pain/Palliative Care Resource Center
  1500 East Duarte Rd.
  Duarte, CA 91010
  626/359-8111 x3829
  626/301-8941 Fax
  Web: http://prc.coh.org

Comfort Assessment Journal. A notebook developed by the Iowa Pain Relief Inititative to answer patients' questions about pain medication and to teach them how to record their pain ratings in the journal. Spanish version available.
Up-to-Date Answers to Questions About Measuring Pain. A 12-page, easy-to-read brochure for patients and family providing broad information about pain and the patient's role in measuring pain. Spanish version available.
Up-to-Date Answers to Questions About Pain Medication. Provides informtation about pain control and is intended to help cancer patients understand their pain and its management.
You, Your Patient, and Purdue. Partners Against Pain. Tools and services for patients and professionals. Order from:
- Purdue Frederick Co.
  1000 Connecticut Avenue
  Norwalk, CT 06850
  Website: http://www.partnersagainstpain.com

Constipation and Opiod Use
Continuous Lumbar Epidural Analgesia
Patient Controlled Analgesia (PCA)
Non-drug Pain Relief
Use of Teaching Guides for Patient Education
Understanding Pain Control and Pain Medicine
Pain management information one-page flyers. Price: Single copy free. Order from:
- James Cancer Hospital and Research Institute
  The Ohio State University James Cancer Hospital and Research Institute
  300 West 10th Avenue, Room 775
  Columbus, OH 43210
  Website: http://www.osu.edu/units/oduhodp/disclaim2.htm

Culture and Nursing Care: A Pocket Guide
- UCSF Nursing Press
  Box 0608
  School of Nursing
  University of California, San Francisco
  521 Parnassus Avenue
  San Francisco, CA 94143-0608
  (415) 476-4992
  (415) 476-6042 Fax
  Website: http://nurseweb.ucsf.edu/www/books.htm

Dyspnea (1996), *Terminal Restlessness* (1997), and *Nausea and Vomiting* (1999). Monographs published by the Hospice and Palliative Nurses Association. To order:
- Hospice and Palliative Nurses Association
  Medical Center East, Suite 375
  211 N. Whitfield Street
  Pittsburgh, PA 15206-3031
  (412) 361-2470
  (412) 361-2425 FAX
  Website: http://www.hpna.org

Education for Physicians on End-of-Life Care Project (EPEC). A train-the-trainer program, supported by the Robert Wood Johnson Foundation and sponsored by the Northwestern University Medical School, designed to educate physicians in the essential clinical competencies in end-of-life care. For more information or to order materials:

- The EPEC Project
  Northwestern University School of Medicine (NUMS)
  680 N. Lake Shore Drive, Suite 912
  Chicago, IL 60611
  (877) 524-EPEC (toll-free)
  or
  (312) 695-4353
  (312) 695-4355 FAX
  Website: http://www.epec.net
  E-mail: info@epec.net

The End of Life: Exploring Death in America. Collection of National Public Radio's transcripts of programs in its ongoing series on death and dying in America. Contact:

- National Public Radio
  635 Massachusetts Ave., NW
  Washington, DC 20001
  (202) 414-2000
  (202) 414-3329 Fax
  Website: http://www.npr.brg/programs/death/
  E-mail: webmaster@npr.org

End-of-Life Care: Ethical Dimensions (monograph #GNE017); *End-of-Life Care for Children and Their Families: Ethical Dimensions* (monograph #GNE070). Provides nurses with information concerning end-of-life issues.

- GlaxoWellcome Inc.
  Research Triangle Park, NC 27709
  (800) 824-2896
  Website: http://www.HELIX.com

End of Life Physician Education Resource Center (EPERC). A center, supported by the Robert Wood Johnson Foundation, for educational materials and information about end of life issues to assist physician educators and others in training materials.

- End of Life Physician Education Resource Center (EPERC)
  Medical College of Wisconsin
  8701 Watertown Plank Road
  414/456-4353
  414/456-6506 FAX
  Website: http://www.eperc.mcw.edu
  E-mail: jrehm@mcw.edu

Get Relief from Cancer Pain. A simple patient education booklet that contains the essential facts about pain control. Quantities are limited to 100. Publication is available free of charge. Available in Spanish only.

Questions and Answers about Pain Control. A guide for people with cancer and their families that contains detailed information about pain control. Quantities are limited to 100. Booklet is available free of charge from:

- National Cancer Institute
  Cancer Information Service
  (800) 422-6237
  Website: http://cis.nci.nih.gov/

or

- The American Cancer Society
  Website: http://cancer.org/index_4up.html

Making Cancer Less Painful: A Handbook for Parents

Pain, Pain, Go Away: Helping Children with Pain. Both booklets available for a nominal cost.

Order from:

- Association for the Care of Children's Health
  7910 Woodmont Avenue, Suite 300
  Bethesda, Maryland 20814
  (800) 808-2224
  Website: http://is.dal.ca/~pedpain/ppga-ti.htm
  E-mail: acch@clark.net

On Our Own Terms: Moyers on Dying in America. A four-part PBS series premiering in Fall 2000 and companion outreach campaign. For more information:

- (703) 827-0783 Fax
  Website: http://www.thirteen.org/onourownterms
  or www.pbs.org/onourownterms

Practice Parameters for Systematic IV Analgesia and Sedation for Adult Patients in the ICU; Sustained Neuromuscular Blockade in the Adult Critically Ill Patient. Practice parameters developed by a task force of the American College of Critical Care Medicine (ACCM) & approved by ACCM Board of Regents and the Society of Critical Care Medicine. To order:

- Society of Critical Care Medicine
  8101 East Kaiser Blvd., Suite 300
  Anaheim, CA 92808-2259
  (714) 282-6056
  (714) 282-6050 Fax
  Website: http://www.sccm.org

Principles of Analgesic Use in the Treatment of Acute Pain and Cancer Pain

- American Pain Society
  4700 W. Lake Avenue
  Glenview, IL 60025
  (708) 966-5595
  Website: http://www.ampainsoc.org

Protocols for Practice: Pain Management in the Acutely Ill (Author: Julie Stanik-Hoff), 1998. Part of a series 6 books of *Protocols for Practice: Creating a Healing Environment.* To order:

- American Association of Critical Care Nurses
  101 Columbia
  Aliso Viejo, CA 92656
  (800) 899-2226
  (949) 362-2000 Fax
  Website: http://www.aacn.org
  E-mail: aacninfo@aacn.org

Quality of Life: A Nursing Challenge Monograph—Pain Management (Volume 4, Issue 4) A journal issue dedicated to the topic of pain management. To order:

- Meniscus Educational Institute
  P.O. Box 2649
  Bala Cynwyd, PA 19004-9292
  Reference # for ordering: GNE057RO
  Website: http://www.meniscus.com/

Note: Monographs can also be ordered from GlaxoWellcome.

The Roxane Pain Institute

- P.O. Box 16532
  Columbus, Ohio 43216
  (614) 276-4000
  (614) 274-0974 Fax
  Website: http://www.roxane.com/pain/library/Newsletters/MDA

Symptom Management Algorithms for Palliative Care

- Intellicard
  P.O. Box 8255
  Yakima, WA 98908
  (509) 965-5447 Fax

Taking Time: Support for People with Cancer and the People Who Care for Them

- National Cancer Institute
  (800)-4-CANCER
  Publication No. 92-2059

Treating Chronic Pain with Implantable Therapies (pamphlet)
Living with Chronic Pain (booklet)
About Living with Chronic Pain (booklet)
All Alone with Chronic Pain (booklet)
Pain Management Strategies (flyer)
10 Hints for Helping your Patients with Chronic Pain (flyer)
Choosing a Pain Clinic or a Pain Specialist (flyer)
Distraction for Pain Management (flyer)
Humor for Pain Management (flyer)

Breathing for Pain Management (flyer)
Heat or Cold for Pain Management (flyer)
Touch and Simple Massage for Relaxation and Pain Management (flyer)
Neuropathy Pain (flyer)
Implantable Pain Management: An Overview (flyer)
Implantable Pain Management: Living with Chronic Pain—Patient Perspective (flyer)
Pain Relief After Surgery: A Patient's Guide (flyer)
Information on chronic pain developed by the National Chronic Pain Outreach Association. To order at no cost, write or call:

- The National Chronic Pain Outreach Association
  PO Box 274
  Millboro, VA 24460
  540/862-9437
  540/862-9485 Fax

JOURNALS

American Journal of Hospice & Palliative Care. A peer-reviewed research journal published bimonthly. Focus on hospice and palliative care news and research.

- Prime National Publishing Corp.
  470 Boston Post Rd.
  Weston, MA 02493
  (781) 899-2702
  (781) 899-4900 Fax
  Website: http://www.pnpco.com

Clinical Journal of Pain—Official Journal of the American Academy of Pain Medicine. A quarterly journal that provides information on all aspects of pain including the psychosocial dimensions and ethical issues of pain management.

- Lippincott Williams & Wilkins
  12107 Insurance Way
  Hagerstown, MD 21740
  (800) 638-3030
  (301) 714-2300
  (301) 714-2398 Fax
  Website: http://www.clinicalpain.com

The European Journal of Palliative Care. Official journal of the European Association for Palliative Care. Published six times a year.

- Hayward Medical Communications
  44 Earlham Street
  London WC2H 9LA, United Kingdom
  +44 (0) 171 240 4493
  +44 (0) 171 240 4479 FAX
  Website: http://www.ejpc.co.uk

Innovations in End-of-Life Care. An online international peer-reviewed journal and forum highlighting promising practices that improve end-of-life care.

- Contact: Stacy A. Piszcz
  (617) 969-7100 X3388
  Website: http://www.edc.org/lastacts
  E-mail: inteleoljournal@edc.org

Journal of Hospice and Palliative Nursing. A quarterly peer-reviewed journal.

- NurseCom, Inc.
  C/o HPNA
  Medical Center East
  211 N. Whitfield Street, Suite 375
  Pittsburgh, PA 15206-3031
  412) 361-2470
  (412) 361-2425 Fax
  NurseCom Phone (for subscription information) (800)242-6757
  NurseCom (215) 545-8107 Fax
  Website: http://www.HPNA.org
  E-mail: HPNA@hpna.org

Hospice Journal. Official journal of the National Hospice and Palliative Care Organization (NHPCO), which promotes and maintains quality care for the terminally ill and their families.

- Haworth Press, Inc.
  10 Alice Street
  Binghamton, NY 13904-1580
  (800) HAWORTH
  (800) 895-0582 Fax
  Website: http://www.haworthpressinc.com
  E-mail: getinfo@haworthpressinc.com

HOSPICE Magazine. A quarterly magazine dedicated to promoting hospice care and end-of-life care issues.

- Editor, HOSPICE
  National Hospice and Palliative Care Organization
  1901 North Moore Street, Suite 901
  Arlington, VA 22209
  (703) 243-5900
  (703) 525-5762 Fax
  Website: http://www.nhpco.org

International Journal of Palliative Nursing. A bimonthly publication that promotes excellence in palliative nursing.

- International Journal of Palliative Nursing
  Mark Allen Group
  Croxted Mews
  286A288 Road
  London, United Kingdom SE24 9BY
  PH: 0181-671 7521
  Website: http://www.markallengroup.com
  E-mail: mark_allen_publishing@compuserve.com

Journal of Palliative Care. A quarterly publication that focuses on issues surrounding palliative care.

- Center for Bioethics
  Clinical Research Institute of Montreal
  110 Pine Avenue West
  Montreal, Quebec H2W 1R7
  Canada
  (514) 987-5617
  (514) 987-5695 Fax
  Website: http://www.allenpress.com
  E-mail: marcot@ircm.umontreal.ca

Journal of Palliative Medicine. The journal covers the team approach to palliative medicine, pain and symptom management, palliative care education, legal, ethical, and reimbursement issues, and more.

- Mary Ann Liebert, Inc. Publishers
  2 Madison Ave.
  Larchmont, NY 10538-1962
  (800) M-LIEBERT
  (914) 834-3100
  (914) 834-3771 Fax
  Web: http://www.liebertpub.com
  E-mail: info@liebertpub.com

Journal of Pain and Symptom Management. Monthly journal that publishes original articles and other clinical papers.

- Elsevier Science Publishing Co., Inc.
  Journals Fulfillment Dept.
  655 6th Avenue
  New York, NY 10010
  (212) 633-3950
  (212) 633-3680 Fax
  Website: http://www.sevier.com

Journal of Pharmaceutical Care in Pain & Symptom Control. Covers innovations in drug development, evaluation, and use for pain and symptom control.

- Haworth Press, Inc.
  10 Alice Street
  Binghamton, NY 13904-1580
  (800) HAWORTH
  (801) 581-5986
  (801) 585-6160 Fax
  E-mail: ALIPMAN@DEANS.PHARM.UTAH.EDU

Journal of Psycho Oncology. Quarterly journal concerned with the psychological, behavioral, and ethical aspects of cancer.

- Journals Subscriptions Department
  John Wiley & Sons, Ltd.
  1 Oldlands Way, Bognor Regis
  West Sussex PO22 9SA, UK
  +44(0) 1243 779777
  +44(0) 1243 843232 Fax
  Website: http://www.wiley.com
  E-mail: cs-journals@wiley.co.uk

Journal of Psychosocial Nursing. Covers current news in psychosocial nursing, updates on psychopharmacology, geopsychiatry, and mental health nursing.

- Journal of Psychosocial Nursing
  6900 Grove Road
  Thorofare, NJ 08086
  (800) 257-8290
  (609) 853-5991 Fax
  Website: http://www.slackinc.com
  E-mail: slackinc.com

PAIN. Official publication of the International Association for the Study of Pain.

- LE Jones
  Executive Officer
  International Association for the Study of Pain
  909 NE 43rd Street, Suite 306
  Seattle, WA 98105
  (206) 547-1703 FAX
  Website: http://www.halcyon.com/iasp
  E-mail: iasp@locke.hs.washington.edu

Palliative Medicine. International journal, published bimonthly, dedicated to improving knowledge and clinical practice in the palliative care of patients with advanced disease.

- Edward Arnold
  338 Euston Road
  London NW1 3BH
  United Kingdom
  +44 (0) 171 873 6355
  +44 (0) 171 873 6325 FAX
  Website: http://www.healthworks.co.uk
  E-mail: arnold@hodder.mhs_compuserve.com

Progress in Palliative Care. Multidisciplinary journal that provides information on all aspects of palliative care.

- WS Maney and Son Ltd
  Hudson Road
  Leeds LS9 7DL
  United Kingdom
  +44 (0) 113 249 7481
  +44 (0) 113 248 6983 FAX
  Website: http://www.leeds.ac.uk/lmi/maneys.html
  E-mail: maney@maney.co.uk

Supportive Care in Cancer. Provides members of the Multinational Association of Supportive Care in Cancer (MASCC) the most recent scientific and social information on aspects of supportive care for cancer patients at all stages of the disease.

- Springer-Verlag, New York, Inc.
  Journal Fulfillment Services Department
  P.O. Box 2485
  Secaucus, NJ 07096-2485
  (800) SPRINGER
  (212) 460-1612 (voicemail)
  (212) 460-5817 Fax
  Website: http://link.springer-ny.com or http://www.springer-ny.com
  E-mail: custserv@springer-ny.com

NEWSLETTERS

ABCD EXCHANGE A newsletter from Americans for Better Care of the Dying (ABCD). ABCD aims to enhance the experience of the last phase of life for all Americans, advocate for the interests of patients and their families, improve communication between providers and patients, involve society in end-of-life care, and demand continuity in services for the seriously ill.

- ABCD
  2175 K Street NW, Suite 820
  Washington DC 20037-1803
  (202) 530-9864
  (202) 530-2336 Fax
  Website: http://www.abcd-caring.com
  E-mail: caring@erols.com

CANCER CARE NEWS. Provides information for people with cancer, their families, and loved ones.

- Cancer Care, Inc. National Office
  1180 Avenue of the Americas
  New York, NY 10036
  (800) 813-HOPE (4673)
  (212) 221-3300
  (212) 719-0263 Fax
  Website: http://www.cancercare.org

CANCER PAIN UPDATE. A quarterly newsletter of the Wisconsin Cancer Pain Initiative.

- Wisconsin Cancer Pain Initiative
  1300 University Avenue, Room 4720
  Madison, Wisconsin 53706
  (608) 262-0978
  (608) 265-4014 Fax
  Website: http://www.wisc.edu/wcpi
  E-mail: wcpi@facstaff.wisc.edu

FANFARE. Official newsletter of the Hospice & Palliative Nurses Association. Published quarterly, *FANFARE*, provides current clinical articles and educational opportunities relevant to hospice nursing.

- FANFARE
  Medical Center East, Suite 375
  211 North Whitfield Street
  Pittsburgh, PA 15206-3031
  Donna J. Carothers
  Managing Editor
  (412) 361-2470
  (412) 361-2425 FAX
  Website: http://www.hpna.org
  E-mail: hnafan@usa.pipeline.com

HEADWAY MIGRAINE. Newsletter (free)

- (800) 377-0282 to subscribe
  Website: http://www.imitrex.com/coping/headway.html

THE HOSPICE PROFESSIONAL. A quarterly publication for members of the National Council of Hospice Professionals. This newsletter emphasizes hospice care and the interdisciplinary team concept. Each issue focuses on a theme.

- National Hospice and Palliative Care Organization
  1901 North Moore Street, Suite 901
  Arlington, VA 22209
  (703) 243-5900
  (703) 525-5762 Fax
  Website: http://www.nhpco.org

IASP NEWSLETTER. International Association for the Study of Pain (IASP). Timely topics in pain research and treatment selected for publication.

- IASP
  909 NE 43rd Street #306
  Seattle, WA 98105
  (206) 547-6409
  (206) 547-1703 Fax
  Website: http://www.halcyon.com/iasp

IPOS NEWSLETTER. The International Psycho-Oncology Society's (IPOS) membership is global and has international discourse to enrich the understanding of psycho-oncologic issues.

- Box 421
  1275 York Avenue
  New York, NY 10021
  (212) 639-6777
  (212) 717-3087 Fax
  Contact: Tony Marchini
  Website: http://www.ipos-aspboa.org

*LAST ACTS: **Care and Caring at the End of Life.*** Published quarterly by the Robert Wood Johnson Foundation.

- LAST ACTS
  c/o Barksdale, Ballard & Company
  1951 Kidwell Drive, Suite 205
  Vienna, VA 22182
  (703) 827-8771
  (703) 827-0783 Fax
  Website: http://www.lastacts.org

LIFELINE. The newsletter of the National Chronic Pain Outreach Association, Inc. (NCPOA). Lifeline welcomes reader correspondence and submissions of articles, book reviews, commentaries, cartoons, artwork, and poetry. Call for information.

- LIFELINE
  P.O. Box 274
  Millboro, VA 24460
  (540) 862-9437
  (540) 862-9485 Fax
  Website: http://www.chronicpain.org
  E-mail: ncpoa@cfw.com

NABCO NEWS. National Alliance of Breast Cancer Organizations (NABCO). A leading, nonprofit central information resource on breast cancer and a network of over 375 breast cancer organizations. NABCO provides information to medical professionals and their organizations, patients and their families, and the media.

- NABCO
  9 East 37th Street, 10th Floor
  New York, NY 10016
  (212) 889-0606 or (888) 80-NABCO
  Website: http://www.nabco.org
  E-mail: NABCOinfo@aol.com

NCCN ADVANTAGE. National Comprehensive Cancer Network (NCCN). Outlines current programs, conferences, and resources.

- NCCN
  50 Huntington Pike #200
  Rockledge, PN 19046
  (215) 728-2577
  (215) 728-4788 Fax
  Website: http://www.nccn.org

NCCS NETWORKER. A quarterly publication of the National Coalition for Cancer Survivorship (NCCS). Provides information about NCCS activities and survivorship issues.

- National Coalition for Cancer Survivorship
  1010 Wayne Ave, Suite 505
  Silver Spring, MD 20910-5600
  (888) 650-9127
  (301) 565-9670 Fax
  Website: http://www.cansearch.org
  E-mail: info@cansearch.org

NHO NEWSLINE. National Hospice and Palliative Care Organization sponsored newsletter, published biweekly, that details the activities of NHPCO and provides a calendar of events along with updates on legislative issues that may impact hospice care.

- National Hospice and Palliative Care Organization
  1901 North Moore Street, Suite 901
  Arlington, VA 22209
  (703) 243-5900
  (703) 525-5762 Fax
  Website: http://www.nhpco.org

NYSCAPI NEWS. New York State Cancer and AIDS Pain Initiative (NYSCAPI). Part of NYSCAPI's goal is to educate health care professionals, patients, and families affected by cancer and AIDS about the management of pain; to develop research that permits better management of pain; and to monitor legislation that might influence clinical management of pain.

- NYSCAPI
  1180 Avenue of the Americas
  New York, NY 10036
  (212) 221-3300
  (212) 719-0263 Fax
  Website: http://www.cancercare.org
  E-mail: info@cancercare.org

PAIN RELIEF PAPERS. Provides patients with information about cancer pain assessment and controlling pain.

- Janssen Pharmaceuticals Research Foundation
  Janssen at Washington Crossing
  1125 Trenton-Harbourton Road
  P.O. Box 200
  Trenton, NJ 08560-0200
  (800) 334-0222
  (856) 423-5007 Fax
  Website: http://us.janssen.com

PALLIATIVE CARE LETTER. Published by Roxane Laboratories, Inc. Contains abstracts of scientific articles.

- Roxane Laboratories, Inc.
  P.O. Box 16532
  Columbus, OH 43216
  (614) 276-4000
  (614) 276-2470 Fax
  Website: http://www.roxane.com
  E-mail: info@Roxane.com

PDIA READER. An interesting and easily accessible source of recent articles on end-of-life issues. Published by the Project on Death in America (PDIA).

- Open Society Institute, PDIA
  400 W. 59th Street
  New York, NY 10019
  (212) 548-0600
  (212) 548-4679 Fax
  Website: http://www.soros.org

PROGRESS IN PALLIATIVE CARE. Multidisciplinary, international journal covers material pertinent to living with chronic or progressive disease and those engaged in end-of-life studies. To order:

- Subscriptions Dept.
  TEL 0171-290-2928 (United Kingdom)

REFLECTIONS. Prepared by the Program for Ethics at Oregon State University. Contains essays by leading participants in public debate regarding legalized assisted suicide.

- Department of Philosophy
  Oregon State University
  Corvallis, OR 97331
  Contact person: Sandra Shockley
  (541) 737-5648
  (541) 737-2571 Fax
  E-mail: pese@orst.edu

SCCPI NEWSLETTER. A newsletter from the Southern California Cancer Pain Initiative that provides individuals with information on pain-related items and upcoming meetings.

- Southern California Cancer Pain Initiative
  c/o City of Hope National Medical Center
  1500 E. Duarte Road
  Duarte, CA 91010
  (626) 359-8111 X3829
  Website: http://www.sccpi.coh.org
  E-mail: sccpi@coh.org

VISTACARE NEWS NETWORK. Published 48 times per year from news compiled by a consortium of hospice organization. For additional information, contact:

- Richard Fitzpatrick, Executive Director
  VistaCare Foundation
  (702) 940-0160
  E-mail: rfitzpatrick@vista-care.com

ORGANIZATIONS

Aging with Dignity
P.O. Box 1661
Tallahassee, FL 32302-1661
(850) 681-2010
(850) 681-2481 Fax
Website: http://www.agingwithdignity.org
E-mail: fivewishes@aol.com

American Academy of Hospice and Palliative Medicine (AAHPM)
11250 Roger Bacon Drive, Suite 8
Reston, VA 20190-5202
(703) 787-7718
(703) 435-4390 Fax
Website: http://www.aahpm.org
E-mail: aahpm@aahpm.org

American Academy of Pain Medicine
4700 W. Lake Avenue
Glenview, IL 60025
(847) 375-4731
(847) 375-6331 Fax
Website: http://www.painmed.org
E-mail: aapm@amctec.com

American Academy of Pediatrics
141 Northwest Point Blvd.
P.O. Box 927
Elk Grove Village, IL 60009-0927
(800) 433-9016
Website: http://www.aap.org/

Americans for Better Care of the Dying (ABCD)
2175 K St., NW #810
Washington, DC 20037
202/530-9864
Website: http://www.abcd-caring.org

American Cancer Society (National Headquarters) (ACS)
1599 Clifton Road, NE
Atlanta, GA 30329
1-800-ACS-2345
Website: http://www.cancer.org

American Chronic Pain Association (ACPA)
P. O. Box 850
Rocklin, CA 95677
(916) 632-0922
(916) 632-3208 Fax
Website: http://www.theacpa.org
E-mail: ACPA@pacbell.net

American Council for Headache Education
19 Mantua Road
Mt. Royal, NJ 08061
(609) 423-0258
(609) 423-0082 Fax
Website: http://www.achenet.org
E-mail: achehq@talley.com

American Holistic Nurses Association
P.O. Box 2130
Flagstaff, AZ 86003-2130
(800) 278-AHNA
Website: http://www.ahna.org

American Pain Foundation
111 South Calvert Street, Suite 2700
Baltimore, MD 21202
Website: http://www.painfoundation.org
E-mail: ampainfoun@aol.com

American Pain Society (APS)
4700 W. Lake Avenue
Glenview, IL 60025
(847) 375-4715
(847) 375-4777 Fax
Website: http://www.ampainsoc.org
E-mail: info@ampainsoc.org

American Society of Pain Management Nurses (ASPMN)
7794 Grow Drive
Pensacola, FL 32514-7072
(850) 473-0233
(850) 484-8762 Fax
Website: http://www.aspmn.org
E-mail: ASPMN@puetzamc.com

Arthritis Foundation
1330 Peachtree Street
Atlanta, GA 30309
(404) 872-7100
Website: http://www.arthritis.org

Association of American Sickle Cell Disease
200 Corporate Point, Suite 495
Culver City, CA 90230-7633
(310) 216-6363
(310) 215-3722 Fax
Website: http://www.sicklecelldisease.org
E-mail: LASCDAA@aol.com

Association for the Care of Children's Health (ACCH)
7910 Woodmont Avenue, Suite 300
Bethesda, MD 20814
(800) 808-2224
Website: http://www.acch.org
E-mail: acch@clark.net

Association of Nurses in AIDS Care (ANAC)
11250 Roger Bacon Drive, Suite 8
Reston, VA 20190-5202
(703) 925-0081
(703) 435-4390 Fax
Website: http://www.anacnet.org
E-mail: AIDSNURSE@aol.com

Association of Oncology Social Work (AOSW)
1910 East Jefferson St.
Baltimore, MD 21205
(410) 614-3990
(410) 614-3991 Fax
Website: http://www.aosw.org

Association of Pediatric Oncology Nurses (APON)
4700 West Lake Avenue
Glenview, IL 60025
(847) 375-4724
(847) 375-4777 Fax
Website: http://www.apon.org
E-mail: apon@amctec.com

Beyond Ordinary Nursing
P.O. Box 8177
Foster City, CA 94404
(650) 570-6157

Cancer Care, Inc.
275 7th Avenue
New York, NY 10001
(800) 813-HOPE (4673) or
(212) 302-2400
(212) 719-0263 Fax
Website: http://www.cancercare.org/

Candlelighters Childhood Cancer Foundation
7910 Woodmont Ave., Suite 460
Bethesda, MD 20814-3015
(800) 366-2223
(301) 657-8401
(301) 718-2686 Fax
Website: http://www.candlelighters.org

CARF—The Rehabilitation Accreditation Commission
4891 East Grant Road
Tucson, AZ 85712
(520) 325-1044
Website: http://www.carf.org

Center to Improve Care of the Dying
c/o George Washington University Medical Center
2175 K Street NW, Suite 820
Washington DC 20037
(202) 467-2222
(202) 467-2271 Fax
Website: http://www.gwu.edu/~cicd
E-mail: cicd@gwi52.circ.gwu.edu

Children's Hospice International
2202 Mt. Vernon Avenue, Suite 3C
Alexandria, VA 22301
(800) 24-CHILD
(703) 684-0330
(703) 684-0226 Fax
Website: http://www.chionline.org

Choice in Dying (CID)
1035 30th Street, NW
Washington, DC 20007
(202) 338-9790
(202) 338-0242 Fax
Website: http://www.choices.org

Compassion in Dying Federation
6312 SW Capitol Hwy, Suite 415
Portland, OR 97201
(503) 221-9556
(503) 228-9160 Fax
Website: http://www.compassionindying.org
E-mail: info@compassionindying.org

The Compassionate Friends, Inc. (TCF)
P.O. Box 3696
Oak Brook, IL 60522-3696
(630) 990-0010
(630) 990-0246 Fax
Website: http://www.compassionatefriends.org

FACCT—The Foundation for Accountability
520 SW Sixth Ave.
Suite 700
Portland, OR 97204
(503) 223-2228
(503) 223-4336 FAX
Website: http://www.facct.org
E-mail: info@facct.org

Fibromyalgia Network
P.O. Box 31750
(800) 853-2929
Website: http://www.fmnetnews.com

Hospice Association of America
228 7th Street SE
Washington DC 20003
(202) 546-4759
(202) 546-9559 Fax
Website: http://www.hospice-america.org

Hospice and Palliative Nurses Association (HPNA)
Medical Center E, Suite 375
211 N. Whitfield
Pittsburgh, PA 15206-3031
(412) 361-2470
(412) 361-2425 Fax
Website: http://www.hpna.org
E-mail: HPNA@hpna.org

International Association for the Study of Pain (IASP)
909 NE 43rd Street, Suite 306
Seattle, WA 98105-6020
(206) 547-6409
(206) 547-1703 Fax
Website: http://www.halcyon.com/iasp/
E-mail: IASP@lock.hs.washington.edu

Leukemia Society of America
600 Third Ave.
New York, NY 10016
(800) 955-4LSA (educational materials)
(212) 573-8484 (general information)
(212) 856-9686 Fax
Website: http://www.leukemia.org

The Mayday Fund
Fenella Rouse JD
Executive Director
c/o UBS AG
10 E. 50th Street, 15th Floor
New York, NY 10022
(212) 838-2904
(212) 838-2896 Fax
Website: http://foundationcenter.org/grantmaker/gws-priv/indiv/mayday.html

Make a Wish Foundation
100 West Claendon, Suite 2200
Phoenix, AZ 85013-3518
(800) 722-WISH
(602) 279-0885 Fax
Website: http://www.wish.org
E-mail: mawfa@wish.org

National Cancer Institute
Public Inquiries Office
Building 31, Room 10A03
31 Center Drive
MSC 2580
Bethesda, MD 20892-2580
(800) 4-CANCER
Website: http://www.nci.nih.gov

National Chronic Pain Outreach Association (NCPOA)
P.O. Box 274
Millboro, VA 24460
540/997-5004
540/997-1305 Fax
Website: http://neurosurgery.mgh.harvard.edu/ncpainoa.htm

National Headache Foundation
5252 North Western Avenue
Chicago, IL 60625
(800) 843-2256
(773) 525-7356 Fax
Website: http://www.headaches.org

National Hospice and Palliative Care Organization (NHPCO)
1700 Diagonal Road, Suite 300
Alexandria, VA 22314
(703) 243-5900
(703) 525-5762 Fax
Website: http://www.nhpco.org

National Prison Hospice Association
P.O. Box 3679
Boulder, CO 80306-0941
(303) 544-1485
(303) 544-9875 Fax
Website: http://www.npha.org
E-mail: npha-news@npha.org

Oncology Nursing Society (ONS)
501 Holiday Drive
Pittsburgh, PA 15220-2749
(412) 921-7373
(412) 921-6565 Fax
Website: http://www.ons.org
E-mail: member@ons.org

Project on Death in America
Open Society Institute
400 W. 59th Street
New York, NY 10019
(212) 548-0150
(212) 548-4613 Fax
Website: http://www.soros.org/death.html
E-mail: pdia@sorosny.org

Reflex Sympathetic Dystrophy Association of California
P.O. Box 771
San Marcos, CA 92019-0771
Phone/Fax: (760) 744-3266
Website: http://www.rsdsa-ca.org

The Resource Center of the American Alliance of Cancer Pain Initiatives
1300 University Avenue
Madison, WI 53706
(608) 265-4013
(608) 265-4014 Fax
Website: http://www.wisc.edu/trc/stcont/stcont.htm
E-mail: alliance@mail.com

Robert Wood Johnson Foundation (RWJF)
P.O. Box 2316
College Road East and Route 1
Princeton, NJ 08543-2316
(609) 452-8701
(609) 452-8701 Fax
Website: http://www.rwjf.org
E-mail: mail@rwjf.org

Southern California Cancer Pain Initiative
C/o City of Hope National Medical Center
1500 E. Duarte Road
Duarte, CA 91010
(626) 359-8111 x3829
(626) 301-8941 Fax
Website: http://sccpi.coh.org
E-mail: SCCPI@coh.org

Supportive Care of the Dying
C/o Sylvia McSkimming, Ph.D., R.N.
Executive Director
Providence Health System
4805 NE Glisan Street, 2E07
Portland, OR 97213
(503) 215-5053
(503) 215-5054 Fax
Website: http://www.careofdying.org
E-mail: smcskimming@providence.org

TMJ Association, Ltd.
P.O. Box 26770
Milwaukee, WI 53226-0770
(414) 259-3223
(414) 259-8112 Fax
Website: http://www.tmj.org

United Hospital Fund of New York
Empire State Building, 350 Fifth Avenue
New York, NY 10118
(212) 494-0700 or (888) 291-4161
(212) 494-0823 FAX
Website: http://www.uhfnyc.org

VZV Research Foundation, Inc.
40 East 72nd Street
New York, NY 10021
800-472-VIRUS
(212) 861-7033 Fax
Website: http://www.vzvfoundation.org
E-mail: VZV@VZVFoundation.org

The Vulvar Pain Foundation
Post Office Drawer 177
Graham, NC 27253
(336) 226-0704
(336) 226-8518 Fax
Website: http://www.vulvarpainfoundation.org

Wisconsin Cancer Pain Initiative
1300 University Avenue, Room 4720
Madison, Wisconsin 53706
(608) 262-0978
(608) 265-4014 Fax
Website: http://www.wisc.edu/wcpi
E-mail: wcpi@facstaff.wisc.edu

SLIDE SET RESOURCES

ASCO:American Society of Clinical Oncology. Cancer Pain Assessment & Treatment Curriculum Guidelines Teaching Syllabus & Slide Sets:

- American Society of Clinical Oncology (ASCO)
  435 N. Michigan Ave., Suite 1717
  Chicago, IL 60611
  312-644-0878
  312-644-8557 Fax

Illinois Cancer Pain Initiative. Cancer Pain Can be Relieved. A 25-slide set with narrative script designed for presentation to the general public. Send check payable to:

- Illinois Cancer Pain Initiative
  P.O. Box 6794
  Villa Park, IL 60181.
  1-800-DUL-PAIN.

Memorial Sloan-Kettering Cancer Center and Psychiatry Services.

Cancer Pain: Principles of Assessment, by Russell Portenoy, MD and Nathan Cherny, MBBS, FRACP.

Cancer Pain Syndromes, by Russell Portenoy, MD and Nathan Cherny, MBBS, FRACP.

Opioid Pharmacotherapy of Cancer Pain, by Russell Portenoy, MD.

The Use of Adjuvant Analgesics in Cancer Pain, by Russell Portenoy, MD.

The Use of Nonopioid and Adjuvant Analgesics in Cancer Pain, by Russell Portenoy, M.D.

Psychiatric Aspects of Cancer Pain Management, by William Breitbart, M.D.

Psychiatric Aspects of HIV/AIDS Pain, by William Breitbart, MD.

The Assessment and Syndromes of Pain in HIV/AIDS, by William Breitbart, M.D.

The Treatment of Pain in HIV/AIDS, by William Breitbart, M.D.

Teaching modules developed by the faculty of the Network Project includes a lecture with references and 25–40 color slides. Each module costs. To order: indicate title of each teaching module and the number of copies. Check payable to: The Network Project, CC 5112, Fund 7045". Send to:

- The Network Project
  Box 421, MSKCC
  1275 York Ave
  New York, NY 10021.
  (212) 639-3164
  (212) 752-7185 Fax

VIDEOTAPES

Before I Die: Medical Care and Personal Choices. Produced by Seminars, Inc., contains scenarios that focus on how three terminal patients and their families cope with the patients' terminal illness. A Fred Friendly Seminar. 1997.

- PBS Home Video
  1320 Braddoch Place
  Alexandria, VA 22314
  (800) 424-7963

Cancer Pain Management, and *New Modalities of Cancer Pain Management.* Produced by Knoll Pharmaceutical Company. The first provides an overview of currently accepted standards of practice in pain assessment and runs approximately 14 min. The second provides a program designed to dispel the patient's fears and clarify the misconceptions related to the treatment of cancer pain and runs approximately 10 min. The third tape provides an in-depth view of PCA. Order from:

- Knoll Pharmaceutical Company
  30 North Jefferson Road
  Whippany, New Jersey 07981
  (800) 526-0221

Cancer Pain Management. Produced by the South Carolina Cancer Pain Initiative. A two-hour presentation of a September 1994 live satellite conference identifying the magnitude of pain problems; myths and errors regarding pain management, and pharmacological and nonpharmacological methods of pain control. Presenters include health care providers and patients. Contact Bud Cooper to order: (803) 792-4971.

The Caring Helper (videotape set with workbook). Teaches helping and self-care skills to volunteer and professional caregivers working with people who face life-threatening illness, dying, and bereavement. To order:

- Applied Vision
  Post Office Box 1344
  San Carlos, CA 94070-7344
  (650) 591-9307
  Website: http://www.appliedvision.com

Communicating About Cancer Pain.

Is Cancer Pain Inevitable? Produced in October 1995 by the Outreach Education Department of University of Wisconsin Hospitals and Clinics in conjunction with the UW Comprehensive Cancer Center and the WCPI. Each tape is ½ hour in length. Single copy of ½-inch VHS available for a minimal cost plus tax, shipping, and handling. Discounts for multiple copies. Also available in ¾-inch VHS master.

Dealing with Chronic Pain. Describes how chronic pain affect many aspects of living, including moods, family relations, and self-esteem. Item #031797A.

To order:

- University of Wisconsin Hospital
  Outreach Education Department
  702 Blackhawk Ave, Suite 215
  Madison, WI 53705
  (800) 757-4354
  Website: http://www.uwhealth.wisc.edu.outreach

Controlling Cancer Pain. Produced by John Hopkins Oncology Center. Developed to help patients and families understand cancer pain. To order:

- John Hopkins Oncology Center
  600 North Wolfe Street
  Baltimore, MD 21287
  (410) 955-1287

End-of-Life Care for Children and Their Families: Ethical Dimensions. Explains principles of shared decision making; describes the role of the nurse as advocate for the child and family; suggests approaches to resolving ethical conflicts; and discusses the impact of a child's death on the parents.

End-of-Life Care: Ethical Dimensions. Provides nurses with practical information concerning end-of-life issues that can be applied in daily practice. To order:

- Glaxo Welcome Inc.
  Research Triangle Park, NC 27709
  (800) 824-2896

Facing Death: Practical Planning & Legal Issues. Produced by Aquarius Productions, Inc. (1997). A nurse attorney and hospice professionals share their thoughts, experiences, and suggestions to help terminally ill patients "make it clear" so that patients have what they want at the end of life.

Facing Death: Providing Physical, Emotional & Spiritual Comfort to Loved Ones. Produced by Aquarius Productions, Inc. (1997). Patients, caregivers, hospice professionals, and social workers share their thoughts, experiences, and specific suggestions to help terminally ill patients and their caregivers comfort each other. Order from:

- Aquarius Productions, Inc.
  5 Powderhouse Lane
  Sherborn, MA 01770
  (508) 651-2963
  (508) 650-4216 Fax
  Website: http://www.aquariousproductions.com
  E-mail: aqvideos@tiac.net

Final Blessings. Examines the spiritual dimensions in the lives of the terminally ill rather than turning away from the unavoidable sadness in these stories. A program about uncovering a place within the soul to begin to understand suffering on a different level and to look forward to what lies ahead. To order:

- The Catholic Communication Campaign
  3321 Fourth St NE
  Washington DC 20017
  (800) 235-8722

Helping to Control Cancer Pain and *I Got My Life Back.* The first is designed to alleviate patients' concerns about cancer pain, teaching patients how to communicate their pain to health care professionals and how to use the comfort assessment journal. Also available in Spanish. In the second video, patients tell how pain affected their lives. Order from:

- Purdue Frederick Co.
  100 Connecticut Avenue
  Norwalk, CT 06850-3590
  (203) 853-0123
  (203) 838-1576 Fax
  Website: http://partnersagainstpain.com

Laughter Therapy. Four Candid Camera videos are mailed to the patient. When the first video is returned, the second video is sent. The process continues until all four have been viewed and returned. Order from:

- Laughter Therapy (funded by Allen Funt)
  Candid Camera, Inc.
  P.O. Box 827
  Monterey, CA 93942
  Website: http://candidcamera.com

Managing Cancer Pain: A Rural Perspective. Virginia Cancer Pain Initiative. A 28-minute video that depicts caregivers'/patients' challenges of pain management in a rural setting. Minimal cost. To order:

- VCPI Videos
  Virginia Cancer Pain Initiative
  PO Box 6359
  Glen Allen, VA 23058-6359
  Website: http://www.vcpi.org

McCaffery on Pain: Nursing Assessment & Management (1991) and *McCaffery: Contemporary Issues in Pain Management* (1994). Each set includes four videotapes, approximately 30 min. each.

Pain in Infants: Confronting the Challenges. A videotape by Bonnie J. Stevens describing assessment strategies and analgesic intervention for neonates and infants.

The Williams and Wilkins Complete Library on Pain. These videotapes (approximately 30 minutes each) concentrate on various aspects of the nursing management of the patient with pain, including pain assessment, use of the three groups of analgesics treatment of pain, pain in the elderly, pain in children, and physiology of pain. Order from:

- Williams & Wilkins Electronic Media Division
  428 E. Preston St.
  Baltimore, MD 21202
  (800) 527-5597
  (410) 528-4422 Fax

My Word Against Theirs. This videotape is produced by Texas Cancer Pain Initiative and contains many moving patient vignettes supporting the need for effective cancer pain management. These vignettes could act as a useful supplement to presentations on cancer pain management to the public and health care professionals. Available for short-term loan through:

- The Resource Center
  1300 University Avenue
  Madison, WI 53706
  (608) 262-0978
  (608) 265-4014 Fax

On the Edge of Being. An intimate view of six physicians who have personally, or in their immediate families, confronted cancer. To order:

- Cerenex Pharmaceuticals, a division of Glaxo Inc.
  Research Triangle Park, NC 27709
  (800) 824-2896

Pain Management 101. (1998). Denice Economou, M.N., R.N., A.O.C.N., and Sandy Sentivany-Collins, R.N. Home study course (9 contact hours) is divided into chapters to enhance your learning experience. To order:

- NurseWeek Publishing
  1156-Aster Avenue
  Sunnyvale, CA 94086
  (408) 249-5877

Pain Management for the Oncology Nurse (March 2000). This videotape is one of four video programs from the *Oncology Nursing Today*™ *2000.* Video contents include: barriers to effective pain management, pain assessment, pharmacological therapies to manage pain, and strategies for improving pain management. Order information:

- Stratos Institute
  E-mail: info@StratosInstitute.com
- **West Cost Office**
  29805 Weatherwood
  Suite 200
  Laguna Niguel, CA 92677-1945 USA
  Tel: (949) 388-2100
  Fax: (949) 249-2885

- **East Coast Office**
  7990 Old Georgetown Road
  Bethesda, MD 20814-2430 USA
  Tel: (301) 652-9400
  Fax: (301) 652-9401

Relieving Cancer Pain. Patient notebook, ¾-inch videotape, and script. Available from:

- Fred Hutchinson Cancer Research Center
  1100 Fairview Avenue North, FM815
  P.O. Box 19024
  Seattle, WA 98109-1024
  (206) 667-5022
  (206) 667-4356 Fax

Walk Me to the Water. Portrays the experiences of three terminally ill cancer patients being cared for at home. Available for rental or purchase. To order:

- Walk Me to the Water
  P.O. Box 55
  New Lebanon, NY 12125
  (518) 794-8081

Why Not Freedom from Cancer Pain? World Health Organization has produced this 14-minute videotape, which is geared for health care professionals as well as the general public, and focuses on the fact that cancer pain can be relieved and that patients and families have the right to adequate medications. Prepayment is required for this video (plus shipping and handling). To order:

- World Health Organization Publishing Center, USA
  49 Sheridan Ave.
  Albany, NY 12210
  (518) 436-9686
  (518) 436-7433 Fax

Winning the Battle and *Control Your Cancer Pain.* Produced by Marshfield Clinic in 1990, with each approximately 12 minutes in length. The first addresses three common myths about cancer pain control; the second corrects common misconceptions about how pain medications work. Order from:

- Marshfield Video Network
  1000 North Oak Avenue
  Marshfield, WI 54449
  (715) 387-5023

WEBSITE/INTERNET RESOURCES

Agency for Healthcare Research and Quality	http://www.ahcpr.gov/
Aging with Dignity	http://www.agingwithdignity.org
American Academy of Hospice and Palliative Medicine	http://www.aahpm.org
American Academy of Pain Medicine	http://www.painmed.org
American Association for Therapeutic Humor	http://www.aath.org
ABCD Americans for Better Care of the Dying	http://www.abcd-caring.com
American Board of Internal Medicine—Care for the Dying, Physician Narratives	http://www.abim.org/pubs/narr001.htm
American Cancer Society	http://www.cancer.org
American Chronic Cancer Pain Association	http://www.theacp.org
American Council for Headache Education	http://www.achenet.org
The American Geriatrics Society	http://www.americangeriatrics.org
American Holistic Nurses Association	http://www.ahna.org
American Massage Therapy Association	http://www.amtamassage.org
American Medical Association	http://www.ama-assn.org.80/about.htm
American Medical Association Education of Physicians on End of Life Care (EPEC)	http://www.ama-assn.org/ethic/epec
American Music Therapy Association	http://www.namt.com
American Pain Foundation	http://www.painfoundation.org
American Pain Society	http://www.ampainsoc.org
American Society for the Advancement of Palliative Care	http://www.asap-care.com
American Society of Anesthesiologists	http://www.asahq.org
American Society for Bioethics and Humanities	http://www.asbh.org
American Society of Clinical Oncology (ASCO)	http://www.asco.org
American Society of Law, Medicine and Ethics	http://www.aslme.org
American Society of Pain Management Nurses	http://www.aspmn.org
Approaching Death: Improving Care at the End of Life	http://www.nap.edu/readingroom/books/approaching/
Arthritis Foundation	http://www.arthritis.org
Association of Cancer Online Resources, Inc.	http://www.medinfo.org;http://www.acor.org
Association of American Sickle Cell Disease	http://www.sicklecelldisease.org
Association of Death Education and Counseling (ADEC)	http://www.adec.org
Association of Nurses in AIDS Care	http://www.anacnet.org
Association of Oncology Social Work (AOSW)	http://www.aosw.org
Association of Pediatric Oncology Nurses (APON)	http://www.apon.org
Before I Die: Medical Care and Personal Choices	http://www.wnet.org/archive/bid
Bereavement and Hospice Support Netline	http://www.ubalt.edu/www/bereavement
Better Health	http://www.BetterHealth.com
Breast Cancer Information Clearinghouse	http://www.nysernet.org/bcic
Cancer Care, Inc.	http://www.cancercare.org
Cancer Library	http://www.medhip.usa.net.cancer.htm
Cancer Links	http://charm.net/-kkdk
Cancer Net	http://cancernet.nci.nih.gov/
Candlelighters Childhood Cancer Foundation	http://www.candlelighters.org
Caregiver Network	http://www.caregiver.on.ca/index.html
Caregiver Survival Resources	http://www.caregiver911.com/
Catholic Health Association of the United States	http://www.chausa.org
Center for Medical Ethics and Mediation	http://www.wh.com/cmem
Center to Improve Care of the Dying	http://www.gwu.edu/~cicd
Children's Hospice International	http://www.chionline.org
Choice in Dying	http://www.choices.org
City of Hope Pain/Palliative Care Resource Center	http://prc.coh.org

The Compassionate Friends	http://www.compassionatefriends.org/
Compassion in Dying	http://www.compassionindying.org
C. Richard Chapman Pain Information Page	http://faculty.washington.edu/crc/
Cultural Guides to Dying, Death & the Afterlife	http://www.indranet.com/bardo/culutral.html
Department of Health and Human Services, Healthfinder	http://www.healthfinder.gov
Dying Well	http://www.dyingwell.org or http://www.dyingwell.com
The Edmonton Palliative Care Program	http://www.palliative.org
Education for Physicians on End of Life Care Project (EPEC)	http://www.epec.net
Elizabeth Kubler Ross, M. D., "On Death and Dying"	http://www.doubleclickd.com/kubler.html
The End of Life: Exploring Death in America	http://www.npr.org/programs/death/
End of Life Physician Education Resource Center (EPERC)	http://www.eperc.mcw.edu
FACCT—The Foundation for Accountability	http://www.facct.org
Family Caregiver Alliance	http://www.caregiver.org
Fibromyalgia Network	http://www.fmnetnews.com
Growth House	http://www.growthhouse.org
History of Body Donation	http://www.com.uci.edu/~anatomy/willed body/wbpol.htm
Hospice Association of America	http://www.hospice-america.org
Hospice and Palliative Nurses Association	http://www.HPNA.org
Hospice Foundation of America	http://www.hospicefoundation.org
Hospice Hands	http://hospice-cares.com
Institute for Healthcare Improvement	http://www.ihi.org
International Association for the Study of Pain	http://www.halcyon.com/iasp
The International Work Group on Death, Dying and Bereavement	http://www.wwdc.com/death/iwg/iwg.html
Last Acts	http://www.lastacts.org
Leukemia Society of America	http://www.leukemia.org
Make a Wish Foundation	http://www.wish.org
Management of Cancer Pain	http://www.ahcpr.gov/consumer/
Medical College of Wisconsin Bioethics	http://www.mcw.edu/bioethics/
Medical College of Wisconsin Palliative Care Programs	http://www.mcw.edu/pallmed/
Memorial Sloan-Kettering Cancer Center	http://www.mskcc.org
The Nathan Cummings Foundation	http://www.ncf.org/ncf/aboutncf/about.html
National Association for Home Care (NAHC)	http://www.nahc.org/
The National Center for Health Statistics	http://www.cdc.gov/nchswww/about/about.htm
National Conference of State Legislatures	htttp://www.ncsl.org/programs/pubs/ednoflife.htm
National Family Caregivers Association	http://www.nfcacares.org/
National Hospice and Palliative Care Organization	http://www.nhpco.org
The National Institute of Aging	http://www.nih.gov/nia/
National Prison Hospice Association – Development of Hospice Care in Correctional Facilities	http://www.npha.org
Neuropathy Association	http://www.neuropathy.org
New York State Partnership for Long-Term Care	http://www.nyspltc.org/about/index.html#3
Not Dead Yet	http://acils.com/NotDeadYet/
On Our Own Terms	http://www.thirteen.org/onourownterms
Oncolink	http://www.oncolink.com
Oncolinks Pain Page	http://oncolink.upenn.edu/specialty/pain
Open Society Institute Project on Death in America	http://www.soros.org/death.html
Oregon Health Sciences University Center for Ethics in Health Care	http://www.ohsu.edu/ethics/
Oncology Nursing Society	http://www.ons.org

Pain Link	http://www.edc.org/PainLink
Pain Net	http://www.painnet.com
The Palliative Medicine Program	http://www.mcw.edu/pallmed
Partners Against Pain	http://www.partnersagainstpain.com
The Patient Education Institute	http://www.patient-education.com
Pediatric Pain	http://is.dal.ca/~pedpain/prohp.html
Pediatric Pain Education for Patients & Families	http://coinfo.nursing.uiowa.edu/sited/pedspain/index .htm
Project on Death in America	http://www.soros.org/death/
Reflex Sympathetic Dystrophy Association of California	http://www.rsdsa-ca.org
Resource Center of the American Alliance of Cancer Pain Initiatives	http://www.wisc.edu/trc/stcont/stcont.htm
The Robert Wood Johnson Foundation	http://www.rwjf.org
Roxane Pain Institute	http://pain.roxane.com
Southern California Cancer Pain Initiative (SCCPI)	http://sccpi.coh.org
Supportive Care of the Dying	http://www.careofdying.org
TMJ Association, Ltd.	http://www.tmj.org
Talarian Map-Cancer Pain	http://www.statscilcom/talaria/talaria.html
Telemedicine Information Exchange	http://tie.telemed.org
United Hospital Fund of New York	http://www.uhfnyc.org
University of Wisconsin Pain & Policy Studies Group	http://www.medsch.wis.edu/painpolicy
VistaCare	http://www.vista-care.com
Wellness Web Cancer Center	http://www.wellweb.com/cancer/cancer.htm
When Death is Sought Assisted Suicide and Euthanasia in the Medical Context	http://www.health.ny.us/nysdoh/provider/death.htm
Wisconsin Cancer Pain Initiative	http://www.wisc.edu/wcpi
Worldwide Congress on Pain	http://www.careofdying.org

Index